SAUNDERS

COMPREHENSIVE
REVIEW *for the*
NCLEX-PN®
EXAMINATION

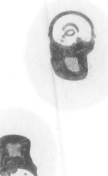

SAUNDERS

EDITION 4

COMPREHENSIVE REVIEW *for the* NCLEX-PN® EXAMINATION

LINDA ANNE SILVESTRI, MSN, RN
Instructor of Nursing
Salve Regina University
Newport, Rhode Island
President
Nursing Reviews, Inc.
and
Professional Nursing Seminars, Inc.
Charlestown, Rhode Island
Instructor: NCLEX-RN® and NCLEX-PN® Review Courses

SAUNDERS

ELSEVIER

SAUNDERS

ELSEVIER

11830 Westline Industrial Drive
St. Louis, Missouri 63146

SAUNDERS COMPREHENSIVE REVIEW FOR THE NCLEX-PN®
EXAMINATION

ISBN: 978-1-4160-4730-8

Notice

Knowledge and best practice in this field are constantly changing. As new research and experience broaden our knowledge, changes in practice, treatment, and drug therapy may become necessary or appropriate. Readers are advised to check the most current information provided (i) on procedures featured or (ii) by the manufacturer of each product to be administered, to verify the recommended dose or formula, the method and duration of administration, and contraindications. It is the responsibility of the practitioner, relying on their own experience and knowledge of the patient, to make diagnoses, to determine dosages and the best treatment for each individual patient, and to take all appropriate safety precautions. To the fullest extent of the law, neither the Publisher nor the Author assumes any liability for any injury and/or damage to persons or property arising out of or related to any use of the material contained in this book.

The Publisher

NCLEX® and NCLEX-PN® are registered trademarks and service marks of the National Council of State Boards of Nursing, Inc.

Library of Congress Cataloging-in-Publication Data

Silvestri, Linda Anne.
   Saunders comprehensive review for the NCLEX-PN examination / Linda Anne Silvestri. – 4th ed.
      p. ; cm.
   Includes bibliographical references and index.
   ISBN 978-1-4160-4730-8 (pbk. : alk. paper) 1. Practical nursing–Examinations, questions, etc.
 2. National Council Licensure Examination for Practical/Vocational Nurses–Study guides.
 I. Title. II. Title: Comprehensive review for NCLEX-PN examination.
   [DNLM: 1. Nursing, Practical–Examination Questions. WY 18.2 S587sb 2010]
   RT62.S53 2010
   610.7306'93076–dc22   2008052894

ISBN: 978-1-4160-4730-8

Managing Editor: Nancy O'Brien
Developmental Editor: Todd McKenzie
Publishing Services Manager: Anne Altepeter
Senior Project Manager: Doug Turner
Multimedia Producer: David Rushing
Designer: Margaret Reid

Printed in Canada

Last digit is the print number: 9   8   7   6   5   4   3   2

To my parents,
*To my mother, **Frances Mary**, and in loving memory of my father, **Arnold Lawrence**,*
who taught me to always love, care, and be the best that I could be.

About the Author

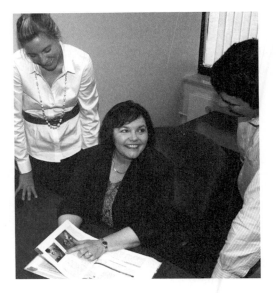

Linda Anne Silvestri

As a child, I dreamed of becoming either a nurse or teacher. Initially I chose to become a nurse because I wanted to help others, especially those who were ill. Then I realized that both of my dreams could come true: I could be a nurse and a teacher. So I pursued my dreams.

I received my diploma in nursing from Cooley Dickinson Hospital School of Nursing in Northampton, Massachusetts. Afterward, I worked at Baystate Medical Center in Springfield, Massachusetts. At Baystate Medical Center, I cared for clients in acute medical-surgical units, the intensive care unit, the emergency department, pediatric units, and other acute care units. Later, I received an associate degree from Holyoke Community College in Holyoke, Massachusetts, my BSN from American International College in Springfield, Massachusetts,

and my MSN from Anna Maria College in Paxton, Massachusetts, with a dual major in Nursing Management and Patient Education. I am currently working on my PhD in Nursing at the University of Nevada, Las Vegas, and am doing research related to success on the NCLEX examination. I am also a member of the Honor Society of Nursing, Sigma Theta Tau International, Phi Kappa Phi, the Western Institute of Nursing, the Eastern Nursing Research Society and the Golden Key International Honour Society.

As a native of Springfield, Massachusetts, I began my teaching career as an instructor of medical-surgical nursing and leadership-management nursing at Baystate Medical Center School of Nursing in 1981. In 1989, I relocated to Rhode Island and began teaching medical-surgical nursing and psychiatric nursing to RN and LPN students at the Community College of Rhode Island. In 1994, I began teaching nursing at Salve Regina University in Newport, Rhode Island, and remain there as an adjunct faculty member.

My experiences as a student, nursing educator, and item writer for the NCLEX exams aided me as I developed a comprehensive review course to prepare nursing students and graduates for the NCLEX examination. In 1991, I established Professional Nursing Seminars, Inc., and in 2000, I started Nursing Reviews, Inc. Both companies are dedicated to conducting review courses for the NCLEX-RN and the NCLEX-PN examinations and assisting nursing graduates to achieve their goals of becoming registered nurses or licensed practical/vocational nurses.

Today I conduct review courses for the NCLEX examinations throughout New England and am the author of numerous successful review products. I am so pleased that you have decided to join me in your journey to success in testing for nursing examinations and for the NCLEX-PN examination!

Contributors

Katrina D. Allen, RN, MSN, CCRN
Nursing Instructor
Faulkner State Community College
Chickasaw, Alabama

Sonya S. Beacham, MSN, RN
Cain, Hale & Associates, Inc.
Wilmington, North Carolina

Joyce Campbell, RN, MSN, CCRN, FNP-C
Associate Professor of Nursing
Chattanooga State Technical Community College
Chattanooga, Tennessee

Brigitte L. Casteel, RN, BSN
Assistant Professor, Program Director
Practical Nursing Program
Mountain Empire Community College
Weber City, Virginia

Faith Chumchal Darilek, RN, MSN
Professor of Nursing
The Victoria College
Victoria, Texas

Mary Joanne Hovey, MSN, RN
Cain, Hale & Associates, Inc.
Wilmington, North Carolina

Misty D. Johnson, LPN
Graduate
Mid-Plains Community College
North Platte, Nebraska

Nancy K. Maebius, PhD, RN
Consultant, Instructor
Galen Health Institute School of Nursing
San Antonio, Texas

Barbara Magenheim, EdD, MSN, BSN, RN, CNE
Nursing Instructor
Chandler-Gilbert Community College
Chandler, Arizona

Victoria Oxendine, RN, MSN, FNPC
Cain, Hale & Associates, Inc.
Wilmington, North Carolina

Elizabeth Pratt, BSN, RNC
Instructor of Women's Health
ADN Program
Southern Arkansas University
Magnolia, Arkansas

Bonnie L. Shipferling, PhD(c), MSN, BSBA, RN
Professor of Nursing
San Jacinto College Central
Pasadena, Texas

Jennifer C. Spencer, RN, BSN
Certified Wound, Ostomy, & Continence Care Nurse
Cain, Hale & Associates, Inc.
Wilmington, North Carolina

Louis M. Stackler, RN, BSN, MS
Nursing Instructor
ARN, NACNS
Tulsa Technology Center
Tulsa, Oklahoma

Jacquelyn Stovall, RN, BSN
Nursing Instructor
Texas Careers School of Vocational Nursing
San Antonio, Texas

Bethany Hawes Sykes, EdD, RN, CEN
Adjunct Faculty
Department of Nursing
Salve Regina University
Newport, Rhode Island

Ruth Chandley Threlkeld, MSN, BSN
Nurse Educator
College of Graduate and Extended Studies
Central Methodist University
Clark, Missouri

Julie Traynor, MS, RN
Nursing Instructor
Lake Region State College
Devils Lake, North Dakota

Laurent W. Valliere, BS
Vice President
Professional Nursing Seminars, Inc.
Charlestown, Rhode Island

Kim Webb, RN, MN
Nursing Chair
Northern Oklahoma College
Tonkawa, Oklahoma

Patricia H. White, BSN, RNC
Certified Neonatal Intensive Care Unit Nurse
Cain, Hale & Associates, Inc.
Wilmington, North Carolina

STUDENT REVIEWERS

Larry Pelland
Elms College
Chicopee, Massachusetts

Angela Silvestri
Salve Regina University
Newport, Rhode Island

The author and publisher would also like to acknowledge the following individuals for their contributions to the previous editions of this book:

Alicia M. Adams, MN, RN, CEN
Roosevelt, Utah

Carol Boswell, EdD, RN
Odessa, Texas

Sharen Brady, MSN, RN
Ogden, Utah

Brenda E. Caranicas, MS, RN
New Town, North Dakota

Jean DeCoffe, MSN, RN
Milton, Massachusetts

Stephanie A. Dupler
Lebanon, Pennslyvania

Mary Ann Hogan, MSN, RN, CS
Amherst, Massachusetts

Lisa Ivers, BSN, RN
Hamilton, Ohio

Lula Johnson, MSN, RN
Detroit, Michigan

Mary T. Kowalski, MSN, BA, RN
Ridgecrest, California

Beverly McNeese, RN
Baton Rouge, Louisiana

Jan H. Mearkle, MSN, RN, CSNP
Summit, Mississippi

Jo Ann Barnes Mullaney, PhD, RN, CS
Newport, Rhode Island

Joann E. Potts Peuterbaugh, MSN, RN
Alton, Illinois

Ann Leiphart Unholz, MS, RN
Highland Springs, Virginia

Paula A. Viau, PhD, RN
Kingston, Rhode Island

Margaret Wafstet, MN, RN
Missoula, Montana

Mary Louise White, MSN, RN
University Center, Michigan

CONSULTANT

Nicole Marie Valliere, BSN, RN
Professional Nurse I—Pediatrics
Hasbro Children's Hospital
Providence, Rhode Island

ANCILLARY CO-AUTHOR

Lois S. Marshall, PhD, RN
Nurse Researcher Scholar in Residence
Honor Society of Nursing, Sigma Theta Tau
  International;
Nurse Education Consultant
LSM Educational Consulting
Miami, Florida

Preface

"To know that even one life has breathed easier because you have lived, this is to have succeeded."

Ralph Waldo Emerson

Welcome to *Saunders Pyramid to Success!*

Saunders Comprehensive Review for the NCLEX-PN® Examination is one in a series of products designed to assist you in achieving your goal of becoming a licensed practical/vocational nurse. This book will provide you with an all-inclusive review of the nursing content areas specifically related to the new 2008 NCLEX-PN test plan as implemented by the National Council of State Boards of Nursing.

ORGANIZATION

Saunders Comprehensive Review for the NCLEX-PN® Examination contains 20 units and 66 chapters. The chapters are designed to identify specific components of nursing content. The chapters contain practice questions that reflect the chapter content and the 2008 NCLEX-PN test plan.

The new test plan identifies a framework based on Client Needs. These Client Needs categories include Safe and Effective Care Environment, Health Promotion and Maintenance, Psychosocial Integrity, and Physiological Integrity. Integrated Processes are also identified as a component of the test plan. These include Caring, Clinical Problem-Solving Process (Nursing Process), Communication and Documentation, and Teaching and Learning. All of the chapters address the components of the test plan framework.

UNIT I: NCLEX-PN® PREPARATION

Chapter 1 provides information about the 2008 NCLEX-PN test plan and the testing procedures related to the examination. This chapter answers all of those questions that you may have regarding the testing procedures.

Chapter 2 provides information to the foreign-educated nurse about the process of obtaining a license to practice as a licensed practical/vocational nurse in the United States.

Chapter 3 discusses the issue of NCLEX-PN preparation from a nonacademic perspective and provides an emphasis on a holistic approach for your individual test preparation. This chapter identifies the components of a structured study plan, anxiety reduction techniques, and personal focus issues.

Nursing students want to hear what other students have to say about their experiences with the NCLEX-PN examination. Chapter 4 is written by a nursing student who recently took the NCLEX-PN examination. The chapter discusses what the examination is all about and includes the student's story of success.

Test-taking strategies are a key component of success in taking such an important examination. Chapter 5, "Test-Taking Strategies," includes important strategies that will help teach you how to read a question, how not to read into a question, and how to use the process of elimination and various other strategies to select the correct response from the choices presented.

UNIT II: ISSUES IN NURSING

Unit II addresses relevant nursing issues reflective of the components of the NCLEX-PN test plan. Chapter 6, "Cultural Diversity," identifies cultures and the related factors that promote the maintenance of cultural identity when caring for culturally diverse clients. Alternative and complementary therapies are also reviewed in this chapter. Chapter 7, "Ethical and Legal Issues," provides a review of the ethical and legal considerations important to the practice of nursing and relevant to the components of the test plan. Chapter 8, "Delegating, Managing, and Prioritizing Care," identifies the leadership and management issues pertinent to the practice of nursing. This chapter emphasizes content related to time management, prioritizing, and assignment-making and the principles related to delegation. Disaster planning and triage are also covered.

UNIT III: NURSING SCIENCES

The chapters in this unit specifically address topics that students have identified as areas of concern requiring review. Chapter 9, "Fluids and Electrolytes," and Chapter 10, "Acid-Base Balance," highlight the key components of human physiology and then introduce the necessary data collection and nursing interventions required for caring for a client with an alteration or an imbalance. Chapter 11, "Laboratory Values," identifies common laboratory studies, normal values, and significant information related to specific laboratory tests. Chapter 12, "Nutritional Components of Care," examines the various food groups and important nutritional components of specific diet therapies. This chapter will assist in your review of which foods to include and which foods to avoid with certain physiological conditions. Chapter 13, "Intravenous Therapy and Blood Administration," focuses on the nurse's role in monitoring these therapies and related complications.

UNIT IV: FUNDAMENTAL SKILLS

Chapter 14, "Hygiene and Safety," addresses nursing care specific to client safety and the measures that promote environmental safety. Standard precautions, transmission-based precautions, and radiation precautions are reviewed. Additionally, chemical and biological warfare agents and their potentially fatal effects are examined. Chapter 15, "Medication and Intravenous Administration," includes the important components related to conversion tables, calculation of medication dosages, and intravenous solutions and flow rates. Chapter 16, "Basic Life Support," reviews the steps in cardiopulmonary resuscitation and abdominal thrusts, as well as the priorities to be addressed in emergency situations. Chapter 17, "Perioperative Nursing Care," covers the key components related to caring for the client who requires surgery. Chapter 18, "Positioning Clients," identifies safe client positions specific to various surgical and diagnostic procedures. Chapter 19, "Care of a Client With a Tube," looks at the common types of tubes used in the clinical setting—such as chest, gastrointestinal, and renal tubes—which have always been very confusing to students, particularly in terms of their purpose and the nursing care involved.

UNITS V, VI, AND VII: MATERNITY NURSING, GROWTH AND DEVELOPMENT ACROSS THE LIFE SPAN, AND PEDIATRIC NURSING

Unit V, "Maternity Nursing," includes chapters that address maternity issues, the care of the newborn, and maternity and newborn medications. Unit VI, "Growth and Development Across the Life Span," examines the common theories of growth and development used in

the profession of nursing, developmental stages and transitions, and content related to caring for the older client. Unit VII, "Pediatric Nursing," focuses on pediatric care and the specifics related to administering medication to the child.

UNITS VIII THROUGH XVIII: ADULT HEALTH

Units VIII through XVIII address the components of adult health and are divided based on specific body systems including the integumentary, endocrine, gastrointestinal, respiratory, cardiovascular, renal, eye and ear, neurological, musculoskeletal, and immune systems. Oncology nursing is also addressed. These chapters incorporate the Integrated Processes and all of the Client Needs components of the NCLEX-PN test plan, with a particular emphasis on Physiological Integrity. Each unit includes a pharmacology chapter that provides a comprehensive review of the medications specific to that body system.

UNIT XIX: MENTAL HEALTH NURSING

This unit primarily addresses the Psychosocial Integrity category of the Client Needs component of the test plan. Specific mental health disorders are addressed. This unit includes a chapter that provides a comprehensive review of psychiatric medications.

UNIT XX: COMPREHENSIVE TEST

Unit XX contains a comprehensive examination with practice questions related to all of the content areas addressed in this book. The Comprehensive Test consists of 85 questions that reflect the percentages identified in the NCLEX-PN test plan. Multiple-choice questions and questions in the alternate item formats are included in this test, as well as in the practice tests found at the end of each chapter.

SPECIAL FEATURES OF THE BOOK

Pyramid Terms

Each content area, either a chapter or unit, begins with *Pyramid Terms* and their definitions. These important terms are significant to the content contained in the chapter or unit. In addition, the *Pyramid Terms* are in bold type throughout the content section.

Pyramid to Success

The *Saunders Pyramid to Success*, which takes the form of a unit or chapter introduction, provides you with an overview, guidance, and direction regarding the focus of review in the particular content area and its relative importance to the 2008 NCLEX-PN test plan. Specific nursing content areas, as detailed by the test plan, are identified. The *Saunders Pyramid to Success* reviews the

Client Needs and the Integrated Processes as they pertain to the content in that unit or chapter. These points are the specific components to keep in mind as you review the chapter outline.

Pyramid Points

Pyramid Points ▲ are the bullets that are placed next to specific content areas throughout the chapters. The *Pyramid Points* provide you with immediate recognition of content that is important in preparation for the NCLEX-PN examination. These icons identify areas of content that typically appear on the NCLEX-PN examination.

Practice Questions

While preparing for the NCLEX-PN examination, it is crucial for students to answer the practice questions. This book contains 1027 practice questions in NCLEX format. The accompanying software includes all of the questions from the book, plus an additional 2673 questions, for a total of 3700 questions.

Multiple-Choice and Alternate Item Format Questions

Each content chapter is followed by a practice test. Each practice test contains several multiple choice questions and one alternate item format question. The alternate item format question may be presented as a fill-in-the-blank, multiple response, prioritizing (ordered response), or chart/exhibit question. These questions provide you with practice in prioritizing and decision-making.

Answer Section

The answer section for each practice question includes the correct answer, rationale, test-taking strategy, question categories, and reference. The structure for the answer section is unique and provides the following information:

Rationale: The rationale provides you with the significant information regarding both correct and incorrect options.

Test-Taking Strategy: The test-taking strategy describes the logical path for selecting the correct option and helps you select an answer to a question on which you must guess. Specific suggestions for review are identified in the test-taking strategy.

Question Categories: Each question is identified based on the categories used by the NCLEX-PN test plan. Additional content categories are provided with each question to assist you in identifying areas in need of review. The categories identified with each practice question include Level of Cognitive Ability, Client Needs, Integrated Process, and the specific nursing Content Area. All categories are identified by their full names so that you do not need to memorize codes or abbreviations.

Reference: A reference, including a page number, is provided so you can easily find the information that you need to review in your nursing textbooks.

PHARMACOLOGY AND MEDICATION CALCULATIONS REVIEW

Students consistently say that pharmacology is an area with which they need assistance. The 2008 NCLEX-PN test plan continues to incorporate pharmacology in the examination. Therefore, pharmacology chapters have been included for your review and practice. This book includes 13 pharmacology chapters, a medication and intravenous calculation chapter, and a pediatric medication calculation chapter. Each of these chapters is followed by a practice test using the same question format described earlier. This book and the accompanying software contain more than 500 pharmacology questions.

NCLEX-PN® REVIEW SOFTWARE

You will find a CD-ROM containing NCLEX-PN review software packaged in the back of this book. This CD also includes a 75-question Assessment Pretest that provides you with feedback on your strengths and weaknesses. The results of your Assessment Pretest will generate an individualized study calendar to guide you in your preparation for the NCLEX-PN. This software contains 3700 practice questions, which include alternate item format questions and lung and heart sound questions. This Windows- and Macintosh-compatible CD-ROM offers the following testing modes for review:

Quiz: Ten randomly chosen questions in a specific selected content area. The answer, rationale, test-taking strategy, question categories, reference source, and results appear after you have answered all 10 questions.

Study: All questions in a specific selected content area. The answer, rationale, test-taking strategy, question categories, and reference source appear after you have answered each question.

Examination: One hundred randomly chosen questions from the entire pool of 3700 questions. The answer, rationale, test-taking strategy, question categories, reference source, and results appear after you have answered all 100 questions.

If you are connected to the Internet while using the companion CD, click the "Check for Updates" button to download and install the most recent version of the program. Any updates to the software or content of this CD will be automatically integrated, keeping you up to date for the entire edition.

HOW TO USE THIS BOOK

Saunders Comprehensive Review for the NCLEX-PN® Examination is especially designed to help you with your successful journey to the peak of the *Saunders Pyramid to Success*, becoming a licensed practical/vocational nurse. As you begin your journey through this book, you will be introduced to all of the important points regarding the 2008 NCLEX-PN examination, the process of testing, and the unique and special tips regarding how to prepare yourself for this very important examination.

You should begin your process through the *Saunders Pyramid to Success* by reading all of Unit I and becoming familiar with the important points regarding the NCLEX-PN examination. Read the chapter from the nursing graduate who recently passed the examination and note what this graduate has to say about it. The test-taking strategy chapter will provide you with important strategies that will help you select the correct answer or narrow your choices when you must guess. Read this chapter and practice these strategies as you proceed through your journey with this book. Continue your journey by reading each of the chapters and content areas. Review the *Pyramid Terms* and the *Saunders Pyramid to Success* and identify the Client Needs and Integrated Processes specific to the test plan in that area. Read each of the content areas, focusing on the *Pyramid Points* that identify those areas most likely to be tested on the NCLEX-PN examination.

As you read each chapter, identify your strengths and those areas in need of further review. Highlight these areas and test your strengths and abilities by taking all of the practice tests provided at the end of the chapters. Be sure to read all of the rationales and the test-taking strategies. The rationale provides you with the significant information regarding both the correct and incorrect options. The test-taking strategy offers you the logical path to selecting the correct option. The strategy also identifies content area that you need to review if you had difficulty with the question. Use the reference source listed so you can easily find the information that you need to review.

After you review all of the chapters in the book, turn to Unit XX, the Comprehensive Test. Take this test and then go over each question, answer, and rationale. Identify any areas requiring further review and then take the time to read through those areas again.

After reviewing the book and taking the Comprehensive Test, proceed to the CD and take the 75-question Assessment Pretest. The results will provide you with feedback on your strengths and weaknesses and will generate a study calendar to guide you in your continued preparation for the NCLEX-PN.

After using this book to review specific content areas, continue on your journey through the *Saunders Pyramid to Success* with the companion book, *Saunders Q&A Review for the NCLEX-PN® Examination*, for additional practice questions. The companion book and its accompanying software offer you more than 3000 practice questions on specific areas outlined by the NCLEX-PN test plan. With practice questions uniquely focused on the Client Needs and the Integrated Processes, you can assess your level of competence.

Additional components of the *Saunders Pyramid to Success* are *Saunders Review Cards for the NCLEX-PN® Examination* and *Saunders Strategies for Success for the NCLEX-PN® Examination*. *Saunders Review Cards for the NCLEX-PN® Examination* provides you with more than 900 practice test questions, including multiple-choice questions and the new alternate item format questions such as fill-in-the-blank, multiple response, prioritizing (ordered response), and image (hot spot) questions. The practice question is located on one side of the review card. The reverse side of the review card contains the correct answer, rationale, and question categories for the practice question on the front of the card. *Saunders Strategies for Success for the NCLEX-PN® Examination* and its accompanying CD provide all of the test-taking strategies that will help you pass your nursing examinations and the NCLEX-PN. The chapters describe these test-taking strategies, include several sample questions that illustrate how to use the strategy, and provide an additional 500 practice questions, including multiple-choice and alternate item formats.

Good luck with your journey through the *Saunders Pyramid to Success*. I wish you continued success throughout your new career as a licensed practical/vocational nurse!

Linda Anne Silvestri, MSN, RN

Acknowledgments

Sincere appreciation and warmest thanks are extended to the many individuals who in their own way have contributed to the publication of this book.

First, I want to thank all of my nursing students at the Community College of Rhode Island in Warwick who approached me in 1991 and persuaded me to help them prepare to take the NCLEX examination. Their enthusiasm and inspiration led to the commencement of my professional endeavors in conducting NCLEX review courses for nursing students. I also thank the numerous nursing students who have attended my review courses for their willingness to share their needs and ideas. Their input has certainly added a special uniqueness to this publication.

I wish to acknowledge all of the nursing faculty who taught in my NCLEX review courses. Their commitment, dedication, and expertise have certainly assisted nursing students in achieving success with the NCLEX examination. Additionally, a special acknowledgment goes to Laurent W. Valliere for his contribution to this publication, for teaching in my NCLEX review courses, and for his commitment and dedication in helping my nursing students prepare for the NCLEX examination from a nonacademic point of view.

I sincerely acknowledge and thank two very important individuals from Elsevier. I thank Nancy O'Brien, managing editor, for all of her assistance throughout the preparation of this edition and for her continuous enthusiasm, support, and expert professional guidance. And I thank Todd McKenzie, my new developmental editor. Todd, who took on with ease a tremendous role as my developmental editor, has outstanding organizational skills and has maintained order for all of the work that I submitted for manuscript production. I also thank Todd for his dedication to my work, his continuous assistance and support, and for keeping me on schedule with manuscript submission.

A special thank you and acknowledgment goes to three important individuals, Dianne E. Ventrice, Lawrence Fiorentino, and Karen Machnacz. They provided continuous support and dedication to my work in both the NCLEX review courses and in reference support for the fourth edition of this book.

I also thank my student reviewers, Angela Silvestri from Salve Regina University in Newport, Rhode Island, and Larry Pelland from Elms College in Chicopee, Massachusetts, for reviewing content and questions and for providing ideas and feedback regarding the book.

I want to acknowledge all of the staff in marketing, especially Bob Boehringer, senior segment marketing director; Dan Hughes, marketing manager; and Kathy Mantz, group segment manager, and all of the additional staff at Elsevier for their tremendous assistance throughout the preparation and production of this publication. A special thank you to all of them.

I thank all of the special people in the production department—Anne Altepeter, publication services manager; Doug Turner, project manager; Margaret Reid, book designer; and Dave Rushing, multimedia producer, all of whom assisted in finalizing this publication.

I would also like to acknowledge Patricia Mieg, former educational sales representative, who encouraged me to submit my ideas and initial work for the first edition of this book to the W.B. Saunders Company.

I want to acknowledge my parents, who opened my door of opportunity in education. I thank my mother, Frances Mary, for all of her love, support, and assistance as I continuously worked to achieve my professional goals. I thank my father, Arnold Lawrence, who always provided insightful words of encouragement. My memories of his love and support will always remain in my heart.

I also thank my sister, Dianne Elodia; my brother, Lawrence Peter; my nieces and nephews, Gina Marie, Angela, Nicole, and Nicholas; and my fiancé, Larry, all of whom were continuously supportive, giving, and helpful during my research and preparation of this publication.

I want to acknowledge all of the contributors and reviewers of this publication for their thoughts and ideas. And a special thank you goes to Misty Johnson, LPN, for providing a chapter to this publication regarding her experiences with the NCLEX-PN examination.

I also need to thank Salve Regina University for the opportunity to educate nursing students in the baccalaureate nursing program and for its support during my research and writing of this publication. I would like to especially thank my colleagues Dr. Peggy Matteson, Dr. JoAnn Mullaney, Dr. Ellen McCarty, and Dr. Bethany Sykes for all of their support and encouragement.

I wish to acknowledge the Community College of Rhode Island, which provided me with the opportunity to educate nursing students in the Associate Degree of Nursing Program, and a special thank you to Patricia Miller, MSN, RN, and Michelina McClellan, MS, RN, from Baystate Medical Center, School of Nursing, in Springfield, Massachusetts, who were my first mentors in nursing education.

Lastly, a very special thank you to all of my nursing students—past, present, and future. Your love for and dedication to the profession of nursing and your commitment to provide health care will bring never-ending rewards!

Linda Anne Silvestri, MSN, RN

Contents

NCLEX-PN® Preparation

CHAPTER 1

The NCLEX-PN® Examination

PYRAMID TO SUCCESS

Welcome to the Pyramid to Success!

Saunders Comprehensive Review for the NCLEX-PN® Examination is specially designed to help you begin your successful journey to the peak of the Pyramid: becoming a licensed practical/vocational nurse!

As you begin your journey, you will be introduced to all of the important aspects of the NCLEX-PN examination, the process of testing, and unique and special tips for preparing yourself for this very important examination. You will read what a nursing graduate, who recently passed NCLEX-PN, has to say about the examination. Many important test-taking strategies are detailed that will guide you to selecting the correct option or to making a logical guess when you are unsure about an answer.

Each of the content areas in this book begins with the Pyramid to Success. The Pyramid to Success addresses specific points related to NCLEX-PN, including the Pyramid Terms, the Client Needs, and the Integrated Processes as identified in the test plan framework for the examination. Pyramid Terms are key words that are defined and that are then boldfaced throughout each chapter to direct your attention to those significant NCLEX-PN points. The Client Needs and Integrated Processes specific to the content of the chapter are identified.

Throughout each chapter, you will find the Pyramid Point bullets that identify the areas that are most likely to be tested on NCLEX-PN. Read each chapter, and identify your strengths and the areas in which you need further review. Test your strengths and abilities by taking all of the practice tests provided in this book. Be sure to read all of the rationales and the test-taking strategies. The rationale provides you with significant information regarding both the correct and incorrect options. The test-taking strategy provides you with the logical path to selecting the correct option. The test-taking strategy also identifies the content area to review, if required. The reference source and page number are provided so that you can easily locate the information that you need to review. Each question is coded on the basis of the Level of Cognitive Ability,

the Client Needs, the Integrated Process, and the Content Area.

After completing the comprehensive review in this book, continue on your journey though the Pyramid to Success with the companion book, *Saunders Q & A Review for the NCLEX-PN® Examination*, which provides you with more than 3000 practice questions based on the NCLEX-PN test plan, and *Saunders Review Cards for the NCLEX-PN® Examination*, which provides you with more than 900 additional practice questions. Also available to you is the *Saunders Strategies to Success for the NCLEX-PN® Examination*. This book provides you with specific test-taking strategies that will assist you with nursing examinations while in nursing school, as well as with the NCLEX-PN. These additional products in Saunders Pyramid to Success can be obtained online at www.elsevierhealth.com or by calling (800) 545-2522.

Let's begin our journey through the Pyramid to Success!

THE EXAMINATION PROCESS

An important step in the Pyramid to Success is becoming as familiar as possible with the examination process. A significant amount of anxiety can occur among candidates facing the challenge of this examination. Knowing what the examination is all about and knowing what you will encounter during the process of testing will assist with alleviating fear and anxiety. The information contained in this chapter addresses the procedures related to the development of the NCLEX-PN test plan, the components of the test plan, and the answers to the questions most commonly asked by nursing students and graduates preparing to take the NCLEX-PN.

The information in this chapter related to the test plan was obtained from the National Council of State Boards of Nursing (NCSBN) Web site (www.ncsbn.org) and from the *2008 Detailed Test Plan for the NCLEX-PN® Examination, National Council of State Boards of Nursing*. Additional information regarding the test and its development can be obtained by accessing the NCSBN

Web site or by writing to the National Council of State Boards of Nursing, 111 E. Wacker Drive, Suite 2900, Chicago, IL 60601-4277.

NCLEX-PN®

The acronym *NCLEX-PN* stands for National Council Licensure Examination for Practical/Vocational Nurses. The NCLEX-PN is a computer-administered examination that the nursing graduate must take and pass to practice in the role of a practical/vocational nurse. This examination measures the competency needed to practice safely and effectively as a newly licensed entry-level practical/vocational nurse.

DEVELOPMENT OF THE TEST PLAN

As an initial step in the test-development process, the NCSBN considers the legal scope of nursing practice as governed by state laws and regulations, including the nurse practice act. The NCSBN uses these laws to define the areas on NCLEX-PN that will assess the competence of the candidates for nurse licensure.

The NCSBN also conducts a practice analysis study to determine the framework for the test plan for the NCLEX-PN. The participants in this study include newly licensed practical and vocational nurses. The participants are provided with a list of nursing activities and asked about the frequency with which they perform these specific activities, the impact of these activities on client safety, and the settings in which the activities are performed. The expert analysis of the data obtained from this study guides the development of a framework for entry-level nurse performance that incorporates specific client needs and the processes that are fundamental to the practice of nursing. The NCLEX-PN test plan is derived from this framework. Because nursing practice continues to change, this study is conducted every 3 years. The results of this study provided the structure for the test plan that was implemented in April 2008.

THE TEST PLAN

The content of the NCLEX-PN reflects the activities that an entry-level practical and vocational nurse must be able to perform to provide clients with safe and effective nursing care. The questions are written to address the Levels of Cognitive Ability, the Client Needs, and the Integrated Processes as identified by the test plan.

Levels of Cognitive Ability

The NCLEX-PN examination consists of questions that are written at the cognitive levels of application and higher. See Box 1-1 for an example of a question at the cognitive level of application.

Client Needs

In the new test plan implemented in April 2008, the NCSBN identified a test-plan framework based on Client Needs. This framework was selected on the basis of the findings in the practice analysis study. In addition, Client Needs provide a structure for defining nursing actions and competencies across all settings for all clients that meet requirements specified by state laws and statutes. The NCSBN identifies four major categories of Client Needs. Some categories are further divided into subcategories, and the percentage of test questions in each subcategory is identified. Table 1-1 identifies these categories and subcategories and the associated percentage of test questions.

Safe and Effective Care Environment

The Safe and Effective Care Environment category includes two subcategories: Coordinated Care and

---

BOX 1-1 Level of Cognitive Ability

A nurse notes blanching, coolness, and edema at the peripheral intravenous (IV) site. On the basis of these findings, the nurse should take which action?
1. Discontinue the IV.
2. Apply a warm compress.
3. Check for a blood return.
4. Measure the area of infiltration.

Answer: 1

This question requires that you focus on the data identified in the question to determine that the client is experiencing an infiltration. You also need to consider the harmful effects of infiltration and to determine the action to take. Because infiltration can be damaging to the surrounding tissue, the most appropriate action is to discontinue the IV to prevent any further damage.

Level of Cognitive Ability: Application

TABLE 1-1 Client Needs and Percentage of NCLEX-PN® Test Questions

Category	Percentage of Test Questions
Safe and Effective Care Environment	
Coordinated Care	12-18
Safety and Infection Control	8-14
Health Promotion and Maintenance	7-13
Psychosocial Integrity	8-14
Physiological Integrity	
Basic Care and Comfort	11-17
Pharmacological Therapies	9-15
Reduction of Risk Potential	10-16
Physiological Adaptation	11-17

From National Council of State Boards of Nursing (Eds.) (2008). *2008 Detailed Test Plan for the NCLEX-PN® Examination, National Council of State Boards of Nursing.* Chicago: Author.

Safety and Infection Control. Coordinated Care (12% to 18%) addresses content related to facilitating effective client care through collaboration with other health care team members. Safety and Infection Control (8% to 14%) addresses content that tests the knowledge, skills, and abilities required to protect clients and health care personnel from health and environmental hazards. Box 1-2 presents examples of questions that address these two subcategories.

Health Promotion and Maintenance

The Health Promotion and Maintenance category (7% to 13%) addresses the principles related to growth, development, and the aging process. This Client Needs category also addresses content that tests the knowledge, skills, and abilities required to assist clients, family members, and significant others with preventing health problems, recognizing alterations in health, and developing health practices that promote and support wellness. See Box 1-3 for an example of a question in this Client Needs category.

BOX 1-2 Safe and Effective Care Environment

Coordinated Care

A nurse is caring for a client who has skeletal traction applied to the left leg. The client complains of severe left-leg pain. The nurse checks the client's alignment in bed and notes that proper alignment is maintained. Which action should the nurse take next?
1. Provide pin care.
2. Medicate the client.
3. Collaborate with the registered nurse.
4. Remove 2 lbs of weight from the traction.

Answer: 3

This question addresses the subcategory of Coordinated Care in the Client Needs category of Safe and Effective Care Environment. On the basis of the data in the question, the nurse has the responsibility to facilitate safe and effective client care through collaboration with other health care team members (in this situation, the registered nurse).

Safety and Infection Control

A nurse is assigned to care for a client with contact precautions who has a nosocomial infection caused by methicillin-resistant *Staphylococcus aureus*. The client has an abdominal wound that requires irrigation and a tracheostomy attached to a mechanical ventilator that requires frequent suctioning. The nurse gathers supplies before entering the client's room and obtains which of the following necessary protective items?
1. Gloves and a gown
2. Gloves, mask, and goggles
3. Gloves, mask, gown, and goggles
4. Gloves, gown, and shoe protectors

Answer: 3

This question addresses the subcategory of Safety and Infection Control in the Client Needs category of Safe and Effective Care Environment. It focuses on content related to protecting oneself from contracting an infection.

Psychosocial Integrity

The Psychosocial Integrity category (8% to 14%) addresses content that tests the knowledge, skills, and abilities required to promote and support the emotional, mental, and social well-being of clients, family members, and significant others. See Box 1-4 for an example of a question in this Client Needs category.

Physiological Integrity

The Physiological Integrity category includes four subcategories: Basic Care and Comfort, Pharmacological Therapies, Reduction of Risk Potential, and Physiological Adaptation. Basic Care and Comfort (11% to 17%) addresses content that tests the knowledge, skills, and abilities required to provide comfort and assistance during the performance of activities of

BOX 1-3 Health Promotion and Maintenance

A nurse is reviewing the record of a client in the labor room and notes that the nurse-midwife has documented that the fetus is at the −1 station. The nurse determines that the fetal presenting part is:
1. 1 inch below the coccyx
2. 1 inch below the iliac crest
3. 1 cm above the ischial spines
4. 1 fingerbreadth below the symphysis pubis

Answer: 3

This question addresses the Client Needs category of Health Promotion and Maintenance, and it focuses on maternity content, specifically the labor process. The station is the relationship of the fetus' presenting part to an imaginary line drawn between the ischial spines. It is measured in centimeters, and it is noted as a negative number above the line and a positive number below the line.

BOX 1-4 Psychosocial Integrity

A client with coronary artery disease has selected guided imagery to help cope with psychological stress. Which statement by the client indicates the best understanding of this stress-reduction measure?
1. "This works for me only if I am alone in a quiet area."
2. "This will help me only if I play music at the same time."
3. "I need to do this only when I lie down in case I fall asleep."
4. "The best thing about this is that I can use it anywhere, anytime."

Answer: 4

This question addresses the Client Needs category of Psychosocial Integrity, and the content addresses coping mechanisms. Guided imagery involves the client creating an image in the mind, concentrating on that image, and gradually becoming less aware of the offending stimulus. It can be done anytime and anywhere. Some clients may use other relaxation techniques or play music when performing this technique.

daily living. Pharmacological Therapies (9% to 15%) addresses content that tests the knowledge, skills, and abilities required to provide care related to the administration of medications and the monitoring of clients receiving parenteral therapies. Reduction of Risk Potential (10% to 16%) addresses content that tests the knowledge, skills, and abilities required to reduce the client's potential for developing complications or health problems related to existing conditions, treatments, or procedures. Physiological Adaptation (11% to 17%) addresses content that tests the knowledge, skills, and abilities required to

participate in providing care to clients with acute, chronic, or life-threatening physical health conditions. See Box 1-5 for examples of questions in this Client Needs category.

Integrated Processes of the Test Plan

The NCSBN has identified four processes that are fundamental to the practice of nursing. These processes are components of the test plan, and they are integrated throughout the categories of Client Needs (Box 1-6).

BOX 1-5   **Physiological Integrity**

Basic Care and Comfort

A client with Parkinson's disease quickly develops akinesia while ambulating, thus increasing the risk for falls. Which suggestion should the nurse provide to the client to alleviate this problem?

1. Use a wheelchair to move around.
2. Stand erect, and use a cane to ambulate.
3. Keep the feet close together while ambulating, and use a walker.
4. Consciously think about walking over imaginary lines on the floor.

Answer: 4

This question addresses the subcategory of Basic Care and Comfort in the Client Needs category of Physiological Integrity, and it focuses on client mobility and promoting assistance with an activity of daily living to maintain safety. Clients with Parkinson's disease can develop bradykinesia (slow movement) or akinesia (freezing or no movement). Having these individuals imagine lines on the floor to step over can keep them moving forward while remaining safe.

Pharmacological Therapies

The nurse is caring for a client who is receiving digoxin (Lanoxin). The nurse monitors the client for which early manifestation of digoxin toxicity?

1. Anorexia
2. Facial pain
3. Photophobia
4. Yellow color perception

Answer: 1

This question addresses the subcategory of Pharmacological Therapies in the Client Needs category of Physiological Integrity. Digoxin is a cardiac glycoside that is used to manage and treat heart failure and to control ventricular rates in clients with atrial fibrillation. The most common early manifestations of toxicity include gastrointestinal disturbances such as anorexia, nausea, and vomiting. Neurological abnormalities can also occur early, and these include fatigue, headache, depression, weakness, drowsiness, confusion, and nightmares. Facial pain, personality changes, and ocular disturbances (e.g., photophobia, light flashes, halos around bright objects, yellow or green color perception) are also signs of toxicity, but they are not early signs.

Reduction of Risk Potential

Magnetic resonance imaging (MRI) is prescribed for a client with a suspected brain tumor. The nurse implements which action to prepare the client for this test?

1. Removes all metal-containing objects from the client
2. Shaves the client's groin for the insertion of a femoral catheter
3. Has the client receive nothing by mouth (NPO) for 6 hours before the test
4. Instructs the client regarding inhalation techniques for the administration of the radioisotope

Answer: 1

This question addresses the subcategory of Reduction of Risk Potential in the Client Needs category of Physiological Integrity, and it focuses on the nurse's responsibilities when preparing the client for the diagnostic test. During MRI, radiofrequency pulses in a magnetic field are converted into pictures. All metal objects (e.g., rings, bracelets, hairpins, watches) should be removed from the client. In addition, a history should be taken to ascertain whether the client has any internal metallic devices, such as orthopedic hardware, pacemakers, or shrapnel. For an abdominal MRI, the client is usually NPO, but NPO status is not necessary for MRI of the head. The groin may be shaved for an angiogram, and the inhalation of a radioisotope may be prescribed with positron emission tomography.

Physiological Adaptation

A nurse is assigned to care for a client with a diagnosis of pheochromocytoma. The nurse is told during report that the client's magnesium level is 7 mEq/L. On the basis of this laboratory result, the nurse recognizes which of the following signs as significant?

1. Hyperpnea
2. Drowsiness
3. Hypertension
4. Hyperactive reflexes

Answer: 2

This question addresses the subcategory of Physiological Adaptation in the Client Needs category of Physiological Integrity. It addresses an alteration in body systems. Neurological manifestations begin to occur at magnesium levels of 6 to 7 mEq/L, and they are noted as symptoms of neurological depression, such as drowsiness, sedation, lethargy, respiratory depression, muscle weakness, and areflexia.

Caring
Clinical Problem-Solving Process (Nursing Process)
Communication and Documentation
Teaching and Learning

TYPES OF QUESTIONS ON THE EXAMINATION

The types of questions that may be administered on the examination include multiple choice, fill-in-the-blank, multiple response, prioritizing (ordered response), chart/exhibit, and questions that contain a figure or illustration (hot spots). Some questions may require you to use the mouse component of the computer system. For example, you may be presented with a visual that displays the arterial vessels of an adult client. In this visual, you may be asked to "point and click" (using the mouse) on the area where the dorsalis pedis pulse could be felt (the hot spot). The NCSBN provides specific directions for you to follow with these questions to guide you during the testing process. Be sure to read these directions as they appear on the computer screen.

Multiple-Choice Questions

Most of the questions that you will be asked to answer will be in the multiple-choice format. These questions will provide you with data about a particular client situation, and you will then be given four answers or options.

Fill-in-the-Blank Questions

These types of questions may ask you to perform a medication calculation, to determine the intravenous flow rate, or to calculate an intake or output record for a client. You will need to type in your answer. Read the directions carefully, because you may be asked to round the answer to the nearest whole number or to the nearest tenth. See Box 1-7 for an example of a fill-in-the-blank question.

Multiple-Response Questions

With this type of question, you will be asked to select or check all of the options, such as the nursing interventions, that relate to the information presented in the question. There is no partial credit given for correct selections. See Box 1-8 for an example of a multiple-response question.

Prioritizing (Ordered-Response) Questions

These questions may ask you to place your nursing actions in order of priority. Information will be

BOX 1-7 **Fill-in-the-Blank Question**

The physician's order reads as follows: Acetaminophen (Tylenol Extra Strength) liquid, 650 mg orally every 4 hours as needed for pain. The medication label reads as follows: 500 mg/15 mL. The nurse prepares how many milliliters to administer one dose?
Answer: 19.5
Formula:

$$\frac{\text{Desired}}{\text{Available}} \times \text{Volume} = \text{mL}$$

$$\frac{650\,\text{mg}}{500\,\text{mg}} \times 15\,\text{mL} = 19.5\,\text{mL}$$

For this question, you need to use the formula for calculating a medication dose. After the dose is determined, you will need to type in your answer. Always follow the specific directions noted on the computer screen when answering any question. In addition, remember that there will be an on-screen calculator on the computer for your use, if needed.

BOX 1-8 **Multiple-Response Question**

A nurse assists with caring for a child who is suspected of having acute epiglottitis. Choose the nursing interventions that apply to the care of this child. Select all that apply.

- ☐ 1. Obtain a throat culture
- ☑ 2. Ensure a patent airway
- ☑ 3. Prepare the child for a chest x-ray
- ☐ 4. Maintain the child in a supine position
- ☑ 5. Obtain a pediatric-size tracheostomy tray
- ☑ 6. Place the child on an oxygen saturation monitor

For a multiple-response question, you will be asked to select or check all of the options, such as the nursing interventions, that relate to the information in the question. To answer this question, recall that acute epiglottitis is a serious obstructive inflammatory process that requires immediate intervention. To reduce respiratory distress, the child should sit upright. Examining the throat with a tongue depressor or attempting to obtain a throat culture is contraindicated because the examination can precipitate further obstruction. The child is placed on an oxygen saturation monitor to observe the oxygenation status. Lateral neck and chest x-rays are obtained to determine the degree of obstruction, if present. Intubation may be necessary if respiratory distress is severe. Remember to follow the specific directions given on the computer screen.

presented in the question, and, on the basis of the data, you will determine what you would do first, second, third, and so on. See Box 1-9 for an example of a prioritizing (ordered-response) question.

Figure or Illustration (Hot-Spot) Questions

This type of question will provide you with a figure or illustration, and you will be asked to answer the

BOX 1-9	Prioritizing (Ordered-Response) Question

A nurse is preparing to suction a client who has a tracheostomy tube and gathers the supplies needed for the procedure. In order of priority, number the actions that the nurse takes to perform this procedure. (Number 1 is the first priority action, and number 6 is the last action.)

1. Place the client in semi-Fowler's position.
2. Turn on the suction device, and set the regulator to 80 mm Hg.
3. Apply gloves, and attach the suction tubing to the suction catheter.
4. Hyperoxygenate the client.
5. Insert the catheter into the tracheostomy until resistance is met, and then pull back 1 cm.
6. Apply intermittent suction, and slowly withdraw the catheter while rotating it back and forth.

This question requires you to list in order of priority the actions that the nurse takes to suction a client who has a tracheostomy tube. The nurse would position the client first, turn the suction device on, and then set the regulator. The nurse then dons gloves and attaches the suction tubing to the suction catheter. The nurse would hyperoxygenate the client both before and after suctioning. At this point, the nurse inserts the catheter into the tracheostomy until resistance is met and then pulls back 1 cm, applies intermittent suction, and slowly withdraws the catheter while rotating it back and forth. Remember that the client and the equipment are prepared before the procedure is performed. In addition, remember that on the NCLEX-PN examination you will use the drag-and-drop feature of the computer mouse to place the actions in order of priority.

BOX 1-10	Figure or Illustration Question

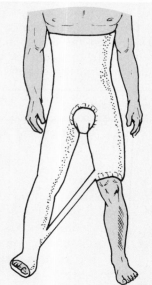

(From Black, J., & Hawks, J. [2009]. *Medical-surgical nursing: Clinical management for positive outcomes*, Vol. 1 [8th ed.]. Philadelphia: Saunders.)

A nurse is providing care to a client with this type of cast. The nurse documents that the client is in a:

1. Long leg cast
2. Short leg cast
3. Hip spica cast
4. Body jacket cast

Answer: 3

For this question, you are provided with a figure and asked to document the type of cast applied to the client. A hip spica cast is used to treat pelvic and femoral fractures. The cast covers the lower torso and extends to one or both of the lower extremities. If only one lower extremity is included, it is called a *single hip spica;* if two are included, it is called a *double hip spica.* Short and long leg casts are applied to the leg. A body jacket cast is applied to the upper torso.

question on the basis of the image. The question could contain, a table, or a figure or illustration. You may also be asked to use the computer mouse and to "point and click" on a specific area (hot spot) of the visual. A visual or image may appear in any type of question, including a multiple-choice question. See Box 1-10 for an example of a figure or illustration question.

Chart/Exhibit Questions

With this type of question, you will be presented with a problem and a client's chart or exhibit. You will need to refer to the information in the chart or exhibit to answer the question. Be sure to read all of the information before answering. See Box 1-11 for an example of a chart or exhibit question.

COMPUTERIZED ADAPTIVE TESTING

The acronym *CAT* stands for computerized adaptive testing. This means that the examination is created as the test-taker answers each question. All of the test questions are categorized on the basis of the test-plan structure and the level of difficulty of the question. As you answer a question, the computer will determine your competency on the basis of the answer that you selected. If you selected a correct answer to a question, the computer scans the question bank and selects a more difficult question. If you selected an incorrect answer, the computer scans the question bank and selects an easier question. This process continues until the test plan requirements are met and a reliable pass-or-fail decision can be made.

When a test question is presented on the computer screen, it must be answered, or the test will not move on. This means that you will not be able to skip questions, go back and review questions, or go back

BOX 1-11 **Chart/Exhibit Question**

A nurse reviews the history and physical examination documented in the medical record of a client who is requesting a prescription for oral contraceptives. The nurse determines that oral contraceptives are contraindicated because of which documented item?

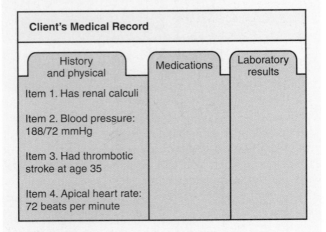

Answer: 3

This chart or exhibit question provides you with data from the client's medical record and asks you to identify the item that is a contraindication to the use of oral contraceptives. Oral contraceptives are contraindicated among women with a history of any of the following: thrombophlebitis and thromboembolic disorders; cardiovascular or cerebrovascular diseases (including stroke); any estrogen-dependent cancer or breast cancer or benign or malignant liver tumors; impaired liver function; hypertension; and diabetes mellitus with vascular involvement. Adverse effects of oral contraceptives include the following: increased risk of superficial and deep venous thrombosis; pulmonary embolism; thrombotic stroke (or other types of strokes); myocardial infarction; and acceleration of preexisting breast tumors.

and change answers. Remember, with a CAT examination, after an answer is recorded, all subsequent questions administered depend to an extent on the answer that you selected for that question. Skipping questions and returning to earlier questions are not compatible with the logical methodology of this type of testing. The inability to skip questions or go back to change previous answers will not be a disadvantage to you. Actually, you will not fall into the "trap" of changing a correct answer to an incorrect one with CAT.

If you are faced with a question that contains unfamiliar content, you may need to guess at the answer. There is no penalty for guessing on this examination. Remember, with the majority of the questions, the answer will be right there in front of you. If you need to guess, use your nursing knowledge to its fullest extent and rely on the test-taking strategies that you will have practiced with this review program.

You do not need any computer experience to take this examination. A keyboard and question tutorial are provided to all test-takers at the beginning of the examination. The tutorial will tell you how to use the on-screen optional calculator and the mouse and how to record your answers for the various question types. A proctor is present to assist with explaining the use of the computer to ensure your full understanding of how to proceed.

REGISTERING TO TAKE THE EXAMINATION

The initial step in the registration process is to submit an application to the state board of nursing of the state in which you intend to obtain licensure. You need to obtain information from the board of nursing regarding the specific registration process, because the process may vary from state to state. In most states, you may register for the examination via the Web, mail, or telephone. The NCLEX-PN candidate Web site is www.vue.com/nclex. Following the registration instructions and completing the registration forms precisely and accurately are important. Registration forms that are not properly completed or that are not accompanied by the proper fees paid by the required method of payment will be returned to you and will delay testing. You must pay a fee for taking the examination, and you also may have to pay additional fees to the board of nursing of the state in which you are applying. You will be sent a confirmation letter indicating that your registration was received. If you do not receive such a confirmation within 4 weeks of submitting your registration, you should contact the candidate services. This contact information can be obtained at the NCLEX-PN candidate Web site at www.vue.com/nclex.

AUTHORIZATION TO TEST FORM

After your eligibility to test has been determined, your registration form is processed, and an Authorization to Test (ATT) form will be sent to you. You cannot make an appointment until you are declared eligible and until you receive this form. The examination will take place at a Pearson Professional Center, and you can make an appointment via the Web (www.vue.com/nclex) or by telephone. You can schedule an appointment at any Pearson Professional Center. You do not have to take the examination in the same state in which you are seeking licensure. A confirmation of your appointment will be sent to you.

The ATT form contains important information, including your test authorization number, your candidate identification number, and an expiration date. Note the expiration date on the form, because you must test by this date. You also need to take your ATT form to the test center on the day of your examination.

You will not be admitted to the examination if you do not have it.

If for any reason you need to cancel or reschedule your appointment to test, you can make the change on the candidate Web site (www.vue.com/nclex) or by calling candidate services. The change needs to be made 1 full business day (24 hours) before your scheduled appointment. If you fail to arrive for the examination or fail to cancel your appointment to test without providing appropriate notice, you will forfeit your examination fee, and your ATT form will be invalidated. This information will be reported to the board of nursing in the state in which you have applied for licensure, and you will be required to register and pay the testing fees again.

It is important that you arrive at the testing center at least 30 minutes before the test is scheduled. If you arrive late for the scheduled testing appointment, you may be required to forfeit your examination appointment. If it is necessary to forfeit your appointment, you will need to reregister for the examination and pay an additional fee. The board of nursing will be notified that you did not test. A few days before your scheduled date of testing, take the time to drive to the testing center to determine its exact location, the length of time required to arrive at your destination, and any potential obstacles that may delay you, such as road construction, traffic, or parking sites.

SPECIAL TESTING CIRCUMSTANCES

If you require special testing accommodations, you should contact the board of nursing before submitting a registration form. The board of nursing will provide the procedures for the request. The board of nursing must authorize special testing accommodations. After approval from the board of nursing has been obtained, the NCSNB reviews the requested accommodations, and it must also approve the request. If the request is approved, the testing appointment must be made by an NCLEX-PN program coordinator, whom you can contact by calling NCLEX-PN candidate services. If it is necessary, you must cancel or reschedule an appointment through an NCLEX-PN program coordinator.

THE TESTING CENTER

The testing center is designed to ensure the complete security of the testing process. Strict candidate identification requirements have been established. To be admitted to the testing center, you must bring your ATT form and two forms of identification. Both forms of identification must be signed and current or nonexpired, and one must include a recent photograph of you. The name on the photograph identification must be the same as the name on the ATT form. A digital fingerprint, signature, and photograph will be taken at the testing center, and these will accompany the NCLEX-PN examination results to confirm your identity. In addition, if you leave the testing room for any reason, you may be required to have your fingerprint taken again to be readmitted to the room.

Personal belongings are not allowed in the testing room. Secure storage will be provided for you; however, storage space is limited, so you must plan accordingly. In addition, the testing center will not assume responsibility for your personal belongings. The testing waiting areas are generally small; therefore, friends or family members who accompany you are not permitted to wait in the testing center while you are taking the examination.

After you have completed the admission process and a brief orientation, the proctor will escort you to your assigned computer. You will be seated at an individual work space that includes computer equipment, appropriate lighting, an erasable note board, and a marker. No items, including unauthorized scratch paper, are allowed into the testing room. Electronic devices such as watches, beepers, and cell phones are not allowed in the testing room. Eating, drinking, and the use of tobacco are not allowed in the testing room. You will be observed at all times by the test proctor while taking the examination. In addition, video and audio recording of all test sessions occurs. Pearson Professional Centers have no control over the sounds made by typing on the computer by others. If these sounds are distracting, raise your hand to summon the proctor. Earplugs are available on request.

You must follow the instructions given by the test center staff, and you must remain seated during the test, except when authorized to leave. If you feel that you have a problem with the computer, that you need an additional note board or to take a break, or that you require the services of the test proctor for any reason, you must raise your hand.

TESTING TIME

The maximum testing time is 5 hours, and this time period includes the tutorial, the sample items, all breaks, and the examination. All breaks are optional. You must leave the testing room during breaks. When you return, you may be required to provide a fingerprint to be readmitted to the testing room.

LENGTH OF THE EXAMINATION

The minimum number of questions that you will need to answer is 85. Of these 85 questions, 60 will be operational (scored) questions, and 25 will be pretest (unscored) questions. The maximum number of questions on the test is 205. Twenty-five of the total number of questions that you answer will be pretest (unscored) questions.

The pretest questions are questions that may be presented as scored questions on future examinations. These pretest questions are not identified as such. In other words, you do not know which questions are the pretest (unscored) questions.

PASS-OR-FAIL DECISIONS

All of the examination questions are categorized by test plan area and level of difficulty. This is an important point to keep in mind when you consider how the computer makes a pass-or-fail decision, because a pass-or-fail decision is not based on a percentage of correctly answered questions.

After the minimum number of questions (85) have been answered, the computer compares the test-taker's ability level with the standard required for passing. The standard required for passing is set on the basis of the expert judgment of several individuals appointed by the NCSBN. If the test-taker is clearly above the passing standard, then the test-taker passes the examination. If the test-taker is clearly below the passing standard, then the test-taker fails the examination. If the computer is not able to determine clearly whether the test-taker has passed or failed because the test-taker's ability is close to the passing standard, then the computer continues asking questions. After each question, the computer determines the test-taker's ability. When it becomes clear on which side of the passing standard the test-taker falls (i.e., above or below the standard), the examination ends. If the test-taker is administered the maximum number of questions (205), the computer will make a pass-or-fail decision by recomputing the test-taker's final ability level on the basis of every question answered and comparing it with the passing standard. If the ability level is above the passing standard, the test-taker passes. If the ability level is not above the passing standard, the test-taker fails.

If the examination ends because you have run out of time, the computer may not have enough information to make a clear pass-or-fail decision. If this is the situation, the computer will review the test-taker's performance during testing. If the test-taker's ability was consistently above the passing standard on the final 60 questions specifically, then the test-taker passes. If the test-taker's ability falls at or below the passing standard, even once, then the test-taker fails.

COMPLETING THE EXAMINATION

When the test is finished, you will complete a brief computer-delivered questionnaire about your testing experience. After this questionnaire is completed, you need to raise your hand to summon the test proctor. The test proctor will collect and inventory all note boards and then permit you to leave.

PROCESSING RESULTS

Every computerized examination is scored twice: once by the computer at the testing center and then again after the examination is transmitted to Pearson Professional Centers. No results are released at the test center. The board of nursing will mail your results to you approximately 1 month after you take the examination. You should not telephone Pearson Professional Centers, the NCSBN, candidate services, or the state board of nursing for results. In some states, results can be obtained via the state Web site or via an NCSBN telephone results service. Information about obtaining NCLEX-PN results by this method can be obtained on the NCSBN Web site (www.ncsbn.org) in the candidate services section.

CANDIDATE PERFORMANCE REPORT

A candidate performance report is provided to any test-taker who failed the examination. This report provides the test-taker with information about their strengths and weaknesses in relation to the test plan, and it provides a guide for studying and retaking the examination. The test-taker should refer to the state board of nursing of the state in which licensure is sought for procedures regarding the time period for retaking the examination.

INTERSTATE ENDORSEMENT

Because the NCLEX-PN examination is a national examination, you can apply to take the examination in any state. After licensure is received, you can apply for Interstate Endorsement, which is the obtaining of another license in another state to practice nursing in that state. The procedures and requirements for Interstate Endorsement may vary from state to state, and these procedures can be obtained from the state board of nursing of the state in which endorsement is sought. You may also be allowed to practice nursing in another state if the state has enacted the nurse licensure compact. The state boards of nursing can be accessed via the NCSBN Web site at www.ncsbn.org.

NURSE LICENSURE COMPACT

It may be possible to hold one license from the state of residency and to practice nursing in another state under the mutual recognition model of nursing licensure if the state has enacted the nurse licensure compact. To obtain information about the Nurse Licensure Compact and the states that entered into this interstate compact, access the NCSBN Web site at www.ncsbn.org.

ADDITIONAL INFORMATION ABOUT THE EXAMINATION

Additional information regarding the NCLEX-PN examination can be obtained from the National Council of State Boards of Nursing, 111 E. Wacker Drive, Suite 2900, Chicago, IL 60601-4277. The telephone number for the testing service is (866) 293-9600, and the Web site is www.ncsbn.org.

REFERENCES

Black, J., & Hawks, J. (2005). *Medical-surgical nursing: Clinical management for positive outcomes* (7th ed.). Philadelphia: Saunders.

Chernecky, C., & Berger, B. (2008). *Laboratory tests and diagnostic procedures* (5th ed.). Philadelphia: Saunders.

Christensen, B., & Kockrow, E. (2006). *Foundations and adult health nursing* (5th ed.). St. Louis: Mosby.

deWit, S. (2009). *Medical-surgical nursing: Concepts & practice.* St. Louis: Saunders.

Hill, S., & Howlett, H. (2005). *Success in practical/vocational nursing: From student to leader* (5th ed.). Philadelphia: Saunders.

Hodgson, B., & Kizior, R. (2008). *Saunders nursing drug handbook 2008,* Philadelphia: Saunders.

Lilley, L., Harrington, S., & Snyder, J. (2007). *Pharmacology and the nursing process* (5th ed.). St. Louis: Mosby.

Linton, A., & Maebius, N. (2007). *Introduction to medical-surgical nursing* (4th ed.). Philadelphia: Saunders.

National Council of State Boards of Nursing (Eds.) (2008). *2008 Detailed Test Plan for the NCLEX-PN® Examination, National Council of State Boards of Nursing.* Chicago: Author.

National Council of State Boards of Nursing. *NCSBN home page.* www.ncsbn.org. Accessed June 2, 2008.

Potter, P., & Perry, A. (2005). *Fundamentals of nursing* (6th ed.). St. Louis: Mosby.

Pagana, K., & Pagana, T. (2005). *Mosby's diagnostic and laboratory test reference* (7th ed.). St. Louis: Mosby.

Preparation for the NCLEX-PN® Examination: Transitional Issues for the Foreign-Educated Nurse

This chapter provides you with information regarding the certification processes that you will have to pursue to become a licensed practical/vocational nurse in the United States. An important factor to consider as you pursue this process is that some of the requirements may vary from state to state. Therefore, as a first step in the process, you need to contact the board of nursing in the state in which you are planning to obtain licensure. You can obtain contact information for each state board of nursing through the National Council of State Boards of Nursing (NCSBN) Web site at www.ncsbn.org. After you have accessed the NCSBN Web site, select the link titled "Boards of Nursing." In addition, you can write to the NCSBN regarding the NCLEX-PN exam at 111 E. Wacker Drive, Suite 2900, Chicago, IL 60601. The telephone number for the NCSBN is (312) 525-3600, and the fax number is (312) 279-1032.

An additional step in the process of obtaining information about becoming a licensed practical/vocational nurse in the United States is to access the NCSBN Web site (www.ncsbn.org) and to look at the information provided for international nurses under the "NCLEX Examinations" link. The NCSBN provides information about some of the data that you will need to obtain as an international nurse seeking licensure as a licensed practical/vocational nurse in the United States and about credentialing agencies.

This chapter provides information about the Commission on Graduates of Foreign Nursing Schools (CGFNS) credentialing program. The NCSBN Web site (www.ncsbn.org) can provide information about additional credentialing agencies. The credentialing agency needs to follow the standards identified by professional credentialing associations such as the National Association of Credential Evaluation Services (www.naces.org). Therefore, it is important to obtain contact information for credentialing agencies from the NCSBN. In addition, because criteria can change, it is recommended that you access the NCSBN Web site to obtain the most up-to-date information about the credentialing process and about obtaining a license to practice as a licensed practical/vocational nurse (LPN/LVN) in the United States.

VISASCREEN

U.S. immigration law requires certain health care professionals to successfully complete a screening program before receiving an occupational visa (§343 of the Illegal Immigration Reform and Immigration Responsibility Act of 1996). Therefore, you are required to obtain a VisaScreen certificate.

The CGFNS is an organization that offers this federal screening program. The International Commission on Health Care Professions, a division of the CGFNS, administers the VisaScreen. The VisaScreen components include an educational analysis, a license verification, an assessment of proficiency in the English language, and an examination that tests nursing knowledge. This chapter describes each of these components. After successfully completing each of the components, the applicant is presented with a VisaScreen certificate. You can obtain information related to the VisaScreen through the CGFNS Web site at www.cgfns.org.

Educational Analysis

The educational analysis component requires the following:
1. The applicant must present proof of the completion of senior secondary school education that is separate from any professional certification.
2. The applicant must present proof of the completion of a government-approved professional health care nursing program.
3. The applicant must provide documentation of the completion of a specified number of clock and/or credit hours in specific theoretical and clinical areas while in nursing school.

Licensure Verification

The applicant must present all current and past licensure for review.

BOX 2-1 **English Language Proficiency Exams and Testing Organizations**

Tests Administered by the Educational Testing Service (ETS) Worldwide
- Test of English as a Foreign Language (TOEFL)
- The Test of English for International Communication (TOEIC)

Contact Information:
Educational Testing Service (ETS)
P.O. Box 6151
Princeton, NJ 08541-6151
Telephone: 609-771-7100
Email: toefl@ets.org
Web site: www.ets.org

International English Language Testing System (IELTS), Jointly Managed by British Council and IELTS Australia
Contact Information:
International English Language Testing System (IELTS)
IELTS Administrator
Cambridge Examinations and IELTS International
100 East Corson Street
Suite 200
Pasadena, CA 91103
Telephone: 626-564-2954
Email: ielts@ceii.org
Web site: www.ielts.org

Proficiency in the English Language

The applicant must submit proof of a passing score on an approved U.S. Department of Education and Health and Human Services English language proficiency examination. Box 2-1 lists English proficiency examinations and testing organizations. The credentialing agency will also provide you with information about English language proficiency examinations.

Examination to Test Nursing Knowledge

An examination to test nursing knowledge includes the following:

1. A qualifying examination that is administered as part of the process for obtaining a CGFNS Certificate tests nursing knowledge; therefore, a CGFNS Certificate provides proof of adequate nursing knowledge. This qualifying examination is described later in this chapter in Components of the CGFNS Certification Program.
2. A foreign-educated nurse who is licensed and practicing nursing in the United States is also required to obtain a VisaScreen; if the nurse does not have a CGFNS Certificate, the nurse may be granted eligibility to take the NCLEX-PN exam to provide proof of nursing knowledge.

STATE REQUIREMENTS

Most states require that you receive certification from the CGFNS or another credentialing agency before you are eligible to take the NCLEX-PN exam. If the state in which you intend to obtain licensure does not require certification, it may require the submission of some of the same documents that the CGFNS or other credentialing agencies require. Therefore, in addition to what the CGFNS or other credentialing agencies require, a state may require the following:

1. Proof of citizenship or lawful alien status
2. Official transcripts of educational credentials sent directly to the agency and board of nursing from the school of nursing
3. Validation of theoretical instruction and clinical practice in a variety of nursing areas including but not limited to medical nursing, surgical nursing, pediatric nursing, maternity and newborn nursing, and mental health nursing; validation of nursing course work may also be required
4. Copy of nursing license and/or diploma
5. Proof of proficiency in the English language
6. Photographs of the applicant
7. Application fees

THE COMMISSION ON GRADUATES OF FOREIGN NURSING SCHOOLS

The CGFNS provides a certification program for nurses who have been educated and licensed outside of the United States.

The certificate program offered by the CGFNS is a requirement of most state boards of nursing, and the certificate may be required before you can take the NCLEX-PN exam. The certificate program ensures that you are eligible and qualified to meet licensure and other practice requirements in the United States, and it also predicts your success on the NCLEX-PN exam. This program also assists you with obtaining your VisaScreen certificate. You can obtain additional information about the CGFNS and its certification program through the CGFNS Web site at www.cgfns.org.

Eligibility for the CGFNS Certification Program

The CGFNS Certification Program is designed for nurses educated outside of the United States who hold both initial and current registrations or licensures as a nurse. According to the CGFNS, the foreign-educated nurse must have obtained theoretical instruction and clinical practice in a variety of nursing areas. These nursing areas include but are not limited to medical nursing, surgical nursing, pediatric nursing, maternity and newborn nursing, and mental health nursing. If a nurse educated outside of the United States does not meet these requirements, then that nurse is not eligible for the Certification Program.

Components of the CGFNS Certification Program

The CGFNS Certification Program contains three parts, and you must complete all parts successfully to be awarded a CGFNS Certificate. The three parts are a credentials review, a qualifying examination that tests nursing knowledge, and an English language proficiency examination. You can take the qualifying and English language proficiency examinations at various locations throughout the world. This provides the applicant with the opportunity to obtain the CGFNS Certificate before coming to the United States or traveling to other countries to take the NCLEX-PN exam. These three parts of the certificate program are described next.

Credentials Review

The CGFNS requires the validation of education and a licensing history of the applicant to ensure that the applicant has the appropriate credentials to seek certification. The CGFNS must receive transcripts and validation documents from the nursing program and the licensing agency. The CGFNS does not accept transcripts and validation documents from the applicant. The specific credentialing requirements are similar to those needed for the VisaScreen certificate and include the following:

1. Completion of a senior secondary school education
2. Graduation from a government-approved nursing program
3. Acquisition of theoretical instruction and clinical practice in the areas of medical nursing, surgical nursing, pediatric nursing, maternity/newborn nursing, and mental health nursing
4. Possession of a full and unrestricted current license or registration to practice as a nurse in the country in which the general nursing education was completed

Qualifying Examination

The qualifying examination tests the applicant's knowledge of nursing in the areas of adult health (medical and surgical), pediatrics, maternity and newborn, and mental health. The examination is designed to ensure that the applicant has the knowledge to provide nursing care to various client groups at the same level as recent U.S. nursing graduates.

English Language Proficiency Examination

The applicant must take and pass an English language proficiency examination. You can take the examination before or after the qualifying examination. The English language proficiency exam needs to be administered by a testing organization that is approved by the CGFNS, and the applicant must apply directly with the testing organization to take the examination. The scores must be sent directly to the CGFNS from the testing organization. The CGFNS will not accept test scores from the applicant. Box 2-1 lists the types of English proficiency examinations, the approved testing organizations, and their contact information. The CGFNS or another credentialing agency will provide you with current information about these approved testing organizations.

The CGFNS or another credentialing agency may identify certain applicants as exempt from the English language proficiency requirement. To be exempt, the applicant must meet all of the following criteria: native language is English; country of nursing education was Australia, Canada (except Quebec), New Zealand, the United Kingdom, or Trinidad and Tobago; and language of instruction and language of textbooks was English. Because these criteria may change, it is recommended that you obtain current information from the credentialing agency.

When you have successfully completed each of the three required components of the CGFNS Certification Program, the CGFNS will issue a certificate of completion. If you have received your VisaScreen certificate, you will then be eligible to take the NCLEX-PN exam, unless the state in which you intend to obtain licensure indicates additional requirements.

REGISTERING TO TAKE THE NCLEX-PN®

If you are planning to take the NCLEX-PN exam in the United States, the initial step in the registration process is to submit an application to the state board of nursing of the state in which you intend to obtain licensure. You need to obtain information from the board of nursing regarding the specific registration process, because the process may vary from state to state. In most states, you may register for the examination via the Web, mail, or telephone. The NCLEX-PN candidate Web site is www.vue.com/nclex. You must follow the registration instructions and complete the registration forms precisely and accurately. Registration forms that are not properly completed or that are not accompanied by the proper fees paid by the required method of payment will be returned to you and will delay testing. You must pay a fee for taking the examination, and you may also have to pay additional fees to the board of nursing of the state in which you are applying. You will be sent a confirmation letter indicating that your registration was received. If you do not receive such a confirmation within 4 weeks of submitting your registration, you should contact the candidate services. You can obtain information about candidate services at the candidate Web site (www.vue.com/nclex).

After the board of nursing of the state in which you request licensure has verified your eligibility to take the examination, it will process your registration form and send you an Authorization to Test (ATT) form. You cannot make an appointment until the board of nursing declares eligibility and you receive an ATT form. The examination will take place at a Pearson Professional Center, and you can make an appointment via the Web or by telephone. You can schedule an appointment at any Pearson Professional Center. You do not have to take the examination in the same state in which you are seeking licensure. A confirmation of your appointment will be sent to you. For additional information regarding the NCLEX-PN exam and testing procedures, refer to Chapter 1. You can also obtain information about the registration process and testing procedures from the NCSBN Web site at www.ncsbn.org.

NCLEX-PN testing abroad is also available in some countries. International sites that currently provide this testing are Australia, Canada, England, Germany, Hong Kong, India, Japan, Mexico, Puerto Rico, South Korea, and Taiwan. These testing sites provide the nurse who is interested in becoming a licensed nurse in the United States with an opportunity to pass the NCLEX-PN before traveling to the United States. Because the location of testing sites may change, it is recommended that you visit the NCLEX Web site for current information about international testing sites.

PREPARING TO TAKE THE NCLEX-PN®

The challenge that is presented to you is one that requires patience and endurance. The positive result of your endeavor certainly will reward you professionally and give you the personal satisfaction of knowing that you have become part of a family of highly skilled and professional LPN/LVNs. You have successfully completed the requirements to become

eligible to take the NCLEX-PN exam, and now you have one more important goal to achieve: passing the exam.

I highly recommend adequate preparation for the NCLEX-PN, because the examination is difficult. You have already taken an important step in that you are using this book. After you have reviewed the content and answered the practice questions, the next step in your journey to success is to use the companion book, *Saunders Q&A Review for the NCLEX-PN® Examination*, which provides you with an additional 3000 practice questions based on the NCLEX-PN examination test plan framework, with a specific focus on Client Needs and Integrated Processes. Additional resources to prepare you for this examination are the *Saunders Strategies for Success for the NCLEX-PN® Examination* and the *Saunders Q & A Review Cards for the NCLEX-PN Examination*, which contains more than 900 practice questions. All of these products can be obtained online by visiting www.elsevierhealth.com or by calling (800)545-2522 for domestic orders or (800) 460-3110 for international orders.

Remember to never lose sight of your goal. Patience and dedication will contribute significantly to your achieving the status of licensed practical/vocational nurse. Remember, success is climbing a mountain, facing the challenges and obstacles, and reaching the top of that mountain. I wish you much success on your journey and with beginning your career as a licensed practical/vocational nurse in the United States of America.

REFERENCES

Commission on Graduates of Foreign Nursing Schools. *CGFNS home page*. www.cgfns.org. Accessed June 2, 2008.

Educational Testing Service. *ETS home page*. www.ets.org. Accessed June 2, 2008.

International English Language Testing System. *IELTS home page*. www.ielts.org. Accessed June 2, 2008.

National Council of State Boards of Nursing. *NCSBN home page*. www.ncsbn.org. Accessed June 2, 2008.

National Council of State Boards of Nursing (Eds.) (2008). *2008 Detailed Test Plan for the NCLEX-PN® Examination, National Council of State Boards of Nursing*. Chicago: Author.

Pathways to Success

LAURENT W. VALLIERE, BS

PYRAMID TO SUCCESS

Preparing to take the NCLEX-PN exam can produce a great deal of anxiety. You may be thinking that the NCLEX-PN is the most important exam that you will ever have to take, and that it reflects the culmination of everything for which you have worked so hard. The NCLEX-PN is an important exam, because receiving that nursing license means that you can begin your career as a licensed practical/vocational nurse. Your success on the NCLEX-PN involves expelling all thoughts from your mind that allow this exam to appear overwhelming and intimidating; such thoughts will take complete control over your destiny. A positive attitude, a structured plan for preparation, and maintaining control of your pathway to success will ensure your achievement of reaching the peak of the Pyramid to Success (Figure 3-1).

PATHWAYS TO SUCCESS (Box 3-1)

The Foundation

The foundation of Pathways to Success begins with a positive attitude, the belief that you will achieve success, and the development of control. It also includes the creation of a list of your personal short- and long-term goals and a plan for preparation. A positive attitude, belief in yourself, control, and a list of personal goals will lead you to becoming a licensed practical/vocational nurse. Without these components, your Pathway to Success leads to nowhere and has no end point. You will expend energy and valuable time in your journey, but you will lack control over where you are heading, and you will experience exhaustion without any accomplishment. Therefore, it is imperative that you take the time to develop that positive attitude and to establish your short- and long-term goals.

Where do you start? To begin this process, find a location that offers solitude. Sit or lie in a comfortable position, close your eyes, relax, inhale deeply, hold your breath to a count of 4, exhale slowly, and, again, relax. Repeat this breathing exercise several times until you begin to feel relaxed, free from anxiety, and in control of your destiny. Allow your mind to become void of all

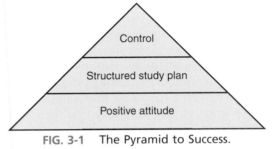

FIG. 3-1   The Pyramid to Success.

of the mind chatter; you are now in control, and your mind can see for miles. Your highway of life has a multitude of destinations to which you may travel. Next, reflect on all that you have accomplished and the path that brought you to where you are today. Journal your reflections as you plan the order of your journey to the Pyramid to Success.

The List

It is time to create "The List." "The List" is your set of short- and long-term goals. At this time, you may or may not have a scheduled date for taking the NCLEX-PN exam. Therefore, begin by developing the goals you wish to accomplish today, tomorrow, over the next month, and into the future. Allow yourself the opportunity to list all that is flowing from your mind. Write your goals in your personal journal. When "The List" is complete, put it away for 2 or 3 days. After that time, retrieve and review "The List," and begin the process of planning for preparing for the NCLEX-PN exam.

The Plan for Preparation

Now that you have "The List" in order, look at the goals that relate to studying for the licensing exam. The first task is to decide what study pattern works best for you. Think about what has worked most successfully for you in the past. There are questions that must be addressed to develop your plan for study. These questions are identified in Box 3-2.

The plan must include a schedule. Use a calendar to plan and document the times and nursing content areas

---

BOX 3-1 **Pathways to Success**

The Foundation
- Maintaining a positive attitude
- Thinking about realistic short- and long-term goals
- Preparing a plan for preparation
- Maintaining control

The List
- Journaling realistic short- and long-term goals

The Plan for Preparation
- Developing a study plan and schedule
- Deciding on the place to study
- Balancing personal and work obligations with the study schedule
- Sharing the study schedule and personal needs with others
- Implementing the study plan

Positive Pampering
- Planning time for exercise and fun activities
- Establishing healthy eating habits
- Including activities in the schedule that provide positive mental stimulation

Final Preparation
- Reviewing goals
- Identifying goals that have been achieved
- Remaining focused to complete the plan of study
- Writing down the date and time of the exam and posting it next to your name with the letters "LPN" or "LVN" after it, along with the word "YES!"
- Taking a test drive to the testing center
- Enjoying relaxing activities on the day before the exam

The Day of the Exam
- Grooming yourself for success
- Eating a healthy and nutritious breakfast
- Maintaining a confident and positive attitude
- Maintaining control
- Meeting the challenges of the day
- Reaching the peak of the Pyramid to Success

Box 3-2 **Developing a Plan of Study**

- Do I work better alone or in a group study environment?
- If I work best in a group, does the group consist of one, two, or more study partners?
- Who are these study partners?
- How long should my study sessions last?
- Does the time of day that I study make a difference for me?
- Do I retain more if I study in the morning?
- How does my work schedule affect my study pattern?
- How do I balance my family obligations with my need to study?
- Do I have a comfortable study area at home, or do I need to find another environment that is more conducive to my study needs?

---

for your study sessions. Establish a realistic schedule that includes your daily, weekly, and future goals, and adhere to it. This consistency will provide advantages to you and to those supporting you. A daily schedule allows you to plan your content areas for study more carefully. Stick to your plan of study. Adherence to the plan helps you develop a rhythm that can only enhance your retention and positive momentum. Those who are supporting you will share this rhythm, and they will be able to schedule their activities and life better because you are consistent with your study schedule. You are moving forward, and you are in control!

The length of the study session will depend on you and your ability to focus and concentrate. What you need to think about is quality rather than quantity when you are determining a realistic amount of time for each session. Plan to schedule 2 hours of daily quality study time at the very least. If you can spend more than 2 hours studying, then by all means do so.

You may be asking yourself, "What do you mean by quality time?" Quality time means spending uninterrupted quiet time focusing on your study session. This may mean that you will have to isolate yourself for these study sessions. Think again about what has worked for you during nursing school when you studied for exams, and select a study place that has also worked for you in the past. If you have a special study room at home that you have always used, then plan your study sessions in that special room. If you have always studied at a library, then plan your study sessions for the library. If you plan to study at home, make the time spent studying uninterrupted and quiet. Sometimes it is difficult to balance your study time with your family obligations and possibly a work schedule, but, if you can, plan your study time for when you know that you will be at home alone. Try to eliminate anything that may be distracting during your study time. For example, unplug your telephone or shut off your cell phone so that you will not be disturbed. If you have small children, plan your study time during their nap time or school hours.

Your plan must include the ways in which you will manage your study needs and the demands of your work, family, and friends. Take time to think about how you will balance your everyday commitments with your plan for study. Your family and friends are key players in your life, and they are going to become a part of your Pyramid to Success. After you have established your study needs, communicate your needs and the importance of your study plan for achieving your goal of becoming a licensed practical/vocational nurse to your family and friends.

A difficult part of the plan may be how you will deal with those family and friends who choose not to participate in your Plan for Success. What if an individual or individuals choose to not be part of your plan? For example, what do you do if a friend asks you to go to a movie during your scheduled study time?

Your friend may say, "Come on. Take some time off. You have plenty of time to study. Study later when we get back!" Then you are faced with a decision. You must weigh all of the factors carefully. You must keep your goals in mind and remember that your need for positive momentum is critical. Your decision may not be an easy one, but it must be one that will help you ensure that your goal of becoming a licensed practical/vocational nurse is achieved. Remember, positive momentum and meeting your goals are most important.

POSITIVE PAMPERING

What is positive pampering? This means that you must continue to care for yourself holistically. Positive momentum can be maintained only if you are properly balanced. Proper exercise, diet, and positive mental stimulation are critical to achieving your goal of becoming a licensed practical/vocational nurse. Just as you have developed a schedule for study, you should have a schedule that includes some fun and some form of physical activity. It is your choice—aerobics, running, walking, weight lifting, bowling, or whatever makes you feel good about yourself. Time spent away from the hard study schedule and devoted to some form of fun and physical exercise pays its rewards 100-fold. You will feel alive and more energetic with a schedule that includes these activities.

Establish healthy eating habits. Stay away from fatty foods, because they will slow you down. Eat lighter meals, and eat more frequently. Include complex carbohydrates in your diet for energy, and be careful to not include too much caffeine in your daily diet. Continue to feel good about yourself, because you are in control.

Take the time to pamper yourself with activities that make you feel even better about who you are. Make dinner reservations at your favorite restaurant with someone who is special and who is supporting your goal of becoming a licensed practical/vocational nurse. Take walks in a place that has a particular tranquillity that enables you to reflect on the positive momentum that you have achieved and maintained. Whatever it is and wherever it takes you, allow yourself the time to do some positive pampering.

FINAL PREPARATION

You have established the foundation of your Pyramid to Success. You have developed your list of goals and your study plan, and you have maintained your positive momentum. You are moving forward, and you are in control. When you receive your date and time for the NCLEX-PN exam, you may immediately think, "I'm not ready!" Stop thinking that way! Reflect on all that you have achieved. Think about your goal achievement and the organization of the positive life momentum with which you have surrounded yourself.

Think about all those individuals who love and support your effort to become a licensed practical/vocational nurse. Believe that the challenge that awaits you is one that you have successfully prepared for and that will lead you to your goal of becoming a licensed practical/vocational nurse!

Take a deep breath, and organize the remaining days so that they support your educational and personal needs. Support your positive momentum with a visual technique. Write your name in large letters, and write the letters "LPN" or "LVN" after it. Post one or more of these visual reinforcements in areas that you frequent. This form of visual motivational technique works for many individuals preparing for this exam.

Through all that you have accomplished to this point, it is imperative that you not fall into the trap of expecting too much of yourself. The idea of perfection must not drive you to a point that causes your positive momentum to hesitate. You must believe in who you are as you are, and you need to stay focused on your goal. Allow yourself the opportunity to continue to carry out your plan in a manner that is the most conducive to who you are. The date and time are in hand. Write down the date and time, and underneath write the word "YES!" Post this next to your note with your name plus "LPN" or "LVN."

You must ensure that you know how to get to the testing center. A test run is a must. Time the drive, and allow for road construction or whatever may occur to slow traffic down. On the test run, when you arrive at the testing facility, you may want to walk into it. Walk in and become familiar with the lobby and the surroundings. This may help to alleviate some of the peripheral nervousness associated with entering an unknown building. Remember, you must do whatever it takes to keep yourself in control. If familiarizing yourself with the facility will help you to maintain positive momentum, then by all means be sure to do so. Who is in control? You are!

It is time to check your study plan and make the necessary adjustments now that a firm date and time are set. Adjust your review so that it flows to your needs and so that your study plan ends 2 days before the exam. Remember that the mind is like a muscle. If it is overworked, it has no strength or stamina. Your strategy is to rest the body and mind on the day before the exam. Your need to stay in control and allow yourself the opportunity to be absolutely fresh and attentive on the day of the exam. This will help you to control the nervousness that is natural, achieve the clear thought processes required, and feel confident that you have done all that is necessary to prepare for and conquer this challenge. The day before the exam is to be one of pleasure. Treat yourself to what you enjoy the most.

Relax! You have prepared yourself well for the challenge of the next day. Allow yourself a good night's sleep, and wake up on the day of the exam knowing that you are absolutely ready to succeed. Look at your name with "LPN" or "LVN" after it next to the word "YES!"

THE DAY OF THE EXAM (Box 3-3)

Wake up believing in yourself and knowing that all you have accomplished is about to propel you to the professional level of becoming a licensed practical/vocational nurse. Allow yourself plenty of time, eat a nutritious breakfast, and groom yourself for success. You are ready to meet the challenges of the day and to overcome any obstacle that may face you. Today will soon be history, and tomorrow will bring you the envelope on which you read your name with the letters "LPN" or "LVN" after it.

Be proud and confident of your achievements. You have worked hard to achieve your goal of becoming

---

Box 3-3 **The Day of the Exam**

Breathe—Inhale deeply, hold your breath to a count of 4, and exhale slowly.
Believe—Think positive thoughts about your achievements today and always.
Control—Yes! You are in command!
Believe—Yes! This is your day!
Visualize—See your name with the letters "LPN" or "LVN" after it!

---

a licensed practical/vocational nurse. If you believe in yourself and your goals, no one person or obstacle can move you off of the pathway that leads to success and to the peak of the Pyramid!

Congratulations! I wish you the very best in your career as a licensed practical/vocational nurse.

The NCLEX-PN® Examination: From a Graduate's Perspective

MISTY D. JOHNSON, LPN

I would first like to welcome you to the world of nursing. You've come a long way!

As a recent graduate of a nursing program, I understand that you may feel a little bit relieved that you are at the point of preparing to take "the big test." You may also feel a little bit overwhelmed with the amount of information that you need to know to embark on your chosen career. It may seem as though you could never know enough, and, to a point, you are correct. You never stop learning or growing in your profession. However, you do learn the basics of becoming a nurse through your nursing program and through your own diligence in studying to become one of the best in your profession.

As a graduate who successfully prepared for the NCLEX-PN, I would like to offer you some tips to help you prepare yourself for the test and hopefully to save you some stress as you do so. Not everyone will prepare for this exam in the same way, but if you at least have some "inside information" about how to prepare, then the purchase of this book will be well worth the cost.

The nursing program that I attended was staffed with some of the best nurses I have ever had the pleasure to meet. I feel especially lucky to have been able to study under them. I have every confidence that they fully prepared me for the NCLEX-PN exam to the best of their—and my—abilities. This nursing program provided me with the foundation that will be the basis for my future as a nurse. These nurse educators not only imparted their technical knowledge to me, but they also somehow conveyed a terrific sense of excitement about what it truly means to be a nurse. This experience cannot be found online or in a book, and it is important enough of a point for me to emphasize to future nurses. The nursing program that prepares you to become a licensed practical/vocational nurse will make a difference throughout your life, so don't take it for granted!

First, let me just say that studying is *not* overrated. During school, many hours were dedicated to memorizing information and to learning about the human body, disease processes, nursing diagnoses, and interventions. Although you may feel that you have a full grasp of this information, the NCLEX-PN may address a content area that you did not really learn enough about. So you need to prepare, but remember that you will not be able to learn everything about everything. Studying diligently for the NCLEX-PN helped immensely with regard to drawing out my weaknesses, and it allowed me to focus on those weaknesses as I prepared for the exam.

There are many, many resources available to the NCLEX-PN candidate. A search on the Internet leads to unlimited options, but beware! Some of these sources are expensive, and they may not provide the level of acuity that you may desire as you prepare. You should be aware of the method of study that worked for you to become successful in nursing school.

While still in my nursing program, I had the idea to purchase an NCLEX-PN question-and-answer book that was broken down by body system. During school, this was one of the best ideas I had. As we would study a system with its associated disease processes and nursing and medical interventions, I would refer to the corresponding section of this book and quiz myself with the types of questions that appear on the NCLEX-PN. This not only helped me in class and with nursing tests, but I feel that I was a bit more prepared for the NCLEX-PN after doing this for a year. I think I had a better feel for what the NCLEX-PN would address. The most important points were brought forward for me to focus on while studying for school and then later for the NCLEX-PN. This was one of the most valuable preparation tools for me! I also used the *Saunders Q&A Review for the NCLEX-PN® Examination.* I felt that this particular book tied everything together for me. It is set up more in the way that the NCLEX-PN is formatted; it is not divided into body systems, as the comprehensive review book is, but rather it is organized into the areas of Client Needs as identified by the NCLEX-PN test plan.

The nursing program I was enrolled in offered standardized testing to students to assess our progress through the program. After this test was graded, an individual analysis was sent to each student with a score; an analysis of strengths and weaknesses with regard to Client Needs, the Nursing Process, and Content Areas; and an average of how the student's score compared with that of other students in the country who took the test. When the results arrived, I received a copy of my answers, the correct answers, and their rationales. This is an important test, and, if your school offers standardized testing, it is important to pay attention to the results to help you with your preparation for the NCLEX-PN.

I was able to schedule the NCLEX-PN for a day that was convenient for me. I tried to schedule a day when my friends were not taking the test. It's always nice to have moral support, but I did not want the distraction of watching my friends finish the exam before me and wondering if I was doing something wrong, if I had failed, or if maybe they had! There were not nearly as many people in the room during the test as I expected there would be. This helped to take some of the pressure off of me. I took my time, read each question thoroughly, eliminated the two obviously wrong answers, and then made my selection on the basis of my knowledge and my experience in the nursing program. I honestly never saw another person leave the room during my test. I focused solely on the screen in front of me, but I had to take a break one time. I did not feel very nervous, because I truly felt prepared for the exam. I knew that I was as prepared as I was going to be and that I had done my best. No matter the outcome, I was proud that I was in that place at that time. Nothing could take that away from me!

If I had to offer NCLEX-PN candidates some study tips, the most important would be that it is never too early to start studying. Everything you learn during your nursing program culminates in the taking of the NCLEX-PN exam. Each time you hear a new concept, think of how that applies to patient care in a clinical setting, and consider whether those all-knowing people who design the NCLEX-PN would find this information important enough to include in an exam in the future. For this reason, I found the question-and-answer book very helpful. It helped me to decide which information was most important for future reference.

In addition, it is important to devise a study plan. Some say that 100 questions per day is acceptable when reviewing with a question-and-answer book. However, I did not feel comfortable setting such a rigid goal for myself. There were times when I did 100 and times when I did not do quite that many. I set aside at least 1 hour each day to review either with books or CDs. I did not stress if I could not get in that hundredth question on a particular day. I was still studying, so it was OK.

Be sure to take some time for yourself the day before the test. Don't get caught up in cramming, stressing, and worrying. You have truly done your best, so enjoy that day, and don't beat yourself up! Go shopping, have lunch with a friend, or spend that extra time with family. Do something for you!

Finally, keep in mind that you are already a winner! You persevered through your nursing program and through all of the hard times and the silly and rewarding moments that you had. Those "nursing moments"—when you realized the true meaning of being a nurse—can carry you through all the bad days, the long days, and the tough times ahead. You should be proud of where you are! You've already won, you're just waiting for your prize!

I wish all of you luck with your NCLEX-PN exams, and, more importantly, I wish you wonderful careers as licensed practical/vocational nurses.

Test-Taking Strategies

I. PYRAMID TO SUCCESS (Box 5-1)
II. THE "WHAT IF ...?" SYNDROME AND HOW
TO AVOID READING INTO THE QUESTION
(Box 5-2)

A. Pyramid points
   1. Avoid asking yourself, "What if ...?" because this will lead you right into the "forbidden" act of reading into the question
   2. Focus only on the information in the question, read every word, and make a decision regarding what the question is asking
   3. Look for the strategic words in the question, such as *side effect* or *toxic effect*; strategic words make a difference with regard to what the question is asking about
   4. For multiple-choice questions, multiple-response questions, or questions that require you to number options in order of priority, read every option presented before selecting your answers
   5. Always use the process of elimination when options are presented; after you have eliminated some options, reread the question before making your final choice or choices
   6. With questions that require you to fill in the blank, focus on the information in the question, and determine what the question is asking; if the question requires you to calculate a medication dose, an intravenous flow rate, or intake and output amounts, recheck your calculations, and always use the on-screen calculator to verify the answer
   7. Remember, avoid asking yourself the "forbidden" question "What if ...?" when determining the answer to a question

B. The Ingredients of a Question (Box 5-3)
   1. The ingredients of a question include the event, which is a client or clinical situation; the event query; and the options or answers; a fill-in-the blank question will not contain options, and some figure or illustration (hot spot) questions may or may not contain options

| BOX 5-1 | **Pyramid to Success** |

Avoid asking yourself "What if ...?," because this will lead you right into reading into the question.

Focus only on the information in the question, read every word, and make a decision regarding what the question is asking.

Look for the strategic words in the question; strategic words make a difference with regard to what the question is asking about.

Always use the process of elimination when options are presented; after you have eliminated some options, reread the question before making your final choice or choices.

Determine if the question contains a positive or negative event query.

Use all of your nursing knowledge, your clinical experiences, and your test-taking skills and strategies to answer the question.

   2. The client or clinical event provides you with the content that you need to think about when answering the question
   3. The event query asks something specific about the client or clinical event
   4. The options are all of the answers provided with the question
   5. With a multiple-choice question, there will be four options, and you must select one; read every option carefully, and think about the client or clinical event and the event query as you use the process of elimination
   6. With a multiple-response question, there will be six options, and you must select all options that apply to the event in the question; visualize the event, and use your nursing knowledge and your clinical experiences to answer the question
   7. With a prioritizing (ordered-response) question, you will be required to list in order of priority (using the computer mouse and dragging and dropping the options) certain nursing interventions or other data; visualize the event, and use your nursing knowledge and clinical experiences to answer the question

BOX 5-2
Practice Question: Avoiding the "What If ...?" Syndrome and Reading Into the Question

A nurse is changing the tapes on a tracheostomy tube. The client coughs, and the tube is dislodged. The initial nursing action is to:

1. Call the physician to reinsert the tube.
2. Ventilate the client using a manual resuscitation bag and face mask.
3. Cover the tracheostomy site with a sterile dressing to prevent infection.
4. Call the respiratory therapy department to reinsert the tracheostomy tube.

Answer: 2

Test-Taking Strategy: Now, you may immediately think, "The tube is dislodged and I need a physician." Read the question carefully, and note the strategic word "initial." Focus on the subject of the tube being dislodged. The question is asking you for a nursing action, so that is what you need to look for as you eliminate the incorrect options. Eliminate options 1 and 4, because they are comparable or alike and delay the initial intervention needed. Eliminate option 3, because this action will block the airway. If the tube is dislodged, the initial nursing action is to ventilate the client using a manual resuscitation bag and face mask. In addition, the use of the ABCs—airway, breathing, and circulation—will direct you to the correct option. Remember, avoid reading into the question!

BOX 5-4 ## Common Strategic Words

- Early
- Late
- Best
- First
- Initial

- Immediately
- Most likely
- Least likely
- Most appropriate
- Least appropriate

---

8. A chart/exhibit question will most likely contain options; read the question carefully and look at all of the information in the chart/exhibit before selecting an answer

III. THE STRATEGIC WORDS (Boxes 5-4 and 5-5)

A. Strategic words focus your attention on a critical point to consider when answering the question and will assist you with eliminating the incorrect options

B. Some strategic words may indicate that all of the options are correct and that it will be necessary to prioritize to select the correct option

C. As you read the question, look for the strategic words; strategic words make a difference with regard to what the question is asking

IV. THE SUBJECT OF THE QUESTION (Box 5-6)

A. The subject of the question is the specific topic that the question is asking about

B. Identifying the subject of the question will assist with eliminating the incorrect options and direct you to the correct option

---

BOX 5-3 ## Multiple-Choice Question: Event, Event Query, and Options

Event: After thoracic surgery, a client has two chest tubes inserted into the right pleural space that are attached to chest drainage systems.

Event Query: To promote optimal respiratory functioning, the nurse plans to implement which of the following?

Options:

1. Milk and strip the chest tubes once per shift.
2. Position the client on the back and the right side.
3. Encourage the client to cough and deep breathe every hour.
4. Maintain the client on bedrest until the chest tubes are removed.

Answer: 3

Test-Taking Strategy: Focus on the subject of promoting optimal respiratory functioning. Option 1 is eliminated first, because milking and stripping a chest tube is done only with a physician's order or when allowed by agency policy. Bedrest (option 4) does not promote respiratory function and is eliminated next. From the remaining options, recalling that positioning is done according to surgeon preference directs you to option 3.

BOX 5-5 ## Practice Question: Strategic Words

A client with a diagnosis of heart failure reports the occurrence of sudden shortness of breath and dyspnea. The nurse takes which immediate action?

1. Calls the physician
2. Administers oxygen
3. Elevates the head of the bed
4. Prepares to administer furosemide (Lasix)

Answer: 3

Test-Taking Strategy: Note the strategic word "immediate." Focusing on this strategic word and the client's symptoms (shortness of breath and dyspnea) will direct you to the correct option. Note that the question is asking for an immediate nursing action, so that is what

---

BOX 5-6 ## The Subject of the Question

The nurse is planning to teach a client in skeletal leg traction about measures to increase bed mobility. Which item would be most helpful for this client?

1. Television
2. Fracture bedpan
3. Overhead trapeze
4. Reading materials

Answer: 3

Test-Taking Strategy: Focus on the subject of increasing bed mobility. Also note the strategic words "most helpful." The use of an overhead trapeze is extremely helpful for assisting a client with moving about in bed and with getting on and off of the bedpan. Television and reading materials are helpful to reduce boredom and provide distraction. A fracture bedpan is useful for reducing discomfort with elimination. Remember to focus on the subject!

V. POSITIVE AND NEGATIVE EVENT QUERIES (Boxes 5-7 and 5-8)

A. A positive event query uses strategic words that ask you to select an option that is correct; for example, the event query may read: "Which statement by a client *indicates an understanding* of the side effects of the prescribed medication?"

B. A negative event query uses strategic words that ask you to select an option that is an incorrect item or statement; for example, the event query may read: "Which statement by a client *indicates a need for further teaching* about the side effects of the prescribed medication?"

VI. QUESTIONS THAT REQUIRE PRIORITIZING

A. Questions in the exam may require you to use the skill of prioritizing nursing actions

B. Look for the strategic words in the question that indicate the need to prioritize (Box 5-9)

C. Remember, when a question requires prioritization, all options may be correct, and you need to determine the correct order of action

D. Strategies to use to prioritize include the ABCs—airway, breathing, and circulation; Maslow's Hierarchy of Needs theory; and the steps of the nursing process (clinical problem-solving process)

E. The ABCs (Box 5-10)
   1. Use the ABCs—airway, breathing, and circulation—when selecting an answer or determining the order of priority
   2. Remember the order of priority: airway, breathing, and circulation
   3. Airway is always the first priority!

F. Maslow's Hierarchy of Needs theory (Box 5-11; Figure 5-1)
   1. According to Maslow's Hierarchy of Needs theory, physiological needs are the priority, followed by safety and security needs, love and belonging needs, self-esteem needs, and, finally, self-actualization needs; therefore, select the option or determine the order of priority by addressing physiological needs first
   2. When a physiological need is not addressed in the question or noted in one of the options, continue to use Maslow's Hierarchy of Needs theory as a guide, and look for the option that addresses safety

---

BOX 5-7 | **Practice Question: Positive Event Query**

The nurse has provided discharge instructions regarding nitroglycerin therapy to the client with angina. Which statement by the client indicates an understanding of the home use of the nitroglycerin?
1. "If I use the nitroglycerin and the pain does not subside in 15 minutes, I should go to the hospital."
2. "When I have pain, I should lie down and place a tablet under my tongue. If unrelieved in 5 minutes, I should take another tablet."
3. "When I have chest pain, I should put a tablet under my tongue. If I have a burning sensation, I should call my doctor immediately."
4. "When I experience chest pain, I can continue what I'm doing. If it doesn't go away in 10 minutes, I should use a nitroglycerin tablet."

Answer: 2

Test-Taking Strategy: This question identifies an example of a positive event query. Note the strategic words "indicates an understanding." The client taking sublingual nitroglycerin should lie down after taking the medication, because lightheadedness and dizziness may occur as a result of postural hypotension. The client should use up to three tablets at 5-minute intervals before seeking medical attention. A burning sensation is a common side effect of nitroglycerin. Nitroglycerin should be taken with the onset of anginal pain. The client should repeat the nitroglycerin dose if relief is not obtained with the first or second dose. Remember, positive event queries ask you to select an option that is a correct item or statement!

BOX 5-8 | **Practice Question: Negative Event Query**

A nurse has provided medication instructions to a client who will be taking warfarin sodium (Coumadin) indefinitely. Which statement by the client indicates a need for further teaching?
1. "I need to use a soft toothbrush."
2. "I need to use a straight razor for shaving."
3. "I need to avoid drinking alcohol while taking this medication."
4. "I need to carry identification about the medication being taken."

Answer: 2

Test-Taking Strategy: This question identifies an example of a negative event query. Note the strategic words "need for further teaching." These strategic words indicate that you need to select an option that identifies an incorrect client statement. Recalling that warfarin sodium is an anticoagulant and that the client is at risk for bleeding will direct you to the correct option. Remember that negative event queries ask you to select an option that is an incorrect item or statement!

BOX 5-9 | **Common Strategic Words That Indicate the Need to Prioritize**

- Best
- Essential
- First
- Highest priority
- Immediate

- Initial
- Most important
- Next
- Primary
- Vital

BOX 5-10 Practice Question: Use of the ABCs

A client with a compound (open) fracture of the radius has a cast applied in the emergency department. The nurse provides home-care instructions and tells the client to seek medical attention if which of the following occurs?

1. Numbness and tingling are felt in the fingers.
2. The cast feels heavy and damp 24 hours after application.
3. The entire cast feels warm during the first 24 hours after application.
4. Bloody drainage is noted on the cast during the first 6 hours after application.

Answer: 1

Test-Taking Strategy: Use the ABCs—airway, breathing, and circulation—as a guide to direct you to the correct option. A limb encased in a cast is at risk for nerve damage and diminished circulation from increased pressure caused by edema. Signs of increased pressure and diminished circulation from the cast include numbness, tingling, and increased pain. Remember to use the ABCs—airway, breathing, and circulation—to prioritize.

BOX 5-11 Practice Question: Maslow's Hierarchy of Needs Theory

A nurse is assigned to care for a client experiencing dystocia. When assisting with planning care, the nurse would consider the highest priority to be frequent:

1. Position changes and providing comfort measures
2. Explanations to family members about what is happening to the client
3. Monitoring for changes in the physical condition of the mother and fetus
4. Reinforcement of breathing techniques learned in childbirth preparatory classes

Answer: 3

Test-Taking Strategy: All of the options presented are correct and would be implemented during the care of this client. However, note the strategic words "highest priority," and use Maslow's Hierarchy of Needs theory to prioritize, remembering that physiological needs come first. Using this guideline will direct you to option 3. In addition, note that option 3 is the only option that addresses both the mother and the fetus.

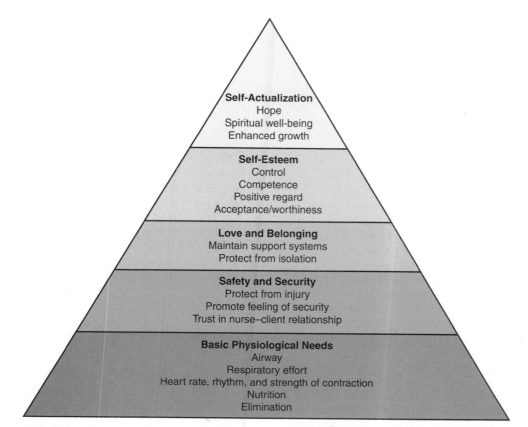

Nursing Priorities from Maslow's Hierarchy

FIG. 5-1   Using Maslow's Hierarchy of Needs theory to establish priorities. (From Harkreader, H., Hogan, M. A., & Thobaben, M. [2007]. *Fundamentals of nursing: Caring and clinical judgment* [3rd ed.]. Philadelphia: Saunders.)

G. Steps of the nursing process (clinical problem-solving process)
   1. Use the steps of the nursing process (clinical problem-solving process) to prioritize
   2. The steps include data collection, planning, implementation, and evaluation and are followed in this order
   3. Data collection
      a. Data collection questions will address the process of gathering subjective and objective data relative to the client, communicating and documenting information gained during data collection, and contributing to the formulation of nursing diagnoses
      b. Remember that data collection is the first step of the nursing process (clinical problem-solving process)
      c. When you are asked a question regarding your initial or first nursing action, look for strategic words in the options that reflect the collection of data relative to the client (Box 5-12)
      d. If an option contains the concept of collection of client data, it is best to select that option (Box 5-13)
      e. If a data-collection action is not one of the options, follow the steps of the nursing process (clinical problem-solving process) as your guide to select your initial or first action
      f. Possible exception to the guideline: If the question presents an emergency situation, read carefully; in an emergency situation, an intervention may be the priority
   4. Planning: Planning questions will require providing input into plan development, assisting with the formulation of the goals of care, and assisting with the development of a plan of care (Box 5-14)
   5. Implementation (Box 5-15)
      a. Implementation questions address the process of assisting with organizing and managing care, providing care to achieve established goals, and communicating and documenting nursing interventions thoroughly and accurately
      b. Focus on a nursing action rather than on a medical action when you are answering a question, unless the question is asking you what prescribed medical action is anticipated
      c. On the NCLEX-PN, the only client that you need to be concerned about is the client in the question that you are answering; avoid the "What if ...?" syndrome, and remember that the client in the question on the computer screen is your only assigned client

---

BOX 5-12   Data Collection: Strategic Words

- Check
- Collect
- Determine
- Find out
- Gather
- Identify
- Monitor
- Observe
- Obtain information
- Recognize

BOX 5-13   Practice Question: The Nursing Process/Data Collection

The nurse develops a plan of care for an older client with diabetes mellitus. The nurse plans to first:
1. Structure menus for adherence to diet.
2. Teach with videotapes showing insulin administration to ensure competence.
3. Encourage dependence on others to prepare the client for the chronicity of the disease.
4. Determine the client's ability to read label markings on syringes and blood glucose monitoring equipment.

Answer: 4

Test-Taking Strategy: Note the strategic word "first." Use the steps of the nursing process to answer the question, remembering that data collection is the first step. The only option that addresses data collection is option 4. Options 1, 2, and 3 address the implementation step of the nursing process. Remember, data collection is the first step in the nursing process.

BOX 5-14   Practice Question: The Nursing Process/Planning

A nurse reviews the plan of care for a client with a cataract and determines that which nursing diagnosis is the priority?
1. *Fear* related to loss of eyesight
2. *Risk for injury* related to decreased vision
3. *Disturbed sensory perception (visual)* related to ocular lens opacity
4. *Social isolation* related to decreased ability to be active in the community

Answer: 3

Test-Taking Strategy: This question relates to the planning of nursing care and asks you to identify the priority nursing diagnosis. Use Maslow's Hierarchy of Needs theory to answer the question. Remembering that physiological needs are the priority will direct you to option 3. *Risk for injury* is a potential rather than an actual problem, and, according to Maslow's Hierarchy of Needs theory, safety is the second priority. *Fear* and *Social isolation* are psychosocial needs. Remember that planning is the second step of the nursing process!

d. Answer the question from a textbook and ideal perspective, and remember that the nurse has all the time and resources needed and readily available at the client's bedside; avoid the "What if ...?" syndrome, and remember that you do not need to run to the treatment room to obtain sterile gauze, because it will be at the client's bedside

6. Evaluation (Box 5-16)

a. Evaluation questions focus on comparing the actual outcomes of care with the expected outcomes and on communicating and documenting findings

b. These questions focus on assisting with determining the client's response to care and on identifying factors that may interfere with achieving expected outcomes

c. With an evaluation question, watch for negative event queries, because they are frequently used with this type of question

BOX 5-15	Practice Question: The Nursing Process/Implementation

A nurse is checking the fundus of a postpartum woman and notes that the uterus is soft and spongy. Which nursing action is appropriate initially?

1. Notify the physician.
2. Encourage the mother to ambulate.
3. Massage the fundus gently until it is firm.
4. Document fundal position, consistency, and height.

Answer: 3

Test-Taking Strategy: Implementation questions address the process of organizing and managing care. Note the strategic word "initially." If the fundus is boggy (soft), it should be massaged gently until firm, and the nurse should observe for increased bleeding or clots. Remember that implementation is the third step of the nursing process!

BOX 5-16	Practice Question: The Nursing Process/Evaluation

A client has just taken a dose of trimethobenzamide (Tigan). The nurse evaluates that the medication has been effective if the client states relief of:

1. Heartburn
2. Constipation
3. Abdominal pain
4. Nausea and vomiting

Answer: 4

Test-Taking Strategy: Note the strategic words "medication has been effective." These words indicate that this is an evaluation-type question. Recalling that this medication is an antiemetic will direct you to option 4. Remember that evaluation is the fourth step of the nursing process!

VII. CLIENT NEEDS

A. Safe and Effective Care Environment

1. These questions test the concepts that the nurse provides nursing care; collaborates with other health care team members to facilitate effective client care; and protects clients, significant others, and health care personnel from environmental hazards

2. Focus on safety with these types of questions, and remember the importance of handwashing, call bells, bed positioning, and the appropriate use of side rails

B. Physiological Integrity

1. These questions test the concepts that the nurse provides comfort and assistance during the performance of activities of daily living; provides care related to the administration of medications; and monitors clients receiving parenteral therapies

2. These questions also address the nurse's ability to reduce the client's potential for developing complications or health problems related to treatments, procedures, or existing conditions and the nurse's role in providing care to clients with acute, chronic, or life-threatening physical health conditions

3. Focus on Maslow's Hierarchy of Needs theory for these types of questions, and remember that physiological needs are a priority and are addressed first

4. Use the ABCs—airway, breathing, and circulation—and the steps of the nursing process (clinical problem-solving process) when selecting an option that addresses physiological integrity

C. Psychosocial Integrity

1. These questions test the concepts that the nurse provides nursing care that promotes and supports the emotional, mental, and social well-being of the client and significant others

2. Content addressed in these questions relates to supporting and promoting the client's or significant others' abilities to cope, adapt, or problem-solve in situations involving illnesses, disabilities, or stressful events such as abuse, neglect, or violence

3. In this Client Needs category, you may be asked communication-type questions that relate to how you would respond to a client, a client's family members or significant others, or other health care team members

4. Use therapeutic communication techniques to answer communication questions because of their effectiveness in the communication process

5. Remember to select the option that focuses on the client's, the client's family members', or the client's significant others' thoughts, feelings, concerns, anxieties, and fears (Box 5-17)

BOX 5-17   Practice Question: Communication

A client with a diagnosis of major depression says to the nurse, "I should have died. I've always been a failure." The nurse should make which therapeutic response to the client?

1. "I see a lot of positive things in you."
2. "You still have a great deal to live for."
3. "Feeling like a failure is part of your illness."
4. "You've been feeling like a failure for some time now?"

Answer: 4

Test-Taking Strategy: Remember the techniques that facilitate therapeutic communication to answer this question. Address the client's feelings and concerns. Option 4 is the only option that is stated in the form of a question and that is open-ended; this will encourage the verbalization of feelings. Remember to use therapeutic communication techniques and to focus on the client.

BOX 5-18   Practice Question: Eliminate Comparable or Alike Options

A nurse instructs an adolescent with iron-deficiency anemia about the administration of oral iron preparations. The nurse tells the adolescent that it is best to take the iron with:

1. Cola
2. Soda
3. Ginger ale
4. Tomato juice

Answer: 4

Test-Taking Strategy: Note that options 1, 2, and 3 are comparable or alike options in that they are carbonated beverages. Iron should be administered with vitamin-C–rich fluids, because vitamin C enhances the absorption of the iron preparation. Tomato juice contains a high content of ascorbic acid (vitamin C), whereas cola, soda, and ginger ale do not contain vitamin C. Remember to eliminate comparable or alike options!

D. Health Promotion and Maintenance
   1. These questions test the concepts that the nurse provides and assists with directing nursing care to promote and maintain health
   2. Content addressed in these questions relates to assisting the client and significant others during the normal expected stages of growth and development from conception through advanced old age and to providing client care related to the prevention and early detection of health problems
   3. Use the Teaching and Learning Theory if the question addresses client teaching, remembering that client willingness, desire, and readiness to learn are the first priorities
   4. Watch for negative event queries, because they are frequently used in questions that address health promotion and maintenance and client education

VIII. ELIMINATE COMPARABLE OR ALIKE OPTIONS (Box 5-18)
A. When reading the options, look for options that are comparable or alike; these options will include a similar concept or nursing action
B. Comparable or alike options can be eliminated as possible answers

IX. ELIMINATE OPTIONS THAT CONTAIN CLOSE-ENDED WORDS (Box 5-19)
A. Close-ended words include *all, always, every, must, none, never,* and *only*
B. Eliminate options with close-ended words, because these words infer a fixed or extreme meaning; these types of options are usually incorrect
C. Options that contain open-ended words such as *may, usually,* and *generally* should be considered as possible correct options

BOX 5-19   Practice Question: Eliminate Options That Contain Close-Ended Words

A client will undergo a barium swallow, and the nurse provides preprocedure instructions to the client. The nurse instructs the client to:

1. Avoid eating or drinking after midnight before the test.
2. Take all routine medications on the morning of the test.
3. Have only a clear-liquid breakfast on the morning of the test.
4. Limit smoking to only two cigarettes on the morning of the test.

Answer: 1

Test-Taking Strategy: Note the close-ended words *all* in option 2 and *only* in options 3 and 4. Remember to eliminate options that contain close-ended words, because these options are usually incorrect. In addition, note that options 2, 3, and 4 are comparable or alike in that they all involve taking in something on the morning of the examination.

X. LOOK FOR THE UMBRELLA OPTION (Box 5-20)
A. When answering a question, look for the umbrella option
B. The umbrella option is one that is a broad or universal statement and that usually contains the concepts of the other options within it
C. The umbrella option will be the correct answer

XI. USE THE GUIDELINES FOR DELEGATING AND ASSIGNMENT MAKING (Box 5-21)
A. You may be asked a question that will require you to decide how you will delegate a task or assign clients to other health care providers
B. Focus on the information in the question and on the task or assignment that is to be delegated

BOX 5-20 **Practice Question: Look for the Umbrella Option**

A nurse is teaching health education classes to a group of expectant parents, and the topic is preventing mental retardation caused by congenital hypothyroidism. The nurse tells the parents that the most effective means of preventing this disorder is by:
1. Vitamin intake
2. Neonatal screening
3. Adequate protein intake
4. Limiting alcohol consumption
Answer: 2

Test-Taking Strategy: Focus on the subject of preventing mental retardation caused by congenital hypothyroidism. Congenital hypothyroidism is the most common preventable cause of mental retardation. Neonatal screening is the only means of the early diagnosis and subsequent prevention of mental retardation. Options 1, 3, and 4 are measures to prevent all birth defects. In addition, note that neonatal screening is the umbrella option. Remember to look for the umbrella option!

C. After you have determined what task or assignment is to be delegated, consider the client's needs, and match the client's needs with the scope of practice of the health care providers identified in the question

D. The nurse practice act and any practice limitations define which aspects of care can be delegated and which must be performed by a nursing assistant, a licensed practical/vocational nurse, or a registered nurse

E. Generally, noninvasive interventions such as skin care, range-of-motion exercises, ambulation, grooming, and hygiene measures can be assigned to a nursing assistant

F. A licensed practical/vocational nurse can perform the tasks that a nursing assistant can in addition to certain invasive tasks such as dressings, suctioning, urinary catheterization, and administering oral, subcutaneous, intramuscular, and some intravenous piggy back medications

G. The registered nurse can perform the tasks that a licensed practical/vocational nurse can and is responsible for assessing, planning and supervising care, and initiating teaching

XII. ANSWERING PHARMACOLOGY QUESTIONS (Box 5-22)
A. If you are familiar with the medication, use your nursing knowledge to answer the question
B. Remember that the question will identify both the generic name and the trade name of the medication
C. If the question identifies a medical diagnosis, then try to make a relationship between the medication and the diagnosis; for example, you can determine that cyclophosphamide (*Cytoxan*) is an antineoplastic medication if the question refers to a client with breast cancer who is taking this medication

BOX 5-21 **Practice Question: Use the Guidelines for Delegating and Assignment Making**

A nurse is planning the client assignments for the day and most appropriately assigns which client to the nursing assistant?
1. A client on strict bedrest
2. A client with dyspnea who is receiving oxygen therapy
3. A client scheduled for transfer to the hospital for surgery
4. A client with a gastrostomy tube who requires tube feedings every 4 hours
Answer: 1

Test-Taking Strategy: Note that the question asks for the assignment to be delegated to the nursing assistant. When asked questions related to delegation, think about the role description of the employee and the needs of the client. A client scheduled for transfer to the hospital for surgery, a client with dyspnea who is receiving oxygen therapy, or a client with a gastrostomy tube who requires tube feedings every 4 hours has both physiological and psychosocial needs that require care by a licensed nurse. The nursing assistant has been trained to care for a client on bedrest. Remember to match the client's needs with the scope of practice of the health care provider!

BOX 5-22 **Practice Question: Answering Pharmacology Questions**

The nurse is preparing to administer atenolol (Tenormin) to a client. The nurse checks which of the following before administering the medication?
1. Temperature
2. Blood pressure
3. Potassium level
4. Blood glucose level
Answer: 2

Test-Taking Strategy: Focus on the name of the medication. Recall that most β-blocker medication names end with the letters -*lol* and that these medications are used to treat hypertension. This will direct you to option 2. Remember to focus on the medication name when answering pharmacology questions!

D. Try to determine the classification of the medication being addressed to assist with answering the question; identifying the classification will help with determining a medication's action and/or side effects; for example, diltiazem (*Cardizem*) is a cardiac medication

E. Recognize the common side effects associated with each medication classification, and then relate the appropriate nursing interventions to each side effect; for example, if a side effect is hypertension, then the associated nursing intervention would be to monitor the blood pressure

F. Learn the medications that belong to a classification by commonalities in their names; for example, medications that are xanthine bronchodilators end with -*line* (e.g., theophyl*line*)

G. Look at the medication name, and use medical terminology to assist with determining the medication action; for example, *Lopressor* lowers *(Lo)* the blood pressure *(pressor)*

H. If the question requires a medication calculation, remember that an on-screen calculator is on the computer; talk yourself through each step to be sure the answer makes sense, and recheck the calculation before answering the question, particularly if the answer seems like an unusual dosage

I. Pyramid points to remember
   1. Generally the client should not take an antacid with medication, because the antacid will affect the absorption of the medication
   2. Enteric-coated and sustained-release tablets should not be crushed, and capsules should not be opened
   3. The client should never adjust or change a medication dose or abruptly stop taking a medication
   4. The nurse never adjusts or changes the client's medication dosage or discontinues a medication
   5. The client needs to avoid taking any over-the-counter medications or herbal preparations unless they are approved for use by the health care provider
   6. The client needs to avoid alcohol and smoking
   7. Medications are never administered if the order is difficult to read or unclear or if it identifies a medication dose that is not a normal one

REFERENCES

deWit, S. (2005). *Fundamental concepts and skills for nursing* (2nd ed.). Philadelphia: Saunders.

Harkreader, H., Hogan, M.A., & Thobaben, M. (2007). *Fundamentals of nursing: Caring and clinical judgment* (3rd ed.). Philadelphia: Saunders.

Hill, S., & Howlett, H. (2005). *Success in practical/vocational nursing: From student to leader* (5th ed.). Philadelphia: Saunders.

Hockenberry, M., & Wilson, D. (2007). *Wong's nursing care of infants and children* (8th ed.). St. Louis: Mosby.

Hodgson, B., & Kizior, R. (2008). *Saunders nursing drug handbook 2008*. Philadelphia: Saunders.

Huber, D. (2006). *Leadership and nursing care management* (3rd ed.). Philadelphia: Saunders.

Lehne, R. (2007). *Pharmacology for nursing care* (6th ed.). St. Louis: Saunders.

Leifer, G. (2005). *Maternity nursing* (9th ed.). Philadelphia: Saunders.

Meiner, S., & Leuckenotte, A. (2006). *Gerontologic nursing* (3rd ed.). St. Louis: Mosby.

Morrison-Valfre, M. (2005). *Foundations of mental health care* (3rd ed.). St. Louis: Mosby.

National Council of State Boards of Nursing (Eds.) (2008). *2008 Detailed Test Plan for the NCLEX-PN® Examination, National Council of State Boards of Nursing*. Chicago: Author.

National Council of State Boards of Nursing. *NCSBN home page*. www.ncsbn.org. Accessed June 4, 2008.

Potter, P., & Perry, A. (2005). *Fundamentals of nursing* (6th ed.). St. Louis: Mosby.

Price, D., & Gwin, J. (2005). *Thompson's pediatric nursing* (9th ed.). Philadelphia: Saunders.

Skidmore-Roth, L. (2008). *Mosby's nursing drug reference* (21st ed.). St. Louis: Mosby.

Issues in Nursing

Cultural Diversity

PYRAMID TERMS

acculturation The process of learning the norms, beliefs, and behavioral expectations of a group other than one's own group.

belief Something accepted as true by a culture.

cultural assimilation The process by which individuals from a minority group are absorbed by the dominant culture and take on the characteristics of the dominant culture.

cultural competence The acquisition of knowledge, understanding, and appreciation of a culture that facilitates the provision of culturally appropriate health care.

cultural diversity The differences among groups of people that result from ethnic, racial, and cultural variables.

cultural imposition The tendency to impose one's own beliefs, values, and patterns of behavior on individuals from other cultures.

culture The dynamic network of knowledge, beliefs, patterns of behavior, ideas, attitudes, values, and norms that are unique to a particular group of people.

dominant culture The group whose values prevail within a society.

ethnic group A group of people within a culture who share an identity based on race, religion, color, national origin, or language.

ethnicity An individual's identification of self as part of an ethnic group.

ethnocentrism An assumption of cultural superiority and an inability to accept another culture's ways.

minority group An ethnic, cultural, racial, or religious group that constitutes less than a numerical majority of the population.

oppression The imposition of the cultural ways of one group on another group.

race A grouping of people that is based on biological similarities. Members of a racial group have similar physical characteristics, such as blood group, facial features, and color of skin, hair, and eyes.

racism Discrimination directed toward individuals or groups who are perceived to be inferior because of biological differences; often accompanied by oppression.

stereotyping An expectation that all people within the same racial, ethnic, or cultural group act alike and share the same beliefs and attitudes.

subculture A group of people with characteristic patterns of behavior that distinguish the group from the larger culture or society.

values Principles and standards that have meaning and worth to an individual, family, group, community, or culture.

PYRAMID TO SUCCESS

Often nurses care for clients who come from ethnic, cultural, or religious backgrounds that are different from their own. Awareness of and sensitivity to the unique health and illness beliefs and practices of others are essential for the delivery of safe and effective care. The acknowledgment and acceptance of cultural differences with a nonjudgmental attitude are essential for providing culturally sensitive care. The belief underlying the NCLEX-PN test plan is that people are unique individuals and that they define their own systems of daily living that reflect their values, motives, and lifestyles. The Integrated Processes addressed in this chapter are Caring, Clinical Problem-Solving Process (Nursing Process), Communication and Documentation, and Teaching and Learning.

CLIENT NEEDS

Safe and Effective Care Environment

Acting as a client advocate

Communicating the need for referrals to members of the health care team

Ensuring ethical practices and legal rights and responsibilities

Establishing priorities

Maintaining confidentiality

Providing continuity of care

Upholding the client's rights

Health Promotion and Maintenance

Considering cultural issues related to family

Identifying changes related to the aging process

Preventing disease

Promoting health and wellness

Respecting lifestyle choices

Psychosocial Integrity

Assisting the client with using coping mechanisms effectively

Identifying cultural diversity issues

Identifying end-of-life care issues

Identifying family dynamics as they relate to the client's culture

Identifying the client's support systems

Respecting religious and spiritual preferences

Using therapeutic communication techniques

Physiological Integrity

Identifying cultural considerations related to alternative and complementary therapies

Identifying cultural issues related to receiving blood and blood products

Implementing therapeutic procedures

Using cultural concepts in illness management

Providing nonpharmacological comfort interventions

Providing nutrition and oral hydration (Boxes 6-1 and 6-2)

I. AFRICAN AMERICANS

A. Communication
   1. Competent in standard English and in Black English, a variation based on pronunciation, grammar, and vocabulary; may use the Black English dialect when speaking with family and friends

---

BOX 6-1 Dietary Preferences of Different Ethnic Groups

African Americans
- Fried foods
- Pork, greens, and rice
- Some pregnant African-American women engage in pica

Asian Americans
- Soy sauce
- Raw fish
- Rice

European-Origin (white) Americans
- Carbohydrates (potatoes)
- Red meat

Hispanic Americans
- Beans
- Fried foods
- Spicy foods
- Tortillas
- Carbonated beverages

American Indians, Aleuts, and Eskimos
- Blue cornmeal
- Fish
- Game
- Fruits and berries
- Navajos prefer meat and blue cornmeal and tend to avoid the consumption of milk

---

BOX 6-2 Dietary Preferences of Different Religions

Seventh-Day Adventist (Church of God)
- Alcohol and caffeinated beverages are prohibited
- Many are lacto-ovo vegetarians; those who eat meat avoid pork
- Overeating is prohibited; 5 to 6 hours between meals without snacking is practiced

Buddhism
- Alcohol is prohibited
- Many are lacto-ovo vegetarians
- Some eat fish, and some avoid only beef

Roman Catholicism
- Avoid meat on Ash Wednesday and Fridays during Lent
- Optional fasting practiced during Lent
- Children, pregnant women, and the ill are exempt from fasting

Church of Jesus Christ of Latter-Day Saints (Mormon)
- Alcohol and caffeinated beverages are prohibited
- Consumption of meat is limited
- First Sunday of the month is optional for fasting

Hinduism
- Many are vegetarians
- Limit the consumption of meat; abstain from some types of meat
- Fasting rituals vary
- Children are not allowed to participate in fasting

Islam
- Pork, birds of prey, alcohol, and any meat product not ritually slaughtered are prohibited
- During the month of Ramadan, fasting occurs during the daytime

Jehovah's Witness
- Any foods to which blood has been added are prohibited
- Can consume animal flesh that has been drained

Judaism
- Dietary kosher laws must be adhered to by Orthodox believers
- Meats allowed include animals that are vegetable eaters, cloven-hoofed animals, and animals that are ritually slaughtered
- Fish that have scales and fins are allowed
- Any combination of meat and milk is prohibited
- During Yom Kippur, 24-hour fasting is observed
- Pregnant women and those who are seriously ill are exempt from fasting
- During Passover, only unleavened bread is eaten

Pentecostal (Assembly of God)
- Alcohol is prohibited
- Avoid consumption of anything to which blood has been added
- Some individuals avoid pork

Eastern Orthodox
- During Lent, all animal products, including dairy products, are forbidden
- Fasting during Advent
- Pregnant women and those who are seriously ill are exempt from fasting

2. Head nodding does not necessarily mean agreement
3. Direct eye contact may be interpreted as rudeness or aggressive behavior
4. Nonverbal communication is very important
5. Personal questions asked on initial contact with a person may be viewed as intrusive

B. Time orientation and personal space preferences
1. Time orientation varies according to age, socio-economics, and subgroups and may include past, present, or future orientation
2. May be late for an appointment because relationships and events may be deemed more important than being on time
3. Comfortable with close personal space when interacting with family and friends

C. Social roles
1. Large extended-family networks are important; older adults are respected
2. Many single-parent, female-headed households
3. Religious **beliefs** and church affiliation are sources of strength

D. Health and illness
1. Religious **beliefs** profoundly affect ideas about health and illness
2. Illness can be prevented by nutritious meals, rest, and cleanliness

E. Health risks
1. Sickle cell anemia
2. Hypertension
3. Heart disease
4. Cancer
5. Lactose intolerance
6. Diabetes mellitus

F. Interventions
1. Recognize the presence of many individual and subgroup variations
2. Build a relationship based on trust
3. Clarify the meaning of the client's verbal and nonverbal behaviors
4. Be flexible and avoid rigidity when scheduling care
5. Encourage family involvement
6. Alternative modes of healing may include herbs, prayer, and laying on of hands

II. **ASIAN AMERICANS**
A. Communication
1. Languages include Chinese, Japanese, Korean, Vietnamese, and English
2. Silence is valued
3. Eye contact may be considered inappropriate or disrespectful
4. Criticism or disagreement is not expressed verbally
5. Head nodding does not necessarily mean agreement
6. The word *no* may be interpreted as disrespect for others

B. Time orientation and personal space preferences
1. Time orientation reflects respect for the past but includes emphasis on the present and the future
2. Prefer a formal personal space, except with family and close friends
3. Usually do not touch others during conversation
4. Touching is unacceptable with members of the opposite sex
5. The head is considered to be sacred; therefore, touching someone on the head is disrespectful

C. Social roles
1. Devoted to tradition
2. Large extended-family networks
3. Loyalty to immediate and extended family and honor are valued
4. Family unit is very structured and hierarchical
5. Men have the power and authority, and women are expected to be obedient
6. Education is viewed as important
7. Religions include Taoism, Buddhism, Islam, and Christianity
8. Social organizations are strong within the community

D. Health and illness
1. Health is a state of physical and spiritual harmony with nature and a balance between positive and negative energy forces (yin and yang)
2. A healthy body is viewed as a gift from ancestors
3. Illness is viewed as an imbalance between yin and yang
4. Believe that diseases and foods are "hot" and "cold," and the diet is adjusted to treat diseases with the appropriate foods; yin foods are cold and yang foods are hot; cold foods are eaten when one has a hot illness, and hot foods are eaten when one has a cold illness; this dietary adjustment may lead to dietary problems if the basic nutritional needs are not met
5. Illness is attributed to prolonged sitting or lying or to overexertion

E. Health risks
1. Hypertension
2. Heart disease
3. Cancer
4. Lactose intolerance
5. Thalassemia

F. Interventions
1. Avoid physical closeness and excessive touching; only touch a client's head when necessary, and inform the client before doing so
2. Limit eye contact
3. Avoid gesturing with hands
4. If possible, a female client prefers a female health care provider
5. Clarify responses to questions and the expectations of the health care provider

6. Be flexible and avoid rigidity when scheduling care
7. Encourage family involvement
8. Alternative modes of healing may include herbs, acupuncture, restoration of balance with foods, massage, and offering prayers and incense

III. EUROPEAN-ORIGIN (WHITE) AMERICANS
A. Communication
   1. Languages include national languages and English
   2. Silence can be used to show respect or disrespect for another, depending on the situation
   3. Eye contact is viewed as indicating trustworthiness
B. Time orientation and personal space preferences
   1. Future oriented
   2. Time is valued; tend to be on time and to be impatient with people who are not on time
   3. May be aloof and tend to avoid close physical contact
   4. Handshakes may be used for formal greetings
C. Social roles
   1. The nuclear family is the basic unit, but the extended family is also important
   2. The man is the dominant figure, but variations of gender roles exist within families and relationships
   3. Religion includes Judeo-Christian **beliefs**
   4. Community social organizations are important
D. Health and illness
   1. Health is usually viewed as an absence of disease or illness
   2. Have a tendency to be stoical when expressing physical concerns
   3. Primarily rely on modern Western health care delivery system
E. Health risks
   1. Cancer
   2. Heart disease
   3. Diabetes mellitus
   4. Injury
F. Interventions
   1. Monitor the client's body language
   2. Respect the client's personal space

IV. HISPANIC AMERICANS
A. Communication
   1. Languages include Spanish and Portuguese
   2. Tend to be verbally expressive, yet confidentiality is important
   3. Avoiding eye contact with a person in authority indicates respect and attentiveness
   4. Direct confrontation is disrespectful, and the expression of negative feelings is impolite
   5. Dramatic body language, such as gestures or facial expressions, is used to express emotion or pain

B. Time orientation and personal space preferences
   1. Oriented more to the present
   2. May be late for an appointment, because relationships and events are valued more than being on time
   3. Comfortable when in close proximity with family, friends, and acquaintances
   4. Very tactile; use embraces and handshakes
   5. Value the physical presence of others
   6. Politeness and modesty are essential
C. Social roles
   1. The nuclear family is the basic unit, and there are large extended-family networks
   2. The extended family is highly regarded
   3. The needs of the family take precedence over individual family members' needs
   4. Depending on age and **acculturation** factors, men are the decision makers and breadwinners, and women are the caretakers and homemakers
   5. Religions include Catholicism, evangelical Christianity, Jehovah's Witness, and Mormonism
   6. Strong church affiliation
   7. Social organizations are strong within the community
D. Health and illness
   1. Health may be a reward from God or a result of good luck
   2. Health results from a state of balance between "hot and cold" forces and "wet and dry" forces
   3. Illness may be viewed as a result of God's punishment for sins
   4. Folk medicine traditions
E. Health risks
   1. Lactose intolerance
   2. Diabetes mellitus
   3. Parasites
   4. Hypertension
   5. Heart disease
F. Interventions
   1. Allow time for the client to discuss treatment options with family members
   2. Protect privacy
   3. Offer to call clergy because of the significance of religious practices related to illnesses
   4. Ask the parent if it is all right to touch the child before examining the child
   5. Be flexible regarding time of arrival for appointments, and avoid rigidity when scheduling care
   6. Alternative modes of healing include herbs, consultation with lay healers, restoration of balance with hot or cold foods, prayer, and religious medals

V. NATIVE AMERICANS
A. Communication
   1. Languages include English, Navajo, and other tribal languages
   2. Silence indicates respect for the speaker

3. Speak in a low tone of voice, and expect others to be attentive
4. Eye contact is viewed as a sign of disrespect
5. Body language is important

B. Time orientation and personal space preferences
1. Oriented more to present
2. Personal space is very important
3. Will lightly touch another person's hand during greetings
4. Massage is used for the newborn infant to promote bonding between the infant and the mother
5. Touching a dead body may be prohibited in some tribes

C. Social roles
1. Very family oriented
2. Basic family unit is the extended family, which often includes people from several households
3. In some tribes, grandparents are viewed as family leaders
4. Elders are honored
5. Children are taught to respect traditions
6. The father does all the work outside of the home, and the mother assumes responsibility for domestic duties
7. Sacred myths and legends provide spiritual guidance
8. Religion and healing practices are integrated
9. Community social organizations are important

D. Health and illness
1. Health is a state of harmony between the person, the family, and the environment
2. Illness is caused by supernatural forces and by disequilibrium between the person and the environment
3. Traditional health and illness **beliefs** may continue to be observed; natural and religious folk medicine traditions may come into play

E. Health risks
1. Alcohol abuse
2. Injury
3. Heart disease
4. Diabetes mellitus
5. Tuberculosis
6. Arthritis
7. Lactose intolerance
8. Gallbladder disease
9. American Eskimos are susceptible to glaucoma

F. Interventions
1. Clarify communication
2. Understand that the client may be attentive, even when eye contact is absent
3. Be attentive to your own use of body language
4. Obtain input from members of the extended family

5. Encourage the client to personalize the space in which health care is delivered; for example, encourage the client to bring personal items or objects to the hospital
6. In the home, check for the availability of running water, and modify infection control and hygiene practices as necessary
7. Alternative modes of healing include herbs, the restoration of balance between the person and the universe, and consultation with traditional healers

VI. THE AMISH SOCIETY

A. Cultural **beliefs** and practices (Box 6-3)
B. Interventions
1. Speak to both the husband and wife regarding health care decisions, because they consider themselves partners in family life
2. Health instructions must be given in a simple, clear language
3. Most Amish need to have church (bishop and community) permission to be hospitalized, because it is the community that will come together to help pay the costs
4. Typically, they do not have health insurance, because it is a "worldly product" and may show a lack of faith in God
5. Barriers to modern health care include distance, lack of transportation, cost, and language (most do not understand scientific jargon)

VII. RELIGION AND END-OF-LIFE ISSUES (Box 6-4)

A. Followers of the Christian Science religion are unlikely to use medical means to prolong life
B. Jewish faith generally opposes prolonging life after irreversible brain damage
C. Autopsy may be prohibited, opposed, or discouraged by Eastern Orthodox religions, Muslims, Jehovah's Witnesses, and Orthodox Jews
D. Organ donation is prohibited by Jehovah's Witnesses and Muslims
E. Buddhists in the United States encourage organ donation and consider it an act of mercy
F. Cremation is discouraged, opposed, or prohibited by the Mormon, Eastern Orthodox, Islamic, and Jewish faiths
G. Hindus prefer cremation and casting the ashes into a holy river
H. Hispanic and Latino groups
1. The family generally makes decisions and may withhold the diagnosis or prognosis from the client
2. Extended family members are often involved in end-of-life care
3. Pregnant women may be prohibited from caring for the dying or attending funerals
4. Several family members may be at the dying client's bedside

BOX 6-3 The Amish Society: Beliefs and Practices

- Maintain a culture distinct and separate from the non-Amish society
- Usually speak a German dialect called Pennsylvania Dutch
- German language is used during worship; English is learned in school
- Men follow the laws of the Hebrew Scriptures with regard to beards (mustaches are not grown because of the long association of mustaches with the military)
- Men usually dress in plain, dark suits; women usually wear plain dresses with long sleeves, bonnets, and aprons
- Women are not allowed to hold positions of power in the congregational organization
- Marriage outside of the faith is not allowed
- Family life has a patriarchal structure
- Although the roles of the women are considered equally important to those of men, they are very unequal in terms of authority
- Unmarried women remain under the authority of their fathers
- Wives are submissive to their husbands
- Generally remain separate from the rest of the world, both physically and socially
- Reject materialism and worldliness
- Some Amish prefer not to be photographed
- Value living simply; may choose to avoid technology, such as electricity and cars
- Highly value responsibility, generosity, and helping others
- Often work as farmers, builders, quilters, and homemakers
- May use traditional and alternative health care, such as healers, herbs, and massage
- Believe that health is a gift from God but that clean living and a balanced diet help maintain it
- Amish have lower risk factors for disease than the general population because of their work in manual labor, consumption of fresh foods, and rare consumption of tobacco and alcohol
- Many choose not to have health insurance and instead maintain mutual aid funds for Amish members who require help with medical costs
- Funerals are conducted in the home without a eulogy, flower decorations, or any other display; caskets are plain and simple, without adornment
- At death, women are usually buried in their bridal dresses
- One is believed to live on after death, with either eternal reward in heaven or punishment in hell

BOX 6-4 Religion and End-of-Life Care

Catholic and Eastern Orthodox
- Anointing of the sick is done by a priest
- Other sacraments before death include reconciliation and holy communion

Protestant
- No last rites (anointing of the sick is accepted by some groups)
- Prayers are given to offer comfort and support

Church of Jesus Christ of Latter-Day Saints (Mormon)
- May administer a sacrament if the client requests it

Jehovah's Witness
- Do not believe in sacraments
- Will be excommunicated if they receive a blood transfusion

Islam
- Second-degree male relatives such as cousins or uncles should be the contact people; they determine whether the client or family should be given information about the client
- Client may choose to face Mecca (west or southwest in the United States)
- The head should be elevated above the body
- Discussions about death are not usually welcomed
- Stopping medical treatment is against the will of Allah (Arabic word for God)
- Grief may be expressed through slapping or hitting the body
- If possible, only a same-gender Muslim should handle the body after death; if not possible, non-Muslims should wear gloves so as to not touch the body

Judaism
- Prolongation of life is important (life support must be maintained for a client until death)
- A dying person should not be left alone (a rabbi's presence is desired)
- Autopsy and cremation are forbidden

Hinduism
- Rituals include tying a thread around the neck or wrist of the dying person, sprinkling the person with special water, or placing a basil leaf on the person's tongue
- After death, the sacred threads are not removed, and the body is not washed

Buddhism
- A shrine to Buddha may be placed in the client's room
- Time for meditation at the shrine is important and should be respected
- Clients may refuse medications that could alter their awareness (e.g., opioids)
- After death, a monk may recite prayers for 1 hour (this need not be done in the presence of the body)

5. Vocal expression of grief and mourning is acceptable and expected
6. Refuse procedures that alter the body, such as organ donation or autopsy
7. Prefer to die at home

I. African Americans
  1. Discuss issues with the spouse or older family member (elders are held in high respect)
  2. Family is highly valued and central to the care of the terminally ill

3. Open displays of emotion are common and accepted
4. Organ and blood donation are usually not allowed
5. Prefer to die at home

J. Chinese Americans
   1. Family members may make decisions about care and often withhold the diagnosis or prognosis from the client
   2. Dying at home may be considered bad luck

K. Native Americans
   1. Family meetings may be held to make decisions about end-of-life issues and the type of treatments that should be pursued
   2. Some tribes avoid contact with the dying
   3. May prefer to die in the hospital

VIII. COMPLEMENTARY AND ALTERNATIVE THERAPIES
A. Description
   1. Therapies used in addition to conventional treatment that provide healing resources and focus on the mind–body connection
   2. Includes high-risk therapies (some that are invasive) and low-risk therapies (those that are noninvasive)
   3. The National Center for Complementary and Alternative Medicine has proposed a classification system that includes five categories of complementary and alternative types of therapy (Box 6-5)

B. Alternative medical systems
   1. Environmental medicine: Focuses on preventing the harmful effects of environmental toxins; interventions include teaching, therapeutic diets, detoxification, immunotherapy, counseling, and the use of environmentally safe products
   2. Traditional Chinese medicine: Focuses on restoring and maintaining a balanced flow of vital energy and on interventions such as acupressure, acupuncture, herbal therapies, diet, meditation, and tai chi and qi gong (exercises that focus on breathing, visualization, and movement)
   3. Ayurveda: Focus is on the balance of the mind, body, and spirit; interventions include diet, medicinal herbs, detoxification, breathing exercises, meditation, and yoga

4. Homeopathy: Focuses on healing; interventions consist of small doses of specially prepared plant and mineral extracts that assist with the body's innate healing process
5. Naturopathy: Focuses on enhancing the body's natural healing responses; interventions include nutrition, herbology, hydrotherapy, homeopathy, acupuncture, physical therapies, counseling, and psychotherapy

C. Mind–body interventions
   1. Focus on controlling physical functions through positive mental processes
   2. Interventions include biofeedback, hypnosis, relaxation therapy, meditation, music or art therapy, qi gong, prayer, and mental healing

D. Biologically based therapies (Box 6-6)
   1. Include natural and biologically derived products, interventions, and practices
   2. Interventions include aromatherapy, herbal therapies, macrobiotic diet, and orthomolecular therapy

E. Manipulative and body-based interventions
   1. Involve the manipulation and movement of the body by a therapist
   2. Include acupressure, movement reeducation techniques, chiropractic therapy, and therapeutic massage

F. Energy therapies
   1. Focus on energy that originates within the body or from other sources
   2. Interventions include therapeutic touch and magnetic therapy

IX. HERBAL THERAPIES (Box 6-7)
A. Description: The use of herbs (plant or a plant part) for therapeutic effect on health
B. Some herbs have been determined to be safe, yet some herbs, even in small amounts, can be toxic

---

BOX 6-5 Categories of Complementary and Alternative Medicine

- Whole medical systems
- Mind–body interventions
- Biological-based therapies
- Manipulative and body-based methods
- Energy therapies

BOX 6-6 Biological-Based Therapies

Aromatherapy
- The use of topical or inhaled oils (plant extracts) to promote and maintain health

Herbal Therapies
- The use of herbs derived from mostly plant sources to maintain and restore balance and health

Macrobiotic Diet
- A diet high in whole-grain cereals, vegetables, beans, sea vegetables, and vegetarian soups
- Meat, animal fat, eggs, poultry, dairy products, sugars, and artificially produced foods are eliminated from the diet

Orthomolecular Therapy
- Focuses on nutritional balance and includes the use of vitamins, essential amino acids, essential fats, and minerals

C. If the client is taking prescription medications, the client should consult with the health care provider regarding the use of herbs, because serious herb–medication interactions can occur

D. Client teaching points

1. Discuss herbal therapies with the health care provider before use
2. Contact the physician if any side effects of the herbal substance occur
3. Contact the health care provider before stopping the use of a prescription medication
4. Avoid using herbs to treat serious medical conditions such as heart disease

---

BOX 6-7 **Commonly Used Herbs**

Aloe: Anti-inflammatory and antimicrobial effects; accelerates wound healing

Angelica: Antispasmodic and vasodilator; balances the effects of estrogen

Bilberry: Improves microcirculation in the eyes

Black cohosh: Produces estrogen-like effects —*menopause*

Cat's claw: Antioxidant; stimulates the immune system and lowers the blood pressure

Chamomile: Antispasmodic and anti-inflammatory; produces a mild sedative effect

Echinacea: Stimulates the immune system

Evening primrose: Helps metabolize fatty acid

Feverfew: Anti-inflammatory; used for migraine headaches, arthritis, and fever

Garlic: Antioxidant; used to lower cholesterol levels

Ginger: Antiemetic; used for nausea and vomiting

Ginkgo biloba: Antioxidant; used to improve memory

Ginseng: Increases physical endurance and stamina; used for stress and fatigue

Glucosamine: Amino acid that assists with the synthesis of cartilage

Goldenseal: Anti-inflammatory and antimicrobial; used to stimulate the immune system; has an anticoagulant effect and may increase blood pressure

Kava: Antianxiety and skeletal muscle relaxant; produces a sedative effect

Lavender: Antiseptic and fragrance; used for its calming mild sedative effect; may be used orally as a tea

Melatonin: Hormone that regulates sleep; used for insomnia

Milk thistle: Antioxidant; stimulates the production of new liver cells and reduces liver inflammation; used for liver and gallbladder disease

Peppermint oil: Antispasmodic; used for irritable bowel syndrome

St. John's wort: Antibacterial, antiviral, and antidepressant

Saw palmetto: Antiestrogen activity; used for urinary tract infections and benign prostatic hypertrophy

Tea tree oil: Used for skin irritations, acne, and athlete's foot; for external use only

Valerian: Used to treat nervous disorders such as anxiety, restlessness, and insomnia

Zinc: Antiviral; stimulates the immune system

5. Avoid taking herbs if pregnant or attempting to get pregnant or if nursing
6. Do not give herbs to infants or young children
7. Purchase herbal supplements only from a reputable manufacturer; the label should contain the scientific name of the herb, name and address of the manufacturer, batch or lot number, date of manufacture, and expiration date
8. Adhere to the recommended dose; if herbal preparations are taken in high doses, they can be toxic
9. Moisture, sunlight, and heat may alter the components of herbal therapy
10. If surgery is planned, the herbal therapy may need to be discontinued 2 to 3 weeks before surgery

X. LOW-RISK THERAPIES

A. Description: Therapies that have no adverse effects that the nurse can use when implementing care

B. Common low-risk therapies

1. Meditation
2. Relaxation techniques
3. Imagery
4. Music therapy
5. Massage
6. Touch
7. Laughter and humor
8. Spiritual measures such as prayer

XI. NURSING CONSIDERATIONS

A. Principle: If health care recommendations, interventions, or treatments do not fit within the client's cultural value system, they will not be followed

B. Data-collection skills: Be alert to cues regarding eye contact, personal space, time concepts, and understanding of the recommended plan of care

C. Knowledge: Learn about the **cultures** of the clients with whom you will be working; additionally, learn from your clients about their health care practices

D. Flexibility: Allow for variation in accomplishing goals of health care; negotiate with the client until a mutually agreed-upon plan is established

E. Communication principles

1. Treat each client and those accompanying the client with respect
2. Appreciate the differences and diversity of **beliefs** about health, illness, and treatment modalities
3. Ask the client who has been consulted about the illness or condition and about what treatments were recommended by the consultant
4. Clarify perceptions of what the client has said or done and perceptions about the client's expectations of the health care provider
5. If language barriers pose a problem, seek an interpreter; avoid using family members as interpreters except as a last resort

PRACTICE QUESTIONS

More questions on the companion CD!

1. A client is diagnosed with cancer and is told that surgery followed by chemotherapy will be necessary. The client states to the nurse, "I have read a lot about complementary therapies. Do you think that I should try any?" The nurse responds by making which appropriate statement?
   1. "You need to ask your physician about it."
   2. "I would try anything that I could if I had cancer."
   3. "No, because it will interact with the chemotherapy."
   4. "There are many different forms of complementary therapies. Let's talk about these therapies."

2. A nurse is preparing to assist a Jewish client with eating lunch. A kosher meal is delivered to the client. Which nursing action is appropriate when assisting the client with the meal?
   1. Unwrapping the eating utensils for the client
   2. Replacing the plastic utensils with metal utensils
   3. Carefully transferring the food from paper plates to glass plates
   4. Asking the client to unwrap the utensils and allowing the client to prepare the meal for eating

3. A nurse is caring for a group of clients who are taking herbal medications at home. Which of the following clients should not be taking herbal medications?
   1. A 60-year-old male client with rhinitis
   2. A 24-year-old male client with a lower back injury
   3. A 10-year-old female client with a urinary tract infection
   4. A 45-year-old female client with a history of migraine headaches

4. The client asks the student nurse about various herbal therapies available for the treatment of insomnia. The student could provide information about which of the following?
   1. Garlic
   2. Valerian
   3. Lavender
   4. Glucosamine

5. A nurse is assisting with collecting data from an African-American client admitted to the ambulatory care unit who is scheduled for a hernia repair. Which of the following information about the client is of least priority during the data collection?
   1. Respiratory
   2. Psychosocial
   3. Neurological
   4. Cardiovascular

6. A nurse is planning to reinforce nutrition instructions to an African-American client. When developing the plan, the nurse is aware that a common dietary practice of clients with African-American heritage is to eat:
   1. Raw fish
   2. Red meat
   3. Fried foods
   4. Rice as the basis for all meals

7. A nurse consults with a dietitian regarding the dietary preferences of an Asian-American client. Which of the following foods would the nurse likely include in the diet plan?
   1. Rice
   2. Fruits
   3. Red meat
   4. Fried foods

8. An antihypertensive medication has been prescribed for a client with hypertension. The client tells the nurse that she would like to take an herbal substance to help lower her blood pressure. The nurse should:
   1. Tell the client that herbal substances are not safe and should never be used.
   2. Advise the client to discuss the use of an herbal substance with the physician.
   3. Teach the client how to take her blood pressure so that it can be monitored closely.
   4. Tell the client that if she takes the herbal substance, she will need to have her blood pressure checked frequently.

9. An Hispanic-American mother brings her child to the clinic for an examination. Which of the following is important when gathering data about the child?
   1. Avoiding eye contact
   2. Using body language only
   3. Avoiding speaking to the child
   4. Touching the child during the examination

ALTERNATE ITEM FORMAT: MULTIPLE RESPONSE

10. A nursing student is asked to identify the practices and beliefs of the Amish society. Select all that apply.
    1. Many choose not to have health insurance.
    2. They believe that health is a gift from God.
    3. The authority of women is equal to that of men.
    4. They remain secluded and avoid helping others.
    5. They use both traditional and alternative health care, such as healers, herbs, and massage.
    6. Funerals are conducted in the home without a eulogy, flower decorations, or any other display; caskets are plain and simple, without adornment.

ANSWERS

1. **4**

Rationale: Complementary (alternative) therapies include a wide variety of treatment modalities that are used in addition to conventional treatment to treat a disease or illness. These therapies complement conventional treatment, but they should be approved by the person's health care provider to ensure that the treatment does not interact with prescribed therapy. Although the physician should approve the use of a complementary therapy and although some of these therapies can interact with the prescribed treatment plan, the statements in options 1 and 3 are inappropriate. Similarly, option 2 is an inappropriate response to the client. Option 4 addresses the client's question and encourages discussion.

Test-Taking Strategy: Use therapeutic communication techniques. Eliminate options 1, 2, and 3, because they are nontherapeutic. Option 4 is the only option that addresses the client's question and encourages discussion. Review therapeutic communication techniques if you had difficulty with this question.

Level of Cognitive Ability: Application
Client Needs: Physiological Integrity
Integrated Process: Communication and Documentation
Content Area: Fundamental Skills
References: Christensen, B., & Kockrow, E. (2006). *Foundations of nursing* (5th ed., p. 427). St. Louis: Mosby.
Jarvis, C. (2008). *Physical examination & health assessment* (5th ed., pp. 58-61). Philadelphia: Saunders.

2. **4**

Rationale: Kosher meals arrive on paper plates and with plastic utensils sealed. Health care providers should not unwrap the utensils or transfer the food to another serving dish. Although the nurse may want to be helpful by assisting the client with the meal, the only appropriate option for this client is option 4.

Test-Taking Strategy: Use the process of elimination and your knowledge regarding the rituals associated with kosher meals. Options 2 and 3 are comparable or alike and can be eliminated first. To choose from the remaining options, it is necessary to be familiar with kosher rituals. If you had difficulty with this question, review the dietary practices of the Jewish client.

Level of Cognitive Ability: Application
Client Needs: Psychosocial Integrity
Integrated Process: Nursing Process/Implementation
Content Area: Fundamental Skills
References: Giger, J., & Davidhizar, R. (2008), *Transcultural nursing assessment & intervention* (5th ed., pp. 609-610). St. Louis: Mosby.
Grodner, M., Long, S., & Walkinshaw, B. (2007). *Foundations and clinical applications of nutrition: A nursing approach* (4th ed., p. 564). St. Louis: Mosby.
Nix, S. (2005). *Williams' basic nutrition and diet therapy* (12th ed., p. 249). St. Louis: Mosby.

3. **3**

Rationale: Children should not be given herbal therapies, especially in the home and without professional supervision.

There are no general contraindications for the clients described in options 1, 2, and 4.

Test-Taking Strategy: Use the process of elimination and your knowledge regarding herbal therapies. Note the age in option 3 to direct you to this option. Options 1, 2, and 4 describe clients for which there are no contraindications and can thus be eliminated. If you had difficulty with this question, review the indications and contraindications for herbal therapies.

Level of Cognitive Ability: Analysis
Client Needs: Safe and Effective Care Environment
Integrated Process: Nursing Process/Data Collection
Content Area: Pharmacology
Reference: Christensen, B., & Kockrow, E. (2006). *Foundations of nursing* (5th ed., p. 427). St. Louis: Mosby.

4. **2**

Rationale: Valerian has been used to treat insomnia, hyperactivity, and stress. It has also been used to treat nervous disorders such as anxiety and restlessness. Garlic is used as an antioxidant and to lower cholesterol levels. Glucosamine is an amino acid that assists with the synthesis of cartilage. Lavender is used as an antiseptic and fragrance for a mild sedative effect.

Test-Taking Strategy: Use the process of elimination and your knowledge regarding herbal therapies to assist with answering this question. Focus on the subject of a substance that may be used to treat insomnia, and remember that valerian has been used to treat insomnia. If you had difficulty with this question, review specific herbal therapies.

Level of Cognitive Ability: Application
Client Needs: Physiological Integrity
Integrated Process: Teaching and Learning
Content Area: Pharmacology
Reference: Christensen, B., & Kockrow, E. (2006). *Foundations of nursing* (5th ed., p. 426). St. Louis: Mosby.

5. **2**

Rationale: The psychosocial data is the least priority during the initial admission data collection. In the African-American culture, it is considered intrusive to ask personal questions during the initial contact or meeting. Additionally, cardiovascular, neurological, and respiratory data include physiological assessments that would be the priority.

Test-Taking Strategy: Note the strategic words "least priority." Use Maslow's Hierarchy of Needs theory to answer the question. Options 1, 3, and 4 address physiological needs. Review the characteristics of the African-American culture if you had difficulty with this question.

Level of Cognitive Ability: Comprehension
Client Needs: Physiological Integrity
Integrated Process: Nursing Process/Data Collection
Content Area: Fundamental Skills
Reference: Giger, J., & Davidhizar, R. (2008). *Transcultural nursing assessment & intervention* (5th ed. pp. 207-208). St. Louis: Mosby.

6. **3**

Rationale: African-American food preferences include chicken, pork, greens, rice, and fried foods. Asian Americans eat raw

fish, rice, and soy sauce. Hispanic Americans prefer beans, fried foods, spicy foods, chili, and carbonated beverages. European Americans prefer carbohydrates and red meat.
Test-Taking Strategy: Use the process of elimination. Recalling that African Americans are at risk for hypertension and coronary artery disease will direct you to option 3. Review the food preferences of the African-American culture if you had difficulty with this question.
Level of Cognitive Ability: Comprehension
Client Needs: Physiological Integrity
Integrated Process: Nursing Process/Planning
Content Area: Fundamental Skills
References: Grodner, M., Long, S., & Walkinshaw, B. (2007). *Foundations and clinical applications of nutrition: A nursing approach* (4th ed., p. 562). St. Louis: Mosby.
Nix, S. (2005). *Williams' basic nutrition and diet therapy* (12th ed., pp. 252-254). St. Louis: Mosby.
Schlenker, E., & Long, S. (2007). *Williams' essentials of nutrition & diet therapy* (9th ed., p. 734). St. Louis: Mosby.

7. **1**
Rationale: Asian-American food preferences include raw fish, rice, and soy sauce. African-American food preferences include chicken, pork, greens, rice, and fried foods. Hispanic Americans prefer beans, fried foods, spicy foods, chili, and carbonated beverages. European Americans prefer carbohydrates and red meat.
Test-Taking Strategy: Knowledge regarding the food practices and preferences related to various cultures is required to answer the question. Correlate rice with Asian Americans to answer questions similar to this one. Review the food preferences associated with the Asian-American culture if you had difficulty with this question.
Level of Cognitive Ability: Comprehension
Client Needs: Physiological Integrity
Integrated Process: Nursing Process/Planning
Content Area: Fundamental Skills
References: Grodner, M., Long, S., & Walkinshaw, B. (2007). *Foundations and clinical applications of nutrition: A nursing approach* (4th ed., p. 563). St. Louis: Mosby.
Nix, S. (2005). *Williams' basic nutrition & diet therapy* (12th ed., p. 255). St. Louis: Mosby.

8. **2**
Rationale: Although herbal substances may have some beneficial effects, not all herbs are safe to use. Clients who are being treated with conventional medication therapy should be advised to avoid herbal substances with similar pharmacological effects, because the combination may lead to an excessive reaction or to unknown interaction effects. Therefore, the nurse would advise the client to discuss the use of the herbal substance with the physician.
Test-Taking Strategy: Use the process of elimination. Eliminate option 1 first because of the close-ended word *never*. Next, eliminate options 3 and 4, because they are comparable or alike. Review the limitations associated with the use of herbal substances if you had difficulty with this question.
Level of Cognitive Ability: Application
Client Needs: Physiological Integrity

Integrated Process: Nursing Process/Implementation
Content Area: Fundamental Skills
Reference: Christensen, B., & Kockrow, E. (2006). *Foundations of nursing* (5th ed., p. 427). St. Louis: Mosby.
Linton, A., & Maebius, N. (2007). *Introduction to medical-surgical nursing* (4th ed., pp. 88-89). Philadelphia: Saunders.

9. **4**
Rationale: In the Hispanic-American culture, eye behavior is significant. It is believed that the "bad/evil eye" can be given to a child if a person looks at and admires a child without touching the child. Therefore, touching the child during the examination is very important. Although avoiding eye contact indicates respect and attentiveness, this is not the most important intervention. Avoiding speaking to the child and using body language only are not therapeutic interventions.
Test-Taking Strategy: Use the process of elimination. Eliminate options 2 and 3 first, because they are comparable or alike. From the remaining options, select the intervention that is most therapeutic, which is touch. Review the characteristics of the Hispanic-American culture if you had difficulty with this question.
Level of Cognitive Ability: Application
Client Needs: Psychosocial Integrity
Integrated Process: Nursing Process/Data Collection
Content Area: Fundamental Skills
Reference: Jarvis, C. (2008). *Physical examination & health assessment* (5th ed., pp. 73-74). Philadelphia: Saunders.

ALTERNATE ITEM FORMAT: MULTIPLE RESPONSE

10. **1, 2, 5, 6**
Rationale: The Amish society maintains a culture that is distinct and separate from the non-Amish society, and members generally remain separate from the rest of the world, both physically and socially. Men usually dress in plain, dark suits; women usually wear plain dresses with long sleeves, bonnets, and aprons. Women are not allowed to hold positions of power in the congregational organization. Family life has a patriarchal structure, and, although the roles of the women are considered equally important to those of men, they are very unequal in terms of authority. Marriage outside of the faith is not allowed, and unmarried women remain under the authority of their fathers. Amish society rejects materialism and worldliness. Members value living simply, and they may choose to avoid technology, such as electricity and cars. They highly value responsibility, generosity, and helping others, and they often work as farmers, builders, quilters, and homemakers. The Amish use traditional health care and alternative health care, such as healers, herbs, and massage. They believe that health is a gift from God but that clean living and a balanced diet help maintain it. They may choose not to have health insurance and instead to maintain mutual aid funds for those members who need help with medical costs. Funerals are conducted in the home without a eulogy, flower decorations, or any other display; caskets are plain and simple, without adornment. At death, women are usually buried in their bridal dresses. The Amish believe that one

lives on after death, either receiving eternal reward in heaven or being punished in hell.

Test-Taking Strategy: Focus on the subject of the Amish society. Read each option, and think about the practices and beliefs of this society to answer the question. Review the characteristics of the Amish society if you had difficulty with this question.

Level of Cognitive Ability: Comprehension
Client Needs: Psychosocial Integrity
Integrated Process: Teaching and Learning
Content Area: Fundamental Skills
Reference: Harkreader, H., Hogan, M. A., & Thobaben, M. (2007). *Fundamentals of nursing: Caring and clinical judgment* (3rd ed., p. 960). St. Louis: Saunders.

REFERENCES

Christensen, B, Kockrow, E. (2003). *Foundations of nursing* (4th ed.). St. Louis: Mosby.

Grodner, M., Long, S., & Walkinshaw, B. (2007). *Foundations and clinical applications of nutrition: A nursing approach* (4th ed.). St. Louis: Mosby.

Giger, J., & Davidhizar, R. (2008). *Transcultural nursing assessment & intervention* (5th ed.). Louis: Mosby.

Harkreader, H., Hogan, M.A., & Thobaben, M. (2007). *Fundamentals of nursing: Caring and clinical judgment* (3rd ed.). St. Louis: Saunders.

Jarvis, C. (2008). *Physical examination & health assessment* (5th ed.). Philadelphia: Saunders.

Linton, A., & Maebius, N. (2007). *Introduction to medical-surgical nursing* (4th ed.). Philadelphia: Saunders.

National Council of State Boards of Nursing (Eds.) (2008). *2008 Detailed Test Plan for the NCLEX-PN® Examination, National Council of State Boards of Nursing.* Chicago: Author.

National Council of State Boards of Nursing. *NCSBN home page.* www.ncsbn.org. Accessed June 4, 2008.

Nix, S. (2005). *Williams' basic nutrition and diet therapy* (12th ed.). St. Louis: Mosby.

Ontario Consultants on Religious Tolerance. *The Amish: History, beliefs, practices, conflicts, etc.* www.religioustolerance.org/amish.htm. Accessed June 4, 2008.

Schlenker, E., & Long, S. (2007). *Williams' essentials of nutrition & diet therapy* (9th ed.). St. Louis: Mosby.

Skidmore-Roth, L. (2006). *Mosby's handbook of herbs & natural supplements* (3rd ed.). St. Louis: Mosby.

Ethical and Legal Issues

PYRAMID TERMS

advance directive A written document, recognized by state law, that provides directions concerning the provision of care when a person is unable to make his or her own treatment choices.

advocacy Acting on behalf of the client and protecting the client's right to make his or her own decisions.

consent A voluntary act by which a person agrees to allow someone else to do something.

ethics Concerns the distinction between right and wrong on the basis of a body of knowledge rather than opinion.

informed consent The client understands the reason for the proposed intervention, with its benefits and risks, and agrees to the treatment by signing a consent form.

law A system composed of general rules governing conduct and the procedures for resolving disputes when the rules are not followed.

malpractice The failure to meet the standards of acceptable care that results in harm to another person.

negligence The failure to provide care that a reasonable person would ordinarily use in a similar situation.

patient's (client's) bill of rights The rights and responsibilities of clients receiving care.

values The beliefs and attitudes that may influence behavior and the process of decision making.

▲ PYRAMID TO SUCCESS

Across all settings in the practice of nursing, nurses are frequently confronted with ethical and legal issues related to client care. It is the responsibility of the professional nurse to be aware of the ethical principles, laws, and guidelines related to providing safe and quality care to clients. In the Pyramid to Success, focus areas include the following: ethical practices; the nurse practice act, client's rights (especially confidentiality and informed consent); advocacy, documentation, and advance directives; and cultural, religious, and spiritual issues. The Integrated Processes addressed in this chapter are Caring, Clinical Problem-Solving Process (Nursing Process), Communication and Documentation, and Teaching and Learning.

CLIENT NEEDS ▲

Safe and Effective Care Environment

Acting as an advocate
Completing incident reports, if necessary
Ensuring that advance directives are in place
Ensuring that informed consent is obtained
Establishing priorities
Implementing ethical practices and legal responsibilities
Maintaining confidentiality
Upholding the client's rights

Health Promotion and Maintenance

Considering developmental stages and transitions when planning care
Respecting lifestyle choices

Psychosocial Integrity

Considering cultural, spiritual, and religious issues related to care
Considering end-of-life issues when providing care
Encouraging the use of coping mechanisms
Identifying abuse and neglect situations
Identifying signs of chemical dependency
Identifying support systems

Physiological Integrity

Monitoring for responses to therapies
Providing palliative/comfort care

I. ETHICS
A. Description: The branch of philosophy that concerns the distinction between right and wrong on the basis of a body of knowledge rather than opinion
B. Morality: Behavior in accordance with customs or tradition and that usually reflects personal or religious beliefs
C. Ethical principles: Codes that direct or govern nursing actions (Box 7-1)

BOX 7-1 **Ethical Principles**

Autonomy: Respect for an individual's right to self-determination

Beneficence: The duty to do good to others and to maintain a balance between benefits and harms; paternalism is an undesirable outcome of beneficence, in which the health care provider decides what is best for the client and attempts to encourage the client to act against his or her own choices

Fidelity: The duty to do what one has promised

Justice: The equitable distribution of potential benefits and tasks; determining the order in which clients should be cared for

Nonmaleficence: The obligation to do or cause no harm to another

Veracity: The obligation to tell the truth

D. **Values**: Beliefs and attitudes that may influence behavior and the process of decision making
E. **Values** clarification: Process of analyzing one's own **values** to better understand what is truly important
F. Ethical codes
   1. Provide broad principles for determining and evaluating client care
   2. Are not legally binding, but, in most states, the board of nursing has authority to reprimand nurses for unprofessional conduct that violates the ethical codes
   3. Specific ethical codes
      a. National Federation of Licensed Practical Nurses (NFLPN) Code for Licensed Practical/Vocational Nurses
      b. NFLPN Nursing Practice Standards
      c. NFLPN Specialized Nursing Practice Standards
      d. National Association of Practical Nurse Education and Service (NAPNES) Code of **Ethics**
      e. NAPNES Standards of Practice for Practical/ Vocational Nurses
G. Ethical dilemma
   1. Occurs when there is a conflict between two or more ethical principles
   2. There is no correct decision
   3. The nurse must make a choice between two alternatives that are equally unsatisfactory
   4. May occur as a result of differences in cultural or religious beliefs
   5. Ethical reasoning is the process of thinking through what one ought to do in an orderly and systematic manner to provide justification for actions on the basis of principles
H. Advocate
   1. A person who speaks up for or acts on the behalf of the client, protects the client's right to make his or her own decisions, and upholds the principle of fidelity (duty)
   2. Represents the client's viewpoint to others

3. Avoids letting personal **values** influence **advocacy** for the client
4. Supports the client's decision, even when it conflicts with his or her own preferences or choices

I. **Ethics** committees
   1. Multidisciplinary approach to facilitate dialogue regarding ethical dilemmas
   2. Develop and establish policies and procedures for the prevention and resolution of dilemmas

II. **REGULATION OF NURSING PRACTICE**
A. Nurse practice act
   1. A series of statutes enacted by each state legislature to regulate the practice of nursing in that state
   2. Nurse practice acts set educational requirements for the nurse, distinguish between nursing practice and medical practice, and define the scope of nursing practice
   3. Additional issues covered by nurse practice acts include licensure requirements for the protection of the public, grounds for disciplinary action, rights of the nurse licensee if a disciplinary action is taken, and related topics
   4. All nurses are responsible for knowing the provisions of the act for the state or province in which they work
B. Standards of care
   1. Guidelines by which the nurse should practice
   2. Guidelines for determining whether nurses have performed duties in an appropriate manner
   3. If a nurse does not perform duties within accepted standards of care, the nurse places him- or herself in jeopardy of legal action and risks possible harm to the client
   4. If a nurse is named as a defendant in a **malpractice** lawsuit, the nurse's legal liability will be clear if it is shown that neither the accepted standards of care outlined by the state or province nursing practice act nor the policies of the employing institution were followed
C. Employee guidelines
   1. Respondent superior: Employer will be held liable for any negligent acts of an employee if the alleged negligent act occurred during the employment relationship and was within the scope of the employee's responsibilities
   2. Contracts
      a. Nurses are responsible for carrying out the terms of contractual agreements with the employee agency and the client
      b. The nurse's role as employee is governed by established employee handbooks and by client-care policies and procedures that create obligations, rights, and duties between the nurse and the client
   3. Institutional policies

a. Written policies and procedures of the employing institution that detail how nurses are to perform their duties

b. Policies and procedures are usually quite specific and located in manuals in most health care facilities

c. Although policies are not **laws**, courts generally rule against nurses who violate policies

d. If the nurse practices in accordance with the client-care policies and procedures established by the employer, functions within the job responsibilities, and provides care consistently in a diligent manner, the potential for liability is minimized

D. Hospital staffing

1. Nurses should not walk out when staffing is inadequate, because charges of abandonment can be made

2. Nurses in short-staffing situations are obligated to notify a nursing supervisor and follow up in writing (per agency policy)

E. Floating: The use of nursing staff on various nursing units or units other than the one that the nurse is normally assigned to work when such units require additional nursing staff

1. An acceptable legal practice used by hospitals to solve their understaffing problems

2. Legally a nurse cannot refuse to float unless a union contract guarantees that the nurse can work only in a specified area or the nurse can prove a lack of knowledge for the performance of assigned tasks

3. Nurses in a floating situation must not assume responsibility beyond their level of experience or qualification

4. Nurses who float should inform the supervisor of any lack of experience with caring for the types of clients on the new nursing unit

5. The nurse should request and be given orientation to the new unit

F. Disciplinary action

1. Boards of nursing may deny, revoke, or suspend any license to practice as a practical/vocational nurse in accordance with their statutory authority

2. Causes for disciplinary action

a. Unprofessional conduct

b. Conduct that could adversely affect the health and welfare of the public

c. Breach of client confidentiality

d. Failure to use sufficient knowledge, skills, or nursing judgment

e. Physically or verbally abusing a client

f. Assuming duties without sufficient preparation

g. Knowingly delegating nursing care to unlicensed personnel that places the client at risk for injury

h. Failure to accurately maintain a record for each client

i. Falsifying a client's record

j. Leaving a nursing assignment without properly notifying appropriate personnel

k. Any felony

III. LEGAL LIABILITY

A. Laws

1. Nurses are governed by civil and criminal law in roles as providers of services, employees of institutions, and private citizens

2. A nurse has a personal and legal obligation to provide a standard of client care expected of a reasonably competent professional nurse

3. Nurses are held responsible (liable) for harm resulting from their negligent acts or their failure to act

B. Sources of laws (Figure 7-1)

C. **Negligence** and **malpractice**

1. Conduct that falls below the standard of care

2. Can include acts of commission (doing an act) as well as acts of omission (not doing an act)

3. If a nurse gives care that does not meet appropriate standards, he or she may be held liable for **negligence**

4. **Malpractice** is **negligence** on the part of a nurse or of another health care professional

5. **Malpractice** is determined if the nurse owed a duty to the client and did not carry out the duty and the client was injured because the nurse failed to perform the duty

6. Proof of liability

a. Duty: At the time of injury, a duty existed between the plaintiff (client) and the defendant (nurse or other health care professional)

b. Breach of duty: The defendant breached the duty of care to the plaintiff

c. Proximate cause: The breach of the duty was the legal cause of injury to the client

d. Damage or injury: The plaintiff experienced injury, damages, or both and can be compensated by law

D. Professional liability insurance

1. Nurses need their own liability insurance for protection against malpractice lawsuits

2. Having personal insurance provides the nurse with protection as an individual and allows the nurse to have an attorney present who has only the nurse's interests in mind

E. Good Samaritan laws

1. Passed by state legislatures; laws may vary from state to state

2. Encourage health care professionals to assist during emergency situations without fear of being sued for the care provided

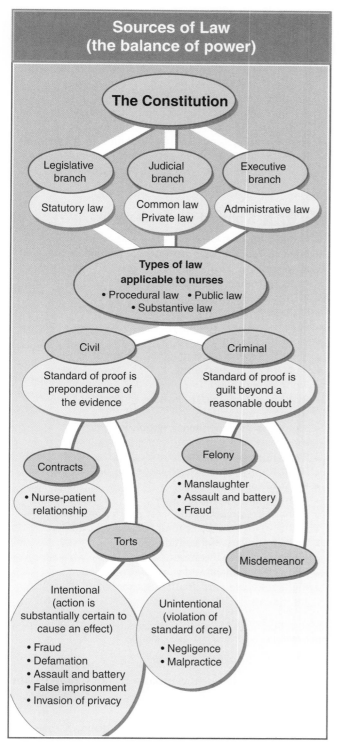

FIG. 7-1 Sources of law for nursing practice. (From Harkreader, H., Hogan, M. A., & Thobaben, M. [2007]. *Fundamentals of nursing: Caring and clinical judgment* [3rd ed.]. Philadelphia: Saunders.)

3. These laws limit liability and offer legal immunity for people who help during an emergency, provided that they give reasonable care
4. Immunity from suit applies only when all conditions of the state law are met; for example, the health care provider receives no compensation for the care provided and the care given is not intentionally negligent

F. Controlled substances
   1. Adhere to facility policies and procedures concerning the administration of controlled substances, which are governed by federal and state laws
   2. Controlled substances must be kept securely locked; only authorized personnel should have access to them

IV. **COLLECTIVE BARGAINING**
A. Formalized decision-making process between representatives of management and representatives of labor (union) to negotiate wages and conditions of employment
B. When collective bargaining breaks down because an agreement cannot be reached, the employees usually call a strike
C. Striking presents a moral dilemma to many nurses, because nursing practice is a service to people

V. **LEGAL RISK AREAS**
A. Assault
   1. Occurs when one person puts another person in fear of a harmful or offensive contact
   2. The victim fears and believes that harm will result from the threat
B. Battery: An intentional touching of another's body without the other's **consent**
C. Invasion of privacy: Includes violating confidentiality, intruding on private client or family matters, and sharing client information with unauthorized persons
D. False imprisonment
   1. Occurs when a client is not allowed to leave a health care facility when there is no legal justification to detain the client
   2. Occurs when restraining devices are used without an appropriate clinical need and **consent**
   3. A client can sign an "Against Medical Advice" form and refuse care if the client is competent to make decisions
   4. Document circumstances in the medical record to avoid allegations by the client that cannot be defended
E. Defamation: A false communication or a careless disregard for the truth that causes damage to someone's reputation, either in writing (libel) or verbally (slander)
F. Fraud: Results from a deliberate deception intended to produce unlawful gains

VI. **CLIENT'S RIGHTS**
A. Description
   1. A document that reflects the acknowledgment of a client's right to participate in his or her health care, with an emphasis on client autonomy

BOX 7-2   Patient's Rights When Hospitalized

- Right to considerate and respectful care
- Right to be informed about illness, possible treatments, and likely outcome and to discuss this information with the physician
- Right to know the names and roles of the people who are involved in care
- Right to consent or refuse a treatment
- Right to have an advance directive
- Right to privacy
- Right to expect that medical records are confidential
- Right to review the medical record and to have information explained
- Right to expect that the hospital will provide necessary health care services
- Right to know if the hospital has relationships with outside parties that may influence treatment or care
- Right to consent or refuse to take part in research
- Right to be told of realistic care alternatives when hospital care is no longer appropriate
- Right to know about hospital rules that affect treatment and about charges and payment methods

Modified from Christensen, B., & Kockrow, E. (2003). *Foundations of nursing* (4th ed.). St. Louis: Mosby.

2. Provides a list of the rights of the client and responsibilities that the hospital cannot violate (Box 7-2)
3. The client's rights affect the relationship between the client and the health care provider and between the client and the health care delivery system, and they protect the client's ability to determine the level and type of care received
4. **Laws** and standards (Box 7-3)

B. Rights for the mentally ill (Box 7-4)
   1. The Mental Health Systems Act of 1980 created rights for the mentally ill
   2. The Joint Commission developed policy statements addressing the rights of the mentally ill
   3. Psychiatric facilities are required to have a **client's bill of rights** posted in a visible area

C. Organ donation and transplantation
   1. The client has the right to decide to become an organ donor and a right to refuse an organ transplant as a treatment option
   2. An individual who is at least 18 years old may indicate his or her wish to become a donor on his or her driver's license (state specific) or in an **advance directive**
   3. The Uniform Anatomical Gift Act provides a list of individuals who can provide **informed consent** for the donation of a deceased individual's organs
   4. Criteria for organ donations are set by the United Network for Organ Sharing
   5. Some organs, such as the heart, lungs, and liver, can only be obtained from a person who was

BOX 7-3   Laws and Standards

American Hospital Association: Issued a patient's bill of rights

American Nurses Association: Developed the Code for Nurses, which defines the nurse's responsibility for upholding the client's rights

The Joint Commission: Developed policy statements addressing the rights of the mentally ill

Mental Health Systems Act: Developed rights for the mentally ill client

BOX 7-4   Rights of the Mentally Ill

- Right to be treated with dignity and respect
- Right to communicate with people outside of the hospital
- Right to keep clothing and personal effects with them
- Right to religious freedom
- Right to be employed
- Right to manage property
- Right to execute wills
- Right to enter into contractual agreements
- Right to make purchases
- Right to education
- Right to habeas corpus (written request for release from the hospital)
- Right to an independent psychiatric examination
- Right to civil service status, including the right to vote
- Right to retain licenses, privileges, or permits
- Right to sue or be sued
- Right to marry or divorce
- Right to treatment in the least restrictive setting
- Right to not be subject to unnecessary restraints
- Right to privacy and confidentiality
- Right to informed consent
- Right to treatment and to refuse treatment
- Right to refuse participation in experimental treatments or research

Modified from Stuart, G., & Laraia, M. (2005). *Principles and practice of psychiatric nursing* (8th ed.). St. Louis: Mosby.

on mechanical ventilation and suffered brain death; other organs or tissues can be removed several hours after death
6. Donor must be free of infectious disease and cancer
7. Requests to the family for organ donation from a deceased family member are usually done by the physician or a nurse specially trained for making such requests
8. The donation of organs does not delay funeral arrangements, there is no obvious evidence that the organs were removed from the body when the body is dressed, and there is no cost to the family for the removal of the donated organs

D. Religious beliefs: Organ donation and transplantation
   1. Catholic Church: Organ donation and transplants are acceptable
   2. Eastern Orthodox Church: Discourages organ donation
   3. Islam: Body parts may not be removed or donated for transplantation
   4. Jehovah's Witness: An organ transplant may be accepted, but the organ must be cleansed with a nonblood solution before transplantation
   5. Orthodox Judaism
      a. All body parts removed during autopsy must be buried with the body, because it is believed that the entire body must be returned to the earth
      b. Organ transplantation may be allowed with the rabbi's approval

▲ VII. INFORMED CONSENT
A. Description
   1. **Consent** is a client's approval (or that of the client's legal representative) to have the client's body touched by a specific individual
   2. **Consents** or releases are legal documents that indicate the client's acceptance of surgery or treatment or that permit information to be given to a third party
   3. Types of **consent** (Box 7-5)
   4. **Informed consent** indicates the client's participation in the decision regarding health care
   5. The client must be informed, in understandable terms, of the risks and benefits of the surgery or treatment, what the consequences are for not having the surgery or procedure performed, treatment options, and the name of the health care provider performing the surgery or procedure
   6. A client's questions about the surgery or procedure must be answered before the **consent** is signed
   7. A **consent** must be freely signed by the client without threat or pressure, and it must be witnessed by another adult
   8. A client who has been medicated with sedating medications or any other medications that can affect his or her cognitive abilities should not be asked to sign a **consent**
   9. Legally the client must be mentally and emotionally competent to give **consent**
   10. If a client is declared mentally or emotionally incompetent, the next of kin, appointed guardian (appointed by the court), or durable power of attorney has legal authority to give **consent** for the client (Box 7-6)
   11. A competent client who is more than 18 years old must sign the **consent**

BOX 7-5 Types of Consent

Admission agreement: Obtained at the time of admission; identifies the health care agency's responsibilities to the client
Blood transfusion consent: Indicates that the client was informed of the benefits and risks of the transfusion; some clients hold religious beliefs that would prohibit receiving a blood transfusion, even in a life-threatening situation
Research consent: Obtains permission from the client regarding participation in a research study; informs the client about the possible risks, consequences, and benefits of the research
Special consents: Required for the use of restraints, photographing of the client, disposal of body parts during surgery, donating organs after death, and performing an autopsy
Surgical consent: Obtained for all surgical or invasive procedures or diagnostic tests that are invasive; the physician, surgeon, or anesthesiologist who performs the surgical or other procedure is responsible for explaining the procedure and its risks, benefits, and possible alternatives

BOX 7-6 Mentally or Emotionally Incompetent Clients

- Declared incompetent
- Unconscious
- Under the influence of alcohol or drugs
- Chronic dementia or other mental deficiency

12. In most states, when a nurse is involved in the **informed consent** process, the nurse is only witnessing the signature of the client on the **informed consent** form
13. An **informed consent** can be waived for urgent medical or surgical intervention as long as institutional policy so indicates
14. A client has the right to refuse information, waive the **informed consent**, and undergo treatment, but this decision must be documented in the medical record
15. A client may withdraw his or her **consent** at any time
B. Minors
   1. A minor is a client who is younger than the legal age of adulthood as defined by state statute (usually less than 18 years old)
   2. A minor may not give legal **consent; consent** must be obtained from a parent or legal guardian
   3. Parental or guardian consent should be obtained before treatment is initiated for a minor, except in an emergency
   4. In certain situations, the **consent** of the minor is sufficient and may include the following: treatment related to substance abuse; treatment

of a sexually transmitted infection; human immunodeficiency virus testing and acquired immunodeficiency syndrome treatment; birth
control services, pregnancy, or psychiatric services; client is an emancipated minor; or if a
court order or other legal authorization has
been obtained (state **laws** need to be followed)
C. Emancipated minor
1. A minor who has established independence
from the parents through marriage, pregnancy,
service in the armed forces, or court order
2. An emancipated minor is considered legally
capable of signing an **informed consent**
VIII. **HEALTH INSURANCE PORTABILITY AND
ACCOUNTABILITY ACT (HIPAA)**
A. Description
1. Describes how personal health information
(PHI) may be used and how the client can
obtain access to the information
2. PHI includes individually identifiable information that relates to the client's past, present, or
future health; treatment; and payment for
health care services
3. HIPAA requires health care agencies to keep
PHI private, provides information to the client
about the legal responsibilities regarding privacy, and explains the client's rights with respect
to PHI
4. The client has various rights as a consumer of
health care under HIPAA, and any client
requests may need to be placed in writing; a
fee may be attached to certain client requests
5. The client may file a complaint if he or she
believes that privacy rights have been violated
B. Client's rights
1. To request a copy of the PHI
2. To ask the health care agency to amend the PHI
that is contained in a record if the PHI is
inaccurate
3. To request a list of disclosures made regarding
the PHI as specified by HIPAA
4. To request to restrict the way the health care
agency uses or discloses the PHI regarding treatment, payment, or health care services unless
information is needed to provide emergency
treatment
5. To request that the health care agency communicates with the client in a certain way or at a
certain location; the request must specify how
or where the client wishes to be contacted
6. To request a paper copy of the HIPAA notice
C. Health care agency use and disclosure of PHI
1. The health care agency obtains the PHI during
the course of providing and/or administering
health insurance benefits for the client and
may use or disclose the PHI when administering benefits

2. Reasons that the use or disclosure of PHI may
occur
a. Health care payment purposes
b. Health care operations purposes
c. Treatment purposes
d. Providing information about health care
services
e. Data aggregation purposes to make health
care benefit decisions
f. Administering health care benefits
3. Additional uses or disclosures of PHI (Box 7-7)
IX. **CLIENT PRIVACY**
A. Client's right to protection against unreasonable
and unwarranted interference into his or her private
affairs
B. Violations (Box 7-8)
X. **CONFIDENTIALITY**
A. Description
1. Client's right to privacy in the health care
system
2. A special relationship exists between the client
and nurse that ensures information discussed
will not be shared with a third party who is
not directly involved in the client's care
B. Nurse's responsibility
1. Nurses are bound to protect client confidentiality
by most nurse practice acts, by ethical principles
and standards, by institutional and agency policies and procedures, and by the **law**
2. The disclosure of confidential information
exposes the nurse to liability for the invasion
of the client's privacy
3. The nurse needs to protect the client from the
indiscriminate disclosure of health care information that may cause harm (Box 7-9)
C. Medical records
1. The medical record is confidential
2. The client has the rights to read the medical
record and to have copies of the record
3. Only staff directly involved in care have legiti-
mate access to a client's record; these staff may
include physicians and nurses caring for the
client, technicians, therapists, social workers,
unit secretaries, client advocates, and adminis-
trators (for statistical analysis, staffing, and quality care review); others must ask permission
from the client to review a record
4. The medical record is sent to the hospital
records or health information department
after the client is discharged
D. Computerized medical records
1. Health care employees have access to the client's record in the nursing unit or work area
only
2. Confidentiality can be protected with the use of
special computer access codes to limit what
employees can find in computer systems

BOX 7-7 Uses or Disclosures of Personal Health Information

- Compliance with legal proceedings or for limited law-enforcement purposes
- May be disclosed:
  - To a family member or significant other in a medical emergency
  - To a personal representative appointed by the client or designated by law
  - For research purposes in limited circumstances
  - To a coroner, medical examiner, or funeral director about a deceased person
  - To an organ procurement organization in limited circumstances
  - To avert a serious threat to the client's health or safety or the health or safety of others
  - To a governmental agency authorized to oversee the health care system or government programs
  - To the U.S. Department of Health and Human Services for the investigation of compliance with the Health Insurance Portability and Accountability Act or to fulfill another lawful request
  - To federal officials for lawful intelligence or national security purposes
  - To protect health authorities for public health purposes
  - To appropriate military authorities if a client is a member of the armed forces
  - In accordance with a valid authorization signed by the client

Modified from U.S. Department of Health and Human Services Office for Civil Rights. (2006). *HIPAA Administration Simplification Regulation Text.* http://www.hhs.gov/ocr/AdminSimpRegtext.pdf.

3. The use of a password or identification code is needed to enter and sign off of a computer system
4. A password or identification code should never be shared with another person
5. Personal passwords should be periodically changed to prevent unauthorized computer access

E. Research: Any information provided by the client will not be reported in any manner that could identify the client or made accessible to anyone outside of the research team

XI. LEGAL SAFEGUARDS
A. Risk management
  1. A planned method to identify, analyze, and evaluate risks followed by a plan for reducing the frequency of accidents and injuries
  2. Programs are based on a systematic reporting system for incidents or unusual occurrences
B. Incident report (Box 7-10)
  1. A tool used as a means of identifying risk situations and improving client care
  2. Follows specific documentation guidelines

BOX 7-8 Invasion of Privacy

- Taking photographs of the client
- Releasing the client's medical information to an unauthorized person, such as a member of the press or a family member, friend, or neighbor of the client, without the client's permission
- Using the client's name or picture for the health care agency's sole advantage
- Intruding into the client's affairs by the health care agency
- Publishing information about the client
- Publishing embarrassing facts about the client
- Publicly disclosing private information about the client
- Leaving the client's curtains or room door open while a treatment or procedure is being performed
- Allowing individuals to observe a treatment or procedure without the client's consent
- Leaving a confused or agitated client sitting in the nursing unit hallway
- Interviewing a client in a room with only a curtain between clients or in another place where conversations can be overheard
- Accessing the client's medical records when unauthorized to do so

BOX 7-9 Maintaining Confidentiality

- Not discussing client issues with other clients or staff uninvolved in the client's care
- Not sharing the client's health care information with others without the client's consent (this includes family members and friends of the client)
- Keeping all information about a client private and not revealing it to someone not directly involved in care
- Sharing client information in private and secluded areas
- Protecting the client's medical record from all unauthorized readers

3. Fill out completely, accurately, and factually
4. The report form should not be copied or placed in the client's record
5. No reference should be made to the incident report form in the client's record
6. Not a substitute for a complete entry in the client's record regarding the incident
C. Safeguarding valuables
  1. The client's valuables should be given to a family member or secured for safekeeping, stored and locked in a designated location, such as the agency's safe; the location of the client's valuables is documented per agency policy
  2. Many health care agencies require a client to sign a release to free the agency of responsibility for lost valuables

Incidents That Need to Be Reported

- Accidental omission of ordered therapies
- Circumstances that led to client injury or to a risk for client injury
- Client falls
- Medication administration errors
- Needlestick injuries
- Procedure- or equipment-related accidents
- Visitor(s) with symptoms of an illness

3. A client's wedding band can be taped in place unless there is a risk of swelling of the hand or fingers
4. Religious items, such as scapulas or religious medals, may be pinned to the client's gown if allowed by agency policy

D. Physician's orders
1. A nurse is obligated to carry out a physician's orders except when the nurse believes an order to be inappropriate
2. A nurse carrying out an inaccurate order may be legally responsible for any harm suffered by the client
3. Clarify an unclear or inappropriate order or an order in question with the physician
4. If no resolution occurs regarding the order in question, contact the nurse manager or supervisor
5. Telephone orders: Follow agency policy (Box 7-11)
6. Medication orders (Box 7-12)

E. Documentation
1. Legally required by accrediting agencies, state licensing laws, and state nurse and medical practice acts
2. Follow agency guidelines and procedures (Box 7-13)

F. Client/family teaching
1. Provide complete instructions in a language that the client or family can understand
2. Document client and family teaching, what was taught, evaluation of understanding, and who was present during the teaching session
3. Inform client of what would happen if information shared during teaching is not followed

XII. LEGAL DOCUMENTS
A. Advance directives
1. A written document (sometimes called a *living will*) recognized by state law that provides directions concerning the provision of care when a client is unable to make his or her own treatment choices
2. May also include the naming of a relative or friend (health care proxy) who will make health care decisions in the event of the client's incapacitation

BOX 7-11 **Telephone Orders**

- Date and time the entry.
- Repeat the order to the physician, and record the order.
- Sign the order; begin with "t.o." (telephone order); write the physician's name, and then add your signature to the order.
- If another nurse witnessed the order, his or her signature follows.
- The physician needs to countersign the order within a certain time frame in accordance with agency policy.

BOX 7-12 **Components of a Medication Order**

- Date and time when the order was written
- Medication name
- Medication dosage
- Route of administration
- Frequency of administration
- Physician or health care provider's signature

B. Patient Self-Determination Act
1. Became a law in the United States in 1990 and was implemented in all health care institutions
2. Clients must be provided with information about their rights to identify written directions about the care they wish to receive in the event that they become incapacitated and unable to make health care decisions
3. On admission to a health care facility, the client is asked about the existence of an advance directive; if one exists, it must be documented and included as part of the medical record
4. If the client signs an advance directive at the time of admission, it must be documented in the client's medical record

C. Living will
1. An advance directive document that lists the medical treatment a client chooses to omit or refuse if he or she becomes unable to make decisions and is terminally ill
2. States have their own requirements for executing living wills but, generally, two witnesses who are not relatives or physicians are needed when the client signs the living will

D. Durable power of attorney: A legal document that appoints a person (health care proxy) chosen by the client to carry out his or her wishes as expressed in the advance directive or to make decisions on his or her behalf if and when he or she can no longer do so

E. "Do not resuscitate" (DNR) orders
1. Orders written by a physician when a client has indicated a desire to be allowed to die if he or she stops breathing or his or her heart stops beating

BOX 7-13   Documentation Guidelines

Narrative Documentation
- Use a black-colored ink pen.
- Date and time entries.
- Provide objective, factual, and complete documentation.
- Document care, medications, treatments, and procedures as soon as possible after completion.
- Document client's responses to interventions.
- Document client's consent for or refusal of treatments.
- Document calls made to other health care providers.
- Do not document or change documentation for other individuals.
- Sign and title each entry.
- Use quotes as appropriate for subjective data.
- Use correct spelling, grammar, and punctuation.
- Avoid unacceptable abbreviations.
- Avoid judgmental or evaluative statements such as "uncooperative client."
- Do not leave blank spaces on documentation forms.
- Follow agency policies when an error is made (i.e., draw one line through the error, initial, and date).
- Follow agency guidelines regarding late entries.

Computerized Documentation
- Use only your own user identification (ID) code, name, or password.
- Never lend your access ID to another individual.
- Maintain the privacy and confidentiality of documented information printed from the computer.

2. The client or his or her legal representative must provide informed consent for the DNR status
3. The DNR order must be clearly defined so that other treatment not refused by the client will be continued
4. The DNR order must be reviewed on a regular basis according to agency policy (usually every 3 days for hospitalized clients and every 60 days for clients in residential health care facilities)
5. All health care personnel must know if a client has a DNR order
6. A nurse who attempts to resuscitate a client who has a DNR order would be acting without the client's consent and committing battery
7. Specific agency guidelines must be followed regarding when and under what circumstances a verbal DNR order is acceptable

F. The nurse's role
1. Discussing advance directives with the client opens the communication channel to establish what is important to the client and what he or she may view as promoting life versus prolonging dying
2. The nurse needs to ensure that the client was provided with information about his or her right to identify written directions about the care he or she wishes to receive
3. On admission to a health care facility, the nurse determines if an advance directive exists and ensures that it is part of the medical record
4. The nurse ensures that the physician was notified of the presence of an advance directive
5. All health care workers need to follow the directions of an advance directive to protect themselves from liability
6. Some agencies have specific policies that prohibit a nurse from signing as a witness to a legal document such as a living will
7. If a nurse witnesses a legal document, he or she must document the event and the factual circumstances surrounding the signing in the medical record
8. Documentation as a witness should include who was present, any significant comments by the client, and the nurse's observations of the client's conduct during this process

XIII. REPORTING RESPONSIBILITIES
A. Requirements: Nurses are required to report certain communicable diseases, criminal activities (e.g., abuse, gunshot or stab wounds, assaults, homicides), and suicides to the appropriate authorities
B. The impaired nurse
1. If a nurse suspects that a coworker is abusing chemicals, the nurse must report the individual to the nursing administration in a confidential manner, with the goal of treatment being the priority issue
2. Nursing administration will investigate and then notify the board of nursing regarding the nurse's behavior
C. Occupational Safety and Health Act
1. Requires that an employer provide a safe workplace for employees according to regulations
2. Employees can confidentially report working conditions that violate regulations
3. An employee who does not report unsafe working conditions can be retaliated against by the employer
D. Sexual harassment
1. Prohibited by state and federal **laws**
2. Includes unwelcome conduct of a sexual nature
3. Follow agency policies and procedures to handle reporting a concern or complaint

XIV. INFORMATION TECHNOLOGY IN HEALTH CARE
A. Telecommunication technologies are changing the way health care is delivered to clients and facilitating information exchange among health care providers
B. Telemedicine is the provision of health care services, clinical information, and education over a distance

using telecommunication technology; this may or may not include methods that require inter-activity

C. Telehealth is the use of telecommunication technology integrated into the practice of health care

D. E-health refers to all forms of electronic health care delivery through the Internet; it includes services provided by professionals, nonprofessionals, businesses, and consumers

E. Uses of telecommunication technology in health care

1. Clinical uses: Client-care applications involving synchronous and asynchronous technologies such as fax machines, Email, virtual chat rooms, videoconferencing, and discussion boards

2. Administrative applications: The use of technology for accounting records and billing services, electronic connections to pharmacies and other units for ordering medications and supplies, verification of medical records for client history and treatments, research applications, and record keeping

3. Remote medical instruments: The use of enhanced computer technology devices to record and process medical information such as robotics, imaging, and other services

4. Educational applications: The use of telecommunication technologies to deliver or assist with providing educational opportunities for both professionals and clients; may also include the use of Internet and web-based applications to provide training and educational opportunities for staff and clients

F. Benefits of telecommunication technologies

1. Reduction in health care costs
2. Enhanced health care access and delivery
3. Improved information and client support
4. Improved information and continuing education training for health care providers
5. Enhanced distribution of health care resources
6. Reduced isolation and stress of health care professionals
7. Increased access to health care information
8. Improved communications between clients and health care professionals

G. Challenges to the use of telecommunication technologies in health care

1. Confidentiality of records: Protection needs to be provided for data
2. **Malpractice** issues related to the delivery of services across state lines and other jurisdictions
3. Staff training: Time consuming, expensive, and difficult

4. Reimbursement issues by Medicare or other third-party payers
5. Acceptance of telecommunications technology use

XV. DOCUMENTATION BY COMPUTER
(see Box 7-13)

A. Computer-based records contain information that is identical to traditional print-based records

B. Eliminates repetitive entries and allows for the information to be accessed as part of a database for future review

C. Provides reduced cost and reduced frequency of documentation errors such as lost charts, illegible notes, or illegible prescription orders

D. Major concerns of using computer-based medical records system are confidentiality and security issues

E. Nurses or other health care professionals using computer documentation should log into the system with a user name and secure password that should be changed periodically (typically monthly); the password should not be shared among other health care providers

F. Printouts of computerized records should be protected; copy logs and the shredding of printouts assist with protecting confidentiality

PRACTICE QUESTIONS

More questions on the companion CD!

11. Which of the following is a recommended guideline for safe computerized charting?
   1. Passwords to the computer system should only be changed if lost.
   2. Computer terminals may be left unattended during client-care activities.
   3. Report accidental deletions from the computerized file to the nursing manager or supervisor.
   4. Copies of printouts from computerized files should be kept on a clipboard at the nurses' station for other nurses to access.

12. A nurse enters a client's room and finds the client sitting on the floor. The nurse checks the client thoroughly and then assists the client back into bed. The nurse completes an incident report and notifies the nursing supervisor and physician of the incident. Which of the following is the next nursing action regarding the incident?
   1. Place the incident report in the client's chart.
   2. Make a copy of the incident report for the physician.
   3. Document a complete entry in the client's record concerning the incident.
   4. Document in the client's record that an incident report has been completed.

13. An unconscious client who is bleeding profusely is brought to the emergency department after a serious accident. Surgery is required immediately to save the client's life. With regard to informed consent for the surgical procedure, which of the following is the best action?
    1. Call the nursing supervisor to initiate a court order for the surgical procedure.
    2. Try calling the client's spouse to obtain telephone consent before the surgical procedure.
    3. Ask the friend who accompanied the client to the emergency department to sign the consent form.
    4. Transport the client to the operating department immediately, as required by the physician, without obtaining an informed consent.

14. A nurse arrives at work and is told to report (float) to the pediatric unit for the day because the unit is understaffed and needs additional nurses to care for the children. The nurse has never worked in the pediatric unit. Which of the following is the appropriate nursing action?
    1. Call the hospital lawyer.
    2. Call the nursing supervisor.
    3. Refuse to float to the pediatric unit.
    4. Report to the pediatric unit and identify tasks that can be safely performed.

15. A nurse enters a client's room and notes that the client's lawyer is present and that the client is preparing a living will. The living will requires that the client's signature be witnessed, and the client asks the nurse to witness the signature. Which of the following is the appropriate nursing action?
    1. Decline from signing the will.
    2. Sign the will as a witness to the signature only.
    3. Call the hospital lawyer before signing the will.
    4. Sign the will, clearly identifying credentials and employment agency.

16. A nurse enters a client's room and finds the client lying on the floor. The nurse checks the client and then calls the nursing supervisor and the physician to inform them of the occurrence. The nurse completes the incident report, understanding that it allows for the analysis of adverse client events through:
    1. Providing clients with necessary stabilizing treatments
    2. A method of promoting quality care and risk management
    3. Determining the effectiveness of interventions in relation to outcomes
    4. The appropriate method of reporting to local, state, and federal agencies

17. A nurse observes that a client received pain medication 1 hour ago from another nurse but that the client still has severe pain. The nurse has previously observed this same occurrence. On the basis of the nurse practice act, the observing nurse plans to do which of the following?
    1. Report the information to the police.
    2. Call the impaired nurse organization.
    3. Talk with the nurse who gave the medication.
    4. Report the information to a nursing supervisor.

18. A client has died, and a nurse asks a family member about the funeral arrangements. The family member refuses to discuss the issue. The nurse's appropriate action is to:
    1. Show acceptance of feelings.
    2. Provide information needed for decision making.
    3. Suggest a referral to a mental health professional.
    4. Remain with the family member without discussing funeral arrangements.

19. A nurse lawyer provides an education session to the nursing staff regarding client rights. A nurse asks the lawyer to describe an example that may relate to invasion of client privacy. A nursing action that indicates a violation of this right is:
    1. Threatening to place a client in restraints
    2. Performing a surgical procedure without consent
    3. Taking photographs of the client without consent
    4. Telling the client that he or she cannot leave the hospital

20. An older woman is brought to the emergency department. When caring for the client, the nurse notes old and new ecchymotic areas on both of the client's arms and buttocks. The nurse asks the client how the bruises were sustained. The client, although reluctant, tells the nurse in confidence that her daughter frequently hits her if she gets in the way. Which of the following is the appropriate nursing response?
    1. "I have a legal obligation to report this type of abuse."
    2. "I promise I won't tell anyone, but let's see what we can do about this."
    3. "Let's talk about ways that will prevent your daughter from hitting you."
    4. "This should not be happening. If it happens again, you must call the emergency department."

21. A client tells the nurse about his decision to refuse external cardiac massage. Which of the following would be the appropriate initial nursing action?
    1. Notify the physician of the client's request.
    2. Discuss the client's request with the family.
    3. Document the client's request in the client's record.
    4. Conduct a client conference to share the client's request.

22. A nurse is documenting information regarding a client's care into the computerized medical record. Which of the following actions by the nurse would be inappropriate?
    1. Change the password for entering computer files at least monthly.
    2. Shred the printout of the nurse's flowchart at the end of the nurse's shift.
    3. Use own user name and password when logging into the computer system.
    4. Leave the computer terminal immediately after logging in to check on the status of a client.

ALTERNATE ITEM FORMAT: MULTIPLE RESPONSE

23. Choose the correct guidelines related to narrative documentation. Select all that apply.
    ☑ 1. Date and time entries.
    ☑ 2. Sign and title each entry.
    ☐ 3. Use a blue-colored ink pen.
    ☑ 4. Avoid judgmental and evaluative statements.
    ☐ 5. Document judgmental information completely.
    ☑ 6. Do not leave blank spaces on documentation forms.

ANSWERS

11. 3
Rationale: After any inadvertent deletions of permanent computerized records, the nurse should type an explanation into the computer file with the date, time, and his or her initials. The nurse should also contact the nursing manager or supervisor with a written explanation of the situation. Options 1, 2, and 4 represent unsafe charting actions. Only option 3 follows the guidelines for safe computer charting
Test-Taking Strategy: Use the process of elimination. Focusing on the subject of a safe guideline will direct you to option 3. Options 1, 2, and 4 represent unsafe charting actions. Review the guidelines for computerized documentation if you had difficulty with this question.
Level of Cognitive Ability: Application
Client Needs: Safe and Effective Care Environment
Integrated Process: Nursing Process/Implementation
Content Area: Fundamental Skills
Reference: Christensen, B., & Kockrow, E. (2006). *Foundations and adult health nursing* (5th ed., p. 120). St. Louis: Mosby.

12. 3
Rationale: The incident report is confidential and privileged information, and it should not be copied, placed in the chart, or have any reference made to it in the client's record. The incident report is not a substitute for a complete entry in the client's record concerning the incident.
Test-Taking Strategy: Use the process of elimination. Eliminate options 1 and 4 first, because they are comparable or alike. Recalling that incident reports should not be copied will direct you to option 3. Review the nursing responsibilities related to incident reports if you had difficulty with this question.
Level of Cognitive Ability: Application
Client Needs: Safe and Effective Care Environment
Integrated Process: Nursing Process/Implementation
Content Area: Fundamental Skills
Reference: Christensen, B., & Kockrow, E. (2006). *Foundations of nursing* (5th ed., pp. 112, 115). St. Louis: Mosby.

13. 4
Rationale: Generally there are only two instances in which the informed consent of an adult client is not needed. One instance is when an emergency is present and delaying treatment for the purpose of obtaining informed consent would result in injury or death to the client. The second instance is when the client waives the right to give informed consent. Options 1, 2, and 3 are inappropriate.
Test-Taking Strategy: Use the process of elimination. Option 3 can easily be eliminated first. Note the strategic words "surgery is required immediately." Options 1 and 2 would delay treatment and should be eliminated. Review the issues surrounding informed consent if you had difficulty with this question.
Level of Cognitive Ability: Application
Client Needs: Safe and Effective Care Environment
Integrated Process: Nursing Process/Implementation
Content Area: Fundamental Skills
Reference: Ignatavicius, D., & Workman, M. (2006). *Medical-surgical nursing: Critical thinking for collaborative care* (5th ed., p. 857). Philadelphia: Saunders.

14. 4
Rationale: Floating is an acceptable legal practice used by hospitals to solve their understaffing problems. Legally a nurse cannot refuse to float unless a union contract guarantees that the nurse can only work in a specified area or the nurse can prove a lack of knowledge for the performance of assigned tasks. When faced with this situation, the nurse should identify potential areas of harm to the client.
Test-Taking Strategy: Use the process of elimination. Options 1 and 3 can be eliminated first, because they are inappropriate. From the remaining options, eliminate option 2, because it is premature to call the nursing supervisor. Review the nursing responsibilities related to floating if you had difficulty with this question.
Level of Cognitive Ability: Application
Client Needs: Safe and Effective Care Environment
Integrated Process: Nursing Process/Implementation
Content Area: Fundamental Skills
Reference: Huber, D. (2006). *Leadership and nursing care management* (3rd ed., p. 426). Philadelphia: Saunders.

15. 1
Rationale: Living wills are required to be in writing and signed by the client. The client's signature either must be witnessed by specified individuals or notarized. Many states prohibit any employee, including a nurse in a facility in which the client is receiving care, from being a witness.
Test-Taking Strategy: Use the process of elimination. Options 2 and 4 are comparable or alike and should be eliminated first. From the remaining options, option 1 is the appropriate action.

Review the legal implications associated with wills if you had difficulty with this question.
Level of Cognitive Ability: Application
Client Needs: Safe and Effective Care Environment
Integrated Process: Nursing Process/Implementation
Content Area: Fundamental Skills
Reference: McHale, J., & Tingle, J. (2007). *Law & nursing* (3rd ed, pp. 234-236). Oxford: Butterworth-Heinemann.

16. **2**
Rationale: Proper documentation of unusual occurrences, incidents, accidents, and the nursing actions taken as a result of the occurrence are internal to the institution or agency. Documentation on the incident report allows the nurse and administration to review the quality of care and to determine any potential risks present. Options 1, 3, and 4 are incorrect.
Test-Taking Strategy: Use the process of elimination. Eliminate options 1 and 3, because incident reports are not routinely filled out for interventions or treatment measures. Eliminate option 4, because incident reports are not used to report occurrences to other agencies; medical records are used for this purpose. Review the purpose of incident reports if you had difficulty with this question.
Level of Cognitive Ability: Application
Client Needs: Safe and Effective Care Environment
Integrated Process: Nursing Process/Implementation
Content Area: Fundamental Skills
Reference: Christensen, B., & Kockrow, E. (2006). *Adult health nursing* (5th ed., pp. 112, 115). St. Louis: Mosby.

17. **4**
Rationale: Nurse practice acts require reporting the suspicion of impaired nurses. The state board of nursing has jurisdiction over the practice of nursing and may develop plans for treatment and supervision. This suspicion needs to be reported to the nursing supervisor, who will then report to the board of nursing. Options 1 and 2 are inappropriate. Option 3 may cause a conflict.
Test-Taking Strategy: Use the principles related to following the channels of communication in a health care agency when answering this question. By reporting the information, the nurse alerts the institution to the potential problem and sets the stage for further investigation and appropriate action. Review the actions to take regarding reporting the suspicion of an impaired nurse if you had difficulty with this question.
Level of Cognitive Ability: Application
Client Needs: Safe and Effective Care Environment
Integrated Process: Nursing Process/Planning
Content Area: Fundamental Skills
Reference: Ignatavicius, D., & Workman, M. (2006). *Medical-surgical nursing: Critical thinking for collaborative care* (5th ed., p. 93). Philadelphia: Saunders.

18. **4**
Rationale: The family member is exhibiting the first stage of grief (denial), and the nurse should remain with the family member. Option 1 is an appropriate intervention for the acceptance or reorganization and restitution stage. Option 2 may be an appropriate intervention for the bargaining stage. Option 3 may be an appropriate intervention for depression.

Test-Taking Strategy: Use therapeutic communication techniques to direct you to option 4. Remember to address client and family feelings first. Review the grieving process and therapeutic communication techniques if you had difficulty with this question.
Level of Cognitive Ability: Application
Client Needs: Psychosocial Integrity
Integrated Process: Caring
Content Area: Fundamental Skills
References: Christensen, B., & Kockrow, E. (2006). *Foundations of nursing* (5th ed., pp. 194-197). St. Louis: Mosby.
Linton, A., & Maebius, N. (2007). *Introduction to medical-surgical nursing* (4th ed., pp. 1240-1241). Philadelphia: Saunders.

19. **3**
Rationale: Invasion of privacy takes place when an individual's private affairs are intruded on unreasonably. Threatening to place a client in restraints constitutes assault. Performing a surgical procedure without consent is an example of battery. Not allowing a client to leave the hospital constitutes false imprisonment.
Test-Taking Strategy: Use the process of elimination. Note the strategic words "invasion of client privacy." These words should direct you to option 3. Review the situations that constitute the invasion of client privacy if you had difficulty with this question.
Level of Cognitive Ability: Comprehension
Client Needs: Safe and Effective Care Environment
Integrated Process: Nursing Process/Implementation
Content Area: Fundamental Skills
Reference: Christensen, B., & Kockrow, E. (2006). *Foundations of nursing* (5th ed., p. 25). St. Louis: Mosby.

20. **1**
Rationale: Confidential issues are not to be discussed with nonmedical personnel or with the client's family or friends without the client's permission. Clients should be assured that information is kept confidential unless it places the nurse under a legal obligation. The nurse must report situations related to child or older adult abuse, gunshot wounds, stabbings, and certain infectious diseases.
Test-Taking Strategy: Use the process of elimination. Option 4 can be eliminated first, because this action does not protect the client from injury. Options 2 and 3 are comparable or alike and should be eliminated next. Review the nursing responsibilities related to reporting obligations if you had difficulty with this question.
Level of Cognitive Ability: Application
Client Needs: Psychosocial Integrity
Integrated Process: Communication and Documentation
Content Area: Fundamental Skills
Reference: McHale, J., & Tingle, J. (2007). *Law & nursing* (3rd ed, pp.144, 158-159). Oxford: Butterworth-Heinemann.

21. **1**
Rationale: External cardiac massage is one type of treatment that a client can refuse. The appropriate initial action is to notify the physician, because a written "do not resuscitate" (DNR) order from the physician must be present. The DNR order must be reviewed or renewed on a regular basis per agency policy.

Test-Taking Strategy: Use the process of elimination. Note the strategic words "appropriate initial nursing action." Although options 2, 3, and 4 may be appropriate, remember that first a written physician's order is necessary. Review DNR procedures if you had difficulty with this question.
Level of Cognitive Ability: Application
Client Needs: Safe and Effective Care Environment
Integrated Process: Nursing Process/Implementation
Content Area: Fundamental Skills
Reference: McHale, J., & Tingle, J. (2007). *Law & nursing* (3rd ed, pp. 236-237). Oxford: Butterworth-Heinemann.

22. **4**
Rationale: Computer terminals should never be left unattended after the nurse has logged on. This could allow unauthorized users to access the personal information of clients, and it represents a breach of confidentiality and of the security of client records. Options 1, 2, and 3 represent actions that are acceptable ways to protect client information.
Test-Taking Strategy: Use the process of elimination, and note the strategic word "inappropriate." Options 1, 2, and 3 represent actions that are acceptable ways to protect client information. Review the guidelines for safe computer charting if you had difficulty with this question.
Level of Cognitive Ability: Application
Client Needs: Safe and Effective Care Environment
Integrated Process: Nursing Process/Implementation
Content Area: Fundamental Skills

Reference: Christensen, B., & Kockrow, E. (2006). *Foundations of adult health nursing* (5th ed., p. 120). St. Louis: Mosby.

ALTERNATE ITEM FORMAT: MULTIPLE RESPONSE

23. **1, 2, 4, 6**
Rationale: The nurse uses a black-colored ink pen to document, because black ink allows the chart to be duplicated with adequate readability for long-term storage. The nurse always dates and times entries and signs and titles each entry. The nurse provides objective, factual, and complete documentation and avoids subjective, judgmental, and evaluative statements. Quotes are used to relate what the client actually said. The nurse avoids leaving blank spaces on documentation forms, because this allows for an area in which notes can be entered by others at a later time. The recording of information in the client's record must be sequential.
Test-Taking Strategy: Read each item carefully. Think about the legal responsibilities related to documentation to select the correct guidelines. Review these guidelines if you had difficulty with this question.
Level of Cognitive Ability: Application
Client Needs: Safe and Effective Care Environment
Integrated Process: Communication and Documentation
Content Area: Fundamental Skills
Reference: Christensen, B., & Kochrow, E. (2006). *Foundations of adult health nursing* (5th ed., pp 99-100, 106-111). St. Louis: Mosby.

REFERENCES

Christensen, B., & Kockrow, E. (2006). *Adult health nursing* (5th ed., pp. 112, 115). St Louis: Mosby.

Christensen, B., & Kockrow, E. (2006). *Foundations and adult health nursing* (5th ed.). St. Louis: Mosby.

Christensen, B., & Kockrow, E. (2003). *Foundations of nursing* (4th ed.). St. Louis: Mosby.

Harkreader, H., Hogan, M.A., & Thobaben, M. (2007). *Fundamentals of nursing: Caring and clinical judgment* (3rd ed.). Philadelphia: Saunders.

Harkreader, H., & Hogan, M.A. (2004). *Fundamentals of nursing* (2nd ed.). Philadelphia: Saunders.

Huber, D. (2006). *Leadership and nursing care management* (3rd ed.). Philadelphia: Saunders.

Ignatavicius, D., & Workman, M. (2006). *Medical-surgical nursing: Critical thinking for collaborative care* (5th ed.). Philadelphia: Saunders.

Linton, A., & Maebius, N. (2007). *Introduction to medical-surgical nursing* (4th ed.). Philadelphia: Saunders.

McHale, J., & Tingle, J. (2007). *Law & nursing* (3rd ed.). Oxford: Butterworth-Heinemann.

National Council of State Boards of Nursing (Eds.) (2008). *2008 Detailed Test Plan for the NCLEX-PN® Examination, National Council of State Boards of Nursing.* Chicago: Author.

National Council of State Boards of Nursing. *NCSBN home page.* www.ncsbn.org. Accessed June 5, 2008.

Stuart, G., & Laraia, M. (2005). *Principles and practice of psychiatric nursing* (8th ed.). St. Louis: Mosby.

U.S. Department of Health and Human Services Office for Civil Rights (2006). *HIPAA Administration Simplification Regulation Text.* http://www.hhs. gov/ocr/AdminSimpRegtext.pdf.

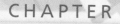

Delegating, Managing, and Prioritizing Client Care

PYRAMID TERMS

accountability A moral concept that involves acceptance by the professional nurse of the consequences of a decision or action.

case management An interdisciplinary health care delivery system designed to promote the appropriate use of hospital personnel and material resources to maximize hospital revenues while providing for optimal outcomes of care.

critical paths Provide effective clinical management systems for monitoring care and for reducing or controlling the length of the hospital stay.

delegation The process of transferring a selected nursing task in a situation to an individual who is competent to perform that specific task.

empowerment An interpersonal process of enabling others to do for themselves.

leadership An interpersonal process that involves motivating and guiding others to achieve goals.

management The accomplishment of tasks either by oneself or by directing others.

prioritizing Ranking needs or problems by their urgency and importance and deciding which of them require immediate action and which ones could be delayed until a later time because they are not urgent.

medication reconciliation The process of avoiding medication errors by comparing a client's medication orders with all of the medications that the client has been taking (Box 8-1).

responsibility The duty to act.

variances The actual deviations or detours from critical paths.

▲ PYRAMID TO SUCCESS

The nurse is both a leader and a manager. As described in the NCLEX-PN test plan, the nurse needs to collaborate with other members of the multidisciplinary health care team to facilitate effective care. Pyramid points focus on the concepts of management and supervision, leadership responsibilities, case management, resource management, making client care assignments, the process of delegation, establishing priorities or tasks required by one client or a group of clients, and the principles of time management. The Integrated Processes addressed in this chapter include Caring, Clinical Problem-Solving Process (Nursing Process), Communication and Documentation, and Teaching and Learning.

CLIENT NEEDS
Safe and Effective Care Environment

Understanding case management concepts
Consulting with members of the health care team
Monitoring for continuous (total) quality improvement and effective client care outcomes
Delegating client care activities
Establishing priorities related to client care activities
Implementing cost-effective measures when providing nursing care
Using leadership skills effectively
Supervising the delivery of client care
Using appropriate health care resources

Health Promotion and Maintenance

Monitoring the client's ability to perform self-care
Promoting health and wellness

Psychosocial Integrity

Identifying available support systems
Considering cultural, spiritual, and religious issues when providing care
Using therapeutic communication techniques when communicating with others

Physiological Integrity

Ensuring that palliative/comfort care is provided to the client
Monitoring for unexpected responses to therapy

I. HEALTH CARE DELIVERY
A. Managed care
   1. Designed to control the cost of health services and to promote a continuum of care through the development and use of integrated services

BOX 8-1 **Medication Reconciliation Process**

- Process of comparing a client's medication orders with all of the medications that the client has been taking
- Helps to avoid medication errors related to omissions, duplications, dosing errors, or drug interactions
- Done at every transition of care in which new medications are ordered or existing orders are rewritten, such as when the client is admitted to, transferred within, or discharged from a health care facility

From The Joint Commission: Using medication reconciliation to prevent errors. *Sentinel Event Alert* 2006;(35):1-4.

2. Uses a select group of providers who agree to a predetermined payment before delivering care
3. Client care is outcome driven and managed by a **case management** process
4. Emphasizes the promotion of health, client education, responsible self-care, early identification of disease, and the use of health care resources

▲ B. **Case management**
   1. An organized system for delivering health care to an individual client or a group of clients through their illness
   2. Includes assessment, the development of a plan of care, the coordination of all services, referral, and follow-up

▲ C. Case manager
   1. A registered nurse, social worker, or other health care professional who assumes **responsibility** for coordinating the client's care from the time of admission until after discharge
   2. Establishes a plan of care with the client, coordinates any consultations and referrals, and facilitates discharge

D. **Critical paths**
   1. A multidisciplinary treatment plan that identifies the clinical interventions for a projected length of stay or a projected time frame for specific case types
   2. All members of the health care team work with one plan to achieve the same client outcomes
   3. The goal of a critical path is to anticipate and recognize negative variance early so that appropriate action can be taken and better client outcomes can result
   4. **Variances**
      a. Actual deviations or detours from the critical path
      b. Positive variance occurs when a client achieves maximum benefit and is discharged earlier than anticipated by his or her critical path

   c. Negative variance occurs when untoward events prevent a timely discharge and the length of hospital stay is longer than planned for a client on a specific critical path
   d. Variance analysis occurs continually as the case manager and other caregivers monitor client outcomes against the critical path
   e. Accurate monitoring of the critical path with variance analysis can estimate the financial impact of client care
   f. If the variance is predictable, negotiation with insurers for an additional length of hospital stay can maximize client care revenues

E. Care maps
   1. Initially developed at the New England Medical Center in Boston
   2. Models for critical paths
   3. Incorporate day-to-day expected client outcomes and those outcomes anticipated at discharge or at the end of a treatment phase
   4. Outline clinical assessments, treatments and procedures, dietary interventions, activity and exercise therapies, client education, and discharge planning

F. Nursing care plan
   1. A written guideline and communication tool that identifies the client's pertinent assessment data, problems, nursing diagnoses, goals, interventions, and expected outcomes
   2. Enhances the continuity of care by identifying specific nursing actions necessary to achieve the goals of care
   3. The client and the family are involved in developing the plan of care, and both short-term and long-term goals are identified
   4. Client problems, goals, interventions, and expected outcomes are documented in the care plan, and the plan provides a framework for the evaluation of the client's response to nursing actions

II. FORMAL ORGANIZATIONS

A. Mission statement: Communicates in broad terms an organization's reason for existence, the geographic area that the organization serves, and the attitudes, beliefs, and values within which the organization functions
B. Goals and objectives: Measurable activities specific to the development of the designated services and programs of an organization
C. Organizational chart: Depicts and communicates how activities are arranged, how authority relationships are defined, and how communication channels are established
D. Procedures and protocols
   1. Guides that define appropriate courses of action
   2. Procedures define a task
   3. Protocols signify the definition of a clinical process

E. Centralization: Decisions are made by a limited number of individuals at the top of the organization or by the managers of a department or unit and thereafter communicated to the employees

F. Decentralization: Authority is distributed throughout the organization to allow for increased **responsibility** and **delegation** in decision making

III. CONTINUOUS (TOTAL) QUALITY IMPROVEMENT

A. A program that focuses on processes or systems that significantly contribute to effective client care outcomes

B. When total quality improvement is part of a health care agency's philosophy, every staff member becomes involved in ways that improve care and outcomes

C. The quality of a health care organization is defined in its mission statement and in the philosophy of the nursing department; these statements identify how nurses are to perform, identify the services that are made available to the client, and provide directions for professional standards and care guidelines that should guarantee excellent client outcomes

D. The Joint Commission describes quality improvement as an approach to the continuous assessment and improvement of the methods of providing health care to meet the needs of others

E. The quality improvement process is similar to the nursing process and involves a multidisciplinary process

F. An outcome indicates whether the interventions are effective, if the client progressed, how well standards are met, and if changes are necessary

G. The evaluation of health care is a process used to determine the quality of care and the service provided to clients

H. The nurse has the **responsibility** of recognizing trends in nursing practice, identifying when recurrent problems occur, and initiating opportunities to improve the quality of care

IV. NURSING DELIVERY SYSTEMS

A. Functional nursing

1. Involves a task approach to client care, with major tasks being delegated by the charge nurse to individual members of the team

2. Goals are concerned with work productivity at the lowest possible cost

B. Team nursing

1. The team is generally led by a registered nurse who is responsible for assessing, developing nursing diagnoses, planning, and evaluating each client's plan of care

2. Each staff member works fully within the realm of his or her educational and clinical expertise

3. Each staff member is accountable for client care and outcomes of care delivered in accordance

with the licensing and practice scope as determined by hospital policy and state law

4. Characterized by a high degree of respect for and maturity of team members and by a high degree of communication and collaboration among members

C. Primary nursing

1. Focuses on client outcomes as opposed to nursing tasks

2. Concerned with keeping the nurse at the bedside and actively involved in client care while planning goal-directed, individualized care

V. PROFESSIONAL RESPONSIBILITIES

A. **Accountability**

1. The process that mandates that individuals are answerable for their actions and that they have an obligation or duty to act

2. Involves assuming only the responsibilities that are within one's scope of practice and not assuming responsibility for activities in which competence has not been achieved

3. Involves admitting mistakes rather than blaming others and evaluating the outcomes of one's own actions

4. Includes a responsibility to the client to be competent, to render nursing services in accordance with standards of nursing practice, and to adhere to the professional ethics code

B. **Leadership**

1. The interpersonal process that involves motivating and guiding others to achieve goals

2. A method of modeling accountable behavior to others

C. Leadership styles

1. Autocratic

a. Leader focused

b. Leader maintains strong control, makes the decisions, and solves all problems

c. Leader dominates the group and commands rather than makes suggestions or seeks input

2. Democratic

a. Also called participative leadership

b. Based on the belief that every group member should have input into the development of goals and problem solving

c. Leader acts primarily as a facilitator and a resource person

d. Leader is concerned for each member of the group

e. A more participative style and much less authoritarian than the autocratic leadership style

3. Laissez-faire

a. Leader assumes a passive, nondirective, and inactive approach

b. Leadership responsibilities are either assumed by the members of the group or completely relinquished

c. All decision making is left to the group, with the leader giving little if any guidance, support, or feedback

d. Some unprofessional behaviors exhibited by the group may be permissible as a result of the leader's lack of limit setting and stated expectations

4. Situational

a. Using a combination of styles based on current circumstances and events

b. Leadership styles are assumed according to the needs of the group and the tasks to be achieved

D. Leadership qualities (Box 8-2)

E. **Management:** The accomplishment of tasks either by oneself or by directing others

F. Problem-solving process

1. Involves obtaining information and using it to reach an acceptable solution to a problem

2. Steps of the problem-solving process are similar to the steps of the clinical problem-solving process (nursing process) (Table 8-1)

VI. EMPOWERMENT

A. An interpersonal process of enabling others to do for themselves

B. Occurs when individuals are better able to influence what happens to them

C. Involves open communication, mutual goal setting, and decision making

D. Nurses can empower clients through advocacy

VII. CONFLICT

A. Description: Arises from a perception of incompatibility or differences in beliefs, attitudes, values, goals, priorities, or decisions

B. Types of conflict

1. Intrapersonal: Occurs within a person

2. Interpersonal: Occurs between and among clients, nurses, and other staff members

3. Organizational: Occurs when an employee confronts policies and procedures of the organization

C. Modes of conflict resolution

1. Avoiding

a. Is unassertive and uncooperative

b. The individual neither pursues his or her needs, goals, or concerns nor assists others with pursuing theirs

c. Postpones the issue

2. Accommodating

a. The individual neglects his or her own needs, goals, or concerns (unassertive) while trying to satisfy those of others

b. The individual obeys and serves others and often feels resentment and disappointment because he or she "gets nothing in return"

3. Competing

a. The individual pursues his or her own needs and goals at the expense of others

b. May also take the form of standing up for rights and defending important principles

4. Compromising

a. Is assertive and cooperative

b. Individuals work creatively and openly to find the solution that most fully satisfies all important goals and concerns to be achieved

VIII. ROLES OF HEALTH TEAM MEMBERS

A. Nurse

1. Collects data, plans, implements, and evaluates client care

2. Promotes client health and disease prevention

3. Provides comfort and care to clients

4. Makes decisions

5. Acts as a client advocate

6. Manages client care

7. Communicator

8. Teaches clients and others

9. Acts as a resource person

10. Allocates resources in a cost-effective manner

B. Nurse practitioner

1. Usually provides care in an outpatient, ambulatory care, or community-based setting.

2. Treats clients on his or her own and writes prescriptions under the direction of a physician

C. Physician: Diagnoses and prescribes treatment for disease

D. Physician assistant

1. Provides assistance to the physician

2. Conducts physical examinations, performs diagnostic procedures, assists in the operating and emergency departments, and performs treatments

E. Physical therapist: Examines, tests, treats, and develops a plan of care for clients to regain maximum possible physical activity and strength

---

BOX 8-2 **Leadership Qualities**

Communication
Credibility
Critical thinking
Initiating action
Risk taking

TABLE 8-1   **Problem-Solving Processes**

Problem-Solving Process	Clinical Problem-Solving Process (Nursing Process)
Identifying a problem and collecting data about the problem	Data collection
Determining a plan of action	Planning
Carrying out the plan	Implementation
Evaluating the plan	Evaluation

F. Occupational therapist: Works with the physical therapist to develop plans to assist clients with resuming activities of daily living after an illness or injury

G. Respiratory therapist: Delivers treatments designed to improve the client's ventilation and oxygenation status

H. Nutritionist: Assists with planning dietary measures to improve or maintain a client's nutritional status

I. Continuing care nurse: Coordinates discharge plans for the client

J. Assistive personnel/nursing assistant: Provides assistance to the nurse with specified tasks and functions

K. Pharmacist: Formulates and dispenses medications

L. Social worker: Counsels clients and families

M. Pastoral care provider: Offers spiritual support and guidance to clients and families

N. Secretarial staff: Provides support to the health care team, organizes and schedules diagnostic tests and procedures, and arranges for services needed by the client and family

IX. HEALTH CARE TEAM COMMUNICATION

A. Client care planning can be accomplished through referral to or consultation with other health care specialists and through client care conferences, which involve members from all health care disciplines

B. Reports

1. Should be factual, accurate, current, complete, organized, and confidential

2. Should include essential background information, subjective data, objective data, any changes in the client's status, nursing diagnoses, treatments and procedures, medication administration, client teaching, discharge planning, family information, the client's response to treatments and procedures, and the client's priority needs

3. Change of shift report (Box 8-3)
   a. Provides continuity of care among nurses who are caring for a client
   b. May be given orally, by audiotape, or by walking rounds at the client's bedside
   c. Describes the client's health status and informs the nurse on the next shift about the client's needs and priorities for care

4. Telephone reports
   a. Used to inform a physician of a client's change in status, to communicate information about a client's transfer to or from another unit or facility, and to obtain results of laboratory or diagnostic tests
   b. The telephone report should be documented and should include when the call was made, who made the call, who was called, to whom information was given, what information was given, and what information was received

5. Transfer reports
   a. Provide continuity of care; may be given by phone or in person (Box 8-4)
   b. Complete the **medication reconciliation** process pertaining to the transfer of clients
   c. The receiving nurse needs to be provided with an opportunity to ask questions about the client's status

X. CONSULTING WITH THE HEALTH CARE TEAM

A. Process in which a specialist is sought to identify methods of care or treatment plans to meet the needs of a client

B. Consultation is needed when the nurse encounters a problem that cannot be solved with nursing knowledge, skills, and available resources

---

BOX 8-3 | **Information Included in the Change-of-Shift Report**

- Room number and bed designation; client name, age, and sex; date of admission and medical diagnoses; and name of primary physician (If a computer census sheet is used that contains some of this information, then only the room number, the name, and any missing data are given.)
- Tests and treatments or therapies performed during the past 24 hours, in addition to client response (e.g., computed tomography scans, surgery, arteriogram); intake and output for the past shift
- Significant changes in client condition
- Scheduled tests; consults or surgery; current intravenous solution, flow rate, and amount remaining; next solution to be hung; oxygen flow rate; equipment in use and current settings (e.g., gastric suction on low)
- Current problems (e.g., dehydration, severe pain, anxiety, depression, insufficient rest, abnormal laboratory values or test results); amount of assistance needed with activities of daily living
- Scheduled treatments; PRN medications given, times given, and client response
- Concerns; need for order changes; teaching; pertinent family dynamics; and emotional status

From deWit, S. (2005). *Fundamental concepts and skills for nursing* (2nd ed., p. 109). Philadelphia: Saunders.

BOX 8-4 | **Transfer Reports**

- Client's name, age, physician, and diagnosis
- Current health status and current plan of care
- Client's needs and priorities for care
- Any data collection or interventions that need to be done after transfer, such as laboratory tests, medication administration, or dressing changes
- Need for any special equipment
- Any additional considerations, such as resuscitation status, precautionary considerations, or family issues

BOX 8-5 **Discharge Teaching**

- How to administer prescribed medications
- Side effects of medications that need to be reported to the physician
- Prescribed dietary and activity measures
- Complications of the medical condition that need to be reported to the physician
- How to perform prescribed treatments
- How to use any prescribed special equipment
- Schedule for any home-care services that are planned
- How to access available community resources
- When to obtain follow-up care

BOX 8-6 **Five Rights of Delegation**

- *Right Task:* A task that can safely be delegated for a specific client, such as a repetitive task that requires little supervision and that is relatively noninvasive
- *Right Circumstances:* The appropriate client, setting, and resources
- *Right Person:* The right person delegates the right task to the most appropriate person to be performed on the right client
- *Right Direction/Communication:* A clear, concise description of the task, including its objective, limits, and expectations
- *Right Supervision:* The appropriate monitoring, evaluation, intervention (as needed), and feedback

From Elkin, M., Perry A., & Potter P. (2004). *Nursing interventions and clinical skills* (3rd ed.) St. Louis: Mosby.

   C. Consultation is also needed when the exact problem remains unclear; a consultant can objectively and more clearly assess and identify the exact nature of the problem

▲ **XI. DISCHARGE PLANNING**
   A. Begins when the client is admitted to the hospital or health care facility
   B. Is a multidisciplinary process that ensures that the client has a plan for continuing care after leaving the health care facility and that assists with the client's transition from one environment to another
   C. All caregivers need to be involved in discharge planning, and referrals to other health care professionals or agencies may be needed; a physician's order may be needed for the referral, and the referral needs to be approved by the client's insurer
   D. The nurse should anticipate the client's discharge needs and suggest making the referral as soon as possible; the client and family should also be involved in the referral process
   E. The nurse needs to reinforce client and family teaching regarding care at home (Box 8-5)
   F. The nurse needs to complete the **medication reconciliation** process pertaining to discharge

▲ **XII. PERFORMANCE IMPROVEMENT (QUALITY ASSURANCE)**
   A. Description
      1. Process of evaluating the outcome of care by measuring it against predetermined standards
      2. Aspects of care that represent the predetermined standards are selected, criteria for achievement of the standards are identified, and methods of monitoring are defined
      3. Compliance with achieving the predetermined standards is measured, and ways to improve compliance are sought, if needed
   B. Retrospective audit: An evaluation method that involves inspecting the medical record for the documentation of compliance with the standards
   C. Concurrent audit: An evaluation method that involves inspecting the nursing staff's compliance with predetermined standards and criteria while the nurses are providing care

   D. Quality assurance staff, a charge nurse, or a nurse educator may perform the review; a peer-review approach may be implemented in which all members of the nursing staff are involved

XIII. DELEGATION AND ASSIGNMENTS ▲
   A. Delegation
      1. Process of transferring a selected nursing task in a situation to an individual who is competent to perform that specific task
      2. Involves achieving outcomes and sharing activities with other individuals who have the authority to accomplish the task
      3. The nurse practice act and any practice limitations may define which aspects of care can be delegated and which must be performed by a registered nurse, a licensed practical/vocational nurse, and unlicensed personnel
      4. Although a task may be delegated to someone, the nurse who delegates maintains accountability for the overall nursing care of the client
      5. Only the task—not the ultimate accountability—may be delegated to another
   B. Principles and guidelines of delegating (Boxes 8-6 and 8-7)
   C. Assignments
      1. Description: Transferring performance of client care activities to specific staff members
      2. Guidelines for client care assignments (Box 8-8)
         a. Always ensure client safety
         b. Be aware of individual variations in work abilities
         c. Determine which tasks can be delegated and to whom
         d. Match the task with the delegatee on the basis of the nurse practice act, appropriate position descriptions, and the delegatee's educational preparation and experience
         e. Provide directions that are clear, concise, accurate, and complete

BOX 8-7 **Principles and Guidelines of Delegating**

- Delegate the right task to the right delegatee: Be familiar with the experience of the delegatee, his or her scope of practice and job description, agency policy and procedures, and the state's nurse practice act
- Provide clear directions about the task, and ensure that the delegatee understands the expectations
- Determine the degree of supervision that may be required
- Provide the delegatee with the authority to complete the task; provide a deadline for the completion of the task
- Evaluate the outcome of the care that has been delegated
- Provide feedback to the delegatee regarding his or her performance
- Generally noninvasive interventions such as skin care, range-of-motion exercises, ambulation, grooming, and hygiene measures can be assigned to a nursing assistant
- An LPN can perform the tasks that a nursing assistant can perform, and he or she can also carry out certain invasive tasks, such as applying dressings, suctioning, urinary catheterization, and administering oral, subcutaneous, and intramuscular injections
- An RN can perform the tasks that a licensed practical nurse can perform, and he or she is responsible for assessment, planning care, initiating teaching, and administering intravenous medications

LPN, Licensed practical nurse; *RN,* registered nurse.

BOX 8-8 **Delegatable Tasks for the Nursing Assistant or Unlicensed Assistive Personnel**

Note: Delegatable tasks are also based on state nurse practice acts and agency policies and procedures.
- Applying a condom catheter
- Applying a hearing aid
- Applying elastic stockings
- Assessing vital signs
- Assisting with ambulation
- Assisting with deep breathing and coughing
- Bathing
- Bed making
- Collecting specimens
- Emptying certain drainage containers
- Feeding
- Filling water pitchers
- Giving an enema
- Giving a sitz bath
- Measuring weight and height
- Performing range-of-motion exercises
- Providing hair care
- Providing some types of skin care
- Providing oral hygiene
- Recording intake and output
- Stocking unit supplies
- Taking specimens to the laboratory
- Toileting clients
- Transferring clients to a chair or bed
- Turning and repositioning clients

From deWit, S. (2005). *Fundamental concepts and skills for nursing* (2nd ed.) Philadelphia: Saunders.

f. Validate the person's understanding of the directions
g. Communicate a feeling of confidence to the delegatee, and provide feedback promptly after the task is performed
h. Maintain continuity of care as much as possible when assigning client care
i. Follow up with the delegatee

▲ XIV. TIME MANAGEMENT
A. Description
1. A technique designed to assist with completing tasks within a definite time period
2. Learning how, when, and where to use one's time and establishing personal goals and time frames
3. Requires an ability to anticipate the day's activities, to combine activities when possible, and to be uninterrupted by nonessential activities
4. Involves efficiency with completing tasks as quickly as possible, effectiveness when deciding on the most important task to perform, and performing it correctly
B. Principles and guidelines
1. Identify tasks, obligations, and activities, and write them down

2. Organize the workday; identify which tasks must be completed in specified time frames
3. Prioritize client needs according to importance and urgency
4. Anticipate the needs of the day, and provide time for unexpected and unplanned tasks that may arise
5. Focus on beginning the daily tasks, and work on the most important and/or urgent ones first while keeping goals in mind; look at the final goal for the day, which will help break down tasks into manageable parts
6. Begin client rounds at the beginning of the shift, and collect data about each assigned client
7. Delegate tasks when appropriate
8. Keep a daily hour-by-hour log to assist with providing structure to the tasks that must be accomplished; cross tasks off the list as they are accomplished
9. Use hospital resources wisely, anticipate resource needs, and gather the necessary supplies before beginning the task
10. Organize paperwork, and continuously document task completion and necessary client data throughout the day

11. At the end of the day, evaluate the effectiveness of time **management**

▲ **XV. PRIORITIZING CARE**

A. **Prioritizing**: Deciding which needs or problems require immediate action and which ones may be delayed until a later time because they are not urgent

▲ B. Guidelines for **prioritizing** (Box 8-9)

C. Setting priorities for reinforcing client teaching
  1. Determine the client's immediate needs
  2. Review the learning objectives established for the client
  3. Determine what the client perceives as important and/or urgent
  4. Determine the client's anxiety level and the time available to teach

D. **Prioritizing** when caring for a group of clients
  1. Identify the problems of each client
  2. Review the nursing diagnoses
  3. Determine which client problems are most urgent on the basis of basic needs, the client's changing or unstable status, and the complexity of the client's problems
  4. Anticipate the time that it may take to care for the priority needs of the client
  5. If possible, combine activities to resolve more than one problem at a time
  6. Involve the client in his or her own care as much as possible

XVI. DISASTERS AND DISASTER PLANNING ▲

A. Description
  1. A disaster is any human-made or natural event that causes destruction and devastation that requires assistance from others (Box 8-10)
  2. With regard to a health care agency, a disaster can be external or internal; external disasters are those that occur outside of the health care agency, and internal disasters are those that occur inside the health care agency
  3. A disaster preparedness plan is a formal plan of action for coordinating the response of a health care agency's staff in the event of a disaster within the health care agency or the surrounding community

---

BOX 8-9 **Guidelines for Prioritizing**

- The nurse and the client mutually rank the client's needs in order of importance on the basis of the client's physical and psychological needs, safety, and the client's own needs and expectations; what the client sees as his or her priority needs may be different from what the nurse sees as the priority
- Priorities are classified as high, intermediate, or low
- Client needs that are life threatening or that could result in harm to the client if they are left untreated are high priorities
- Nonemergency and non–life-threatening client needs are intermediate priorities
- Client needs that are not directly related to the client's illness or prognosis are low priorities
- When providing care, the nurse needs to decide which needs or problems require immediate action and which ones could be delayed until a later time because they are not urgent
- Client problems that involve actual or life-threatening concerns are considered before potential health-threatening concerns
- When prioritizing care, the nurse must consider time constraints and available resources
- Problems identified as important by the client must be given high priority
- The ABCs—airway, breathing, and circulation—can be used as a guide when determining priorities; client needs related to maintaining a patent airway are always the priority
- Maslow's Hierarchy of Needs theory can be used as a guide for determining priorities; this theory identifies the levels of physiological needs, safety, love and belonging, self-esteem, and self-actualization; basic needs are met before moving on to other needs in the hierarchy
- The steps of the clinical problem-solving process (nursing process) can be used as a guide when determining priorities; remember that data collection is the first step of the nursing process

---

BOX 8-10 **Types of Disasters**

Human-Made Disasters
- Dam failures that result in flooding
- Hazardous substance accidents, such as pollution, chemical spills, and toxic gas leaks
- Accidents that result in the release of radiological materials
- Resource shortages, such as those involving food, water, and electricity
- Structural collapse, fire, and explosions
- Terrorist attacks, such as bombing, riots, and bioterrorism
- Transportation accidents

Natural Disasters
- Blizzards
- Communicable disease epidemics
- Cyclones
- Droughts
- Earthquakes
- Floods
- Forest fires
- Hailstorms
- Hurricanes
- Landslides
- Mudslides
- Tornadoes
- Tsunamis (tidal waves)
- Volcanic eruptions

B. American Red Cross (ARC)
1. Has been given authority by the federal government to provide disaster relief
2. All ARC disaster relief assistance is free; local offices are located across the United States
3. Participates with the government to develop and test community disaster plans
4. Identifies and trains personnel for disaster response
5. Works with businesses and labor organizations to identify resources and people for disaster work
6. Educates the public about ways to prepare for a disaster
7. Operates shelters, provides assistance to meet immediate emergency needs, and provides disaster health services, including emotional and mental health support
8. Handles inquiries from family members
9. Coordinates relief activities with other agencies
10. Nurses are directly involved with the ARC and may be managers, supervisors, or first-aid educators; they also participate in disaster preparedness and disaster relief programs and provide other services such as blood collection drives and immunization programs

C. Phases of disaster **management**
1. The Federal Emergency Management Agency (FEMA) identifies four disaster **management** phases: mitigation, preparedness, response, and recovery
2. Mitigation
   a. Refers to actions or measures that can either prevent the occurrence of a disaster or reduce the damaging effects of a disaster
   b. Involves determining the community hazards and risks (actual and potential threats) that may be present if a disaster occurs
   c. Involves awareness of available community resources and community health personnel, which will facilitate the mobilization of activities and minimize chaos and confusion if a disaster occurs
   d. Includes determining the resources available for care to infants, older adults, disabled clients, and those with chronic health problems
3. Preparedness
   a. Involves plans for rescuing, evacuating, and caring for disaster victims
   b. Involves plans for training disaster personnel and gathering resources, equipment, and other materials needed for dealing with the disaster
   c. Includes identifying specific responsibilities for various disaster response personnel
   d. Includes establishing a community disaster plan and an effective public communication system

   e. Involves setting up an emergency medical system and a plan for activation
   f. Includes checking for the proper functioning of emergency equipment
   g. Involves making anticipatory provisions and setting up a location for distributing food, water, clothing, shelter, needed medicine, and other supplies
   h. Includes checking supplies on a regular basis and replenishing outdated supplies
   i. Includes practicing community disaster plans (mock disaster drills)
4. Response
   a. Includes putting disaster planning services into action, such as the actions taken to save lives and to prevent further damage
   b. Primary concerns include the safety, physical health, and mental health of the victims and the members of the disaster response team
5. Recovery
   a. Includes actions taken to return to a normal situation after the disaster
   b. Includes the prevention of debilitating effects and the restoration of personal, economic, and environmental health and stability to the community

D. Levels of disaster: FEMA identifies three levels of disaster, and the level determines the FEMA response (Box 8-11)
1. After a federal emergency has been declared, the Federal Response Plan may take effect and activate emergency support functions (ESFs)
2. ESFs of the ARC include sheltering, feeding, performing emergency first aid, providing a disaster welfare information system, and coordinating the bulk distribution of emergency relief supplies
3. Disaster medical assistant teams (teams of specially trained personnel) can be activated and sent to a disaster site to provide triage and medical care to victims until the victims can be evacuated to a hospital

BOX 8-11 Levels of Disaster

Level III Disaster
Considered a minor disaster and involves a minimal level of damage; could result in a presidential declaration of an emergency

Level II Disaster
Considered a moderate disaster; will likely result in a presidential declaration of an emergency, with moderate federal assistance

Level I Disaster
Considered a massive disaster and involves significant damage; results in a presidential disaster declaration, with major federal involvement and full engagement of federal, regional, and national resources

BOX 8-12 Emergency Plans and Supplies

- Plan a meeting place for family members
- Identify where to go if an evacuation is necessary
- Determine when and how to turn off water, gas, and electricity at main switches
- Locate safe areas in the home for each type of disaster
- Have a 3-day supply of water available (1 gallon per person per day)
- Have a 3-day supply of nonperishable food available
- Replace the water supply every 3 months and the food supply every 6 months
- Keep emergency supplies on hand: Clothing and blankets; first-aid kit; adequate supply of prescription medication; battery-operated radio; flashlight and batteries; credit card, cash, or traveler's checks; extra set of car keys and full tank of gas in the car; sanitation supplies for washing, toileting, and disposing of trash; extra pair of eyeglasses; special items for infants, older adults, and disabled individuals; pet supplies, such as food, water, leash, kitty litter, and litter box; important documents in a waterproof and fireproof case

BOX 8-13 Triage Rating Systems

Five-Tier System (Most Often Used in Military Triage)
- *Victim is dead or will die*
- *Life threatening (emergent):* Victim has life-threatening injuries, but they are readily correctable
- *Urgent:* Victim must be treated within 1 to 2 hours
- *Delayed (nonurgent):* Victim is noncritical or ambulatory; no immediate treatment is necessary
- *No injury:* No treatment is necessary

Four-Tier System
- *Immediate (emergent):* Victim is seriously injured but has a reasonable chance for survival
- *Delayed (nonurgent):* Victim can wait for care after simple first aid is given
- *Expectant:* Victim is extremely critical and dying
- *Minimal (nonurgent):* Victim has no impairment of function and can either treat him- or herself or be treated by a nonprofessional

Three-Tier System (Commonly Used in Health Care Agencies)
- *Life threatening (emergent):* Victim has life-threatening injuries, but they are readily correctable
- *Urgent:* Victim must be treated within 1 to 2 hours
- *Delayed (nonurgent):* Victim has no injury and is noncritical or ambulatory

Two-Tier System
- *Immediate:* Includes victims who have life-threatening injuries that are readily correctable on the scene (emergent) and victims who must be treated within 1 to 2 hours (urgent)
- *Delayed (nonurgent):* Victims who have no injuries, who have noncritical injuries, or who are ambulatory, dying, or dead

Modified from Mosby. (2002). *Mosby's medical, nursing, and allied health dictionary* (6th ed., p. 1747). St. Louis: Mosby.

E. Nurse's role in disaster planning
  1. Personal and professional preparedness
     a. Make personal and family preparations (Box 8-12)
     b. Be aware of the disaster plan at one's place of employment and in the community
     c. Maintain certification in disaster training and cardiopulmonary resuscitation
     d. Participate in mock disaster drills
     e. Prepare professional emergency response items, such as a copy of one's nursing license, personal health care equipment (e.g., a stethoscope), cash, warm clothing, record-keeping materials, and other nursing care supplies
  2. Disaster response
     a. In the heath care agency setting, if a disaster occurs, the agency disaster preparedness plan (emergency response plan) is immediately activated, and the nurse responds by following the directions identified in the plan
     b. In the community setting, if the nurse is the first responder to a disaster, the nurse cares for the victims by attending to those with life-threatening problems first; when rescue workers arrive at the scene, immediate plans for triage should begin
F. Triage
  1. In a disaster or war: Classifying victims according to the severity of the injury, the urgency of treatment, and the place for treatment
  2. In an emergency department: Classifying clients according to their need for care and establishing priorities of care—the type of illness, the severity of the problem, and the resources available govern the process
     a. Triage rating systems: Various rating system categories are used in clinical settings; the nurse must be familiar with the rating system that is used in the health care agency in which he or she is employed (Box 8-13)
     b. Emergency department triage system
        (1) A commonly used rating system in an emergency department is a three-tiered system that uses the categories of emergent, urgent, and nonurgent; these categories may also be identified by color coding or numbers (Box 8-14)
        (2) The nurse needs to be familiar with the health care agency's triage system
        (3) When caring for the client who has died, the nurse needs to recognize the

BOX 8-14	Emergency Department Triage System

Emergent (Red): Priority 1 (Highest)
Given to clients who have life-threatening injuries and who need immediate attention and continuous evaluation but who have a high probability for survival after stabilization
Such clients include those with trauma, chest pain, severe respiratory distress, cardiac arrest, limb amputation, acute neurological deficits, and chemical splashes to the eyes
Urgent (Yellow): Priority 2
Given to clients who require treatment and whose injuries have complications that are not life threatening, provided that they are treated within 1 to 2 hours; these clients require continuous evaluation every 30 to 60 minutes after treatment
Such clients include those with simple fractures, asthma without respiratory distress, fever, hypertension, abdominal pain, and renal stones
Nonurgent (Green): Priority 3
Given to clients with local injuries who do not have immediate complications and who can wait several hours for medical treatment; these clients require evaluation every 1 to 2 hours after treatment
Such clients include those with conditions such as minor lacerations, sprains, and cold symptoms

importance of family rituals and to provide support to loved ones
    (4) The organ donation procedures of the health care agency need to be addressed, if appropriate
▲ G. Client data collection in the emergency department
  1. Primary data collection
    a. The purpose is to identify any client problem that poses an immediate or potential threat to life
    b. Information is gathered primarily through objective data, and, if any abnormalities are found, immediate interventions are initiated
    c. The nurse uses the ABCs—airway, breathing, and circulation—as a guide for assessing the client's needs, and he or she assesses any clients who sustained traumatic injuries for signs of head or cervical spine injuries
  2. Secondary data collection
    a. Performed after the primary data collection and after treatment for any problems identified
    b. Performed to identify any other life-threatening problems that the client may be experiencing
    c. Both subjective and objective data are obtained with the use of a history, a general overview, a vital sign measurement, a neurological assessment, a pain assessment, and a complete or focused physical assessment

PRACTICE QUESTIONS

More questions on the companion CD!

24. A nurse is recording an end-of-shift report for a client. What information needs to be included?
  1. As-needed medications given that shift
  2. Normal vital signs that have been normal since admission
  3. All of the tests and treatments the client has had since admission
  4. Total number of scheduled medications that the client received on that shift
25. A licensed practical nurse is planning the client assignments for the day. Which of the following is the most appropriate assignment for the nursing assistant?
  1. A client who requires a wound irrigation
  2. A client who requires frequent ambulation
  3. A client who is receiving continuous tube feedings
  4. A client who requires frequent vital signs after a cardiac catheterization
26. A nurse employed in a long-term care facility is planning the client assignments for the shift. Which of the following clients would the nurse appropriately assign to the nursing assistant?
  1. A client who requires a 24-hour urine collection
  2. A client who requires twice-daily dressing changes
  3. A diabetic client who requires daily insulin and the reinforcement of dietary measures
  4. A client who is on a bowel management program and requires rectal suppositories and a daily enema
27. A nurse is assigned to care for four clients. When planning client rounds, which client would the nurse check first?
  1. A client on a ventilator
  2. A client in skeletal traction
  3. A postoperative client preparing for discharge
  4. A client admitted on the previous shift who has a diagnosis of gastroenteritis
28. A nurse employed in an emergency department is assigned to assist with the triage of clients arriving to the emergency department for treatment on the evening shift. The nurse would assign the highest priority to which of the following clients?
  1. A client complaining of muscle aches, a headache, and malaise
  2. A client who twisted her ankle when she fell while rollerblading
  3. A client with a minor laceration on the index finger sustained while cutting an eggplant
  4. A client with chest pain who states that he just ate pizza that was made with a very spicy sauce

29. A nurse is assigned to care for four clients. When planning client rounds, which client would the nurse collect data from first?
    1. A client scheduled for a chest x-ray
    2. A client requiring daily dressing changes
    3. A postoperative client preparing for discharge
    4. A client receiving oxygen via nasal cannula who had difficulty breathing during the previous shift

30. A licensed practical nurse is attending an agency orientation meeting about the nursing model of practice implemented in the facility. The nurse is told that the nursing model is a team nursing approach. The nurse understands that which of the following is a characteristic of this type of nursing model of practice?
    1. A task approach method is used to provide care to clients.
    2. Managed care concepts and tools are used when providing client care.
    3. Nursing staff are led by a registered nurse when providing care to a group of clients.
    4. A single registered nurse is responsible for providing nursing care to a group of clients.

31. A client experiences a cardiac arrest. The nurse leader quickly responds to the emergency and assigns clearly defined tasks to the work group. In this situation, the nurse is implementing which leadership style?
    1. Autocratic
    2. Situational
    3. Democratic
    4. Laissez-faire

32. A nurse has delegated several nursing tasks to staff members. The nurse's primary responsibility after the delegation of the tasks is to:
    1. Document that the task was completed.
    2. Assign the tasks that were not completed to the next nursing shift.
    3. Allow each staff member to make judgments when performing the tasks.
    4. Perform follow up with each staff member regarding the performance of the task and the outcomes related to the implementation of the task.

ALTERNATE ITEM FORMAT: PRIORITIZING (ORDERED RESPONSE)

33. The nurse on the day shift is assigned to care for the following six clients. List in order of priority how the nurse would plan to check the assigned clients. (Number 1 is the client whom the nurse would check first, and number 6 is the last client.)

    _2_ Client who requires before-breakfast insulin

    _4_ Client who requires medications at 10:00 AM

    _6_ Client who is scheduled for physical therapy in the afternoon

    _1_ Client who has a tracheostomy and is on a mechanical ventilator

    _3_ Client who is scheduled for a cardiac catheterization at 9:00 AM

    _5_ Client who has been diagnosed with diabetes mellitus and who is scheduled for discharge to home

ANSWERS

24. 1

Rationale: End-of-shift report needs to be an efficient and accurate account of the client's condition during the last shift. It needs to include pertinent information about the client, such as tests and treatments; as-needed medications given or therapies performed during the past 24 hours, including the client's response to them; changes in the client's condition; scheduled tests and treatments; current problems; and any other special concerns. The total number of medications given or a list of all the tests and treatments that the client has had since admission are not necessary to include. Only significant vital signs need to be included.

Test-Taking Strategy: Remember that the purpose of end-of-shift reports is to communicate accurate and pertinent information about the client. The reporter does not have time to discuss extraneous or repetitive information, and the listener does not have time to listen to reports that include unneeded information. Review the information included in the end-of-shift report if you had difficulty with this question.

Level of Cognitive Ability: Application
Client Needs: Safe and Effective Care Environment
Integrated Process: Nursing Process/Implementation
Content Area: Leadership/Management

Reference: deWit, S. (2005). *Fundamental concepts and skills for nursing* (2nd ed., p. 109). Philadelphia: Saunders.

25. 2

Rationale: The nurse must determine the most appropriate assignment on the basis of the skills of the staff member and the needs of the client. In this case, the most appropriate assignment for a nursing assistant would be to care for the client who requires frequent ambulation. The nursing assistant is skilled in this task. The client who had a cardiac catheterization will require specific monitoring in addition to that of the vital signs. Wound irrigations and tube feedings are not performed by unlicensed personnel.

Test-Taking Strategy: Note the strategic words "most appropriate." Use the process of elimination, and recall the principles of delegation and the supervision of the work of others. Remember that work delegated to others must be done in a way that is consistent with the individual's level of expertise and that individual's licensure or lack of licensure. Review the principles of delegation if you had difficulty with this question.

Level of Cognitive Ability: Application
Client Needs: Safe and Effective Care Environment
Integrated Process: Nursing Process/Planning

Content Area: Leadership/Management
Reference: Huber, D. (2006). *Leadership and nursing care management* (3rd ed., pp. 545-546). Philadelphia: Saunders

26. 1
Rationale: The assignment of tasks needs to be implemented on the basis of the job description of the individual, the individual's level of clinical competence, and state law. Options 2, 3, and 4 involve care that requires the skill of a licensed nurse.
Test-Taking Strategy: Use the process of elimination and your knowledge regarding tasks that can be safely delegated to a nursing assistant. Eliminate options 2, 3, and 4, because these clients require care that needs to be provided by a licensed nurse. Review the principles related to assignments and delegation if you had difficulty with this question.
Level of Cognitive Ability: Application
Client Needs: Safe and Effective Care Environment
Integrated Process: Nursing Process/Planning
Content Area: Leadership/Management
Reference: deWit, S. (2009). *Medical-surgical nursing: Concepts & practice* (3rd ed., pp. 3-4). St. Louis: Saunders.

27. 1
Rationale: The airway is always a high priority, and the nurse first checks the client on a ventilator. The clients described in options 2, 3, and 4 have needs that would be identified as intermediate priorities.
Test-Taking Strategy: Use Maslow's Hierarchy of Needs theory and the ABCs—airway, breathing, and circulation—to answer the question. Remember that the airway is always the first priority. Review the principles related to prioritizing if you had difficulty with this question.
Level of Cognitive Ability: Application
Client Needs: Safe and Effective Care Environment
Integrated Process: Nursing Process/Planning
Content Area: Delegating/Prioritizing
Reference: deWit, S. (2009). *Medical-surgical nursing: Concepts & practice* (3rd ed., p. 28). St. Louis: Saunders.

28. 4
Rationale: In an emergency department, triage involves classifying clients according to their need for care, and it includes establishing priorities of care. The type of illness, the severity of the problem, and the resources available govern the process. Clients with trauma, chest pain, severe respiratory distress, cardiac arrest, limb amputation, or acute neurological deficits and those who sustained a chemical splash to the eyes are classified as emergent, and these clients are the number 1 priority. Clients with conditions such as simple fractures, asthma without respiratory distress, fever, hypertension, abdominal pain, or renal stones have urgent needs, and these clients are classified as the number 2 priority. Clients with conditions such as minor lacerations, sprains, or cold symptoms are classified as nonurgent, and they are the number 3 priority.
Test-Taking Strategy: Note the strategic words "highest priority." Use the ABCs—airway, breathing, and circulation—to direct you to option 4. A client who is experiencing chest pain is always classified as priority number 1 until a myocardial infarction has been ruled out. Review the triage classification system commonly

used in the hospital emergency department if you had difficulty with this question.
Level of Cognitive Ability: Application
Client Needs: Safe and Effective Care Environment
Integrated Process: Nursing Process/Implementation
Content Area: Delegating/Prioritizing
Reference: Fultz, J., & Sturt, P. (2005). *Emergency nursing reference* (3rd ed., p. 86). St. Louis: Mosby.

29. 4
Rationale: The airway is always a high priority, and the nurse would attend to the client who has been experiencing an airway problem first. The clients described in options 1, 2, and 3 would have intermediate priority.
Test-Taking Strategy: Use the ABCs—airway, breathing, and circulation—to answer the question. Remember that the airway is always the first priority. Review the prioritizing principles if you had difficulty with this question.
Level of Cognitive Ability: Application
Client Needs: Safe and Effective Care Environment
Integrated Process: Nursing Process/Planning
Content Area: Delegating/Prioritizing
Reference: Huber, D. (2006). *Leadership and nursing care management* (3rd ed., pp. 486-487). Philadelphia: Saunders

30. 3
Rationale: In team nursing, nursing personnel are led by a registered nurse when providing care to a group of clients. Option 1 identifies functional nursing. Option 2 identifies a component of case management. Option 4 identifies primary nursing.
Test-Taking Strategy: Note that the subject of the question relates to team nursing. Keep this subject in mind, and use the process of elimination. Option 3 is the only option that identifies the concept of a team approach. Review the various types of nursing delivery systems if you had difficulty with this question.
Level of Cognitive Ability: Comprehension
Client Needs: Safe and Effective Care Environment
Integrated Process: Nursing Process/Implementation
Content Area: Leadership/Management
References: Christensen, B., & Kockrow, E. (2006). *Foundations of nursing* (5th ed., p. 1261). St. Louis: Mosby.
Huber, D. (2006). *Leadership and nursing care management* (3rd ed., pp. 317, 322). Philadelphia: Saunders

31. 1
Rationale: Autocratic leadership is an approach in which the leader retains all authority and is primarily concerned with task accomplishment. It is an effective leadership style to implement in an emergency or crisis situation. The leader assigns clearly defined tasks and establishes one-way communication with the work group, and he or she makes all decisions independently. Situational leadership is a comprehensive approach that incorporates the leader's style, the maturity of the work group, and the situation at hand. Laissez-faire leadership is a permissive style in which the leader gives up control and delegates all decision making to the work group. Democratic leadership is a people-centered approach that is primarily concerned with human relations and teamwork. This leadership style facilitates goal accomplishment and contributes to the growth and development of the staff.

Test-Taking Strategy: Use the process of elimination. Focusing on the data in the question and the nurse leader's actions will direct you to option 1. Review the various leadership styles if you had difficulty with this question.
Level of Cognitive Ability: Application
Client Needs: Safe and Effective Care Environment
Integrated Process: Nursing Process/Implementation
Content Area: Leadership/Management
References: Christensen, B., & Kockrow, E. (2006). *Foundations of nursing* (5th ed., pp. 1259-1260). St. Louis: Mosby.
Huber, D. (2006). *Leadership and nursing care management* (3rd ed., pp. 157-158). Philadelphia: Saunders

32. **4**
Rationale: The ultimate responsibility for a task lies with the person who delegated it. Therefore, it is the nurse's primary responsibility to follow up with each staff member regarding the performance of the task and the outcomes related to implementing the task. Not all staff members have the education, knowledge, and ability to make judgments about tasks being performed. The nurse documents that the task has been completed, but this would not be done until follow-up was implemented and outcomes were identified. It is not appropriate to assign the tasks that were not completed to the next nursing shift.
Test-Taking Strategy: Use the process of elimination, and note the strategic words "primary responsibility." Recalling that the ultimate responsibility for a task lies with the person who delegated it will direct you to option 4.
Review the guidelines related to delegating if you had difficulty with this question.
Level of Cognitive Ability: Application
Client Needs: Safe and Effective Care Environment

Integrated Process: Nursing Process/Implementation
Content Area: Leadership/Management
Reference: Huber, D. (2006). *Leadership and nursing care management* (3rd ed., pp. 546-548). Philadelphia: Saunders

ALTERNATE ITEM FORMAT: PRIORITIZING (ORDERED RESPONSE)

33. **2, 4, 6, 1, 3, 5**
Rationale: The airway is always a high priority, and the nurse first assesses the client who has a tracheostomy and is on a mechanical ventilator. The remaining order of priority is guided by time guidelines. Therefore, the nurse next administers before-breakfast insulin, assesses the client who is scheduled for a cardiac catheterization at 9:00 AM, and then administers medications scheduled for 10:00 AM. Finally, the nurse checks the client who is scheduled for discharge, and this is followed by checking the client who is scheduled for physical therapy in the afternoon.
Test-Taking Strategy: Use Maslow's Hierarchy of Needs theory and the ABCs—airway, breathing, and circulation. Focus only on the data identified in the question. Remember that the airway is always the first priority. Next, use time guidelines to plan the order of the remaining clients. Review the principles related to prioritizing if you had difficulty with this question.
Level of Cognitive Ability: Application
Client Needs: Safe and Effective Care Environment
Integrated Process: Nursing Process/Planning
Content Area: Delegating/Prioritizing
Reference: Huber, D. (2006). *Leadership and nursing care management* (3rd ed., p. 167). Philadelphia: Saunders

REFERENCES

Christensen, B., & Kockrow, E. (2006). *Foundations of nursing* (5th ed.). St. Louis: Mosby.
deWit, S. (2005). *Fundamental concepts and skills for nursing* (2nd ed.). Philadelphia: Saunders.
deWit, S. (2009). *Medical-surgical nursing: Concepts & practice* (3rd ed.). St. Louis: Saunders.
Elkin, M., Perry, A., & Potter, P. (2004). *Nursing interventions and clinical skills* (3rd ed.). St. Louis: Mosby.

Fultz, J., & Sturt, P. (2005). *Emergency nursing reference* (3rd ed.). St. Louis: Mosby.
Huber, D (2006). *Leadership and nursing care management* (3rd ed.). Philadelphia: Saunders.
National Council of State Boards of Nursing (Eds.) (2008). *2008 Detailed Test Plan for the NCLEX-PN® Examination, National Council of State Boards of Nursing*. Chicago: Author.
National Council of State Boards of Nursing. *NCSBN home page*. www.ncsbn.org. Accessed May 30, 2008.

Nursing Sciences

CHAPTER 9

Fluids and Electrolytes

PYRAMID TERMS

calcium A mineral element needed for the process of bone formation, coagulation of blood, excitation of cardiac and skeletal muscle, maintenance of muscle tone, conduction of neuromuscular impulses, and synthesis and regulation of the endocrine and exocrine glands.

fluid volume deficit Dehydration in which the body's fluid intake is not sufficient to meet the body's fluid needs.

fluid volume excess Fluid intake or fluid retention that exceeds the body's fluid needs; also called *overhydration or fluid overload*.

homeostasis The tendency of biological systems to maintain relatively constant conditions in the internal environment while continuously interacting with and adjusting to changes originating within or outside of the system.

hypercalcemia A serum calcium level that exceeds 10 mg/dL.

hyperkalemia A serum potassium level that exceeds 5.1 mEq/L.

hypermagnesemia A serum magnesium level that exceeds 2.6 mg/dL.

hypernatremia A serum sodium level that exceeds 145 mEq/L.

hyperphosphatemia A serum phosphorus level that exceeds 4.5 mg/dL.

hypocalcemia A serum calcium level less than 8.6 mg/dL.

hypokalemia A serum potassium level less than 3.5 mEq/L.

hypomagnesemia A serum magnesium level less than 1.6 mg/dL.

hyponatremia A serum sodium level less than 135 mEq/L.

hypophosphatemia A serum phosphorus level less than 2.7 mg/dL.

magnesium An element concentrated in the bone, cartilage, and within the cell itself that is required for the use of adenosine triphosphate as a source of energy. It is necessary for the action of numerous enzyme systems, such as carbohydrate metabolism, protein synthesis, nucleic acid synthesis, and the contraction of muscular tissue. It also regulates neuromuscular activity and the clotting mechanism.

potassium A principal electrolyte of intracellular fluid and the primary buffer within the cell itself; it is needed for nerve conduction, muscle function, acid–base balance, and osmotic pressure. In addition to calcium and magnesium, it controls the rate and force of contraction of the heart and, thus, cardiac output.

phosphorus An element needed for the generation of bony tissue; it functions in the metabolism of glucose and lipids, in the maintenance of acid–base balance, and in the storage and transfer of energy from one site in the body to another. Phosphorus levels are evaluated in relation to calcium levels because of their inverse relationship: when calcium levels are decreased, phosphorus levels are increased, and when phosphorus levels are decreased, calcium levels are increased.

sodium An abundant electrolyte that maintains osmotic pressure and acid–base balance and that transmits nerve impulses.

PYRAMID TO SUCCESS

Pyramid points focus primarily on the collection of data related to a fluid and electrolyte imbalance, interventions, and the evaluation of the expected outcomes. Fluid and electrolytes constitute a content area that is complex and sometimes difficult to understand. It is important to understand cell functions and properties and the concepts related to body fluids as outlined in this chapter. Review this content. Pyramid points also focus on the common fluid and electrolyte disturbances. Focus on the pyramid points related to the causes of imbalances or disturbances, data collection, and related treatments. The Integrated Processes addressed in this chapter are the Nursing Process (Clinical Problem-Solving Process), Caring, Communication and Documentation, and Teaching and Learning.

CLIENT NEEDS

Safe and Effective Care Environment

Consulting with members of the health care team

Establishing priorities for care

Handling hazardous and infectious materials to prevent injury to health care personnel and others

Maintaining medical and surgical asepsis and preventing infection in the client when samples for laboratory studies are obtained or when intravenous solutions are administered

Maintaining standard, transmission-based, and other precautions to prevent the transmission of infection to self and others

Preventing accidents and ensuring the safety of the client when an imbalance exists, particularly when changes in cardiovascular, respiratory, gastrointestinal, neuromuscular, renal, or central nervous systems occur or when the client is at risk for complications such as seizures, respiratory depression, or dysrhythmias

Health Promotion and Maintenance

Implementing health screening and determining the potential risk for a fluid and electrolyte imbalance

Providing education related to medication and diet management

Providing education related to the potential risk for a fluid and electrolyte imbalance, measures to prevent an imbalance, signs and symptoms of an imbalance, and actions to take if signs and symptoms develop

Psychosocial Integrity

Providing reassurance to the client who is experiencing a fluid or electrolyte imbalance

Providing support and continuously informing the client of the purposes of prescribed interventions

Physiological Integrity

Assessing for expected and unexpected responses to therapeutic interventions and documenting findings

Assisting with managing emergencies

Identifying clients who are at risk for a fluid or electrolyte imbalance

Monitoring for complications related to the imbalance

Monitoring laboratory values

I. CELL PROPERTIES (Box 9-1)
II. CONCEPTS OF FLUID AND ELECTROLYTE BALANCE
A. Electrolytes
   1. Description: When a substance is dissolved in solution and some of its molecules split or dissociate into electrically charged atoms or ions (see Box 9-1)
   2. Measurement
     a. To measure volumes of fluids, the metric system is used: liters (L) or milliliters (mL)
     b. The unit of measure that expresses the combining activity of an electrolyte is the milliequivalent (mEq)
B. Body fluid compartments (Box 9-2)
   1. Fluid in each of the body compartments contains electrolytes
   2. Each compartment has a particular composition of electrolytes that differs from that of other compartments

---

BOX 9-1 Cell Properties

Anion: An ion that has gained electrons and therefore carries a negative charge. When an ion has gained or taken on electrons, it assumes a negative charge, and the result is a negatively charged ion.

Atom: The smallest part of an element that still has the properties of the element and that is composed of particles known as *protons* (positive charge), *neutrons* (neutral), and *electrons* (negative charge). Protons and neutrons are in the nucleus of the atom; therefore, the nucleus is positively charged. Electrons carry a negative charge and revolve around the nucleus. As long as the number of electrons is the same as the number of protons, there is no net charge on the atom—that is, it is neither positive nor negative. Atoms may gain, lose, or share electrons, and then they are no longer neutral.

Cation: An ion that carries a positive charge because it has given away or lost electrons. The result is fewer electrons than protons and a positive charge.

Ion: An atom that carries an electrical charge because it has either gained or lost electrons. Some ions carry a negative electrical charge, and some carry a positive charge.

Molecule: Two or more atoms that have combined to form a substance.

BOX 9-2 Body Fluid Compartments

Extracellular compartment: Refers to all fluid outside of the cells.

Interstitial fluids: Fluid that is between the cells and the blood vessels.

Intracellular compartment: Refers to all fluid inside of the cells. Most body fluids are inside of the cells.

Intravascular compartment: Fluid that is within blood vessels.

---

   3. To function normally, body cells must have fluids and electrolytes in the right compartments and in the right amounts
   4. Whenever an electrolyte moves out of a cell, another electrolyte moves in to take its place
   5. Compartments are separated by semipermeable membranes
C. Third-spacing
   1. The accumulation and sequestration of trapped extracellular fluid in an actual or potential body space as a result of disease or injury
   2. The trapped fluid represents a volume loss and is unavailable for normal physiological processes
   3. Fluid may be trapped in body spaces such as the pericardial, pleural, peritoneal, or joint cavities; the bowel; or the abdomen or within soft tissues after trauma or burns
   4. Assessing the intravascular fluid loss is difficult; it may not be reflected in weight changes or

intake and output (I&O) records, and it may not become apparent until after organ malfunction occurs

D. Edema
  1. An excess accumulation of fluid in the interstitial spaces
  2. Localized edema occurs as a result of traumatic injury from accidents or surgery, local inflammatory processes, or burns
  3. Generalized edema, also called *anasarca*, is an excessive accumulation of fluid in the interstitial space throughout the body as a result of a condition such as cardiac, renal, or liver failure

E. Body fluid
  1. Description
     a. Provides the transportation of nutrients to the cells and carries waste products from the cells
     b. Total body fluid amounts to about 60% of body weight
     c. A loss of 10% of body fluid in the adult is serious
     d. A loss of 20% of the body fluid in the adult is fatal
  2. Constituents of body fluids
     a. Body fluids consist of water and dissolved substances
     b. The largest single fluid constituent of the body is water

F. Body fluid transport (Figure 9-1)
  1. Diffusion
     a. The movement of particles in all directions through a solution
     b. Diffusion occurs within fluid compartments and from one compartment to another if the barrier between the compartments is permeable to the diffusing substances
     c. Diffusion of a solute (substance that is dissolved) spreads the molecules from an area of high concentration to an area of lower concentration
     d. A permeable membrane allows substances to pass through it without restriction
     e. A selectively permeable membrane allows some solutes to pass through without restriction but prevents other solutes from passing freely
  2. Osmosis
     a. Osmotic pressure is the force that draws the water from a less concentrated solution through a selectively permeable membrane into a more concentrated solution
     b. If a membrane is permeable to water but not to all of the solutes present, it is a selective or semipermeable membrane

c. When the solvent (solution in which the solvent is dissolved) or water moves across the membrane, the process is called *osmosis*

3. Filtration
   a. Filtration is the movement of solutes and solvents by hydrostatic pressure
   b. Hydrostatic pressure is the force exerted by the weight of a solution
   c. The movement is from an area of greater pressure to an area of lesser pressure

4. Osmolality
   a. Refers to the number of osmotically active particles per kilogram of water
   b. In the body, osmotic pressure is measured in milliosmols (mOsm)
   c. The normal osmolality of plasma is 280 to 294 mOsm/kg

5. Hydrostatic pressure
   a. The force exerted by the weight of a solution
   b. When there is a difference in the hydrostatic pressure on two sides of a membrane, water and diffusible solutes move out of the solution that has the higher hydrostatic pressure by the process of filtration
   c. At the arterial end of the capillary, the hydrostatic pressure is greater than the osmotic pressure; therefore, fluids and diffusible solutes move out of the capillary
   d. At the venous end, the osmotic pressure or pull is greater than the hydrostatic pressure, and fluids and some solutes move into the capillary

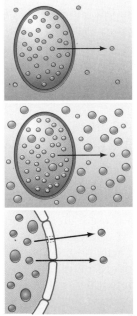

FIG. 9-1 Passive transport processes: diffusion, osmosis, and filtration. (From Christensen, B., & Kockrow, E. [2006]. *Foundations and adult health nursing* [5th ed., p. 669]. St. Louis: Mosby.)

e. The excess fluid and solutes that remain in the interstitial spaces are returned to the intravascular compartment by the lymph channels

G. Movement of body fluid
 1. Description
  a. Cell membranes separate the interstitial fluid from the intravascular fluid
  b. Cell membranes are selectively permeable; that is, the cell membrane and the capillary wall allow water and some solutes free passage through them
  c. Several forces affect the movement of water and solutes through the walls of cells and capillaries
  d. The greater the number of particles in the concentrated solution, the more pull there will be to move the water through the membrane
  e. If the body loses more electrolytes than fluids, as can happen with diarrhea, then the extracellular fluid will contain fewer electrolytes or less solute than the intracellular fluid
  f. Fluids and electrolytes must be kept in balance for health; when they remain out of balance, death can occur
 2. Isotonic solutions (Table 9-1)
  a. When the solutions on both sides of a selectively permeable membrane have established equilibrium or are equal in concentration, they are then isotonic
  b. Isotonic solutions are isotonic to human cells, and thus there will be very little osmosis
 3. Hypotonic solutions (see Table 9-1)
  a. When a solution contains a lower concentration of salt or solute than other solutions, it is hypotonic
  b. A hypotonic solution has less salt or more water than an isotonic solution
  c. Hypotonic solutions are hypotonic to the cells; therefore, osmosis would continue

in an attempt to bring about balance or equality
 4. Hypertonic solutions: A solution that has a higher concentration of solutes than another solution is a hypertonic solution (see Table 9-1)
 5. Osmotic pressure
  a. The force that draws the solvent from a solution with more solvent activity through a selectively permeable membrane to a solution with less solvent activity
  b. When the solutions on each side of a selectively permeable membrane are equal in concentration, they are isotonic
  c. A hypotonic solution has less solute than an isotonic solution, whereas a hypertonic solution contains more solute
 6. Active transport
  a. If an ion is to move through a membrane from an area of low concentration to an area of higher concentration, an active transport system is necessary
  b. An active transport system moves molecules or ions uphill against concentration and osmotic pressure
  c. Metabolic processes in the cell supply the energy for active transport
  d. Substances that are actively transported through the cell membrane include ions of **sodium, potassium, calcium,** iron, and hydrogen; some sugars; and amino acids

H. Body fluid excretion (Table 9-2)
 1. Description
  a. Fluids leave the body by several routes, including the skin, lungs, gastrointestinal (GI) tract, and kidneys
  b. The kidneys excrete the largest quantity of fluid
  c. As long as all organs are functioning normally, the body can maintain balance in its fluid content
 2. Skin
  a. Water is lost through the skin by diffusion in the amount of approximately 400 mL/day and by perspiration
  b. The amount of water lost by perspiration will vary according to the temperature of

TABLE 9-1 **Tonicity of Intravenous Fluids**

Solution	Tonicity
0.45% saline (½ normal saline [NS])	Hypotonic
0.9% saline (NS)	Isotonic
5% dextrose in water (D_5W)	Isotonic
5% dextrose in 0.225% saline (D_5/¼ NS)	Isotonic
Lactated Ringer's solution	Isotonic
5% dextrose in lactated Ringer's solution	Hypertonic
5% dextrose in 0.45% saline (D_5/½ NS)	Hypertonic
5% dextrose in 0.9% saline (D_5/NS)	Hypertonic
10% dextrose in water ($D_{10}W$)	Hypertonic

TABLE 9-2 **Daily Body Fluid Excretion or Loss**

Where Fluid Is Lost or Excreted	Amount Lost or Excreted (mL)
Skin (by diffusion)	400
Skin (by perspiration)	100
Lungs	350
Feces	150
Kidneys	1500

the environment and of the body, but the average amount of loss is 100 mL/day

c. Water lost through the skin by diffusion is called *insensible loss* (the individual is unaware of losing that water)

3. Lungs
   a. Water is lost from the lungs through expired air that is saturated with water vapor
   b. The amount of water lost from the lungs will vary with the rate and the depth of respiration
   c. The average amount of water lost from the lungs is approximately 350 mL/day
   d. Water lost from the lungs is called *insensible loss*

4. GI tract
   a. Large quantities of water are secreted into the GI tract, but almost all of this fluid is reabsorbed
   b. A very large volume of electrolyte-containing liquids moves into the GI tract and then returns again into the extracellular fluid
   c. The average amount of water lost in the feces is 150 mL/day, which is equal to the amount of water gained through the oxidation of foods
   d. Severe diarrhea will result in the loss of large quantities of fluids and electrolytes

5. Kidneys
   a. Play a major role in regulating the fluid and electrolyte balance
   b. Normal kidneys can adjust the amount of water and electrolytes leaving the body
   c. The quantity of fluid excreted by the kidneys is determined by the amount of water ingested and the amount of waste and solutes excreted
   d. The usual urine output is approximately 1500 mL/day; however, this will vary greatly, depending on fluid intake, the amount of perspiration, and other factors

I. Body fluid replacement
1. Description: Water enters the body through three sources: oral liquids, water in foods, and water formed by the oxidation of foods
2. Amounts
   a. The average total amount of water taken into the body by all three sources is 2500 mL/day
   b. About 10 mL of water is released by the metabolism of each 100 calories of fat, carbohydrates, or proteins
3. Electrolytes
   a. Electrolytes are present in both foods and liquids
   b. With a normal diet, an excess of essential electrolytes is taken in, and the unused electrolytes are excreted

J. Maintaining fluid and electrolyte balance
1. Description
   a. *Homeostasis* is a term that indicates the relative stability of the internal environment
   b. The concentration and composition of body fluids must be nearly constant
   c. In a client, when one of the substances (either fluid or electrolyte) is deficient, it must be replaced normally by the intake of food and water or by therapy such as intravenous (IV) administration and/or medications
   d. When the client has an excess of fluid or electrolytes, therapy is directed toward assisting the body with eliminating the excess
2. Kidneys: Play a major role in controlling all types of balance of fluid and electrolytes
3. Adrenal glands: Through the secretion of aldosterone, the adrenal glands also help with controlling the extracellular fluid volume by regulating the amount of **sodium** reabsorbed by the kidneys
4. Antidiuretic hormone from the pituitary gland regulates the osmotic pressure of extracellular fluid by regulating the amount of water reabsorbed by the kidney

III. FLUID VOLUME DEFICIT
A. Description
1. Dehydration in which the body's fluid intake is not sufficient to meet the body's fluid needs
2. The goal of treatment is to restore fluid volume, replace electrolytes as needed, and eliminate the cause of the **fluid volume deficit**
B. Causes
1. Vomiting and/or diarrhea
2. Continuous GI irrigation
3. GI suctioning
4. Ileostomy or colostomy drainage
5. Draining wounds, burns, or fistulas
6. Increased urine output from the use of diuretics
C. Data collection
1. Thirst
2. Poor skin turgor and dry mucous membranes
3. Increased heart rate, thready pulse, and postural hypotension
4. Rapid weight loss
5. Flat neck or hand veins
6. Dizziness or weakness
7. Decrease in urine volume and dark, concentrated urine
8. Increased specific gravity of the urine
9. Confusion
10. Increased hematocrit level
D. Interventions
1. The cause of the **fluid volume deficit** is treated, and fluids are replaced (lactated Ringer's solution, 0.9% normal saline) as prescribed

2. Monitor vital signs
3. Check mucous membranes and skin turgor
4. Monitor weight daily
5. Monitor I&O
6. Test urine for specific gravity
7. Monitor hematocrit and electrolyte levels

IV. FLUID VOLUME EXCESS

A. Description
   1. Fluid intake or retention exceeds the body's fluid needs
   2. Also called *overhydration* or *fluid overload*
   3. The goals of treatment are to restore fluid balance; to correct electrolyte imbalances, if present; and to eliminate or control the underlying cause of the overload
B. Data collection
   1. Cough and dyspnea
   2. Lung crackles
   3. Increased respirations and heart rate
   4. Increased blood pressure and bounding pulse
   5. Pitting edema
   6. Weight gain
   7. Neck and hand vein distention
   8. Decreased hematocrit level
   9. Confusion
C. Interventions
   1. Monitor vital signs
   2. Position client in semi-Fowler's position
   3. Check for edema
   4. Monitor I&O
   5. Monitor weight
   6. Administer diuretics as prescribed
   7. Monitor hematocrit and electrolyte levels
   8. Restrict fluids as prescribed
   9. Provide a low-**sodium** diet as prescribed

V. HYPOKALEMIA (Table 9-3)

A. Description (Box 9-3)
   1. A serum **potassium** level less than 3.5 mEq/L
   2. **Potassium** deficit is the most common electrolyte imbalance and is potentially life threatening
B. Interventions
   1. Monitor vital signs
   2. Monitor neuromuscular activity
   3. Monitor I&O
   4. Check renal function before administering **potassium**
   5. Administer **potassium** supplements as prescribed (orally or monitor by IV)
   6. Oral **potassium** chloride has an unpleasant taste and should be taken with juice or other desired liquid
   7. Oral **potassium** preparations can cause GI irritation and should not be taken on an empty stomach
   8. If the client complains of abdominal pain, distention, nausea, vomiting, diarrhea, or GI

bleeding, the oral **potassium** may need to be discontinued
   9. When **potassium** is added to an IV solution, shake the bag and invert it to ensure that the **potassium** is evenly distributed
   10. An IV bolus injection of concentrated **potassium** is never administered; it is always diluted

TABLE 9-3 Potassium Imbalances

Hypokalemia	Hyperkalemia
Causes	**Causes**
Use of non–potassium-sparing diuretics	Renal failure
Diarrhea	Intestinal obstruction
Vomiting	Cell damage
Inadequate intake of potassium	Excessive oral or parenteral administration of potassium
Excessive gastric suction	Metabolic acidosis
Excessive fistula drainage	Addison's disease
Cushing's syndrome	Excessive use of potassium-based salt substitutes
Chronic use of corticosteroids	Transfusion of stored blood (the breakdown of older red blood cells releases potassium)
Renal disease	
Parenteral nutrition	
Uncontrolled diabetes	
Alkalosis	
Signs and Symptoms	**Signs and Symptoms**
Leg and abdominal cramps	Muscle weakness
Lethargy and weakness	Paresthesias
Shallow respirations and thready pulse	Hypotension
	Diarrhea
Confusion	Hyperactive bowel sounds
Decreased or absent reflexes	Wide, flat P waves; widened QRS complex; prolonged PR interval; depressed ST segment; and narrow, peaked T waves
Hypoactive bowel sounds and ileus	
Postural hypotension	
Peaked P waves; flat T waves; depressed ST segment and U waves	

BOX 9-3 Potassium

Normal Value
   3.5 to 5.1 mEq/L
Common Food Sources
   Avocados
   Bananas
   Cantaloupes
   Carrots
   Fish
   Mushrooms
   Oranges
   Potatoes
   Pork, beef, and veal
   Raisins
   Spinach
   Strawberries
   Tomatoes

11. A client receiving more than 10 mEq/hr should be placed on a cardiac monitor; the infusion is controlled by an infusion device
12. Monitor for cardiac changes during the administration of **potassium**
13. Monitor electrolyte values
14. Monitor the IV site; if phlebitis or infiltration occurs, the IV should be stopped immediately and restarted at another site
15. Instruct the client not to use salt substitutes containing **potassium** unless prescribed by the physician

VI. HYPERKALEMIA (see Table 9-3)
A. Description: A serum **potassium** level that exceeds 5.1 mEq/L (see Box 9-3)
B. Interventions
1. Monitor vital signs
2. Monitor for cardiac changes
3. Decrease **potassium** intake
4. Administer **potassium**-excreting diuretics as prescribed
5. Monitor I&O
6. Monitor laboratory values
7. Emergency treatment includes the rapid IV administration of dextrose with regular insulin to move excess **potassium** into the cells
8. Administer **sodium** polystyrene sulfonate (Kayexalate) orally or by enema as prescribed, which releases **sodium** ions in exchange for primarily **potassium** ions and absorbs the **potassium** into the GI tract for excretion
9. Monitor for **calcium** and **magnesium** loss when using Kayexalate
10. Monitor renal function
11. Prepare for peritoneal dialysis or hemodialysis as prescribed
12. When blood transfusions are prescribed for a client with a **potassium** imbalance, the client should receive fresh blood, if possible; transfusions of stored blood may elevate the **potassium** level, because the breakdown of older blood cells releases **potassium**
13. Instruct the client to avoid foods high in **potassium**
14. Instruct the client to avoid the use of salt substitutes or other **potassium**-containing substances

VII. HYPONATREMIA (Table 9-4)
A. Description: A serum **sodium** level less than 135 mEq/L (Box 9-4)
B. Interventions
1. Monitor vital signs
2. Monitor I&O
3. Monitor weight
4. Assess skin turgor and mucous membranes
5. Restrict water intake and avoid tap-water enemas

6. Use normal saline solution rather than sterile water for irrigation
7. Administer **sodium** replacement as prescribed and monitor electrolyte values
8. Encourage foods high in **sodium**

TABLE 9-4	Sodium Imbalances
Hyponatremia	**Hypernatremia**
Causes	**Causes**
Inadequate sodium intake (nothing by mouth)	Decreased water intake
Gastrointestinal suction	Fever
Excessive intake of water	Excessive perspiration
Irrigation of gastrointestinal tubes with plain water	Dehydration
Potent diuretics	Hyperventilation
Increased perspiration	Watery diarrhea
Draining skin lesions	Enteral nutrition and parental nutrition deplete the cells of water
Burns	Diabetes insipidus
Nausea and vomiting	Cushing's syndrome
Diabetic ketoacidosis	Impaired renal function
Syndrome of inappropriate antidiuretic hormone secretion	Use of corticosteroids
Retention of fluid, such as with kidney or heart failure	Excessive administration of sodium bicarbonate
Signs and Symptoms	**Signs and Symptoms**
Rapid, thready pulse	Dry mucous membranes
Postural blood pressure changes	Loss of skin turgor
Weakness	Thirst
Abdominal cramping	Flushed skin
Poor skin turgor	Elevated temperature
Muscle twitching and seizures	Oliguria
Apprehension	Muscle twitching
	Fatigue
	Confusion
	Seizures

BOX 9-4	Sodium

Normal Value
135 to 145 mEq/L
Common Food Sources
Bacon
Butter
Canned foods
Cheese, such as American or cottage cheese
Hot dogs
Ketchup
Lunch meats
Milk
Mustard
Processed foods
Snack foods
Soy sauce
Table salt
White and whole-wheat bread

9. If the client is taking lithium, monitor the lithium level, because **hyponatremia** can cause diminished lithium excretion that can result in toxicity

VIII. HYPERNATREMIA (see Table 9-4)

A. Description: A serum **sodium** level that exceeds 145 mEq/L (see Box 9-4)

B. Interventions
 1. Monitor vital signs
 2. Monitor I&O
 3. Monitor electrolyte levels
 4. Increase water intake orally; provide water between meals or tube feedings and encourage the client to drink 8 to 10 glasses of water daily

IX. HYPOCALCEMIA (Table 9-5) — *Chvostek sign*

A. Description: A serum **calcium** level less than 8.6 mg/dL (Box 9-5)

B. Interventions
 1. Monitor vital signs
 2. Monitor for the presence of Chvostek's and Trousseau's signs (Figure 9-2)
 3. Provide a quiet environment and avoid overstimulation

BOX 9-5 Calcium

Normal Value
 8.6 to 10 mg/dL *8-10*
Common Food Sources
 Cheese
 Collard greens
 Milk and soy milk
 Rhubarb
 Sardines
 Spinach
 Tofu
 Yogurt

TABLE 9-5 Calcium Imbalances

Hypocalcemia	Hypercalcemia
Causes	**Causes**
Inadequate dietary intake of calcium	Excessive intake of calcium supplements, milk, and antacid products that contain calcium
Inhibited absorption of calcium from the intestinal tract	Excessive intake of vitamin D
Inadequate vitamin D consumption	Increased bone resorption or destruction from conditions such as bone tumors, fractures, osteoporosis, and immobility
Diarrhea	
Long-term immobilization and bone demineralization	
Excessive gastrointestinal losses from diarrhea or wound draining	Decreased excretion of calcium
End-stage renal disease	Renal failure
Calcium-excreting medications such as diuretics, caffeine, anticonvulsants, heparin, laxatives, and nicotine	Use of thiazide diuretics
	Hyperparathyroidism
	Use of lithium
	Use of glucocorticoids
Decreased secretion of parathyroid hormone	Adrenal insufficiency
Acute pancreatitis	**Signs and Symptoms**
Crohn's disease	Increased heart rate and blood pressure
Excessive administration of blood	Bounding pulse
Signs and Symptoms	Bradycardia (late stage)
Tachycardia	Shortened QT interval and widened T wave
Hypotension	Muscle weakness (hypotonicity)
Paresthesias	
Twitching	Diminished deep tendon reflexes
Cramps	
Tetany	Nausea and vomiting
Positive Chvostek's or Trousseau's sign	Constipation
	Abdominal distention
Diarrhea	Confusion, lethargy, and coma
Hyperactive bowel sounds	
Prolongation of QT interval	

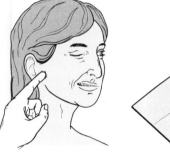
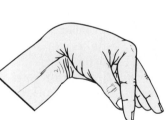
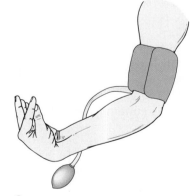

FIG. 9-2 Tests for hypocalcemia. **A,** Chvostek's sign is a contraction of facial muscles in response to a light tap over the facial nerve in front of the ear. **B,** Trousseau's sign is a carpal spasm induced by **C,** inflating a blood pressure cuff above the systolic pressure for a few minutes. (From Christensen, B., & Kockrow, E. [2006]. *Foundations and adult health nursing* [5th ed., p. 676.] St. Louis: Mosby.)

4. Initiate seizure precautions
5. Administer **calcium** orally or monitor IV **calcium** administration as prescribed
6. Administer vitamin D as prescribed to aid in the absorption of **calcium** from the intestinal tract
7. Administer **calcium** supplements 1 to 2 hours after meals to maximize intestinal absorption
8. Keep 10% **calcium** gluconate available for acute **calcium** deficit
9. Monitor **calcium** levels closely after thyroid surgery
10. Instruct the client who is taking **calcium**-excreting medications to have serum **calcium** levels checked periodically
11. Teach the client about the proper use of antacids or laxatives
12. Instruct the client to consume foods high in **calcium**

X. HYPERCALCEMIA (see Table 9-5)

A. Description: A serum **calcium** level that exceeds 10 mg/dL (see Box 9-5)

B. Interventions
1. Monitor vital signs
2. Monitor for dysrhythmias
3. Restrict **calcium** intake
4. Increase mobility
5. Assist with passive range-of-motion exercises when ambulation is not possible
6. Move clients carefully
7. Monitor for the development of pathological fractures
8. Monitor for severe flank or abdominal pain and strain urine to check for urinary stones
9. Monitor level of consciousness
10. Monitor for confusion and neurological changes
11. Avoid large doses of vitamin D supplements
12. Avoid the use of thiazide diuretics
13. Prepare for the administration of phosphate as prescribed
14. Prepare for the administration of calcitonin (Calcimar) as prescribed to increase the incorporation of **calcium** into the bones

XI. HYPOMAGNESEMIA (Table 9-6)

A. Description: A serum **magnesium** level less than 1.6 mg/dL (Box 9-6)

B. Interventions
1. Monitor vital signs
2. Monitor for dysrhythmias
3. Monitor for neuromuscular changes
4. Monitor I&O
5. Initiate seizure precautions
6. Administer **magnesium** supplements and monitor laboratory values
7. Monitor serum **magnesium** levels every 12 to 24 hours when client is receiving **magnesium** by IV

8. Monitor for reduced deep tendon reflexes that suggest **hypermagnesemia** during the administration of **magnesium**
9. Instruct the client to eat food that is high in **magnesium**

TABLE 9-6 Magnesium Imbalances

Hypomagnesemia	Hypermagnesemia
Causes	**Causes**
Malnutrition	Overuse of antacids or
Diarrhea	laxatives that contain
Celiac disease	magnesium
Crohn's disease	Renal insufficiency and renal
Alcoholism	failure
Prolonged gastric suctioning	Treatment of preeclampsia
Ileostomy, colostomy, or	with magnesium
intestinal fistulas	**Signs and Symptoms**
Acute pancreatitis	Hypotension
Diabetic ketoacidosis	Bradycardia
Eclampsia	Weak pulse
Chemotherapy	Sweating and flushing
Sepsis	Respiratory depression
Signs and Symptoms	Loss of deep tendon reflexes
Twitching	Prolonged PR interval and
Paresthesias	widened QRS complexes
Hyperactive reflexes	
Irritability	
Confusion	
Positive Chvostek's or	
Trousseau's sign	
Shallow respirations	
Tetany	
Seizures	
Tachycardia	
Tall T waves and depressed	
ST segment	

BOX 9-6 Magnesium

Normal Value
1.6 to 2.6 mg/dL
Common Food Sources
Avocados
Canned white tuna fish
Cauliflower
Oatmeal
Green leafy vegetables, such as spinach and broccoli
Yogurt
Milk
Peanut butter
Peas
Pork, beef, and chicken
Potatoes
Raisins

▲ **XII. HYPERMAGNESEMIA** (see Table 9-6)

A. Description: A serum **magnesium** level that exceeds 2.6 mg/dL (see Box 9-6)

B. Interventions

1. Monitor vital signs
2. Monitor for respiratory depression
3. Monitor for hypotension, bradycardia, and dysrhythmias
4. Monitor neurological and muscular activity
5. Monitor level of consciousness
6. Remove the source of the excess **magnesium**
7. Monitor laboratory values
8. Increase renal excretion by increasing oral fluids or administering loop diuretics as prescribed
9. Instruct the client to avoid the use of laxatives and antacids that contain **magnesium**

XIII. HYPOPHOSPHATEMIA (Table 9-7)

A. Description: A serum **phosphorus** level less than 2.7 mg/dL (Box 9-7)

B. Interventions

1. Monitor vital signs
2. Monitor respiratory status
3. Move the client carefully
4. Administer phosphate as prescribed
5. Check the renal system before administering ▲ phosphate
6. Monitor **calcium, phosphorus, sodium,** and chloride levels
7. Administer vitamin D
8. Monitor for decreased neuromuscular activity
9. Monitor for **calcium** excess and kidney stones
10. Monitor for hematological changes
11. Decrease intake of **calcium**-rich foods and increase intake of meats and whole grains that contain **phosphorus**
12. Instruct the client regarding the use of antacids

XIV. HYPERPHOSPHATEMIA (see Table 9-7)   ▲

A. Description: A serum **phosphorus** level that exceeds 4.5 mg/dL (see Box 9-7)

B. Interventions

1. Increase the fecal excretion of **phosphorus** by binding **phosphorus** from food in the GI tract with the use of aluminum hydroxide gel
2. Monitor laboratory values
3. Prepare for dialysis if prescribed
4. Monitor for signs of **hypocalcemia**   ▲
5. Administer **calcium** as prescribed if **hypocalcemia** exists   ▲
6. Monitor for neuromuscular irritability   ▲
7. Monitor for hyperreflexia, tetany, and seizures   ▲
8. Monitor for Trousseau's and Chvostek's signs   ▲
9. Instruct the client to avoid phosphate-containing medications, including laxatives and enemas
10. Instruct the client to decrease intake of foods high in **phosphorus**
11. Instruct the client regarding how to take phos-   ▲ phate-binding medications, emphasizing that these should be taken with meals or immediately after meals

TABLE 9-7 Phosphorus Imbalances	
Hypophosphatemia	**Hyperphosphatemia**
Causes	**Causes**
Decreased nutritional intake of phosphorus and malnutrition	Excessive dietary intake of phosphorus
Use of magnesium-based or aluminum-hydroxide–based antacids	Overuse of phosphate-containing laxatives or enemas
Renal failure	Vitamin D intoxication
Hyperparathyroidism	Hypoparathyroidism
Malignancy	Renal insufficiency
Hypercalcemia	Chemotherapy
Alcohol withdrawal	**Signs and Symptoms**
Diabetic ketoacidosis	Neuromuscular irritability
Respiratory alkalosis	Muscle weakness
Signs and Symptoms	Hyperactive reflexes
Confusion	Tetany
Seizures	Positive Chvostek's or Trousseau's sign
Weakness	
Decreased deep tendon reflexes	
Shallow respirations	
Increased bleeding tendency	
Immunosuppression	
Bone pain	

BOX 9-7   Phosphorus

Normal Value
2.7 to 4.5 mg/dL
Common Food Sources
Fish
Organ meats
Nuts
Pork, beef, and chicken
Whole-grain breads and cereals

PRACTICE QUESTIONS

More questions on the companion CD!

34. A nurse is caring for a client with cirrhosis. The nurse notes that the client is dyspneic and that crackles are heard on auscultation of the lungs; fluid volume excess is suspected. What additional signs would the nurse expect to note in this client if a fluid volume excess is present?

1. Flat hand and neck veins
2. A weak and thready pulse
3. An increased urine output
4. An increase in blood pressure

35. The nurse is reviewing the health records of assigned clients. The nurse plans care knowing that which client is at risk for a potassium deficit?
    1. The client with renal disease
    2. The client with Addison's disease
    3. The client with metabolic acidosis
    4. The client receiving nasogastric suction

36. A nurse reviews a client's electrolyte results and notes a potassium level of 5.5 mEq/L. The nurse understands that a potassium value at this level would be noted with which condition?
    1. Colitis
    2. Traumatic burn
    3. Cushing's syndrome
    4. Overuse of laxatives

37. A nurse reviews a client's electrolyte results and notes that the potassium level is 5.4 mEq/L. Which of the following would the nurse note on the cardiac monitor as a result of this laboratory value?
    1. ST elevation
    2. Peaked P wave
    3. Prominent U wave
    4. Narrow, peaked T waves

38. A nurse is reading the physician's progress notes in the client's record and sees that the physician has documented "insensible fluid loss of approximately 800 mL daily." The nurse understands that this type of fluid loss can occur through:
    1. The skin
    2. Urinary output
    3. Wound drainage
    4. The gastrointestinal tract

39. A nurse is reviewing the health records of assigned clients. The nurse plans care knowing that which client is at the lowest risk for the development of third-spacing?
    1. The client with sepsis
    2. The client with cirrhosis
    3. The client with renal failure
    4. The client with diabetes mellitus

40. A nurse is reviewing the health records of assigned clients. The nurse plans care knowing that which client is at risk for fluid volume deficit?
    1. The client with cirrhosis
    2. The client with a colostomy
    3. The client with decreased kidney function
    4. The client with congestive heart failure (CHF)

41. A nurse is caring for a client who has been taking diuretics on a long-term basis. A fluid volume deficit is suspected. Which finding would be noted in the client with this condition?
    1. Gurgling respirations
    2. Increased blood pressure

3. Decreased hematocrit level
4. Increased specific gravity of the urine

42. A nurse reviews electrolyte values and notes a sodium level of 130 mEq/L. The nurse understands that this sodium level would be noted in a client with which condition?
    1. The client with watery diarrhea
    2. The client with diabetes insipidus
    3. The client with an inadequate daily water intake
    4. The client with the syndrome of inappropriate secretion of antidiuretic hormone (SIADH)

43. A nurse is caring for a client with leukemia and notes that the client has poor skin turgor and flat neck and hand veins. The nurse suspects hyponatremia. What additional signs would the nurse expect to note in this client if hyponatremia is present?
    1. Intense thirst
    2. Slow bounding pulse
    3. Dry mucous membranes
    4. Postural blood pressure changes

44. A nurse is caring for a client with a diagnosis of hyperparathyroidism. Laboratory studies are performed, and the serum calcium level is 12.0 mg/dL. On the basis of this laboratory value, the nurse takes which action?
    1. Documents the value in the client's record
    2. Informs the registered nurse of the laboratory value
    3. Places the laboratory result form in the client's record
    4. Reassures the client that the laboratory result is normal

45. A nurse reviews the client's serum calcium level and notes that the level is 8.0 mg/dL. The nurse understands that which condition would cause this serum calcium level?
    1. Renal disease
    2. Prolonged bedrest
    3. Hyperparathyroidism
    4. Excessive ingestion of vitamin D

46. A nurse is caring for a client with a suspected diagnosis of hypercalcemia. Which of the following signs would be an indication of this diagnosis?
    1. Twitching
    2. Positive Trousseau's sign
    3. Hyperactive bowel sounds
    4. Generalized muscle weakness

47. A nurse is instructing a client on how to decrease the intake of calcium in the diet. The nurse tells the client that which food item contains the least amount of calcium?
    1. Milk
    2. Butter
    3. Spinach
    4. Collard greens

48. A nurse is caring for a client with hyperparathyroidism and notes that the client's serum calcium level is 13 mg/dL. Which medication would the nurse prepare to administer as prescribed to the client?
    1. Calcium chloride
    2. Calcium gluconate
    3. Calcitonin (Miacalcin)
    4. Large doses of vitamin D
49. A nurse is instructing a client on how to decrease the intake of potassium in the diet. The nurse tells the client that which food contains the least amount of potassium?
    1. Lettuce
    2. Potatoes
    3. Apricots
    4. Avocados
50. The nurse is caring for a client with renal failure. The laboratory results reveal a magnesium level of 3.6 mg/dL. Which of the following signs would the nurse expect to note in the client based on this magnesium level?
    1. Twitching
    2. Irritability
    3. Hyperactive reflexes
    4. Loss of deep tendon reflexes
51. The nurse reviews the client's serum phosphorus level and notes that the level is 2.0 mg/dL. The

nurse understands that which condition caused this serum phosphorus level?
    1. Alcoholism
    2. Chemotherapy
    3. Hypoparathyroidism
    4. Vitamin D intoxication
52. A nurse is instructing a client regarding how to decrease the intake of phosphorus in the diet. The nurse tells the client that which food item contains the least amount of phosphorus?
    1. Fish
    2. Oranges
    3. Almonds
    4. Whole-grain bread

ALTERNATE ITEM FORMAT: MULTIPLE RESPONSE

53. The nurse is told in report that the client has a positive Chvostek's sign. What data would the nurse expect to note during the data collection? Select all that apply.
    ☐ 1. Coma
    ☑ 2. Tetany
    ☑ 3. Diarrhea
    ☑ 4. Possible seizure activity
    ☐ 5. Hypoactive bowel sounds
    ☑ 6. A positive Trousseau's sign

ANSWERS

34. 4
Rationale: Findings associated with fluid volume excess include cough, dyspnea, crackles, tachypnea, tachycardia, an elevated blood pressure, a bounding pulse, an elevated central venous pressure, weight gain, edema, neck and hand vein distention, an altered level of consciousness, and a decreased hematocrit level.
Test-Taking Strategy: Use the process of elimination. Note that options 1, 2, and 3 are comparable or alike. Each of these signs relates to a decrease in fluid volume. Option 4 reflects an increase. If you had difficulty with this question, review the signs noted in clients with fluid volume excess.
Level of Cognitive Ability: Comprehension
Client Needs: Physiological Integrity
Integrated Process: Nursing Process/Data Collection
Content Area: Fundamental Skills
References: Ignatavicius, D., & Workman, M. (2006). *Medical-surgical nursing: Critical thinking for collaborative care* (5th ed., p. 1375). Philadelphia: Saunders.
Linton, A., & Maebius, N. (2007). *Introduction to medical-surgical nursing* (4th ed., p. 193). Philadelphia: Saunders.

35. 4
Rationale: Potassium-rich gastrointestinal (GI) fluids are lost through GI suction, which places the client at risk for hypokalemia. The client with renal disease, Addison's disease, and metabolic acidosis is at risk for hyperkalemia.
Test-Taking Strategy: Read the question carefully, and note that it asks for the client who is at risk for hypokalemia.

Read each option, and think about the electrolyte loss that can occur with each condition. Option 4 clearly identifies a loss of body fluid. If you had difficulty with this question, review the causes of hypokalemia.
Level of Cognitive Ability: Analysis
Client Needs: Physiological Integrity
Integrated Process: Nursing Process/Planning
Content Area: Fundamental Skills
Reference: Linton, A., & Maebius, N. (2007). *Introduction to medical-surgical nursing* (4th ed., pp. 194-195). Philadelphia: Saunders.

36. 2
Rationale: A serum potassium level that exceeds 5.1 mEq/L is indicative of hyperkalemia. Clients who experience the cellular shifting of potassium, as in the early stages of massive cell destruction (i.e., with trauma, burns, sepsis, or metabolic or respiratory acidosis), are at risk for hyperkalemia. The client with Cushing's syndrome or colitis and the client who has been overusing laxatives are at risk for hypokalemia.
Test-Taking Strategy: Use the process of elimination, and eliminate options 1 and 4 first, because they are comparable or alike and reflect a gastrointestinal loss. From the remaining options, recalling that cell destruction causes potassium shifts will direct you to the correct option. Remember that Cushing's syndrome presents a risk for hypokalemia and that Addison's disease presents a risk for hyperkalemia. Review the causes of hyperkalemia if you had difficulty with this question.

Level of Cognitive Ability: Analysis
Client Needs: Physiological Integrity
Integrated Process: Nursing Process/Data Collection
Content Area: Fundamental Skills
References: Chernecky, C., & Berger, B. (2008). *Laboratory tests and diagnostic procedures* (5th ed., pp 891-893). Philadelphia: Saunders.
Linton, A., & Maebius, N. (2007). *Introduction to medical-surgical nursing* (4th ed., p. 196). Philadelphia: Saunders.

37. 4
Rationale: A serum potassium level of 5.4 mEq/L is indicative of hyperkalemia. Cardiac changes include a wide, flat P wave; a prolonged PR interval; a widened QRS complex; narrow, peaked T waves; and a depressed ST segment.
Test-Taking Strategy: From the information in the question, you need to determine that this condition is a hyperkalemic one. From this point, it is necessary to know the cardiac changes that are expected when hyperkalemia exists. Review these cardiac changes if you had difficulty with this question.
Level of Cognitive Ability: Analysis
Client Needs: Physiological Integrity
Integrated Process: Nursing Process/Data Collection
Content Area: Fundamental Skills
References: Linton, A., & Maebius, N. (2007). *Introduction to medical-surgical nursing* (4th ed., p. 196). Philadelphia: Saunders.
Pagana, K., & Pagana, T. (2005). *Mosby's diagnostic and laboratory test reference* (7th ed., p. 733). St. Louis: Mosby.

38. 1
Rationale: Sensible losses are those that the person is aware of, such as those that occur through wound drainage, GI tract losses, and urination. Insensible losses may occur without the person's awareness. Insensible losses occur daily through the skin and the lungs.
Test-Taking Strategy: Note that the subject of the question is insensible fluid loss. Use the process of elimination, and note that options 2, 3, and 4 are comparable or alike. These types of losses can be measured for accurate output. Fluid loss through the skin cannot be accurately measured, only approximated. If you had difficulty with this question, review the differences between sensible and insensible fluid loss.
Level of Cognitive Ability: Comprehension
Client Needs: Physiological Integrity
Integrated Process: Nursing Process/Data Collection
Content Area: Fundamental Skills
References: Black, J., & Hawks, J. (2005). *Medical-surgical nursing: Clinical management for positive outcomes* (7th ed., p. 230). Philadelphia: Saunders.
Linton, A., & Maebius, N. (2007). *Introduction to medical-surgical nursing* (4th ed., p. 188). Philadelphia: Saunders.

39. 4
Rationale: Fluid that shifts into the interstitial spaces and remains there is referred to as *third-space fluid*. Common sites for third-spacing include the abdomen, pleural cavity, peritoneal cavity, and pericardial sac. Third-space fluid is physiologically useless, because it does not circulate to provide nutrients for the cells. Risk factors include liver or kidney disease, major trauma, burns, sepsis, wound healing, major surgery, malignancy, malabsorption syndrome, malnutrition, alcoholism, and older age.
Test-Taking Strategy: Note the strategic words "lowest risk." These words indicate a negative event query and ask you to select the client who is at least risk for third-spacing. Eliminate options 2 and 3 first, because it is likely that fluid balance disturbances will occur with these conditions. From the remaining options, sepsis is the option that is the most acute and therefore the most similar to options 2 and 3. Review the risk factors associated with third-spacing if you had difficulty with this question.
Level of Cognitive Ability: Analysis
Client Needs: Physiological Integrity
Integrated Process: Nursing Process/Planning
Content Area: Fundamental Skills
Reference: Black, J., & Hawks, J. (2005). *Medical-surgical nursing: Clinical management for positive outcomes* (7th ed., pp. 213-219). Philadelphia: Saunders.

40. 2
Rationale: Causes of a fluid volume deficit include vomiting, diarrhea, conditions that cause increased respirations or increased urinary output, insufficient intravenous fluid replacement, draining fistulas, ileostomy, and colostomy. A client with cirrhosis, CHF, or decreased kidney function is at risk for fluid volume excess.
Test-Taking Strategy: Read the question carefully, and note that it asks for the client who is at risk for a deficit. Read each option, and think about the fluid imbalance that can occur in each client. The clients presented in options 1, 3, and 4 retain fluid. The only condition that can cause a fluid volume deficit is the condition noted in option 2. If you had difficulty with this question, review the causes of fluid volume deficit.
Level of Cognitive Ability: Analysis
Client Needs: Physiological Integrity
Integrated Process: Nursing Process/Planning
Content Area: Fundamental Skills
Reference: Linton, A., & Maebius, N. (2007). *Introduction to medical-surgical nursing* (4th ed., pp. 191, 399). Philadelphia: Saunders.

41. 4
Rationale: Findings in a client with a fluid volume deficit include increased respirations and heart rate, decreased central venous pressure, weight loss, poor skin turgor, dry mucous membranes, decreased urine volume, increased specific gravity of the urine, dark-colored and odorous urine, an increased hematocrit level, and an altered level of consciousness. The signs in options 1, 2, and 3 are seen in a client with fluid volume excess.
Test-Taking Strategy: Use the process of elimination. Eliminate options 1 and 2 first. Gurgling respirations and increased blood pressure are noted in clients with fluid volume excess. Remember that the specific gravity of urine is increased in a client with a fluid volume deficit. If you had difficulty with this question, review the findings noted in a client with a fluid volume deficit.
Level of Cognitive Ability: Comprehension
Client Needs: Physiological Integrity

Integrated Process: Nursing Process/Data Collection
Content Area: Fundamental Skills
Reference: Linton, A., & Maebius, N. (2007). *Introduction to medical-surgical nursing* (4th ed, p. 192). Philadelphia: Saunders.

42. 4
Rationale: Hyponatremia is a serum sodium level less than 135 mEq/L. Hyponatremia can result secondary to SIADH. The client with an inadequate daily water intake, watery diarrhea, or diabetes insipidus is at risk for hypernatremia.
Test-Taking Strategy: Knowledge regarding the normal sodium level and the causes of hyponatremia are required to answer the question. Remember that hyponatremia can result secondary to SIADH. Review the causes of hyponatremia if you had difficulty with this question.
Level of Cognitive Ability: Analysis
Client Needs: Physiological Integrity
Integrated Process: Nursing Process/Data Collection
Content Area: Fundamental Skills
References: Ignatavicius, D., & Workman, M. (2006). *Medical-surgical nursing: Critical thinking for collaborative care* (5th ed., pp. 1469-1470). Philadelphia: Saunders.
Linton, A., & Maebius, N. (2007). *Introduction to medical-surgical nursing* (4th ed., pp. 192-193). Philadelphia: Saunders.

43. 4
Rationale: Postural blood pressure changes occur in the client with hyponatremia. Dry mucous membranes and intense thirst are seen in clients with hypernatremia. A slow, bounding pulse is not indicative of hyponatremia. In a client with hyponatremia, a rapid thready pulse is noted.
Test-Taking Strategy: Use the process of elimination, and note the information provided in the question. Eliminate options 1 and 3 first, because they are comparable or alike (a client with dry mucous membranes is likely to have intense thirst). From the remaining options, it is necessary to recall the signs of hyponatremia. Review the signs associated with hyponatremia if you had difficulty with this question.
Level of Cognitive Ability: Analysis
Client Needs: Physiological Integrity
Integrated Process: Nursing Process/Data Collection
Content Area: Fundamental Skills
Reference: Linton, A., & Maebius, N. (2007). *Introduction to medical-surgical nursing* (4th ed., pp. 192-193). Philadelphia: Saunders.

44. 2
Rationale: The normal serum calcium level ranges from 8.6 to 10.0 mg/dL. The client is experiencing hypercalcemia, and the nurse would inform the registered nurse of the laboratory value. Because the client is experiencing hypercalcemia, options 1, 3, and 4 are incorrect.
Test-Taking Strategy: Focus on the laboratory value in the question to determine that the client is experiencing hypercalcemia. Note that options 1, 3, and 4 are comparable or alike and indicate that no action would be taken to report the value. Review the normal calcium level if you had difficulty with this question.
Level of Cognitive Ability: Application
Client Needs: Physiological Integrity

Integrated Process: Nursing Process/Implementation
Content Area: Fundamental Skills
Reference: Linton, A., & Maebius, N. (2007). *Introduction to medical-surgical nursing* (4th ed., p 393). Philadelphia: Saunders.

45. 2
Rationale: The normal serum calcium level is 8.6 to 10.0 mg/dL. A client with a serum calcium level of 8.0 mg/dL is experiencing hypocalcemia. The excessive ingestion of vitamin D, renal disease, and hyperparathyroidism are causative factors associated with hypercalcemia. Although immobilization can initially cause hypercalcemia, the long-term effect of prolonged bedrest is hypocalcemia.
Test-Taking Strategy: Knowledge regarding the normal serum calcium level will assist you with determining that the client is experiencing hypocalcemia. This should help you to eliminate option 4. Recalling the causative factors associated with hypocalcemia is necessary to select the correct option from those remaining. Remember that the long-term effect of prolonged bedrest is hypocalcemia. If you had difficulty with the question, review the causative factors associated with hypocalcemia.
Level of Cognitive Ability: Analysis
Client Needs: Physiological Integrity
Integrated Process: Nursing Process/Data Collection
Content Area: Fundamental Skills
Reference: Christensen, B., & Kockrow, E. (2006). *Foundations of nursing* (5th ed., p. 675). St. Louis: Mosby.

46. 4
Rationale: Generalized muscle weakness is seen in clients with hypercalcemia. Options 1, 2, and 3 identify signs of hypocalcemia.
Test-Taking Strategy: Use the process of elimination. Note that options 1, 2, and 3 are comparable or alike, because they all reflect a hyperactivity of body systems. The option that is different is option 4. Review the signs of hypercalcemia if you had difficulty with this question.
Level of Cognitive Ability: Analysis
Client Needs: Physiological Integrity
Integrated Process: Nursing Process/Data Collection
Content Area: Fundamental Skills
Reference: Monahan, F., Marek, J., Neighbors, M., & Green, C., (2007). *Phipps' medical-surgical nursing: Health and illness perspectives* (8th ed., pp. 380-381). St. Louis: Mosby.

47. 2
Rationale: Butter comes from milk fat and does not contain significant amounts of calcium. Milk, spinach, and collard greens are calcium-containing foods and should be avoided by the client on a calcium-restricted diet.
Test-Taking Strategy: Note the strategic words "least amount." These words indicate a negative event query and ask you to select the item that is lowest in calcium. Option 1 can be easily eliminated first. Eliminate options 3 and 4 next, because they are comparable or alike. Review the foods that are high and low in calcium if you had difficulty with this question.
Level of Cognitive Ability: Application
Client Needs: Health Promotion and Maintenance

Integrated Process: Teaching and Learning
Content Area: Fundamental Skills
Reference: Schlenker, E. & Long, S. (2007). *Williams' essentials of nutrition & diet therapy* (9th ed., pp. 147-152). St. Louis: Mosby.

48. **3**
Rationale: The normal serum calcium level is 8.6 to 10.0 mg/dL. This client is experiencing hypercalcemia. Calcium gluconate and calcium chloride are medications used for the treatment of tetany, which occurs as a result of acute hypocalcemia. In hypercalcemia, large doses of vitamin D need to be avoided. Calcitonin, a thyroid hormone, decreases the plasma calcium level by inhibiting bone resorption and lowering the serum calcium concentration.
Test-Taking Strategy: Recalling the normal serum calcium level will assist you with determining that the client is experiencing hypercalcemia. With this knowledge, you can easily eliminate options 1 and 2, because you would not administer medication that adds calcium to the body. Remembering that excessive vitamin D is a causative factor of hypercalcemia will assist you with eliminating option 4. If you had difficulty with this question, review the treatment of hypercalcemia.
Level of Cognitive Ability: Application
Client Needs: Physiological Integrity
Integrated Process: Nursing Process/Planning
Content Area: Pharmacology
Reference: Hodgson, B., & Kizior, R. (2008). *Saunders nursing drug handbook 2008* (p. 173). Philadelphia: Saunders.

49. **1**
Rationale: Lettuce contains less than 100 mg of potassium. Potatoes, apricots, and avocados are potassium-containing foods and should be avoided by the client on a potassium-restricted diet.
Test-Taking Strategy: Note the strategic words "least amount." These words indicate a negative event query and ask you to select the item that is lowest in potassium. Recalling the foods high in potassium will direct you to option 1. Review the foods that are high in potassium if you had difficulty with this question.
Level of Cognitive Ability: Application
Client Needs: Health Promotion and Maintenance
Integrated Process: Teaching and Learning
Content Area: Fundamental Skills
Reference: Schlenker, E., & Long, S. (2007). *Williams' essentials of nutrition & diet therapy* (9th ed., pp. 159, 162). St. Louis: Mosby.

50. **4**
Rationale: The normal magnesium level is 1.6 to 2.6 mg/dL. A client with a magnesium level of 3.6 mg/dL is experiencing hypermagnesemia. Options 1, 2, and 3 would be noted in a client with hypomagnesemia.
Test-Taking Strategy: Knowledge regarding the normal magnesium level and the associated signs related to an imbalance are helpful for answering this question. Use the process of elimination, and note that options 1, 2, and 3 are comparable or alike, because they reflect neurological excitability. Review

the signs of magnesium imbalance if you had difficulty with this question.
Level of Cognitive Ability: Analysis
Client Needs: Physiological Integrity
Integrated Process: Nursing Process/Data Collection
Content Area: Fundamental Skills
Reference: Linton, A., & Maebius, N. (2007), *Introduction to medical-surgical nursing* (4th ed., p. 196). Philadelphia: Saunders.

51. **1**
Rationale: The normal serum phosphorus level is 2.7 to 4.5 mg/dL. The client in this question is experiencing hypophosphatemia. Causative factors relate to decreased nutritional intake and malnutrition. A poor nutritional state is associated with alcoholism. Hypoparathyroidism, chemotherapy, and vitamin D intoxication are causative factors of hyperphosphatemia.
Test-Taking Strategy: Knowledge regarding the normal phosphorus level is required to determine the condition that this client is experiencing. From this point, it is necessary to know the causes of hypophosphatemia. Remember that causative factors relate to decreased nutritional intake and malnutrition. Review the causative factors associated with hypophosphatemia if you had difficulty with this question.
Level of Cognitive Ability: Analysis
Client Needs: Physiological Integrity
Integrated Process: Nursing Process/Data Collection
Content Area: Fundamental Skills
References: Chernecky, C., & Berger, B. (2008). *Laboratory tests and diagnostic procedures* (5th ed., pp. 876-877). Philadelphia: Saunders.
Linton, A., & Maebius, N. (2007). *Introduction to medical-surgical nursing* (4th ed., p. 124). Philadelphia: Saunders.

52. **2**
Rationale: An orange contains the least amount of phosphorus. Foods high in phosphorus include fish, pork, beef, chicken, organ meats, nuts, whole-grain breads, and cereals.
Test-Taking Strategy: Note the strategic words "least amount." These words indicate a negative event query and ask you to select the food that contains the least amount of phosphorus. Recalling the foods that are high and low in phosphorus will direct you to option 2. Review these foods if you had difficulty with this question.
Level of Cognitive Ability: Application
Client Needs: Health Promotion and Maintenance
Integrated Process: Teaching and Learning
Content Area: Fundamental Skills
Reference: Schlenker, E., & Long, S. (2007). *Williams' essentials of nutrition & diet therapy* (9th ed., pp. 154, 161). St. Louis: Mosby.

ALTERNATE ITEM FORMAT: MULTIPLE RESPONSE

53. **2, 3, 4, 6**
Rationale: A positive Chvostek's sign is indicative of hypocalcemia. Other signs and symptoms include tachycardia,

hypotension, paresthesias, twitching, cramps, tetany, a positive Trousseau's sign, diarrhea, seizures, hyperactive bowel sounds, and a prolonged QT interval.

Test-Taking Strategy: Focus on the data in the question, and recall that a positive Chvostek's sign indicates hypocalcemia. Next, recalling the signs of hypocalcemia will direct you to the correct options. Review the signs and symptoms of calcium imbalances if you had difficulty with this question.

Level of Cognitive Ability: Analysis
Client Needs: Physiological Integrity
Integrated Process: Nursing Process/Data Collection
Content Area: Fundamental Skills
Reference: Christensen, B., & Kockrow, E. (2006). *Foundations of nursing* (5th ed.. p. 675). St. Louis: Mosby.

REFERENCES

Black, J., & Hawks, J. (2005). *Medical-surgical nursing: Clinical management for positive outcomes* (7th ed.). Philadelphia: Saunders.

Chernecky, C., & Berger, B. (2008). *Laboratory tests and diagnostic procedures* (5th ed.). Philadelphia: Saunders.

Christensen, B., & Kochrow, E. (2006). *Foundations of nursing* (5th ed.). St. Louis: Mosby.

Hodgson, B., & Kizior, R. (2008). *Saunders nursing drug handbook 2008.* Philadelphia: Saunders.

Ignatavicius, D., & Workman, M. (2006). *Medical-surgical nursing: Critical thinking for collaborative care* (5th ed.). Philadelphia: Saunders.

Lilley, L., Harrington, S., & Snyder, J. (2007). *Pharmacology and the nursing process* (5th ed.). St. Louis: Mosby.

Linton, A., & Maebius, N. (2007). *Introduction to medical-surgical nursing* (4th ed.). Philadelphia: Saunders.

National Council of State Boards of Nursing (Eds.) (2008). *2008 Detailed Test Plan for the NCLEX-PN® Examination, National Council of State Boards of Nursing.* Chicago: Author.

National Council of State Boards of Nursing. *NCSBN home page.* www.ncsbn.org. Accessed June 9, 2008.

Pagana, K., & Pagana, T. (2005). *Mosby's diagnostic and laboratory test reference* (7th ed.). St. Louis: Mosby.

Monahan, F., Marek, J., Neighbors, M., & Green, C. (2007). *Phipps' medical-surgical nursing: Health and illness perspectives* (8th ed.). St. Louis: Mosby.

Schlenker, E., & Long, S. (2007). *Williams' essentials of nutrition & diet therapy* (9th ed.). St. Louis: Mosby.

Acid-Base Balance

PYRAMID TERMS

Allen's test A test for determining collateral circulation to the hand by evaluating the patency of the radial and ulnar arteries.

metabolic acidosis The total concentration of buffer base is lower than normal, with a relative increase in the hydrogen ion concentration. It results from losing buffer bases or retaining too much acid without sufficient base. It occurs as a result of conditions such as renal failure and diabetic ketoacidosis, the production of lactic acid, and the ingestion of toxins such as aspirin.

metabolic alkalosis A deficit or loss of hydrogen ions or acids or an excess of base (bicarbonate). It results from an accumulation of base or a loss of acid without a comparable loss of base in the body fluids. It is caused by conditions that result in hypovolemia, the loss of gastric fluid, excessive bicarbonate intake, massive transfusion of whole blood, and hyperaldosteronism.

respiratory acidosis The total concentration of buffer base is lower than normal, with a relative increase in hydrogen ion concentration; thus, a greater number of hydrogen ions are circulating in the blood than can be absorbed by the buffer system. It is caused by primary defects in the function of the lungs or by changes in normal respiratory patterns as a result of secondary problems. Any condition that causes an obstruction of the airway or depresses respiratory status can cause respiratory acidosis.

respiratory alkalosis A deficit of carbonic acid or a decrease in hydrogen ion concentration; it results from an accumulation of base or a loss of acid without a comparable loss of base in the body fluids. It is caused by conditions that cause overstimulation of the respiratory status.

▲ PYRAMID TO SUCCESS

Acid-base imbalance is a content area that is sometimes viewed as difficult to comprehend. It is important to understand the description of each imbalance and to then review the causes of each disorder to correlate the pathophysiology with each cause. At this point, the signs and symptoms related to each disorder and the treatment associated with the clinical manifestations can be noted. The maintenance of a patent airway is a priority. The nurse also needs to monitor the vital signs, cardiovascular status, neurological status, intake and output, laboratory values, and arterial blood gas values. Remember that safety and seizure precautions

may need to be initiated. The Integrated Processes addressed in this chapter are Clinical Problem-Solving Process (Nursing Process), Caring, Communication and Documentation, and Teaching and Learning.

CLIENT NEEDS ▲

Safe and Effective Care Environment

Establishing priorities

Maintaining medical and surgical asepsis

Maintaining standard, transmission-based, and other precautions

Obtaining informed consent for invasive procedures

Preventing accidents

Providing safety for the client during the implementation of various treatments for the acid-base imbalance

Health Promotion and Maintenance

Identifying clients at risk for an acid-base imbalance

Performing data-collection techniques

Teaching the client and family about the prevention, early detection, and treatment measures of health disorders

Psychosocial Integrity

Identifying support systems

Monitoring for sensory and perceptual alterations

Providing emotional support to the client and family

Physiological Integrity

Administering and monitoring medications, intravenous fluids, and other therapeutic interventions

Assisting with diagnostic tests

Monitoring for alterations in body systems

Monitoring for changes in status and complications

Monitoring for the expected effects of pharmacological and parenteral therapies

Monitoring laboratory values

Providing wound care when blood is obtained for an arterial blood gas study

Reducing the likelihood that an acid-base imbalance will occur

I. HYDROGEN IONS, ACIDS, AND BASES
A. Hydrogen (H^+) ions
　1. Vital to life, because H^+ ions determines the pH of the body, which must be maintained in a narrow range
　2. Expressed as pH; the pH scale is determined by the number of H^+ ions and goes from 1 to 14; 7 is considered neutral
　3. The number of H^+ ions in the body fluid determines whether it is acid (acidic), alkaline (alkalosis), or neutral
　4. The pH of body fluid is normally alkaline (between 7.35 and 7.45)
B. Acids
　1. Produced as end products of metabolism
　2. Contain H^+ ions
　3. Are H^+ ion donors; they give up H^+ ions to neutralize or decrease the strength of an acid or to form a weaker base
C. Bases
　1. Contain no H^+ ions
　2. Are H^+ ion acceptors; they accept H^+ ions from acids to neutralize or decrease the strength of a base or to form a weaker acid
　3. Normal serum levels of bicarbonate (HCO_3^-) are 22 to 27 mEq/L

II. REGULATORY SYSTEMS FOR HYDROGEN CONCENTRATION IN THE BLOOD
A. Buffers
　1. The fastest-acting regulatory system
　2. Provide immediate protection against changes in H^+ ion concentration in the extracellular fluid (i.e., absorb or release H^+ ions as needed)
　3. Serve as a transport mechanism that carries excess H^+ ions to the lungs
　4. After the primary buffer systems react, they are consumed, and this leaves the body less able to withstand further stress until they are replaced
B. Primary buffer systems in extracellular fluid
　1. Hemoglobin system
　　a. In the red blood cells
　　b. Maintains the acid-base balance by a process called *chloride shift*
　　c. Chloride shifts in and out of the red blood cells in response to the levels of oxygen (O_2) and HCO_3^- in the blood
　2. Plasma proteins system
　　a. Functions in conjunction with the liver to vary the amount of H^+ ions in the chemical structure of protein
　　b. Plasma proteins have the ability to attract or release H^+ ions as the body needs them

　3. Carbonic acid–HCO_3^- system
　　a. Maintains a pH of 7.4, with a ratio of 20 parts HCO_3^- to 1 part carbonic acid (20:1)
　　b. This 20:1 ratio determines the concentration of H^+ ions in body fluid
　　c. The carbonic acid concentration is controlled by the excretion of carbon dioxide (CO_2) by the lungs; the rate and depth of respirations change in response to CO_2 levels
　　d. HCO_3^- concentration is controlled by the kidneys, which selectively retain or secrete HCO_3^- in response to body needs
　4. Phosphate buffer system
　　a. Present in the cells and body fluids
　　b. Especially active in the kidneys
　　c. Acts like HCO_3^- and clears excess H^+
C. Lungs
　1. The body's second defense; interacts with the buffer system to maintain the acid-base balance
　2. In acidosis, the pH goes down and the respiratory rate and depth go up in an attempt to blow off acids; the carbonic acid created by the neutralizing action of HCO_3^- can be carried to the lungs, where it is reduced to CO_2 and water and exhaled; thus, H^+ ions are inactivated
　3. In alkalosis, the pH goes up and the respiratory rate and depth go down; CO_2 is retained, and the carbonic acid concentration increases to neutralize and decrease the strength of excess HCO_3^-
　4. The action of the lungs is reversible for controlling an excess or deficit
　5. The lungs can hold H^+ ions until the deficit is corrected; they can also inactivate H^+ ions, changing the ions to water molecules to be exhaled along with CO_2, thereby correcting the excess
　6. The lungs can inactivate only H^+ ions carried by carbonic acid; excess H^+ ions created by other problems must be excreted by the kidneys
D. Kidneys
　1. The ultimate correction of acid-base disturbances is dependent on the kidneys, although the renal excretion of acids and alkali (bases) occurs more slowly
　2. Compensation requires a few hours to several days; however, it is a more thorough and selective process than that of other regulators
　3. In acidosis, the pH goes down; excess H^+ ions are secreted into the tubules, where they combine with buffers for excretion in the urine
　4. In alkalosis, the pH goes up; HCO_3^- ions move into the tubules, combine with sodium, and are excreted in the urine
　5. Selective regulation of HCO_3^- in the kidneys
　　a. The kidneys restore HCO_3^- by releasing H^+ ions and holding onto HCO_3^- ions

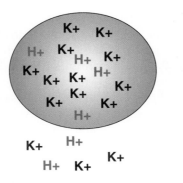 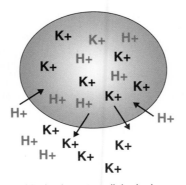 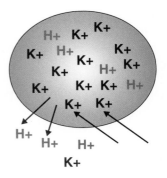

Under normal conditions, the intracellular potassium content is much greater than that of the extracellular fluid. The concentration of hydrogen ions is low in both compartments.

In acidosis, the extracellular hydrogen ion content increases, and the hydrogen ions move into the intracellular fluid. To keep the intracellular fluid electrically neutral, an equal number of potassium ions leave the cell, creating a relative hyperkalemia.

In alkalosis, more hydrogen ions are present in the intracellular fluid than in the extracellular fluid. Hydrogen ions move from the intracellular fluid into the extracellular fluid. To keep the intracellular fluid electrically neutral, potassium ions move from the extracellular fluid into the intracellular fluid, creating a relative hypokalemia.

FIG. 10-1 Movement of potassium in response to changes in the extracellular fluid hydrogen ion concentration. (From Ignatavicius, D., & Workman, M. [2006]. *Medical-surgical nursing: Critical thinking for collaborative care* [5th ed., p. 286]. Philadelphia: Saunders. © M. Linda Workman. All rights reserved.)

b. Extra H^+ ions are excreted in the urine in the form of phosphoric acid
c. The alteration of certain amino acids in the renal tubules results in the diffusion of ammonia into the kidneys; the ammonia combines with extra H^+ ions and is excreted into the urine
E. Potassium (Figure 10-1)
   1. Plays an exchange role in maintaining the acid-base balance
   2. The body changes the potassium (K) level by drawing H^+ ions into the cell or by pushing them out of the cell
   3. In acidosis, the body protects itself from the acid state by moving H^+ ions into the cell; therefore, K moves out to make room for H^+ ions; the K serum level increases
   4. In alkalosis, the cells release H^+ ions into the blood in an attempt to increase the acidity of the blood and to combat the alkalinity; the K moves into the cells, and the K serum level decreases
III. RESPIRATORY ACIDOSIS
A. Description: The total concentration of buffer base is lower than normal, with a relative increase in H^+ ion concentration; thus, a greater number of H^+ ions are circulating in the blood than can be absorbed by the buffer system
B. Causes (Box 10-1)
   1. Caused by primary defects in the function of the lungs or by changes in normal respiratory patterns from secondary problems

BOX 10-1   **Causes of Respiratory Acidosis**

- Asthma
- Atelectasis
- Brain trauma
- Bronchiectasis
- Bronchitis
- Central nervous system depression
- Emphysema
- Hypoventilation
- Medications
- Pneumonia
- Pulmonary edema
- Respiratory failure or depression

   2. Remember that any condition that causes an obstruction of the airway or that depresses respiratory status can cause **respiratory acidosis**
C. Data collection
   1. In an attempt to compensate, the respiratory rate and depth increase
   2. The pH is less than 7.35, and the partial pressure of CO_2 (Pco_2) is greater than 45 mm Hg
   3. Headache
   4. Restlessness
   5. Mental status changes, such as drowsiness and confusion
   6. Visual disturbances
   7. Diaphoresis
   8. Cyanosis as the hypoxia becomes more acute
   9. Hyperkalemia

BOX 10-2   Causes of Respiratory Alkalosis

- Anxiety
- Fever
- Hyperventilation
- Hypoxia
- Hysteria
- Overventilation by mechanical ventilators
- Pain

BOX 10-3   Causes of Metabolic Acidosis

- Diabetes mellitus or diabetic ketoacidosis
- Excessive ingestion of acetylsalicylic acid (aspirin)
- Gastrointestinal fistulas
- High-fat diet
- Insufficient metabolism of carbohydrates
- Lactic acidosis
- Malnutrition
- Renal insufficiency or renal failure
- Severe diarrhea
- Starvation

10. Rapid, irregular pulse
11. Dysrhythmias leading to ventricular fibrillation

D. Interventions
1. Maintain a patent airway
2. Monitor for signs of respiratory distress
3. Administer O_2 as prescribed
4. Place the client in semi-Fowler's position unless contraindicated
5. Encourage and assist the client to turn, cough, and deep breathe
6. Prepare to administer chest physiotherapy and postural drainage as prescribed
7. Encourage hydration to thin secretions unless excess fluid intake is contraindicated
8. Suction the client as necessary
9. Monitor electrolyte values
10. Avoid the use of tranquilizers, opioids, and sedatives/hypnotics, because they further depress respirations
11. Administer antibiotics for infection or other medications (e.g., bronchodilators, opioid antagonists) as prescribed

IV. RESPIRATORY ALKALOSIS
A. Description: A deficit of carbonic acid or a decrease in H^+ ion concentration; results from the accumulation of base or the loss of acid without a comparable loss of base in the body fluids
B. Causes: Conditions that cause overstimulation of the respiratory status (Box 10-2)
C. Data collection
1. Initially hyperventilation and respiratory stimulation cause abnormal rapid and deep respirations (tachypnea); in an attempt to compensate, the respiratory rate and depth then decrease
2. The pH is less than 7.45, and the P_{CO_2} is less than 35 mm Hg
3. Headache
4. Lightheadedness, vertigo
5. Mental status changes
6. Paresthesias, such as tingling of the fingers and toes
7. Hypokalemia, hypocalcemia
8. Tetany, convulsions
D. Interventions
1. Maintain a patent airway
2. Provide emotional support and reassurance to the client

3. Encourage appropriate breathing patterns
4. Assist with breathing techniques and breathing aids as prescribed
   a. Voluntary holding of breath or slowed breathing
   b. Rebreathing exhaled CO_2 by methods such as using a paper bag or a rebreathing mask as prescribed
5. Provide cautious care with ventilator clients so that they are not forced to take breaths too deeply or rapidly
6. Monitor electrolyte values, particularly K and calcium levels
7. Administer medications (antianxiety or antipyretic) as prescribed
8. Prepare to assist with administering calcium gluconate for tetany as prescribed

V. METABOLIC ACIDOSIS
A. Description: The total concentration of buffer base is lower than normal, with a relative increase in the H^+ ion concentration; this occurs as a result of losing buffer bases or retaining too much acid without sufficient base
B. Causes (Box 10-3)
1. Diabetes mellitus–diabetic ketoacidosis: An insufficient supply of insulin causes increased fat metabolism, which leads to an excess accumulation of ketones or other acids; HCO_3^- then ends up being depleted
2. Renal insufficiency or failure
   a. Increased waste products of protein metabolism are retained
   b. Excessive acids build up, and HCO_3^- cannot maintain the acid-base balance
3. Insufficient metabolism of carbohydrates: When an insufficient supply of O_2 is available for the proper burning of carbohydrates, the lactic acid concentration increases, and lactic acidosis results
4. Excessive ingestion of acetylsalicylic acid (aspirin): Causes an increase in the H^+ ion concentration
5. Severe diarrhea: Intestinal and pancreatic secretions are normally alkaline; therefore, excessive loss of base leads to acidosis

6. Malnutrition/starvation: Improper metabolism of nutrients causes fat catabolism, which leads to an excess buildup of ketones and acids
7. High-fat diet: A high intake of fat causes the waste products of fat metabolism to be accumulated much too rapidly, which leads to a buildup of ketones and acids

C. Data collection
1. In an attempt to blow off the extra CO_2 and compensate for the acidosis, hyperpnea with Kussmaul's respirations (deep and fast) occurs
2. The pH is less than 7.35, and the HCO_3^- ion level is less than 22 mEq/L
3. Headache
4. Nausea, vomiting, diarrhea
5. Fruity-smelling breath as a result of improper fat metabolism
6. Central nervous system (CNS) depression: mental dullness, drowsiness, stupor, coma
7. Hypotension
8. Hyperkalemia

D. Interventions
1. Based on the cause of the acidosis
2. Maintain a patent airway
3. Assess the level of consciousness for CNS depression
4. Monitor intake and output, and assist with fluid and electrolyte replacement as prescribed
5. Initiate safety and seizure precautions
6. Monitor the serum K level closely; when acidosis is being treated, K will move back into the cell, and the serum K level will drop
7. Give medications as prescribed, depending on cause (e.g., antidiarrheals if diarrhea is the cause)

E. Interventions for diabetes mellitus–diabetic ketoacidosis
1. Insulin is given to hasten the movement of serum glucose into the cell, thereby decreasing the concurrent ketosis
2. When glucose is being properly metabolized, the body stops converting fats to glucose
3. Monitor for circulatory collapse caused by polyuria, which can result from the hyperglycemic state; polyuria or diuresis may lead to extracellular volume deficit

F. Interventions for renal failure
1. Dialysis may be used to remove protein and waste products, thereby decreasing the acidosis
2. A diet low in protein and high in calories will decrease the amount of protein waste products; this in turn will lessen the acidosis

VI. METABOLIC ALKALOSIS
A. Description: A deficit or loss of H^+ or acids or an excess of base (HCO_3^-); results from the accumulation of base or from the loss of acid without a comparable loss of base in the body fluids

B. Causes (Box 10-4)
C. Data collection
1. In an attempt to compensate, respiratory rate and depth decrease to conserve CO_2
2. Nausea, vomiting
3. Dizziness
4. Numbness and tingling in the extremities
5. Twitching in the extremities
6. Hypokalemia, hypocalcemia
7. Dysrhythmia: tachycardia

D. Interventions
1. Maintain a patent airway
2. Monitor K and calcium serum blood levels
3. Institute safety precautions
4. Prepare to administer medications as prescribed to promote the excretion of HCO_3^- by the kidneys
5. Prepare to replace K chloride as prescribed

VII. ARTERIAL BLOOD GASES (Box 10-5)
A. Description: Levels reflect the ability of the lungs to exchange O_2 and CO_2, the effectiveness of the kidneys for balancing the retention and elimination of HCO_3^-, and the effectiveness of the heart as a pump
B. Obtaining an arterial blood gas specimen
1. Obtain vital signs
2. Perform **Allen's test** to determine the presence of collateral circulation (Box 10-6)
3. Identify factors that may affect the accuracy of the results, such as changes in the O_2 settings on respiratory assistive devices, suctioning within the past 20 minutes, and client activities
4. Assist with the specimen draw by preparing a heparinized syringe
5. Provide emotional support to the client

BOX 10-4 **Causes of Metabolic Alkalosis**
- Diuretics
- Excessive vomiting or gastrointestinal suctioning
- Excessive intake of antacids
- Hyperaldosteronism
- Ingestion or parenteral injection of excess sodium bicarbonate
- Massive transfusion of whole blood

BOX 10-5 **Normal Blood Gas Values**
- pH: 7.35 to 7.45
- Pco_2: 35 to 45 mm Hg
- HCO_3^-: 22 to 27 mEq/L
- Po_2: 80 to 100 mm Hg

Po_2, Partial pressure of oxygen.

6. Apply pressure immediately to the puncture site for 5 minutes or for 10 minutes if the client is taking anticoagulants
7. Record the client's temperature and the type of supplemental O_2 that the client is receiving on the laboratory form
8. Appropriately label the specimen, and transport it on ice to the laboratory

C. Respiratory imbalances (Table 10-1)
1. Remember that the respiratory function indicator is the P_{CO_2}
2. In a respiratory imbalance, there is an opposite relationship between the pH and the P_{CO_2}: the pH will be up when the P_{CO_2} is down (alkalosis), or the pH will be down in the presence of an elevated P_{CO_2} (acidosis)
3. Remember that the pH is down in an acidotic condition and elevated in an alkalotic condition
4. Look at the pH and the P_{CO_2} to determine if the condition is a respiratory problem
5. **Respiratory acidosis**
   a. The pH is down
   b. The P_{CO_2} is up
6. **Respiratory alkalosis**
   a. The pH is up
   b. The P_{CO_2} is down

D. Metabolic imbalances (see Table 10-1)
1. Remember that the metabolic function indicator is the HCO_3^- ion

---

BOX 10-6   Performing Allen's Test

Apply direct pressure over the client's ulnar and radial arteries simultaneously.

While pressure is applied, ask the client to open and close the hand repeatedly; the hand should blanch.

Release pressure from the ulnar artery while still compressing the radial artery, and assess the color of the extremity distal to the pressure point.

If pinkness fails to return within 6 seconds, the ulnar artery is insufficient, which indicates that the radial artery should not be used for obtaining a blood specimen.

---

2. In a metabolic imbalance, you will find a corresponding relationship between the pH and the HCO_3^-: the pH will be up and the HCO_3^- will be up (alkalosis), or the pH will be down and the HCO_3^- will be down (acidosis)
3. Remember that the pH is down in an acidotic condition and elevated in an alkalotic condition
4. Look at the pH and the HCO_3^- concentration to determine if the condition is a metabolic problem
5. **Metabolic acidosis**
   a. The pH is down
   b. The HCO_3^- is down
6. **Metabolic alkalosis**
   a. The pH is up
   b. The HCO_3^- is up

E. Steps for analyzing arterial blood gas results (Box 10-7)

BOX 10-7   Analyzing Arterial Blood Gas Results

If you can remember the following pyramid points and steps, you will be able to analyze any blood gas report.

Pyramid Points

In acidosis, the pH is down.

In alkalosis, the pH is up.

The respiratory function indicator is the partial pressure of carbon dioxide (P_{CO_2}) value.

The metabolic function indicator is the bicarbonate (HCO_3^-) level.

Pyramid Steps

Look at the blood gas report.

Pyramid Step 1

Look at the pH. Is it up or down? If it is up, it reflects alkalosis. If it is down, it reflects acidosis.

Pyramid Step 2

Look at the P_{CO_2} level. Is it up or down? If it reflects an opposite relationship to the pH, then you know that the condition is a respiratory imbalance. If it does not reflect an opposite relationship to the pH, then move on to pyramid step 3.

Pyramid Step 3

TABLE 10-1   Acid-Base Imbalances: Significant Laboratory Value Changes That Normally Occur

Imbalance	pH	HCO_3^-	Pa_{O_2}	Pa_{CO_2}	K^+
Respiratory acidosis	Decreased	Increased	Decreased	Increased	Increased
Respiratory alkalosis	Increased	Decreased	Normal	Decreased	Decreased
Metabolic acidosis	Decreased	Decreased	Normal	Normal or decreased	Increased
Metabolic alkalosis	Increased	Increased	Normal	Normal or increased	Decreased

HCO_3^-, Bicarbonate; K^+, potassium; Pa_{O_2}, partial pressure of oxygen in arterial blood; Pa_{CO_2}, partial pressure of carbon dioxide in arterial blood.

PRACTICE QUESTIONS

🔘 More questions on the companion CD!

54. A client has the following laboratory values: a pH of 7.55, an HCO_3^- level of 22 mm Hg, and a P_{CO_2} of 30 mm Hg. What should the nurse do?
    1. Perform Allen's test.
    2. Prepare the client for dialysis.
    3. Administer insulin as ordered.
    4. Encourage the client to slow down breathing.

55. The nurse is told that the blood gas results indicate a pH of 7.55 and a P_{CO_2} of 30 mm Hg. The nurse determines that these results indicate:
    1. Metabolic acidosis
    2. Metabolic alkalosis
    3. Respiratory acidosis
    4. Respiratory alkalosis

56. A client is scheduled for blood to be drawn from the radial artery for an arterial blood gas (ABG) determination. A nurse assists with performing Allen's test before drawing the blood to determine the adequacy of the:
    1. Ulnar circulation
    2. Carotid circulation
    3. Femoral circulation
    4. Brachial circulation

57. A nurse is caring for a client with a nasogastric tube that is attached to low suction. The nurse monitors the client closely for which acid-base disorder that is most likely to occur in this situation?
    1. Metabolic acidosis
    2. Metabolic alkalosis   *[handwritten: vomitting & suctioning is alkalosis]*
    3. Respiratory acidosis
    4. Respiratory alkalosis

58. A nurse is caring for a client with severe diarrhea. The nurse monitors the client closely, understanding that this client is at risk for developing which acid-base disorder?
    1. Metabolic acidosis
    2. Metabolic alkalosis
    3. Respiratory acidosis
    4. Respiratory alkalosis

59. A nurse is caring for a client with diabetic ketoacidosis and documents that the client is experiencing Kussmaul's respirations. Based on this documentation, which of the following did the nurse most likely observe?
    1. Respirations that cease for several seconds *[handwritten: apnea]*
    2. Respirations that are regular but abnormally slow *[handwritten: Bradypnea]*

[handwritten: hyperpnea]
    3. Respirations that are labored and increased in depth and rate
    4. Respirations that are abnormally deep, regular, and increased in rate

60. A nurse is caring for a client with a diagnosis of chronic obstructive pulmonary disease (COPD). The nurse monitors the client for which acid-base imbalance that most likely occurs in clients with this condition?
    1. Metabolic acidosis
    2. Metabolic alkalosis
    3. Respiratory acidosis
    4. Respiratory alkalosis

61. The registered nurse reviews the results of the arterial blood gases with the licensed practical nurse (LPN) and tells the LPN that the client is experiencing respiratory acidosis. The LPN would expect to note which of the following on the laboratory result form?
    1. pH 7.50, P_{CO_2} 52 mm Hg
    2. pH 7.35, P_{CO_2} 40 mm Hg
    3. pH 7.25, P_{CO_2} 50 mm Hg
    4. pH 7.50, P_{CO_2} 30 mm Hg

62. A nurse is caring for a client with respiratory insufficiency. The arterial blood gas results indicate a pH of 7.50 and a P_{CO_2} of 30 mm Hg, and the nurse is told that the client is experiencing respiratory alkalosis. Which of the following additional laboratory values would the nurse expect to note?
    1. A sodium level of 145 mEq/L
    2. A potassium level of 3.2 mEq/L
    3. A magnesium level of 2.4 mg/dL
    4. A phosphorus level of 4.0 mg/dL

ALTERNATE ITEM FORMAT: PRIORITIZING (ORDERED RESPONSE)

63. A client is scheduled for an arterial blood gas specimen to be drawn, and the nurse assists with performing Allen's test on the client. Number the steps for performing Allen's test in order of priority. (Number 1 is the first step, and number 6 is the last step.)
    ___6___ Document the findings.
    ___1___ Explain the procedure to the client.
    ___4___ Release pressure from the ulnar artery.
    ___2___ Apply pressure over the ulnar and radial arteries.
    ___3___ Ask the client to open and close the hand repeatedly.
    ___5___ Assess the color of the extremity distal to the pressure point.

ANSWERS

54. 4

Rationale: The client is in respiratory alkalosis based on the laboratory results of a high pH and a low P_{CO_2} level. Interventions for respiratory alkalosis are the voluntary holding of breath or slowed breathing and the rebreathing of exhaled CO_2 by methods such as using a paper bag or a rebreathing mask as prescribed. Option 1 would be contraindicated, because the blood specimen has already been drawn, and the laboratory results have been completed. Options 2 and 3 are interventions for metabolic acidosis.

Test-Taking Strategy: First determine the laboratory results. Because the pH is high, the P_{CO_2} level is low, a respiratory problem is occurring. Using the process of elimination, you can determine that only one intervention deals with respirations. Review the interventions for respiratory alkalosis if you had difficulty with this question.

Level of Cognitive Ability: Analysis
Client Needs: Physiological Integrity
Integrated Process: Nursing Process/Implementation
Content Area: Adult Health/Respiratory
Reference: Zerwekh, J., Claborn, J., Gaglione, T., & Miller, C. (2006). *Mosby's fluid and electrolytes memory notecards* (p. 98). St. Louis: Mosby.

55. 4

Rationale: The normal pH is 7.35 to 7.45. In a respiratory condition, an opposite relationship will be seen between the pH and the P_{CO_2}, as is seen in option 4. In an alkalotic condition, the pH is increased. Options 1 and 3 indicate acidosis, and option 2 indicates a metabolic conditions.

Test-Taking Strategy: Remember that with a respiratory condition, you will find an opposite relationship between the pH and the P_{CO_2} level. Therefore, options 1 and 2 can be eliminated. Remembering that the pH is increased in an alkalotic condition helps you to eliminate option 3. Review the steps related to reading blood gas values if you had difficulty with this question.

Level of Cognitive Ability: Analysis
Client Needs: Physiological Integrity
Integrated Process: Nursing Process/Data Collection
Content Area: Adult Health/Respiratory
References: Linton, A., & Maebius, N. (2007). *Introduction to medical-surgical nursing* (4th ed., p. 639). Philadelphia: Saunders.
Pagana, K., & Pagana, T. (2005). *Mosby's diagnostic and laboratory test reference* (7th ed., p. 119). St. Louis: Mosby.

56. 1

Rationale: Before performing a radial puncture to obtain an arterial specimen for ABGs, Allen's test should be performed to determine adequate ulnar circulation. Failure to assess collateral circulation could result in severe ischemic injury to the hand if damage to the radial artery occurs with arterial puncture. Options 2, 3, and 4 are not associated with this test.

Test-Taking Strategy: Use the process of elimination. Note the relationship between the words "radial artery" in the question and option 1. Review Allen's test if you had difficulty with this question.

Level of Cognitive Ability: Analysis
Client Needs: Physiological Integrity

Integrated Process: Nursing Process/Evaluation
Content Area: Adult Health/Cardiovascular
Reference: Chernecky, C., & Berger, B. (2008). *Laboratory tests and diagnostic procedures* (5th ed., p. 213). Philadelphia: Saunders.

57. 2

Rationale: The loss of gastric fluid via nasogastric suction or vomiting causes metabolic alkalosis as a result of the loss of hydrochloric acid; this results in an alkalotic condition. Options 3 and 4 deal with respiratory problems. Option 1 relates to acidosis.

Test-Taking Strategy: Remember that hydrochloric acid is lost when the client is receiving nasogastric suctioning. This will direct you to the options that identify an alkalotic condition. Because the question addresses a situation other than a respiratory one, the acid-base disorder would be a metabolic condition. Review the causes of metabolic alkalosis if you had difficulty with this question.

Level of Cognitive Ability: Analysis
Client Needs: Physiological Integrity
Integrated Process: Nursing Process/Data Collection
Content Area: Adult Health/Gastrointestinal
Reference: Monahan, F., Marek, J., Neighbors, M., & Green, C., (2007). *Phipps' medical-surgical nursing: Health and illness perspectives* (8th ed., p. 396). St. Louis: Mosby.

58. 1

Rationale: Intestinal secretions high in bicarbonate may be lost through enteric drainage tubes, an ileostomy, or diarrhea. The decreased bicarbonate level creates the actual base deficit of metabolic acidosis. Options 2, 3, and 4 are unlikely to occur in a client with severe diarrhea.

Test-Taking Strategy: Note that the condition described in the question is a gastrointestinal disorder; this will direct you to thinking about a metabolic disorder. Remembering that intestinal fluids are primarily alkaline will assist you with selecting the correct option. When excess bicarbonate is lost, acidosis will result. Review the causes of metabolic acidosis if you had difficulty with this question.

Level of Cognitive Ability: Analysis
Client Needs: Physiological Integrity
Integrated Process: Nursing Process/Data Collection
Content Area: Adult Health/Gastrointestinal
References: Lewis, S., Heitkemper, M., Dirksen, S., & Bucher, L. (2007). *Medical-surgical nursing: Assessment and management of clinical problems* (7th ed., p. 335). St. Louis: Mosby.
Linton, A., & Maebius, N. (2007). *Introduction to medical-surgical nursing* (4th ed., p.199). Philadelphia: Saunders.

59. 4

Rationale: Kussmaul's respirations are abnormally deep, regular, and increased in rate. In bradypnea, respirations are regular but abnormally slow. In hyperpnea, respirations are labored and increased in depth and rate. In apnea, respirations cease for several seconds.

Test-Taking Strategy: Knowledge regarding the descriptions of alterations in breathing patterns is required to answer this question. Remember that Kussmaul's respirations occur in clients with diabetic ketoacidosis. Review the data collection findings in diabetic ketoacidosis if you had difficulty with this question.

Level of Cognitive Ability: Comprehension
Client Needs: Physiological Integrity
Integrated Process: Nursing Process/Data Collection
Content Area: Fundamental Skills
References: Lewis, S., Heitkemper, M., Dirksen, S., & Bucher, L. (2007). *Medical-surgical nursing: Assessment and management of clinical problems* (7th ed., p. 335). St. Louis: Mosby.
Linton, A., & Maebius, N. (2007). *Introduction to medical-surgical nursing* (4th ed., p. 512). Philadelphia: Saunders.

60. **3**
Rationale: Respiratory acidosis most often occurs as a result of primary defects in the function of the lungs or changes in normal respiratory patterns from secondary problems. Chronic respiratory acidosis is most commonly caused by COPD. Acute respiratory acidosis also occurs in clients with COPD when superimposed respiratory infection or concurrent respiratory disease increases the work of breathing. Options 1, 2, and 4 are not likely to occur unless other conditions complicate the COPD.
Test-Taking Strategy: Use the process of elimination. Remembering that primary defects in the function of the lungs result in respiratory acidosis will direct you to the correct option. Review the causes of respiratory acidosis if you had difficulty with this question.
Level of Cognitive Ability: Comprehension
Client Needs: Physiological Integrity
Integrated Process: Nursing Process/Data Collection
Content Area: Fundamental Skills
References: Lewis, S., Heitkemper, M., Dirksen, S., & Bucher, L. (2007). *Medical-surgical nursing: Assessment and management of clinical problems* (7th ed., p. 335). St. Louis: Mosby.
Linton, A., & Maebius, N. (2007). *Introduction to medical-surgical nursing* (4th ed., pp. 197-198, 553). Philadelphia: Saunders.

61. **3**
Rationale: The normal pH is 7.35 to 7.45, and the normal Pco_2 value is 35 to 45 mm Hg. In respiratory acidosis, the pH is down and the Pco_2 is up. Option 3 is the only option that reflects an acidotic condition. Options 1 and 4 reflect an elevated pH, which indicates an alkalotic condition. Option 2 reflects a normal blood gas result.
Test-Taking Strategy: Remember that with a respiratory imbalance, you will find an opposite relationship between the pH and the Pco_2 value. In addition, remember that the pH is down in an acidotic condition. Review the interpretation of arterial blood gas results if you had difficulty with this question.
Level of Cognitive Ability: Analysis
Client Needs: Physiological Integrity
Integrated Process: Nursing Process/Data Collection
Content Area: Adult Health/Neurological
References: Chernecky, C., & Berger, B. (2008). *Laboratory tests and diagnostic procedures* (5th ed., p. 211). Philadelphia: Saunders.
Pagana, K., & Pagana, T. (2005). *Mosby's diagnostic and laboratory test reference* (7th ed., pp. 119-120). St. Louis: Mosby.

62. **2**
Rationale: Clinical manifestations of respiratory alkalosis include tachypnea, mental status changes, dizziness, pallor around the mouth, spasms of the muscles of the hands, and hypokalemia. Options 1, 3, and 4 identify normal laboratory results.
Test-Taking Strategy: Recalling the clinical manifestations of respiratory alkalosis and the normal laboratory values will assist you with answering this question. By the process of elimination, you can then determine that the only abnormal laboratory value is the potassium level. Review the clinical manifestations of respiratory alkalosis if you had difficulty with this question.
Level of Cognitive Ability: Analysis
Client Needs: Physiological Integrity
Integrated Process: Nursing Process/Data Collection
Content Area: Adult Health/Respiratory
Reference: Monahan, F., Marek, J., Neighbors, M., & Green, C. (2007). *Phipps' medical-surgical nursing: Health and illness perspectives* (8th ed., pp. 392-393). St. Louis: Mosby.

ALTERNATE ITEM FORMAT: PRIORITIZING (ORDERED RESPONSE)
63. **6, 1, 4, 2, 3, 5**
Rationale: Allen's test is performed before obtaining an arterial blood specimen from the radial artery to determine the presence of adequate collateral circulation and the adequacy of the ulnar artery. Failure to determine the presence of adequate collateral circulation could result in severe ischemic injury to the hand if damage to the radial artery occurs with arterial puncture. The nurse would first explain the procedure to the client. To perform the test, the nurse applies direct pressure over the client's ulnar and radial arteries simultaneously. While pressure is applied, the nurse asks the client to open and close the hand repeatedly; the hand should blanch. The nurse then releases pressure from the ulnar artery while compressing the radial artery and assesses the color of the extremity distal to the pressure point. If pinkness fails to return within 6 seconds, the ulnar artery is insufficient, which indicates that the radial artery should not be used for obtaining a blood specimen. Finally, the nurse documents the findings.
Test-Taking Strategy: Recalling that Allen's test needs to be explained to the client will assist you with determining the first action. Next, think about the purpose and reason for performing this test, and visualize the procedure. This will help you to determine the steps for performing the test. Review Allen's test if you had difficulty with this question.
Level of Cognitive Ability: Application
Client Needs: Physiological Integrity
Integrated Process: Nursing Process/Data Collection
Content Area: Fundamental Skills
References: Chernecky, C., & Berger, B. (2008). *Laboratory tests and diagnostic procedures* (5th ed., pp. 213-214). Philadelphia: Saunders.
Linton, A., & Maebius, N. (2007). *Introduction to medical-surgical nursing* (4th ed., p. 521). Philadelphia: Saunders.

REFERENCES

Chernecky, C., & Berger, B. (2008). *Laboratory tests and diagnostic procedures* (5th ed.). Philadelphia: Saunders.

Lewis, S., Heitkemper, M., Dirksen, S., & Bucher, L. (2007). *Medical-surgical nursing: Assessment and management of clinical problems* (7th ed.). St. Louis: Mosby.

Linton, A., & Maebius, N. (2007). *Introduction to medical-surgical nursing* (4th ed.). Philadelphia: Saunders.

Monahan, F., Marek, J., Neighbors, M., & Green, C. (2007). *Phipps' medical-surgical nursing: Health and illness perspectives* (8th ed.). St. Louis: Mosby.

National Council of State Boards of Nursing (Eds.) (2008). *2008 Detailed Test Plan for the NCLEX-PN® Examination, National Council of State Boards of Nursing.* Chicago: Author.

National Council of State Boards of Nursing. *NCSBN home page.* www.ncsbn.org. Accessed June 12, 2008.

Pagana, K., & Pagana, T. (2005). *Mosby's diagnostic and laboratory test reference* (7th ed.). St. Louis: Mosby.

Zerwekh, J., Claborn, J., Gaglione, T., & Miller, C. (2006). *Mosby's fluid and electrolytes memory notecards.* St. Louis: Mosby.

Laboratory Values

PYRAMID TERMS

blood The liquid pumped by the heart through the arteries, veins, and capillaries. It is composed of a clear yellow fluid (plasma) and cell types with different functions (Figure 11-1).

blood cell Any of the formed elements of the blood, including red cells (erythrocytes), white cells (leukocytes), and platelets (thrombocytes).

plasma The fluid ground substance; what remains after the cells have been removed from a sample of whole blood. The watery, straw-colored fluid part of the lymph and blood in which the formed elements (blood cells) are suspended. It is made up of water, electrolytes, protein, glucose, fats, bilirubin, and gases, and it is essential for carrying the cellular elements of the blood through the circulation.

serum The clear and thin fluid part of the blood that remains after coagulation. Serum contains no blood cells, platelets, or fibrinogen.

venipuncture Puncture into a vein to obtain a blood specimen for testing; the antecubital veins are the veins of choice because of ease of access.

▲ PYRAMID TO SUCCESS

This chapter identifies the normal adult values for the most common laboratory tests. If you are familiar with the normal values, you will be able to determine if an abnormality exists when a laboratory value is presented in a question. It is unlikely that a question on the NCLEX-PN will simply ask you what a normal value may be. The questions on the NCLEX-PN related to laboratory values will require you to identify whether the laboratory value is normal or abnormal, and then you will be required to think about the effects of the laboratory value in terms of the client. Pyramid points focus on knowledge of the normal values for the most common laboratory tests, the therapeutic serum levels of commonly prescribed medications, and interventions based on the findings. When a question is presented on the NCLEX-PN regarding a specific laboratory value, note the disorder presented in the question and the associated body organ that is affected as a result of the disorder. This process will assist you with determining the correct answer. For example, if the question is asking you about the immune status of a client who is receiving chemotherapy, the assessment of the laboratory values will focus on the white blood cell (WBC) count and on the neutrophils, because this client may be at risk for infection. For the client who is receiving chemotherapy and who has a low WBC count, the plan of care focuses on the immune system and the protection of the client from infection. Implementation focuses on preventive interventions related to infection, perhaps even protective isolation measures. Evaluation may focus on the maintenance of a normal temperature in the client. Integrated Processes addressed in this chapter are the Clinical Problem-Solving Process (Nursing Process), Caring, Communication and Documentation, and Teaching and Learning. Box 11-1 lists the abbreviations used in laboratory values.

CLIENT NEEDS ▲

Safe and Effective Care Environment

Applying principles of infection control
Ensuring medical and surgical asepsis when obtaining a specimen
Implementing procedures for handling hazardous and infectious materials
Maintaining confidentiality
Maintaining standard, transmission-based, and other precautions
Obtaining informed consent for specific procedures
Verifying the identity of the client

Health Promotion and Maintenance

Discussing the importance of follow-up laboratory studies
Identifying community resources available for the follow-up
Implementing posttest procedures
Monitoring for signs and symptoms that indicate the need to notify the health care provider
Preparing the client for the laboratory test

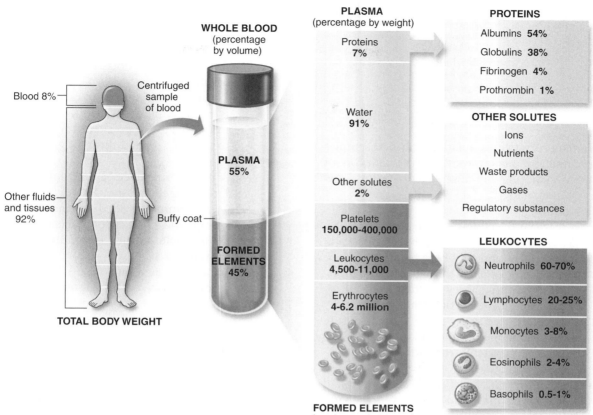

FIG. 11-1 Approximate values for the components of blood in a normal adult. (Modified from Thibodeau, G.A., & Patton, K.T. [2005]. *The human body in health and disease* [4th ed.]. St. Louis: Mosby.)

BOX 11-1 Pyramid Abbreviations

Abbreviation	Description
g/dL	Grams per deciliter
mcg/dL	Micrograms per deciliter
mg/dL	Milligrams per deciliter
mEq/L	Milliequivalents per liter
units/L	Units per liter
mm/hr	Millimeters per hour
IU/L	International units per liter
mcg/mL	Micrograms per milliliter
ng/mL	Nanograms per milliliter
microunits/mL	Microunits per milliliter
mL/kg	Milliliters per kilogram
mm^3	Millimeters cubed
μL	Microliters

Psychosocial Integrity

Communicating the purpose of the laboratory test to the client

Communicating with the client regarding the laboratory results

Describing specific interventions or home-care measures required based on the results

Providing emotional support during testing

Physiological Integrity

Determining the need to implement specific actions based on the laboratory results

Identifying normal values for the most common laboratory tests

Identifying therapeutic serum medication levels of commonly prescribed medications

Monitoring for clinical manifestations associated with an abnormal laboratory value

Monitoring for potential complications related to a test

Providing comfort measures

Reporting significant laboratory values

I. ELECTROLYTES (Table 11-1)
A. **Serum** sodium
  1. Description
    a. A major cation of extracellular fluid
    b. Maintains osmotic pressures and acid-base balance and assists with the transmission of nerve impulses
    c. Absorbed from the small intestine and excreted in the urine in amounts that depend on dietary intake
    d. Minimum daily requirement of sodium is approximately 15 mEq

TABLE 11-1 Normal Adult Electrolyte Values

Electrolyte	Value
Sodium	135-145 mEq/L
Potassium	3.5-5.1 mEq/L
Chloride	98-107 mEq/L
Bicarbonate (venous)	22-29 mEq/L

2. Nursing consideration: Drawing **blood** samples proximal to the intravenous (IV) infusion of sodium chloride will falsely elevate results

B. **Serum** potassium (K)
   1. Description
      a. A major intracellular cation; regulates cellular water balance, electrical conduction in muscle cells, and acid-base balance
      b. The body obtains K through dietary ingestion, and the kidneys either preserve or excrete K, depending on cellular need
      c. K levels are used to evaluate cardiac function, renal function, gastrointestinal function, and the need for IV replacement therapy
   2. Nursing considerations
      a. Use of a tourniquet and clenching and unclenching the hand before venous sampling can increase the value
      b. Do not draw **blood** from an IV infusion site
      c. If the client is receiving K supplementation, note this on the laboratory form
      d. Clients with elevated WBC and platelet counts may have falsely elevated K levels

C. **Serum** chloride
   1. Description
      a. Most abundant body anion in the extracellular fluid
      b. Functions to counterbalance cations (e.g., sodium) and acts as a buffer during oxygen and carbon dioxide exchange in red **blood cells** (RBCs)
      c. Aids in digestion and maintaining osmotic pressure and water balance
   2. Nursing considerations
      a. Draw **blood** from an extremity that does not have normal saline infusing into it
      b. Do not allow the client to clench and unclench the hand before a **blood** draw
      c. Any condition accompanied by prolonged vomiting, diarrhea, or both will alter levels

D. **Serum** bicarbonate
   1. Description: Is part of the bicarbonate–carbonic acid buffering system; mainly responsible for regulating the pH of body fluids
   2. Nursing considerations
      a. Ingestion of acidic or alkaline solutions may cause increased or decreased results, respectively
      b. Prolonged tourniquet application before the **blood** draw increases the **serum** bicarbonate level

II. COAGULATION STUDIES
A. Activated partial thromboplastin time (aPTT)
   1. Description
      a. Evaluates how well the coagulation sequence is functioning by measuring the amount of time it takes for recalcified, citrated **plasma** to clot after partial thromboplastin is added to it
      b. Screens for deficiencies and inhibitors of all factors except VII and XIII
      c. Most commonly used to monitor heparin therapy and to screen for coagulation disorders
   2. Value: 20 to 36 seconds, depending on the type of activator used
   3. Nursing considerations
      a. If the client is receiving intermittent heparin therapy, draw the **blood** sample 1 hour before the next scheduled dose
      b. Do not draw samples from an arm into which heparin is infusing
      c. Transport the specimen to the laboratory immediately
      d. The aPTT should be between 1.5 and 2.5 times normal when the client is receiving heparin therapy; if the value is prolonged, initiate bleeding precautions

B. Prothrombin time (PT) and international normalized ratio (INR)
   1. Description
      a. Prothrombin is a vitamin K–dependent glycoprotein produced by the liver that is necessary for firm fibrin clot formation
      b. Each laboratory establishes a normal or control PT value based on the method used to perform the test
      c. The PT measures the amount of time it takes for clot formation; it is used to monitor response to warfarin sodium (Coumadin) therapy or to screen for dysfunction of the extrinsic system that results from liver disease, vitamin K deficiency, or disseminated intravascular coagulation
      d. A PT value within 2 seconds (plus or minus) of the control value is considered normal
      e. The INR standardizes the PT ratio; it is calculated in the laboratory setting by raising the observed PT ratio to the power of the international sensitivity index specific to the thromboplastin reagent used
      f. The INR measures the effects of oral anticoagulants
   2. Values
      a. PT: 9.6 to 11.8 seconds (adult male); 9.5 to 11.3 seconds (adult female)

b. INR: 2 to 3 for standard warfarin sodium (Coumadin) therapy

c. INR: 3 to 4.5 for high-dose warfarin sodium (Coumadin) therapy

3. Nursing considerations

a. Baseline PT should be determined before anticoagulation therapy is started; note the time of collection on the laboratory form

b. Apply direct pressure to the **venipuncture** site for 3 to 5 minutes if a coagulation defect is present

c. Concurrent warfarin sodium (Coumadin) therapy with heparin therapy can lengthen the PT for up to 5 hours after dosing

d. Diets high in green leafy vegetables can increase the absorption of vitamin K, which shortens the PT

e. Oral anticoagulation therapy usually maintains the PT at 1.5 to 2 times the laboratory control value

f. A PT longer than 30 seconds places the client at risk for hemorrhage

C. Clotting time

1. Description: Measures the time required for the interaction of all factors involved in the clotting process

2. Value: 8 to 15 minutes

3. Nursing considerations

a. The client should not receive heparin therapy for 3 hours before specimen collection, because the heparin therapy will affect the results

b. The test result is prolonged by any anticoagulant therapy, test-tube agitation, or high temperature changes that may affect the specimen

D. Platelet count

1. Description

a. Platelets function in hemostatic plug formation, clot retraction, and coagulation factor activation

b. Platelets are produced by the bone marrow to function in hemostasis

2. Value: 150,000 to 400,000 cells/μL

3. Nursing considerations

a. Monitor the **venipuncture** site for bleeding in clients with known thrombocytopenia

b. High altitudes, chronic cold weather, and exercise increase platelet counts

c. Bleeding precautions should be instituted in clients with low platelet counts

III. ERYTHROCYTE STUDIES

A. Erythrocyte sedimentation rate

1. Description

a. The rate at which erythrocytes settle out of anticoagulated **blood** in 1 hour

TABLE 11-2 Normal Adult Hemoglobin, Hematocrit, Iron, and Red Blood Cell Levels

Blood Component	Normal Value
Hemoglobin	
Male adult	14-16.5 g/dL
Female adult	12-15 g/dL
Hematocrit	
Male adult	42%-52%
Female adult	35%-47%
Iron	
Male adult	65-175 mcg/dL
Female adult	50-170 mcg/dL
Red Blood Cells	
Male adult	4.5-6.2 million cells/μL
Female adult	4.0-5.5 million cells/μL

b. Not diagnostic of any particular disease but indicates that an inflammatory process is ongoing

2. Value: 0 to 30 mm/hour, depending on the age of the client

3. Nursing consideration: Fasting is not necessary, but a fatty meal may cause **plasma** alterations

B. Hemoglobin and hematocrit (Table 11-2)

1. Description

a. Hemoglobin is the main component of erythrocytes and serves as the vehicle for the transportation of oxygen and carbon dioxide

b. Hemoglobin determinations are important for identifying anemia

c. Hematocrit represents RBC mass and is an important measurement in the identification of anemia or polycythemia

2. Nursing consideration: Fasting is not required

C. **Serum** iron

1. Description

a. Iron is mostly found in hemoglobin

b. Iron acts as a carrier of oxygen from the lungs to the tissues and indirectly aids in the return of carbon dioxide to the lungs

c. Helps with diagnosing anemias and hemolytic disorders

2. Values

a. Male: 65 to 175 mcg/dL

b. Female: 50 to 170 mcg/dL

3. Nursing consideration: Level will be increased if the client has ingested iron before the test

D. RBC count

1. Description

a. RBCs function in hemoglobin transport, which results in the delivery of oxygen to the body tissues

b. RBCs are formed by red bone marrow, have a life span of 120 days, and are removed from the **blood** by the liver, spleen, and bone marrow

    c. Helps with diagnosing anemias and **blood** dyscrasias

    d. Evaluates the body's ability to produce RBCs in sufficient numbers

  2. Values

    a. Female: 4 to 5.5 million cells/μL

    b. Male: 4.5 to 6.2 million cells/μL

  3. Nursing consideration: Fasting is not required

IV. SERUM ENZYMES/CARDIAC MARKERS (Table 11-3)

A. Creatine kinase (CK)

  1. Description

    a. An enzyme found in muscle and brain tissue; it reflects tissue breakdown resulting from cell trauma

    b. The test is performed to detect myocardial or skeletal muscle damage or central nervous system damage; the normal CK value is 26 to 174 units/L

    c. Isoenzymes include CK-MB (cardiac), CK-BB (brain), and CK-MM (muscle)

    d. CK-MB is found mainly in cardiac muscle, CK-BB is found mainly in brain tissue, and CK-MM is found mainly in skeletal muscle

  2. Values

    a. CK-MB: 0% to 5% of total CK value

    b. CK-MM: 95% to 100% of total CK value

    c. CK-BB: 0% of CK value

  3. Nursing considerations

    a. If the test is performed to evaluate skeletal muscle, instruct the client to avoid strenuous physical activity for 24 hours before the test

    b. Instruct the client to avoid the ingestion of alcohol for 24 hours before the test

    c. Invasive procedures and intramuscular injections may falsely elevate CK levels

B. Lactate dehydrogenase (LDH)

  1. Description

    a. The isoenzymes that are particularly affected by acute myocardial infarction are LDH_1 and LDH_2

    b. The LDH level begins to increase approximately 24 hours after myocardial infarction and peaks in 48 to 72 hours; it returns to normal thereafter, usually within 7 to 14 days

    c. The presence of an LDH flip (i.e., when LDH_1 is higher than LDH_2) is helpful for diagnosing a myocardial infarction

  2. Nursing considerations

    a. LDH isoenzyme levels should be interpreted in view of the clinical findings

    b. Testing should be repeated on 3 consecutive days

TABLE 11-3	Normal Adult Serum Enzyme and Cardiac Marker Values
Serum Enzyme	**Normal Value**
Creatine kinase (CK)	26-174 units/L
CK isoenzymes	
CK-MB	0%-5% of total
CK-MM	95%-100% of total
CK-BB	0%
Lactate dehydrogenase	140-280 units/L
Lactate dehydrogenase isoenzymes	
LDH_1	14%-26%
LDH_2	29%-39%
LDH_3	20%-26%
LDH_4	8%-16%
LDH_5	6%-16%
Troponins	
Troponin I	<0.6 ng/mL
	>1.5 ng/mL indicates myocardial infarction
Troponin T	>0.1-0.2 ng/mL indicates myocardial infarction
Myoglobin	<90 mcg/L; an elevation could indicate myocardial infarction

C. Troponins

  1. Description

    a. Troponins are regulatory proteins found in striated (skeletal and myocardial) muscle

    b. Increased amounts of troponins are released into the bloodstream when an infarction causes damage to the myocardium.

    c. Levels elevate as early as 3 hours after myocardial injury; troponin I levels may remain elevated for 7 to 10 days, and troponin T levels may remain elevated for up to 10 to 14 days

    d. Serial measurements are important to compare with a baseline test

  2. Values

    a. Troponin I: Usually less than 0.6 ng/mL; greater than 1.5 ng/mL is consistent with a myocardial infarction

    b. Troponin T: Greater than 0.1 to 0.2 ng/mL is consistent with a myocardial infarction

  3. Nursing considerations:

    a. Client does not need to be fasting; testing repeated after 12 hours and followed by daily testing for 3 to 5 days

    b. Rotate **venipuncture** sites

D. Myoglobin

  1. Description

    a. An oxygen-binding protein found in striated (cardiac and skeletal) muscle that releases oxygen at very low tensions

    b. Any injury to skeletal muscle will cause a release of myoglobin into the **blood**

  2. Values: Normal value is less than 90 mcg/L; an elevation could indicate myocardial infarction

3. Nursing considerations
   a. The level can rise as early as 2 hours after a myocardial infarction, with a rapid decline in the level seen after 7 hours
   b. Because the myoglobin level is not cardiac specific and rises and falls so rapidly, its use for diagnosing myocardial infarction may be limited

V. SERUM GASTROINTESTINAL STUDIES

A. Albumin
   1. Description
      a. A main **plasma** protein of **blood**
      b. Maintains oncotic pressure and transports bilirubin, fatty acids, medications, hormones, and other substances that are insoluble in water
      c. Increased in conditions such as dehydration, diarrhea, and metastatic carcinoma; decreased in conditions such as acute infection, ascites, and alcoholism
      d. The presence of detectable albumin or protein in the urine is indicative of abnormal renal function
   2. Value: 3.4 to 5 g/dL
   3. Nursing considerations: Draw from an extremity that does not have an IV infusing into it

B. Alkaline phosphatase
   1. Description
      a. An enzyme normally found in bone, liver, intestine, and placenta
      b. The level rises during periods of bone growth, liver disease, and bile duct obstruction
   2. Value: 4.5 to 13 King-Armstrong units/dL
   3. Nursing considerations
      a. The client may need to fast 12 hours before the test
      b. Hepatotoxic medications administered within 12 hours before specimen collection can cause false values
      c. Transport the specimen to the laboratory immediately

C. Ammonia
   1. Description
      a. A waste product from nitrogen breakdown during protein metabolism
      b. Metabolized by the liver and excreted by the kidneys as urea
      c. Elevated levels resulting from hepatic dysfunction may lead to encephalopathy
      d. Not a reliable indicator of hepatic coma
   2. Value: 35 to 65 mcg/dL
   3. Nursing considerations
      a. Instruct the client to fast (except for water) and to refrain from smoking for 8 to 10 hours before the test
      b. Place the specimen in ice and transport it to the laboratory immediately

D. Amylase
   1. Description
      a. An enzyme produced by the pancreas and salivary glands that aids in the digestion of complex carbohydrates and that is excreted by the kidneys
      b. In acute pancreatitis, the amylase level is greatly increased; the level starts rising 3 to 6 hours after the onset of pain, peaks at about 24 hours, and returns to normal 2 to 3 days after the onset of pain
   2. Value: 25 to 151 units/L
   3. Nursing considerations
      a. On the laboratory form, list medications that the client has taken during the 24 hours before the test
      b. Note that many medications may cause false-positive or false-negative results
      c. Results are invalidated if the specimen was obtained less than 72 hours after cholecystography with radiopaque dyes

E. Lipase
   1. Description
      a. A pancreatic enzyme that changes fats and triglycerides into fatty acids and glycerol
      b. Elevated lipase levels occur in pancreatic disorders; elevations may not occur until 24 to 36 hours after the onset of illness and may remain elevated for up to 14 days
   2. Value: 10 to 10 units/L
   3. Nursing considerations: Endoscopic retrograde cholangiopancreatography may increase lipase activity

F. Bilirubin
   1. Description
      a. Produced by the liver, spleen, and bone marrow; also a byproduct of hemoglobin breakdown
      b. Total bilirubin can be broken down into direct bilirubin, which is primarily excreted via the intestinal tract, and indirect bilirubin, which circulates primarily in the bloodstream
      c. Total bilirubin levels rise with any type of jaundice, whereas direct and indirect levels rise depending on the cause of the jaundice
   2. Values
      a. Bilirubin, direct: 0 to 0.3 mg/dL
      b. Bilirubin, indirect: 0.1 to 1 mg/dL
      c. Bilirubin, total: Less than 1.5 mg/dL
   3. Nursing considerations
      a. Instruct the client to eat a diet low in yellow foods (e.g., carrots, yams, yellow beans, pumpkins) for 3 to 4 days before the **blood** is drawn
      b. Instruct the client to fast for 4 hours before the **blood** is drawn

c. Results will be elevated with the ingestion of alcohol or the administration or ingestion of morphine sulfate, theophylline, ascorbic acid (vitamin C), or aspirin

d. Results are invalidated if the client has undergone a radioactive scan within 24 hours before the test

G. Lipids

1. Description

a. **Blood** lipids consist primarily of cholesterol, triglycerides, and phospholipids

b. Lipid assessment includes total cholesterol, high-density lipoprotein (HDL), low-density lipoprotein (LDL), and triglycerides

c. Cholesterol is present in all body tissues and is a major component of LDLs, brain and nerve cells, cell membranes, and some gallbladder stones

d. Triglycerides constitute a major part of very low-density lipoproteins (VLDLs) and a small part of LDLs

e. Triglycerides are synthesized in the liver from fatty acids, protein, and glucose and they are obtained from the diet

f. Increased cholesterol, LDL, and triglyceride levels place the client at risk for coronary artery disease

g. HDLs help protect against the risk of coronary artery disease

2. Values

a. Cholesterol: 140 to 199 mg/dL

b. LDLs: Less than 130 mg/dL

c. HDLs: 30 to 70 mg/dL

d. Triglycerides: Less than 200 mg/dL

3. Nursing considerations

a. Oral contraceptives may increase the lipid level

b. Instruct the client to abstain from foods and fluid (except for water) for 12 to 14 hours before the test and from alcohol for 24 hours before the test

c. Instruct the client that the evening meal before the test should be free from high-cholesterol foods

H. Protein

1. Description

a. Reflects the total amount of albumin and globulins in the **serum**

b. Regulates osmotic pressure and comprises coagulation factors for hemostasis, enzymes, hormones, tissue growth and repair, and pH buffers

c. Increased in conditions such as Addison's disease, autoimmune collagen disorders, chronic infection, and Crohn's disease

d. Decreased in conditions such as burns, cirrhosis, edema, and severe hepatic disease

2. Value: 6 to 8 g/dL

3. Nursing considerations

a. Do not draw in an extremity with an IV infusion

b. Instruct the client to avoid a high-fat diet for 8 hours before the test

I. Uric acid

1. Description

a. Formed as the purines adenine and guanine; is continuously metabolized during the formation and degradation of DNA and RNA and from the metabolism of dietary purines

b. Elevated amounts deposit in joints and soft tissue and cause gout

c. Fast cell turnover and the slowed renal excretion of uric acid may cause uricemia

d. Elevated amounts of urinary uric acid form precipitates of urate stones in the kidneys

2. Values

a. Male: 4.5 to 8 mg/dL

b. Female: 2.5 to 6.2 mg/dL

3. Nursing considerations

a. Instruct the client to fast for 8 hours before the test

b. Aminophylline, caffeine, and vitamin C may cause falsely elevated results

VI. GLUCOSE STUDIES

A. Fasting **blood** glucose

1. Description

a. Glucose is a monosaccharide found in fruits and formed from the digestion of carbohydrates and the conversion of glycogen by the liver

b. Glucose is the body's main source of cellular energy, and it is essential for brain and erythrocyte function

c. Fasting **blood** glucose levels are used to help diagnose diabetes mellitus and hypoglycemia (Table 11-4)

2. Nursing considerations

a. Instruct the client to fast for 8 to 12 hours before the test

b. Instruct a client with diabetes mellitus to withhold morning insulin or oral

TABLE 11-4 Normal Adult Glucose Values	
Point of Measurement	Normal Value
Glucose, fasting	70-110 mg/dL
Glucose monitoring (capillary blood)	60-110 mg/dL
Glucose tolerance test, oral	
Baseline fasting	70-110 mg/dL
30-minute fasting	110-170 mg/dL
60-minute fasting	120-170 mg/dL
90-minute fasting	100-140 mg/dL
120-minute fasting	70-120 mg/dL
Glucose, 2-hour postprandial	<140 mg/dL

hypoglycemic medication until after the **blood** is drawn

B. Glucose tolerance test (see Table 11-4)
1. Description
   a. Aids in the diagnosis of diabetes mellitus
   b. If the glucose levels peak at higher than normal at 1 to 2 hours after the injection or ingestion of glucose and are slower than normal to return to fasting levels, then diabetes mellitus is confirmed
2. Nursing considerations
   a. Instruct the client to eat a high-carbohydrate (200- to 300-g) diet for 3 days before the test
   b. Instruct the client to avoid alcohol, coffee, and smoking for 36 hours before the test
   c. Instruct the client to fast for 10 to 16 hours before the test
   d. Instruct the client to avoid strenuous exercise for 8 hours before and after the test
   e. Instruct the client with diabetes mellitus to withhold morning insulin or oral hypoglycemic medication
   f. Instruct the client that the test will take 3 to 5 hours and that it requires the IV or oral administration of glucose and multiple **blood** samples

C. Glycosylated hemoglobin
1. Description
   a. Glycosylated hemoglobin is **blood** glucose that is bound to hemoglobin
   b. Glycosylated hemoglobin A (HbA_{1c}) is a reflection of how well **blood** glucose levels have been controlled for up to the past 3 to 4 months
   c. Hyperglycemia in diabetic clients is usually a cause of an increase in the HbA_{1c} level
2. Values
   a. Values are expressed as a percentage of the total hemoglobin
   b. Diabetics with good control: 7% or less
   c. Diabetics with fair control: 7% to 8%
   d. Diabetics with poor control: 8% or more
3. Nursing considerations: Fasting is not required before the test

D. Glycosylated **serum** albumin (fructosamine)
1. Description
   a. Reflects the average **serum** glucose levels over a period of 2 to 3 weeks
   b. More sensitive to recent changes than the HbA_{1c} test
2. Values: Normal ranges vary according to method of testing used; for the nondiabetic client, normal is 1.5 to 2.7 mmol/L, and for the diabetic client, normal is 2.0 to 5.0 mmol/L
3. Nursing considerations: The client needs to fast for 12 hours before the test

VII. RENAL FUNCTION STUDIES
A. **Serum** creatinine
1. Description
   a. Very specific indicator of renal function
   b. Elevated levels indicate a slowing of the glomerular filtration rate
2. Value: 0.6 to 1.3 mg/dL
3. Nursing considerations: Instruct the client to avoid excessive exercise for 8 hours before the test and excessive red meat intake for 24 hours before the test

B. **Blood** urea nitrogen
1. Description
   a. Urea nitrogen is the nitrogen portion of urea, which is a substance formed in the liver through an enzymatic protein breakdown process
   b. Urea is normally freely filtered through the renal glomeruli, with a small amount reabsorbed in the tubules and the remainder excreted into the urine
   c. Elevated levels indicate a slowing of the glomerular filtration rate
2. Value: 8 to 25 mg/dL
3. Nursing considerations: Both creatinine levels and urea nitrogen levels should be analyzed when renal function is evaluated

VIII. ELEMENTS
A. Calcium
1. Description
   a. A cation that is absorbed into the bloodstream from dietary sources and that functions in bone formation, nerve impulse transmission, and the contraction of myocardial and skeletal muscles
   b. Aids in **blood** clotting by converting prothrombin to thrombin
2. Value: 8.6 to 10 mg/dL
3. Nursing considerations
   a. Instruct the client to eat a diet with normal calcium levels (800 mg/day) for 3 days before the test
   b. Instruct the client that fasting may be required for 8 hours before the test

B. Magnesium
1. Description
   a. Used as an index to determine metabolic activity and renal function
   b. Magnesium is needed for the **blood**-clotting process; it regulates neuromuscular activity, acts as a cofactor that modifies the activity of many enzymes, and has an effect on the metabolism of calcium
2. Value: 1.6 to 2.6 mg/dL
3. Nursing considerations
   a. Prolonged use of magnesium products will cause increased levels

b. Long-term parenteral nutrition therapy or excessive loss of body fluids may cause decreased levels

C. Phosphorus
1. Description
   a. Important in bone formation, energy storage and release, urinary acid–base buffering, and carbohydrate metabolism
   b. Absorbed from food and excreted by the kidneys
   c. High concentrations of phosphorus are stored in bone and skeletal muscle
2. Value: 2.7 to 4.5 mg/dL
3. Nursing considerations: Instruct the client to fast before the test

IX. THYROID STUDIES
A. Description
1. Performed if a thyroid disorder is suspected
2. Helpful to differentiate primary thyroid disease from secondary causes and from abnormalities in thyroxine-binding globulin levels
B. Values
1. Thyroid-stimulating hormone (thyrotropin): 0.2 to 5.4 microunits/mL
2. Thyroxine: 5 to 12 mcg/dL
3. Thyroxine, free: 0.8 to 2.4 ng/dL
4. Triiodothyronine: 80 to 230 ng/dL
C. Nursing considerations: Test results may be invalid if the client has undergone a recent radionuclide scan

X. WHITE BLOOD CELL COUNT
A. Description
1. WBCs function in the body's immune defense system
2. The WBC count assesses leukocyte distribution
B. Value: 4500 to 11,000 cells/mm^3 (Table 11-5)
C. Nursing considerations
1. A "shift to the left" means that there is an increased number of immature neutrophils in the peripheral **blood**
2. A low total WBC count with a left shift indicates a recovery from bone marrow depression or an infection of such intensity that the demand for neutrophils in the tissue is greater than the capacity of the bone marrow to release them into the circulation

3. A high total WBC count with a left shift indicates an increased release of neutrophils by the bone marrow in response to an overwhelming infection or inflammation
4. A "shift to the right" means that cells have more than the usual number of nuclear segments; this is found with liver disease, Down syndrome, and megaloblastic and pernicious anemia

XI. HEPATITIS TESTS
A. Description
1. Tests include radioimmunoassay, enzyme-linked immunosorbent assay (ELISA), and microparticle enzyme immunoassay
2. Serologic tests for specific hepatitis virus markers assist with defining the specific type of hepatitis
B. Values
1. The presence of immunoglobulin M (IgM) antibody to hepatitis A virus (IgM anti-HAV) and total antibody to hepatitis A virus (total anti-HAV) identify the disease
2. The detection of core antigen, envelope antigen, and surface antigen or their corresponding antibodies constitutes hepatitis B assessment
3. Hepatitis C is confirmed by the presence of antibodies to hepatitis C
4. Serologic hepatitis delta virus (HDV) determination is made by the detection of the hepatitis D antigen early during the course of the infection and by the detection of anti-HDV antibody in later disease stages
5. Specific serologic tests for hepatitis E virus include the detection of IgM and immunoglobulin G antibodies to hepatitis E
6. Hepatitis G virus (HGV) has been found in some **blood** donors, IV drug users, hemodialysis clients, and clients with hemophilia; however, HGV does not appear to cause significant liver disease
C. Nursing considerations: If the radioimmunoassay technique is being used, the injection of radionuclides within 1 week before the **blood** test may falsely elevate results

XII. HUMAN IMMUNODEFICIENCY VIRUS (HIV) AND ACQUIRED IMMUNODEFICIENCY SYNDROME (AIDS) TESTING
A. Description
1. Detects HIV, which cause AIDS
2. Tests that are used to determine the presence of antibodies to HIV include ELISA, Western blot (WB), and immunofluorescence assay (IFA)
3. A single reactive ELISA test by itself cannot be used to diagnose HIV and should be repeated in duplicate with the same blood sample; if the result is repeatedly reactive, follow-up tests using WB or IFA should be done
4. A positive WB or IFA is considered confirmatory for HIV

TABLE 11-5 **Normal Adult White Blood Cell Differential Count**

Cell Type	Percentage and Count
Neutrophils	56%; 1800-7800 cells/mm^3
Bands	3%; 0-700 cells/mm^3
Eosinophils	2.7%; 0-450 cells/mm^3
Basophils	0.3%; 0-200 cells/mm^3
Lymphocytes	34%; 1000-4800 cells/mm^3
Monocytes	4%; 0-800 cells/mm^3

5. A positive ELISA that fails to be confirmed by WB or IFA should not be considered negative, and repeat testing should take place in 3 to 6 months

B. CD4 T-cell counts
1. Monitor the progression of HIV
2. As the disease progresses, there is usually a decrease in the CD4$^+$ T-cell count and a resultant decrease in immunity
3. The normal CD4$^+$ T-cell count is between 500 and 1600 cells/mm^3
4. Generally the immune system remains healthy with CD4$^+$ T-cell counts greater than 500 cells/mm^3
5. Immune system problems occur when the CD4$^+$ T-cell count is between 200 and 499 cells/mm^3
6. Severe immune system problems occur when the CD4$^+$ T-cell count is less than 200 cells/mm^3

C. CD4$^+$ to CD8$^+$ ratio
1. Monitors the progression of the disease
2. The normal ratio is approximately 2:1

D. Viral culture: Involves placing the infected client's **blood cells** in a culture medium and measuring the amount of reverse transcriptase activity during a specified period of time

E. Viral load testing: Measures the presence of HIV viral genetic material (RNA) or other viral protein in the client's **blood**

F. p24 antigen assay: Quantifies the amount of HIV viral core protein in the client's **serum**

G. Oral testing for HIV
1. Uses a device that is placed against the gum and cheek for 2 minutes
2. Fluid (not saliva) is drawn into an absorbable pad; this fluid contains antibodies in an HIV-positive individual
3. The pad is placed in a solution, and a specified observable change is noted if the test is positive
4. If the result is positive, a **blood** test is needed to confirm the results

H. Home test kits for HIV
1. A drop of **blood** is placed on a test card with a special code number; the card is mailed to the laboratory for testing for HIV antibodies
2. The individual receives the results by calling a special telephone number and entering the special code number; test results are then given

I. Nursing considerations
1. Maintain issues of confidentiality surrounding HIV and AIDS testing
2. Follow prescribed state regulations and protocols related to reporting positive test results

XIII. **URINE TESTS** (Table 11-6)

XIV. **THERAPEUTIC SERUM MEDICATION LEVELS** (Table 11-7)

A. If the result is below the therapeutic level, the client may not be compliant with the medicine regimen

TABLE 11-6   Normal Adult Values: Urine Tests

Name of Test	Value
Color	Pale yellow
Odor	Specific aromatic odor similar to ammonia
Turbidity	Clear
pH	4.5-7.8
Specific gravity	1.016-1.022
Glucose	<0.5 g/day
Ketones	None
Protein	0.8 mg/dL
Bilirubin	None
Casts	None to few
Crystals	None
Bacteria	<1000 colonies/mL
Red blood cells	0-2
White blood cells	0-5
Chloride	110-250 mEq/24 hours
Magnesium	7.3-12.2 mg/dL per day
Potassium	25-125 mEq/24 hours
Sodium	40-220 mEq/24 hours
Uric acid	250-750 mg/24 hours

TABLE 11-7   Therapeutic Serum Medication Levels

Medication	Therapeutic Range
Acetaminophen (Tylenol)	10-20 mcg/mL
Carbamazepine (Tegretol)	5-12 mcg/mL
Digoxin (Lanoxin)	0.5-2 ng/mL
Gentamicin (Garamycin)	5-10 mcg/mL
Lithium (Lithobid)	0.5-1.3 mEq/L
Magnesium sulfate	4-7 mg/dL
Phenytoin (Dilantin)	10-20 mcg/mL
Salicylates	100-250 mcg/mL
Theophylline	10-20 mcg/mL
Tobramycin (Nebcin)	5-10 mcg/mL
Valproic acid (Depakene)	50-100 mcg/mL

or the dose may need to be increased; notify the registered nurse (RN) or physician

B. If the result is within the range, the medication can be administered as prescribed

C. If the result is above the therapeutic level (toxic), the dose is too high or the client did not understand the medicine regimen and is taking too much; hold the dose and notify the RN or physician

PRACTICE QUESTIONS

More questions on the companion CD!

64. A nurse is told that the laboratory result for the serum digoxin level is 2.4 ng/mL. The nurse plans to do which of the following?
1. Hold the medication.
2. Check the client's last respiratory rate.

3. Record the normal value on the client's flow sheet.
4. Administer the next dose of the medication as scheduled.

65. A client with atrial fibrillation who is receiving maintenance therapy with warfarin sodium (Coumadin) has a prothrombin time (PT) of 30 seconds. The nurse anticipates that which of the following will be prescribed?
    1. Adding a dose of heparin
    2. Holding the next dose of warfarin sodium
    3. Increasing the next dose of warfarin sodium
    4. Administering the next dose of warfarin sodium

66. An adult client who has had preadmission testing before surgery has had blood drawn for the determination of serum electrolyte levels. The nurse identifies which of the following as an abnormal value?
    1. Sodium, 148 mEq/L
    2. Chloride, 101 mEq/L
    3. Potassium, 3.8 mEq/L
    4. Bicarbonate, 26 mEq/L

67. An adult client with a critically high potassium level has received sodium polystyrene sulfonate (Kayexalate). The nurse determines that the medication has brought the potassium level back into normal range when the serum potassium level is:
    1. 3.3 mEq/L
    2. 4.9 mEq/L
    3. 5.8 mEq/L
    4. 6.2 mEq/L

68. The adult client with a history of cardiac disease is due for a morning dose of furosemide (Lasix). The nurse reviews the client's record and reports which of the following serum potassium levels before administering the dose of furosemide?
    1. 3.2 mEq/L
    2. 3.8 mEq/L
    3. 4.2 mEq/L
    4. 4.8 mEq/L

69. A client with diabetes mellitus has a sample drawn for the determination of a fasting blood glucose level. The nurse identifies which of the following results as a critical value?
    1. 150 mg/dL
    2. 200 mg/dL
    3. 220 mg/dL
    4. 340 mg/dL

70. An adult client with a history of gastrointestinal bleeding has a platelet count of 300,000 cells/mL. Which of the following actions by the nurse is most appropriate after reading this report?
    1. Report the abnormally low count.
    2. Report the abnormally high count.
    3. Place the client on bleeding precautions.
    4. Place the normal report in the client's medical record.

71. A nurse is reviewing the laboratory results of an adult client with Addison's disease. The nurse determines that the magnesium level is normal if it is which of the following? *1.6 – 2.6*
    1. 2 mg/dL
    2. 3 mg/dL
    3. 4 mg/dL
    4. 5 mg/dL

72. An adult male client has had laboratory work done as part of a routine physical examination. The nurse reviews the client's record and determines that the client may have a mild degree of renal insufficiency if which of the following serum creatinine levels is found?
    1. 0.6 mg/dL
    2. 1.1 mg/dL
    3. 1.9 mg/dL
    4. 3.5 mg/dL

73. A client with a seizure disorder is taking phenytoin (Dilantin). A sample for a serum phenytoin level is drawn, and the nurse determines that the medication therapy is effective if the laboratory result is: *10–20 mcg/ml*
    1. 3 mcg/mL
    2. 8 mcg/mL
    3. 16 mcg/mL
    4. 24 mcg/mL

74. An adult client with hepatic cirrhosis has been consuming a diet with optimal amounts of protein. The nurse evaluates the client's status as most satisfactory if the total protein level is which of the following values?
    1. 0.4 g/dL
    2. 3.7 g/dL
    3. 6.4 g/dL
    4. 9.8 g/dL

75. An adult client was diagnosed with acute pancreatitis 9 days ago. The nurse interprets that the client is recovering from this episode if the serum lipase level drops to which of the following values, which is just beneath the upper limit of normal? *10–140*
    1. 20 units/L
    2. 80 units/L
    3. 135 units/L
    4. 250 units/L

76. A client arrives in the emergency department complaining of chest pain that began 4 hours ago. A troponin T blood specimen is obtained, and the results indicate a level of 0.6 ng/mL. The nurse interprets that this result indicates:
    1. A normal level
    2. A low value that indicates possible gastritis
    3. A level that indicates a myocardial infarction
    4. A level that indicates the presence of possible angina

77. An adult female client has a hemoglobin level of 10.8 g/dL. The nurse interprets that this result is most likely the result of which of the following factors in the client's history?
    1. Heart failure
    2. Dehydration
    3. Iron deficiency anemia
    4. Chronic obstructive pulmonary disease (COPD)

78. An adult male client admitted with dehydration has received fluid volume replacement. The nurse determines that the client has had adequate fluid resuscitation if the client's repeat hematocrit level has decreased to which of the following values in the normal range?
    1. 34%   *Male -42-52*
    2. 39%
    3. 48%
    4. 56%

79. A client with diabetes mellitus has a glycosylated hemoglobin A (HbA$_{1c}$) level of 8%. Based on this test result, the nurse plans to reinforce teaching measures with the client about the need to:
    1. Avoid infection.
    2. Prevent hyperglycemia.

3. Take in adequate fluids.
4. Increase iron for anemia.

80. A nurse is caring for a client with a diagnosis of cancer who is immunosuppressed. The nurse knows that neutropenic precautions will be implemented if the client's white blood cell (WBC) count is:
    1. 2000 cells/mm^3
    2. 5800 cells/mm^3
    3. 8400 cells/mm^3
    4. 11,500 cells/mm^3

ALTERNATE ITEM FORMAT: MULTIPLE RESPONSE

81. A nurse is reviewing the laboratory results of several clients. Which laboratory tests indicate that the nurse can administer the medication as ordered? Select all that apply.
    ☐ 1. Digoxin (Lanoxin) 3 ng/mL
    ☐ 2. Phenytoin (Dilantin) 28 mcg/mL
    ☐ 3. Tobramycin (Nebcin) 20 mcg/mL
    ☑ 4. Gentamicin (Garamycin) 8 mcg/mL
    ☑ 5. Theophylline (Theo-Dur) 10 mcg/mL
    ☑ 6. Carbamazepine (Tegretol) 10 mcg/mL

ANSWERS

64. 1
Rationale: The normal therapeutic range for digoxin is 0.5 to 2 ng/mL. A value of 2.4 ng/mL exceeds the therapeutic range and could be toxic to the client. The nursing action is to hold further doses of digoxin. Option 3 is incorrect, because the value is not normal. Option 4 would cause the client to become more toxic. The next dose should not be administered automatically. Checking the client's respiratory rate is not applicable at this time.
Test-Taking Strategy: Recall that the normal therapeutic range for digoxin is 0.5 to 2 ng/mL. Noting that the value is high will direct you to option 1. Review this therapeutic level if you had difficulty with this question.
Level of Cognitive Ability: Application
Client Needs: Physiological Integrity
Integrated Process: Nursing Process/Implementation
Content Area: Fundamental Skills
Reference: Chernecky, C., & Berger, B. (2008). *Laboratory tests and diagnostic procedures* (5th ed., p. 448). Philadelphia: Saunders.

65. 2
Rationale: The normal PT is 9.6 to 11.8 seconds for the adult male and 9.5 to 11.3 seconds for the adult female. Because the value stated is extremely high (and perhaps near the critical range), the nurse should anticipate that the client would not receive further doses at this time. If the level were too high, then the antidote (vitamin K) may be prescribed. Options 1, 3, and 4 would make the client more toxic and prone to bleeding.

Test-Taking Strategy: Note that the PT is 30 seconds. Noting that the PT value is high will direct you to option 2. Review this laboratory value if you had difficulty with this question.
Level of Cognitive Ability: Application
Client Needs: Physiological Integrity
Integrated Process: Nursing Process/Planning
Content Area: Fundamental Skills
References: Chernecky, C., & Berger, B. (2008). *Laboratory tests and diagnostic procedures* (5th ed., pp. 927-928). Philadelphia: Saunders.
Pagana, K., & Pagana, T. (2005). *Mosby's diagnostic and laboratory test reference* (7th ed., pp. 768-770). St. Louis: Mosby.

66. 1
Rationale: The normal serum electrolyte ranges for adults are as follows: sodium, 135 to 145 mEq/L; potassium, 3.5 to 5.1 mEq/L; chloride, 98 to 107 mEq/L; and bicarbonate (venous), 22 to 29 mEq/L. The only abnormal value identified is the serum sodium level.
Test-Taking Strategy: Focus on the subject of an abnormal value. Recalling the normal serum electrolyte values will direct you to option 1. Review the normal electrolyte values if you had difficulty with this question.
Level of Cognitive Ability: Comprehension
Client Needs: Physiological Integrity
Integrated Process: Nursing Process/Data Collection
Content Area: Fundamental Skills
Reference: Chernecky, C., & Berger, B. (2008). *Laboratory tests and diagnostic procedures* (5th ed., p. 1022). Philadelphia: Saunders.

67. 2
Rationale: The normal serum potassium level in the adult is 3.5 to 5.1 mEq/L. Option 2 is the only option that reflects a normal potassium value.
Test-Taking Strategy: Note the strategic words "critically high." You would expect that this medication is administered to lower the potassium level. Recalling the normal serum potassium level will direct you to option 2. Review this normal level if you had difficulty with this question.
Level of Cognitive Ability: Comprehension
Client Needs: Physiological Integrity
Integrated Process: Nursing Process/Evaluation
Content Area: Fundamental Skills
Reference: Chernecky, C., & Berger, B. (2008). *Laboratory tests and diagnostic procedures* (5th ed., p. 891). Philadelphia: Saunders.

68. 1
Rationale: The normal adult serum potassium level is 3.5 to 5.1 mEq/L. Option 1 is the only value that falls below the therapeutic range. Administering furosemide (Lasix) to a client with a low potassium level and a cardiac history could precipitate ventricular dysrhythmias in the client.
Test-Taking Strategy: Use the process of elimination. Recalling the normal serum potassium level will assist you with identifying the value that is not within normal range. This will direct you to option 1. Review the normal adult serum potassium level if you had difficulty with this question.
Level of Cognitive Ability: Comprehension
Client Needs: Physiological Integrity
Integrated Process: Nursing Process/Implementation
Content Area: Fundamental Skills
References: Chernecky, C., & Berger, B. (2008). *Laboratory tests and diagnostic procedures* (5th ed., p. 891). Philadelphia: Saunders.
Pagana, K., & Pagana, T. (2005). *Mosby's diagnostic and laboratory test reference* (7th ed., p. 733). St. Louis: Mosby.

69. 4
Rationale: The normal fasting blood glucose level is 70 to 110 mg/dL in the adult client. A critical level is considered to be one that exceeds 300 mg/dL. This makes option 4 the correct option.
Test-Taking Strategy: Use the process of elimination and your knowledge of the normal fasting blood glucose level to answer the question. Noting the strategic words "critical value" will direct you to option 4. Review this laboratory test if you had difficulty with this question.
Level of Cognitive Ability: Comprehension
Client Needs: Physiological Integrity
Integrated Process: Nursing Process/Data Collection
Content Area: Fundamental Skills
References: Chernecky, C., & Berger, B. (2008). *Laboratory tests and diagnostic procedures* (5th ed., p. 578). Philadelphia: Saunders.
Pagana, K., & Pagana, T. (2005). *Mosby's diagnostic and laboratory test reference* (7th ed., p. 482). St. Louis: Mosby.

70. 4
Rationale: A normal platelet count ranges from 150,000 to 400,000 cells/μL. The nurse should place the report that contains the normal laboratory value into the client's medical record.
Test-Taking Strategy: Use the process of elimination. Remember that options that are comparable or alike are not likely to be correct. With this in mind, eliminate options 1 and 3 first. From the remaining options, recalling the normal range for this laboratory test will direct you to option 4. Review the normal platelet count if you had difficulty with this question.
Level of Cognitive Ability: Application
Client Needs: Physiological Integrity
Integrated Process: Nursing Process/Implementation
Content Area: Fundamental Skills
Reference: Chernecky, C., & Berger, B. (2008). *Laboratory tests and diagnostic procedures* (5th ed., p. 883). Philadelphia: Saunders.

71. 1
Rationale: The normal magnesium level in an adult client is 1.6 to 2.6 mg/dL. Options 2, 3, and 4 indicate elevated values.
Test-Taking Strategy: Knowledge regarding the normal magnesium level in an adult client is required to answer this question. Remember that the normal magnesium level in an adult client is 1.6 to 2.6 mg/dL. Review this laboratory test if you had difficulty with this question.
Level of Cognitive Ability: Comprehension
Client Needs: Physiological Integrity
Integrated Process: Nursing Process/Data Collection
Content Area: Fundamental Skills
Reference: Chernecky, C., & Berger, B. (2008). *Laboratory tests and diagnostic procedures* (5th ed., p. 744). Philadelphia: Saunders.

72. 3
Rationale: The normal serum creatinine level is 0.6 to 1.3 mg/dL. The client with a mild degree of renal insufficiency would have a slightly elevated level, which would be the value of 1.9 mg/dL. Creatinine levels of 3.5 mg/dL may be associated with acute or chronic renal failure.
Test-Taking Strategy: Note the strategic word "mild." This tells you that the correct option will be an abnormal value but perhaps not the most abnormal of all of the options. Use your knowledge of the normal serum creatinine level to direct you to option 3. Review the normal value of this laboratory test if you had difficulty with this question.
Level of Cognitive Ability: Analysis
Client Needs: Physiological Integrity
Integrated Process: Nursing Process/Data Collection
Content Area: Fundamental Skills
Reference: Pagana, K., & Pagana, T. (2005). *Mosby's diagnostic and laboratory test reference* (7th ed., pp. 326-327). St. Louis: Mosby.

73. 3
Rationale: The therapeutic range for serum phenytoin (Dilantin) level is 10 to 20 mcg/mL. If the level is below the therapeutic range, as in options 1 and 2, then the client may continue to experience seizure activity. If the level is too high, as in option 4, the client could experience phenytoin toxicity.
Test-Taking Strategy: Focus on the subject of effective medication therapy. Remember that the therapeutic range for serum phenytoin (Dilantin) level is 10 to 20 mcg/mL. Review this normal range if you had difficulty with this question.

Level of Cognitive Ability: Comprehension
Client Needs: Physiological Integrity
Integrated Process: Nursing Process/Evaluation
Content Area: Fundamental Skills
References: Black, J., & Hawks, J. (2005). *Medical-surgical nursing: Clinical management for positive outcomes* (7th ed., p. 2307). Philadelphia: Saunders.
Chernecky, C., & Berger, B. (2008). *Laboratory tests and diagnostic procedures* (5th ed., p. 872). Philadelphia: Saunders.

74. 3
Rationale: The normal range for the protein level in the adult client is 6 to 8 g/dL, which makes option 3 the correct option. Options 1 and 2 indicate low levels. Option 4 indicates an elevated level.
Test-Taking Strategy: Note the strategic words "most satisfactory." Recalling the normal protein level will direct you to option 3. Review this normal level if you had difficulty with this question.
Level of Cognitive Ability: Comprehension
Client Needs: Physiological Integrity
Integrated Process: Nursing Process/Evaluation
Content Area: Fundamental Skills
Reference: Chernecky, C., & Berger, B. (2008). *Laboratory tests and diagnostic procedures* (5th ed., p. 920). Philadelphia: Saunders.

75. 3
Rationale: The normal serum lipase level is 10 to 140 units/L. Option 3 is the only option that contains a value just beneath the upper limit of normal. The client who is recovering from acute pancreatitis usually has elevated lipase levels for approximately 10 days after the onset of symptoms. This makes lipase a valuable test for monitoring the client's pancreatic function.
Test-Taking Strategy: Note the strategic words "just beneath the upper limit of normal." Recalling the normal lipase level will direct you to option 3. Review this normal level if you had difficulty with this question.
Level of Cognitive Ability: Comprehension
Client Needs: Physiological Integrity
Integrated Process: Nursing Process/Evaluation
Content Area: Fundamental Skills
References: Chernecky, C., & Berger, B. (2008). *Laboratory tests and diagnostic procedures* (5th ed., p. 713). Philadelphia: Saunders.
Pagana, K., & Pagana, T. (2005). *Mosby's diagnostic and laboratory test reference* (7th ed., p. 588). St. Louis: Mosby.

76. 3
Rationale: Troponins are regulatory proteins that are found in striated muscle. The troponins function together in the contractile apparatus for striated muscle in the skeletal muscle and in the myocardium. Increased amounts of troponins are released into the bloodstream when an infarction causes damage to the myocardium. A troponin T level greater than 0.1 to 0.2 ng/mL is consistent with a myocardial infarction. A normal troponin I level is less than 0.6 ng/mL, whereas a level greater than 1.5 ng/mL is consistent with a myocardial infarction. A level of 0.6 is not normal, so option 1 is incorrect.

Troponin T does not test for angina or gastritis; thus options 2 and 4 are incorrect.
Test-Taking Strategy: Note that the subject of the question relates to the troponin T level. Recalling that a level greater than 0.1 to 0.2 ng/mL is consistent with a myocardial infarction will direct you to option 3. Review this diagnostic test if you had difficulty with this question.
Level of Cognitive Ability: Analysis
Client Needs: Physiological Integrity
Integrated Process: Nursing Process/Evaluation
Content Area: Adult Health/Cardiovascular
Reference: Pagana, K., & Pagana, T. (2005). *Mosby's diagnostic and laboratory test reference* (7th ed., pp. 941-943). St. Louis: Mosby.

77. 3
Rationale: The normal hemoglobin level for an adult female client is 12 to 15 g/dL. A low hemoglobin level usually indicates anemia. Iron deficiency anemia can result in lower hemoglobin levels. Options 1, 2, and 4 may increase hemoglobin. Heart failure and COPD may increase the hemoglobin level as a result of the body's need for more oxygen-carrying capacity. Dehydration may increase the hemoglobin level by hemoconcentration.
Test-Taking Strategy: Use the process of elimination. Evaluate each condition presented in the options with regard to whether it is likely to raise or lower the hemoglobin level. This will direct you to option 3. Review the normal hemoglobin level and the causes of a low level if you had difficulty with this question.
Level of Cognitive Ability: Analysis
Client Needs: Physiological Integrity
Integrated Process: Nursing Process/Data Collection
Content Area: Fundamental Skills
References: Chernecky, C., & Berger, B. (2008). *Laboratory tests and diagnostic procedures* (5th ed., pp. 617-618). Philadelphia: Saunders.
Pagana, K., & Pagana, T. (2005). *Mosby's diagnostic and laboratory test reference* (7th ed., pp. 514-515). St. Louis: Mosby.

78. 3
Rationale: The normal hematocrit level for an adult male is 42% to 52%. Thus, option 3 is the only correct choice. The client who is dehydrated has an elevated level as a result of hemoconcentration. The client's level may be expected to drift back down to within the normal range after the fluid volume has been adequately restored. Option 4 is too high, and options 1 and 2 are low. *Test-Taking Strategy:* Use the process of elimination, and note the strategic words "normal range." Recalling the normal hematocrit level for an adult male will direct you to option 3. Review this normal value if you had difficulty with this question.
Level of Cognitive Ability: Comprehension
Client Needs: Physiological Integrity
Integrated Process: Nursing Process/Evaluation
Content Area: Fundamental Skills
Reference: Pagana, K., & Pagana, T. (2005). *Mosby's diagnostic and laboratory test reference* (7th ed., pp. 511-513). St. Louis: Mosby.

79. 2

Rationale: Elevations of the HbA$_{1c}$ value indicate a need for teaching related to the prevention of hyperglycemic episodes. The HbA$_{1c}$ value measures the amount of glucose that has become permanently bound to the red blood cells. Elevations in blood glucose levels will cause elevations in the amount of glycosylation. Thus, this test is useful for detecting clients who have periods of hyperglycemia that are undetected in other ways. Values are expressed as a percentage of total hemoglobin and include the following: diabetic client with good control, 7.5% or less; diabetic client with fair control, 7.6% to 8.9%; and diabetic client with poor control, 9% or greater. Option 1 relates to a low white blood cell count rather than the HbA$_{1c}$ level. Option 3 relates to an increased hematocrit level rather than the HbA$_{1c}$ level. Option 4 relates to a low red blood cell count and hemoglobin level rather than the HbA$_{1c}$ level. HbA$_{1c}$ relates to glucose.

Test-Taking Strategy: Use the process of elimination, and focus on the level identified in the question. Recalling the expected values related to the HbA$_{1c}$ test and their significance will assist you with answering correctly. Review the HbA$_{1c}$ test if you had difficulty with this question.

Level of Cognitive Ability: Application
Client Needs: Physiological Integrity
Integrated Process: Teaching and Learning
Content Area: Fundamental Skills
Reference: Pagana, K., & Pagana, T. (2005). *Mosby's diagnostic and laboratory test reference* (7th ed., pp. 496-497). St. Louis: Mosby.

80. 1

Rationale: The normal WBC count ranges from 4500 to 11,000 cells/mm^3. The client who is immunosuppressed has a decrease in the number of circulating WBCs. The nurse implements neutropenic precautions when the client's values fall sufficiently below the low-normal level. Options 2 and 3 are within normal limits, and option 4 is elevated.

Test-Taking Strategy: Knowledge regarding the normal WBC count and the purpose of neutropenic precautions will direct you to option 1. Remember that the normal WBC count ranges from 4500 to 11,000 cells/mm^3. Review this laboratory test if you had difficulty with this question.

Level of Cognitive Ability: Comprehension
Client Needs: Safe and Effective Care Environment
Integrated Process: Nursing Process/Implementation
Content Area: Fundamental Skills
Reference: Pagana, K., & Pagana, T. (2005). *Mosby's diagnostic and laboratory test reference* (7th ed., p. 944). St. Louis: Mosby.

ALTERNATE ITEM FORMAT: MULTIPLE RESPONSE

81. 4, 5, 6

Rationale: Options 4, 5, and 6 are the only ones within the normal therapeutic range; all other results are abnormal (too high). Therapeutic medication levels include the following: carbamazepine (Tegretol), 5 to 12 mcg/mL; digoxin (Lanoxin), 0.5 to 2 ng/mL; gentamicin (Garamycin), 5 to 10 mcg/mL; phenytoin (Dilantin), 10 to 20 mcg/mL; theophylline, 10 to 20 mcg/mL; and tobramycin (Nebcin), 5 to 10 mcg/mL.

Test-Taking Strategy: Note the strategic words "can administer the medication." This phrase implies that you need to select the options that indicate normal levels. Use your knowledge of therapeutic levels to answer this question. Review these therapeutic serum medication levels if you had difficulty with this question.

Level of Cognitive Ability: Analysis
Client Needs: Physiological Integrity
Integrated Process: Nursing Process/Planning
Content Area: Fundamental Skills
Reference: Pagana, K., & Pagana, T. (2005). *Mosby's diagnostic and laboratory test reference* (7th ed., pp. 894-895). St. Louis: Mosby.

REFERENCES

Black, J., & Hawks, J. (2005). *Medical-surgical nursing: Clinical management for positive outcomes* (7th ed.). Philadelphia: Saunders.

Chernecky, C., & Berger, B. (2008). *Laboratory tests and diagnostic procedures* (5th ed.). Philadelphia: Saunders.

National Council of State Boards of Nursing (Eds.) (2008). *2008 Detailed Test Plan for the NCLEX-PN® Examination, National Council of State Boards of Nursing.* Chicago: Author.

National Council of State Boards of Nursing. *NCSBN home page.* www.ncsbn.org. Accessed June 16, 2008.

Pagana, K., & Pagana, T. (2005). *Mosby's diagnostic and laboratory test reference* (7th ed.). St. Louis: Mosby.

CHAPTER 12

Nutritional Components of Care

PYRAMID TERMS

absorption The passage of digested nutrients through the wall of the stomach or small intestine into the blood or lymph system.

enteral nutrition The administration of nutrition with liquefied foods into the gastrointestinal tract via a tube.

fat emulsion (lipids) The administration of lipids during parenteral nutrition therapy to prevent fatty-acid deficiency.

malnutrition A deficiency of the nutrients required for the development and maintenance of the human body.

metabolism An ongoing chemical process within the body that converts digested nutrients into energy for the functioning of body cells.

nutrients Substances, including carbohydrates, fats or lipids, proteins, vitamins, minerals, and water, that must be supplied in adequate amounts to provide energy, growth, development, and maintenance of the human body.

parenteral nutrition The administration of nutrition through a central or peripheral intravenous catheter.

peripheral parenteral nutrition Parenteral nutrition administered through a peripheral vein in an extremity; also called *peripheral venous nutrition.*

total parenteral nutrition Parenteral nutrition administered intravenously through a central vein, such as the subclavian vein; also called *central parenteral nutrition.*

PYRAMID TO SUCCESS

Nutrition is a basic need that must be met for all clients. Nurses must have the knowledge required to educate and care for both healthy clients and clients with nutritional needs or disorders that require alterations in dietary measures. The NCLEX-PN will address the dietary measures required for basic needs and for particular body-system alterations. When presented with a question related to nutrition, consider the client's diagnosis and the particular requirement or restriction necessary for the treatment of the disorder. Pyramid points focus on the common types of therapeutic diets, nutrients contained in food items, enteral feedings, and parenteral nutrition (PN). The Integrated Processes addressed in this chapter include Clinical Problem-Solving

Process (Nursing Process), Caring, Communication and Documentation, and Teaching and Learning.

CLIENT NEEDS

Safe and Effective Care Environment

Consulting with members of the health care team, such as the dietitian

Discussing home safety for storing and cooking foods

Handling hazardous and infectious materials

Maintaining medical and surgical asepsis to prevent infection

Maintaining standard, transmission-based, and other precautions

Obtaining informed consent for invasive procedures

Health Promotion and Maintenance

Performing data collection techniques

Providing client and family education regarding the administration of PN at home

Providing dietary teaching about diet and foods to avoid or increase

Psychosocial Integrity

Considering cultural and religious preferences and lifestyle choices related to nutritional patterns

Discussing role changes related to the need for PN at home

Identifying coping mechanisms

Identifying support systems in the home

Physiological Integrity

Assessing elimination patterns

Checking for adverse, expected, and side effects of PN and enteral therapy for nutrition

Monitoring for alterations in body systems

Monitoring enteral feedings and the client's ability to tolerate feedings

Monitoring for expected effects of nutritional therapy

Monitoring the fluid and electrolyte balance
Monitoring laboratory values
Monitoring nutritional intake and oral hydration
Monitoring for potential complications of nutritional therapy
Providing assistive devices for eating

I. NUTRIENTS

A. Carbohydrates (Box 12-1)
1. Preferred source of energy
2. Include sugars, starches, and cellulose
3. Provide 4 cal/g
4. Promote normal fat **metabolism,** spare protein, and enhance lower gastrointestinal (GI) function
5. Major food sources include milk, grains, fruits, and vegetables
6. Inadequate carbohydrate intake affects **metabolism**

B. Fats (Box 12-2)
1. Provide a concentrated source and a stored form of energy
2. Protect internal organs and maintain body temperature
3. Enhance the **absorption** of the fat-soluble vitamins
4. Provide 9 cal/g
5. Inadequate fat intake leads to clinical manifestations of sensitivity to cold, skin lesions, increased risk of infection, and amenorrhea in women
6. Diets high in fat can lead to obesity and increase the risk of cardiovascular disease and some cancers

C. Proteins (Box 12-3)
1. Made from amino acids, which are critical to all aspects of the growth and development of body tissues
2. Provide 4 cal/g
3. Build and repair body tissues, regulate fluid balance, maintain acid-base balance, produce antibodies, provide energy, and produce enzymes and hormones
4. Essential amino acids (EAAs) are required in the diet because the body cannot manufacture them
5. High-quality proteins or complete proteins such as eggs, dairy products, meat, fish, and poultry contain adequate amounts of EAAs
6. Foods that do not contain EAAs in sufficient amounts are lower-quality or incomplete proteins; these can be combined to provide the EAAs.
7. Inadequate protein intake can cause protein energy **malnutrition** and severe wasting of fat and muscle tissue

D. Vitamins (Box 12-4)
1. Facilitate the **metabolism** of proteins, fats, and carbohydrates; act as catalysts for metabolic functions; promote life and growth processes; and maintain and regulate body functions
2. Fat-soluble vitamins A, D, E, and K can be stored in the body, so an excess can cause toxicity
3. The B vitamins and vitamin C are water soluble, are not stored in the body, and can be excreted in the urine
4. Vitamin K acts as a catalyst for facilitating blood-clotting factors, especially prothrombin
5. Vitamin C produces collagen, which is a vital component in wound healing
6. Vitamin A maintains eyesight and epithelial linings
7. Folic acid helps prevent neural-tube birth defects

BOX 12-1 **Carbohydrate Food Sources**

Glucose	Fructose	Fiber	Lactose
Grapes	Honey	Bran	Milk
Oranges	Fruits	Apples	
Dates		Beans	
Carrots		Cabbage	

Sucrose	Starch/Complex Carbohydrates
Granulated table sugar	Wheat
Molasses	Corn
Apricots	Oats
Peaches	Rye
Plums	Barley
Honeydew and cantaloupe	Potatoes and pasta
	Beets, carrots, and peas

BOX 12-2 **Fat Food Sources**

Saturated Fats	Monounsaturated Fats
Beef	Duck and goose
Luncheon meats	Eggs
Hard yellow cheeses	Olive and peanut oils
Butter	
Coconut oil	
Palm oil	
Polyunsaturated Fats	Cholesterol
Safflower oil	Animal products
Corn oil	Egg yolks
Sunflower oil	Liver and organ meats

BOX 12-3 **Protein Food Sources**

- Meats: beef, poultry, pork, and fish
- Eggs
- Dairy products
- Bread and cereal products
- Dried beans

E. Minerals (Box 12-5)
  1. Components of hormones, cells, tissues, and bones
  2. Act as catalysts for chemical reactions and enhancers of cell function
  3. Almost all foods contain some form of minerals
  4. Deficiency of minerals can occur in chronically ill or hospitalized clients
II. MYPYRAMID FOOD GUIDE
A. Provides individualized guidance for healthy eating and physical activity
B. Emphasizes the importance of finding a balance between food and physical activity
C. Food groups include grains, vegetables, fruits, milk, and meat and beans
D. Provides recommendations regarding physical activity and the amounts and types of foods for each food group
E. Developed as a Web-based, interactive, informational nutritional tool
F. Used for healthy adults; there is a different pyramid for children and for pregnant and breast-feeding women
G. Web site: http://www.mypyramid.gov
III. THERAPEUTIC DIETS
A. Clear liquid diet
  1. Indications
    a. Serves the primary function of providing fluids and electrolytes to prevent dehydration
    b. Initial feeding after complete bowel rest

c. Used initially to feed a malnourished person or a person who has not had any oral intake for some time
d. Bowel preparation for surgery or tests
e. Postsurgical diet
f. Diarrhea
  2. Nursing considerations
    a. Clear liquid is deficient in energy and most **nutrients**
    b. The body digests and absorbs clear liquids easily

BOX 12-4 Food Sources of Vitamins

Water Soluble
- Folic acid: Green, leafy vegetables; liver, beef, and fish; legumes; grapefruit and oranges
- Niacin: Meats, poultry, fish, beans, peanuts, grains
- Vitamin B1 (thiamine): Pork, nuts, whole-grain cereals, legumes
- Vitamin B2 (riboflavin): Milk, lean meats, fish, grains
- Vitamin B6 (pyridoxine): Yeast, corn, meat, poultry, fish
- Vitamin B12 (cobalamin): Meat, liver (only found in animal products)
- Vitamin C (ascorbic acid): Citrus fruits, tomatoes, broccoli, cabbage

Fat Soluble
- Vitamin A: Liver, egg yolk, whole milk, green or orange vegetables, fruits
- Vitamin D: Fortified milk, fish oils, cereals
- Vitamin E: Vegetable oils; green, leafy vegetables; cereals; apricots; apples; peaches
- Vitamin K: Green, leafy vegetables; cauliflower; cabbage

BOX 12-5 Food Sources of Minerals

Calcium
- Broccoli
- Carrots
- Cheese
- Collard greens
- Green beans
- Low-fat yogurt
- Milk
- Rhubarb
- Spinach
- Tofu

Chloride
- Salt

Magnesium
- Avocados
- Canned white tuna
- Cauliflower
- Cooked rolled oats
- Green, leafy vegetables
- Low-fat yogurt
- Milk
- Peanut butter
- Peas
- Pork, beef, chicken
- Potatoes
- Raisins

Phosphorus
- Fish
- Nuts
- Organ meats
- Pork, beef, chicken
- Whole-grain breads and cereals

Potassium
- Avocados
- Bananas
- Cantaloupe
- Carrots

- Fish
- Mushrooms
- Oranges
- Pork, beef, veal
- Potatoes
- Raisins
- Spinach
- Strawberries
- Tomatoes

Sodium
- American cheese
- Bacon
- Butter
- Canned food
- Cottage cheese
- Cured pork
- Frankfurters
- Ketchup
- Lunch meat
- Milk
- Mustard
- Processed food
- Snack food
- Soy sauce
- Table salt
- White and whole-wheat bread

Iron
- Breads and cereals
- Dark green vegetables
- Egg yolk
- Liver
- Meats

Zinc
- Eggs
- Green, leafy vegetables
- Meats
- Protein-rich foods

c. Contributes to little or no residue in the GI tract

d. Can be unappetizing and boring

e. Client should not stay on a clear liquid diet for more than a day or two

f. Consists of foods that are relatively transparent to light and clear and that liquefy at body or room temperature

g. Foods include such items as water, bouillon, clear broth, carbonated beverages, gelatin, hard candy, lemonade, popsicles, and regular or decaffeinated coffee or tea

h. The nurse should limit the amount of caffeine consumed by the client, because caffeine can cause an upset stomach and sleeplessness

i. Client may have salt or sugar

j. Dairy products are not allowed

B. Full liquid diet

1. Indication: May be used as a second diet after clear liquids after surgery or for a client who is unable to chew or swallow

2. Nursing considerations

a. Nutritionally deficient in energy and most **nutrients**

b. Includes both clear and opaque liquid foods and those that liquefy at body temperature

c. Foods include all clear liquids and such items as plain ice cream, sherbet, breakfast drinks, milk, pudding, custard, soups that are strained, and strained vegetable juices

C. Mechanically altered diet

1. Indications

a. Provides foods that have been mechanically altered in texture to require minimal chewing

b. Used for clients who have difficulty chewing but who tolerate more variety in texture than a liquid diet offers

c. Used for clients who have dental problems, who have undergone surgery of the head or neck, or who have dysphagia (requires swallowing evaluation and may require thickened liquids)

2. Nursing considerations

a. Degree of texture modification depends on individual need, including puréed, mashed, ground, or chopped

b. Foods to be avoided in mechanically altered diets include nuts; dried fruit; raw fruits and vegetables; fried foods; chocolate candy; tough, smoked, or salted meats; and foods with coarse textures

D. Soft diet

1. Indications

a. Used for clients with difficulty chewing or swallowing

b. Used for clients with ulcerations of the mouth or gums, broken jaws, or dysphagia and for those who have experienced oral surgery, plastic surgery of the head or neck, or stroke

2. Nursing considerations

a. Clients with mouth sores should be served foods at cooler temperatures

b. Clients who have difficulty chewing and swallowing because of the reduced flow of saliva can increase salivary flow by sucking on sour candy

c. Encourage the client to eat a variety of foods

d. Provide plenty of fluids with meals to make the chewing and swallowing of foods easier

e. Sucking fluids through a straw may be easier than drinking from a cup or glass

f. All foods and seasonings are permitted; however, liquid, chopped, or puréed foods or regular foods with a soft consistency are tolerated best

g. Avoid foods that contain nuts or seeds, which can easily become trapped in the mouth and cause discomfort

h. Raw fruits and vegetables, fried foods, and whole grains are avoided

E. Low-residue, low-fiber diet

1. Indications

a. Supplies foods that are least likely to form an obstruction when the intestinal tract is narrowed by inflammation or scarring or when GI motility is slowed

b. Used for inflammatory bowel disease, partial obstructions of the intestinal tract, gastroenteritis, diarrhea, or other GI disorders

2. Nursing considerations

a. Foods high in carbohydrates are usually low in residue; they include white bread, cereals, and pasta

b. Foods to be avoided are raw fruits (except bananas), vegetables, seeds, plant fiber, and whole grains

c. Dairy products are limited to two servings a day

F. High-residue, high-fiber diet

1. Indications

a. Used for clients with constipation; irritable bowel syndrome, when the primary symptom is alternating constipation and diarrhea; and asymptomatic diverticular disease

b. Helps regulate blood glucose in clients with diabetes mellitus

c. Helps control blood cholesterol in clients with heart disease

2. Nursing considerations

a. Provides 20 to 25 g of dietary fiber daily

b. Adds volume and weight to the stool and speeds the movement of undigested materials through the intestine
c. Consists of fruits, vegetables, and whole-grain products
d. Increase fiber gradually and provide adequate fluids to reduce possible undesirable side effects such as abdominal cramps, bloating, diarrhea, and dehydration
e. Gas-forming foods should be limited (Box 12-6)

G. Cardiac diet (see Box 12-2 and Box 12-7)
1. Indications
   a. Indicated for atherosclerosis, diabetes mellitus, hyperlipidemia, hypertension, myocardial infarction, nephrotic syndrome, and renal failure
   b. Reduces the risk of heart disease
2. Nursing considerations: Limit the total amount of fats (polyunsaturated fats, monounsaturated fats, saturated fats, and trans fats), cholesterol, and sodium

H. Fat-restricted diet
1. Indications
   a. Used to reduce symptoms of abdominal pain, steatorrhea, flatulence, and diarrhea associated with high intakes of dietary fat and to decrease nutrient losses caused by the ingestion of dietary fat in individuals with malabsorptive disorders
   b. Used for clients with malabsorption disorders, pancreatitis, gallbladder disease, and gastroesophageal reflux
2. Nursing considerations
   a. Restricts the amount of total fat, including saturated fats, trans fats, polyunsaturated fats, and monounsaturated fats
   b. Clients with malabsorption may also have difficulty tolerating fiber and lactose
   c. Vitamin and mineral deficiencies may occur in clients with diarrhea or steatorrhea
   d. A fecal-fat test indicates fat malabsorption with the excretion of more than 6 to 8 g fat (or more than 10% of the fat consumed) per day during the 3 days after the test

I. High-calorie, high-protein diet
1. Indications: Severe stress, burns, cancer, human immunodeficiency virus infection, acquired immunodeficiency syndrome, chronic obstructive pulmonary disease, respiratory failure, or any other type of debilitating disease
2. Nursing considerations
   a. Encourage nutrient-dense, high-calorie, high-protein foods such as whole milk and milk products, peanut butter, nuts, seeds, beef, chicken, fish, pork, and eggs.

BOX 12-6 Gas-Forming Foods *SATA*

- Apples
- Artichokes
- Barley
- Beans
- Bran
- Broccoli
- Brussels sprouts
- Cabbage
- Celery
- Cherries
- Coconuts
- Eggplant
- Figs
- Honey
- Melons
- Milk
- Molasses
- Nuts
- Onions
- Radishes
- Soybeans
- Wheat
- Yeast

BOX 12-7 Sodium-Free Spices and Flavorings *SATA*

- Allspice
- Almond extract
- Bay leaves
- Caraway seeds
- Cinnamon
- Curry powder
- Garlic and garlic powder
- Ginger
- Lemon extract
- Maple extract
- Marjoram
- Mustard powder
- Nutmeg

b. Some high-calorie foods include sugar, cream, gravy, oil, butter, mayonnaise, dried fruit, avocados, and honey
c. Encourage snacks between meals, such as milkshakes, instant breakfasts, and nutritional supplements

J. Carbohydrate-consistent diet
1. Indications: Diabetes mellitus, hypoglycemia, hyperglycemia, and obesity
2. Nursing considerations
   a. The Exchange System for Meal Planning, developed by the American Dietetic Association and the American Diabetes Association, is a food guide that may be recommended
   b. The Exchange System groups foods according to the amounts of carbohydrates, fats, and proteins that they contain
   c. Major food groups include the carbohydrate group, the meat and meat substitute group, and the fat group

K. Sodium-restricted diet
1. Indications: Hypertension, heart failure, renal disease, cardiac disease, and cirrhosis of the liver

2. Nursing considerations (see Box 12-7)
   a. Individualized; can include 4 g of sodium daily (no-added-salt diet), 2 to 3 g of sodium daily (moderate restriction), 1 g of sodium daily (strict restriction), or 500 mg of sodium daily (severe and seldom prescribed)
   b. Encourage the intake of fresh rather than processed foods, which contain higher amounts of sodium
   c. Canned, frozen, instant, smoked, pickled, and boxed items usually contain higher amounts of sodium
   d. Lunch meats, soy sauce, salad dressings, fast foods, soups, and snacks such as potato chips and pretzels also contain large amounts of sodium
   e. Certain medications contain significant amounts of sodium
   f. Salt substitutes may be used to improve palatability; most salt substitutes contain large amounts of potassium and should not be used by clients with renal disease
L. Protein-restricted diet
   1. Indications: Acute renal failure, chronic renal disease, cirrhosis of the liver, and hepatic coma
   2. Nursing considerations
      a. Provides enough protein to maintain nutritional status but not an amount that will allow the buildup of waste products from protein **metabolism** (40 to 60 g of protein daily)
      b. The smaller the amount of protein allowed, the more important it becomes that all protein included in the diet be of high quality
      c. An adequate total energy intake from foods is critical for clients on protein-restricted diets (protein will be used for energy rather than for protein synthesis)
      d. Special low-protein products, such as pastas, bread, cookies, wafers, and gelatin made with wheat starch, can improve energy intake and add variety to the diet
      e. Carbohydrates in powdered or liquid form can also provide additional energy
      f. Vegetables and fruits contain some protein; for very low-protein diets, these foods must be calculated into the diet
      g. Foods from the milk, meat, bread, and starch exchanges are limited
M. Renal diet (see Boxes 12-3 and 12-5)
   1. Indications: Acute and chronic renal failure, hemodialysis, peritoneal dialysis
   2. Nursing considerations
      a. Controlled amounts of protein, sodium, phosphorus, calcium, potassium, and fluids may be prescribed; may also require

BOX 12-8 Measures to Relieve Thirst

1. Chew gum or suck hard candy.
2. Freeze fluids so that they take longer to consume.
3. Add lemon juice to water to make it more refreshing.
4. Gargle with refrigerated mouthwash.

modifications of the amounts of fiber, cholesterol, and fat based on individual requirements
      b. Most clients who are receiving dialysis need to restrict fluids (Box 12-8)
N. Potassium-modified diet (see Box 12-5)
   1. Indications
      a. A low-potassium diet is indicated for hyperkalemia, which may be the result of impaired renal function, hypoaldosteronism, Addison's disease, angiotensin-converting enzyme inhibitor medications, immunosuppressive medications, potassium-sparing diuretics, and chronic hyperkalemia
      b. A high-potassium diet is indicated for hypokalemia, which may be the result of renal tubular acidosis, GI losses (diarrhea, vomiting), intracellular shifts, potassium-wasting diuretics, antibiotics, mineralocorticoid or glucocorticoid excess caused by primary or secondary aldosteronism, Cushing's syndrome, or exogenous steroid use.
   2. Nursing considerations
      a. Foods that are low in potassium include applesauce, green beans, cabbage, lettuce, peppers, grapes, blueberries, cooked summer squash, cooked turnip greens, fresh pineapple, and raspberries
      b. Refer to Box 12-5 for foods that are high in potassium
O. High-calcium diet
   1. Indications: Calcium is needed during bone growth and in adulthood to prevent osteoporosis and to facilitate vascular contraction and vasodilation, muscle contraction, and nerve transmission
   2. Nursing considerations
      a. Primary dietary sources of calcium are dairy products (see Box 12-5)
      b. Clients with lactose intolerance need to incorporate sources of calcium other than dairy products into their dietary patterns regularly
P. Low-purine diet
   1. Indications: Gout, kidney stones, and elevated uric acid levels
   2. Nursing considerations
      a. Purine is a precursor of uric acid, which forms stones and crystals

b. Foods to restrict include anchovies, herring, mackerel, sardines, scallops, glandular meats, gravies, meat extracts, wild game, goose, and sweetbreads

Q. High-iron diet
   1. Indication: Anemia
   2. Nursing considerations
      a. The high-iron diet addresses an iron deficit caused by inadequate intake or loss
      b. The diet includes organ meats; meat; egg yolks; whole-wheat products; dark green, leafy vegetables; dried fruit; and legumes (see Box 12-5)

R. Miscellaneous diets: See Chapter 9, Boxes 9-3, 9-4, 9-5, 9-6, and 9-7 for foods high in potassium, sodium, calcium, magnesium, and phosphorus

IV. VEGETARIAN DIETS

A. Types (Box 12-9)
B. Nursing considerations
   1. Ensure that the client eats a sufficient amount of varied foods to meet normal nutrient and energy needs
   2. Clients should be educated about consuming complementary proteins over the course of each day to ensure that all EAAs are provided
   3. Potential deficiencies in vegetarian diets include energy, protein, vitamin B12, zinc, iron, calcium, omega-3 fatty acids, and vitamin D (if limited exposure to sunlight)
   4. To enhance the **absorption** of iron, vegetarians should include a good source of iron and vitamin C with each meal
   5. Foods commonly eaten include tofu, tempeh, soy milk and soy products, meat analogues, legumes, nuts, seeds, sprouts, and a variety of fruits and vegetables
   6. Soy protein is considered equivalent in quality to animal proteins

V. ENTERAL NUTRITION

A. Description: Provides liquefied foods to the GI tract via a tube
B. Indications
   1. When the GI tract is functional but oral intake is not feasible
   2. Used for clients with swallowing problems, burns, major trauma, liver failure, or severe **malnutrition**
C. Nursing considerations
   1. Clients with lactose intolerance (diarrhea, bloating, cramping) need to be placed on lactose-free formulas
   2. See Chapter 19 for information about the administration of GI tube feedings
D. Complications of **enteral nutrition** (Box 12-10)

VI. PARENTERAL NUTRITION

A. Description
   1. Supplies necessary **nutrients** via the veins.

BOX 12-9 Types of Vegetarian Diets

Lacto-Ovo Vegetarian
Consumes eggs and dairy products but excludes meat, poultry, and seafood
Lacto Vegetarian
Consumes dairy products but excludes eggs, meat, poultry, and seafood
Vegan
Refrains from eating animal products
Pesco Vegetarian
Consumes seafood but excludes meat, poultry, eggs, and dairy products

---

BOX 12-10 Complications of Enteral Feeding

- Aspiration
- Diarrhea
- Displacement of tube
- Nasal and mouth mucosal damage
- Obstruction of tube

---

   2. Supplies carbohydrates in the form of dextrose; fats in a special emulsified form; proteins in the form of amino acids; vitamins; minerals; electrolytes; and water
   3. Prevents subcutaneous fat and muscle protein from being catabolized by the body for energy
B. Indications
   1. Clients with severely dysfunctional or nonfunctional GI tracts who are unable to process **nutrients** may benefit from **PN**
   2. Clients who can take some oral nutrition (but not enough to meet their nutrient requirements) may benefit from **PN**
   3. Clients with multiple GI surgeries, GI trauma, severe intolerance to enteral feedings, or intestinal obstructions or those who need to rest the bowel for healing may benefit from **PN**
   4. Clients with acquired immunodeficiency syndrome, cancer, burn injuries, or **malnutrition** or those who have received chemotherapy may benefit from **PN**
   5. **PN** is the least desirable form of nutrition; it is used when there is no other alternative
C. Types of PN (Figure 12-1)
   1. **Total parenteral nutrition (TPN)**
      a. **TPN** is administered through central access when the client requires a larger concentration of carbohydrates (>10% glucose concentration)

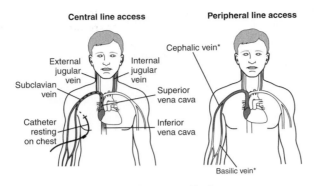

Central line access   Peripheral line access

Cephalic vein*

External jugular vein
Internal jugular vein
Subclavian vein
Superior vena cava
Catheter resting on chest
Inferior vena cava

Basilic vein*

* Access points for catheter (long line) peripheral feeding.
Peripheral feeding using a cannula device may be administered through any vein

FIG. 12-1 Parenteral nutrition access routes. (From Byron, S. E. [2002]. *Pocket guide to nutrition & dietetics* [p. 60]. Edinburgh: Churchill Livingstone.)

> ### BOX 12-11 Signs of an Adverse or Allergic Reaction to Lipids
>
> - Chills
> - Fever
> - Flushing
> - Diaphoresis
> - Dyspnea
> - Cyanosis
> - Chest and back pain
> - Nausea and vomiting
> - Headache
> - Pressure over the eyes
> - Thrombophlebitis
> - Vertigo

b. The subclavian or internal jugular vein is used when **TPN** is a short-term intervention (<4 weeks)

c. When **TPN** is anticipated for an extended period (>4 weeks), a more permanent catheter (e.g., a peripherally inserted central catheter line), a tunneled catheter, or an implanted vascular access device is used

2. **Peripheral parenteral nutrition (PPN)**

a. **PPN** is administered through a peripheral vein, typically in the arm

b. **PPN** is used for short periods (5 to 7 days) and when the client needs only small concentrations of carbohydrates, fats, and proteins

c. **PPN** is used to deliver isotonic or mildly hypertonic solutions; the delivery of highly hypertonic solutions into peripheral veins can cause sclerosis, phlebitis, or swelling

D. **Fat emulsion (lipids)**

1. **Lipids** provide nonprotein calories and prevent or correct fatty-acid deficiency

2. Lipid solutions are isotonic and therefore can be administered through a peripheral or central vein

3. Most **fat emulsions** are prepared from soybean or safflower oil with egg yolk to provide emulsification; the primary components are linoleic, oleic, palmitic, linolenic, and stearic acids

4. **Lipids** contain egg yolk phospholipids and should not be given to clients with egg allergies

5. Glucose-intolerant clients or clients with diabetes mellitus may benefit from receiving a larger percentage of their **PN** from **lipids**; this can help control blood glucose levels and lower insulin requirements as a result of decreased infused dextrose

6. Examine the bottle for the separation of the emulsion into layers, fat globules, and the accumulation of froth; if observed, do not use the solution and return it to the pharmacy

7. Additives should not be put into the **fat emulsion** solution

8. Infuse the solution initially at 1 mL/minute, monitor the vital signs every 10 minutes, and observe for adverse reactions for the first 30 minutes; if signs of an adverse reaction occur, stop the infusion and notify the physician (Box 12-11)

9. If no adverse reaction occurs, adjust the flow rate to the prescribed rate

10. Monitor serum **lipids** 4 hours after discontinuing the infusion

VII. COMPLICATIONS (Table 12-1)

VIII. NURSING CONSIDERATIONS

A. Always check the PN solution with the physician's order to ensure that the prescribed components are contained in the solution

B. To prevent infection and solution incompatibility, intravenous medications and blood are not given through the PN line

C. Monitor the partial thromboplastin time and the prothrombin time for clients receiving anticoagulants

D. Monitor electrolytes, albumin, and liver and renal function studies

E. In severely dehydrated clients, the albumin level may drop initially as the treatment restores hydration

F. With severely malnourished clients, monitor for "refeeding syndrome" (i.e., a rapid drop in the potassium, magnesium, and phosphate serum levels)

G. Abnormal liver function values may indicate intolerance to or an excess of **fat emulsion** or problems with the **metabolism** of glucose and protein

TABLE 12-1   Complications of Parenteral Nutrition

Complication	Possible Cause	Signs/Symptoms	Intervention	Prevention
Air embolism	• Catheter system is opened • IV tubing is disconnected • Air entry occurs on IV tubing changes	• Apprehension • Chest pain • Dyspnea • Hypotension • Loud churning sound heard over the pericardium on auscultation • Rapid and weak pulse • Respiratory distress	• Clamp the catheter • Place the client in a left-side-lying position with the head lower than the feet • Notify the physician • Administer oxygen	• Make sure all catheter connections are secure • Clamp the catheter when not in use • Instruct the client in Valsalva's maneuver for tubing and cap changes • For tubing and cap changes, place the client in Trendelenburg's position (if not contraindicated) with the head turned in the opposite direction of the insertion site
Hyperglycemia	• Client is receiving solution too quickly • Not enough insulin • Infection	• Coma (when severe) • Confusion • Diaphoresis • Elevated blood glucose level (>200 mg/dL) • Excessive thirst • Fatigue • Kussmaul's respirations • Restlessness • Weakness	• Notify the physician • May need to slow the infusion rate • Administer regular insulin as prescribed • Monitor blood glucose levels	• Assess the client for a history of glucose intolerance • Assess the client's medication history • Begin infusion at a slow rate as prescribed • Monitor blood glucose levels • Use strict aseptic technique
Hypervolemia	• Excessive fluid administration or administration of fluid too rapidly • Renal dysfunction • Heart failure • Hepatic failure	• Bounding pulse • Crackles on lung auscultation • Headache • Increased blood pressure • Jugular vein distension • Weight gain greater than desired	• Slow or stop the IV infusion • Fluid restriction • Diuretics • Dialysis (in extreme cases)	• Assess the client's history for risk for hypervolemia • Administer solution via an electronic infusion device • Monitor intake and output • Monitor weight daily
Hypoglycemia	• PN is abruptly discontinued • Too much insulin is being administered	• Anxiousness • Diaphoresis • Hunger • Low blood glucose level (<70 mg/dL) • Shakiness • Weakness	• Intravenous dextrose is administered • Monitor blood glucose levels	• Gradually decrease PN solution when discontinuing it • Infuse 10% dextrose at the same rate as the PN to prevent hypoglycemia when the PN solution is discontinued • Monitor glucose levels when insulin is being given
Infection	• Poor aseptic technique • Catheter contamination • Contamination of solution	• Chills • Fever • Elevated white blood cell count • Erythema or drainage at the insertion site	• Remove catheter • Send the catheter tip to the laboratory for culture • Prepare to obtain blood cultures • Prepare for antibiotic administration	• Use strict aseptic technique • Monitor temperature • Assess the IV site for signs of infection • Change site dressing, solution, and tubing as specified by agency policy • Do not disconnect tubing unnecessarily
Pneumothorax	• Incorrect catheter placement	• Absence of breath sounds on affected side • Chest or shoulder pain • Sudden shortness of breath • Tachycardia • Cyanosis	• Small pneumothorax may resolve • Larger pneumothorax may require chest tube	• Monitor for signs of pneumothorax • Obtain a chest x-ray after the insertion of the catheter to ensure proper placement • PN is not initiated until correct catheter placement is verified and the absence of pneumothorax is confirmed

IV, Intravenous; *PN,* parenteral nutrition.

H. Abnormal renal function tests may indicate an excess of amino acids

I. PN solutions should be refrigerated and administered within 24 hours from the time that they were prepared (remove from the refrigerator 0.5 to 1 hour before use)

J. PN solutions that are cloudy or darkened should not be used and should be returned to the pharmacy

K. Additions to **PN** solutions should be made in the pharmacy and not in the nursing unit

L. Discontinuing **PN** therapy
   1. Gradually decrease the flow rate for 1 to 2 hours while increasing oral intake (this assists with the prevention of hypoglycemia)
   2. After catheter removal, change the dressing daily until the wound heals
   3. Encourage oral nourishment
   4. Record oral intake, body weight, and laboratory results of serum electrolyte and glucose levels

IX. HOME-CARE INSTRUCTIONS (Box 12-12)

PRACTICE QUESTIONS

More questions on the companion CD!

82. A client is having problems with blood clotting. Which food item would the nurse encourage the client to eat?
   1. Legumes
   2. Citrus fruits
   3. Vegetable oils
   4. Green, leafy vegetables

83. A client has acute diverticulitis. Which principle should the nurse keep in mind while planning care for this client?
   1. Avoid fiber intake. _rest bowel — can cause diarrhea_
   2. Use a fluid-restricted diet.
   3. Increase seed and nut intake.
   4. Follow the Exchange List for diet.

84. A client is a lacto vegetarian. Which food item would the nurse remove from the tray?
   1. Eggs
   2. Milk
   3. Cheese
   4. Broccoli

85. A low-sodium diet has been prescribed for a client with hypertension. Which of the following foods, if selected from the menu by the client, would indicate an understanding of this diet?
   1. Baked turkey
   2. Tomato soup
   3. Boiled shrimp
   4. Chicken gumbo

86. A nurse is providing dietary instructions to a client with gout. The nurse tells the client to avoid which food item?
   1. Scallops
   2. Chocolate

   3. Corn bread
   4. Macaroni products

87. A clear liquid diet has been prescribed for a client with gastroenteritis. Which item would be the most appropriate to offer to the client?
   1. Soft custard
   2. Orange juice
   3. Fat-free broth
   4. Strained soup

88. A client with heart disease is instructed regarding a low-fat diet. The nurse determines that the client understands the diet if the client states that a food item to avoid is:
   1. Apples
   2. Cheese
   3. Oranges
   4. Skim milk

89. A nurse instructs a client to increase the amount of riboflavin in the diet. The nurse tells the client to select which food item that is high in riboflavin?
   1. Milk
   2. Tomatoes
   3. Citrus fruits
   4. Green, leafy vegetables

90. A client with a burn injury is transferred to the nursing unit, and a regular diet has been prescribed. The nurse encourages the client to eat which dietary items to promote wound healing?
   1. Veal, potatoes, gelatin, and orange juice
   2. Chicken breast, broccoli, strawberries, and milk

3. Peanut butter and jelly sandwich, cantaloupe, and tea
4. Spaghetti with tomato sauce, garlic bread, and ginger ale

91. A nurse has completed diet teaching for a client who has been prescribed a low-sodium diet to treat hypertension. The nurse determines that further teaching is necessary when the client makes which of these statements?
    1. "This diet will help lower my blood pressure."
    2. "Fresh foods such as fruits and vegetables are high in sodium."
    3. "This diet is not a replacement for my antihypertensive medications."
    4. "The reason I need to lower my salt intake is to reduce fluid retention."

92. A client who is receiving parenteral nutrition may begin to take small amounts of clear liquids today. The nurse's priority is to collect data regarding which of the following before giving the client anything by mouth?
    1. The client's appetite
    2. The client's current weight
    3. The presence of the swallow reflex
    4. Adequate pulse and blood pressure readings

93. A nurse is asked to assist with preparing a client who will be receiving a parenteral nutrition (PN) solution via a central line. The nurse plans to obtain which essential piece of equipment for this procedure?
    1. Urine test strips
    2. Blood glucose meter
    3. Electronic infusion pump
    4. Noninvasive blood pressure monitor

94. A client who is receiving parenteral nutrition (PN) complains of a headache. The nurse notes that the client has an increased blood pressure and a bounding pulse. The nurse reports the findings knowing that these signs are indicative of which complication of this therapy?
    1. Sepsis
    2. Air embolism
    3. Fluid overload
    4. Hyperglycemia

95. A newly pregnant client is asking how to prevent neural-tube birth defects. What food choice should the nurse recommend?
    1. Milk
    2. Peanuts
    3. Egg yolks
    4. Grapefruit

ALTERNATE ITEM FORMAT: MULTIPLE RESPONSE

96. A nurse needs to increase the calcium in the diet of a client who is lactose intolerant. Which food items should the nurse encourage? Select all that apply.
    - ☐ 1. Milk
    - ☑ 2. Tofu
    - ☐ 3. Cheese
    - ☑ 4. Broccoli
    - ☑ 5. Sardines
    - ☑ 6. Mustard greens

ANSWERS

82. 4

Rationale: Green, leafy vegetables are high in vitamin K, which acts as a catalyst for facilitating blood-clotting factors. Vegetable oil is high in vitamin E, which acts as an antioxidant. Legumes are high in folic acid and thiamine. Citrus fruits are high in vitamin C, which helps with wound healing.
Test-Taking Strategy: This question requires a two-step process. First, focus on the client's problem, and recall that vitamin K is involved in the clotting process. Next, determine the food sources that are high in vitamin K. Review the functions of vitamin K and the foods that are high in vitamin K if you had difficulty with this question.
Level of Cognitive Ability: Application
Client Needs: Physiological Integrity
Integrated Process: Teaching and Learning
Content Area: Fundamental Skills
Reference: Grodner, M., Long, S., & Walkingshaw, B. (2007). *Foundations and clinical applications of nutrition: A nursing approach* (4th ed., pp. 131, 149-151). St. Louis: Mosby.

83. 1

Rationale: Diet therapy for acute diverticulitis involves allowing the bowel to rest by avoiding fiber foods. Fluids are encouraged rather than restricted. Seeds and nuts are to be avoided so that they do not become trapped in the diverticula and cause irritation. The Exchange List is a food guide that is used to guide healthy living, specifically for the client with diabetes mellitus.
Test-Taking Strategy: Use the process of elimination, and focus on the client's diagnosis of acute diverticulitis. Recalling foods that are allowed and not allowed when a client has diverticulitis will direct you to option 1. Review diet therapy for diverticulitis if you had difficulty with this question.
Level of Cognitive Ability: Comprehension
Client Needs: Physiological Integrity
Integrated Process: Nursing Process/Planning
Content Area: Adult Health/Gastrointestinal
Reference: Grodner, M., Long, S., & Walkingshaw, B. (2007). *Foundations and clinical applications of nutrition: A nursing approach* (4th ed., pp. 400-401). St. Louis: Mosby.

84. 1

Rationale: Eggs are not consumed by lacto vegetarians. Other dairy and plant products are eaten by lacto vegetarians.
Test-Taking Strategy: Note the words "remove from the tray." This indicates that the food item in question is not appropriate for a lacto vegetarian. Of the options listed, eggs are the food items that are not consumed by lacto vegetarians; however, they are eaten by lacto-ovo vegetarians. Review vegetarian diets if you had difficulty with this question.

Level of Cognitive Ability: Application
Client Needs: Physiological Integrity
Integrated Process: Nursing Process/Implementation
Content Area: Fundamental Skills
Reference: Grodner, M., Long, S., & Walkingshaw, B. (2007). *Foundations and clinical applications of nutrition: A nursing approach* (4th ed., p. 119). St. Louis: Mosby.

85. 1
Rationale: Regular soup (1 cup) contains 900 mg of sodium. Fresh shellfish (1 oz) contains 50 mg of sodium. Poultry (1 oz) contains 25 mg of sodium.
Test-Taking Strategy: Use the process of elimination. Eliminate options 2 and 4 first, because they are comparable or alike. Also, recall that canned foods are high in sodium. From the remaining options, select option 1 over option 3, remembering that shellfish is also high in sodium. Review the foods that are high in sodium if you had difficulty with this question.
Level of Cognitive Ability: Analysis
Client Needs: Health Promotion and Maintenance
Integrated Process: Teaching and Learning
Content Area: Fundamental Skills
References: Nix, S. (2005). *Williams' basic nutrition and diet therapy* (12th ed., pp. 358-359). St. Louis: Mosby.
Schlenker, E. & Long, S. (2007). *Williams' essentials of nutrition & diet therapy* (9th ed., p. 513). St. Louis: Mosby.

86. 1
Rationale: Scallops should be omitted from the diet of a client who has gout because of the high purine content. The food items identified in options 2, 3, and 4 have a negligible purine content and may be consumed by the client with gout.
Test-Taking Strategy: Use the process of elimination, and focus on the client's diagnosis of gout. Recalling the food items that are high in purine will direct you to option 1. Review the foods that are high in purine if you had difficulty with this question.
Level of Cognitive Ability: Application
Client Needs: Physiological Integrity
Integrated Process: Teaching and Learning
Content Area: Fundamental Skills
References: Linton, A., & Maebius, N. (2007). *Introduction to medical-surgical nursing* (4th ed., p. 908). Philadelphia: Saunders.
Nix, S. (2005). *Williams' basic nutrition and diet therapy* (12th ed., p. 405-406). St. Louis: Mosby.

87. 3
Rationale: A clear liquid diet consists of foods that are relatively transparent. The food items in options 1, 2, and 4 would be included in a full liquid diet.
Test-Taking Strategy: Remember that a clear liquid diet consists of foods that are relatively transparent. By the process of elimination, you should easily select option 3, because this is the only food item that is transparent. Review the food items that are allowed on clear liquid and full liquid diets if you had difficulty with this question.
Level of Cognitive Ability: Application
Client Needs: Physiological Integrity
Integrated Process: Nursing Process/Implementation

Content Area: Fundamental Skills
Reference: Grodner, M., Long, S., & Walkingshaw, B. (2007). *Foundations and clinical applications of nutrition: A nursing approach* (4th ed., pp. 323-324, 551). St. Louis: Mosby.

88. 2
Rationale: Fruits, vegetables, and skim milk contain minimal amounts of fat. Cheese is high in fat.
Test-Taking Strategy: Use the process of elimination and your knowledge regarding the fat content of fruits to eliminate options 1 and 3. Recalling that cheese is high in fat will direct you to option 2. Review the foods that are high in fat if you had difficulty with this question.
Level of Cognitive Ability: Comprehension
Client Needs: Health Promotion and Maintenance
Integrated Process: Nursing Process/Evaluation
Content Area: Fundamental Skills
Reference: Grodner, M., Long, S., & Walkingshaw, B. (2007). *Foundations and clinical applications of nutrition: A nursing approach* (4th ed., p. 96). St. Louis: Mosby.

89. 1
Rationale: Food sources of riboflavin include milk, lean meats, fish, and grains. Tomatoes and citrus fruits are high in vitamin C. Green, leafy vegetables are high in folic acid.
Test-Taking Strategy: Knowledge regarding food items that are high in riboflavin is required to answer this question. Remember that milk is a food source of riboflavin. Review the foods that contain riboflavin if you had difficulty with this question.
Level of Cognitive Ability: Application
Client Needs: Health Promotion and Maintenance
Integrated Process: Teaching and Learning
Content Area: Fundamental Skills
Reference: Grodner, M., Long, S., & Walkingshaw, B. (2007). *Foundations and clinical applications of nutrition: A nursing approach* (4th ed., pp. 135, 144). St. Louis: Mosby.

90. 2
Rationale: Protein and vitamin C are necessary for wound healing. Poultry and milk are good sources of protein. Broccoli and strawberries are good sources of vitamin C. Peanut butter is a source of niacin. Gelatin and jelly have no nutrient value. Spaghetti is a complex carbohydrate.
Test-Taking Strategy: Focus on the subject of promoting wound healing, and recall that protein and vitamin C are necessary for wound healing. Eliminate options 1 and 3 first, because jelly and gelatin have no nutrient value related to healing. From the remaining options, select option 2 over option 4 because of the greater nutrient value of the foods listed in option 2. Review the foods that are high in protein and vitamin C if you had difficulty with this question.
Level of Cognitive Ability: Application
Client Needs: Physiological Integrity
Integrated Process: Nursing Process/Implementation
Content Area: Fundamental Skills
References: Grodner, M., Long, S., & Walkinshaw, B. (2007). *Foundations and clinical applications of nutrition: A nursing approach* (4th ed., pp. 115, 141, 144, 353). St. Louis: Mosby.
Schlenker, E., & Long, S. (2007). *Williams' essentials of nutrition & diet therapy* (9th ed., p. 125). St. Louis: Mosby.

91. 2

Rationale: A low-sodium diet is used as an adjunct to antihypertensive medications for the treatment of hypertension. Sodium retains fluid, which leads to hypertension secondary to increased fluid volume. Fresh foods such as fruits and vegetables are low in sodium.

Test-Taking Strategy: Use the process of elimination, and note the strategic words "further teaching is necessary." These words indicate a negative event query and ask you to select an option that is an incorrect statement. Eliminate options 1, 3, and 4, because these are accurate statements related to hypertension. In addition, remember that fresh foods are low in sodium. Review the purpose of a low-sodium diet if you had difficulty with this question.

Level of Cognitive Ability: Analysis
Client Needs: Physiological Integrity
Integrated Process: Teaching and Learning
Content Area: Fundamental Skills
Reference: Grodner, M., Long, S., & Walkinshaw, B. (2007). *Foundations and clinical applications of nutrition: A nursing approach* (4th ed., p. 172). St. Louis: Mosby.

92. 3

Rationale: The nurse ensures that the client has intact gag and swallow reflexes. The nurse would also check for the presence of bowel sounds. The pulse, blood pressure, and weight require ongoing monitoring, but they are not the most important items given the wording of the question. The client may be expected to have a poor appetite after being without oral intake for a period of time.

Test-Taking Strategy: Focus on the subject of the question, and note the strategic word "priority." Option 3 is most closely associated with the subject of the question (feeding the client), and it addresses the prevention of aspiration. Review the nursing care measures for the client resuming an oral intake if you had difficulty with this question.

Level of Cognitive Ability: Application
Client Needs: Physiological Integrity
Integrated Process: Nursing Process/Data Collection
Content Area: Fundamental Skills
References: deWit, S. (2009). *Medical-surgical nursing: Concepts & practice* (p. 63). St. Louis: Saunders.
Linton, A., & Maebius, N. (2007). *Introduction to medical-surgical nursing* (4th ed., p. 120). Philadelphia: Saunders.

93. 3

Rationale: The nurse obtains an electronic infusion pump in preparation for the administration of PN. It is necessary to use an infusion pump to ensure that the solution does not infuse too rapidly or fall too far behind. Because the client's blood glucose level is monitored every 6 to 8 hours during the administration of PN, a blood glucose meter will also be needed, but this is not the most essential item. Urine test strips may be needed to measure glucose. A noninvasive blood pressure cuff is unnecessary for this procedure.

Test-Taking Strategy: Note that the question contains the strategic words "central line" and "essential." Use your knowledge of the method of administration of a fluid via a central line to eliminate each incorrect option. Remember that an electronic infusion pump is required. Review the principles related to

the administration of PN if you had difficulty with this question.

Level of Cognitive Ability: Application
Client Needs: Physiological Integrity
Integrated Process: Nursing Process/Planning
Content Area: Fundamental Skills
Reference: deWit, S. (2009). *Medical-surgical nursing: Concepts & practice* (p. 62). St. Louis: Saunders.

94. 3

Rationale: The client's signs and symptoms are consistent with fluid overload. The increased intravascular volume increases the blood pressure, whereas the pulse rate increases as the heart tries to pump the extra fluid volume. A fever would be present in a client with sepsis. Signs and symptoms of an air embolus include confusion, pallor, lightheadedness, tachycardia, tachypnea, hypotension, anxiety, and unresponsiveness. Polyuria, polydipsia, and polyphagia are manifestations of hyperglycemia.

Test-Taking Strategy: Use the process of elimination. Focus on the data in the question, and recall the complications of PN and their manifestations. This will direct you to option 3. Review the PN-related complications and their manifestations if you had difficulty with this question.

Level of Cognitive Ability: Analysis
Client Needs: Physiological Integrity
Integrated Process: Nursing Process/Data Collection
Content Area: Fundamental Skills
References: Grodner, M., Long, S., & Walkinshaw, B. (2007). *Foundations and clinical applications of nutrition: A nursing approach* (4th ed., p. 332). St. Louis: Mosby.
Monahan, F., Sands, J., Marek, J., Neighbors, M., & Green, C. (2007). *Phipps' medical-surgical nursing: Health and illness perspectives* (8th ed., p. 1236). St. Louis: Mosby.

95. 4

Rationale: Folic acid (folate) helps prevent neural-tube birth defects; it is found in green, leafy vegetables; liver, beef, and fish; legumes; and grapefruit and oranges. Peanuts are high in protein and niacin. Milk is high in carbohydrates and vitamin D. Egg yolks are high in vitamin A, iron, and cholesterol.

Test-Taking Strategy: Knowledge regarding the food items that are high in folic acid (folate) is necessary to answer this question. Remember that green, leafy vegetables; grapefruit; and oranges are high in this vitamin. Review the foods that are high in folic acid (folate) if you had difficulty with this question.

Level of Cognitive Ability: Application
Client Needs: Health Promotion and Maintenance
Integrated Process: Teaching and Learning
Content Area: Fundamental Skills
Reference: Grodner, M., Long, S., & Walkingshaw, B. (2007). *Foundations and clinical applications of nutrition: A nursing approach* (4th ed., pp. 138-139). St. Louis: Mosby.

ALTERNATE ITEM FORMAT: MULTIPLE RESPONSE

96. 2, 4, 5, 6

Rationale: Tofu, broccoli, mustard greens, and sardines are foods that are high in calcium that do not come from dairy sources. Lactose-intolerant clients should not eat dairy products. Therefore, these clients need high-calcium foods from nondairy sources. Although milk and cheese are high in calcium, they are dairy products, which lactose-intolerant clients need to avoid.

Test-Taking Strategy: There are two knowledge elements to this question: lactose intolerance and foods that are high in calcium. Because lactose-intolerant clients cannot digest dairy products properly, choose nondairy foods that are high in calcium. Options 1 and 3 are dairy products and can thus be eliminated. Review high-calcium foods and lactose intolerance if you had difficulty with this question.

Level of Cognitive Ability: Application
Client Needs: Physiological Integrity
Integrated Process: Nursing Process/Implementation
Content Area: Fundamental Skills
Reference: Grodner, M., Long, S., & Walkingshaw, B. (2007). *Foundations and clinical applications of nutrition: A nursing approach* (4th ed., pp. 68, 165). St. Louis: Mosby.

REFERENCES

deWit, S. (2009). *Medical-surgical nursing: Concepts & practice*, St. Louis: Saunders.

Grodner, M., Long, S., & Walkinshaw, B. (2007). *Foundations and clinical applications of nutrition: A nursing approach* (4th ed.). St. Louis: Mosby.

Linton, A., & Maebius, N. (2007). *Introduction to medical-surgical nursing* (4th ed.). Philadelphia: Saunders.

Monahan, F., Sands, J., Marek, J., Neighbors, M., & Green, C. (2007). *Phipps' medical-surgical nursing: Health and illness perspectives* (8th ed.). St. Louis: Mosby.

National Council of State Boards of Nursing (Eds.) (2008). *2008 Detailed Test Plan for the NCLEX-PN® Examination, National Council of State Boards of Nursing*, Chicago: Author.

National Council of State Boards of Nursing. *NSCBN home page*. www.ncsbn.org. Accessed June 17, 2008.

Nix, S. (2005). *Williams' basic nutrition and diet therapy* (12th ed.). St. Louis: Mosby.

Schlenker, E., & Long, S. (2007). *Williams' essentials of nutrition & diet therapy* (9th ed.). St. Louis: Mosby.

CHAPTER 13

Intravenous Therapy and Blood Administration

PYRAMID TERMS

ABO A type of antigen system; the ABO type of the donor should be compatible with the recipient's

air embolism Caused by a bolus of air that enters the vein through an inadequately primed intravenous line, from a loose connection, or during a tubing change or the removal of the intravenous catheter

compatibility Determined by two different types of antigen systems—ABO and Rh—that are present on the membrane surface of the red blood cells (Table 13-1)

crossmatching The testing of the donor's blood and the recipient's blood for compatibility

fluid (circulatory) overload A complication that results from the infusion of blood at a rate that is too rapid for the body size, cardiac status, or clinical condition of the recipient

infiltration The seepage of intravenous fluid out of the vein and into the surrounding interstitial spaces

phlebitis An inflammation of the vein that can occur from either mechanical or chemical (medication) trauma or from a local infection

Rh factor Rh stands for Rhesus factor. The presence or absense of Rh antigens on the surface of the red blood cells (RBCs) determines the classification as Rh positive or Rh negative. A person who has the factor is Rh positive; a person who lacks the factor is Rh negative

transfusion reaction A hemolytic transfusion reaction is caused by blood type or Rh factor incompatibility; an allergic transfusion reaction is most often seen among clients with a history of allergy; a febrile transfusion reaction most commonly occurs among clients with antibodies directed against the transfused white blood cells; a bacterial transfusion reaction occurs after the transfusion of contaminated blood products

▲ PYRAMID TO SUCCESS

The nurse is responsible for monitoring clients who are receiving parenteral therapies. The pyramid points focus on safety related to monitoring an infusion rate and monitoring for complications related to the intravenous (IV) line. Focus on the signs and symptoms of infiltration, phlebitis, circulatory overload, and air embolism and the treatment measures associated with each. The pyramid points also focus on safety related to monitoring a client who is receiving a blood transfusion and

| TABLE 13-1 | Compatibility Chart for Red Blood Cell Transfusions |

Donor	Recipient			
	A	B	AB	O
A	X		X	
B		X	X	
AB			X	
O	X	X	X	X

From Ignatavicius, D., & Workman, M. (2006). *Medical-surgical nursing* (5th ed.). Philadelphia: Saunders.

monitoring for complications related to the transfusion. Focus on the signs and symptoms of a transfusion reaction and the immediate interventions that should be employed if a transfusion reaction occurs. The documentation of the expected and unexpected effects of the therapy is also a pyramid point. The primary Integrated Processes addressed in this chapter are Caring, Clinical Problem-Solving Process (Nursing Process), Communication and Documentation, and Teaching and Learning.

CLIENT NEEDS ▲

Safe and Effective Care Environment

Establishing priorities
Handling hazardous or infectious materials
Implementing standard, transmission-based, and other precautions
Maintaining asepsis
Monitoring the client during the IV infusion
Obtaining informed consent for therapy
Preventing errors in the monitoring of IV lines
Providing continuity of care

Health Promotion and Maintenance

Considering lifestyle choices related to the transfusion
Implementing techniques for the collection of physical data
Teaching about the signs of a transfusion reaction

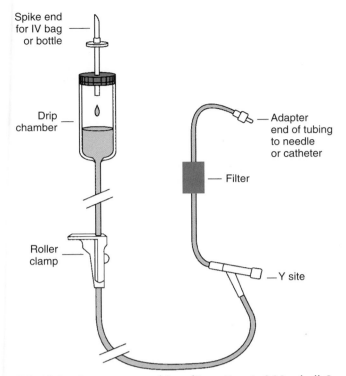

Psychosocial Integrity

Considering religious, spiritual, and cultural matters related to blood administration

Communicating regarding the procedure for IV infusion and blood administration

Identifying coping mechanisms and support systems for the client

Physiological Integrity

Ensuring the safe administration of the IV infusion and the blood transfusion

Monitoring for complications

Monitoring for expected effects

Monitoring IV infusion sites and rates

Monitoring laboratory values

Documenting the client's response to treatment

I. INTRAVENOUS THERAPY (see Chapter 9, Table 9-1)

A. Used to sustain clients who are unable to take substances orally

B. Replaces water, electrolytes, and nutrients more rapidly than oral administration

C. Provides immediate access to the vascular system for the rapid delivery of specific solutions without the time that is required for gastrointestinal tract absorption

D. Provides a vascular route for the administration of medication or blood components

II. INTRAVENOUS DEVICES

A. IV cannulas

1. Butterfly set (winged)
   a. Used when the infusion time will be short and primarily for drawing blood
   b. **Infiltration** is more common with these devices as a result of their stiffness
   c. May commonly be used with children and older clients, whose veins are likely to be small or fragile; an armboard may be needed for a short infusion

2. Plastic cannulas (over-the-needle catheter)
   a. Used in place of a stainless steel needle or a butterfly set when a longer infusion time is expected
   b. Can cause a catheter embolism if the tip of the cannula breaks

B. IV gauges

1. The smaller the gauge number, the larger the outside diameter of the cannula

2. The gauge size used depends on the solution to be administered and the diameter of the available vein

3. For rapid emergency fluid administration, blood products, or anesthetics, a large needle (e.g., 14-, 16-, 18-, or 19-gauge) is used

FIG. 13-1 Intravenous tubing. (From Kee, J., & Marshall, S. [2009]. *Clinical calculations: With applications to general and specialty areas* [6th ed.]. Philadelphia: Saunders.)

4. For standard IV fluid, a 22- or 24-gauge needle is used

5. If the client has very small veins, a 24- to 25-gauge needle is used

C. IV containers

1. May be glass or plastic

2. Squeeze the plastic bag to ensure that it is intact; check the glass bottle for any punctures or cracks

3. Do not write on the plastic IV bag with a marking pen, because the ink may be absorbed through the plastic into the solution.

4. Use a label and a ballpoint pen for marking the bag, and place the label onto the bag

5. The expiration date of IV fluid and all supplies should be checked

D. IV tubing (Figure 13-1)

1. Contains a spike end for the bag or bottle, a drip chamber, a roller clamp, a Y site, and an adapter end for attachment to the needle

2. Extension tubing may be attached to the IV tubing for children, clients who are restless, or clients who have special mobility needs

3. Shorter secondary tubing is used for piggyback solutions to connect them to the injection sites nearest to the drip chamber (Figure 13-2)

4. Vented and nonvented tubing is available
   a. A vent allows air to enter the IV container as the fluid leaves

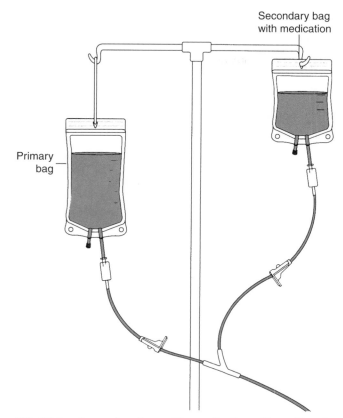

FIG. 13-2 Secondary bag with medication. (From Kee, J., & Marshall, S. [2009]. *Clinical calculations: With applications to general and specialty areas* [6th ed.]. Philadelphia: Saunders.)

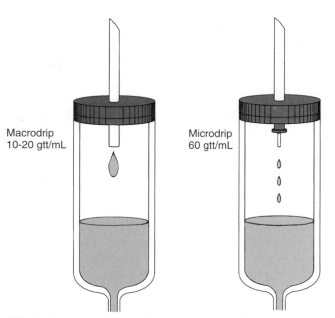

FIG. 13-3 Macrodrip and microdrip sets. (From Kee, J., & Marshall, S. [2009]. *Clinical calculations: With applications to general and specialty areas* [6th ed.]. Philadelphia: Saunders.)

b. A vented adapter can be used to add a vent to a nonvented IV tubing system
c. Use nonvented tubing for flexible containers
d. Use vented tubing for glass or rigid plastic containers to allow air to enter and displace the fluid as it leaves; fluid will not flow from a rigid IV container unless it is vented

E. Drip chambers (Figure 13-3)
1. Microdrip chamber
   a. Normally has a short, vertical, metal piece where the drop forms
   b. Delivers about 60 gtt/mL
   c. Read the tubing package to determine how many drops per milliliter are delivered (drop factor)
   d. Used if fluid will be infused at a slow rate (less than 50 mL/hour), if the solution contains medication, and in the pediatric client
2. Macrodrip chamber
   a. Used if the solution is thick or needs to infuse rapidly
   b. Drop factor varies from 10 to 20 gtt/mL
   c. Read the tubing package to determine how many drops per milliliter are delivered (drop factor)

F. Filters: May be used in IV lines to trap small particles and to provide protection by preventing particles from entering the client's veins
G. Needleless systems: Include recessed needles, plastic cannulas, or one-way valves that decrease exposure to contaminated needles
H. Intermittent infusion sets: Used when intravascular accessibility is desired for the intermittent administration of medications or solutions

III. **LATEX ALLERGY**
A. Ask the client about an allergy to latex
B. IV supplies that may contain latex include IV catheters, IV tubing, IV ports (particularly IV rubber injection ports), rubber stoppers on multidose vials, and adhesive tape
C. Latex-safe IV supplies need to be used for clients with latex allergy
D. Refer to Chapter 60 for additional information about latex allergy

IV. **PERIPHERAL IV SITES**
A. The most frequently used sites are the veins of the forearm, because the bones of the forearm act as a natural support and splint
B. Veins in the lower extremities are not suitable because of the risk of thrombus formation and possible pooling in areas of decreased venous return (Box 13-1)
C. Veins in the scalp and feet may be suitable sites for infants
D. Bending the elbow on the arm with an IV may easily obstruct the flow of the solution, thereby causing **infiltration**, which could lead to thrombophlebitis

BOX 13-1 Peripheral Intravenous Sites to Avoid

- Edematous extremity
- An arm that is weak, traumatized, or paralyzed
- The arm on the same side as a mastectomy
- An arm that has an arteriovenous fistula or a shunt for dialysis
- An infected area

E. Avoid checking the blood pressure on the arm receiving the IV infusion
F. Do not place restraints over the venipuncture site
G. An armboard may be prescribed when the venipuncture site is located in an area of flexion

V. ADMINISTERING IV SOLUTIONS
A. The IV solution should be checked against the physician's orders for the type, amount, percentage of solution, and rate of flow
B. Wash hands thoroughly and use sterile technique when working with an IV
C. When preparing a new solution for administration, clamp the tubing, attach the spike end of the tubing to the IV bag, and then prime the tubing to remove air from the tubing and IV system
D. Change the IV tubing every 24 to 72 hours, depending on agency policy
E. Do not let an IV bag or bottle hang for more than 24 hours
F. Do not allow the IV tubing to touch the floor
G. Change the IV dressing every 72 hours, when the dressing is wet or contaminated, or as specified by agency policy
H. Label the tubing, dressing, and solution bags clearly, including the date and time when changed

VI. PRECAUTIONS
A. Can cause initial pain and discomfort for the client on insertion
B. Provides a route of entry for microorganisms into the body
C. **Fluid (circulatory) overload** or electrolyte imbalances can occur from an excessive or too-rapid infusion of fluids; an IV infusion should be checked at least once per hour in an adult client
D. Incompatibilities between certain solutions can occur
E. Clients with cardiac, respiratory, renal, or liver diseases and older and very young clients cannot tolerate an excessive fluid volume; the risk of **fluid (circulatory) overload** exists with these clients
F. A client with congestive heart failure is usually not given a saline solution, because this type of fluid encourages the retention of water and therefore exacerbates heart failure by increasing **fluid overload**

TABLE 13-2 Signs of Complications of Intravenous Therapy

Complication	Signs
Phlebitis	Heat, redness, and tenderness at site
	Not swollen or hard
	Sluggish IV infusion
Thrombophlebitis	Hard, cord-like vein
	Heat, redness, and tenderness at site
	Sluggish IV infusion
Infiltration	Edema, pain, and coolness at site
	May or may not have a blood return
Catheter embolism	Decrease in BP
	Pain along vein
	Weak, rapid pulse
	Cyanosis of nail beds
	Loss of consciousness
Fluid overload	Increased BP
	Rapid breathing
	Dyspnea
	Moist cough and crackles
Air embolism	Tachycardia
	Dyspnea
	Cyanosis
	Hypotension
	Decreased level of consciousness

BP, Blood pressure; *IV*, intravenous.

G. A client with diabetes mellitus does not typically receive dextrose (glucose) solutions
H. Lactated Ringer's solution contains potassium and should not be administered to clients with renal failure

VII. COMPLICATIONS (Table 13-2)
A. Infection
1. Description
a. The entry of microorganisms into the body through the venipuncture site
b. Venipuncture interrupts the integrity of the skin, which is the first line of defense against infection
c. The longer the therapy continues, the greater the risk of infection
2. At-risk clients
a. Clients who are immunocompromised as a result of diseases such as cancer or acquired immunodeficiency syndrome
b. Clients receiving treatments such as chemotherapy who have an altered or lowered white blood cell count
c. Older clients, because aging alters the effectiveness of the immune system
3. Prevention and interventions
a. Maintain strict asepsis when caring for the IV site
b. Monitor the vital signs, particularly the temperature

c. Monitor for local inflammation at the IV site

d. Check fluid containers for cracks, leaks, cloudiness, or other evidence of contamination

e. Change the tubing and site dressing every 24 to 72 hours, according to agency policy

f. Antimicrobial ointment is used at the IV site

g. Ensure that the IV solution is not hanging for more than 24 hours

h. Monitor for systemic infection; this includes malaise, headache, chills, fever, nausea, vomiting, backache, and tachycardia

i. If infection occurs, the IV is discontinued and the physician is notified; blood cultures may be ordered

B. **Phlebitis** and thrombophlebitis

1. Description

a. An inflammation of the vein that can occur from mechanical or chemical (medication) trauma or local infection

b. **Phlebitis** can cause the development of a clot (thrombophlebitis)

2. Prevention and interventions

a. An IV cannula smaller than the vein is used, and very small veins or veins over an area of flexion are avoided

b. Anchor the cannula and loop of tubing securely with tape

c. Use an armboard or splint as prescribed if the client is restless or active

d. If **phlebitis** occurs, the IV device is removed immediately

e. The physician is notified if **phlebitis** is suspected, and warm, moist compresses are applied if prescribed

C. **Infiltration**

1. Description

a. A form of tissue damage; also called *extravasation*

b. Seepage of the IV fluid out of the vein and into the surrounding tissues

c. Occurs when an IV device has become dislodged or perforates the wall of the vein

2. Prevention and interventions

a. IV sites over an area of flexion are avoided

b. Anchor the cannula and loop of tubing securely with tape

c. Use an armboard or splint as prescribed if the client is restless or active

d. Monitor the IV site for pain, edema, or coolness, and compare it with the opposite extremity

e. Monitor the IV rate for a decrease or halt in flow

f. If **infiltration** has occurred, the IV device is removed immediately

g. Do not rub an infiltrated area, because this can cause the development of a hematoma

h. If **infiltration** has occurred, the extremity is elevated, and compresses (warm or cool, depending on the physician's preference or agency policy) are applied over the affected area

D. Catheter embolism

1. Description: The tip of the catheter breaks off during IV insertion or removal, which results in the possibility of an embolus

2. Prevention and interventions

a. Remove the IV catheter carefully, and inspect the catheter when removed

b. If the catheter tip has broken off, the physician is notified; a tourniquet is placed high on the limb of IV site as prescribed, an x-ray study is obtained, and the client may require surgery to remove the catheter pieces

E. **Fluid (circulatory) overload**

1. Description: Results from the administration of fluids too rapidly or in a client who is at risk for **fluid overload**

2. Prevention and interventions

a. Identify clients who are at risk for **fluid overload**

b. Calculate and monitor the drip rate frequently

c. An infusion controller device may be used for clients who are at risk for **fluid overload**

d. If **fluid overload** occurs, the physician is notified

F. **Air embolism**

1. Description: A bolus of air enters the vein through an inadequately primed IV line, from a loose connection, or during a tubing change or the removal of the IV

2. Prevention and interventions

a. Prime the tubing with fluid before use, and monitor for any air bubbles in the tubing

b. Secure all connections

c. Replace IV fluid before the bag or bottle is empty

d. If an **air embolism** is suspected, the tubing is clamped, the client is turned on his or her left side with the head of the bed lowered to trap the air in the right atrium, and the physician is notified

VIII. CENTRAL VENOUS CATHETERS (Figure 13-4)

A. Description

1. Used to deliver hyperosmolar solutions, measure central venous pressure, and infuse parenteral nutrition and multiple IV infusions or medications

2. Catheter position is determined by x-ray study after insertion

3. May have a single, double, or triple lumen

4. May be inserted peripherally and threaded through the basilic or cephalic vein into the

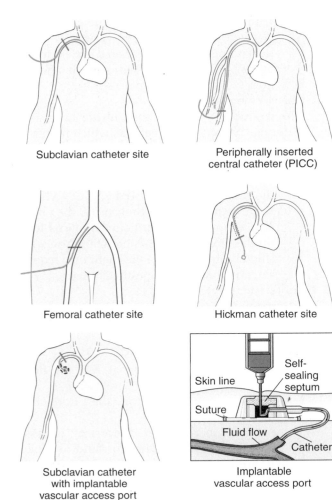

Subclavian catheter site

Peripherally inserted central catheter (PICC)

Femoral catheter site

Hickman catheter site

Subclavian catheter with implantable vascular access port

Implantable vascular access port

Skin line

Self-sealing septum

Suture

Fluid flow

Catheter

FIG. 13-4 Central venous access sites and access port. (From Kee, J., & Marshall, S. [2009]. *Clinical calculations: With applications to general and specialty areas* [6th ed.]. Philadelphia: Saunders.)

superior vena cava, inserted centrally through the internal jugular or subclavian veins, or surgically tunneled through subcutaneous tissue into the cephalic vein
5. With multilumen catheters, more than one medication can be administered at the same time without incompatibility problems, and there is only one insertion site for care
6. For central line insertion, tubing change, and line removal, place the client in Trendelenburg's position (if not contraindicated) or a supine position, and instruct the client to perform Valsalva's maneuver to increase pressure in the central veins when the IV system is open
B. Tunneled central venous catheters
1. A more permanent type of catheter (e.g., Hickman, Broviac, Groshong) used for long-term IV therapy
2. May be single or multilumen

3. Inserted in the operating room; the catheter is threaded into the lower part of the vena cava at the entrance of the right atrium
4. The catheter will be fitted with an intermittent infusion device to allow access as needed and to keep the system closed and intact
5. Patency is maintained by flushing with a diluted heparin solution or a normal saline solution, depending on the type of catheter and according to agency policy
C. Vascular access ports (implantable ports)
1. Surgically implanted under the skin (e.g., Port-a-Cath, Mediport, Infusaport); used for the long-term administration of repeated IV therapy
2. For access, requires palpation and injection through the skin into the self-sealing port with a noncoring needle (e.g., a Huber-point needle)
3. Patency is maintained by periodic flushing with a diluted heparin solution as prescribed and per agency policy
D. Peripherally inserted central catheter line
1. Used for long-term IV therapy, frequently in the home
2. The basilic vein is usually used, but the median cubital and cephalic veins in the antecubital area can also be used
3. Threaded so that the catheter tip may terminate in either the axillary or subclavian vein or the superior vena cava
4. A small amount of bleeding may occur at the time of insertion and continue for 24 hours, but bleeding thereafter is not expected
5. **Phlebitis** is a common complication
6. Insertion is below the heart level; therefore, **air embolism** is not common
IX. **BLOOD ADMINISTRATION**
A. Types of blood components
1. Red blood cells (RBCs)
a. Used to replace erythrocytes
b. Evaluation of an effective response is based on the resolution of the symptoms of anemia and an increase of the erythrocyte count
2. Platelets
a. Platelets are used to treat thrombocytopenia and platelet dysfunctions
b. **Crossmatching** is not required but is usually done (platelet concentrates contain few RBCs)
c. Evaluation of an effective response is based on the improvement of the platelet count
3. Fresh-frozen plasma
a. May be used to provide clotting factors or volume expansion; contains no platelets
b. **Rh factor** and **ABO compatibility** are required for the transfusion of plasma products
c. Evaluation of an effective response is assessed by monitoring coagulation studies

B. **Compatibility**
1. To ensure proper identification, client blood samples are drawn and labeled at the bedside; the client is asked to state his or her name, which is compared with the identification bracelet
2. The recipient's **ABO** and **Rh factor** are identified
3. An antibody screen is done to determine the presence of antibodies
4. **Crossmatching** testing is done, in which donor RBCs are combined with the recipient's serum and Coombs' serum; **crossmatching** is compatible if no RBC agglutination occurs
5. The universal RBC donor is O negative; the universal recipient is AB positive

C. Interventions
1. The client's temperature is checked before beginning a transfusion; a fever may be a cause for delaying the transfusion; in addition, a fever will mask a possible symptom of an acute **transfusion reaction**
2. During the transfusion, the client is monitored for signs and symptoms of a **transfusion reaction**; the first 15 minutes of the transfusion are the most critical, and the nurse must stay with client; if a major **ABO** incompatibility exists or a severe allergic reaction occurs, it is usually evident within the first 50 mL of the transfusion
3. The client is instructed to immediately report anything unusual
4. If a reaction occurs, the transfusion is stopped, and the physician is notified; the blood bag and tubing are returned to the blood bank
5. If a reaction occurs, the client is monitored for any life-threatening symptoms, and the appropriate blood and urine samples are obtained as prescribed
6. Document the client's tolerance to the administration of the blood product

D. **Transfusion reactions**
1. Immediate **transfusion reaction**
   a. Chills and diaphoresis
   b. Muscle aches, back pain, or chest pain
   c. Rashes, hives, itching, and swelling
   d. Rapid, thready pulse
   e. Dyspnea, cough, or wheezing
   f. Pallor and cyanosis
   g. Apprehension
   h. Tingling and numbness
   i. Headache
   j. Nausea, vomiting, abdominal cramping, and diarrhea
2. Delayed **transfusion reaction**
   a. Reactions can occur days to years after a transfusion
   b. Signs include fever, mild jaundice, and a decreased hematocrit level

PRACTICE QUESTIONS

More questions on the companion CD!

97. A nurse is assisting with caring for a client who will receive a unit of blood. Just before the infusion, it is most important for the nurse to assess the client's:
   1. Vital signs
   2. Skin color
   3. Oxygen saturation
   4. Latest hematocrit level

98. A client who is receiving a blood transfusion rings the call bell for the nurse. When entering the room, the nurse notes that the client is flushed, dyspneic, and complaining of generalized itching. The nurse interprets that the client is experiencing:
   1. Bacteremia
   2. Fluid overload
   3. Hypovolemic shock
   4. A transfusion reaction

99. A client who was receiving a blood transfusion has experienced a transfusion reaction. The nurse sends the blood bag that was used for the client to which of the following areas?
   1. The pharmacy
   2. The laboratory
   3. The blood bank
   4. The risk-management department

100. A nurse takes a client's temperature before giving a blood transfusion. The temperature is 100° F orally. The nurse reports the finding to the registered nurse and anticipates that which of the following actions will take place?
   1. The transfusion will begin as prescribed.
   2. The blood will be held, and the physician will be notified.
   3. The transfusion will begin after the administration of an antihistamine.
   4. The transfusion will begin after the administration of 600 mg of acetaminophen (Tylenol).

101. A nurse is assisting with caring for a client who has received a transfusion of platelets. The nurse determines that the client is benefiting most from this therapy if the client exhibits which of the following?
   1. An increased hematocrit level
   2. An increased hemoglobin level
   3. A decline of the temperature to normal
   4. A decrease in oozing from puncture sites and gums

102. A client has an order to receive 1000 mL of 5% dextrose in 0.45% sodium chloride. After gathering the appropriate equipment, the nurse takes which action first before spiking the IV bag with the tubing?
   1. Uncaps the distal end of the tubing
   2. Uncaps the spike portion of the tubing

3. Opens the roller clamp on the IV tubing
4. Closes the roller clamp on the IV tubing

103. A nurse is doing a routine assessment of a client's peripheral IV site. The nurse notes that the site is cool, pale, and swollen and that the IV has stopped running. The nurse determines that which of the following has probably occurred?
1. Phlebitis
2. Infection
3. Infiltration
4. Thrombosis

104. A nurse is assigned to care for a client with a peripheral IV infusion. The nurse is providing hygiene care to the client and would avoid which of the following while changing the client's hospital gown?
1. Using a hospital gown with snaps at the sleeves
2. Disconnecting the IV tubing from the catheter in the vein
3. Checking the IV flow rate immediately after changing the hospital gown
4. Putting the bag and tubing through the sleeve, followed by the client's arm

105. A nurse is making a worksheet and listing the tasks that need to be performed for assigned adult clients during the shift. The nurse writes on the plan to check the IV of an assigned client who is receiving fluid replacement therapy at least every:
1. 1 hour
2. 2 hours
3. 3 hours
4. 4 hours

106. A nurse is checking the insertion site of a peripheral IV catheter. The nurse notes the site to be reddened, warm, painful, and slightly edematous in the area of the vein proximal to the IV catheter. The nurse interprets that this is likely the result of:
1. Phlebitis of the vein
2. Infiltration of the IV line
3. Hypersensitivity to the IV solution
4. An allergic reaction to the IV catheter material

107. A nurse has been instructed to discontinue an IV line. The nurse removes the catheter by withdrawing the catheter while applying pressure to the site with a(n):
1. Band-Aid
2. Alcohol swab
3. Betadine swab
4. Sterile 2 × 2 gauze

108. A nurse is preparing an IV solution and tubing for a client who requires IV fluids. While preparing to prime the tubing, the tubing drops and hits the top of the medication cart. The nurse should plan to do which of the following?
1. Change the IV tubing.
2. Wipe the tubing with Betadine.
3. Scrub the tubing with an alcohol swab.
4. Scrub the tubing before attaching it to the IV bag.

109. A client is going to be transfused with a unit of packed red blood cells. The nurse understands that it is necessary to remain with the client for what time period after the transfusion is started?
1. 5 minutes
2. 15 minutes
3. 30 minutes
4. 45 minutes

110. A nurse is assisting with caring for a client who is receiving a unit of packed red blood cells. The nurse tells the client that it is most important to report which of the following signs immediately?
1. Sore throat or earache
2. Chills, itching, or rash
3. Unusual sleepiness or fatigue
4. Mild discomfort at the catheter site

ALTERNATE ITEM FORMAT: MULTIPLE RESPONSE

111. Which of these clients are most likely to develop fluid (circulatory) overload? Select all that apply.
☐ 1. A premature infant
☐ 2. A 101-year-old man
☑ 3. The client on renal dialysis
☐ 4. The client with diabetes mellitus
☐ 5. A 29-year-old woman with pneumonia
☑ 6. The client with congestive heart failure

ANSWERS

97. 1
Rationale: A change in the vital signs may indicate that a transfusion reaction is occurring. The nurse assesses the client's vital signs before the procedure to obtain a baseline, every 15 minutes for the first half hour after beginning the transfusion, and every half hour thereafter.
Test-Taking Strategy: Note the strategic words "just before" and "most important." This tells you that more than one option may be partially or totally correct. Recalling the signs of a blood transfusion reaction will direct you to option 1. In addition, option 1 is the umbrella option. Review the blood infusion procedure if you had difficulty with this question.
Level of Cognitive Ability: Application
Client Needs: Physiological Integrity
Integrated Process: Nursing Process/Data Collection
Content Area: Fundamental Skills
References: Linton, A., & Maebius, N. (2007). *Introduction to medical-surgical nursing* (4th ed., p. 580). Philadelphia: Saunders.

Potter, P., & Perry, A. (2005). *Fundamentals of nursing* (6th ed., p. 1191). St. Louis: Mosby.

98. 4

Rationale: The signs and symptoms exhibited by the client are consistent with a transfusion reaction. With fluid overload, the client would have crackles in addition to dyspnea. With bacteremia, the client would have a fever, which is not part of the clinical picture presented. There is no correlation between the signs mentioned in the question and hypovolemic shock. The signs identified in the question are indicative of an allergic reaction, which is one type of blood transfusion reaction.

Test-Taking Strategy: Use the process of elimination, and focus on the data in the question. Recalling the signs of a transfusion reaction will direct you to option 4. Review the complications of blood administration and the signs of a transfusion reaction if you had difficulty with this question.

Level of Cognitive Ability: Analysis
Client Needs: Physiological Integrity
Integrated Process: Nursing Process/Data Collection
Content Area: Fundamental Skills
References: Christensen, B., & Kockrow, E. (2006). *Foundations of nursing* (5th ed., pp. 551-552). St. Louis: Mosby.
Potter, P., & Perry, A. (2005). *Fundamentals of nursing* (6th ed., p. 1192). St. Louis: Mosby.

99. 3

Rationale: The nurse prepares to return the blood transfusion bag containing any remaining blood to the blood bank. This allows the blood bank to complete any follow-up testing procedures that are needed after a transfusion reaction has been documented. Options 1, 2, and 4 are incorrect.

Test-Taking Strategy: Use the process of elimination. Recalling that blood is obtained from the blood bank will help you to eliminate each of the incorrect options. Review the procedures to follow when a blood transfusion reaction occurs if you had difficulty with this question.

Level of Cognitive Ability: Application
Client Needs: Physiological Integrity
Integrated Process: Nursing Process/Implementation
Content Area: Fundamental Skills
References: Christensen, B., & Kockrow, E. (2006). *Foundations of nursing* (5th ed., p. 552). St. Louis: Mosby.
Potter, P., & Perry, A. (2005). *Fundamentals of nursing* (6th ed., p. 1193). St. Louis: Mosby.

100. 2

Rationale: If the client has a temperature of 100° F or more, the unit of blood should be held until the physician is notified and has the opportunity to give further orders. The other options are incorrect.

Test-Taking Strategy: Use the process of elimination. Eliminate options 1, 3, and 4, because they are comparable or alike. Remember that if the temperature is elevated, the physician needs to be notified before a blood transfusion is initiated. Review the procedures related to the administration of a blood transfusion if you had difficulty with this question.

Level of Cognitive Ability: Application
Client Needs: Physiological Integrity
Integrated Process: Nursing Process/Implementation
Content Area: Fundamental Skills

Reference: Ignatavicius, D., & Workman, M. (2006). *Medical-surgical nursing: Critical thinking for collaborative care* (5th ed., p. 913). Philadelphia: Saunders.

101. 4

Rationale: Platelets are necessary for proper blood clotting. The client with insufficient platelets may exhibit frank bleeding or the oozing of blood from puncture sites, wounds, and mucous membranes. The client's temperature would decline to normal after the infusion of granulocytes if those transfused cells were then instrumental in fighting infection in the body. Increased hemoglobin and hematocrit levels would be seen when the client has received a transfusion of red blood cells.

Test-Taking Strategy: Use the process of elimination. Recalling that bleeding is a concern when the platelets are low will easily direct you to option 4. Review the action of platelets if you had difficulty with this question.

Level of Cognitive Ability: Analysis
Client Needs: Physiological Integrity
Integrated Process: Nursing Process/Evaluation
Content Area: Fundamental Skills
Reference: Ignatavicius, D., & Workman, M. (2006). *Medical-surgical nursing: Critical thinking for collaborative care* (5th ed., p. 915). Philadelphia: Saunders.

102. 4

Rationale: The nurse should first clamp the tubing to prevent the solution from running freely through the tubing after it is attached to the IV bag. The nurse should next uncap the proximal (spike) portion of the tubing and attach it to the IV bag. The roller clamp is then opened slowly, and the fluid is allowed to flow through the tubing in a controlled fashion to prevent air from remaining in parts of the tubing.

Test-Taking Strategy: Use the process of elimination, and note the strategic word "first." This question tests a specific procedure related to IV therapy. Visualize this procedure to answer the question correctly. Review the intravenous infusion procedure if you had difficulty with this question.

Level of Cognitive Ability: Application
Client Needs: Physiological Integrity
Integrated Process: Nursing Process/Implementation
Content Area: Fundamental Skills
References: Christensen, B., & Kockrow, E. (2006). *Foundations of nursing* (5th ed., p. 542). St. Louis: Mosby.
Potter, P., & Perry, A. (2005). *Fundamentals of nursing* (6th ed., p. 1184). St. Louis: Mosby.

103. 3

Rationale: An infiltrated IV is one that has dislodged from the vein and that is lying in subcutaneous tissue. The pallor, coolness, and swelling are the result of IV fluid being deposited into the subcutaneous tissue. When the pressure in the tissues exceeds the pressure in the tubing, the flow of the IV solution will stop. The other three options identify complications that are likely to be accompanied by warmth at the site rather than coolness.

Test-Taking Strategy: Focus on the data in the question, and note the strategic word "cool." Recalling that coolness occurs at the site of IV infiltration will direct you to option 3. Review the signs of infiltration if you had difficulty with this question.

Level of Cognitive Ability: Analysis
Client Needs: Physiological Integrity
Integrated Process: Nursing Process/Data Collection
Content Area: Fundamental Skills
References: Linton, A., & Maebius, N. (2007). *Introduction to medical-surgical nursing* (4th ed., pp. 285, 287). Philadelphia: Saunders.
Potter, P., & Perry, A. (2005). *Fundamentals of nursing* (6th ed., p. 1189). St. Louis: Mosby.

104. **2**
Rationale: The tubing should not be removed from the IV catheter. With each break in the system, there is an increased chance of introducing bacteria into the system, which can lead to infection. Options 1 and 4 are appropriate. The flow rate should be checked immediately after changing the hospital gown, because the position of the roller clamp may have been affected during the change.
Test-Taking Strategy: Use the process of elimination, and note the strategic word "avoid." This word indicates a negative event query and asks you to select an incorrect action. Visualize this procedure, and use your knowledge of the basic principles related to IV therapy and asepsis to direct you to option 2. Review these principles if you had difficulty with this question.
Level of Cognitive Ability: Application
Client Needs: Safe and Effective Care Environment
Integrated Process: Nursing Process/Implementation
Content Area: Fundamental Skills
References: Christensen, B., & Kockrow, E. (2006). *Foundations of nursing* (5th ed., p. 547). St. Louis: Mosby.
Potter, P., & Perry, A. (2005). *Fundamentals of nursing* (6th ed., p. 1181). St. Louis: Mosby.

105. **1**
Rationale: Safe nursing practice includes monitoring an IV infusion at least once per hour for an adult client. Options 2, 3, and 4 do not provide time frames that are safe or acceptable.
Test-Taking Strategy: Use the process of elimination. To answer this question accurately, it is necessary to be familiar with the specific time frames indicated for this nursing procedure. For questions similar to this one, it is best to select the most frequently occurring time frame. Review the precautions related to the administration of IV fluid if you had difficulty with this question.
Level of Cognitive Ability: Application
Client Needs: Physiological Integrity
Integrated Process: Communication and Documentation
Content Area: Fundamental Skills
Reference: Linton, A., & Maebius, N. (2007). *Introduction to medical-surgical nursing* (4th ed., p. 283). Philadelphia: Saunders.

106. **1**
Rationale: Phlebitis at an IV site results in discomfort at the site and redness, warmth, and swelling proximal to the IV catheter. The IV catheter should be removed, and a new IV line should be inserted at a different site. The remaining options are incorrect.

Test-Taking Strategy: Use the process of elimination. Remember that comparable or alike options are not likely to be correct. In this case, options 3 and 4 are comparable or alike and are therefore eliminated. Recalling that warmth occurs at the site of phlebitis will direct you to option 1. Review the signs of phlebitis if you had difficulty with this question.
Level of Cognitive Ability: Analysis
Client Needs: Physiological Integrity
Integrated Process: Nursing Process/Data Collection
Content Area: Fundamental Skills
References: Christensen, B., & Kockrow, E. (2006). *Foundations of nursing* (5th ed., pp. 549-550). St. Louis: Mosby.
Linton, A., & Maebius, N. (2007). *Introduction to medical-surgical nursing* (4th ed., p. 287). Philadelphia: Saunders.

107. **4**
Rationale: A dry, sterile dressing such as a sterile 2 × 2 gauze is used to apply pressure to the site while the catheter is discontinued and removed. This material is absorbent, sterile, and nonirritating to the site. A Betadine or alcohol swab would irritate the opened puncture site and would not stop the blood flow. A Band-Aid may be used to cover the site after hemostasis has occurred.
Test-Taking Strategy: Use the process of elimination. Visualize this procedure, and think about each of the items identified in the options to answer the question. Noting the word "sterile" in option 4 will assist with directing you to this option. Review the discontinuation of an IV line if you had difficulty with this question.
Level of Cognitive Ability: Application
Client Needs: Safe and Effective Care Environment
Integrated Process: Nursing Process/Implementation
Content Area: Fundamental Skills
References: Christensen, B., & Kockrow, E. (2006). *Foundations of nursing* (5th ed., p. 558). St. Louis: Mosby.
Potter, P., & Perry, A. (2005). *Fundamentals of nursing* (6th ed., p. 1190). St. Louis: Mosby.

108. **1**
Rationale: The nurse should change the IV tubing. The tubing has become contaminated, and, if used, it could result in a systemic infection in the client. Wiping or scrubbing the tubing is insufficient to prevent systemic infection.
Test-Taking Strategy: Use your knowledge of basic infection control measures and IV therapy concepts to answer this question. Note that options 2, 3, and 4 are comparable or alike, and eliminate these options. Review aseptic technique and IV therapy if you had difficulty with this question.
Level of Cognitive Ability: Application
Client Needs: Safe and Effective Care Environment
Integrated Process: Nursing Process/Implementation
Content Area: Fundamental Skills
References: Christensen, B., & Kockrow, E. (2006). *Foundations of nursing* (5th ed., p. 555). St. Louis: Mosby.
Linton, A., & Maebius, N. (2007). *Introduction to medical-surgical nursing* (4th ed., p. 287). Philadelphia: Saunders.

109. **2**
Rationale: The nurse must remain with the client for the first 15 minutes of a transfusion, which is the most likely time that a transfusion reaction will occur. This enables the nurse to detect

a reaction and intervene quickly. The nurse engages in safe nursing practice by obtaining coverage for the other clients during this time. Options 1, 3, and 4 are incorrect.

Test-Taking Strategy: Use the process of elimination and your knowledge regarding blood transfusion procedures to answer this question. Remember, the client must be directly monitored for the first 15 minutes of the transfusion. Review the nursing responsibilities involved when beginning a blood transfusion if you had difficulty with this question.

Level of Cognitive Ability: Application
Client Needs: Physiological Integrity
Integrated Process: Nursing Process/Planning
Content Area: Fundamental Skills
References: Christensen, B., & Kockrow, E. (2006). *Foundations of nursing* (5th ed., p. 550). St. Louis: Mosby.
Linton, A., & Maebius, N. (2007). *Introduction to medical-surgical nursing* (4th ed., p. 580). Philadelphia: Saunders.

110. 2

Rationale: The client is told to report chills, itching, or rash immediately, because these could possibly be signs of a transfusion reaction. Mild discomfort at the catheter site may be indicative of a problem, or it could result from the size of the IV catheter required to infuse the blood product. Sleepiness, fatigue, sore throat, and earache are unrelated to a transfusion reaction.

Test-Taking Strategy: Note the strategic words "most important" and "immediately." These tell you that more than one or all of the options may be partially or totally correct. With the knowledge that a transfusion reaction is of greatest concern to the nurse, prioritize and select the option that characterizes this problem. Review the signs of a transfusion reaction if you had difficulty with this question.

Level of Cognitive Ability: Application
Client Needs: Physiological Integrity
Integrated Process: Nursing Process/Implementation
Content Area: Fundamental Skills
References: Linton, A., & Maebius, N. (2007). *Introduction to medical-surgical nursing* (4th ed., p. 581). Philadelphia: Saunders.
Potter, P., & Perry, A. (2005). *Fundamentals of nursing* (6th ed., pp. 1190-1192). St. Louis: Mosby.

ALTERNATE ITEM FORMAT: MULTIPLE RESPONSE

111. 1, 2, 3, 6

Rationale: Clients with cardiac, respiratory, renal, or liver diseases and older and very young clients cannot tolerate an excessive fluid volume; the risk of fluid (circulatory) overload exists with these clients.

Test-Taking Strategy: Focus on the subject of fluid (circulatory) overload. Thinking about the physiology associated with each client described in the options will assist you with answering correctly. Review the concepts related to fluid overload if you had difficulty with this question.

Level of Cognitive Ability: Analysis
Client Needs: Physiological Integrity
Integrated Process: Nursing Process/Data Collection
Content Area: Fundamental Skills
Reference: Chernecky, C., & Macklin, D. (2004). *Real world survival guide: IV therapy* (1st ed., p. 147). St. Louis: Saunders.

REFERENCES

Chernecky, C., & Macklin, D. (2004). *Real world survival guide: IV therapy* (1st ed.). St. Louis: Saunders.

Christensen, B., & Kockrow, E. (2006). *Foundations of nursing* (5th ed.). St. Louis: Mosby.

Ignatavicius, D., & Workman, M. (2006). *Medical-surgical nursing: Critical thinking for collaborative care* (5th ed.). Philadelphia: Saunders.

Linton, A., & Maebius, N. (2007). *Introduction to medical-surgical nursing* (4th ed.). Philadelphia: Saunders.

National Council of State Boards of Nursing (Eds.) (2008). *2008 Detailed Test Plan for the NCLEX-PN® Examination, National Council of State Boards of Nursing.* Chicago: Author.

National Council of State Boards of Nursing. *NCSBN home page.* www.ncsbn.org. Accessed June 19, 2008.

Potter, P., & Perry, A. (2005). *Fundamentals of nursing* (6th ed.). St. Louis: Mosby.

Fundamental Skills

Hygiene and Safety

PYRAMID TERMS

chemical restraints Medications given to inhibit a specific behavior or movement

environmental safety Many physical and psychosocial factors that influence or affect the life and survival of clients

health care–associated infections Previously referred to as *nosocomial infections*; infections acquired while clients are receiving health care; may be endogenous (from a client's flora) or exogenous (from outside the client; often the result of the hands of health care workers)

physical hazards Hazards that place clients at risk for accidental injury and death

physical restraints (security devices) Devices that are applied to restrict a client's movement

poison Any substance that impairs health or destroys life when ingested, inhaled, or otherwise absorbed by the body

sentinel events The official reporting of an incident, event, irregular occurrence, or variance

standard precautions Guidelines used by all health care providers with all clients to reduce the risk of infection for both clients and caregivers

transmission-based precautions Guidelines that are used in addition to standard precautions; used for specific syndromes that are highly suggestive of infection until a diagnosis is confirmed

warfare agent Substance that may be biological, chemical, or radioactive in nature that can cause mass destruction and fatality

PYRAMID TO SUCCESS

Safety and Infection Control is a subcategory of the Safe and Effective Care Environment component of the Client Needs section of the test plan for the NCLEX-PN. The pyramid points focus on maintaining environmental safety, preventing accidents, the medication reconciliation process, using restraints, priority nursing actions in the event of a disaster, and biological and chemical warfare agents. The pyramid points also focus on standard and transmission-based precautions and the measures required to handle hazardous or infectious materials. The Integrated Processes addressed in this chapter include Caring, Communication and Documentation,

the Clinical Problem-Solving Process (Nursing Process), and Teaching and Learning.

CLIENT NEEDS

Safe and Effective Care Environment

Ensuring that clients' rights are upheld, including informed consent

Establishing priorities

Following guidelines regarding the use of restraints

Following guidelines related to disaster planning and biological and chemical warfare agents

Handling hazardous and infectious materials safely

Maintaining precautions to prevent accidents

Using standard, transmission-based, and other infection-control precautions

Health Promotion and Maintenance

Assisting clients and families with identifying environmental hazards in the home

Teaching clients and families about accident prevention

Teaching clients and families about measures to be implemented during an emergency or disaster

Teaching clients and families about preventing the spread of infection

Psychosocial Integrity

Assessing the client for sensory or perceptual alterations

Identifying cultural and religious lifestyles

Identifying support systems

Physiological Integrity

Assisting the client with activities of daily living

Implementing priority nursing actions during an emergency or disaster

Managing and providing care to clients with infectious diseases

Providing comfort and assistance to the client

Using assistive devices to prevent injury

I. HYGIENE

A. Description

1. The activity of providing care or promoting self-care, which includes bathing and grooming
2. Includes care of the skin, hair, nails, mouth, teeth, eyes, ears, nasal cavities, and perineal and genital areas
3. Personal hygiene is the activity of self-care, including bathing and grooming

B. General principles

1. Wash hands and wear gloves
2. Ensure privacy
3. Explain procedures to the client
4. Determine and treat pain
5. Determine the client's health status and readiness for hygiene procedures
6. Determine the client's routine hygiene practices
7. Use proper body mechanics during bathing and hygiene activities
8. Use time spent with client as an opportunity to determine the client's mental health status and to implement communication and teaching
9. Maintain and encourage independence as much as possible

II. ENVIRONMENTAL SAFETY

A. Fire safety (Box 14-1)

1. Keep open spaces free of clutter
2. Clearly mark fire exits
3. Know the locations of all fire alarms, exits, and extinguishers (Table 14-1; Box 14-2)
4. Know the telephone number for reporting fires
5. Know the agency's fire drill and evacuation plan
6. Never use the elevator in the event of a fire

BOX 14-1 **Priority Actions in the Event of a Fire**

Remember the mnemonic *RACE* to set priorities in the event of a fire:

R Rescue: Remove all clients from the vicinity of the fire.

A Alarm: Activate the fire alarm, and report the fire before attempting to extinguish it.

C Confine: Close the doors and windows when a fire is detected.

E Extinguish: Extinguish the fire using the appropriate fire extinguisher.

TABLE 14-1 **Types of Fire Extinguishers**

Type	Class of Fires
A	Wood, cloth, upholstery, paper, rubbish, and plastic
B	Flammable liquids or gases, grease, tar, and oil-based paint
C	Electrical equipment

Note: Certain extinguishers may be appropriate for more than one type of fire.

---

7. Turn off oxygen and appliances in the vicinity of the fire
8. In the event of a fire, if a client is on life support, maintain the client's respiratory status manually with an Ambu bag until the client is moved away from the threat of the fire
9. In the event of a fire, ambulatory clients can be directed to walk by themselves to a safe area; in some cases, they may be able to assist with moving clients who are in wheelchairs
10. Bedridden clients are generally moved from the scene of a fire by stretcher, bed, or wheelchair
11. If a client must be carried from the area of a fire, appropriate transfer techniques should be used
12. If fire department personnel are at the scene of the fire, they can help evacuate clients

B. Electrical safety

1. Electrical equipment must be maintained in good working order and should be grounded
2. Use a three-pronged electrical cord
3. In a three-pronged electrical cord, the third, longer prong of the cord is the ground; the other two prongs carry the power to the piece of electrical equipment
4. Any electrical equipment that the client brings into the health care facility must be inspected for safety before use
5. Check electrical cords and outlets for exposed, frayed, or damaged wires
6. Avoid overloading any circuit
7. Read warning labels on all equipment; never operate unfamiliar equipment
8. Use safety extension cords only when absolutely necessary, and tape them to the floor with electrical tape
9. Never run electrical wiring under carpets
10. Never pull a plug by using the cord; always grasp the plug itself
11. Never use electrical appliances near sinks, bathtubs, or other water sources
12. Always disconnect a plug from the outlet before cleaning equipment or appliances
13. If a client receives an electrical shock, turn off the electricity before touching the client

C. Radiation safety

1. Know the health care agency's protocols and guidelines
2. Label potentially radioactive material

BOX 14-2 **Using a Fire Extinguisher**

Remember the mnemonic *PASS* when using a fire extinguisher:

P Pull the pin.

A Aim at the base of the fire.

S Squeeze the handles.

S Sweep the fire from side to side.

3. To reduce exposure to radiation:
   a. The time spent near the source should be limited
   b. The distance from the source should be as great as possible
   c. A shielding device such as a lead apron should be used
4. Monitor radiation exposure with a film (dosimeter) badge
5. Place the client who has a radiation implant in a private room
6. Never touch dislodged implants

D. Magnetic resonance imaging safety
   1. Know the protocols and guidelines of the health care agency
   2. Obtain informed consent
   3. Food or fluid restrictions may not be necessary
   4. Contraindicated for clients with cardiac pacemakers and other implanted pumps or metal devices
   5. Tell client that the procedure is noisy and that earplugs are available
   6. If in a "closed" unit, tell the client that he or she will lie on a hard surface inside a hollow tube
   7. Make sure that no metallic objects are allowed in the room, including any metal on the client or on the clothes of medical personnel

E. Disposal of infectious wastes
   1. Handle all infectious materials as a hazard
   2. Dispose of waste in designated areas only, and use proper containers for disposal
   3. Ensure that infectious material is properly labelled
   4. Needles should not be recapped, bent, or broken
   5. Dispose of all sharps immediately after use in closed, puncture-resistant disposal containers that are leakproof and labelled or color coded

F. Falls (Box 14-3 lists measures to prevent falls)
G. Medication errors (Box 14-4)
H. Restraints (security devices)
   1. Protective devices used to limit the physical activity of a client or to immobilize a client or an extremity
   2. Guidelines for protective devices applied to clients with a mental health diagnosis may be governed by state mental health code standards
   3. **Physical restraints**: Restrict client movement through the application of a device
   4. **Chemical restraints**: Medications given to inhibit a specific behavior or movement
   5. Interventions
      a. When restraints are necessary, the physician's orders should state the type of restraint, identify specific client behaviors for which restraints are to be used, and identify a limited time frame for use
      b. Physician's orders for restraints should be renewed within a specific time frame, according to agency policy
      c. Restraints are not to be ordered on an as-needed basis
      d. The reason for the restraints should be given to the client and family, and their permission should be sought
      e. Restraints should not interfere with any treatments or affect the client's health problem
      f. Make sure that restraints are applied appropriately and according to the manufacturer's instructions
      g. Use a half-bow or safety knot to secure the device to the bed frame or chair and not to the side rails (provides for quick release)
      h. Because there are several different types of restraints, ensure that there is enough slack on the straps to allow some movement of the body part

---

BOX 14-3 **Measures to Prevent Falls**

- Assess the client's risk for falling.
- Ensure that the client at risk for falling is in a room near the nurses' station.
- Be alert to clients who are at risk for falling.
- Orient the client to his or her physical surroundings.
- Instruct the client to seek assistance when getting up.
- Explain the use of the call-bell system.
- Keep the bed in the low position with three side rails up. (Having four side rails up is considered a restraint and requires a physician's order and monitoring standards.)
- Lock all beds, wheelchairs, and stretchers.
- Keep personal items within reach.
- Eliminate clutter and obstacles in the client's room.
- Provide adequate lighting, including subdued lighting at night.
- Reduce bathroom hazards.
- Maintain the client's toileting schedule throughout the day.

BOX 14-4 **National Patient Safety Goals to Reduce the Risk of Medication Errors**

- Improve the accuracy of client identification.
- Improve the effectiveness of communication among caregivers.
- Improve safety after high-alert medications.
- Eliminate wrong-site, wrong-client, and wrong-procedure surgery.
- Improve the safety of the use of infusion pumps.
- Improve the effectiveness of clinical alarm systems.
- Reduce the risk of health care–associated (nosocomial) infections.

From The Joint Commission: *www.jointcommission.org/PatientSafety/ NationalPatientSafetyGoals/09_hap_npsgs.htm.* Accessed October 20, 2008.

i. Restraints with plastic quick-release buckles should not be knotted

j. Assess skin integrity and neurovascular and circulatory status every 30 minutes, and remove the restraint at least every 2 hours to permit muscle exercise and promote circulation

k. Continually assess and document the need for the restraints (Box 14-5)

6. Alternatives to restraints
   a. Orient the client and family to surroundings
   b. Explain all procedures and treatments to the client and family
   c. Encourage family and friends to stay with the client, and use sitters for clients who need supervision
   d. Assign confused and disoriented clients to rooms near the nurses' station
   e. Provide appropriate visual and auditory stimuli to the client (e.g., clock, calendar, television, radio)
   f. Place familiar items (e.g., family pictures) near the client's bedside
   g. Maintain toileting routines
   h. Eliminate bothersome treatments (e.g., tube feedings) as soon as possible
   i. Evaluate all medications that the client is receiving
   j. Use relaxation techniques with the client
   k. Institute exercise and ambulation schedules as the client's condition allows

I. **Poisons**

1. Any substance that impairs health or destroys life when ingested, inhaled, or otherwise absorbed by the body
2. Specific antidotes or treatments are available for only some types of **poisons**
3. The capability of body tissue to recover from a **poison** determines the reversibility of the effect
4. **Poison** can impair the respiratory, circulatory, central nervous, hepatic, gastrointestinal, and renal systems of the body
5. Toddlers, preschoolers, and young school-age children must be protected from accidental poisoning

6. In older adults, diminished eyesight and impaired memory may result in the accidental ingestion of poisonous substances or an overdose of prescribed medications
7. A **poison** control center phone number should be visible on the telephone in homes with small children; in all cases of suspected poisoning, the number should be called immediately
8. Interventions
   a. Remove any obvious materials from the mouth, eye, or body area immediately
   b. Identify the type and amount of substance ingested
   c. Call the **poison** control center before attempting an intervention
   d. If the victim vomits or vomiting is induced, save the vomitus if requested to do so, and deliver it to the **poison** control center
   e. If instructed by the **poison** control center to take the poisoned person to the emergency department, call an ambulance
   f. Vomiting is never induced after the ingestion of lye, household cleaners, grease, or petroleum products
   g. Vomiting is never induced in an unconscious victim

III. **HEALTH CARE–ASSOCIATED INFECTIONS** (Box 14-6)
A. Previously referred to as *nosocomial infections*
B. Infections acquired in a hospital or other health care facility that were not present or incubating at the time of a client's admission
C. Illness impairs the body's normal defense mechanisms
D. The health care environment provides exposure to a variety of virulent organisms that the client has not been exposed to in the past; therefore, the client has not developed resistance to these organisms
E. Infections can be transmitted by health care personnel who fail to practice proper handwashing procedures or to change gloves between client contacts
F. Health care agencies usually have dispensers mounted at the entrance to each client's room that contain an alcohol-based solution for hand rubs

IV. **STANDARD PRECAUTIONS**
A. Description
   1. Must be practiced with all clients in any setting, regardless of the diagnosis or the presumed infectiousness

---

BOX 14-5 **Documentation Points With the Use of a Restraint (Security Device)**

- Reason for restraint
- Method of restraint
- Date and time of the application of restraint
- Duration of use of restraint and the client's response
- Release from restraint with periodic exercise and circulatory, neurovascular, and skin assessment
- Determination of the continued need for restraint
- Evaluation of the client's response

BOX 14-6 **Common Drug-Resistant Health Care–Associated Infections**

- Vancomycin-resistant enterococci
- Methicillin-resistant *Staphylococcus aureus*
- Multidrug-resistant tuberculosis

2. Promote handwashing and the use of gloves, masks, eye protection, and gowns, when appropriate, during client contact
3. These precautions apply to blood, all body fluids, secretions, and excretions, regardless of whether they contain blood, nonintact skin, or mucous membranes

B. Interventions
   1. Handle all blood and body fluids from all clients as if they were contaminated
   2. An alcohol-based hand rub or a soap-and-water hand wash to decontaminate the hands is necessary before having direct contact with a client
   3. The hands are also washed between client contacts; after contact with blood, body fluids, secretions, or excretions and after contact with equipment or articles contaminated by them; and immediately after gloves are removed
   4. Gloves are worn when blood, body fluids, secretions, excretions, nonintact skin, mucous membranes, or contaminated items are touched; gloves should be removed and hands washed between client care contacts
   5. Masks, eye protection, or face shields are worn if client care activities may generate splashes or sprays of blood or body fluid
   6. Gowns are worn if the soiling of clothing is likely from contact with blood or body fluid; wash hands after removing a gown
   7. Client care equipment is properly cleaned and reprocessed, and single-use items are discarded
   8. Contaminated linens are placed in leakproof bags and handled to prevent skin and mucous membrane exposure
   9. All sharp instruments and needles are discarded in a puncture-resistant container; needles are disposed of uncapped
   10. Use needleless devices or special needle safety devices whenever possible to reduce the risk to health care workers of needle sticks and sharps injuries
   11. Spills of blood or body fluids are cleaned with a solution of bleach and water (diluted 1:10) or an agency-approved disinfectant
   12. A private room is unnecessary unless the client's hygiene is unacceptable; the nurse should consult with an infection-control professional

▲ V. TRANSMISSION-BASED PRECAUTIONS
A. Airborne precautions
   1. Diseases
      a. Measles
      b. Chickenpox (varicella)
      c. Disseminated varicella zoster
      d. Tuberculosis

   2. Barrier protection for airborne precautions
      a. Single room maintained under negative pressure; door kept closed except when someone is entering or exiting the room
      b. Negative airflow pressure in the room, with a minimum of 6 to 12 air exchanges per hour, depending on the health care agency
      c. Use of ultraviolet germicide irradiation or a high-efficiency particulate air filter in the room
      d. Use of a mask or a personal respiratory protection device
      e. Place a mask on the client when the client needs to leave the room; the client leaves the room only if necessary

B. Droplet precautions
   1. Diseases
      a. Adenovirus
      b. Diphtheria (pharyngeal)
      c. Epiglottitis
      d. Influenza
      e. Meningitis
      f. Mumps
      g. Mycoplasma pneumonia or meningococcal pneumonia
      h. Parvovirus B19
      i. Pertussis
      j. Pneumonia
      k. Rubella
      l. Scarlet fever
      m. Sepsis
      n. Streptococcal pharyngitis
   2. Barrier protection
      a. Private room or cohort client
      b. Use of a mask
      c. Place a mask on the client when the client is out of the room; the client leaves the room only if necessary

C. Contact precautions
   1. Diseases
      a. Colonization or infection with a multidrug-resistant organism
      b. Enteric infections such as *Clostridium difficile*
      c. Respiratory infections such as respiratory syncytial virus
      d. Wound infections
      e. Skin infections such as cutaneous diphtheria, herpes simplex, impetigo, pediculosis, scabies, *Staphylococcus*, varicella zoster
      f. Eye infections such as conjunctivitis
   2. Barrier protection
      a. Private room or cohort client
      b. Use of gloves and a gown when in contact with the client

VI. DISASTERS

▲ A. Know the agency's disaster plan

B. Internal disasters are those in which the agency is in danger

C. External disasters occur in the community, and victims will be brought to the health care facility for care

D. When the health care agency is notified of a disaster, the nurse would follow the guidelines specified in the agency's disaster plan

E. See Chapter 8 for additional information about disaster planning

VII. BIOLOGICAL WARFARE AGENTS

A. Anthrax

1. Caused by *Bacillus anthracis;* can be contracted through the digestive system, abrasions in the skin, or inhalation

2. Transmitted by direct contact with the bacteria and its spores; spores are dormant encapsulated bacteria that become active when they enter a living host (no person-to-person spread; Box 14-7)

3. Carried to the lymph nodes and then spread to the rest of the body via the blood and lymph; high levels of toxins lead to shock and death

4. In the lungs, anthrax can cause a buildup of fluid, tissue decay, and death; it is fatal if untreated

5. A blood test is available to detect anthrax; this test magnifies DNA from the blood sample and matches it with anthrax DNA

6. Treated with ciprofloxacin (Cipro), doxycycline, or penicillin

7. Vaccine has limited availability

B. Smallpox

1. Transmitted in air droplets and by handling contaminated materials

2. Highly contagious

3. Symptoms include fever, back pain, vomiting, malaise, and headache

4. Papules develop 2 days after symptoms develop and progress to pustular vesicles, which are initially abundant on the face and extremities

5. A vaccine is available to those at risk for exposure to smallpox

C. Botulism

1. Serious paralytic illness caused by a nerve toxin that is produced by the bacterium *Clostridium botulinum;* an infected client can die within 24 hours

2. Spores are found in the soil and can spread through the air or food (particularly improperly canned food) or via a contaminated wound

3. Cannot be spread from person to person

4. Symptoms include abdominal cramps, diarrhea, nausea, vomiting, double vision, blurred vision, drooping eyelids, difficulty

---

| **BOX 14-7** | **Transmission and Symptoms of Anthrax** |

Skin

Spores enter the skin through cuts and abrasions and are contracted by handling contaminated animal skin products.

The infection starts with an itchy bump like a mosquito bite that progresses to a small, liquid-filled sac.

The sac becomes a painless ulcer with an area of black, dead tissue in the middle.

Toxins destroy the surrounding tissue.

Gastrointestinal System

Infection occurs after the ingestion of contaminated, undercooked meat.

Symptoms begin with nausea, loss of appetite, and vomiting.

The infection progresses to severe abdominal pain, the vomiting of blood, and severe diarrhea.

Inhalation

Infection is caused by the inhalation of bacterial spores, which multiply in the alveoli.

Symptoms begin with the same symptoms as influenza, including fever, muscle aches, and fatigue.

Symptoms suddenly become more severe with the development of breathing problems and shock.

Toxins cause hemorrhage and the destruction of lung tissue.

---

swallowing or speaking, dry mouth, and muscle weakness

5. Can progress to paralysis of the arms, legs, trunk, or respiratory muscles; mechanical ventilation becomes necessary

6. If diagnosed early, foodborne and wound botulism can be treated with an antitoxin that blocks the action of the toxin circulating in the blood

7. Other treatments include the induction of vomiting, enemas, and penicillin

8. No available vaccine

D. Plague

1. Caused by *Yersinia pestis,* which is a bacteria found in rodents and fleas

2. Contracted by being bitten by a rodent or flea carrying the plague bacterium, the ingestion of contaminated meat, or the handling of an animal infected with the bacteria

3. Transmitted by direct person-to-person spread

4. Forms include bubonic (most common), pneumonic, and septicemic (most deadly)

5. Begins with a fever, chest pain, lymph node swelling, and productive cough (hemoptysis)

6. Rapidly progresses to dyspnea, stridor, and cyanosis; death occurs as a result of respiratory failure, shock, and bleeding

7. Antibiotics are only effective if administered immediately; medications of choice include streptomycin and gentamicin (Garamycin)

8. Vaccine is available

E. Tularemia
1. Infectious disease of animals caused by the bacillus *Francisella tularensis;* also called deerfly fever or rabbit fever
2. Transmitted by ticks, deerflies, or contact with an infected animal
3. Symptoms include fever, headache, ulcerated skin lesion with localized lymph node enlargement, eye infection, gastrointestinal ulceration, and pneumonia
4. Treated with antibiotics
5. Recovery produces lifelong immunity
6. Vaccine is available

F. Hemorrhagic fever
1. Caused by several viruses, including Marburg, Lassa, Junin, and Ebola
2. Virus is carried by rodents and mosquitoes
3. Can be transmitted by direct person-to-person spread via body fluids
4. Symptoms include fever, headache, malaise, conjunctivitis, nausea, vomiting, hypotension, hemorrhage of tissues and organs, and organ failure
5. No known specific treatment is available; treatment is symptomatic

VIII. CHEMICAL AND RADIOACTIVE WARFARE AGENTS
A. Sarin
1. A highly toxic nerve gas that can cause death within minutes of exposure
2. Enters the body through the eyes and skin; acts by paralyzing the respiratory muscles
B. Phosgene: Colorless gas normally used in chemical manufacturing; if inhaled at high concentrations for a long enough period, leads to severe respiratory distress, pulmonary edema, and death
C. Mustard gas: Yellow to brown in color and has a garlic-like odor that irritates the eyes and causes skin burns and blisters
D. Ionizing radiation
1. Acute radiation poisoning develops after substantial exposure to radiation
2. Can occur from external radiation or internal absorption
3. Symptoms depend on the amount of exposure to the radiation; range from nausea and vomiting, diarrhea, fever, electrolyte imbalances, and neurological and cardiovascular impairment to leukopenia, purpura, hemorrhage, and death

IX. NURSING RESPONSIBILITIES IN THE EVENT OF EXPOSURE TO BIOLOGICAL OR CHEMICAL AGENTS
A. Be aware that, at first, a bioterrorism attack may resemble a naturally occurring outbreak
B. Nurses and other health care workers must be prepared to determine what happened, the number of clients who may be affected, and how and when clients will be expected to arrive

C. It is essential to recognize any changes to the microorganism that may increase its virulence or make it resistant to conventional antibiotics or vaccines

PRACTICE QUESTIONS

More questions on the companion CD!

112. A mother calls a neighborhood nurse and tells the nurse that her 3-year-old child has just ingested liquid furniture polish. The nurse would direct the mother to immediately:
1. Induce vomiting.
2. Call an ambulance.
3. Call the poison control center.
4. Bring the child to the emergency department.

113. An emergency department nurse receives a telephone call and is informed that a tornado has hit a local residential area and that numerous casualties have occurred. The victims will be brought to the emergency department. Which of the following would be the initial nursing action?
1. Prepare the triage rooms.
2. Activate the agency disaster plan.
3. Obtain additional supplies from the central supply department.
4. Obtain additional nursing staff to assist with treating the casualties.

114. A nurse is caring for a client with a health care–associated infection caused by methicillin-resistant *Staphylococcus aureus* who is on contact precautions. The nurse prepares to provide colostomy care to the client. Which of the following protective items will be required to perform this procedure?
1. Gloves and a gown
2. Gloves and goggles
3. Gloves, a gown, and goggles
4. Gloves, a gown, and shoe protectors

115. A nurse is preparing a client for a magnetic resonance imaging (MRI) exam. What is the most important action to be taken by the nurse?
1. Make sure that informed consent has been obtained.
2. Make sure that the client wears dark glasses during the exam.
3. Have the client take nothing by mouth for at least 8 hours before the test.
4. Make sure that the client ingests contrast material 1 hour before the exam.

116. A nurse enters a client's room and finds that the wastebasket is on fire. The nurse immediately assists the client out of the room. The next nursing action would be to:
1. Call for help.
2. Extinguish the fire.
3. Activate the fire alarm.
4. Confine the fire by closing the room door.

117. A nurse enters the nursing lounge and discovers that a chair is on fire. The nurse activates the alarm, closes the lounge door, and obtains the fire extinguisher to extinguish the fire. The nurse pulls the pin on the fire extinguisher. The next action would be to:
    1. Aim at the base of the fire.
    2. Squeeze the handle on the extinguisher.
    3. Sweep the fire from side to side with the extinguisher.
    4. Sweep the fire from top to bottom with the extinguisher.

118. A nurse obtains an order from the physician to restrain a client using a jacket restraint and instructs the nursing assistant to apply the restraint to the client. Which of the following observations, if made by the nurse, would indicate the inappropriate application of the restraint?
    1. A safety knot in the restraint strap
    2. The restraint straps are safely secured to the side rails.
    3. The jacket restraint strap does not tighten when force is applied against it.
    4. The jacket restraint is secure, and two fingers can easily slide between the restraint and the client's skin.

119. A nurse is caring for a client who has hand restraints. The nurse assesses the skin integrity of the restrained hands:
    1. Every 2 hours
    2. Every 3 hours
    3. Every 4 hours
    4. Every 30 minutes

120. A nurse is assisting with planning care for a client with an internal radiation implant. Which of the following is an inappropriate component for the nurse to include in the plan of care?
    1. Wearing gloves when emptying the client's bedpan
    2. Keeping all linens in the room until the implant is removed
    3. Wearing a lead apron when providing direct care to the client
    4. Placing the client in a semiprivate room at the end of the hallway

ALTERNATE ITEM FORMAT: MULTIPLE RESPONSE

121. A community health nurse is conducting a teaching session about terrorism with members of the community and discussing information regarding anthrax. The nurse tells those attending that anthrax can be transmitted via which route(s)? Select all that apply.
    ☑ 1. Skin
    ☐ 2. Kissing
    ☑ 3. Inhalation
    ☑ 4. Gastrointestinal
    ☐ 5. Direct contact with an infected individual
    ☐ 6. Sexual contact with an infected individual

ANSWERS

112. **3**

Rationale: If a poisoning occurs, the poison control center should be contacted immediately. Vomiting should not be induced if the victim is unconscious or if the substance ingested is a strong corrosive or petroleum product. Bringing the child to the emergency department or calling an ambulance would not be the initial action, because this would delay treatment. The poison control center may advise the mother to bring the child to the emergency department; if this is the case, the mother should call an ambulance.

Test-Taking Strategy: Use the process of elimination. Note the strategic word "immediately" in the question. Eliminate options 2 and 4, because these options will delay treatment. Recalling that vomiting should not be induced if a corrosive substance was ingested will assist you with eliminating option 1. Review poison control measures if you had difficulty with this question.

Level of Cognitive Ability: Application
Client Needs: Physiological Integrity
Integrated Process: Nursing Process/Implementation
Content Area: Child Health
References: Christensen, B., & Kockrow, E. (2006). *Foundations and adult health nursing* (5th ed., p. 367). St. Louis: Mosby.

Price, D., & Gwin, J. (2008). *Pediatric nursing: An introductory text* (10th ed., p. 216). St. Louis: Saunders.

113. **2**

Rationale: During a widespread disaster, many people will be brought to the emergency department for treatment. Although options 1, 3, and 4 may be components of preparing for the casualties, the initial nursing action must be to activate the disaster plan.

Test-Taking Strategy: Note the strategic word "initial," and note that option 2 is the umbrella option. Review the procedures related to the management of a disaster if you had difficulty with this question.

Level of Cognitive Ability: Application
Client Needs: Safe and Effective Care Environment
Integrated Process: Nursing Process/Implementation
Content Area: Fundamental Skills
References: Christensen, B., & Kockrow, E. (2006). *Foundations of nursing* (5th ed., pp. 365-367). St. Louis: Mosby.
Linton, A., & Maebius, N. (2007). *Introduction to medical-surgical nursing* (4th ed., pp. 241-242, 244). Philadelphia: Saunders.

114. 3

Rationale: Goggles are worn to protect the mucous membranes of the eye during interventions that may produce splashes of blood, body fluids, secretions, and excretions. In addition, contact precautions require the use of gloves, and a gown should be worn if direct client contact is anticipated. Shoe protectors are not necessary.

Test-Taking Strategy: Note the strategic words "contact precautions" and "colostomy." Use the process of elimination to determine the items required to care for this client. Review contact precautions if you had difficulty with this question.

Level of Cognitive Ability: Application
Client Needs: Safe and Effective Care Environment
Integrated Process: Nursing Process/Implementation
Content Area: Fundamental Skills
References: Christensen, B., & Kockrow, E. (2006). *Foundations of nursing* (5th ed., p. 295). St. Louis: Mosby.
Linton, A., & Maebius, N. (2007). *Introduction to medical-surgical nursing* (4th ed., pp. 171-172). Philadelphia: Saunders.

115. 1

Rationale: Informed consent must be obtained before an MRI can be performed. The client may not need to fast. Contrast material and dark glasses are not required for this test.

Test-Taking Strategy: Note the strategic words "most important." Use the process of elimination to determine what is necessary for this test, and remember that informed consent is required. Review the preparation for MRI if you had difficulty with this question.

Level of Cognitive Ability: Application
Client Needs: Safe and Effective Care Environment
Integrated Process: Nursing Process/Implementation
Content Area: Fundamental Skills
Reference: Ignatavicius, D., and Workman, M. (2006). *Medical-surgical nursing: Critical thinking for collaborative care* (5th ed., p. 941). St. Louis: Saunders.
Pagana, K., & Pagana, T. (2005). *Mosby's diagnostic and laboratory test reference* (7th ed., pp. 632-636). St. Louis: Mosby.

116. 3

Rationale: The order of priority in the event of a fire is to rescue the clients who are in immediate danger. The next step is to activate the fire alarm. The fire is then confined by closing all doors. Finally, the fire is extinguished.

Test-Taking Strategy: Note the strategic word "next." Remember the mnemonic *RACE* to help you to prioritize in the event of a fire: *R* = Rescue clients who are in immediate danger; *A* = Alarm, sound the alarm; *C* = Confine the fire by closing all doors; *E* = Extinguish or evacuate. Review fire safety procedures if you had difficulty with this question.

Level of Cognitive Ability: Application
Client Needs: Safe and Effective Care Environment
Integrated Process: Nursing Process/Implementation
Content Area: Delegating/Prioritizing
Reference: Christensen, B., & Kockrow, E. (2006). *Foundations of nursing* (5th ed., pp. 364-365). St. Louis: Mosby.

117. 1

Rationale: A fire can be extinguished by using a fire extinguisher. To use the extinguisher, the pin is pulled first.

The extinguisher should then be aimed at the base of the fire. The handle of the extinguisher is squeezed, and the fire is extinguished by sweeping from side to side to coat the area evenly.

Test-Taking Strategy: Note the strategic word "next." Remember the mnemonic *PASS* to prioritize in the use of a fire extinguisher: *P* = Pull the pin; *A* = Aim at the base of the fire; *S* = Squeeze the handle; *S* = Sweep from side to side to coat the area evenly. Review the procedures related to the use of a fire extinguisher if you had difficulty with this question.

Level of Cognitive Ability: Application
Client Needs: Safe and Effective Care Environment
Integrated Process: Nursing Process/Implementation
Content Area: Fundamental Skills
Reference: Christensen, B., & Kockrow, E. (2006). *Foundations of nursing* (5th ed., p. 365). St. Louis: Mosby.

118. 2

Rationale: A half-bow or safety knot should be used when applying a restraint, because it does not tighten when force is applied against it, and it allows for the quick and easy removal of the restraint in case of an emergency. The restraint strap is secured to the bed frame (never to the side rail) to avoid accidental injury in case the side rail is released. The jacket restraint should be secure, and one to two fingers should easily slide between the restraint and the client's skin.

Test-Taking Strategy: Note the strategic word "inappropriate." This indicates that you are looking for an option that identifies an inaccurate measure related to the application of restraints. The words "secured to the side rails" in option 2 should direct you to this option as an inappropriate action. Review the guidelines related to the application of restraints if you had difficulty with this question.

Level of Cognitive Ability: Comprehension
Client Needs: Safe and Effective Care Environment
Integrated Process: Teaching and Learning
Content Area: Fundamental Skills
References: Linton, A., & Maebius, N. (2007). *Introduction to medical-surgical nursing* (4th ed., pp. 304-305). Philadelphia: Saunders.
Potter, P., & Perry, A. (2005). *Fundamentals of nursing* (6th ed., p. 985). St. Louis: Mosby.

119. 4

Rationale: The nurse needs to assess restraints and skin integrity every 30 minutes. Agency guidelines regarding the use of restraints should always be followed.

Test-Taking Strategy: Use the process of elimination. In this situation, it is best to select the option that identifies the most frequent time frame. Review the guidelines related to the use of restraints if you had difficulty with this question.

Level of Cognitive Ability: Application
Client Needs: Safe and Effective Care Environment
Integrated Process: Nursing Process/Implementation
Content Area: Fundamental Skills
References: Linton, A., & Maebius, N. (2007). *Introduction to medical-surgical nursing* (4th ed., p. 304). Philadelphia: Saunders.
Potter, P., & Perry, A. (2005). *Fundamentals of nursing* (6th ed., p. 987). St. Louis: Mosby.

120. 4

Rationale: A private room with a private bath is essential if a client has an internal radiation implant. This is necessary to prevent the accidental exposure of other clients to radiation. Options 1, 2, and 3 are accurate interventions for a client with a radiation implant.

Test-Taking Strategy: Use the process of elimination, and note the strategic word "inappropriate." This word indicates a negative event query and asks you to select an option that is an incorrect action. Option 1 can be eliminated first, because this is a component of standard precautions for all clients. Options 2 and 3 can be eliminated next, because they directly relate to radiation safety. Review radiation safety principles if you had difficulty with this question.

Level of Cognitive Ability: Application
Client Needs: Safe and Effective Care Environment
Integrated Process: Nursing Process/Planning
Content Area: Fundamental Skills
Reference: Linton, A., & Maebius, N. (2007). *Introduction to medical-surgical nursing* (4th ed., p. 392). Philadelphia: Saunders.

ALTERNATE ITEM FORMAT: MULTIPLE RESPONSE

121. **1, 3, 4**

Rationale: Anthrax is caused by *Bacillus anthracis*, and it can be contracted through the digestive system, abrasions in the skin, or inhalation. It cannot be spread from person to person.

Test-Taking Strategy: Knowledge regarding the methods of contracting anthrax is needed to answer this question. Remember that it is not spread by person-to-person contact. Review information related to anthrax infection if you had difficulty with this question.

Level of Cognitive Ability: Application
Client Needs: Safe and Effective Care Environment
Integrated Process: Teaching and Learning
Content Area: Fundamental Skills
Reference: Christensen, B., & Kockrow, E. (2006). *Foundations of nursing* (5th ed., pp. 274, 369). St. Louis: Mosby.

REFERENCES

Christensen, B., & Kockrow, E. (2006). *Foundations of nursing* (5th, ed.). St. Louis: Mosby.

Ignatavicius, D., & Workman, M. (2006). *Medical-surgical nursing: Critical thinking for collaborative care* (5th, ed.). St. Louis: Saunders.

Linton, A., & Maebius, N. (2007). *Introduction to medical-surgical nursing,* (4th, ed.). Philadelphia: Saunders.

National Council of State Boards of Nursing (Eds.). (2008). 2008 Detailed Test Plan for the NCLEX-PN Examination, National Council of State Boards of Nursing. Chicago: Author .

National Council of State Boards of Nursing. NCSBN home page. www.WCSBN.org. Accassed June 19, 2008.

Pagana, K., & Pagana, T. (2005). *Mosby's diagnostic and laboratory test reference* (7th, ed.). St. Louis: Mosby.

Price, D., & Gwin, J. (2008). *Pediatric nursing: An introductory text* (10th ed.). St. Louis: Saunders.

Perry, A., & Potter, P. (2006). *Clinical nursing skills & techniques* (6th ed.). St. Louis: Mosby.

The Joint Commission. http://www.jointcommission.org/PatientSafety/NationalPatientSafetyGoals/09_hap_Npsgs.htm. Accessed October 20, 2008.

CHAPTER 15

Medication and Intravenous Administration

PYRAMID TERMS

conversion The first step in the calculation of a medication problem.

generic name The common or chemical name of a medication; printed on the label in small letters, usually under the trade name.

milliequivalent(s) Abbreviated as *mEq*; one thousandth of a chemical equivalent; the concentration of electrolytes in a certain volume of solution.

parenteral Given by injection; may be intravenous, intramuscular, or subcutaneous.

reconstitution Dissolving a powder in a sterile diluent before use; usually sterile water or normal saline is used.

trade name Also called the *brand name*; usually printed on the label in large, bold letters.

unit A measurement of a medication in terms of its action rather than its physical weight.

▲ PYRAMID TO SUCCESS

When a medication or intravenous (IV) calculation question is presented, a nurse should always use the appropriate formula to solve the problem. Shortcuts should not be used when making these calculations. The problem and the answer should be expressed in the correct units of measure. Be careful with decimal points. It is important to place the decimal points in the correct places, or the answer will be incorrect. When solving a medication calculation problem, the nurse determines whether the answer is within reason and makes sense. In the clinical setting, the nurse should always seek assistance if he or she is unsure about the accuracy of a calculation.

On the NCLEX-PN, the fill-in-the-blank questions may require that you calculate a medication dose or an IV flow rate. You will be provided with an optional on-screen calculator for these medication and IV problems. Even if you use the calculator to calculate dosages and flow rates, it is important to check the calculation before selecting an option or typing in the answer. Follow the formula, place the decimal points in the

correct places, and check the accuracy of the calculation. Remember, practice makes perfect!

The Integrated Processes addressed in this chapter are Caring, the Clinical Problem-Solving Process (Nursing Process), Communication and Documentation, and Teaching and Learning.

CLIENT NEEDS

Safe and Effective Care Environment

Calculating medication doses and IV flow rates
Maintaining clients' rights
Handling hazardous or infectious materials
Maintaining medical and surgical asepsis
Maintaining standard and other precautions
Preventing errors

Health Promotion and Maintenance

Collecting physical data
Preventing disease
Respecting lifestyle choices
Teaching the client about prescribed medication(s) or
    IV therapy

Psychosocial Integrity

Identifying support systems
Identifying the cultural, religious, and spiritual influ-
    ences on health
Interacting therapeutically with the client and family
Identifying the use of coping mechanisms

Physiological Integrity

Administering medications and IV therapy
Identifying the adverse effects of and contraindications
    to medication or IV therapy
Monitoring for the expected and unexpected effects of
    pharmacological therapy
Monitoring laboratory values

I. MEDICATION ADMINISTRATION (Box 15-1)
II. DRUG-MEASUREMENT SYSTEMS
A. Metric system (Box 15-2)
  1. The basic **units** of metric measurement are meter, liter, and gram
  2. Meter measures length
  3. Liter measures volume
  4. Gram measures weight
B. Apothecary and household systems (Box 15-3)
  1. Apothecary measures such as dram and minim are not commonly used in the clinical setting.
  2. In the apothecary system, equivalents include: 1 grain (gr) = 60 mg; 5 gr = 325 mg; 15 gr = 1000 mg
C. Additional common drug measures
  1. **Milliequivalent** (mEq)
    a. One thousandth of a chemical equivalent; the concentration of electrolytes in a certain volume of solution
    b. For example: 5 mEq of potassium
  2. **Unit**
    a. Measures a medication in terms of its action rather than its physical weight
    b. For example: Penicillin, heparin sodium, and insulin are measured in **units**
III. CONVERSIONS
A. **Conversion** between metric **units** (Box 15-4)
  1. The metric system is a decimal system; therefore, **conversions** between the **units** in this system can be done by either dividing or multiplying by 1000 or by moving the decimal point three places to the right or three places to the left
  2. In the metric system, to convert larger to smaller, multiply by 1000 or move the decimal point three places to the right; for example, 1g = 1000 mg
  3. In the metric system, to convert smaller to larger, divide by 1000 or move the decimal point three places to the left; for example, 1000 mg = 1 g
B. **Conversion** between household and metric systems
  1. **Conversions** between the metric and household systems are equivalent—not equal—measures
  2. **Conversion** to equivalent measures between systems is necessary when a medication order is written in one system but the medication label is given in another
  3. Medications are not always ordered and prepared in the same system of measurement; it

---

BOX 15-1   Medication Administration

Check the medication order.
Ask the client about a history of allergies.
Determine the client's current condition and the purpose of the prescribed medication or intravenous solution.
Determine the client's understanding regarding the purpose of the prescribed medication or intravenous solution.
Plan to teach the client about the medication and about self-administration at home.
Identify and address social, cultural, and religious concerns that the client may have about taking the medication.
Determine the need for conversion when preparing a dose of medication for administration to the client.
Check the six rights: right medication, right dose, right client, right route, right time and frequency, and right documentation.
Check the client's vital signs before administering the medication.
Document the administration of the prescribed therapy and client's response to the therapy.

BOX 15-2   Metric System

Abbreviations/Symbols	Equivalents
meter: m	1 mg = 1000 mcg or 0.001 g
liter: L	1 g = 1000 mg
gram: g, gm, Gm	1 mL = 0.001 L
milligram: mg	1 kg = 1000 g
microgram: mcg	1 mcg = 0.000001 g
kilogram: kg, Kg	
milliliter: mL	1 kg = 2.2 lb

BOX 15-3   Household Systems

Household (volume)
  1 gallon = 4 quarts
  1 quart = 2 pints or 1 liter or 32 fl oz
  1 pint = 500 mL or 16 fl oz
  1 cup = 240 mL 8 fl oz
  2 tablespoons = 30 mL or 1 fl oz
  1 tablespoon = 15 mL or 3 teaspoons
  1 teaspoon = 4 to 5 mL or 60 gtt
  60 microdrops = 1 mL
Household (weight)
  2.2 pounds = 1 kilogram
  1 pound = 0.45 kilograms or 16 oz
Household (length)
  1 inch = 2.5 centimeters

BOX 15-4   Conversion Between Metric Units

PROBLEM 1:
  Convert 2 grams (g) to milligrams (mg).
Solution:
  Change a larger unit to a smaller unit.
  2.000 g = 2000 mg (move the decimal three places to the right)
PROBLEM 2:
  Convert 250 milliliters (mL) to liters (L).
Solution:
  Change a smaller unit to a larger unit.
  250 mL = 0.25 L (move the decimal three places to the left)

is therefore necessary to convert **units** from one system to another

4. **Conversion** is the first step in the calculation of dosages

5. Calculating equivalents between two systems may be done by using the method of ratio and proportion (Box 15-5)

IV. CELSIUS AND FAHRENHEIT TEMPERATURES (Box 15-6)

A. To convert Fahrenheit to Celsius, first subtract 32, and then divide the result by 1.8

B. To convert Celsius to Fahrenheit, first multiply by 1.8, and then add 32

V. MEDICATION LABELS

A. A medication label will contain both the **generic name** and the **trade name** of the medication

B. Each medication has only one official name, but it may have several **trade names,** each for the exclusive use of a company that manufactures the medication

C. Always check the expiration dates on medication labels

VI. MEDICATION ORDERS (Box 15-7)

A. In a medication order, the name of the medication is written first, followed by the dosage, route, and frequency

B. If there are any questions about or inconsistencies in the written order, the person who wrote the order must be contacted immediately, and the order must be verified

VII. ORAL MEDICATIONS

A. Scored tablets contain an indented mark to be used for breaking the tablet into partial dosages; when necessary, scored tablets (those marked for division) can be divided into halves or quarters

B. Enteric-coated tablets and sustained-released capsules delay absorption until the medication reaches the small intestine; these medications should not be crushed

C. Capsules contain a powdered or oily medication in a gelatin cover

D. Oral liquids are supplied in solution form and contain a specific amount of medication in a given amount of solution, as stated on the label

E. The medicine cup (Figure 15-1)
1. Has a capacity of 30 mL or 1 ounce
2. Used for oral liquids
3. Calibrated to measure teaspoons, tablespoons, and drams
4. To pour accurately, hold the medication cup at eye level, and then line up the measure that is needed and pour

F. Volumes of less than 5 mL are measured by using a syringe with the needle removed

G. A calibrated dropper is used for giving medicine to children or to adults in hospice care and for adding small amounts of liquid to water or juice; calibrations are in milliliters, cubic centimeters, or drops

---

BOX 15-5 **Calculating Equivalents Between Two Systems by Ratio and Proportion**

Formula:
H (on hand) : V (vehicle) :: (=) (desired dose) : (unknown)
To solve a ratio and proportion problem, the middle numbers (means) are multiplied and the end numbers (extremes) are multiplied.
Problem:
The physician orders nitroglycerin, grain (gr) 1/150. The medication label reads 0.4 milligram (mg) per tablet. The nurse prepares to administer how many tablets to the client?
Solution:
gr 1:60 mg = gr 1/150:X mg
60/150 × 1 = 60/150 = 0.4
X = 0.4 mg (1 tablet)

BOX 15-6 **Celsius and Fahrenheit Temperature**

Converting Fahrenheit to Celsius
To convert Fahrenheit to Celsius, subtract 32, and divide the result by 1.8.
Formula: Celsius = (Fahrenheit − 32) divided by 1.8
Converting Celsius to Fahrenheit
To convert Celsius to Fahrenheit, multiply by 1.8, and add 32.
Formula: Fahrenheit = (1.8 × Celsius) + 32

BOX 15-7 **Medication Orders**

Name of client
Date and time when order is written
Name of medication to be given
Dosage of medication
Medication route
Time and frequency of administration
Signature of person who wrote the order

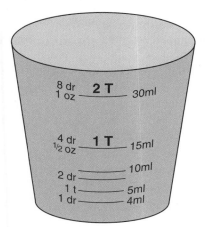

FIG. 15-1 Medicine cup. (From Kee, J., & Marshall, S. [2009]. *Clinical calculations: With applications to general and specialty areas* [6th ed.]. Philadelphia: Saunders.)

VIII. PARENTERAL MEDICATIONS

A. *Parenteral* always means injection route, and **parenteral** medications are administered by IV, intramuscular, or subcutaneous routes

B. **Parenteral** medications are packaged in single-use ampules, in single- and multiple-use rubber-stoppered vials, and in premeasured syringes and cartridges

C. The nurse should not administer more than 3 mL per intramuscular injection site or 1 mL per subcutaneous injection site; larger volumes are difficult for an injection site to absorb and, if prescribed, need to be verified

D. Always question and verify excessively large or small volumes of medication

E. The standard 3-mL syringe is used to measure most injectable medications; it is calibrated in tenths (0.1) of a milliliter (Figure 15-2)

F. The calibrations on a syringe are read from the top black ring on the syringe (i.e., not the middle section and not the bottom ring)

G. Prefilled medication cartridge (Figure 15-3)
  1. The medication cartridge slips into the cartridge holder, which provides a plunger for the injection of the medication
  2. Designed to provide sufficient capacity to allow for the addition of a second medication when combined dosages are prescribed
  3. The prefilled medication cartridge is to be used once and discarded; if a nurse is to give less than the full single dose provided, he or she needs to discard the extra amount before giving the client the injection, in accordance with agency policies and procedures

H. Standard medication doses for adults are to be rounded to the nearest tenth (0.1) of a milliliter and measured on the milliliter scale; for example, 1.25 mL is rounded to 1.3 mL

I. When volumes of more than 3 mL are required, a 5-, 6-, 10-, or 12-mL syringe may be used; these syringes are calibrated in fifths (Figure 15-4)

J. Syringes larger than 12 mL are calibrated in full milliliter measures

K. Tuberculin syringe (Figure 15-5)
  1. Holds a total capacity of 1 mL; used to measure small or critical amounts of medication, such as allergen extract, vaccine, or a child's medication

2. It is calibrated in hundredths (0.01) of a milliliter, with each one tenth (0.1) marked on the metric scale

L. Insulin syringe (Figure 15-6)
  1. The standard **unit**-100 insulin syringe is used to measure **unit**-100 insulin only; it is calibrated for a total of 100 **units** or 1 mL
  2. Insulin should not be measured in any other type of syringe
  3. When the insulin order states to combine regular and neutral protamine Hagedorn (NPH) insulin, remember to draw regular insulin first and then to draw the NPH insulin

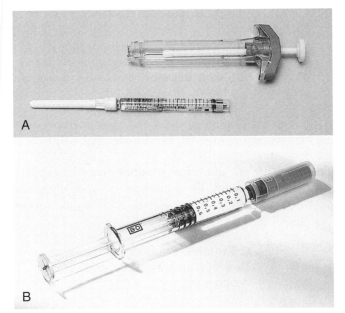

FIG. 15-3 **A,** Tubex syringe with cartridge. **B,** BD Hypak prefilled syringe. (From Kee, J., & Marshall, S. [2000]. *Clinical calculations: With applications to general and specialty areas* [4th ed.]. Philadelphia: Saunders. **A,** Courtesy of Wyeth-Ayerst Laboratories, Philadelphia, PA. **B,** Courtesy of Becton, Dickinson, and Company, Franklin Lakes, NJ.)

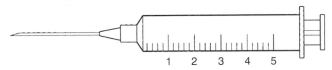

FIG. 15-4 Five-mL syringe. (From Kee, J., & Marshall, S. [2009]. *Clinical calculations: With applications to general and specialty areas* [6th ed.]. Philadelphia: Saunders.)

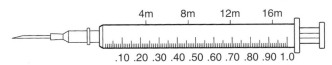

FIG. 15-5 Tuberculin syringe. (From Kee, J., & Marshall, S. [2009]. *Clinical calculations: With applications to general and specialty areas* [6th ed.]. Philadelphia: Saunders.)

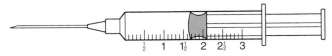

FIG. 15-2 Three-mL syringe. (From Kee, J., & Marshall, S. [2009]. *Clinical calculations: With applications to general and specialty areas* [6th ed.]. Philadelphia: Saunders.)

M. Safety needles: Contain shielding devices to reduce the incidence of needle-stick injuries (Figure 15-7)

IX. INJECTABLE MEDICATIONS IN POWDER FORM

A. Some medications become unstable when stored in solution form and are therefore packaged in powder form

B. Powders must be dissolved with a sterile diluent before use; usually sterile water or normal saline is used; the dissolving procedure is called *reconstitution* (Box 15-8)

X. CALCULATING THE CORRECT DOSAGE (Box 15-9)

A. When calculating dosages of oral medications, check the calculation, and question the order if the calculation calls for more than three tablets

B. When calculating dosages of **parenteral** medications, check the calculation, and question the order if the amount to be given is too large a dose

C. Regardless of the source of the error, if a nurse gives an incorrect dose, he or she is legally responsible for the action

D. Be sure that all measures are in the same system and that all **units** are in the same size, converting them

10 20 30 40 50 60 70 80 90 100
UNITS
5 15 25 35 45 55 65 75 85 95

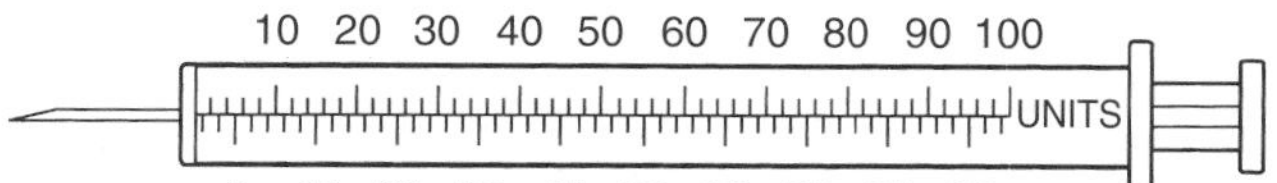

FIG. 15-6   Insulin syringe. (From Kee, J., & Marshall, S. [2009]. *Clinical calculations: With applications to general and specialty areas* [6th ed.]. Philadelphia: Saunders.)

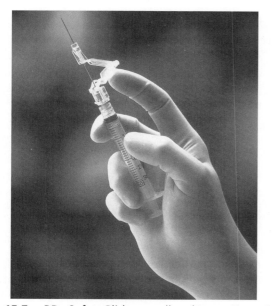

FIG. 15-7   BD SafetyGlide needle. (From Kee, J., & Marshall, S. [2009]. *Clinical calculations: With applications to general and specialty areas* [6th ed.]. Philadelphia: Saunders. Courtesy of Becton, Dickinson, and Company, Franklin Lakes, NJ.)

when necessary; carefully consider the reasonable amount of the medication that should be administered

E. Round standard injection doses to tenths, and measure in a 3-mL syringe

F. Round small, critical, or children's doses to hundredths, and measure in a 1-mL tuberculin syringe

XI. INTRAVENOUS FLOW RATES (Box 15-10)

A. Monitor IVs at least every hour for adults and every 15 minutes for children

B. If an IV is running behind schedule, collaborate with the physician to determine the client's ability to tolerate an increased flow rate, particularly if the client has cardiac, pulmonary, renal, or neurological conditions

C. The nurse should never increase the rate of an IV if the IV is running behind schedule

D. Whenever a prescribed IV rate is increased, the nurse should assess the client for increased heart rate, increased respirations, or increased lung congestion, which could indicate fluid overload

E. IV fluids are most frequently ordered on the basis of milliliters (mL) per hour to be administered

F. The volume per hour ordered is administered by adjusting the rate at which the IV infuses, which is counted in drops (gtt) per minute

G. Most flow-rate calculations involve changing mL/hour into gtt/minute

---

BOX 15-8   Reconstitution

When reconstituting a medication, locate the instructions on the label or in the vial package insert, and read and follow the directions carefully.

The instructions will state the volume of diluent to be used and the resulting volume of the reconstituted medication.

Often a powdered medication adds volume to the solution in addition to the amount of diluent added.

When reconstituting a multiple-dose vial, label the medication vial with the date and time of preparation, your initials, and the date of expiration.

It is also important to label the strength per volume.

The total volume of the prepared solution will always exceed the volume of the diluent added.

BOX 15-9   Formula for Calculating a Medication Dosage

$$\frac{\text{Desired}}{\text{Available}} \times \text{Quantity} = X$$

Desired = The dosage that the physician ordered

Available = The dosage strength as stated on the medication label

Quantity = The volume or form in which the dosage strength is available, such as tablets, capsules, or milliliters

---

| BOX 15-10 | Formulas for Intravenous Calculations |

Flow Rates

$$\frac{\text{Total volume} \times \text{drop (gtt) factor}}{\text{Time in minutes}} = \text{gtt/minute}$$

Infusion Time

$$\frac{\text{Total volume to infuse}}{\text{mL/hour being infused}} = \text{infusion time}$$

Number of mL/hour

$$\frac{\text{Total volume in mL}}{\text{Number of hours}} = \text{number of mL/hour}$$

H. IV tubing
   1. Calibrated in gtt/mL; this calibration is needed for calculating flow rates
   2. A standard or macrodrip set is used for routine adult IV administrations; depending on the manufacturer and type of tubing, it requires 10, 15, or 20 gtt to equal 1 mL
   3. A minidrip or microdrip set is used when more exact measurements are needed, such as in intensive care and pediatric units
   4. In a minidrip or microdrip set, 60 gtt is equal to 1 mL
   5. The calibration, in gtt/mL, is written on the IV tubing package

XII. **ELECTRONIC INTRAVENOUS FLOW-RATE REGULATORS**
A. Controller
   1. Works on the same principle of gravity as a regular IV drip, with the rate of flow being maintained by the rapid compression and decompression of the IV tubing by the machine
   2. The desired flow rate is set on the controller in mL/hour
   3. Because controllers work by gravity, the height of the solution bag is critical; it must be maintained at a minimum of 36 inches above the controller
   4. The nurse should continue to assess the amount of IV solution in the IV container and to monitor the controller to ensure the proper functioning of the machine
B. Pump (Figure 15-8)
   1. A pump is different from a controller in that it physically pumps fluids against resistance
   2. Gravity is not a factor in the use of a pump, and the height of the IV solution container is not a critical factor
   3. The flow rate on a pump is set in mL/hour
   4. The nurse should continue to assess the amount of IV solution in the IV container and to monitor the pump to ensure the proper functioning of the machine

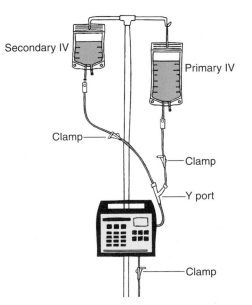

FIG. 15-8 Infusion pump. (From Kee, J., & Marshall, S. [2009]. *Clinical calculations: With applications to general and specialty areas* [6th ed.]. Philadelphia: Saunders.)

PRACTICE QUESTIONS

More questions on the companion CD!

The practice questions below are presented in either multiple-choice or alternate item (fill-in-the-blank) format.

122. A physician's order reads hydromorphone hydrochloride (Dilaudid), 3 mg intramuscular every 4 hours as needed. The medication label reads hydromorphone hydrochloride (Dilaudid), 4 mg/1 mL. The nurse prepares to administer how many mL to the client? (Round answer to nearest tenth position.)

Answer: 0.75 mL / 0.8

123. A physician's order reads digoxin (Lanoxin), 0.25 mg orally daily. The medication label reads digoxin (Lanoxin), 0.125 mg/tablet. The nurse prepares how many tablet(s) to administer the dose?

Answer: 2 tablet(s)

124. A physician orders heparin sodium (Liquaemin), 650 units subcutaneously every 12 hours. The medication vial reads heparin sodium (Liquaemin), 1000 units/mL. The nurse prepares how many milliliters to administer one dose? (Round to the nearest tenth position.)

Answer: 0.65 mL / 0.7

125. A physician orders trimethobenzamide hydrochloride (Tigan), 250 mg intramuscularly as needed. The medication label reads trimethobenzamide hydrochloride (Tigan), 200 mg/2 mL. The nurse plans to prepare how much medication to administer the dose?

Answer: 2.5 mL

126. A physician orders meperidine hydrochloride (Demerol), 35 mg intramuscularly, immediately. The medication label states meperidine hydrochloride (Demerol), 50 mg/mL. The nurse plans to prepare how much medication to administer the dose?

Answer: _0.7_ mL

127. A physician orders prochlorperazine (Compazine), 20 mg intramuscular every 4 hours as needed. The medication label states prochlorperazine (Compazine), 10 mg/mL. The nurse prepares how much medication to administer the dose?

Answer: _2_ mL

128. A physician orders atropine sulfate, 0.4 mg intramuscularly, immediately. The medication label states atropine sulfate, 0.3 mg/0.5 mL. The nurse prepares how much medication to administer the dose? (Round to the nearest tenth position.)

Answer: _0.7_ mL

129. A physician orders levodopa (Dopar), 1 g orally, twice daily. The medication label states levodopa (Dopar), 500-mg tablets. The nurse prepares to administer how many tablets at the evening dose?

Answer: _2_ tablet(s)

130. A physician orders zidovudine (AZT), 0.2 g orally every 4 hours. The medication label states zidovudine (AZT), 100-mg tablets. The nurse prepares to administer how many tablets for one dose?

Answer: _2_ tablet(s)

131. A physician orders atropine sulfate, 0.4 mg. The medication label states atropine sulfate, 0.5 mg/0.5 mL. How many milliliters will the nurse prepare to administer to the client?

Answer: _0.4_ mL

132. A physician's order states to administer Tylenol (acetaminophen) 650 mg orally for a temperature of more than 38° C. The medication bottle states Tylenol (acetaminophen), 325 mg. The nurse takes the client's temperature and notes that it is 101° F. The nurse plans to take which of the following actions?
   1. Administer two Tylenol tablets.
   2. Administer three Tylenol tablets.
   3. Do not administer the Tylenol at this time.
   4. Check the client's temperature in 30 minutes.

133. A physician's order reads aminophylline (theophylline), 250 mg in 500 mL normal saline, infuse at 50 mL/hr. How many milligrams of aminophylline will the client receive every hour?
   1. 50 mg
   2. 25 mg
   3. 2.5 mg
   4. 5.0 mg

134. A physician orders 1000 mL of 0.9% normal saline to run over 12 hours. The drop factor is 15 gtt/1 mL. The nurse plans to adjust the flow rate to how many gtt/minute? (Round answer to the nearest whole number)

Answer: _21_ gtt/minute

135. A physician orders an intramuscular dose of 400,000 units of penicillin G benzathine (Bicillin). The label on the 10-mL ampule sent from the pharmacy reads penicillin G benzathine (Bicillin) 300,000 units/mL. The nurse prepares how much medication to administer the correct dose? (Round answer to the nearest tenth position.)

Answer: _1.3_ mL

136. A physician orders 3000 mL of 5% dextrose to run over a 24-hour period. The drop factor is 10 gtt/1 mL. The nurse plans to adjust the flow rate to how many gtt/minute? (Round answer to the nearest whole number.)

Answer: _21_ gtt/minute

137. A physician's order reads phenytoin (Dilantin) 0.2 g orally, twice daily. The medication label states 100-mg capsules. How many capsule(s) will the nurse prepare to administer one dose?

Answer: _2_ capsule(s)

138. A physician orders 1000 mL of 0.5% normal saline to run over 8 hours. The drop factor is 15 gtt/1 mL. The nurse plans to adjust the flow rate to how many gtt/minute? (Round to the nearest whole number)

Answer: _31_ gtt/minute

139. A physician's order reads levothyroxine (Synthroid), 150 mcg orally daily. The medication label reads levothyroxine, 0.1 mg/tablet. The nurse prepares to administer how many tablet(s) to the client?

Answer: _1.5_ tablet(s)

140. A physician orders 1000 mL of 5% dextrose to run at 125 mL/hour. The nurse calculates the infusion rate knowing that it will take how many hours for 1 L to infuse?

Answer: _8_ hours

141. A physician orders one unit of packed red blood cells to infuse over 4 hours. One unit of blood contains 250 mL, and the drop factor is 10 gtt/1 mL. The registered nurse asks the licensed practical nurse (LPN) to assist with monitoring the flow rate during the infusion. The LPN monitors the flow rate knowing that how many gtt/minute should infuse? (Round answer to the nearest whole number)

Answer: _10_ gtt/minute

ANSWERS

122. **0.8**

Rationale: Follow the formula for dosage calculation.

Formula:

$$\frac{Desired}{Available} \times mL = mL/dose$$

$$\frac{3 \text{ mg}}{4 \text{ mg}} \times 1 \text{ mL} = 0.75 \text{ or } 0.8 \text{ mL}$$

Test-Taking Strategy: Follow the formula for the calculation of the correct dose. Focus on the strategic information: 4 mg/1 mL. After you have performed the calculation, verify your answer using a calculator and round to the nearest tenth. Review medication calculations if you had difficulty with this question.
Level of Cognitive Ability: Application
Client Needs: Physiological Integrity
Integrated Process: Nursing Process/Planning
Content Area: Fundamental Skills
Reference: Kee, J., & Marshall, S. (2009). *Clinical calculations: With applications to general and specialty areas* (6th ed., p. 86). Philadelphia: Saunders.

123. **2**

Rationale: Follow the formula for dosage calculation.

Formula:

$$\frac{Desired}{Available} \times tablet = number \text{ of tablets per dose}$$

$$\frac{0.25 \text{ mg}}{0.125 \text{ mg}} \times 1 \text{ tablet} = 2 \text{ tablets}$$

Test-Taking Strategy: Follow the formula for the calculation of the correct dose. Focus on the strategic information: 0.125 mg/tablet. After you have performed the calculation, verify your answer using a calculator. Review medication calculations if you had difficulty with this question.
Level of Cognitive Ability: Application
Client Needs: Physiological Integrity
Integrated Process: Nursing Process/Planning
Content Area: Fundamental Skills
Reference: Kee, J., & Marshall, S. (2009). *Clinical calculations: With applications to general and specialty areas* (6th ed., p. 86). Philadelphia: Saunders.

124. **0.7**

Rationale: Follow the formula for dosage calculation.

Formula:

$$\frac{Desired}{Available} \times mL = mL/dose$$

$$\frac{650 \text{ units}}{1000 \text{ units}} \times 1 \text{ mL} = 0.65 \text{ or } 0.7 \text{ mL}$$

Test-Taking Strategy: Follow the formula for the calculation of the correct dose. Focus on the strategic information: 1000 units/mL. After you have performed the calculation, verify your answer using a calculator, and remember to round to the nearest tenth. Review medication calculations if you had difficulty with this question.
Level of Cognitive Ability: Application
Client Needs: Physiological Integrity
Integrated Process: Nursing Process/Planning

Content Area: Fundamental Skills
Reference: Kee, J., & Marshall, S. (2009). *Clinical calculations: With applications to general and specialty areas* (6th ed., p. 86). Philadelphia: Saunders.

125. **2.5**

Rationale: Follow the formula for dosage calculation.

Formula:

$$\frac{Desired}{Available} \times mL = mL/dose$$

$$\frac{250 \text{ mg}}{200 \text{ mg}} \times 2 \text{ mL} = 2.5 \text{ mL}$$

Test-Taking Strategy: Follow the formula for the calculation of the correct dose. Focus on the strategic information: 200 mg/2 mL. After you have performed the calculation, verify your answer using a calculator. Review medication calculations if you had difficulty with this question.
Level of Cognitive Ability: Application
Client Needs: Physiological Integrity
Integrated Process: Nursing Process/Planning
Content Area: Fundamental Skills
Reference: Kee, J., & Marshall, S. (2009). *Clinical calculations: With applications to general and specialty areas* (6th ed., p. 86). Philadelphia: Saunders.

126. **0.7**

Rationale: Follow the formula for dosage calculations.

Formula:

$$\frac{Desired}{Available} \times mL = mL/dose$$

$$\frac{35 \text{ mg}}{50 \text{ mg}} \times 1 \text{ mL} = 0.7 \text{ mL}$$

Test-Taking Strategy: Follow the formula for the calculation of the correct dose. Focus on the strategic information: 50 mg/mL. After you have performed the calculation, verify your answer using a calculator. Review medication calculations if you had difficulty with this question.
Level of Cognitive Ability: Application
Client Needs: Physiological Integrity
Integrated Process: Nursing Process/Planning
Content Area: Fundamental Skills
Reference: Kee, J., & Marshall, S. (2009). *Clinical calculations: With applications to general and specialty areas* (6th ed., p. 86). Philadelphia: Saunders.

127. **2**

Rationale: Follow the formula for dosage calculation.

Formula:

$$\frac{Desired}{Available} \times mL = mL/dose$$

$$\frac{20 \text{ mg}}{10 \text{ mg}} \times 1 \text{ mL} = 2 \text{ mL}$$

Test-Taking Strategy: Follow the formula for the calculation of the correct dose. Focus on the strateric information: 10 mg/mL. After you have performed the calculation, verify your answer using a calculator. Review medication calculations if you had difficulty with this question.

Level of Cognitive Ability: Application
Client Needs: Physiological Integrity
Integrated Process: Nursing Process/Planning
Content Area: Fundamental Skills
Reference: Kee, J., & Marshall, S. (2009). *Clinical calculations: With applications to general and specialty areas* (6th ed., p. 86). Philadelphia: Saunders.

128. **0.7**
Rationale: Follow the formula for dosage calculation.
Formula:

$$\frac{Desired}{Available} \times mL = mL/dose$$

$$\frac{0.4\ mg}{0.3\ mg} \times 0.5\ mL = 0.66\ or\ 0.7\ mL$$

Test-Taking Strategy: Follow the formula for the calculation of the correct dose. Focus on the strategic information: 0.3 mg/ 0.5 mL. After you have performed the calculation, verify your answer using a calculator, and remember to round to the nearest tenth. Review medication calculations if you had difficulty with this question.
Level of Cognitive Ability: Application
Client Needs: Physiological Integrity
Integrated Process: Nursing Process/Planning
Content Area: Fundamental Skills
Reference: Kee, J., & Marshall, S. (2009). *Clinical calculations: With applications to general and specialty areas* (6th ed., p. 86). Philadelphia: Saunders.

129. **2**
Rationale: Convert 1 g to milligrams. In the metric system, to convert larger to smaller, multiply by 1000, or move the decimal three places to the right. Therefore, 1 g = 1000 mg
Formula:

$$\frac{Desired}{Available} \times tablet = number\ of\ tablets\ per\ dose$$

$$\frac{1000\ mg}{500\ mg} \times tablet = 2\ tablets$$

Test-Taking Strategy: For this medication calculation problem, it is necessary to first convert grams to milligrams. Follow the formula for conversion, and read the question carefully. After you have performed the calculation, verify your answer using a calculator. Review medication calculations and conversions if you had difficulty with this question.
Level of Cognitive Ability: Application
Client Needs: Physiological Integrity
Integrated Process: Nursing Process/Planning
Content Area: Fundamental Skills
Reference: Kee, J., & Marshall, S. (2009). *Clinical calculations: With applications to general and specialty areas* (6th ed., p. 86). Philadelphia: Saunders.

130. **2**
Rationale: Convert 0.2 g to mg. In the metric system, to convert larger to smaller, multiply by 1000, or move the decimal three places to the right. Therefore, 0.2 g = 200 mg.

Formula:

$$\frac{Desired}{Available} \times tablet = number\ of\ tablets/dose$$

$$\frac{200\ mg}{100\ mg} \times 1\ tablet = 2\ tablets$$

Test-Taking Strategy: For this medication calculation problem, it is necessary to first convert grams to milligrams. Follow the formula for conversion, and read the question carefully. After you have performed the calculation, verify your answer using a calculator. Review medication calculations and conversions if you had difficulty with this question.
Level of Cognitive Ability: Application
Client Needs: Physiological Integrity
Integrated Process: Nursing Process/Planning
Content Area: Fundamental Skills
Reference: Kee, J., & Marshall, S. (2009). *Clinical calculations: With applications to general and specialty areas* (6th ed., p. 86). Philadelphia: Saunders.

131. **0.4**
Rationale: Follow the formula for dosage calculation.
Formula:

$$\frac{Desired}{Available} \times mL = mL/dose$$

$$\frac{0.4\ mg}{0.5\ mg} \times 0.5\ mL = 0.4\ mL$$

Test-Taking Strategy: Follow the formula for the calculation of the correct dose. Focus on the strategic information: 0.5 mg/0.5 mL. After you have performed the calculation, verify your answer using a calculator. Review medication calculations if you had difficulty with this question.
Level of Cognitive Ability: Application
Client Needs: Physiological Integrity
Integrated Process: Nursing Process/Planning
Content Area: Fundamental Skills
Reference: Kee, J., & Marshall, S. (2009). *Clinical calculations: With applications to general and specialty areas* (6th ed., p. 86). Philadelphia: Saunders.

132. **1**
Rationale: Convert Fahrenheit to Celsius, and then calculate the dose to be administered.
Step 1: Conversion of Fahrenheit to Celsius
Formula: To convert Fahrenheit to Celsius, subtract 32, and divide the result by 1.8:
C = (101 − 32) divided by 1.8; C = (69) divided by 1.8; C = 38.3°
Step 2: Dosage calculation

$$\frac{Desired}{Available} \times tablet = number\ of\ tablets/dose$$

$$\frac{650}{325} \times 1\ tablet = 2\ tablets$$

Test-Taking Strategy: Focus on what the question is asking you to determine. For this medication calculation problem, it is necessary to convert Fahrenheit to Celsius. Follow the formula for conversion, and read the question carefully. After you have

performed the calculation, verify your answer using a calculator. Review these formulas if you had difficulty with this question.
Level of Cognitive Ability: Application
Client Needs: Physiological Integrity
Integrated Process: Nursing Process/Planning
Content Area: Fundamental Skills
Reference: Asperheim, M. (2005). *Introduction to pharmacology* (10th ed., p. 13). Philadelphia: Saunders.

133. **2**
Rationale: Use ratio and proportion to solve this problem, and then solve for X.
Formula:

$$250 \text{ mg} : 500 \text{ mL} :: \text{ X mg} : 50 \text{ mL}$$
Change the ratio and proportion to a fraction:
$$500X = 12,500$$
$$X = 25$$

Test-Taking Strategy: Follow the process to solve for X by ratio and proportion equation. After you have performed the calculation, verify your answer using a calculator. Review medication calculations if you had difficulty with this question
Level of Cognitive Ability: Application
Client Needs: Physiological Integrity
Integrated Process: Nursing Process/Planning
Content Area: Fundamental Skills
Reference: Kee, J., & Marshall, S. (2009). *Clinical calculations: With applications to general and specialty areas* (6th ed., p. 88). Philadelphia: Saunders.

134. **21**
Rationale: The prescribed 1000 mL is to be infused over 12 hours. Follow the formula, and multiply 1000 mL by 15 (gtt factor). Then divide the result by 720 minutes (12 hours × 60 minutes). The infusion is to run at 20.8 or 21 gtt/minute.
Formula:

$$\frac{\text{Total volume (in mL)} \times \text{gtt factor}}{\text{Time in minutes}} = \text{flow rate in gtt/minute}$$

$$\frac{1000 \text{ mL} \times 15 \text{ gtt}}{720 \text{ minutes}} = \frac{15,000}{720} = 20.8 \text{ or } 21 \text{ gtt/minute}$$

Test-Taking Strategy: Follow the formula for calculating an infusion rate for an IV. Be sure to change 12 hours to minutes. After you have performed the calculation, verify your answer using a calculator. Review the formula for calculating infusion rates if you had difficulty with this question.
Level of Cognitive Ability: Application
Client Needs: Physiological Integrity
Integrated Process: Nursing Process/Planning
Content Area: Fundamental Skills
Reference: Kee, J., & Marshall, S. (2009). *Clinical calculations: With applications to general and specialty areas* (6th ed., p. 223). Philadelphia: Saunders.

135. **1.3**
Rationale: Follow the formula for dosage calculation.
Formula:

$$\frac{\text{Desired}}{\text{Available}} \times \text{mL} = \text{mL/dose}$$

$$\frac{400,000 \text{ units}}{300,000 \text{ units}} \times 1 \text{ mL} = 1.3 \text{ mL}$$

Test-Taking Strategy: Follow the formula for the calculation the correct dose. Focus on the strategic information: 300,000 units/mL. After you have performed the calculation, verify your answer using a calculator. Review medication calculations if you had difficulty with this question.
Level of Cognitive Ability: Application
Client Needs: Physiological Integrity
Integrated Process: Nursing Process/Implementation
Content Area: Fundamental Skills
Reference: Kee, J., & Marshall, S. (2009). *Clinical calculations: With applications to general and specialty areas* (6th ed., p. 86). Philadelphia: Saunders.

136. **21**
Rationale: The prescribed 3000 mL is to be infused over 24 hours. Follow the formula, and multiply 3000 mL by 10 (gtt factor). Then divide the result by 1440 minutes (24 hours × 60 minutes). The infusion is to run at 20.8 or 21 gtt/minute.
Formula:

$$\frac{\text{Total volume (in mL)} \times \text{gtt factor}}{\text{Time in minutes}} = \text{flow rate in gtt/minute}$$

$$\frac{3000 \text{ mL} \times 10 \text{ gtt}}{1440 \text{ minutes}} = \frac{30,000}{1440} = 20.8 \text{ or } 21 \text{ gtt/minute}$$

Test-Taking Strategy: Follow the formula for calculating the infusion rate for an IV. Be sure to change 24 hours to minutes. After you have performed the calculation, verify your answer using a calculator, and remember to round the answer to the nearest whole number. Review the formula for calculating infusion rates if you had difficulty with this question.
Level of Cognitive Ability: Application
Client Needs: Physiological Integrity
Integrated Process: Nursing Process/Planning
Content Area: Fundamental Skills
Reference: Kee, J., & Marshall, S. (2009). *Clinical calculations: With applications to general and specialty areas* (6th ed., p. 223). Philadelphia: Saunders.

137. **2**
Rationale: Convert 0.2 g to milligrams. In the metric system, to convert larger to smaller, multiply by 1000, or move the decimal three places to the right. Therefore, 0.2 g = 200 mg.
Formula:

$$\frac{\text{Desired}}{\text{Available}} \times \text{capsules} = \text{capsules per dose}$$

$$\frac{200 \text{ mg}}{100 \text{ mg}} \times 1 \text{ capsules} = 2 \text{ capsules}$$

Test-Taking Strategy: For this medication calculation problem, it is necessary to first convert grams to milligrams. Follow the formula for conversion, and read the question carefully. After you have performed the calculation, verify your answer using a calculator. Review medication calculations and conversions if you had difficulty with this question.
Level of Cognitive Ability: Application
Client Needs: Physiological Integrity
Integrated Process: Nursing Process/Implementation
Content Area: Fundamental Skills
Reference: Kee, J., & Marshall, S. (2009). *Clinical calculations: With applications to general and specialty areas* (6th ed., p. 88). Philadelphia: Saunders.

138. **31**
Rationale: The prescribed 1000 mL is to be infused over 8 hours. Follow the formula, and multiply 1000 mL by 15 (gtt factor). Then divide the result by 480 minutes (8 hours × 60 minutes). The infusion is to run at 31.2 or 31 gtt/minute.
Formula:

$$\frac{\text{Total volume in mL} \times \text{gtt factor}}{\text{Time in minutes}} = \text{flow rate in gtt/minute}$$

$$\frac{1000\text{ mL} \times 15\text{ gtt}}{480\text{ minutes}} = \frac{15,000}{480} = 31.2 \text{ or } 31 \text{ gtt/minute}$$

Test-Taking Strategy: Follow the formula for calculating the infusion rate for an IV. Be sure to change 8 hours to minutes. After you have performed the calculation, verify your answer using a calculator and round answer to nearest whole number. Review the formula for calculating infusion rates if you had difficulty with this question.
Level of Cognitive Ability: Application
Client Needs: Physiological Integrity
Integrated Process: Nursing Process/Planning
Content Area: Fundamental Skills
Reference: Kee, J., & Marshall, S. (2009). *Clinical calculations: With applications to general and specialty areas* (6th ed., p. 223). Philadelphia: Saunders.

139. **1.5**
Rationale: Convert 150 mcg to milligrams. In the metric system, to convert smaller to larger, divide by 1000, or move the decimal three places to the left. Therefore, 150 mcg = 0.15 mg.
Formula:

$$\frac{\text{Desired}}{\text{Available}} \times \text{tablet(s)} = \text{tablet(s)/dose}$$

$$\frac{0.15\text{ mg}}{0.1\text{ mg}} \times 1 \text{ tablet} = 1.5 \text{ tablets}$$

Test-Taking Strategy: For this medication calculation problem, it is necessary to first convert micrograms to milligrams. Follow the formula, and, after you have performed the calculation, verify your answer using a calculator. Review medication calculations and conversions if you had difficulty with this question.

Level of Cognitive Ability: Application
Client Needs: Physiological Integrity
Integrated Process: Nursing Process/Planning
Content Area: Fundamental Skills
Reference: Kee, J., & Marshall, S. (2009). *Clinical calculations: With applications to general and specialty areas* (6th ed., p. 86). Philadelphia: Saunders.

140. **8**
Rationale: To determine how many hours it will take for 1 L to infuse, first recall that 1 L is equal to 1000 mL. Next, divide the 1000 mL by the amount being delivered in 1 hour.
Formula:

$$\frac{\text{Total volume in mL}}{\text{mL/hour}} = \text{infusion time in hours}$$

$$\frac{1000\text{ mL}}{125\text{ mL}} = 8 \text{ hours}$$

Test-Taking Strategy: Focus on the subject of the question: how many hours it takes for 1 L to infuse. Follow the formula, and, after you have performed the calculation, verify your answer using a calculator. Review the formula for determining the infusion time if you had difficulty with this question.
Level of Cognitive Ability: Application
Client Needs: Physiological Integrity
Integrated Process: Nursing Process/Implementation
Content Area: Fundamental Skills
Reference: Asperheim, M. (2005). *Introduction to pharmacology* (10th ed., p. 38). Philadelphia: Saunders.

141. **10**
Rationale: The prescribed 250 mL is to be infused over 4 hours. Follow the formula, and multiply 250 mL by 10 (gtt factor). Then divide the result by 240 minutes (4 hours × 60 minutes). The infusion is to run at 10.4 or 10 gtt/minute.
Formula:

$$\frac{\text{Total volume (in mL)} \times \text{gtt factor}}{\text{Time in minutes}} = \text{flow rate in gtt/minute}$$

$$\frac{250\text{ mL} \times 10\text{ gtt}}{240\text{ minutes}} = \frac{2500}{240} = 10.4 \text{ or } 10 \text{ gtt/minute}$$

Test-Taking Strategy: Follow the formula for calculating the infusion rate for an IV. Be sure to change 4 hours to minutes. After you have performed the calculation, verify your answer using a calculator and round answer to the nearest whole number. Review the formula for calculating infusion rates if you had difficulty with this question.
Level of Cognitive Ability: Application
Client Needs: Physiological Integrity
Integrated Process: Nursing Process/Implementation
Content Area: Fundamental Skills
Reference: Kee, J., & Marshall, S. (2009). *Clinical calculations: With applications to general and specialty areas* (6th ed., p. 223). Philadelphia: Saunders.

REFERENCES

Asperheim, M. (2005). *Introduction to pharmacology* (10th ed.). Philadelphia: Saunders.

Kee, J., & Marshall, S. (2009). *Clinical calculations: With applications to general and specialty areas* (6th ed.). Philadelphia: Saunders.

Lilley, L., Harrington, S., & Snyder, J. (2005). *Pharmacology and the nursing process* (4th ed.). St. Louis: Mosby.

National Council of State Boards of Nursing (Eds.) (2008). *2008 Detailed Test Plan for the NCLEX-PN® Examination, National Council of State Boards of Nursing*. Chicago: Author.

National Council of State Boards of Nursing. *NCSBN home page*. www.ncsbn.org. Accessed June 23, 2008.

Potter, P., & Perry, A. (2009). *Fundamentals of nursing* (7th ed.). St. Louis: Mosby.

Basic Life Support

PYRAMID TERMS

abdominal thrusts (Heimlich maneuver) A method to relieve a foreign-body airway obstruction.

automated external defibrillator (AED) A machine that converts ventricular fibrillation into a perfusing rhythm and that allows for early defibrillation by first responders.

basic life support (BLS) A method that provides oxygen to the brain, heart, and other vital organs until help arrives.

cardiopulmonary resuscitation (CPR) Another term for basic life support.

head tilt–chin lift The preferred method for opening a victim's airway.

jaw thrust maneuver The method used to open a victim's airway if a neck injury is suspected.

▲ THE PYRAMID TO SUCCESS

The Pyramid to Success focuses on the emergency measures related to performing basic life support (BLS) measures. Focus on the points related to the breath-to-compression ratio for one-person and two-person adult cardiopulmonary resuscitation (CPR) and CPR in the infant and child. The pyramid points focus on airway management in CPR and on relieving a foreign-body airway obstruction (Heimlich maneuver). Focus on the correct hand placement for cardiac compressions and on the differences between the adult, the child, and the infant. For the health care provider (HCP), the initial action is to determine unresponsiveness before beginning CPR. Remember the ABCDs—airway, breathing, circulation, and defibrillation or definitive treatment—when performing CPR. The Integrated Processes addressed in this chapter include Caring, Communication and Documentation, the Clinical Problem-Solving Process (Nursing Process), and Teaching and Learning.

▲ CLIENT NEEDS

Safe and Effective Care Environment

Acting as an advocate for the client's wishes
Considering ethical and legal responsibilities

Establishing priorities
Following advance directives regarding the client's documented requests
Implementing standard, transmission-based, and other precautions
Upholding the client's rights

Health Promotion and Maintenance

Performing the techniques of data collection
Providing health promotion programs
Teaching significant others about how to perform CPR and how to relieve choking (foreign-body airway obstruction)

Psychosocial Integrity

Considering the client's cultural, religious, and spiritual preferences
Discussing end-of-life, grief, and loss issues
Providing emotional support to significant others

Physiological Integrity

Administering emergency treatments
Documenting the client's response to BLS measures
Handling medical emergencies
Identifying alterations in the cardiopulmonary system
Performing CPR or foreign-body airway obstruction measures
Using special equipment

I. BASIC LIFE SUPPORT (Box 16-1)
A. **BLS** provides oxygen to the brain, heart, and other vital organs until help arrives
B. Also known as **CPR**
II. ADULT CARDIOPULMONARY RESUSCITATION GUIDELINES FOR THE HEALTH CARE PROVIDER (Box 16-2; Table 16-1)
A. Description: An adult can be defined as a person who is an adolescent or older (for lay rescuers, adults are defined as those 8 years of age or older)

B. Airway
1. Remember, for the HCP, assessment is the first step of the nursing process; assessing a victim of sudden illness or accident for unconsciousness is the initial action (assess for 5 to 10 seconds)
2. Gently shake the victim's shoulders and ask, "Are you OK?"; be alert to the potential for a head or neck injury
3. Call the emergency response number when the victim is found unconscious; if asphyxial arrest is likely, call after 5 cycles (2 minutes) of **CPR**
4. Place the victim in a supine position on a firm, flat surface (logroll the victim using spine precautions)
   a. One-person rescue: The rescuer is positioned on his or her knees, perpendicular to the victim's sternum and facing the victim
   b. Two-person rescue: One rescuer faces the victim and is kneeling perpendicular to the victim's head while maintaining an open airway, monitoring the carotid pulse, and performing the rescue breathing; the second rescuer moves to the opposite side and faces the victim, kneeling perpendicular to the victim's sternum and performing the chest compressions
   c. When two rescuers are present during **CPR,** the rescuers should rotate the compressor role every 2 minutes
   d. The rescuers apply gloves and face shields, if available
5. Open the airway
6. The **head tilt–chin lift** is the preferred method for opening the airway; if the victim has a neck injury, use the **jaw thrust maneuver** to open the airway (see Figure 16-1 for the head tilt-chin lift)
7. Look for any foreign material, liquids, or solids in the victim's mouth; wipe out any foreign material with a hooked index or middle finger

C. Breathing
1. Assess breathing and maintain an open airway
2. The rescuer places his or her ear over the victim's nose and mouth and looks for the chest to rise and fall, listens for air moving in and out of the lungs, and feels for the flow of air
3. For the breathing victim, do the following:
   a. Place the victim on his or her side if no cervical trauma is suspected; logroll the victim

onto his or her side as a unit (without twisting) to help maintain an open airway and to decrease the risk of aspiration
   b. If trauma or injury is suspected, do not move the victim
4. For the nonbreathing victim, do the following:
   a. Maintain the **head tilt–chin lift**; pinch the nostrils closed, and give two effective breaths at 1 second per breath
   b. Avoid delivering breaths that are too large or too forceful
   c. Attempt to use a resuscitation bag or mouth if available, and ensure an adequate air seal; allow the victim to exhale fully between breaths
   d. If unsuccessful at giving the breath, reposition the victim's head, and try again (improper chin and head positions are the most common causes of difficulty with ventilating the victim)
   e. If still unsuccessful, check the victim's mouth for a foreign body or for loose dentures (remove the dentures only if they interfere with the mouth seal), clear the airway, and try to ventilate again
   f. Be alert for gastric distention when giving ventilations
5. Mouth to nose: This method is recommended when ventilating through the victim's mouth is impossible, when the mouth cannot be opened or is seriously injured, or when a tight mouth-to-mouth seal is difficult to achieve
6. Mouth to stoma (advanced airway)
   a. This method is used for the victim who has had a laryngectomy or who has a temporary tracheostomy; to be effective, an adequate seal over the victim's mouth and nose is necessary
   b. With an advanced airway (i.e., endotracheal tube, laryngeal airway, tracheostomy, esophageal–tracheal Combitube), 8 to 10 breaths per minute are delivered (i.e., 1 breath every 6 to 8 seconds)

D. Circulation
1. Palpate the carotid artery to assess circulation; always check for the absence of a pulse before

TABLE 16-1	Summary of Basic Life Support ABCD Maneuvers for Infants, Children, and Adults		
Maneuver*	Adult†	Child‡	Infant§
Activate (call) emergency response number (one rescuer)	Call when victim is found unresponsive HCP: If asphyxial arrest is likely, call after five cycles (2 minutes) of CPR	Call after performing five cycles of CPR For sudden, unwitnessed collapse, call after verifying that victim is unresponsive	Call after performing five cycles of CPR For sudden, unwitnessed collapse, call after verifying that victim is unresponsive
Airway Breaths			
	Head tilt–chin lift (HCP: If trauma is suspected, use jaw thrust) Two effective breaths at 1 sec/breath	Head tilt–chin lift HCP: If trauma is suspected, use jaw thrust Two effective breaths at 1 sec/breath	Head tilt–chin lift (HCP: If trauma is suspected, use jaw thrust) Two effective breaths at 1 sec/breath
HCP: Rescue breathing without chest compressions	10-12 breaths/min (1 breath every 5-6 sec)	12-20 breaths/min (1 breath every 3-5 sec)	12-20 breaths/min (1 breath every 3-5 sec)
HCP: Rescue breathing for CPR with advanced airway	8-10 breaths/min (1 breath every 6-8 sec)	8-10 breaths/min (1 breath every 6-8 sec)	8-10 breaths/min (1 breath every 6-8 sec)
Foreign-body airway obstruction	Abdominal thrusts	Back slaps and chest thrusts	Back slaps and chest thrusts
Circulation			
HCP: Pulse check (10 seconds or less)	Carotid artery	HCP can use femoral artery in child	Brachial or femoral artery
Compression landmarks	Center of chest, between nipples	Center of chest, between nipples	Just below nipple line
Compression method: Push hard and fast, and allow for complete recoil	Two hands: Heel of one hand, other hand on top	Two hands: Heel of one hand with second on top *or* One hand: Heel of one hand only	One rescuer: Two fingers HCP or two rescuers: Two-thumb/encircling hands technique
Compression depth	1½ to 2 inches	Approximately one third to one half the depth of the chest	Approximately one third to one half the depth of the chest
Compression rate	Approximately 100/min	Approximately 100/min	Approximately 100/min
Compression-to-ventilation ratio	30:2 (one or two rescuers)	30:2 (single rescuer) HCP: 15:2 (two rescuers)	30:2 (single rescuer) HCP: 15:2 (two rescuers)
Defibrillation			
AED	Use adult pads; do not use child pads or a child system HCP: For out-of-hospital response, you may provide five cycles (2 min) of CPR before shock if response time is longer than 4-5 min and arrest was not witnessed	HCP: Use AED as soon as possible for sudden and in-hospital collapse. All: Use AED after five cycles of CPR (out of hospital); use child pads and system for child 1-8 years old, if available; if child pads and system are not available, use adult AED and pads	No recommendations for infants less than 1 year old

AED, Automatic external defibrillator; *CPR*, cardiopulmonary resuscitation; *HCP*, health care provider.
*Maneuver performed only by HCP.
†For lay rescuers, adults are defined as those 8 years old and older; for HCPs, adults are adolescents and older.
‡For lay rescuers, children are those 1 to 8 years old; for HCPs, children are those 1 year old to adolescents.
§For all rescuers, infants are defined as those younger than 1 year old.
With permission from American Heart Association. (Winter 2005-2006). Highlights of the 2005 American Heart Association Guidelines for Cardiopulmonary Resuscitation and Emergency Cardiovascular Care. *Currents in Emergency Cardiovascular Care*, 16(4), 15.

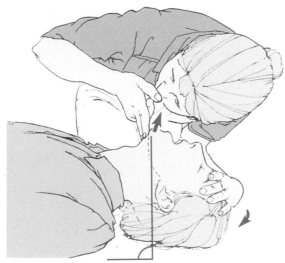

FIG. 16-1 Head tilt–chin lift maneuver. (From Christensen, B., & Kockrow, E. [2006]. *Foundations and adult health nursing* [5th ed.]. St. Louis: Mosby.)

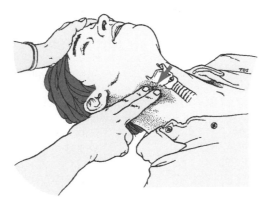

FIG. 16-2 Feeling for the carotid pulse. (From Harkreader, H., & Hogan, M. A. [2004]. *Fundamentals of nursing: Caring and clinical judgment* [2nd ed.]. Philadelphia: Saunders.)

beginning chest compressions on the victim (Figure 16-2)
2. Maintain an open airway, and palpate for a carotid pulse for 10 seconds or less
3. If there is a pulse, continue to give 10 to 12 breaths per minute
4. If there is no pulse, chest compressions should begin
E. Chest compression landmarks: center of the chest, between the nipples
F. Chest compression method
1. The rescuer uses two hands; the heel of one hand is placed on the landmark, and the other hand is placed on top
2. The rescuer should push hard and fast and avoid interrupted compressions (every time chest compressions are stopped, blood flow stops as well)
3. The rescuer should allow for complete recoil between compressions

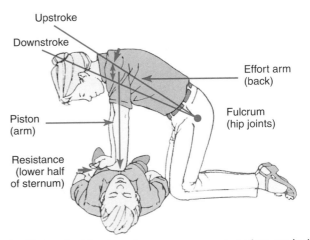

FIG. 16-3 Positioning for proper compression techniques. (From Christensen, B., & Kockrow, E. [2006]. *Foundations and adult health nursing* [5th ed.]. St. Louis: Mosby.)

4. Compression depth should be 1½ to 2 inches (Figure 16-3)
5. The compression rate is approximately 100 times per minute
6. The compression-to-ventilation ratio is 30:2 for both one and two rescuers
G. Complications of chest compressions
1. Laceration of internal organs
2. Punctured lungs
3. Fractured ribs or sternum
III. **PEDIATRIC CARDIOPULMONARY RESUSCITATION GUIDELINES FOR THE HEALTH CARE PROVIDER**
A. Description
1. For HCPs, a child is defined as a person between the ages of 1 year and adolescence; for lay rescuers, children are those individuals between 1 and 8 years old
2. For both HCPs and lay rescuers, an infant is defined as a person who is less than 1 year old
3. For an unresponsive infant or child, the lone HCP (i.e., one rescuer) should perform five cycles (about 2 minutes of **CPR**) and then call the emergency response number; the HCP must assess the most likely cause of the arrest
4. If the infant or child has a sudden witnessed collapse, the collapse is likely to be cardiac in origin (hypoxic cardiac arrest); in this situation, the HCP should call the emergency response number after verifying that the victim is unresponsive
B. Airway
1. Assess unresponsiveness
2. Use the **head tilt–chin lift** to open the airway (the HCP would use the **jaw thrust maneuver** if neck trauma is suspected)
C. Breathing
1. Breathing victim: Keep the airway open

2. Nonbreathing victim
   a. Deliver two initial effective breaths (breaths that cause a visible chest rise) to the infant or child at 1 second per breath; then 12 to 20 breaths per minute are delivered (1 breath every 3 to 5 seconds)
   b. With the infant, provide ventilations by mouth to mouth and nose
   c. With the larger child, provide ventilations by mouth to mouth
   d. For the child or infant with an advanced airway, 8 to 10 breaths per minute are delivered (i.e., 1 breath every 6 to 8 seconds)

D. Circulation
   1. Assess the circulation for no more than 10 seconds
   2. If the victim is more than 1 year old, assess the circulation via the carotid or femoral pulse
   3. If the victim is less than 1 year old, assess the circulation via the brachial pulse
   4. If there is a pulse, continue to give 12 to 20 breaths per minute (i.e., 1 breath every 3 to 5 seconds)
   5. If there is no pulse, chest compressions should begin
   6. Chest compression landmarks
      a. Child: Center of the chest between the nipples
      b. Infant: Just below the nipple line
   7. Chest compression method
      a. Child: Use two hands with the heel of one hand on the chest and the second hand on top or use one hand with the heel of that one hand only on the chest
      b. Infant: One rescuer uses two fingers; two rescuers use the two-thumb/encircling hands technique
      c. Compression depth: One third to one half the depth of the chest
      d. Compression rate: Approximately 100 per minute
      e. Compression-to-ventilation ratio: 30:2 for a single rescuer; 15:2 for two rescuers

IV. AUTOMATED EXTERNAL DEFIBRILLATOR AND THE HEALTH CARE PROVIDER
A. Description
   1. The **automated external defibrillator (AED)** is used to convert ventricular fibrillation into a perfusing rhythm
   2. The **AED** differentiates nonventricular fibrillation rhythms and allows for early defibrillation by first responders
   3. The use of **AEDs** is recommended for children in cardiac arrest who are 1 year old and older; it is not recommended for infants less than 1 year old

4. For a sudden witnessed arrest in a child or adult in an out-of-hospital setting, the HCP should phone the emergency response number, retrieve the **AED,** and return to the victim to perform CPR and use the **AED**

B. Adult
   1. Adult pads need to be used (child pads or a child system cannot be used on an adult)
   2. Out-of-hospital response: Provide five cycles (2 minutes) of **CPR** before defibrillating if the response time was longer than 4 to 5 minutes and the arrest was not witnessed

C. Child
   1. Child pads and a child system are used for the child 1 to 8 years old, if available; if child pads and a child system are not available, an adult **AED** and pads are used
   2. Out-of-hospital response: Provide five cycles of **CPR** before defibrillating

D. Interventions
   1. Attach **AED** pads to the victim
   2. Turn on the **AED** and push the button to activate the analyzer
   3. Follow the instructions given for the **AED,** which are usually to "assess," "stand back," "shock," and "reassess"
   4. **CPR** guidelines to treat cardiac arrest associated with ventricular fibrillation or pulseless ventricular tachycardia recommend the delivery of single shocks followed immediately by a period of **CPR**; interruptions of chest compressions to check circulation should not be done until about 5 cycles or approximately 2 minutes of **CPR** have been provided after the shock

V. FOREIGN-BODY AIRWAY OBSTRUCTION
A. General guidelines
   1. The HCP needs to distinguish choking victims who require treatment (**abdominal thrusts** or back slaps and chest thrusts) from those who do not (*mild* versus *severe* airway obstruction)
   2. Signs of severe airway obstruction include poor air exchange and increased breathing difficulty, a silent cough, cyanosis, or the inability to speak or breathe
   3. Every time the airway is opened (with a **head tilt–chin lift**) to deliver rescue breaths, the rescuer should look in the mouth and remove an object if one is seen
   4. Blind finger sweeps of the mouth should not be performed
   5. **Abdominal thrusts** are used for the adult; back slaps and chest thrusts are used for both the child and the infant

B. Conscious adult
   1. Ask the victim, "Are you choking?"; the victim will not be able to speak or cough if he or she is

choking, but if he or she nods, then help is needed

2. Relieve the obstruction with **abdominal thrusts** (**Heimlich maneuver**; Box 16-3 and Figure 16-4)
3. Continue **abdominal thrusts** until the object is dislodged or the victim becomes unconscious

C. Unconscious adult
1. Assess unconsciousness
2. Call for help
3. Perform the **head tilt–chin lift** technique
4. Open the airway and look in the mouth; remove an object if one is seen
5. Attempt ventilation
6. Reposition the head if unsuccessful; reattempt ventilation
7. Relieve the obstruction with five **abdominal thrusts**
8. To perform **abdominal thrusts,** straddle the victim's thighs, place the heel of one hand on top of the other between the umbilicus and the xiphoid process, and give five **abdominal thrusts** in and up with the heel of the bottom hand
9. Reattempt ventilation

BOX 16-3 **Abdominal Thrusts (Heimlich Maneuver)**

1. Stand behind the victim.
2. Place your arms around the victim's waist.
3. Make a fist.
4. Place the thumb side of your fist just above the umbilicus (belly button) and well below the xiphoid process.
5. Perform five quick in and up abdominal thrusts (between the umbilicus and the xiphoid process).
6. Use chest thrusts for the obese victim or for the victim in the late stages of pregnancy.

---

10. Repeat the sequence of **head tilt–chin lift,** breaths, and **abdominal thrusts** until successful
11. Be sure to assess the victim's carotid pulse, and look for the presence of spontaneous respirations
12. Perform rescue breathing or **CPR,** if required

D. Choking child or infant
1. Foreign-body airway obstruction requiring intervention occurs when signs of severe airway obstruction exist
2. For the conscious child:
   a. Assess for obstruction by asking the child, "Are you choking?"; if the victim nods, help is needed
   b. Relieve the obstruction by **abdominal thrusts** until the obstruction is dislodged or the child becomes unconscious
3. For the unconscious child, do the following:
   a. Assess unconsciousness
   b. Open the airway using the **head tilt–chin lift** technique
   c. Check for breathing, and look for a foreign object (remove one if seen)
   d. Attempt ventilation
   e. If unsuccessful, reposition the head; reattempt ventilation
   f. Relieve the obstruction with **abdominal thrusts**
   g. Look in the mouth and remove a foreign object if one is seen
   h. Reattempt ventilation
   i. Repeat the sequence
4. For the conscious infant, do the following:
   a. Assess for obstruction, and note if mild or severe airway obstruction exists
   b. Relieve the obstruction with five back slaps and five chest thrusts (Figure 16-5)
   c. Straddle the infant over the arm, place the infant's head lower than the trunk, and support the head firmly, holding the jaw

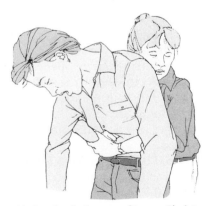

FIG. 16-4 Abdominal thrusts. (From Christensen, B., & Kockrow, E. [2006]. *Foundations and adult health nursing* [5th ed.]. St. Louis: Mosby.)

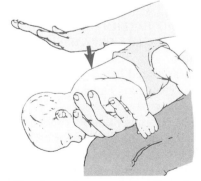

FIG. 16-5 Clearing airway obstruction in an infant. (From Christensen, B., & Kockrow, E. [2006]. *Foundations and adult health nursing* [5th ed.]. St. Louis: Mosby.)

d. Give five back slaps with the heel of the hand between the shoulder blades

e. Turn the infant; place the head lower than the trunk

f. Give five chest thrusts at the same location as for chest compressions

g. Check for the object, and remove it if it is visible

h. Continue until the object is removed or the infant becomes unconscious

5. For the unconscious infant, do the following:

a. Assess unconsciousness with gentle taps

b. Open the airway with the **head tilt–chin lift** technique, and check for breathing

c. Look in the mouth, and remove any visualized foreign object every time the airway is opened

d. Attempt ventilation

e. Reposition the head, if unsuccessful; reattempt ventilation

f. Relieve the obstruction with five back slaps and five chest thrusts

g. Reattempt ventilation, and repeat the sequence

VI. PREGNANT OR OBESE VICTIM

A. Relieving a foreign-body airway obstruction

1. Place the arms under the woman's axilla and across the chest

2. Place the thumb side of a clenched fist against the middle of the sternum, and place the other hand over the fist

3. Perform backward chest thrusts until the foreign body is expelled or until the woman becomes unconscious

4. If she becomes unconscious, place her on her back; a wedge, such as a pillow or a rolled blanket, should be placed under the right abdominal flank and hip to displace the uterus to the left side of the abdomen

5. If unable to ventilate, position the hands as for chest compressions, and deliver chest thrusts firmly to remove the obstruction

B. Defibrillation in the pregnant client: If defibrillation is needed, place the paddles one rib interspace higher than usual, because the heart is displaced slightly by the enlarged uterus

PRACTICE QUESTIONS

More questions on the companion CD!

142. A nursing instructor asks a nursing student to describe the procedure for relieving an airway obstruction on an unconscious pregnant woman at 8 months' gestation. The student describes the procedure correctly if the student states to:
   1. Place the hands in the pelvis to perform the thrusts.

2. Perform abdominal thrusts until the object is dislodged.
   3. Perform left lateral abdominal thrusts until the object is dislodged.
   4. Place a rolled blanket under the right abdominal flank and hip area.

143. A nurse on the day shift walks into a client's room and finds the client unresponsive. The client is not breathing and does not have a pulse, and the nurse immediately calls out for help. The next nursing action is which of the following?
   1. Open the airway.
   2. Give the client oxygen.
   3. Start chest compressions.
   4. Ventilate with a mouth-to-mask device.

144. A nurse witnesses a neighbor's husband sustain a fall from the roof of his house. The nurse rushes to the victim and determines the need to open the airway. The nurse opens the airway in this victim with the use of which method?
   1. Flexed position
   2. Head tilt–chin lift
   3. Jaw thrust maneuver
   4. Modified head tilt–chin lift

145. A nurse understands that which of the following is a correct guideline for adult cardiopulmonary resuscitation (CPR) for a health care provider?
   1. One breath should be given for every five compressions.
   2. Two breaths should be given for every 15 compressions.
   3. Initially, two quick breaths should be given as rapidly as possible.
   4. Each rescue breath should be given over 1 second and should produce a visible chest rise.

146. A nurse attempts to relieve an airway obstruction on a 3-year-old conscious child. The nurse performs this maneuver by placing the hands between:
   1. The groin and the abdomen
   2. The umbilicus and the groin
   3. The lower abdomen and the chest
   4. The umbilicus and the xiphoid process

147. A nurse is performing cardiopulmonary resuscitation (CPR) on a 7-year-old child. The nurse delivers how many breaths per minute to the child?
   1. 6
   2. 8
   3. 10
   4. 20

148. A nurse is performing cardiopulmonary resuscitation (CPR) on an infant. When performing chest compressions, the nurse understands that the compression rate is at least:
   1. 60 times per minute
   2. 80 times per minute

3. 100 times per minute
4. 160 times per minute

149. Which of the following is the most appropriate location for assessing the pulse of an infant who is less than 1 year old?
   1. Radial
   2. Carotid
   3. Brachial
   4. Popliteal

150. A nurse is teaching cardiopulmonary resuscitation to a group of nursing students. The nurse asks a student to describe the reason why blind finger sweeps are avoided in infants. The nurse determines that the student understands the reason if the student makes which statement?
   1. "The object may have been swallowed."
   2. "The infant may bite down on the finger"
   3. "The mouth is too small to see the object."
   4. "The object may be forced back further into the throat."

151. A nurse is performing cardiopulmonary resuscitation (CPR) on an adult client. The nurse understands that when performing chest compressions, one should depress the sternum:
   1. ¾ to 1 inch
   2. ½ to ¾ inch
   3. 1½ to 2 inches
   4. 2½ to 3 inches

ALTERNATE ITEM FORMAT: PRIORITIZING (ORDERED RESPONSE)

152. A nursing student is asked to describe the correct steps for performing adult cardiopulmonary resuscitation (CPR). Number the steps of adult CPR in order of priority. (Number 1 is the first step, and number 6 is the last step.)
   _4_ Initiate breathing.
   _2_ Open the client's airway.
   _3_ Determine breathlessness.
   _6_ Perform chest compressions.
   _5_ Check for a pulse at the carotid artery.
   _1_ Determine unconsciousness by shaking the client and asking, "Are you OK?"

ANSWERS

142. 4
Rationale: To relieve an airway obstruction on an unconscious woman in an advanced stage of pregnancy, place the woman on her back. Place a wedge, such as a pillow or rolled blanket, under the right abdominal flank and hip to displace the uterus to the left side of the abdomen. Options 1, 2, and 3 are incorrect and can cause harm to the woman and the fetus.
Test-Taking Strategy: Use the process of elimination, and note that the client is an unconscious pregnant woman at 8 months' gestation. Recall the concepts associated with hypotension and vena cava syndrome to assist with directing you to option 4. Review the principles associated with relieving an airway obstruction on a pregnant woman if you had difficulty with this question.
Level of Cognitive Ability: Analysis
Client Needs: Physiological Integrity
Integrated Process: Nursing Process/Evaluation
Content Area: Maternity/Antepartum
Reference: Lowdermilk, D., & Perry, A. (2004). *Maternity & woman's health care* (8th ed., pp. 917-918) St. Louis: Mosby.

143. 1
Rationale: The next nursing action would be to open the airway. Ventilation cannot be initiated unless the airway is opened. One starts chest compressions after opening the airway and initiating ventilation. Oxygen may be helpful at some point, but the airway is opened first.
Test-Taking Strategy: Visualize the steps of basic life support (BLS) to answer the question. Recalling the ABCDs—airway, breathing, circulation, defibrillation or definitive treatment—will assist with directing you to option 1. Review the steps of BLS if you had difficulty with this question.
Level of Cognitive Ability: Application
Client Needs: Physiological Integrity
Integrated Process: Nursing Process/Implementation

Content Area: Delegating/Prioritizing
Reference: Ignatavicius, D., & Workman, M. (2006). *Medical-surgical nursing: Critical thinking for collaborative care* (5th ed., p. 161). Philadelphia: Saunders.

144. 3
Rationale: If a neck injury is suspected, the jaw thrust maneuver is used to open the airway. The head tilt–chin lift produces hyperextension of the neck and could cause complications if a neck injury is present. A flexed position is an inappropriate position for opening the airway.
Test-Taking Strategy: Use the process of elimination. Eliminate options 2 and 4 first, because they are comparable or alike. Next, eliminate option 1, because this position would not open the airway. If you had difficulty with this question, review the appropriate methods for opening an airway.
Level of Cognitive Ability: Application
Client Needs: Physiological Integrity
Integrated Process: Nursing Process/Implementation
Content Area: Adult Health/Neurological
Reference: Perry, A., & Potter, P. (2006). *Clinical nursing skills & techniques* (6th ed., p. 890). St. Louis: Mosby.

145. 4
Rationale: During adult CPR, each rescue breath should be given over 1 second and should produce a visible chest rise. Excessive ventilation (too many breaths per minute or breaths that are too large or forceful) may be harmful and should not be performed. Health care providers should employ a 30-compression-to-2-ventilation ratio for the adult victim. Options 1, 2, and 3 are incorrect.
Level of Cognitive Ability: Comprehension
Client Needs: Physiological Integrity
Integrated Process: Nursing Process/Implementation
Content Area: Fundamental Skills

Reference: American Heart Association. (Winter 2005-2006). Highlights of the 2005 American Heart Association Guidelines for Cardiopulmonary Resuscitation and Emergency Cardiovascular Care. *Currents in Emergency Cardiovascular Care, 16*(4), 13.

146. 4

Rationale: To relieve an airway obstruction in a child, the rescuer stands behind the victim and places the arms directly under the victim's axillae and around the victim. The rescuer places the thumb side of one fist against the victim's abdomen in the midline slightly above the umbilicus and well below the tip of the xiphoid process. The rescuer grasps the fist with the other hand and delivers up to five thrusts. One must take care to not touch the xiphoid process or the lower margins of the rib cage, because force applied to these structures may damage the internal organs. Options 1, 2, and 3 are incorrect hand placements.

Test-Taking Strategy: Use the process of elimination, and note the age of the child. Eliminate options 1 and 2 first, because they are comparable or alike. From the remaining options, considering the anatomic location and the effect of the maneuver for dislodging an obstruction will direct you to option 4. If you had difficulty with this question, review the correct hand placement for relieving an airway obstruction.

Level of Cognitive Ability: Application
Client Needs: Physiological Integrity
Integrated Process: Nursing Process/Implementation
Content Area: Child Health
References: Ignatavicius, D., & Workman, M. (2006). *Medical-surgical nursing: Critical thinking for collaborative care* (5th ed., p. 570). Philadelphia: Saunders.
Hockenberry, M., Wilson, D., & Winkelstein, M. (2005). *Wong's essentials of pediatric nursing* (7th ed., p. 836.). St. Louis: Mosby.

147. 4

Rationale: For a child between the ages of 1 and 8 years, 12 to 20 breaths per minute are delivered. Options 1, 2, and 3 are incorrect.

Test-Taking Strategy: Use the process of elimination, and note the age of the child. Recalling the normal respiratory rate of a child at this age will assist with directing you to option 4. If you had difficulty with this question, review the CPR guidelines for a child.

Level of Cognitive Ability: Application
Client Needs: Physiological Integrity
Integrated Process: Nursing Process/Implementation
Content Area: Child Health
References: McKinney, E., James, S., Murray, S., & Ashwill, J. (2005). *Maternal-child nursing* (2nd ed., pp. 861, 863). St. Louis: Saunders.
Perry, A., & Potter, P. (2006). *Clinical nursing skills & techniques* (6th ed., p. 888). St. Louis: Mosby.

148. 3

Rationale: For an infant, the rate of chest compressions is at least 100 per minute. Options 1 and 2 identify rates that are too low, and option 4 identifies a rate that is too high.

Test-Taking Strategy: Use the process of elimination, and consider the normal heart rate of an infant. Eliminate options 1 and 2 because of the low rates identified in the options.

Eliminate option 4, because this rate would be much too rapid for an infant. Review the CPR guidelines for an infant if you had difficulty with this question.

Level of Cognitive Ability: Application
Client Needs: Physiological Integrity
Integrated Process: Nursing Process/Implementation
Content Area: Child Health
References: McKinney, E., James, S., Murray, S., & Ashwill, J. (2005). *Maternal-child nursing* (2nd ed., p. 863). St. Louis: Saunders.
Perry, A., & Potter, P. (2006). *Clinical nursing skills & techniques* (6th ed., p. 888). St. Louis: Mosby.

149. 3

Rationale: To assess a pulse in an infant (i.e., a child <1 year old), the pulse is checked at the brachial artery. The infant's relatively short, fat neck makes palpation of the carotid artery difficult. The popliteal and radial pulses are also difficult to palpate in an infant.

Test-Taking Strategy: Use the process of elimination and your knowledge regarding circulatory assessment in an infant. Considering the body structure of an infant will assist with directing you to option 3. Review cardiac assessment and basic life support for an infant if you had difficulty with this question.

Level of Cognitive Ability: Comprehension
Client Needs: Physiological Integrity
Integrated Process: Nursing Process/Data Collection
Content Area: Child Health
Reference: McKinney, E., James, S., Murray, S., & Ashwill, J. (2005). *Maternal-child nursing* (2nd ed., p. 862). St. Louis: Saunders.

150. 4

Rationale: Blind finger sweeps are not recommended for infants and children because of the risk of forcing the object further down into the airway. Options 1, 2, and 3 are not related directly to the subject of the question.

Test-Taking Strategy: Use the ABCDs—airway, breathing, circulation, and defibrillation or definitive treatment—to answer this question. Option 4 addresses the concern of airway patency. Review the management of an obstructed airway in an infant or a child if you had difficulty with this question.

Level of Cognitive Ability: Comprehension
Client Needs: Physiological Integrity
Integrated Process: Nursing Process/Evaluation
Content Area: Child Health
References: McKinney, E., James, S., Murray, S., & Ashwill, J. (2005). *Maternal-child nursing* (2nd ed., p. 862). St. Louis: Saunders.
Perry, A., & Potter, P. (2006). *Clinical nursing skills & techniques* (6th ed., p. 888). St. Louis: Mosby.

151. 3

Rationale: When performing CPR on an adult client, the sternum is depressed 1½ to 2 inches. Options 1 and 2 identify compression depths that would be ineffective for an adult, and option 4 identifies a depth that could cause injury to the client.

Test-Taking Strategy: Note the strategic word "adult" in the question. Consider the normal body structure of an adult to assist with directing you to option 3. Review the procedure for performing adult CPR if you had difficulty with this question.

Level of Cognitive Ability: Application
Client Needs: Physiological Integrity
Integrated Process: Nursing Process/Implementation
Content Area: Adult Health/Cardiovascular
Reference: Perry, A., & Potter, P. (2006). *Clinical nursing skills & techniques* (6th ed., p. 888). St. Louis: Mosby.

ALTERNATE ITEM FORMAT: PRIORITIZING (ORDERED RESPONSE)

152. **4, 2, 3, 6, 5, 1**

Rationale: The sequence for basic CPR for health care providers is as follows. After determining unconsciousness, the airway is opened, and breathlessness is determined. Next, the health care provider delivers effective breaths that produce a visible rise in the chest, and this is followed by assessing the carotid artery for presence of a pulse. In the absence of any pulse, chest compressions are provided at an adequate rate and depth that will allow for adequate chest recoil with minimal interruptions in chest compressions.

Test-Taking Strategy: Remember that determining unresponsiveness is the first action. Next, use the ABCs—airway, breathing, and circulation—to determine the correct order of action. Review the procedure for performing CPR if you had difficulty with this question.

Level of Cognitive Ability: Application
Client Needs: Physiological Integrity
Integrated Process: Nursing Process/Implementation
Content Area: Delegating/Prioritizing
Reference: American Heart Association. (Winter 2005-2006). Highlights of the 2005 American Heart Association Guidelines for Cardiopulmonary Resuscitation and Emergency Cardiovascular Care. *Currents in Emergency Cardiovascular Care, 16*(4), 11.

REFERENCES

American Heart Association. (Winter 2005-2006). Highlights of the 2005 American Heart Association Guidelines for Cardiopulmonary Resuscitation and Emergency Cardiovascular Care. *Currents in Emergency Cardiovascular Care, 16*(4).

Hockenberry, M., Wilson, D., & Winkelstein, M. (2005). *Wong's essentials of pediatric nursing* (7th ed.). St. Louis: Mosby.

Ignatavicius, D., & Workman, M. (2006). *Medical-surgical nursing: Critical thinking for collaborative care* (5th ed.). Philadelphia: Saunders.

Lowdermilk, D., & Perry, A. (2004). *Maternity & woman's health care* (8th ed.). St. Louis: Mosby.

McKinney, E., James, S., Murray, S., & Ashwill, J. (2005). *Maternal-child nursing* (2nd ed.). St. Louis: Saunders.

National Council of State Boards of Nursing (Eds.). (2008). *2008 Detailed Test Plan for the NCLEX-PN® Examination, National Council of State Boards of Nursing.* Chicago: Author.

National Council of State Boards of Nursing. *NSCBN home page.* www.ncsbn.org. Accessed June 25, 2008.

Perry, A., & Potter, P. (2006). *Clinical nursing skills & techniques* (6th ed.). St. Louis: Mosby.

Perioperative Nursing Care

PYRAMID TERMS

atelectasis A collapsed or airless state of the lung that may be the result of airway obstruction caused by accumulated secretions or the failure of the client to deep breathe; a common postoperative complication that usually occurs 1 to 2 days after surgery.

extended postoperative stage The period of at least 1 to 4 days after surgery.

immediate postoperative stage The period of 1 to 4 hours after surgery.

intermediate postoperative stage The period of 4 to 24 hours after surgery.

perioperative nursing Nursing care given before (preoperative), during (intraoperative), and after (postoperative) surgery.

wound dehiscence A separation or opening of the wound edges.

wound evisceration A protrusion of the internal organs through an opening of the wound edges.

▲ PYRAMID TO SUCCESS

The pyramid points focus on reinforcing instructions to the client, family, and significant others during the preoperative stage; medication reconciliation; preparing the client for the operative procedure; and ensuring that prescribed preoperative procedures have been performed, that the results are within the expected range, and that they have been documented. During the postoperative stage, the pyramid points focus on monitoring for surgical complications and on the implementation of initial nursing measures if a complication arises. They also focus on preparing the client for discharge, reinforcing instructions related to the prescribed treatments, and identifying the need for home-care support services. The Integrated Processes addressed in this chapter include Caring, Communication and Documentation, the Clinical Problem-Solving Process (Nursing Process), and Teaching and Learning.

CLIENT NEEDS   ▲

Safe and Effective Care Environment

Ensuring that advance directive documents are in the client's medical record
Establishing priorities
Informing the client about the surgical process
Maintaining confidentiality
Maintaining standard and other precautions
Maintaining surgical asepsis
Obtaining informed consent for the surgical procedure
Preventing a surgical infection
Providing safety to the medicated client
Upholding client's rights

Health Promotion and Maintenance

Discussing expected body-image changes
Identifying lifestyle choices
Performing techniques of data collection
Providing client and family teaching related to the prescribed discharge plan
Providing health and wellness teaching to prevent complications

Psychosocial Integrity

Assessing psychosocial concerns
Assisting the client with the development of coping methods
Communicating therapeutically
Identifying support systems
Identifying unexpected body-image changes
Promoting an environment that will allow the client to express concerns

Physiological Integrity

Administering preoperative and postoperative medications safely

Initiating nursing interventions when surgical complications arise

Monitoring for unexpected responses to treatments and procedures

Monitoring for surgical complications

Monitoring for wound infection

Providing basic care and comfort

Providing respiratory therapy

I. PREOPERATIVE CARE

A. Obtaining informed consent
1. The surgeon is responsible for obtaining the consent for surgery
2. No sedation should be administered to the client before he or she signs the consent form
3. Minors (<18 years old) may need a parent or legal guardian to sign the consent form
4. Older clients may need a legal guardian to sign the consent form
5. The nurse may witness the client signing the preoperative consent form
6. The nurse needs to document the witnessing of the signing of the operative consent form after the client acknowledges understanding the procedure

B. Nutrition
1. Check the physician's orders regarding nothing by mouth (NPO) status before surgery
2. Solid foods and liquids are generally withheld for 6 to 8 hours before general anesthesia and for 3 hours before surgery with local anesthesia to avoid aspiration
3. Monitor intravenous (IV) fluids, if prescribed
4. Note that parenteral nutrition may be prescribed for clients who are malnourished, who have protein or metabolic deficiencies, or who cannot ingest foods

C. Elimination
1. If the client is to have intestinal or abdominal surgery, an enema, laxative, or both may be prescribed the night before surgery
2. The client should void immediately before surgery
3. Prepare to insert a Foley catheter, if prescribed
4. If there is a Foley catheter in place, it should be emptied immediately before surgery, and the amount and quality of urine output should be documented

D. Surgical site
1. Prepare to clean the surgical site with a mild antiseptic soap the night before surgery, as prescribed
2. Inform the client about the procedure for shaving the operative site (the hair is shaved only if it will interfere with the surgical procedure and only if prescribed)

E. Reinforcing preoperative instructions
1. Inform the client about what to expect after surgery
2. Tell the client to notify the nurse if he or she experiences any postoperative pain and that pain medication will be prescribed to be given as the client requests
3. Instruct the client to use noninvasive pain relief techniques such as relaxation or guided imagery before the pain occurs and as soon as the pain is noticed
4. Reinforce instructions about the use of a client-controlled analgesia pump, if its use is prescribed
5. Inform the client that requesting an opioid after surgery will not make the client a drug addict, and explain the difference between analgesic need and psychological dependence
6. The client should be instructed to not smoke for at least 24 hours before surgery and to refrain from taking daily aspirin, selected vitamins, and complementary therapies unless they are approved by the surgeon
7. Instruct the client in deep-breathing and coughing techniques, the use of incentive spirometry, and the importance of performing the techniques after surgery to prevent the development of pneumonia and **atelectasis** (Box 17-1, Figure 17-1)
8. Instruct the client in leg and foot exercises to prevent venous stasis of blood and to facilitate venous blood return (Figure 17-2; see Box 17-1)
9. Instruct the client about how to splint an incision and how to turn and reposition (Figure 17-3; see Box 17-1)
10. Inform the client of any invasive devices that may be needed after surgery, such as tubes, drains, Foley catheters, or IV lines
11. Tell the client to not pull on any of the invasive devices and that they will be removed as soon as possible

F. Psychosocial preparation
1. Be alert to the client's anxiety level
2. Ask the client about questions or concerns that he or she may have regarding surgery
3. Allow time for privacy for the client to prepare psychologically for surgery
4. Provide support and assistance as needed (Box 17-2)

G. Preoperative checklist
1. Ensure that the client is wearing an identification bracelet
2. Check for client allergies (see Chapter 60 for information about latex allergy)
3. Review the preoperative checklist to be sure that each item is addressed before the client is transported to surgery

BOX 17-1 Preoperative Instructions

Deep-Breathing and Coughing Exercises

Instruct the client that a sitting position provides the best lung expansion for coughing and deep-breathing exercises.

Instruct the client to breathe deeply three times by inhaling through the nostrils and exhaling slowly through pursed lips.

Instruct the client that the third breath should be held for 3 seconds; then the client should cough deeply three times.

The client should perform this exercise every 2 hours.

Incentive Spirometry

Instruct the client to assume a sitting or upright position.

Instruct the client to place the mouth tightly around the mouthpiece.

Instruct the client to inhale slowly to raise and maintain the flow rate indicator between the 600 and 900 marks.

Instruct the client to hold his or her breath for 5 seconds and then to exhale through pursed lips.

Instruct the client to repeat this process 10 times every hour.

Leg and Foot Exercises

Gastrocnemius (calf) pumping: Instruct the client to move both ankles by pointing the toes up and then down.

Quadriceps (thigh) setting: Instruct the client to press the back of the knees against the bed and then to relax the knees; this contracts and relaxes the thigh and calf muscles to prevent thrombus formation.

Foot circles: Instruct the client to rotate each foot in a circle.

Hip and knee movements: Instruct the client to flex the knee and thigh, straighten the leg, and hold the position for 5 seconds before lowering. (This should not performed if the client is having abdominal surgery or if the client has a back problem.)

Splinting the Incision

If the surgical incision is abdominal or thoracic, instruct the client to place a pillow or one hand with the other hand on top over the incisional area.

During deep breathing and coughing, the client presses gently against the area of the incision to splint or support it.

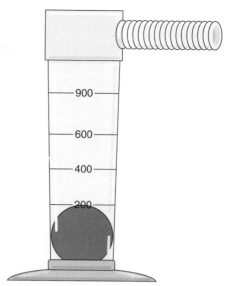

FIG. 17-1 Incentive spirometer. (From Monahan, F., Sands, J., Neighbors, M., Marek, J., & Green, C. [2007]. *Phipps' medical-surgical nursing: Health and illness perspectives* [8th ed.]. St. Louis: Mosby.)

Essential
Gastrocnemius (calf) pumping

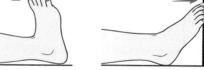

Quadriceps (thigh) setting

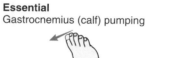

Desirable
Foot circles

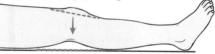

Hip and knee movements

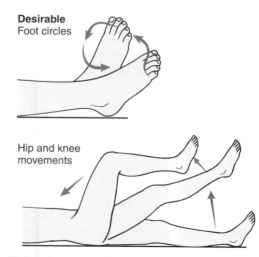

FIG. 17-2 Postoperative leg exercises. (From Lewis, S., Heitkemper, M., & Dirksen, S. [2004]. *Medical-surgical nursing: Assessment and management of clinical problems* [6th ed.]. St. Louis: Mosby.)

4. Ensure that consent forms have been signed for the operative procedure, anesthesia, any blood transfusions, the disposal of a limb, or surgical sterilization procedures

5. Ensure that a history and physical examination were completed and documented in the client's record (Box 17-3)

6. Ensure that the consultations prescribed were completed and documented in the client's record

7. Ensure that the prescribed laboratory test results are documented in the client's record

8. Ensure that electrocardiography and chest radiography reports are noted in the client's record

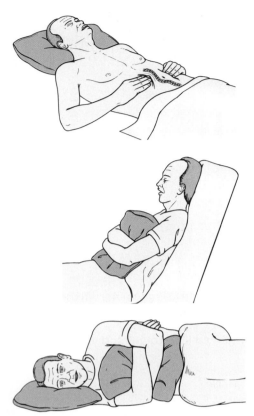

FIG. 17-3 Techniques for splinting a wound when coughing. (From Lewis, S., Heitkemper, M., & Dirksen, S. [2004]. *Medical-surgical nursing: Assessment and management of clinical problems* [6th ed.]. St. Louis: Mosby.)

9. Ensure that blood type and screen or type and crossmatch are noted in the client's record
10. Document that the client has voided before surgery
11. Remove the client's jewelry, makeup, dentures, hairpins, nail polish, glasses, and any prostheses
    a. Religious medals or scapulars may be pinned to the pillow
    b. Hearing aids or glasses may be removed at the last possible moment before surgery
    c. Clients with language or hearing concerns need to have access to translators until anesthesia induction
12. Document that valuables were given to the client's family members or locked in the hospital safe
13. Document that the prescribed preoperative medication was given (Box 17-4)
14. Monitor and document the client's vital signs
15. Document the last time that the client ate or drank
H. Preoperative medications
    1. Prepare to administer preoperative medications as prescribed or to have them be administered in the operating room immediately before the surgery

BOX 17-2 **Cultural Aspects of Perioperative Nursing Care**

Cultural assessment includes questions related to:
- Primary language spoken
- Feelings related to surgery and pain
- Pain management
- Expectations
- Support systems
- Feelings toward self

Allow a family member to be present, if appropriate.
Secure the help of a professional interpreter to communicate with non–English speaking clients.
Use pictures or phrase cards to communicate and assess the non–English speaking client's perception of pain or other feelings.
Provide preoperative and postoperative educational materials in the appropriate language.

Modified from Potter, P. & Perry, A. (2009). *Fundamentals of nursing* (7th ed.). St. Louis: Mosby.

BOX 17-3 **Medical Conditions That Increase the Risk of Surgery**

- Bleeding disorders, such as thrombocytopenia and hemophilia
- Diabetes mellitus
- Chronic pain
- Heart disease, such as a recent myocardial infarction, dysrhythmia, congestive heart failure, and peripheral vascular disease
- Obstructive sleep apnea
- Upper respiratory infection
- Liver disease
- Fever
- Chronic respiratory disease, such as emphysema, bronchitis, or asthma
- Immunological disorders, such as leukemia, acquired immunodeficiency syndrome, bone marrow depression, and the use of chemotherapy or immunosuppressive agents
- The abuse of street drugs

Modified from Potter, P. & Perry, A. (2009). *Fundamentals of nursing* (7th ed.). St. Louis: Mosby.

2. Instruct the client that he or she will feel drowsy after the medications are given
3. After administering the preoperative medications, keep the client in bed with the side rails up (per agency policy)
4. Place the call bell next to the client; instruct the client to not get out of bed and to call for assistance if needed
I. Arrival at the operating room
    1. When the client arrives to the operating room, the operating room nurse will verify the identification bracelet with the client's verbal response and review the client's chart (Boxes 17-5 and 17-6)

BOX 17-4 Substances That Can Affect the Surgical Client

Antibiotics
These potentiate the action of anesthetic agents.

Anticholinergics
Medications with anticholinergic effects increase the potential for confusion.

Anticoagulants
These alter normal clotting factors and increase the risk of hemorrhaging.
Aspirin (acetylsalicylic acid) and nonsteroidal anti-inflammatory drugs are commonly used medications that can alter clotting mechanisms.
Complementary remedies such as garlic and ginseng may also alter normal clotting factors.
These medications should be discontinued at least 48 hours before surgery.

Anticonvulsants
The long-term use of certain anticonvulsants can alter the metabolism of anesthetic agents.

Antidepressants
These may lower the blood pressure during anesthesia.
Complementary remedies such as St. John's wort may also lower blood pressure.

Antidysrhythmics
These reduce cardiac contractility and impair cardiac conduction during anesthesia.

Antihypertensives
These can interact with anesthetic agents and cause bradycardia, hypotension, and impaired circulation.

Corticosteroids
These cause adrenal atrophy and reduce the body's ability to withstand stress.
Before and during surgery, dosages may be temporarily increased.

Diuretics
These potentiate electrolyte imbalances after surgery.

Herbal Substances
These can interact with anesthesia and cause a variety of adverse effects. These substances may need to be stopped at a specific time before surgery. During the preoperative period, the client needs to be asked if he or she is taking any herbal substances.

Insulin
The need for insulin after surgery in a diabetic client may either be reduced, because the client's nutritional intake is decreased, or be increased, because of the stress response and the intravenous administration of glucose solutions.

Modified from Potter, P. & Perry, A. (2009). *Fundamentals of nursing* (7th ed.). St. Louis: Mosby.

BOX 17-5 The Joint Commission's Protocol for Preventing Wrong-Site, Wrong-Procedure, and Wrong-Person Surgery

Preoperative Client Verification
At least two client identifiers must be used to verify the client's identity (e.g., full name, date of birth).
Confirm and verify the following:
- Client's name on the identification band
- Date of birth
- Medical record number
- Consent forms
- Scheduled procedure and marked surgical site
- Availability of implant, if needed
- Availability of blood
- Radiologic examinations

Site Marking
Site verification is required for all procedures that involve laterality, multiple structures, or multiple levels.
The site is marked with a permanent marker that is visible after the skin is prepped and draped.
The operating surgeon marks the site with his or her initials before the client enters the operating suite.
The site is marked in accordance with client participation (i.e., verbal confirmation or pointing).
The client has the right to refuse to mark the site. Each institution will determine the policy for these situations.

Modified from Monahan, F., Sands, J., Neighbors, M., Marek, J., & Green, C. (2007). *Phipps' medical-surgical nursing: Health and illness perspectives* (8th ed.). St. Louis: Mosby.

BOX 17-6 Time-Out Procedure

A time-out occurs in the operating room after the client has been prepped and draped. The entire team must verbally verify their agreement about the following:
- The client's name
- The procedure to be performed
- The surgical site
- Laterality, implants, and radiologic examinations, if applicable

The documentation of the time-out should indicate that the following were verified:
- Correct client
- Correct site and side
- Agreement to proceed
- Correct client position
- Availability of implants or special equipment

From Monahan, F., Sands, J., Neighbors, M., Marek, J., & Green, C. (2007). *Phipps' medical-surgical nursing: Health and illness perspectives* (8th ed.). St. Louis: Mosby.

2. The operating room nurse will confirm the operative procedure and the site to be operated on (the client may be asked to mark the operative site)
3. The client's chart will be checked for completeness

4. The client's chart will be reviewed for consent forms, history and physical examination, and allergic reaction information
5. The physician's orders will be reviewed and their completion verified

6. The IV line may be initiated at this time, if prescribed
7. The anesthesia team will administer the prescribed anesthesia

II. POSTOPERATIVE CARE

A. **Immediate postoperative stage**
1. Description: The period of 1 to 4 hours after surgery
2. Respiratory system
   a. Monitor vital signs
   b. Monitor airway patency and adequate ventilation, because prolonged mechanical ventilation during anesthesia may affect postoperative lung function
   c. Remember that extubated clients who are lethargic may not be able to maintain an airway
   d. Monitor for secretions and remove them by suctioning if the client is unable to clear the airway by coughing
   e. Observe chest movements for symmetry and the use of accessory muscles
   f. Monitor oxygen administration, if prescribed
   g. Monitor pulse oximetry, as prescribed
   h. Encourage coughing and deep-breathing exercises as soon as possible
   i. Note the rate, depth, and quality of respirations; the respiratory rate should be more than 10 and less than 30 breaths per minute
3. Cardiovascular system
   a. Check the client's color
   b. Observe capillary refill, mucous membranes, and sclerae
   c. Check peripheral pulses and for peripheral edema
   d. Monitor for bleeding
   e. Check the pulse for rate and rhythm; a bounding pulse may indicate hypertension, fluid overload, or anxiety
   f. Monitor for signs of hypertension and hypotension
   g. Monitor for cardiac irregularities
   h. Checking for Homans' sign may be helpful for clients who are predisposed to developing deep vein thrombosis (i.e., clients who are in the lithotomy position during surgery)
4. Musculoskeletal system
   a. Check the client for moving extremities
   b. Check the physician's orders regarding client positioning or restrictions
   c. Unless contraindicated, place the client in a low Fowler's position after surgery to increase the size of the thorax
   d. Avoid positioning the client in a supine position until the pharyngeal reflexes have returned
   e. If the client is comatose or semicomatose, position on his or her side, unless contraindicated
5. Neurological system
   a. Check the level of consciousness
   b. Closely monitor the client who may be drowsy or unconscious
   c. Frequent periodic attempts to awaken the client should continue until the client awakens
   d. Orient the client to the environment
   e. Speak in a soft tone, and filter out extraneous noises in the environment
   f. Maintain the client's body temperature and prevent heat loss by providing the client with warm blankets and raising the room temperature as necessary
6. Temperature control
   a. Monitor the temperature
   b. Monitor for signs of hypothermia that may result from anesthesia, a cool operating room, and exposure of the skin and internal organs during surgery
   c. Apply warm blankets and continue oxygen, as prescribed, if the client is shivering
7. Integumentary system
   a. Check the surgical site, drains, and wound dressings (Figure 17-4)
   b. Monitor for and document any drainage or bleeding from the surgical site
   c. Check the skin for redness, abrasions, or breakdown that may have resulted from surgical positioning
8. Fluid and electrolyte balance
   a. Monitor IV administration, as prescribed
   b. Accurately record input and output
9. Gastrointestinal system
   a. Monitor for nausea and vomiting
   b. Maintain the patency of nasogastric tube, if present
   c. Monitor for abdominal distention (the return of bowel sounds is unlikely during the **immediate postoperative stage**)
10. Renal system
    a. Check the bladder for distention
    b. Monitor the color, quantity, and quality of urine output if a Foley catheter is present
    c. Expect the client to void 6 to 8 hours after the surgical procedure, depending on the type of anesthesia administered
11. Pain management
    a. Check for pain
    b. Note the type of anesthetic used, the preoperative medication that the client received, and if the client received any pain medications during the postanesthesia period

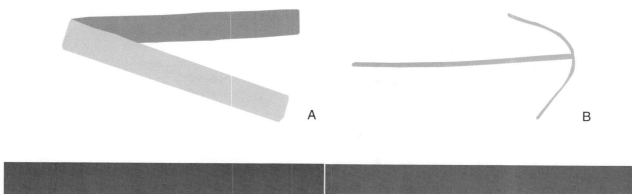

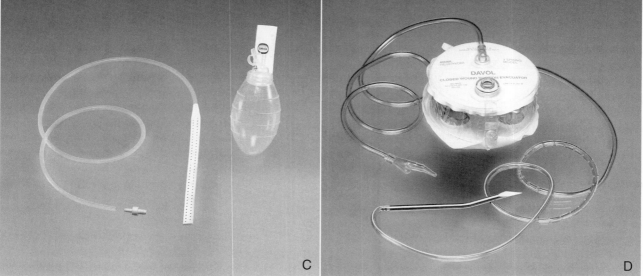

FIG. 17-4 Types of surgical drains. Gravity drains drain directly through a tube from the surgical area. **A,** Penrose. **B,** T-tube. With closed-wound drains, drainage collects in a collecting vessel by means of the compression and reexpansion of the system. **C,** Jackson-Pratt. **D,** Hemovac. (From Ignatavicius, **D.,** & Workman, L. [2006]. *Medical-surgical nursing: Critical thinking for collaborative care* [5th ed.]. St. Louis: Saunders. **C** and **D** Courtesy of C. R. Bard, Inc., Covington, GA.)

c. Ask the client to rate the degree of pain on a scale of 1 to 10, with 10 being the most severe

d. Monitor such objective data as facial expressions, body gestures, pulse rate, blood pressure, and respirations

e. Inquire about the effectiveness of the last pain medication

f. If an opioid has been prescribed, during the initial administration, check the client every 30 minutes for respiratory rate and pain relief

g. Noninvasive measures to relieve postoperative pain such as distraction, comfort measures, positioning, back rubs, and providing a quiet and restful environment during the **immediate postoperative stage** should not detract from medication administration

h. Document the effectiveness of pain medication

B. **Intermediate postoperative stage**

1. Description

a. The period of 4 to 24 hours after surgery

b. Nursing care implemented during the **immediate postoperative stage** is continued

2. Respiratory system: Encourage coughing and deep breathing

3. Cardiovascular system: Encourage the use of antiembolism stockings and an automated intermittent pulsatile compression device, if prescribed, to promote venous return, strengthen muscle tone, and prevent the pooling of blood in the legs

4. Musculoskeletal system

a. Before ambulation, instruct the client to sit at the edge of the bed with the feet supported

b. If the client is unable to walk, turn the client every 1 to 2 hours

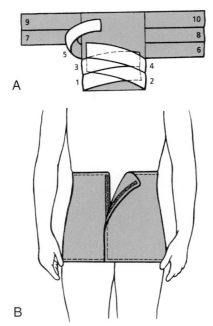

FIG. 17-5 Abdominal binders. **A,** Scultetus: Binder with flaps that wrap over each other. **B,** Straight binder with Velcro. (From Elkin, M., Perry, A., & Potter, P. [2008]. *Nursing interventions & clinical skills* [4th ed.]. St. Louis: Mosby.)

5. Neurological system: Check the level of consciousness
6. Integumentary system
   a. Monitor wound for signs of infection
   b. Maintain a dry and intact dressing
   c. Reinforce with a sterile dressing, if necessary, and notify the primary health care provider if bleeding from the site occurs
   d. Change dressings as prescribed, noting the amount of bleeding or drainage, any odor, and the intactness of sutures or staples
   e. Use an abdominal binder for obese and debilitated individuals to prevent rupture of the incision (Figure 17-5)
   f. Drains should be patent, and there should be minimal bleeding or drainage
   g. Prepare to assist with the removal of drains as prescribed by the physician when the drainage amount becomes insignificant
7. Gastrointestinal system
   a. Turn the unconscious client to a side-lying position if vomiting occurs, and have suctioning equipment available and ready to use
   b. Administer frequent mouth care
   c. Maintain the client's NPO status until the gag reflex and peristalsis return
   d. Assess for bowel sounds over the ileocecal valve area; if no sounds are heard, then assess for bowel sounds in all four quadrants

   e. When oral fluids are permitted, start with ice chips and water
   f. Ensure that the client advances to clear liquids and then to a regular diet, as prescribed
   g. Monitor the client for flatus and encourage ambulation, as prescribed
8. Renal system
   a. Monitor the urinary output (should be >30 mL/hour)
   b. If the client does not have a Foley catheter, he or she is expected to void within 6 to 8 hours after the surgical procedure; ensure that the amount is at least 200 mL
9. Pain management: Continue with data collection and interventions, as during the **immediate postoperative stage**
C. **Extended postoperative stage**
   1. Description: The period of at least 1 to 4 days after the surgical procedure
   2. Interventions
      a. Continue to check and observe the client's body systems during this stage
      b. Monitor for signs of infection, such as redness, swelling, and tenderness at the surgical site; fever; and leukocytosis
      c. Encourage active range-of-motion exercises every 2 hours
      d. Continue to encourage ambulation, which will promote peristalsis and the passage of fluid and flatus
      e. Increase ambulation every day to increase muscle strength
      f. Encourage the client to perform as many activities of daily living as possible
      g. Instruct the client to eat foods that are high in protein and vitamin C content to promote wound healing
III. **PNEUMONIA AND ATELECTASIS** (Figure 17-6; Box 17-7)
A. Description
   1. Pneumonia, which is an inflammation of the alveoli caused by an infectious process, may develop 3 to 5 days after the surgical procedure because of infection, aspiration, or immobility
   2. **Atelectasis,** which is a collapse of the alveoli with retained mucous secretions, is the most common postoperative complication; it usually occurs 1 to 2 days after the surgical procedure
B. Data collection
   1. Dyspnea and increased respiratory rate
   2. Elevated temperature
   3. Productive cough and chest pain
   4. Crackles over involved lung area
   5. Delirium in the older client
   6. Hyperglycemia in diabetic clients

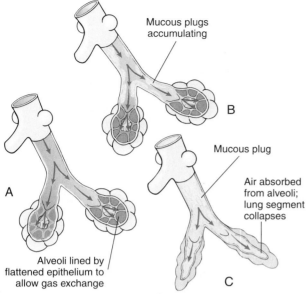

FIG. 17-6 Postoperative atelectasis. **A,** Normal bronchiole and alveoli. **B,** Mucous plug in bronchiole. **C,** Collapse of alveoli as a result of atelectasis after the absorption of air. (Lewis, S., Heitkemper, M., & Dirksen, S. [2004]. *Medical-surgical nursing: Assessment and management of clinical problems* [6th ed.]. St. Louis: Mosby.)

C. Interventions
1. Monitor temperature
2. Encourage ambulation
3. Reposition the client every 1 to 2 hours
4. Encourage the client to use an incentive spirometer and to cough and deep breathe
5. Check the lung sounds, and suction to clear secretions if the client is unable to cough
6. Encourage fluid intake

IV. HYPOXIA (see Box 17-7)
A. Description: An inadequate concentration of oxygen in the arterial blood
B. Data collection
1. Restlessness and agitation
2. Confusion
3. Dyspnea
4. Increased heart rate and blood pressure
5. Diaphoresis
6. Cyanosis
C. Interventions
1. Monitor for signs of hypoxia, eliminate the cause of hypoxia, and notify the registered nurse and/or physician immediately
2. Monitor pulse oximetry
3. Administer oxygen, as prescribed
4. Encourage coughing, deep breathing, and the use of incentive spirometry
5. Turn and reposition the client frequently

V. PULMONARY EMBOLISM (see Box 17-7)
A. Description: An embolus blocking the pulmonary artery and disrupting the blood flow to one or more lobes of the lung

BOX 17-7 **Postoperative Complications**

- Constipation
- Hemorrhage
- Hypoxia
- Paralytic ileus
- Pneumonia and atelectasis
- Pulmonary embolism
- Shock
- Thrombophlebitis
- Urinary retention
- Wound dehiscence
- Wound evisceration
- Wound infection

Note: The licensed practical vocational nurse always notifies the registered nurse and/or the physician if signs of complications are noted.

B. Data collection
1. Dyspnea
2. Sudden sharp chest or upper abdominal pain
3. Increased heart rate and a decrease in blood pressure
4. Cyanosis
C. Interventions
1. Notify the registered nurse and/or physician immediately
2. Establish IV access
3. Monitor vital signs

VI. HEMORRHAGE (see Box 17-7)
A. Description: The loss of a large amount of blood externally or internally during a short period of time
B. Data collection
1. Restlessness
2. Weak, rapid pulse and hypotension
3. Cool, clammy skin
4. Tachypnea
5. Reduced urine output
C. Interventions
1. Apply pressure to the site of bleeding
2. Notify the registered nurse and/or physician immediately
3. Establish IV access

VII. SHOCK (see Box 17-7)
A. Description: A loss of circulatory fluid volume that is usually caused by hemorrhage
B. Data collection: Similar to data collection findings of hemorrhage
C. Interventions
1. If shock develops, elevate the legs
2. If the client has had spinal anesthesia, do not elevate the legs any higher than placing them on the pillow; otherwise, diaphragm muscles could be impaired
3. Notify the registered nurse and/or physician immediately
4. Establish IV access

▲ VIII. THROMBOPHLEBITIS (see Box 17-7)
  A. Description
      1. An inflammation of a vein, often accompanied by clot formation
      2. Veins in the legs are most commonly affected
  B. Data collection
      1. Aching or cramping leg pain
      2. Vein inflammation; vein feels hard and cord-like and is tender to touch
      3. Elevated temperature
  ▲ 4. Positive Homans' sign may be an unreliable finding
  C. Interventions
      1. Monitor legs for swelling, inflammation, cyanosis, pain, tenderness, and venous distention
      2. Elevate the extremity 30 degrees without allowing any pressure on the popliteal area
      3. Encourage the client to perform "foot pumps" while on bedrest
      4. Encourage the use of antiembolism stockings, as prescribed, removing them twice a day to wash and inspect the legs
      5. Use intermittent pulsatile compression devices, as prescribed (Figure 17-7)
      6. Perform passive range of motion every 2 hours if the client is on bedrest
      7. Do not allow the client's legs to dangle
      8. Instruct the client to not sit in one position for an extended period of time
      9. Heparin sodium or warfarin (Coumadin) may be prescribed

▲ IX. URINARY RETENTION (see Box 17-7)
  A. Description
      1. The involuntary accumulation of urine in the bladder from a loss of muscle tone
      2. Occurs as a result of the effects of anesthetics and opioid analgesics
      3. Appears 6 to 8 hours after surgery
  B. Data collection
      1. Restlessness and diaphoresis
      2. Lower abdominal pain
      3. Inability to void and a distended bladder
      4. Elevated blood pressure
      5. On percussion, the bladder sounds like a drum
  C. Interventions
      1. Monitor for voiding, and check for a distended bladder with an ultrasound bladder scanner, if available
      2. Encourage fluid intake unless contraindicated
      3. Assist the client to void by helping him or her to stand
      4. Provide privacy
      5. Pour warm water over the perineum or allow the client to hear running water to promote voiding
      6. Catheterize the client, as prescribed, after all noninvasive techniques have been attempted

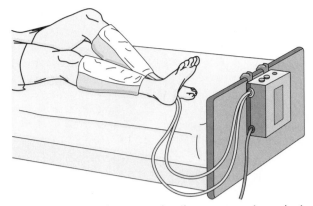

FIG. 17-7 Intermittent pulsatile compression device. (From Monahan, F., Sands, J., Neighbors, M., Marek, J., & Green, C. [2007]. *Phipps' medical-surgical nursing: Health and illness perspectives* [8th ed.]. St. Louis: Mosby.)

X. CONSTIPATION (see Box 17-7) ▲
  A. Description
      1. The abnormal and infrequent passage of stool
      2. When the client resumes a solid diet after surgery, failure to pass stool within 48 hours is a cause for concern
  B. Data collection
      1. Abdominal distention
      2. Absence of bowel movements
      3. Anorexia, headache, and nausea
  C. Interventions
      1. Check bowel sounds
      2. Encourage fluid intake up to 3000 mL/day unless contraindicated
      3. Encourage early ambulation
      4. Encourage the consumption of fiber-rich foods unless contraindicated
      5. Administer stool softeners and laxatives, as prescribed
      6. Provide privacy and adequate time for bowel elimination

XI. PARALYTIC ILEUS (see Box 17-7) ▲
  A. Description
      1. A failure of the appropriate forward movement of bowel contents
      2. May occur as a result of anesthetic medications or the manipulation of the bowel during the surgical procedure
  B. Data collection
      1. Postoperative nausea and vomiting
      2. Abdominal distention
      3. Absence of bowel sounds, bowel movement, or flatus
  C. Interventions
      1. Maintain NPO status until bowel sounds return
      2. Maintain the patency of the nasogastric tube, if present
      3. Encourage ambulation
      4. Monitor IV fluids, as prescribed

5. Administer medications, as prescribed, to increase gastrointestinal motility and secretions
6. If ileus occurs, it is first treated nonsurgically with bowel decompression by the insertion of a nasogastric tube attached to intermittent or constant suction

XII. WOUND INFECTION (see Box 17-7)

A. Description
1. Often caused by poor aseptic technique or a wound that was contaminated before surgical exploration
2. Usually occurs 3 to 6 days after surgery
3. Purulent material may exit from the drains or separated wound edges

B. Data collection
1. Fever and chills
2. Warm, tender, painful, and inflamed incision site
3. Edematous skin at the incision and tight skin sutures
4. Elevated white blood cell count

C. Interventions
1. Monitor the temperature
2. Monitor the incision site for approximation of the suture line, edema, bleeding, and signs of infection (*REEDA: Redness, Erythema, Ecchymosis, Drainage,* and *Approximation of the wound edges*)
3. Maintain the patency of any drains, and keep drains and tubes away from the incision line
4. Monitor drains, and assess drainage amount, color, and consistency
5. Change dressings, as prescribed
6. Administer antibiotics, as prescribed

XIII. WOUND DEHISCENCE (Figure 17-8; see Box 17-7)

A. Description
1. The separation of the wound edges at the suture line
2. Usually occurs 6 to 8 days after surgery

B. Data collection
1. Increased drainage
2. Opened wound edges
3. The appearance of underlying tissues through the wound

C. Interventions
1. Notify the registered nurse and/or physician immediately
2. Place the client in a low Fowler's position with the knees bent to prevent abdominal tension on abdominal wounds
3. Cover the wound with a sterile normal saline dressing
4. Prevent wound infection
5. Administer antiemetics, as prescribed, to prevent vomiting and further strain on the incision

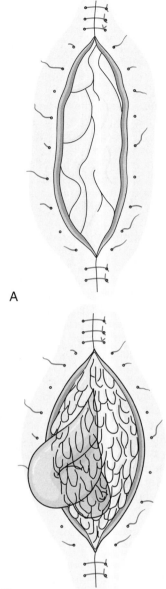

A

B

FIG. 17-8 **A,** Wound dehiscence. **B,** Wound evisceration. (From Monahan, F., Sands, J., Neighbors, M., Marek, J., & Green, C. [2007]. *Phipps' medical-surgical nursing: Health and illness perspectives* [8th ed.]. St. Louis: Mosby.)

6. Instruct the client to splint the incision when coughing

XIV. WOUND EVISCERATION (see Box 17-7 and Figure 17-8)

A. Description
1. The protrusion of the internal organs and tissues through an opening in the wound edges
2. Most common among obese clients, clients who have had abdominal surgery, or those who have poor wound-healing ability
3. Usually occurs 6 to 8 days after surgery
4. **Wound evisceration** is an emergency

B. Data collection

BOX 17-8 **Reinforcing Discharge Instructions**

Determine the client's readiness to learn, educational level, and desire to change or modify his or her lifestyle.

Determine the need for resources for home care.

Demonstrate the care of the incision and how to change the dressing.

Instruct the client to cover the incision with plastic if showering is allowed.

Be sure that the client is provided with a 48-hour supply of dressings for home use.

Instruct the client about the importance of returning to the physician's office for follow-up visits.

Instruct the client that sutures are usually removed in the physician's office 7 to 10 days after surgery.

Inform the client that staples are removed 7 to 14 days after surgery and that the skin may become slightly reddened when they are ready to be removed.

Steri-Strips may be applied to provide extra support after the sutures are removed.

Instruct the client regarding the use of medications and their purposes, doses, administration, and side effects.

Instruct the client regarding proper diet and to drink 6 to 8 glasses of liquid per day.

Instruct the client regarding activity levels and to resume normal activities gradually.

Instruct the client to avoid lifting for 6 weeks if a major surgical procedure was performed.

Instruct the client with an abdominal incision to not lift anything weighing 10 lbs or more and to not engage in any activities that involve pushing or pulling.

Clients usually can return to work after 6 to 8 weeks, as prescribed by the physician.

Instruct the client regarding the signs and symptoms of complications and when to call a physician.

1. The discharge of serosanguineous fluid from a previously dry wound
2. The appearance of loops of bowel or other abdominal contents through the wound
3. The client may report feeling a popping sensation after coughing or turning

C. Interventions
1. Notify the registered nurse and/or physician immediately
2. Place the client in a low Fowler's position with the knees bent to prevent abdominal tension
3. Cover the wound with a sterile normal saline dressing
4. Prevent wound infection
5. Administer antiemetics, as prescribed, to prevent vomiting and further strain on the incision
6. Instruct the client to splint the incision when coughing

XV. AMBULATORY SURGERY
A. Criteria for client discharge
1. Is alert and oriented
2. Has voided

3. Has no respiratory distress
4. Vital signs and oxygen saturation are within normal limits
5. Is able to ambulate, swallow, and cough
6. Has minimal pain
7. Is not vomiting
8. Has minimal (if any) bleeding from the incision site
9. A responsible adult is available to drive the client home
10. The surgeon has signed a release form

B. Reinforcing discharge instructions (Box 17-8)
1. Should be performed before the date of the scheduled procedure
2. Provide written instructions to the client and family regarding the specifics of care
3. Instruct the client and family about postoperative complications that can occur
4. Suggest appropriate resources for home-care support
5. Instruct the client to not drive for 24 hours if he or she has had a general anesthetic
6. Inform the client to call the surgeon, ambulatory center, or emergency department if postoperative problems occur
7. Instruct the client to keep follow-up appointments with the surgeon

PRACTICE QUESTIONS

More questions on the companion CD!

153. A nurse is developing a plan of care for a client who is scheduled for surgery. The nurse would include which of the following activities in the nursing care plan for the client on the day of surgery?
   1. Have the client void immediately before surgery.
   2. Avoid oral hygiene and rinsing with mouthwash.
   3. Verify that the client has not eaten for the last 24 hours.
   4. Report immediately any slight increase in blood pressure or pulse.

154. A nurse is caring for a client who is scheduled for surgery. The client is concerned about the surgical procedure. To alleviate the client's fears and misconceptions about surgery, the nurse should:
   1. Tell the client that preoperative fear is normal.
   2. Explain all nursing care and possible discomfort that may result.
   3. Ask the client to discuss information known about the planned surgery.
   4. Provide explanations about the procedures involved in the planned surgery.

155. A nurse is collecting data from a client who is scheduled for surgery in 1 week in the ambulatory

care surgical center. The nurse notes that the client has a history of arthritis and has been taking acetylsalicylic acid (aspirin). The nurse reports the information to the physician and anticipates that the physician will prescribe which of the following?

1. Discontinue the aspirin immediately.
2. Continue to take the aspirin as prescribed.
3. Discontinue the aspirin 48 hours before the scheduled surgery.
4. Decrease the dose of the aspirin to half of what is normally taken.

156. A nurse obtains the vital signs on a postoperative client who just returned to the nursing unit. The client's blood pressure (BP) is 100/60 mm Hg, the pulse is 90 beats per minute, and the respiration rate is 20 breaths per minute. On the basis of these findings, which of the following nursing actions should be performed?

1. Shake the client gently to arouse.
2. Continue to monitor the vital signs.
3. Call the registered nurse immediately.
4. Cover the client with a warm blanket.

157. A client arrives to the surgical nursing unit after surgery. The initial nursing action is to check the:

1. Patency of the airway
2. Dressing for bleeding
3. Tubes or drains for patency
4. Vital signs to compare with preoperative measurements

158. A nurse is monitoring an adult client for postoperative complications. Which of the following would be the most indicative of a potential postoperative complication that requires further observation?

1. A urinary output of 20 mL/hour
2. A temperature of 37.6° C (99.6° F)
3. A blood pressure of 100/70 mm Hg
4. Serous drainage on the surgical dressing

159. A nurse monitors the postoperative client frequently for the presence of secretions in the lungs, knowing that accumulated secretions can lead to:

1. Pneumonia
2. Fluid imbalance
3. Pulmonary edema
4. Carbon dioxide retention

160. A nurse is caring for a postoperative client who has a drain inserted into the surgical wound. Which of the following nursing actions would be inappropriate for the care of the drain?

1. Check the drain for patency.
2. Observe for bright red, bloody drainage.
3. Maintain aseptic technique when emptying.
4. Secure the drain by curling or folding it and taping it firmly to the body.

161. A nurse checks the client's surgical incision for signs of infection. Which of the following would be indicative of a potential infection?

1. The presence of serous drainage
2. The presence of purulent drainage
3. A temperature of 98.8° F (37.1° C)
4. The client complaining of feeling cold

162. A nurse is checking a client's surgical incision and notes an increase in the amount of drainage, a separation of the incision line, and the appearance of underlying tissue. Which of the following is the initial action?

1. Cover the wound with a Betadine-soaked dressing.
2. Apply a sterile dressing soaked with normal saline to the wound.
3. Leave the incision open to the air to assist with drying the drainage.
4. Clean the wound using aseptic technique, and apply a sterile, dry dressing.

163. A nurse monitors a postoperative client for signs of complications. Which of the following signs would the nurse determine to be indicative of a potential complication?

1. Increasing restlessness
2. A negative Homans' sign
3. Faint bowel sounds heard in all four quadrants
4. A blood pressure of 120/70 mm Hg with a pulse of 90 beats per minute

164. A nurse is explaining the concept of "time-out" in the perioperative area. The purpose of "time out" is:

1. To give the client an opportunity to refuse the operative procedure
2. To provide a quiet time for the nurse to discuss discharge instructions with the client
3. To give the surgeon an opportunity to discuss the surgery and potential complications with the client
4. To allow the surgical team a chance to verbally verify their agreement about the client's name, the surgical procedure, and the site

165. A nurse is explaining the Joint Commission's (TJC's) universal protocol for preventing wrong-site, wrong-procedure, and wrong-person surgery to a group of nursing students. The nurse explains that site marking involves:

1. The surgeon marking the area of the operative procedure
2. The circulating nurse marking the area of the operative procedure
3. Marking the site of the operative procedure during the "time-out" period
4. Marking the site of the operative procedure at the completion of the procedure to measure any increase in swelling

ALTERNATE ITEM FORMAT: MULTIPLE RESPONSE

166. A client who had abdominal surgery complains of feeling as though "something gave way" in the incisional site. The nurse removes the dressing and notes the presence of a loop of bowel protruding through the incision. Select all nursing interventions that the nurse would take.

- ☑ **1.** Notify the registered nurse.
- ☑ **2.** Document the client's complaint.
- ☑ **3.** Instruct the client to remain quiet.
- ☑ **4.** Prepare the client for wound closure.
- ☐ **5.** Place a sterile saline dressing and ice packs over the wound.
- ☐ **6.** Place the client in a supine position without a pillow under the head.

ANSWERS

153. **1**
Rationale: The nurse would assist the client with voiding immediately before surgery so that the bladder will be empty. Oral hygiene is allowed, but the client should not swallow any water. The client usually has a restriction of food and fluids for 8 hours before surgery rather than 24 hours. A slight increase in blood pressure and pulse is common during the preoperative period; this is generally the result of anxiety.
Test-Taking Strategy: Use the process of elimination, and read each option carefully. Eliminate option 3, knowing that the client should receive nothing by mouth for 8 hours before surgery. Eliminate option 4 because of the words "immediately" and "slight." There is no useful reason for option 2; in fact, oral hygiene may make the client feel more comfortable. Review general preoperative care if you had difficulty with this question.
Level of Cognitive Ability: Application
Client Needs: Physiological Integrity
Integrated Process: Nursing Process/Planning
Content Area: Fundamental Skills
References: Perry, A., & Potter, P. (2006). *Clinical nursing skills & techniques* (6th ed., p. 1202). St. Louis: Mosby.
Potter, P., & Perry, A. (2005). *Fundamentals of nursing* (6th ed., pp. 1606, 1609). St. Louis: Mosby.

154. **3**
Rationale: Explanations should begin with the information that the client knows. Option 1 is a block to communication, and options 2 and 4 may produce additional anxiety in the client.
Test-Taking Strategy: Use the process of elimination. Remember to always focus on the client's feelings first; this will direct you to option 3. Additionally, option 3 is the only option that addresses Data Collection, which is the first step of the Nursing Process. Review the psychosocial aspects related to the preoperative client if you had difficulty with this question.
Level of Cognitive Ability: Application
Client Needs: Psychosocial Integrity
Integrated Process: Caring
Content Area: Fundamental Skills
References: Christensen, B., & Kockrow, E. (2006). *Adult health nursing* (5th ed. pp. 23-24). St. Louis: Mosby.
Potter, P., & Perry, A. (2005). *Fundamentals of nursing* (6th ed., p. 1604). St. Louis: Mosby.

155. **3**
Rationale: Anticoagulants alter normal clotting factors and increase the risk of hemorrhage. Aspirin has properties that can alter the clotting mechanism and should thus be discontinued at least 48 hours before surgery.
Test-Taking Strategy: Use the process of elimination. Remembering that aspirin has properties that can alter normal clotting factors and that it should be discontinued at least 48 hours before surgery will assist with directing you to option 3. Review the medications that affect the preoperative client if you had difficulty with this question.
Level of Cognitive Ability: Application
Client Needs: Physiological Integrity
Integrated Process: Nursing Process/Planning
Content Area: Fundamental Skills
References: Linton, A. (2007). *Introduction to medical-surgical nursing* (4th ed., p. 248). Philadelphia: Saunders.
Potter, P., & Perry, A. (2005). *Fundamentals of nursing* (6th ed., p. 1602). St. Louis: Mosby.

156. **2**
Rationale: A slightly lower-than-normal BP and an increased pulse rate are common after surgery. Warm blankets are applied to maintain the client's body temperature. The level of consciousness can be determined by checking the client's response to light touch and verbal stimuli rather than by shaking the client. There is no reason to contact the registered nurse immediately.
Test-Taking Strategy: Focus on the data in the question. Noting that the vital signs are within normal limits will direct you to option 2. Review expected postoperative findings if you had difficulty with this question.
Level of Cognitive Ability: Application
Client Needs: Physiological Integrity
Integrated Process: Nursing Process/Implementation
Content Area: Fundamental Skills
References: Christensen, B., & Kockrow, E. (2006). *Adult health nursing* (5th ed., pp. 51-52). St. Louis: Mosby.
Linton, A. (2007). *Introduction to medical-surgical nursing* (4th ed., pp. 264, 266-267). Philadelphia: Saunders.

157. **1**
Rationale: If the airway is not patent, immediate measures must be taken for the survival of the client. After checking the client's airway, the nurse would then check the client's vital signs, and this would be followed by checking the dressings, tubes, and drains.

Test-Taking Strategy: Use the ABCs—airway, breathing, and circulation. Maintaining the airway patency is the first action to be taken. Options 2, 3, and 4 are all nursing actions that should be performed after a patent airway has been established. Review the care of the postoperative client if you had difficulty with this question.
Level of Cognitive Ability: Application
Client Needs: Physiological Integrity
Integrated Process: Nursing Process/Implementation
Content Area: Delegating/Prioritizing
References: Linton A. (2007). *Introduction to medical-surgical nursing* (4th ed., p. 264). Philadelphia: Saunders.
Potter, P., & Perry, A. (2005). *Fundamentals of nursing* (6th ed., p. 1632). St. Louis: Mosby.

158. 1
Rationale: Urine output is maintained at a minimum of at least 30 mL/hour for an adult. An output of less than 30 mL/hour for each of two consecutive hours should be reported to the physician. A temperature more than 37° C (100° F) or less than 36.1° C (97° F) and a falling systolic blood pressure less than 90 mm Hg are to be reported. The client's preoperative or baseline blood pressure is used to make informed postoperative comparisons. Moderate or light serous drainage from the surgical site is considered normal.
Test-Taking Strategy: Knowledge of the normal ranges for temperature, blood pressure, urinary output, and wound drainage is necessary to determine the correct option. Use the process of elimination to determine that the urinary output is the only observation that is not within the normal range. Review expected postoperative findings if you had difficulty with this question.
Level of Cognitive Ability: Analysis
Client Needs: Physiological Integrity
Integrated Process: Nursing Process/Data Collection
Content Area: Fundamental Skills
References: Christensen, B., & Kockrow, E. (2006). *Adult health nursing* (5th ed. p. 56). St. Louis: Mosby.
Linton, A. (2007). *Introduction to medical-surgical nursing* (4th ed., p. 274). Philadelphia: Saunders.

159. 1
Rationale: The most common postoperative respiratory problems are atelectasis, pneumonia, and pulmonary emboli. Pneumonia is the inflammation of lung tissue that causes a productive cough, dyspnea, and crackles. Pulmonary edema usually results from left-sided heart failure, and it can be caused by medications, fluid overload, and smoke inhalation. Carbon dioxide retention results from the inability to exhale carbon dioxide in clients with conditions such as chronic obstructive pulmonary disease. Fluid imbalance can be a deficit or excess related to fluid loss or overload.
Test-Taking Strategy: Use the process of elimination, and note the strategic words "presence of secretions in the lungs." Focus on the subject of the postoperative client to direct you to option 1. Options 2, 3, and 4 most commonly occur with other conditions. Review postoperative complications if you had difficulty with this question.
Level of Cognitive Ability: Comprehension
Client Needs: Physiological Integrity

Integrated Process: Nursing Process/Data Collection
Content Area: Fundamental Skills
References: Linton, A. (2007). *Introduction to medical-surgical nursing* (4th ed., p. 272). Philadelphia: Saunders.
Potter, P., & Perry, A. (2005). *Fundamentals of nursing* (6th ed., p. 1636). St. Louis: Mosby.

160. 4
Rationale: Aseptic technique must be used when emptying the drainage container or changing the dressing to avoid contamination of the wound. Usually drainage from the wound is pale, red, and watery, whereas active bleeding will be bright red in color. The drain should be checked for patency to provide an exit for the fluid or blood to promote healing. The nurse needs to ensure that drainage flows freely and that there are no kinks in the drains. Curling or folding the drain prevents the flow of the drainage.
Test-Taking Strategy: Use the process of elimination, and note the strategic word "inappropriate." Remember that the nurse needs to ensure that drainage flows freely from a drain. Review the care of the surgical client with a drain if you had difficulty with this question.
Level of Cognitive Ability: Application
Client Needs: Physiological Integrity
Integrated Process: Nursing Process/Implementation
Content Area: Fundamental Skills
References: Christensen, B., & Kockrow, E. (2006). *Adult health nursing* (5th ed., p. 52). St. Louis: Mosby.
Ignatavicius, D., & Workman, M. (2006). *Medical-surgical nursing: Critical thinking for collaborative care* (5th ed., p. 346). Philadelphia: Saunders.
Lewis, S., Heitkemper, M., Dirksen, S., & Bucher, L., (2007). *Medical-surgical nursing: Assessment and management of clinical problems* (7th ed., p. 393). St. Louis: Mosby.

161. 2
Rationale: Signs and symptoms of a wound infection include warm, red, and tender skin around the incision. The client may have fever and chills. Purulent material may exit from drains or from separated wound edges. Infection may be caused by poor aseptic technique or a wound that was contaminated before surgical exploration; it appears 3 to 6 days after surgery. Serous drainage is not indicative of a wound infection. A temperature of 98.8° F is not an abnormal finding in a postoperative client. The fact that a client feels cold is not indicative of an infection, although chills and fever are signs of infection.
Test-Taking Strategy: Use the process of elimination. Noting the word "purulent" in option 2 will direct you to this option. Review the signs of a wound infection if you had difficulty with this question.
Level of Cognitive Ability: Comprehension
Client Needs: Physiological Integrity
Integrated Process: Nursing Process/Data Collection
Content Area: Fundamental Skills
References: Linton, A. (2007). *Introduction to medical-surgical nursing* (4th ed., pp. 271-272). Philadelphia: Saunders.
Potter, P., & Perry, A. (2005). *Fundamentals of nursing* (6th ed., p. 1640). St. Louis: Mosby.

162. **2**

Rationale: Wound dehiscence is the separation of the wound edges at the suture line. Signs and symptoms include increased drainage and the appearance of underlying tissues. It usually occurs as a complication 6 to 8 days after surgery. The client should be instructed to remain quiet and to avoid coughing or straining, and he or she should be positioned to prevent further stress on the wound. Sterile dressings soaked with sterile normal saline should be used to cover the wound. The physician needs to be notified.

Test-Taking Strategy: Use the process of elimination. Eliminate option 3 first, because this action would expose the open wound and the underlying tissues to infection. Eliminate options 1 and 4 next, because a dry dressing and a dressing soaked with Betadine will irritate the exposed body tissues. Review emergency care when dehiscence or evisceration occurs if you had difficulty with this question.

Level of Cognitive Ability: Application
Client Needs: Physiological Integrity
Integrated Process: Nursing Process/Implementation
Content Area: Fundamental Skills
References: Christensen, B., & Kockrow, E. (2006). *Adult health nursing* (5th ed., p. 52). St. Louis: Mosby.
Linton, A. (2007). *Introduction to medical-surgical nursing* (4th ed., p. 263). Philadelphia: Saunders.

163. **1**

Rationale: Increasing restlessness noted in a client is a sign that requires continuous and close monitoring, because it could be a potential indication of a complication such as hemorrhage or shock. A negative Homans' sign is normal. However, a positive Homans' sign may be indicative of thrombophlebitis. Faint bowel sounds heard in all four quadrants is a normal occurrence. A blood pressure of 120/70 mm Hg with a pulse of 90 beats per minute is a relatively normal sign.

Test-Taking Strategy: Use the process of elimination. Eliminate options 2, 3, and 4, because these are normal and expected findings. Review the normal and expected postoperative findings if you had difficulty with this question.

Level of Cognitive Ability: Analysis
Client Needs: Physiological Integrity
Integrated Process: Nursing Process/Data Collection
Content Area: Fundamental Skills
References: Christensen, B., & Kockrow, E. (2006). *Adult health nursing* (5th ed. p. 52). St. Louis: Mosby.
Potter, P., & Perry, A. (2005). *Fundamentals of nursing* (6th ed., p. 1636). St. Louis: Mosby.

164. **4**

Rationale: The time-out occurs in the perioperative area after the client has been prepped and draped. The entire team must verbally verify their agreement regarding the client's name, the procedure to be performed, and the surgical site. Options 1, 2, and 3 are incorrect, because they do not occur during the intraoperative period in the perioperative area.

Test-Taking Strategy: Note the strategic words "perioperative area." Recalling the procedures that occur during this period will assist you with eliminating options 1, 2, and 3. Review the definition of a time-out and the procedures that occur during the intraoperative period if you had difficulty with this question.

Level of Cognitive Ability: Application
Client Needs: Physiological Integrity
Integrated Process: Nursing Process/Implementation
Content Area: Fundamental Skills
Reference: Phipps, W., Monahan, F., Marek, J., Neighbors, M., & Green, C., (2007). *Medical-surgical nursing: Health and illness perspectives* (8th ed., p. 259). St. Louis: Mosby.

165. **1**

Rationale: The surgeon is responsible for verifying the operative site, and he or she must mark the operative site before the client is brought into the operating suite. The client will be asked to verify the site that requires surgery. The client may refuse to have the site marked and is asked about marking the site. Although the nurse may also verify the site, this procedure is a primary responsibility of the physician. Verification of the site should be done both before and during the time-out period. The verification of the surgical site is not done at the completion of the procedure.

Test-Taking Strategy: Focus on the subject of surgical site marking, and remember that it is the physician's responsibility to verify the surgical site. Review TJC's universal protocol for preventing wrong-site, wrong-procedure, and wrong-person surgery if you had difficulty with this question.

Level of Cognitive Ability: Application
Client Needs: Safe and Effective Care Environment
Integrated Process: Nursing Process/Implementation
Content Area: Fundamental Skills
Reference: Phipps, W., Monahan, F., Marek, J., Neighbors, M., & Green, C. (2007). *Medical-surgical nursing: Health and illness perspectives* (8th ed., pp. 258-259). St. Louis: Mosby.

ALTERNATE ITEM FORMAT: MULTIPLE RESPONSE

166. **1, 2, 3, 4**

Rationale: Wound dehiscence is the separation of the wound edges, and wound evisceration is the protrusion of the internal organs through an incision. If wound dehiscence or evisceration occurs, the registered nurse is notified, and he or she then contacts the surgeon immediately. The client is placed in a low Fowler's position, kept quiet, and instructed to not cough. Protruding organs are covered with a sterile, saline dressing. Ice packs are not applied. The treatment for evisceration is immediate wound closure under local or general anesthesia.

Test-Taking Strategy: Focus on the information in the question to determine that the client is experiencing wound evisceration. Visualizing this occurrence will assist you with determining that the client would not be placed supine and that ice packs would not be placed on the incision. Review wound evisceration if you had difficulty with this question.

Level of Cognitive Ability: Application
Client Needs: Physiological Integrity
Integrated Process: Nursing Process/Implementation
Content Area: Fundamental Skills
References: Christensen, B., & Kockrow, E. (2006). *Adult health nursing* (5th ed., p. 52). St. Louis: Mosby.
Monahan, F., Marek, J., Neighbors, M., & Green, C., (2007). *Phipps' medical-surgical nursing: Health and illness perspectives* (8th ed., pp. 319, 328). St. Louis: Mosby.

REFERENCES

Christensen, B., & Kockrow, E. (2006). *Adult health nursing* (5th ed.). St. Louis: Mosby.

Ignatavicius, D., & Workman, M. (2006). *Medical-surgical nursing: Critical thinking for collaborative care* (5th ed.). Philadelphia: Saunders.

Lewis, S., Heitkemper, M., Dirksen, S., & Bucher, L. (2007). *Medical-surgical nursing: Assessment and management of clinical problems* (7th ed.). St. Louis: Mosby.

Linton, A. (2007). *Introduction to medical-surgical nursing* (4th ed.). Philadelphia: Saunders.

Monahan, F., Marek, J., Neighbors, M., & Green, C. (2007). *Phipps' medical-surgical nursing: Health and illness perspectives* (8th ed.). St. Louis: Mosby.

National Council of State Boards of Nursing (Eds.) (2008). *2008 Detailed Test Plan for the NCLEX-PN® Examination, National Council of State Boards of Nursing.* Chicago: Author.

National Council of State Boards of Nursing. *NCSBN home page.* www.ncsbn.org. Accessed June 26, 2008.

Perry, A., & Potter, P. (2006). *Clinical nursing skills & techniques* (6th ed.). St. Louis: Mosby.

Potter, P., & Perry, A. (2005). *Fundamentals of nursing* (6th ed.). St. Louis: Mosby.

Positioning Clients

PYRAMID TERMS

ergonomic principles The anatomical, physiological, and mechanical principles affecting the effecient and safe use of an individual's energy.

Fowler's position The client is supine, and the head of the bed is elevated to 45 to 60 degrees.

high Fowler's position The client is supine, and the head of the bed is elevated to 90 degrees; the knees of the bed are often slightly raised to prevent client sliding and shear injuries.

lateral (side-lying) position The client is lying on the side, and the head and shoulders are aligned with the hips and the spine parallel to the edge of the mattress; the head, neck, and upper arm are supported by a pillow; the lower shoulder is pulled forward slightly and, along with the elbow, it is flexed at 90 degrees; the legs are flexed or extended, and a pillow is placed to support the back.

lithotomy position The client is lying on his or her back with the hips and knees flexed at right angles and the feet in stirrups.

prone position The client is lying on his or her abdomen with the head turned to the side.

reverse Trendelenburg's position The bed is tilted so that the foot of the client's bed is lower than the head of the bed.

semi-Fowler's position (low Fowler's position) The client is supine, and the head of the bed is elevated approximately 30 degrees.

Sims' position The client is lying on his or her side with the body turned prone at 45 degrees; the lower leg is extended with the upper leg flexed at the hip and knee at a 45- to 90-degree angle.

supine position The client is lying on his or her back; the head and shoulders are usually slightly elevated with a small pillow; the arms and legs are extended, and the legs are slightly abducted; an open airway should be preserved in clients with decreased levels of consciousness.

Trendelenburg's position The bed is tilted so that the head of the client's bed is lower than the foot of the bed; this position is contraindicated for clients with head injuries, increased intracranial pressure, spinal cord injuries, and certain cardiac and respiratory disorders.

PYRAMID TO SUCCESS

Nursing responsibilities include positioning clients in a safe and appropriate manner to provide safety and comfort. Knowledge regarding the client's position required for a certain procedure or condition is expected. It is the nurse's responsibility to reduce the likelihood and prevent the development of complications related to an existing condition, a prescribed treatment, or a medical or surgical procedure. It is imperative that the nurse review the physician's orders after treatments or procedures and that he or she take note of instructions regarding positioning and mobility (Figures 18-1 and 18-2). The nurse must also be aware of the various body pressure points when clients are positioned in lying or sitting positions (Figure 18-3). The Integrated Processes addressed in this chapter include Caring, Communication and Documentation, the Clinical Problem-Solving Process (Nursing Process), and Teaching and Learning.

CLIENT NEEDS

Safe and Effective Care Environment

Preventing accidents and injuries
Positioning the client appropriately and safely
Ensuring environmental and personal safety
Establishing priorities
Ensuring home safety
Providing protective measures
Using equipment safely
Using ergonomic principles and body mechanics when moving a client

Health Promotion and Maintenance

Providing information regarding the need for prescribed therapies
Performing the techniques of data collection

Psychosocial Integrity

Assisting the client with the use of coping mechanisms
Keeping the family informed about the client's progress
Providing support to the client

Physiological Integrity

Providing comfort measures for rest and sleep
Assessing the client's mobility and immobility levels
Preventing the complications of immobility
Providing nutrition and oral intake
Providing personal hygiene to the client as needed
Using assistive devices

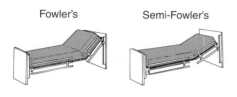

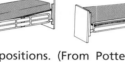

Fowler's   Semi-Fowler's

Trendelenburg's   Reverse Trendelenburg's   Flat

FIG. 18-1 Common bed positions. (From Potter, P., & Perry, A. [2005]. *Fundamentals of nursing* [6th ed.]. St. Louis: Mosby.)

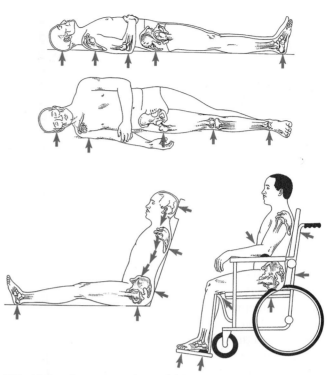

FIG. 18-3 Pressure points of lying and sitting positions. (From Elkin, M., Perry, A., & Potter, P. [2008]. *Nursing interventions and clinical skills* [4th ed.]. St. Louis: Mosby.)

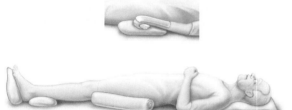

Supine position

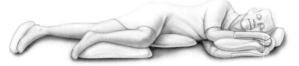

Lateral (side-lying) position

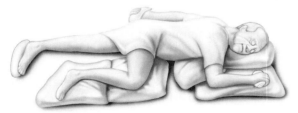

Semiprone (Sims' or forward side-lying) position

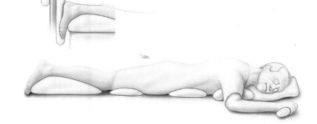
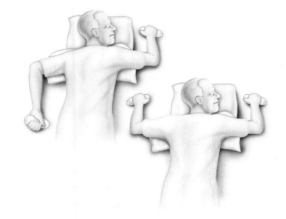

Prone position

FIG. 18-2 Common client positions. (From Harkreader, H. & Hogan, M. [2004]. *Fundamentals of nursing: Caring and clinical judgment* [2nd ed.]. Philadelphia: Saunders.)

I. GUIDELINES FOR POSITIONING

A. Principles of body movement for clients
   1. Body movement and alignment are important for clients; many clients are unable to change position or move in bed independently
   2. Basic principles include maintaining correct anatomical position and changing the position frequently
B. Position in a safe and appropriate manner to provide safety, alignment, and comfort
C. Review the physician's orders, especially after treatments or procedures, and take note of instructions regarding positioning and mobility
D. Select a position that will prevent the development of complications related to an existing condition, a prescribed treatment, or a medical or surgical procedure

II. ERGONOMIC PRINCIPLES RELATED TO BODY MECHANICS (Box 18-1)

III. POSITIONS TO ENSURE SAFETY AND COMFORT

A. Integumentary system
   1. Autograft: After surgery, the site is immobilized for approximately 3 to 7 days to provide the time needed for the graft to adhere and attach to the wound bed
   2. Burns of the face and head: Elevate the head of the bed to prevent or reduce facial, head, and tracheal edema
   3. Circumferential burns of the extremities: Elevate the extremities above the level of the heart to prevent or reduce dependent edema
   4. Skin graft: Elevate and immobilize the graft site to prevent the movement and shearing of the graft and the disruption of tissue; avoid weight bearing
B. Reproductive system
   1. Mastectomy
      a. Position the client with the head of the bed elevated at least 30 degrees, with the affected arm elevated on a pillow to promote lymphatic fluid return after the removal of axillary lymph nodes
      b. Turn the client only to the back and the unaffected side
   2. Perineal and vaginal procedures: Place the client in the **lithotomy position** (Figure 18-4)
C. Endocrine system
   1. Hypophysectomy: Elevate the head of the bed to prevent increased intracranial pressure
   2. Thyroidectomy
      a. Place the client in **semi-Fowler's position** to reduce swelling and edema in the neck area
      b. Sandbags or pillows may be used to support the client's head or neck
D. Gastrointestinal system
   1. Hemorrhoidectomy: Assist the client to a **lateral (side-lying) position** to prevent pain and bleeding

---

BOX 18-1	**Body Mechanics for Health Care Workers**

Action
1. When planning to move a client, arrange for adequate help. Use mechanical aids if help is unavailable.
2. Encourage the client to assist as much as possible.
3. Keep your back, neck, pelvis, and feet aligned. Avoid twisting.
4. Flex your knees, and keep your feet wide apart.
5. Position yourself close to the client or to the object being lifted.
6. Use your arms and legs rather than your back.
7. Slide the client toward yourself using a pull sheet. When transferring a client onto a stretcher, a slide board is more appropriate.
8. Set (tighten) your abdominal and gluteal muscles in preparation for the move.
9. The person with the heaviest load should coordinate the efforts of the team involved by counting to three.

Modified from Elkin, M., Perry, A., & Potter, P. (2004) *Nursing interventions and clinical skills* (3rd ed., p. 111). St. Louis: Mosby.

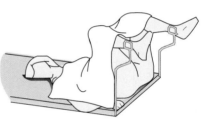

FIG. 18-4 Lithotomy position for examination. (From Potter, P., & Perry, A. [2005]. *Fundamentals of nursing* [6th ed.]. St. Louis: Mosby.)

   2. Gastroesophageal reflux disease: **Reverse Trendelenburg's position** may be prescribed to promote gastric emptying and prevent esophageal reflux
   3. Liver biopsy
      a. During the procedure
         (1) Position the client supine with the right side of the upper abdomen exposed
         (2) The client's right arm is raised and extended over the left shoulder behind the head
         (3) The liver is located on the right side, and this position provides for maximal exposure of the right intercostal spaces
      b. After the procedure
         (1) Assist the client into a right **lateral (side-lying) position**
         (2) Place a small pillow or folded towel under the puncture site for at least 3 hours to provide pressure to the site and prevent bleeding

4. Nasogastric tube
   a. Insertion
      (1) Position the client in **high Fowler's position** with the head tilted forward
      (2) This position will help close the trachea and open the esophagus
   b. Irrigations and tube feedings
      (1) Keep the head of the bed elevated 30 degrees (**semi-Fowler's position**) to prevent aspiration
      (2) Maintain head elevation for 1 hour after an intermittent feeding
      (3) The head of the bed should remain elevated for continuous feedings
5. Rectal enemas or irrigations: Place the client in left **Sims' position** to allow the solution to flow by gravity in the natural direction of the colon
6. Sengstaken-Blakemore tube: Maintain the elevation of the head of the bed to increase lung expansion and reduce portal blood flow, thereby permitting the effective compression of the esophageal varices

E. Respiratory system
   1. Chronic obstructive pulmonary disease: For the client with advanced disease, place the client in a sitting position, leaning forward, with the arms over several pillows or on an overbed table; this position will help the client to breathe easier
   2. Laryngectomy (radical neck dissection): Place the client in **semi-Fowler's** or **Fowler's position** to maintain a patent airway and minimize edema
   3. Bronchoscopy postprocedure: Place the client in a **semi-Fowler's position** to prevent choking or aspiration resulting from an impaired ability to swallow
   4. Postural drainage: The lung segment to be drained should be in the uppermost position; **Trendelenburg's position** may be used
   5. Thoracentesis
      a. During the procedure: To facilitate the removal of fluid from the chest wall, position the client sitting on the edge of the bed and leaning over the bedside table with the feet supported on a stool or lying in bed on the unaffected side with the head of the bed elevated approximately 45 degrees (**Fowler's position**)
      b. After the procedure: Assist the client to a position of comfort
   6. Thoracotomy: Check the physician's orders regarding positioning

F. Cardiovascular system
   1. Abdominal aneurysm resection
      a. After surgery, limit the elevation of the head of the bed to 45 degrees (**Fowler's position**) to avoid flexion of the graft
      b. The client may be turned from side to side
   2. Amputation of the lower extremity
      a. During the first 24 hours after amputation, elevate the foot of the bed to reduce edema; the stump is supported with pillows but not elevated because of the risk of flexion contractures
      b. Consult with the physician and then position the client prone twice a day for a 20- to 30-minute period to stretch muscles and prevent flexion contractures of the hip
   3. Arterial vascular grafting of an extremity
      a. To promote graft patency after the procedure, bedrest is usually maintained for approximately 24 hours, and the client's affected extremity is kept straight
      b. Limit movement and avoid flexion of the client's hip and knee
   4. Cardiac catheterization
      a. If the femoral artery was used, the client is maintained on bedrest for approximately 3 to 4 hours; the client may turn from side to side
      b. The client's affected extremity is kept straight and the head elevated no more than 30 degrees until hemostasis is adequately achieved
   5. Congestive heart failure and pulmonary edema: Position the client upright (**high Fowler's position**), preferably with the bed in a chair-sitting position, to decrease venous return and lung congestion
   6. Peripheral arterial disease
      a. Obtain the physician's order for positioning
      b. Because swelling can prevent arterial blood flow, clients may be advised to elevate their feet when at rest; they should not raise their legs above the level of the heart, because extreme elevation slows arterial blood flow; some clients may be advised to maintain a slightly dependent position to promote perfusion
   7. Deep vein thrombosis
      a. If the extremity is red, edematous, and painful and traditional heparin therapy is initiated, bedrest with leg elevation may be prescribed for the client
      b. Clients receiving low-molecular-weight heparin can usually be out of bed after 24 hours, if the pain level permits
   8. Varicose veins: Leg elevation above the level of the heart is usually prescribed; the client is also advised to minimize prolonged sitting or standing during daily activities
   9. Venous insufficiency and leg ulcers: Leg elevation is usually prescribed

G. Sensory system
   1. Cataract surgery: Postoperatively, elevate the head of the bed (**semi-Fowler's** to **Fowler's**

position), and position the client on the back or the nonoperative side to prevent the development of edema at the operative site

2. Retinal detachment
   a. If the detachment is large, bedrest and bilateral eye patching may be prescribed to minimize eye movement and prevent the extension of the detachment
   b. Restrictions in activity and positioning after the repair of the detachment depend on the physician's preference and the surgical procedure performed

H. Neurological system
   1. Autonomic dysreflexia: Elevate the head of the bed to a **high Fowler's position** to help with adequate ventilation and the prevention of hypertensive stroke
   2. Cerebral aneurysm: Bedrest is maintained with the head of the bed elevated 30 to 45 degrees (**semi-Fowler's** to **Fowler's position**) to prevent pressure on the aneurysm site
   3. Cerebral angiography
      a. Maintain bedrest for 12 to 24 hours, as prescribed
      b. The extremity into which the contrast medium is injected is kept straight and immobilized for approximately 8 hours
   4. Brain attack (stroke)
      a. In clients with hemorrhagic strokes, the head of the bed is usually elevated to 30 degrees to reduce intracranial pressure and facilitate venous drainage
      b. For clients with ischemic strokes, the head of the bed is usually kept flat
      c. Maintain the client's head in a midline, neutral position to facilitate venous drainage from the head
      d. Avoid extreme hip and neck flexion; extreme hip flexion may increase intrathoracic pressure, whereas extreme neck flexion prohibits venous drainage from the brain
   5. Craniotomy
      a. The client should not be positioned on the site that was operated on, especially if the bone flap has been removed, because the brain has no bony covering over the affected site
      b. Elevate the head of the bed 30 to 45 degrees (**semi-Fowler's** to **Fowler's position**), and maintain the head in a midline, neutral position to facilitate venous drainage from the head
      c. Avoid extreme hip and neck flexion
   6. Traumatic head injury: Elevate the head of the bed
   7. Laminectomy
      a. Logroll the client
      b. When the client is out of bed, the client's back is kept straight (the client is placed in

a straight-backed chair) with the feet resting comfortably on the floor

8. Increased intracranial pressure
   a. Elevate the head of the bed 30 to 45 degrees (**semi-Fowler's** to **Fowler's position**), and maintain the head in a midline, neutral position to facilitate venous drainage from the head
   b. Avoid extreme hip and neck flexion
9. Lumbar puncture
   a. During the procedure: Assist the client to the **lateral (side-lying) position**, with the back bowed at the edge of the examining table, the knees flexed up to the abdomen, and the head bent so that the chin is resting on the chest
   b. After the procedure: Place the client in the **supine position** for 4 to 12 hours, as prescribed
10. Myelogram postprocedure
    a. The head position varies according to the dye used
    b. The head is usually elevated if an oil-based or water-soluble contrast agent is used; the head is usually positioned lower than the trunk if air contrast is used
11. Spinal cord injury
    a. Immobilize the client on a spinal backboard with the head in a neutral position to prevent an incomplete injury from becoming complete
    b. Prevent head flexion, rotation, or extension; the head is immobilized with a firm, padded cervical collar
    c. Logroll the client; no part of the body should be twisted or turned, and the client should not be allowed to assume a sitting position

I. Musculoskeletal system
   1. Total hip replacement
      a. Positioning depends on the surgical techniques used, the method of implantation, and the prosthesis
      b. Avoid extreme internal and external rotation
      c. Avoid adduction; a side-lying position on the operative side is not allowed (unless specifically prescribed by the physician)
      d. Maintain abduction when the client is in a **supine position** or positioned on the unoperative side
      e. Place a pillow between the client's legs to maintain abduction; instruct the client to not cross the legs
      f. Check the physician's orders regarding the elevation of the head of the bed; flexion is usually limited to 60 degrees during the first postoperative week and then to 90 degrees for 2 to 3 months thereafter
   2. Devices used for proper positioning (Box 18-2)

BOX 18-2 Devices Used for Proper Positioning

Pillows
Pillows provide support, elevate body parts, splint incisional areas, and reduce postoperative pain during activity, coughing, or deep breathing. They should be the appropriate size for the body part to be positioned.

Foot Boots
Foot boots are made of rigid plastic or heavy foam, and they keep the foot flexed at the proper angle. They should be removed two or three times a day to assess skin integrity and joint mobility.

Trochanter Rolls
These rolls prevent the external rotation of the legs when the client is in the supine position. To form a roll, use a cotton bath blanket or a sheet folded lengthwise to a width that extends from the greater trochanter of the femur to the lower border of the popliteal space.

Sandbags
Sandbags are filled plastic tubes that can be shaped to body contours to provide support. They immobilize the extremities and maintain specific body alignment.

Hand Rolls
Hand rolls maintain the fingers in a slightly flexed and functional position, and they keep the thumb slightly adducted in opposition to the fingers.

Hand–Wrist Splints
These splints are individually molded for the client to maintain the proper alignment of the thumb in slight adduction and the wrist in slight dorsiflexion.

Trapeze Bar
This bar descends from a securely fastened overhead bar attached to the bed frame. It allows the client to use the upper extremities to raise the trunk off of the bed, to assist with transfer from the bed to a wheelchair, and to perform upper-arm strengthening exercises.

Side Rails
These bars, which are positioned along the sides of the length of the bed, ensure client safety and are useful for increasing mobility. They also provide assistance to the client with rolling from side to side or sitting up in bed.

Bed Boards
These plywood boards are placed under the entire surface area of the mattress. They are useful for increasing back support and body alignment.

Wedge Pillow
This triangular-shaped pillow is made of heavy foam, and it is used to maintain the legs in abduction after total hip replacement surgery.

Modified from Potter, P., & Perry, A. (2001). *Fundamentals of nursing* (5th ed., p. 1456). St. Louis: Mosby.

PRACTICE QUESTIONS

More questions on the companion CD!

167. A nurse is preparing to reposition a dependent client who weighs more than 250 pounds. What intervention is best for the nurse to consider when moving this client?
   1. Get help.
   2. Keep elbows close and work close to the body.

3. First, place the client in Trendelenburg's position
4. Administer oral pain medication 5 minutes before moving the client.

168. A nurse is assigned to assist with caring for a client after cardiac catheterization. The nurse plans to maintain bedrest with:
   1. High Fowler's position
   2. Bathroom privileges only
   3. Head elevation of 45 degrees
   4. Head elevation of no more than 30 degrees

169. A nurse is reinforcing home-care instructions to a client and family regarding care after cataract removal from the right eye. Which of the following statements, if made by the client, would indicate an understanding of the instructions?
   1. "I will not sleep on my left side."
   2. "I will not sleep on my right side."
   3. "I will take aspirin if I have any pain."
   4. "I will not wear my glasses until my physician says it is OK."

170. After a liver biopsy, the nurse places the client in which of the following positions?
   1. Prone
   2. Supine
   3. A left side-lying position with a small pillow or folded towel under the puncture site
   4. A right side-lying position with a small pillow or folded towel under the puncture site

171. A nurse is administering a cleansing enema to a client with a fecal impaction. Before administering the enema, the nurse assists the client to which of the following positions?
   1. Left Sims' position
   2. Right Sims' position
   3. On the left side of the body with the head of the bed elevated 45 degrees
   4. On the right side of the body with the head of the bed elevated 45 degrees

172. A client is being prepared for a thoracentesis. The nurse assigned to care for the client assists the client to which of the following positions for the procedure?
   1. Sims' position with the head of the bed flat
   2. Prone with the head turned to the side supported by a pillow
   3. Lying in bed on the affected side with the head of the bed elevated 45 degrees
   4. Lying in bed on the unaffected side with the head of the bed elevated 45 degrees

173. A nurse is assisting with the insertion of a nasogastric tube into a client. The nurse places the client in which position for insertion?
   1. Right side
   2. Low Fowler's position

3. High Fowler's position

4. Supine with the head flat

174. A nurse is assisting with caring for a client after a craniotomy. The nurse plans to position the client in a:

1. Prone position

2. Supine position

3. Semi-Fowler's position

4. Dorsal recumbent position

175. A nurse is turning a postoperative client who had extensive back surgery yesterday. What turning intervention or position would be best for repositioning this client?

1. Logrolling

2. Semi-Fowler's

3. Sims' (semi-prone)

4. 30-degree lateral (side-lying)

ALTERNATE ITEM FORMAT: MULTIPLE RESPONSE

176. The nurse is caring for a client after a supratentorial craniotomy in which a large tumor was removed from the left side. Choose the positions in which the nurse can safely place the client. Select all that apply.

☐ **1.** On the left side

☐ **2.** With the neck flexed

☐ **3.** Supine on the left side

☐ **4.** With extreme hip flexion

☑ **5.** In a semi-Fowler's position

☑ **6.** With the head in a midline position

ANSWERS

167. 1

Rationale: Although it is possible to move and position clients independently, getting help first is the best intervention. Lower back strain is a common injury among health care workers. In addition, the shearing of the client's skin over bony prominences may occur when health care workers move clients independently. Administering oral pain medication is necessary, but oral medications need to be given at least 30 to 45 minutes before clients are moved. Keeping the elbows close and working close to the body are useful techniques, but they would not be enough when independently moving a 250-pound client. This client is dependent, so he or she is probably not able to help much, if any.

Test-Taking Strategy: Focus on the data in the question. This client's dependent condition and weight make him or her too difficult for one person to move. Review the procedures and interventions for moving and positioning clients if you had difficulty with this question.

Level of Cognitive Ability: Application

Client Needs: Physiological Integrity

Integrated Process: Nursing Process/Planning

Content Area: Fundamental Skills

References: deWit, S. (2005). *Fundamental concepts and skills for nursing* (2nd ed., p. 246). St. Louis: Saunders.

Christensen, B., & Kockrow, E. (2006). *Foundations of nursing* (5th ed., p. 396). St. Louis: Mosby.

168. 4

Rationale: After cardiac catheterization, the extremity into which the catheter was inserted is kept straight for the prescribed time period. The client may turn from side to side. The head of the bed is not elevated to more than 30 degrees to keep the affected leg straight at the groin and to prevent arterial occlusion. Bathroom privileges are not allowed during the immediate postcatheterization period. For the high Fowler's position, the head of the bed is elevated 90 degrees.

Test-Taking Strategy: Use the process of elimination. Recalling that concerns after this procedure are bleeding and arterial occlusion will direct you to option 4. Review the care of the client after cardiac catheterization if you had difficulty with this question.

Level of Cognitive Ability: Application

Client Needs: Physiological Integrity

Integrated Process: Nursing Process/Planning

Content Area: Fundamental Skills

References: Chernecky, C., & Berger, B. (2008). *Laboratory tests and diagnostic procedures* (5th ed., p. 297). Philadelphia: Saunders.

Monahan, F., Marek, J., Neighbors, M., & Green, C., (2007). *Phipps' medical-surgical nursing: Health and illness perspectives* (8th ed., p. 742). St. Louis: Mosby.

169. 2

Rationale: After cataract surgery, the client should not sleep on the side of the body that was operated on. Clients should be instructed not to take aspirin or any medications that contain aspirin. Acetaminophen (Tylenol) can be taken as needed for pain. Clients may wear their glasses.

Test-Taking Strategy: Use the process of elimination. If you can remember to instruct clients to stay off of the operative side, this will assist you with answering questions related to cataract surgery. Review the care of the client after cataract surgery if you had difficulty with this question.

Level of Cognitive Ability: Comprehension

Client Needs: Physiological Integrity

Integrated Process: Nursing Process/Evaluation

Content Area: Fundamental Skills

Reference: Linton, A. (2007). *Introduction to medical-surgical nursing* (4th ed., p. 1177). Philadelphia: Saunders.

170. 4

Rationale: After a liver biopsy, the client is assisted with assuming a right side-lying position with a small pillow or folded towel under the puncture site for at least 3 hours. Options 1, 2, and 3 are incorrect positions.

Test-Taking Strategy: Knowledge regarding the anatomy of the body will assist you with answering this question. Remember that the liver is on the right side of the body and that the application of pressure on the right side will minimize the escape of blood or bile through the puncture site.

Review the care of the client after a liver biopsy if you had difficulty with this question.
Level of Cognitive Ability: Application
Client Needs: Physiological Integrity
Integrated Process: Nursing Process/Implementation
Content Area: Fundamental Skills
Reference: Chernecky, C., & Berger, B. (2008). *Laboratory tests and diagnostic procedures* (5th ed., p. 722). Philadelphia: Saunders.

171. **1**
Rationale: When administering an enema, the client is placed in a left Sims' position so that the enema solution can flow by gravity in the natural direction of the colon. The head of the bed is not elevated.
Test-Taking Strategy: Recalling the anatomy of the bowel will assist you with eliminating options 2 and 4. Option 3 can be eliminated next, because the head of the bed should be flat during enema administration. Review the procedure for enema administration if you had difficulty with this question.
Level of Cognitive Ability: Application
Client Needs: Physiological Integrity
Integrated Process: Nursing Process/Implementation
Content Area: Fundamental Skills
Reference: Christensen, B., & Kockrow, E. (2006). *Foundations of nursing* (5th ed., pp. 598-599). St. Louis: Mosby.

172. **4**
Rationale: To facilitate the removal of fluid from the chest, the client is positioned sitting on the edge of the bed, leaning over a bedside table, with the feet supported on a stool or lying in bed on the unaffected side with the head of the bed elevated 45 degrees (Fowler's position). Options 1, 2, and 3 are incorrect.
Test-Taking Strategy: Visualize this procedure. Option 3 can be eliminated because, if the client was lying on the affected side, it would be very difficult to perform the procedure. Option 1 can be eliminated, because, the Sims' position is primarily used for rectal enemas or irrigations. In the prone position, the client is lying on his or her abdomen, which is not an appropriate position for this procedure. Review the procedure for the removal of fluid from the chest if you had difficulty with this question.
Level of Cognitive Ability: Application
Client Needs: Physiological Integrity
Integrated Process: Nursing Process/Implementation
Content Area: Fundamental Skills
Reference: Chernecky, C., & Berger, B. (2008). *Laboratory tests and diagnostic procedures* (5th ed., pp. 1062-1064). Philadelphia: Saunders.

173. **3**
Rationale: During the insertion of a nasogastric tube, the client is placed in a sitting or high Fowler's position to reduce the risk of pulmonary aspiration if the client should vomit. Options 1, 2, and 4 do not facilitate the insertion of the tube or prevent aspiration.
Test-Taking Strategy: Use the process of elimination. Recalling that a concern with the insertion of a nasogastric tube is pulmonary aspiration will direct you to option 3. Review the procedure for inserting a nasogastric tube if you had difficulty with this question.

Level of Cognitive Ability: Application
Client Needs: Physiological Integrity
Integrated Process: Nursing Process/Implementation
Content Area: Fundamental Skills
References: Christensen, B., & Kockrow, E. (2006). *Foundations of nursing* (5th ed., p. 653). St. Louis: Mosby.
Linton, A. (2007). *Introduction to medical-surgical nursing* (4th ed., p. 740). Philadelphia: Saunders.

174. **3**
Rationale: After a craniotomy, the head of the bed is elevated 30 to 45 degrees (semi-Fowler's to Fowler's position), and the client's head is maintained in a midline, neutral position to facilitate venous drainage. Options 1, 2, and 4 are incorrect positions.
Test-Taking Strategy: Focus on the surgical procedure. Recalling that a goal of care after this surgery is to facilitate venous drainage will direct you to option 3. Review the care of the client after a craniotomy if you had difficulty with this question.
Level of Cognitive Ability: Application
Client Needs: Physiological Integrity
Integrated Process: Nursing Process/Planning
Content Area: Fundamental Skills
Reference: Linton, A. (2007). *Introduction to medical-surgical nursing* (4th ed., p. 430). Philadelphia: Saunders.

175. **1**
Rationale: Logrolling is used to maintain neck and spinal alignment after injury or surgery. A minimum of three to four staff members is recommended to prevent injury to the client, and a draw or pull sheet is also suggested. Options 2, 3, and 4 do not maintain proper spinal alignment and could be harmful.
Test-Taking Strategy: Focus on the type of surgery performed and the need to maintain proper spinal alignment; this will direct you to option 1. Review the care of the client after spinal surgery or injury if you had difficulty with this question.
Level of Cognitive Ability: Application
Client Needs: Physiological Integrity
Integrated Process: Nursing Process/Implementation
Content Area: Fundamental Skills
References: Elkin, M., Perry, A., & Potter, P., (2004). *Nursing interventions and clinical skills* (3rd ed., p. 118). St. Louis: Mosby.
Monahan, F., Marek, J., Neighbors, M., & Green, C., (2007). *Phipps' medical-surgical nursing: Health and illness perspectives* (8th ed., p. 1599). St. Louis: Mosby.

ALTERNATE ITEM FORMAT: MULTIPLE RESPONSE

176. **5, 6**
Rationale: Clients who have undergone supratentorial surgery should have the head of the bed elevated 30 degrees to promote venous drainage from the head. The client is positioned to avoid extreme hip or neck flexion, and the head is maintained in a midline, neutral position. If a large tumor has been removed, the client should be placed on the nonoperative side to prevent the displacement of the cranial contents.

Test-Taking Strategy: Focus on the data in the question. Remember that a primary concern is the risk for increased intracranial pressure. Therefore, use concepts related to preventing increased intracranial pressure to answer this question. In addition, remember that, with "supra"tentorial surgery, the head is kept "up," and the client is placed on the nonoperative side. Review the positioning of a client after craniotomy if you had difficulty with this question.

Level of Cognitive Ability: Application
Client Needs: Physiological Integrity
Integrated Process: Nursing Process/Implementation
Content Area: Adult Health/Neurological
Reference: Ignatavicius, D., & Workman, M. (2006). *Medical-surgical nursing: Critical thinking for collaborative care* (4th ed., p. 1058). Philadelphia: Saunders.

REFERENCES

Chernecky, C., & Berger, B. (2008). *Laboratory tests and diagnostic procedures* (5th ed.). Philadelphia: Saunders.

Christensen, B., & Kockrow, E. (2006). *Foundations of nursing* (5th ed.). St. Louis: Mosby.

Christensen, B., & Kockrow, E. (2006). *Adult health nursing* (5th ed.). St. Louis: Mosby.

deWit, S. (2005). *Fundamental concepts and skills for nursing* (2nd ed.). St. Louis: Saunders.

Elkin, M., Perry, A., & Potter, P. (2004). *Nursing interventions and clinical skills* (3rd ed.). St. Louis: Mosby.

Ignatavicius, D., & Workman, M. (2006). *Medical-surgical nursing: Critical thinking for collaborative care* (4th ed.). Philadelphia: Saunders.

Linton, A. (2007). *Introduction to medical-surgical nursing* (4 ed.). Philadelphia: Saunders.

Monahan, F., Marek, J., Neighbors, M., & Green, C. (2007). *Phipps' medical-surgical nursing: Health and illness perspectives* (8th ed.). St. Louis: Mosby.

National Council of State Boards of Nursing (Eds.) (2008). *2008 Detailed Test Plan for the NCLEX-PN® Examination, National Council of State Boards of Nursing.* Chicago: Author.

National Council of State Boards of Nursing. *NCSBN home page.* www.ncsbn.org. Accessed June 27, 2008.

CHAPTER 19

Care of a Client With a Tube

PYRAMID TERMS

chest tube A tube that returns negative pressure to the intrapleural space; it is used to remove abnormal accumulations of air and fluid from the pleural space.

endotracheal tube A tube used to maintain a patent airway that is indicated when the client needs mechanical ventilation.

Sengstaken-Blakemore tube A triple-lumen gastric tube with an inflatable esophageal balloon, an inflatable gastric balloon, and a gastric aspiration lumen; it is used as a treatment modality for the client with esophageal varices.

tracheostomy An artificial opening created in the trachea to establish an airway.

▲ PYRAMID TO SUCCESS

The Pyramid to Success focuses on the common types of tubes used in the clinical setting. The NCLEX-PN examination is likely to address content areas related to the appropriate care of certain tubes and the immediate interventions required if a complication arises. Focus on the specific data-collection points related to the specific type of tube. Review the procedures for verifying the correct placement of a tube and the procedures for administering medications or feedings through a tube, if appropriate. The pyramid points also focus on interventions associated with complications or emergencies that may occur. The Integrated Processes addressed in this chapter include Caring, Clinical Problem-Solving Process (Nursing Process), Communication and Documentation, and Teaching and Learning.

▲ CLIENT NEEDS

Safe and Effective Care Environment

Acting as a client advocate
Collaborating with members of the health care team
Ensuring that advance directives are in the client's medical record
Ensuring client's rights
Establishing priorities
Handling infectious materials

Maintaining medical and surgical asepsis
Maintaining standard and other precautions
Obtaining informed consent for invasive procedures

Health Promotion and Maintenance

Assisting the client with accepting lifestyle changes
Preventing disease
Providing client and family education regarding care at home
Performing techniques of data collection

Psychosocial Integrity

Discussing situational role changes
Discussing unexpected body-image changes
Identifying support systems
Monitoring for sensory/perceptual alterations
Providing home-care services

Physiological Integrity

Administering medications
Initiating emergency interventions for complications
Implementing measures to ensure basic care and comfort
Monitoring for potential complications associated with the tube
Monitoring laboratory values
Preparing for diagnostic tests to confirm the accurate placement of the tube
Providing nutrition and oral hydration
Providing respiratory care

I. NASOGASTRIC TUBES
  A. Description
    1. Short tubes used to intubate the stomach
    2. Inserted from the nose to the stomach
  B. Types of tubes and routes (Figure 19-1)
    1. Levin
      a. Single-lumen nasogastric (NG) tube
      b. Used to remove gastric contents via intermittent suction or to provide tube feedings

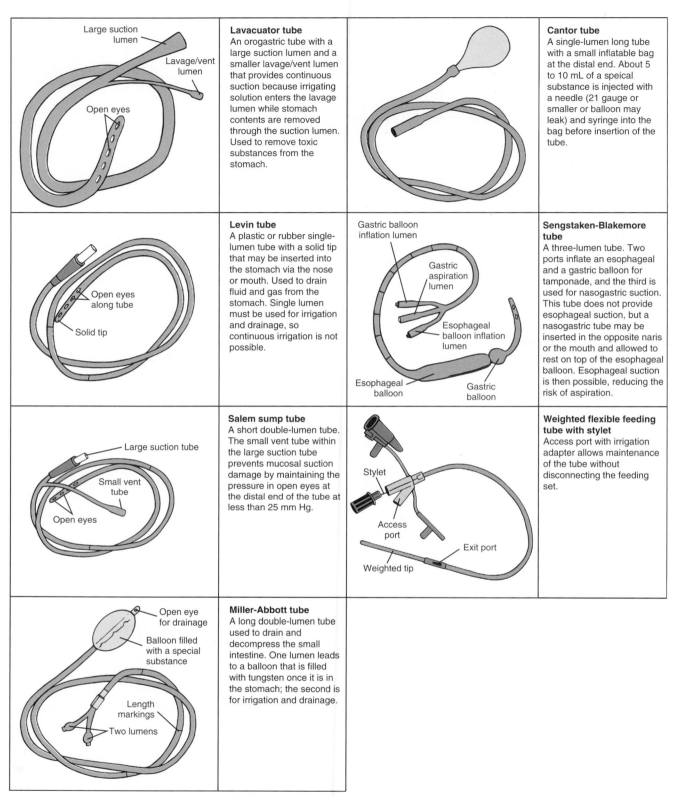

Lavacuator tube
An orogastric tube with a large suction lumen and a smaller lavage/vent lumen that provides continuous suction because irrigating solution enters the lavage lumen while stomach contents are removed through the suction lumen. Used to remove toxic substances from the stomach.

Cantor tube
A single-lumen long tube with a small inflatable bag at the distal end. About 5 to 10 mL of a speical substance is injected with a needle (21 gauge or smaller or balloon may leak) and syringe into the bag before insertion of the tube.

Levin tube
A plastic or rubber single-lumen tube with a solid tip that may be inserted into the stomach via the nose or mouth. Used to drain fluid and gas from the stomach. Single lumen must be used for irrigation and drainage, so continuous irrigation is not possible.

Sengstaken-Blakemore tube
A three-lumen tube. Two ports inflate an esophageal and a gastric balloon for tamponade, and the third is used for nasogastric suction. This tube does not provide esophageal suction, but a nasogastric tube may be inserted in the opposite naris or the mouth and allowed to rest on top of the esophageal balloon. Esophageal suction is then possible, reducing the risk of aspiration.

Salem sump tube
A short double-lumen tube. The small vent tube within the large suction tube prevents mucosal suction damage by maintaining the pressure in open eyes at the distal end of the tube at less than 25 mm Hg.

Weighted flexible feeding tube with stylet
Access port with irrigation adapter allows maintenance of the tube without disconnecting the feeding set.

Miller-Abbott tube
A long double-lumen tube used to drain and decompress the small intestine. One lumen leads to a balloon that is filled with tungsten once it is in the stomach; the second is for irrigation and drainage.

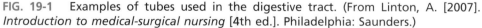

FIG. 19-1 Examples of tubes used in the digestive tract. (From Linton, A. [2007]. *Introduction to medical-surgical nursing* [4th ed.]. Philadelphia: Saunders.)

2. Salem sump
   a. Double-lumen NG tube with an air vent (pigtail)
   b. Air vent is not to be clamped and is to be kept above the level of the stomach
   c. If leakage occurs through the air vent, instill 30 mL of air into the air vent, and irrigate the main lumen with normal saline (NS) per agency policy
C. Determining placement
   1. Note that the most reliable method for determining placement is by x-ray study, which should be performed after initial placement
   2. Determine tube placement every 4 hours and before administering feedings or medications
   3. Determine tube placement by aspirating gastric contents and measuring the pH, which should be 4 or lower (pH values >6 indicate intestinal placement)
   4. Inserting 5 to 10 mL of air into the NG tube and listening for the rush of air over the stomach with a stethoscope is an alternative method for determining placement, but it should not be the sole method of determining placement as a result of unreliability
   5. Secure the tube to the client's nose with adhesive tape
D. Checking the residual
   1. Check residual volumes every 4 hours, before each feeding, or before giving medications
   2. Aspirate all stomach contents (residual) and measure amount
   3. Reinstill residual feeding to prevent excessive fluid and electrolyte losses unless the residual volume exceeds 100 mL, appears abnormal, or per agency policy
   4. Usually, if the residual is less than 100 mL, the feeding is administered (the physician's orders and agency policy are followed)
   5. Aspiration from some small-caliber, soft-walled tubes may not be possible
E. Irrigating
   1. Perform irrigation every 4 hours to check the patency of the tube
   2. Check placement before irrigating
   3. Gently instill 30 to 50 mL of water or NS (depending on agency policy) with an irrigation syringe
   4. Pull back on the syringe plunger to withdraw the fluid to check patency; repeat if the tube remains sluggish
F. Removal of an NG tube: Ask the client to take a deep breath and hold; remove the tube slowly and evenly over the course of 3 to 6 seconds (coil the tube around the hand as it is being removed)

II. GASTROINTESTINAL TUBE FEEDINGS
A. Tubes (Figure 19-2)
   1. NG: Nose to stomach

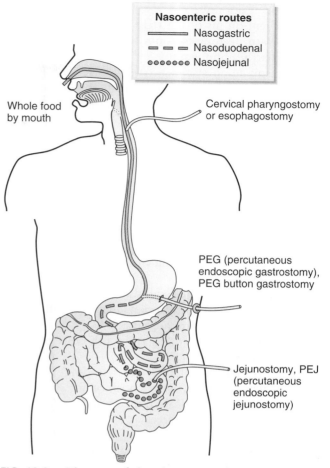

FIG. 19-2 Diagram of the placement of enteral feeding tubes. (From Linton, A. [2007]. *Introduction to medical-surgical nursing* [4th ed.]. Philadelphia: Saunders.)

   2. Gastrostomy: Stomach
   3. Jejunostomy: Jejunum
B. Types of administration
   1. Intermittent (bolus)
      a. Resembles normal meal feeding patterns
      b. Approximately 300 to 400 mL of formula is administered over a 30- to 60-minute period every 3 to 6 hours
   2. Continuous
      a. Administered continuously for 24 hours
      b. An infusion pump regulates the flow
   3. Cyclical
      a. Administered either during the day- or nighttime for 8 to 16 hours
      b. An infusion pump regulates the flow
      c. Feedings at night allow for more freedom during the day
C. Administering feedings
   1. If feedings are prescribed, x-ray confirmation should be performed before initiating feedings after the insertion of the tube
   2. Keep the head of the bed elevated at least 30 degrees at all times, even if no feeding is

being administered; also, position the comatose client on his or her right side

3. Warm feeding to room temperature to prevent diarrhea and cramps

4. Aspirate all stomach contents (residual), measure the amount, and return the contents to the stomach to prevent electrolyte imbalances (unless the residual exceeds 100 mL or as defined by agency policy)

5. Check the physician's orders and agency policy regarding residual amounts; usually, if the residual is less than 100 mL, the feeding is administered; large-volume aspirates indicate delayed gastric emptying and place the client at risk for aspiration

6. Check tube placement by aspirating gastric contents and measuring the pH (should be 4 or lower)

7. Check the bowel sounds; the feeding may be held and the physician may be notified if bowel sounds are absent

8. Use a feeding pump for continuous or cyclic feedings

9. For an intermittent (bolus) feeding, leave the client in a high Fowler's position for 30 minutes after feeding, followed by a semi-Fowler's position (30 to 45 degrees)

10. For a continuous feeding, keep the client in a semi-Fowler's position at all times

D. Precautions

1. Change the feeding container and tubing every 24 hours

2. Do not allow the solution to hang for more than 4 hours to prevent bacterial growth in the solution, per agency policy

3. Check the expiration date on the formula before administering it

4. Shake the formula well before inserting it into the feeding bag

5. Always check the placement of the tube before a feeding

6. Always check the bowel sounds; feedings can not be administered if bowel sounds are absent

7. Administer the feeding at the prescribed rate or via gravity flow (intermittent bolus feedings) with a 60-mL syringe with the plunger removed

8. Gently flush with 30 to 50 mL water or NS (depending on agency policy) with an irrigation syringe after feeding

III. MEDICATIONS VIA NASOGASTRIC OR GASTROSTOMY TUBE

A. Crush medications or use elixir forms of medications

B. Ensure that the medication ordered can be crushed or that the capsule can be opened

C. Dissolve crushed medication or capsule contents in 5 to 10 mL of water

D. Do not administer bulk fiber products or enteric-coated medications through an NG tube

E. Note that administering medications through a small-caliber NG tube may be difficult

F. Check the tube placement and the residual before instilling medications

G. Draw up the medication into a catheter-tip syringe, clear the excess air, and insert the medication into the tube

H. Flush with 30 to 50 mL of water or NS (depending on agency policy)

I. Clamp the tube for 30 to 60 minutes (depending on the medication and agency policy)

IV. INTESTINAL TUBES

A. Description

1. Passed nasally into the small intestine

2. Used to decompress the bowel or to remove intestinal contents

3. Designed to enter the small intestine through the pyloric sphincter with the use of the weight of a small bag of a special substance at the end

B. Types of tubes (see Figure 19-1)

1. Cantor or Harris tube, (single lumen)

2. Miller-Abbott tube (double lumen)

C. Interventions

1. Position the client on the right side to facilitate the passage of the small bag within the tube through the pylorus of the stomach and into the small intestine

2. Do not secure the tube to the client's face with tape until it has reached its final placement in the intestines; this may take several hours

3. An x-ray study is performed to verify desired placement

4. Monitor drainage from the tube

5. If the tube becomes blocked, the registered nurse and physician are notified; a small amount of air injected into the lumen may be prescribed to clear the tube

6. Check the abdomen and measure the abdominal girth

V. ESOPHAGEAL AND GASTRIC TUBES

A. Description

1. Used to apply pressure against the esophageal veins to control bleeding

2. Not used if the client has ulceration or necrosis of the esophagus or has had previous esophageal surgery

B. **Sengstaken-Blakemore tube** (see Figure 19-1)

1. Triple-lumen gastric tube with an inflatable esophageal balloon, an inflatable gastric balloon, and a gastric aspiration lumen

2. The gastric balloon applies pressure at the cardioesophageal junction to compress the gastric varices directly and to decrease blood flow to the esophageal varices; traction is applied to maintain the gastric balloon in position

3. The esophageal balloon directly compresses the esophageal varices
4. An x-ray study of the upper abdomen and chest confirms placement
5. Gastric contents are aspirated by gastric lavage or intermittent suction via the gastric aspiration port
6. With the **Sengstaken-Blakemore tube,** an NG tube is also inserted into the opposite naris to collect secretions that accumulate above the esophageal balloon

C. Interventions
1. The patency and integrity of all balloons are checked before insertion, and each lumen is labeled
2. The client is placed in an upright or Fowler's position for insertion
3. Prepare the client for an x-ray study immediately after insertion to verify placement
4. Maintain head elevation after the tube is in place

5. The balloon ports are double-clamped to prevent air leaks
6. Scissors are kept at the bedside at all times
7. The client is monitored for respiratory distress; if it occurs, notify the registered nurse immediately; the tubes will be cut to deflate the balloons
8. Monitor for increased bloody drainage that may indicate persistent bleeding
9. Monitor for signs of esophageal rupture, including a drop in blood pressure, increased heart rate, and back and upper abdominal pain (esophageal rupture is an emergency and must be reported immediately)

VI. **URINARY AND RENAL TUBES**
A. Types: Single lumen, double lumen, and triple lumen (Figure 19-3)
B. Routine urinary catheter care
1. Use gloves, and wash the perineal area with warm soapy water

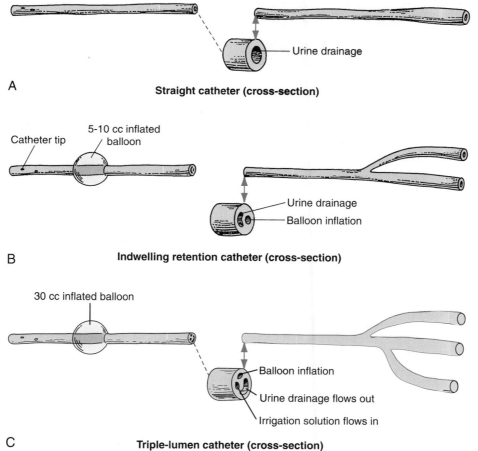

A   **Straight catheter (cross-section)**

B   **Indwelling retention catheter (cross-section)**

C   **Triple-lumen catheter (cross-section)**

FIG. 19-3   Types of urinary catheters: **A,** Straight catheter (cross-section). **B,** Indwelling retention catheter (cross-section). **C,** Triple-lumen catheter (cross-section). (From Elkin, M., Perry, A., & Potter, P. [2008]. *Nursing interventions & clinical skills* [4th ed.]. St. Louis: Mosby.)

2. With the nondominant hand, pull back the labia or foreskin to expose the meatus (in the adult male, return the foreskin to its normal position)
3. Clean along the catheter with soap and water
4. Anchor the catheter to the thigh
5. Maintain the catheter bag below the level of the bladder

C. Ureteral and nephrostomy tubes
   1. Never clamp the tubes
   2. Maintain patency
   3. Monitor output closely; urine output of less than 30 mL/hour or a lack of output for more than 15 minutes should be reported immediately

VII. RESPIRATORY SYSTEM TUBES
   A. **Endotracheal tubes** (Figure 19-4)
      1. Description
         a. Used to maintain a patent airway
         b. Indicated when the client needs mechanical ventilation
         c. If the client requires an artificial airway for longer than 10 to 14 days, a tracheostomy may be created to avoid the mucosal and vocal cord damage that can be caused by the endotracheal tube
      2. Orotracheal
         a. Inserted through the mouth; allows for the use of a larger-diameter tube and reduces the work of breathing
         b. Indicated when the client has a nasal obstruction or a predisposition to epistaxis
         c. Uncomfortable and can be manipulated by the tongue, thus causing airway obstruction; an oral airway may be needed to prevent the client from biting on the tube

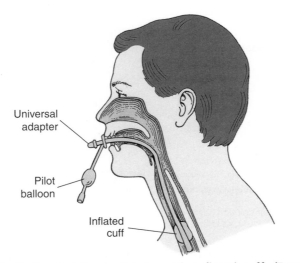

Universal adapter

Pilot balloon

Inflated cuff

FIG. 19-4 Endotracheal tube with inflated cuff. (From Perry A., & Potter P. [2004]. *Clinical nursing skills and nursing techniques* [5th ed]. St. Louis: Mosby.)

3. Nasotracheal
   a. Inserted through the nose; requires the use of a smaller-sized tube, which increases both resistance and the client's work of breathing
   b. Discouraged for clients with bleeding disorders
   c. More comfortable for the client; he or she is unable to manipulate the tube with the tongue
4. Interventions
   a. Placement is confirmed by a chest x-ray study (correct placement is 1 to 2 cm above the carina) and by auscultating both sides of chest while manually ventilating with a resuscitation (Ambu) bag; if breath sounds and chest wall movement are absent on the left side, the tube may be in the right main stem bronchus
   b. If the tube is in the stomach, louder breath sounds will be heard over the stomach than over the chest, and abdominal distention will be present
   c. The tube is secured immediately after intubation with adhesive tape
   d. Monitor the position of the tube at the lip or nose
   e. Monitor the skin and mucous membranes
   f. Suction the tube only when needed
   g. The oral tube needs to be moved to the opposite side of the mouth daily to prevent pressure and necrosis of the lip and mouth area, to prevent nerve damage, and to facilitate the inspection and cleaning of the mouth; moving the tube to the opposite side of the mouth should be done by two health care providers
   h. To prevent dislodgment, prevent pulling or tugging on the tube; suction, coughing, and speaking attempts by the client place extra stress on the tube and can cause dislodgment
   i. Keep a resuscitation (Ambu) bag at the bedside at all times
   j. Cuff inflation is maintained to create a seal and to allow for the complete mechanical control of respirations
5. Extubation
   a. Hyperoxygenate the client, and suction the endotracheal tube and the oral cavity
   b. Place the client in semi-Fowler's position
   c. The cuff is deflated; have the client inhale; at peak inspiration, the tube is removed, and the airway is suctioned through the tube as it is pulled out
   d. After removal, instruct the client to cough and deep breathe to assist with the removal of accumulated secretions from the throat
   e. Apply oxygen therapy, as prescribed

f. Monitor for respiratory difficulty; contact the registered nurse and physician if respiratory difficulty occurs

g. Inform the client that hoarseness or a sore throat is normal and that he or she should limit talking if it occurs

B. Tracheostomy

1. Description
   a. A tracheotomy is a surgical incision into the trachea for the purpose of establishing an airway
   b. The tracheostomy is the stoma or opening that results from the tracheotomy; it can be temporary or permanent

2. Single-cannula tube: Has an outer but no inner cannula; used for client with a thick neck or longer trachea in whom a standard tube will not enter the trachea

3. Cuffed tube: Has an outer and inner cannula, an obturator, and a cuff

4. Cuffless tube
   a. Has an outer cannula, an open and plugged inner cannula, and an obturator
   b. Used over the long term for evaluating the client's ability to breathe through the upper airway and for the client who is no longer at risk for aspiration

5. Fenestrated tube (Figure 19-5)
   a. Has an opening along the posterior wall of the outer cannula
   b. When the tube is capped, the client can breathe through the upper airway and speak
   c. The cuff is always deflated before the tube is capped

6. Foam-cuffed tube
   a. Cuff is larger than the standard cuffed tube
   b. Filled with foam, which may apply less pressure to the tracheal mucosa

7. Interventions
   a. Monitor the respirations and for bilateral breath sounds
   b. Monitor the pulse oximetry
   c. Encourage coughing and deep breathing
   d. Maintain a semi-Fowler's to high Fowler's position
   e. Monitor for bleeding, difficulty breathing, and crepitus, which are indications of hemorrhage, pneumothorax, and subcutaneous emphysema
   f. Provide respiratory treatments, as prescribed
   g. Suction as needed; hyperoxygenate the client before suction (see Chapter 48 for the suctioning procedure)
   h. If the client is allowed to eat, sit him or her up for meals, and ensure that the cuff is inflated (if the tube is not capped) for meals and for 1 hour after meals

   i. Assess the stoma and secretions for blood or purulent drainage
   j. Follow the physician's orders and agency policy for cleaning the tracheostomy site and the inner cannula; half-strength hydrogen peroxide is usually used
   k. Administer humidified oxygen, as prescribed; the normal humidification process is bypassed in a client with a tracheostomy
   l. Obtain assistance with changing the tracheostomy ties; after placing the new ties, cut and remove the old ties that are holding the tracheostomy tube in place (tracheostomy ties with Velcro fasteners may be managed by a single nurse)
   m. Never insert a decannulation plug into a tracheostomy tube until the cuff is deflated and the inner cannula is removed; prior insertion prevents airflow to the client
   n. Keep a resuscitation (Ambu) bag, an obturator, clamps, and a spare tracheotomy set at the bedside
   o. Provide frequent mouth care, to reduce the risk of pneumonia

8. Complications of a tracheostomy (Table 19-1 and Box 19-1)

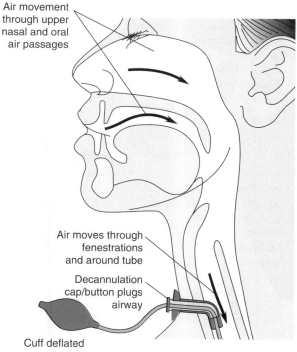

Air movement through upper nasal and oral air passages

Air moves through fenestrations and around tube

Decannulation cap/button plugs airway

Cuff deflated

FIG. 19-5 Breathing through a fenestrated tracheostomy tube with a cap in place and the cuff deflated. (From Ignatavicius, D., & Workman, M. [2006]. *Medical-surgical nursing: Critical thinking for collaborative care* [5th ed.]. St. Louis: Saunders.)

TABLE 19-1   Complications of a Tracheostomy

Complications and Description	Manifestations	Management	Prevention
Tracheomalacia: Consistent pressure exerted by the cuff causes tracheal dilation and the erosion of cartilage.	An increased amount of air is required in the cuff to maintain the seal. A larger tracheostomy tube is required to prevent an air leak at the stoma. Food particles are seen in tracheal secretions. The client does not receive the set tidal volume on the ventilator.	No special management is needed unless bleeding occurs.	Use an uncuffed tube as soon as possible. Monitor the cuff pressure and air volumes closely to detect changes.
Tracheal stenosis: A narrowed tracheal lumen is the result of scar formation from irritation of the tracheal mucosa by the cuff.	Stenosis is usually seen after the cuff is deflated or after the tracheostomy tube is removed. The client has increased coughing, an inability to expectorate secretions, or difficulty breathing or talking.	Tracheal dilation or surgical intervention is used.	Prevent the pulling of and traction on the tracheostomy tube. Properly secure the tube in the midline position. Maintain proper cuff pressure. Minimize oronasal intubation time.
Tracheoesophageal fistula: Excessive cuff pressure causes erosion of the posterior wall of the trachea. A hole is created between the trachea and the anterior esophagus. The client at highest risk also has a nasogastric tube present.	Similar to tracheomalacia: • Food particles are seen in the tracheal secretions. • Increased air is needed in the cuff to achieve a seal. • The client has increased coughing and choking while eating. • The client does not receive the set tidal volume on the ventilator.	Manually administer oxygen by mask to prevent hypoxemia. Use a small, soft feeding tube instead of a nasogastric tube for tube feedings. A gastrostomy or jejunostomy may be performed. Monitor the client with a nasogastric tube closely; assess for tracheoesophageal fistula and aspiration.	Maintain cuff pressure. Monitor the amount of air needed for inflation and detect changes. Progress to a deflated cuff or a cuffless tube as soon as possible.
Trachea-innominate artery fistula: A malpositioned tube causes its distal tip to push against the lateral wall of the tracheostomy. Continued pressure causes the necrosis and erosion of the innominate artery. *This is a medical emergency*.	The tracheostomy tube pulsates in synchrony with the heartbeat. There is heavy bleeding from the stoma. *This is a life-threatening complication*.	Remove the tracheostomy tube immediately. Apply direct pressure to the innominate artery at the stoma site. Prepare the client for immediate repair surgery.	Correct the tube size, length, and midline position. Prevent the pulling of or tugging on the tracheostomy tube. Immediately notify the physician regarding the pulsating tube.

Modified from Ignatavicius, D., & Workman, M. (2006). *Medical-surgical nursing* (5th ed.). St. Louis: Saunders.

BOX 19-1   Complications of a Tracheostomy

Tube Obstruction
Data Collection
Difficulty breathing
Noisy respirations
Difficulty inserting the suction catheter
Thick, dry secretions
Unexplained peak pressures if the client is on a
   mechanical ventilator
Prevention and Interventions
Assist the client to cough and deep breathe.
Provide humidification and suctioning.
Clean the inner cannula regularly.
The physician repositions or replaces the tube if
   obstruction occurs as a result of cuff prolapse over the
   end of the tube.
Tube Dislodgment
Prevention and Interventions
Secure the tube in place.
Minimize the manipulation of and traction on the
   tube.
Ensure that the client does not pull on the tube.
Ensure that a tracheostomy tube of the same type and
   size is at the client's bedside.
Be familiar with facility policy regarding the replacement
   of a tracheostomy tube as a nursing procedure.
During the first 72 hours after the surgical placement of
   the tracheostomy:
  • The nurse manually ventilates the client with
    the use of a manual resuscitation (Ambu) bag
    while another nurse calls the resuscitation team for
    help.
More than 72 hours after the surgical placement of the
   tracheostomy:
  • Extend the client's neck and open the tissues of the
    stoma to secure the airway.
  • Grasp the retention sutures (if they are present) to
    spread the opening.
  • Use a tracheal dilator (curved clamp) to hold the
    stoma open.
  • Prepare to assist with the insertion of the
    tracheostomy tube; place an obturator into
    tracheostomy tube, replace the tube, and remove
    the obturator.
  • Maintain ventilation with the use of a resuscitation
    (Ambu) bag.
  • Check the airflow, and check for bilateral breath
    sounds.
  • If unable to secure an airway, call the resuscitation
    team and the anesthesiologist.

VIII. CHEST-TUBE DRAINAGE SYSTEM (Figure 19-6)
A. Description
   1. Returns negative pressure to the intrapleural space
   2. Used to remove abnormal accumulations of air
      and fluid from the pleural space
   3. Closed **chest-tube** placement (Figure 19-7)

B. Collection chamber
   1. Where the **chest tube** from the client connects
      to the system
   2. Drainage from the tube drains into and collects
      in a series of calibrated columns in this chamber
C. Water-seal chamber
   1. The tip of the tube is underwater, thus allowing
      fluid and air to drain from the pleural space and
      preventing air from entering the pleural space
   2. Water oscillates (i.e., moves up as the client
      inhales and moves down as the client exhales)
   3. Continuous bubbling indicates an air leak in
      the **chest-tube** system
D. Suction-control chamber
   1. Provides suction, which can be controlled to
      provide negative pressure to the chest
   2. Filled with various levels of water to achieve the
      desired level of suction; without this control,
      lung tissue could be sucked into the **chest tube**
   3. Gentle bubbling indicates that there is suction;
      it does not indicate that air is escaping from the
      pleural space
E. Dry-suction system
   1. Because this is a dry-suction system, the absence
      of bubbling is noted in the suction-control
      chamber
   2. A knob on the collection device is used to set
      the prescribed amount of suction; then the wall-
      suction source dial is turned until a small
      orange floater valve appears in the window on
      the device; when the orange floater valve is in
      the window, the correct amount of suction has
      been applied
F. Interventions
   1. Collection chamber
      a. Monitor the drainage; the physician is noti-
         fied if the drainage is more than 100 mL/hr
         or if drainage becomes bright red or
         increases suddenly
      b. Mark the **chest-tube** drainage in the collec-
         tion chamber at 1- to 4-hour intervals with
         the use of a piece of tape
   2. Water-seal chamber
      a. Monitor for the fluctuation of the fluid level
         in the water-seal chamber
      b. Fluctuation in the water-seal chamber stops
         if the tube is obstructed, if a dependent loop
         exists, if the suction is not working properly,
         or if the lung has re-expanded
      c. If the client has a known pneumothorax,
         intermittent bubbling in the water-seal
         chamber is expected as air is drained from
         the chest; continuous bubbling indicates an
         air leak in the system
      d. Notify the registered nurse and physician if
         there is continuous bubbling in the water-
         seal chamber

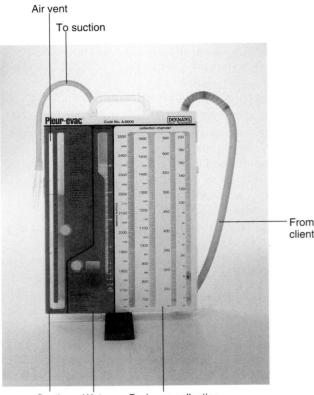

FIG. 19-6   The Pleur-Evac drainage system, a commercial three-bottle chest drainage device. (From Ignatavicius, D., & Workman, M. [2006]. *Medical-surgical nursing: Critical thinking for collaborative care* [5th ed.] St. Louis: Saunders.)

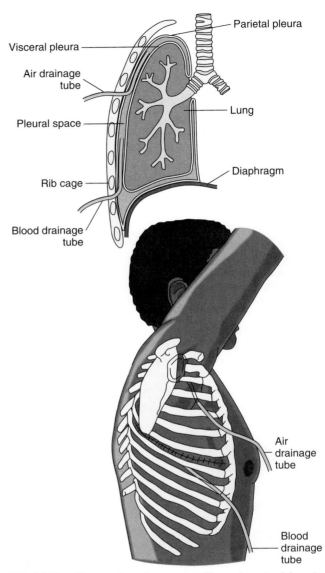

FIG. 19-7   Chest tube placement. (From Ignatavicius, D., & Workman, M. [2006]. *Medical-surgical nursing: Critical thinking for collaborative care* [5th ed.]. St. Louis: Saunders.)

3. Suction-control chamber: Gentle bubbling should be noted in the suction-control chamber; vigorous bubbling indicates an air leak, and the registered nurse and physician should be notified
4. An occlusive sterile dressing is maintained at the insertion site
5. A chest radiograph assesses the position of the tube and determines whether the lung has re-expanded
6. Monitor the respiratory status and listen to the lung sounds
7. Monitor for the signs of an extended pneumothorax or hemothorax
8. Keep the drainage system below the level of the chest and the tubes free of kinks, dependent loops, or other obstructions
9. Ensure that all connections are secure
10. Encourage coughing and deep breathing
11. Change the client's position frequently to promote drainage and ventilation
12. Stripping or milking a **chest tube** is not done unless specifically ordered by a physician and if agency policy allows

13. Keep a clamp and a sterile occlusive dressing at the bedside at all times
14. A **chest tube** is never clamped without a written order from the physician; also, determine agency policy for clamping **chest tubes**
15. If the drainage system cracks or breaks, insert the **chest tube** into a bottle of sterile water; the cracked or broken system is removed and replaced with a new system
16. If the **chest tube** is accidentally pulled out of the chest, pinch the skin opening together, apply an occlusive sterile dressing, cover the dressing with overlapping pieces of 2-inch tape, and notify the registered nurse and the physician immediately

17. When the **chest tube** is removed, the client is asked to take a deep breath and hold it, and the tube is removed; a dry sterile dressing, petroleum gauze dressing, or Telfa dressing (depending on the physician's preference) is taped in place after the removal of the **chest tube**

18. Depending on the physician's preference, when the **chest tube** is removed, the client may be asked to take a deep breath, exhale, and bear down (i.e., Valsalva's maneuver)

PRACTICE QUESTIONS

177. A nurse is preparing to administer an intermittent tube feeding to a client. The nurse aspirates 90 mL of residual tube feeding. What should the nurse do with the aspirated feeding?
    1. Hold the feeding.
    2. Contact the physician.
    3. Reinstill the residual and administer the feeding.
    4. Deduct the amount of the residual from the new feeding and administer that amount to the client.

178. A nurse is providing endotracheal suctioning to a client who is mechanically ventilated when the client becomes restless and tachycardic. What should the nurse do?
    1. Notify the physician immediately.
    2. Finish the suctroning sucitioing as quickly as possible.
    3. Contact the respiratory department to suction the client.
    4. Discontinue suctioning until the client is stabilized and monitor vital signs.

179. A nurse is checking a client for the correct placement of a nasogastric (NG) tube. The nurse aspirates the client's stomach contents and checks their pH level. Which of the following pH values indicates the correct placement of the tube?
    1. 4.0
    2. 7.0
    3. 7.5
    4. 7.35

180. A licensed practical nurse (LPN) is preparing to assist a registered nurse (RN) with removing a nasogastric (NG) tube from the client. The LPN would instruct the client to do which of the following?
    1. Exhale.
    2. Inhale and exhale quickly.
    3. Take and hold a deep breath.
    4. Perform Valsalva's maneuver.

181. A nurse is preparing to administer medication through a nasogastric (NG) tube that is connected to suction. Which of the following indicates the accurate procedure for medication administration?
    1. Position the client supine to assist with medication absorption.
    2. Clamp the NG tube for 30 minutes after medication administration.
    3. Aspirate the NG tube after medication administration to maintain patency.
    4. Change the suction setting to low intermittent suction for 30 minutes after medication administration.

182. A nurse is assigned to assist with caring for a client with esophageal varices who has a Sengstaken-Blakemore tube inserted. The nurse checks the client's room to ensure that which priority item is at the bedside?
    1. An obturator
    2. A Kelly clamp
    3. An irrigation set
    4. A pair of scissors

183. A nurse is inserting an indwelling urinary catheter into a male client. As the catheter is inserted into the urethra, urine begins to flow into the tubing. At this point, the nurse:
    1. Immediately inflates the balloon
    2. Inserts the catheter 2.5 to 5 cm and inflates the balloon
    3. Inserts the catheter until resistance is met and inflates the balloon
    4. Withdraws the catheter approximately 1 inch and inflates the balloon

184. A nurse is assigned to assist with caring for a client who has a chest tube. The nurse notes fluctuations of the fluid level in the water-seal chamber. Based on this observation, which action would be appropriate?
    1. Empty the drainage.
    2. Encourage the client to deep breathe.
    3. Continue to monitor, because this is an expected finding.
    4. Encourage the client to hold his or her breath periodically.

185. A nurse is assigned to assist the physician with the removal of a chest tube. The nurse instructs the client to do which of the following during this process?
    1. Stay very still.
    2. Exhale slowly.
    3. Inhale and exhale quickly.
    4. Perform Valsalva's maneuver.

186. A nurse is preparing to begin a continuous tube feeding on a client with a nasogastric tube. The nurse positions the client:
    1. Supine
    2. Supine on the right side
    3. With the head elevated 15 degrees
    4. With the head elevated 45 degrees

187. A nurse is preparing to administer an intermittent tube feeding to a client with a nasogastric tube. The nurse checks the residual and obtains an amount of 200 mL. The nurse would:
    1. Hold the feeding.
    2. Administer the feeding.
    3. Flush the tubing with 30 mL of water.
    4. Elevate the head of the bed to 90 degrees and administer the feeding.

188. A nurse is assisting in caring for a client with a chest tube. The nurse understands that which of the following is an incorrect action for the care of the client?
    1. Pin the tubing to the bedclothes.
    2. Be sure all connections are taped.
    3. Be sure all connections remain airtight.
    4. Do not allow the tubing to become kinked or obstructed by the weight of the client.

189. A nurse is assigned to care for a client who has a chest tube. The nurse is told to monitor the client for subcutaneous emphysema. The nurse monitors the client for this complication by:
    1. Monitoring for pain
    2. Monitoring respirations hourly
    3. Checking the blood pressure every 2 hours
    4. Palpating for the leakage of air into the subcutaneous tissues

190. A nurse is told that an assigned client will have a fenestrated tracheostomy tube inserted. The nurse prepares the client for the procedure, knowing that this type of tube:
    1. Enables the client to speak
    2. Prevents the client from speaking
    3. Is necessary for mechanical ventilation
    4. Prevents air from being inhaled through the tracheostomy opening

ALTERNATE ITEM FORMAT: MULTIPLE RESPONSE

191. A nurse is assisting with monitoring the functioning of a chest-tube drainage system in a client who just returned from the recovery room after a thoracotomy with wedge resection. Which findings would the nurse expect to note? Select all that apply.
    ☐ 1. Excessive bubbling in the water-seal chamber
    ☐ 2. Vigorous bubbling in the suction-control chamber
    ☑ 3. 50 mL of drainage in the drainage-collection chamber
    ☑ 4. The drainage system is maintained below the client's chest.
    ☑ 5. An occlusive dressing is in place over the chest-tube insertion site.
    ☑ 6. Fluctuation of water in the tube of the water-seal chamber during inhalation and exhalation

ANSWERS

177. 3
Rationale: Unless otherwise instructed, an amount of less than 100 to 150 mL may be reinstituted; then a normal amount of tube feeding is administered. It is important to return the contents to the stomach to prevent electrolyte imbalances.
Test-Taking Strategy: Use the process of elimination. Option 1 could cause an electrolyte imbalance. The physician does not need to be notified for this normal occurrence. To prevent dehydration, clients need to get the correct amount of feeding prescribed. Review tube-feeding administration if you had difficulty with this question.
Level of Cognitive Ability: Application
Client Needs: Physiological Integrity
Integrated Process: Nursing Process/Implementation
Content Area: Fundamental Skills
Reference: Linton, A. (2007). *Introduction to medical-surgical nursing* (4th ed., pp. 740, 742). Philadelphia: Saunders.

178. 4
Rationale: If a client becomes cyanotic or restless or develops tachycardia, bradycardia, or another abnormal heart rhythm, the nurse must discontinue suctioning until the client is stabilized. It is also important to monitor the vital signs and the pulse oximetry. If the client's condition continues to deteriorate, then the respiratory department and physician may need to be notified.

Test-Taking Strategy: Use the process of elimination. Focusing on the data in the question will direct you to option 4. Review endotracheal suctioning if you had difficulty with this question.
Level of Cognitive Ability: Application
Client Needs: Physiological Integrity
Integrated Process: Nursing Process/Implementation
Content Area: Fundamental Skills
Reference: Monahan, F., Marek, J., Neighbors, M., & Green, C. (2007). *Phipps' medical-surgical nursing: Health and illness perspectives* (8th ed., pp. 618-619). St. Louis: Mosby.

179. 1
Rationale: If the NG tube is in the stomach, the pH of the contents will be acidic. Option 2 indicates a slightly acidic pH. Option 3 indicates an alkaline pH. Option 4 indicates a neutral pH.
Test-Taking Strategy: Use the process of elimination. Recalling that gastric contents are acidic will direct you to option 1. Review the procedure for checking NG tube placement if you had difficulty with this question.
Level of Cognitive Ability: Comprehension
Client Needs: Physiological Integrity
Integrated Process: Nursing Process/Evaluation*Content Area:* Fundamental Skills
Reference: Christensen, B., & Kockrow, E. (2006). *Foundations of nursing* (5th ed., p. 591). St. Louis: Mosby.

180. 3
Rationale: When the RN removes the NG tube, the client is instructed to take and hold a deep breath. This will close the epiglottis, and the airway will be temporarily obstructed during the tube removal. This allows for the easy withdrawal of the tube through the esophagus into the nose. The RN removes the tube with one very smooth, continuous pull. Options 1, 2, and 4 are incorrect.
Test-Taking Strategy: Use the process of elimination, and focus on the subject of removing an NG tube. Visualize the procedure, and consider what each client action identified in the options would produce. Review the removal of an NG tube if you had difficulty with this question.
Level of Cognitive Ability: Application
Client Needs: Physiological Integrity
Integrated Process: Nursing Process/Implementation
Content Area: Fundamental Skills
Reference: Christensen, B., & Kockrow, E. (2006). *Foundations of nursing* (5th ed., p. 595). St. Louis: Mosby.

181. 2
Rationale: If a client has an NG tube connected to suction, the nurse should wait up to 30 minutes before reconnecting the tube to the suction apparatus to allow adequate time for medication absorption. Aspirating the NG tube will remove the medication that has just been administered. Low intermittent suction will also remove the medication. The client should not be placed in the supine position because of the risk for aspiration.
Test-Taking Strategy: Use the process of elimination. Eliminate options 3 and 4 first, because these actions are comparable or alike and will produce the same effect. Recalling that the client should not be placed in a supine position will assist you with eliminating option 1. Review the administration of medications through an NG tube if you had difficulty with this question.
Level of Cognitive Ability: Application
Client Needs: Physiological Integrity
Integrated Process: Nursing Process/Implementation
Content Area: Fundamental Skills
References: Monahan, F., Marek, J., Neighbors, M., & Green, C. (2007). *Phipps' medical-surgical nursing: Health and illness perspectives* (8th ed., p. 1234). St. Louis: Mosby.
Perry, A., & Potter, P. (2006). *Clinical nursing skills & techniques* (6th ed., p. 645). St. Louis: Mosby.
Potter, P., & Perry, A. (2005). *Fundamentals of nursing* (6th ed., p. 464). St. Louis: Mosby.

182. 4
Rationale: When the client has a Sengstaken-Blakemore tube, a pair of scissors must be kept at the client's bedside at all times. The client needs to be observed for sudden respiratory distress, which occurs if the gastric balloon ruptures and the entire tube moves upward. If this occurs, the registered nurse is notified immediately, and the balloon lumens will be cut. An obturator and a Kelly clamp are kept at the bedside of a client with a tracheostomy. An irrigation set may also be kept at the bedside, but it is not the priority item.
Test-Taking Strategy: Use your knowledge of the structure, function, and placement of a Sengstaken-Blakemore tube to answer this question. Note the strategic word "priority" in the question; this should assist you with eliminating options 1, 2, and 3. Review the care of a client with a Sengstaken-Blakemore tube if you had difficulty with this question.
Level of Cognitive Ability: Application
Client Needs: Safe and Effective Care Environment
Integrated Process: Nursing Process/Implementation
Content Area: Fundamental Skills
References: Black, J., & Hawks, J. (2005). *Medical-surgical nursing: Clinical management for positive outcomes* (7th ed., p. 1345). Philadelphia: Saunders.
Lewis, S., Heitkemper, M., Dirksen, S., & Bucher, L., (2007). *Medical-surgical nursing: Assessment and management of clinical problems* (7th ed., p. 1114). St. Louis: Mosby.

183. 2
Rationale: The catheter's balloon is behind the opening at the insertion tip. The catheter is inserted 2.5 to 5 cm after urine begins to flow to provide sufficient space to inflate the balloon. Inserting the catheter the extra distance will ensure that the balloon is inflated inside the bladder and not in the urethra, which could produce trauma.
Test-Taking Strategy: Visualize the proper procedure for inserting an indwelling urinary catheter to assist you with answering this question. Note the strategic words "urine begins to flow." Options 3 and 4 can easily be eliminated. Eliminate option 1 next because of the word "immediately." Review bladder catheterization if you had difficulty with this question.
Level of Cognitive Ability: Application
Client Needs: Physiological Integrity
Integrated Process: Nursing Process/Implementation
Content Area: Fundamental Skills
References: Christensen, B., & Kockrow, E. (2006). *Foundations of nursing* (5th ed., p. 577). St. Louis: Mosby.
Potter, P., & Perry, A. (2005). *Fundamentals of nursing* (6th ed., p. 1355). St. Louis: Mosby.

184. 3
Rationale: The presence of fluctuations in the fluid level in the water-seal chamber indicates a patent drainage system. With normal breathing, the water level rises with inspiration and falls with expiration. The apparatus and all connections must remain airtight at all times, and the drainage is never emptied. Encouraging the client to deep breathe is unrelated to this observation. The client is not told to hold his or her breath.
Test-Taking Strategy: Focus on the subject of the question—the fluctuation of the fluid level in the water-seal chamber; this will assist you with eliminating options 1, 2, and 4. Review the expected and unexpected findings when caring for a client with a chest tube if you had difficulty with this question.
Level of Cognitive Ability: Application
Client Needs: Physiological Integrity
Integrated Process: Nursing Process/Implementation
Content Area: Fundamental Skills
References: Christen, B., & Kockrow, E. (2006). *Adult health nursing* (5th ed. pp. 438, 440). St. Louis: Mosby.
Linton, A. (2007). *Introduction to medical-surgical nursing* (4th ed., p. 529). Philadelphia: Saunders.

185. 4
Rationale: When the chest tube is removed, the client is asked to perform Valsalva's maneuver (i.e., take a deep breath, exhale,

and bear down), the tube is quickly withdrawn, and an airtight dressing is taped in place. An alternative instruction is to ask the client to take a deep breath and hold the breath while the tube is removed. Options 1, 2, and 3 are incorrect client instructions.
Test-Taking Strategy: Use the process of elimination. Visualize the procedure and the client instructions given in each option as you answer the question; this will direct you to option 4. Review the procedure for the removal of a chest tube if you had difficulty with this question.
Level of Cognitive Ability: Application
Client Needs: Physiological Integrity
Integrated Process: Nursing Process/Implementation
Content Area: Fundamental Skills
References: Lewis, S., Heitkemper, M., Dirksen, S., & Bucher, L. (2007). *Medical-surgical nursing: Assessment and management of clinical problems* (7th ed., p. 592). St. Louis: Mosby.
Potter, P., & Perry, A. (2005). *Fundamentals of nursing* (6th ed., p. 403). St. Louis: Mosby.

186. **4**
Rationale: When a tube feeding is administered, the client is placed in a high Fowler's position for a bolus feeding and in a semi-Fowler's position (30 to 45 degrees) to allow gravity to help the flow of formula and to prevent reflux and aspiration. Options 1, 2, and 3 are inappropriate positions during a tube feeding.
Test-Taking Strategy: Use the process of elimination. Eliminate options 1 and 2 first, because they are comparable or alike. Recalling the risks associated with the administration of a tube feeding will direct you to option 4. Review the administration of tube feedings if you had difficulty with this question.
Level of Cognitive Ability: Application
Client Needs: Physiological Integrity
Integrated Process: Nursing Process/Implementation
Content Area: Fundamental Skills
References: Christensen, B., & Kockrow, E. (2006). *Foundations of nursing* (5th ed., p. 653). St. Louis: Mosby.
Potter, P., & Perry, A. (2005). *Fundamentals of nursing* (6th ed., p. 658). St. Louis: Mosby.

187. **1**
Rationale: When 200 mL of residual formula are obtained, the feeding is held and the physician is notified, because this is an indication that the feeding is not being absorbed. If the residual is less than 100 mL, the feeding is usually administered; large-volume aspirates indicate delayed gastric emptying and place the client at risk for aspiration. Always check the physician's orders and agency policy regarding residual amounts. Elevating the head of the bed to 90 degrees and flushing the tubing are not appropriate actions.
Test-Taking Strategy: Use the process of elimination. Eliminate options 2 and 4 first, because they are comparable or alike. Recalling that the feeding is held when more than 100 mL of residual are obtained will direct you to option 1. Review the procedure for administering intermittent tube feedings if you had difficulty with this question.
Level of Cognitive Ability: Application
Client Needs: Physiological Integrity
Integrated Process: Nursing Process/Implementation

Content Area: Fundamental Skills
Reference: Christensen, B., & Kockrow, E. (2006). *Foundations of nursing* (5th ed., pp. 653, 657). St. Louis: Mosby.

188. **1**
Rationale: Chest-tube tubing is never pinned to the bed-clothes, because this presents the risk of accidental dislodgment of the tube when the client moves. Options 2, 3, and 4 are appropriate interventions for the plan of care for a client with a chest tube.
Test-Taking Strategy: Note the strategic word "incorrect" in the question. This word indicates a negative event query and asks you to select an incorrect action. Use the process of elimination, and recall the complications associated with a chest tube. Review the care of the client with a chest tube if you had difficulty with this question.
Level of Cognitive Ability: Application
Client Needs: Physiological Integrity
Integrated Process: Nursing Process/Implementation
Content Area: Fundamental Skills
Reference: Potter, P., & Perry, A. (2005). *Fundamentals of nursing* (6th ed., pp. 1118-1119). St. Louis: Mosby.

189. **4**
Rationale: Subcutaneous emphysema is also known as *crepitus*. It presents as a "puffed-up" appearance that is caused by the leakage of air into the subcutaneous tissues. It is monitored by palpating, and it feels like bubble wrap when palpated. Although options 1, 2, and 3 may be components of the plan of care for a client with a chest tube, these actions will not identify subcutaneous emphysema.
Test-Taking Strategy: Use the process of elimination. Note the similarity between the words "subcutaneous emphysema" in the question and "subcutaneous tissues" in the correct option. Review subcutaneous emphysema if you had difficulty with this question.
Level of Cognitive Ability: Application
Client Needs: Physiological Integrity
Integrated Process: Nursing Process/Data Collection
Content Area: Fundamental Skills
References: Black, J., & Hawks, J. (2005). *Medical-surgical nursing: Clinical management for positive outcomes* (7th ed., p. 1780). Philadelphia: Saunders.
Ignatavicius, D., & Workman, M. (2006). *Medical-surgical nursing: Critical thinking for collaborative care* (5th ed., p. 670). St. Louis: Saunders.
Monahan, F., Marek, J., Neighbors, M., & Green, C. (2007). *Phipps' medical-surgical nursing: Health and illness perspectives* (8th ed., p. 653). St. Louis: Mosby.

190. **1**
Rationale: A fenestrated tube has a small opening in the outer cannula that allows some air to escape through the larynx; this type of tube enables the client to speak. Options 2, 3, and 4 are incorrect with regard to this type of tube.
Test-Taking Strategy: Knowledge regarding the design and purpose of a fenestrated tracheostomy tube will direct you to option 1. Review the purpose of a fenestrated tube if you had difficulty with this question.
Level of Cognitive Ability: Comprehension
Client Needs: Physiological Integrity

Integrated Process: Nursing Process/Planning
Content Area: Fundamental Skills
Reference: Lewis, S., Heitkemper, M., Dirksen, S., & Bucher, L. (2007). *Medical-surgical nursing: Assessment and management of clinical problems* (7th ed., p. 544). St. Louis: Mosby.

ALTERNATE ITEM FORMAT: MULTIPLE RESPONSE

191. **3, 4, 5, 6**
Rationale: The bubbling of water in the water-seal chamber indicates air drainage from the client. This is usually seen when intrathoracic pressure is greater than atmospheric pressure, and it may occur during exhalation, coughing, or sneezing. Excessive bubbling in the water-seal chamber may indicate an air leak, which is an unexpected finding. The fluctuation of water in the tube in the water-seal chamber during inhalation and exhalation is expected; an absence of fluctuation may indicate that the chest tube is obstructed, that the lung has re-expanded, or that no more air is leaking into the pleural space. Gentle (not vigorous) bubbling should be noted in the suction-control chamber. A total of 50 mL of drainage is not excessive in a client returning to the nursing unit from the recovery room; however, drainage of more than 100 mL/hr is considered excessive and requires physician notification. The chest-tube insertion site is covered with an occlusive (airtight) dressing to prevent air from entering the pleural space. Positioning the drainage system below the client's chest allows gravity to drain the pleural space.
Test-Taking Strategy: Thinking about the physiology associated with the functioning of a chest-tube drainage system will help you to answer this question. The words "excessive bubbling" and "vigorous bubbling" will assist you with eliminating options 1 and 2. Review the care of the client with a chest-tube drainage system if you had difficulty with this question.
Level of Cognitive Ability: Analysis
Client Needs: Physiological Integrity
Integrated Process: Nursing Process/Data Collection
Content Area: Adult Health/Respiratory
References: Christensen, B., & Kockrow, E. (2006). *Adult health nursing* (5th ed., pp. 438-440). St. Louis: Mosby.
Linton, A. (2007). *Introduction to medical-surgical nursing* (4th ed., pp. 529-530). Philadelphia: Saunders.
Potter, P., & Perry, A. (2005). *Fundamentals of nursing* (6th ed., p. 1120). St. Louis: Mosby.

REFERENCES

Black, J., & Hawks, J. (2005). *Medical-surgical nursing: Clinical management for positive outcomes* (7th ed.). Philadelphia: Saunders.

Christensen, B., & Kockrow, E. (2006). *Adult health nursing* (5th ed.). St. Louis: Mosby.

Christensen, B., & Kockrow, E. (2006). *Foundations of nursing* (5th ed.). St. Louis: Mosby.

Ignatavicius, D., & Workman, M. (2006). *Medical-surgical nursing: Critical thinking for collaborative care* (5th ed.). St. Louis: Saunders.

Lewis, S., Heitkemper, M., Dirksen, S., & Bucher, L. (2007). *Medical-surgical nursing: Assessment and management of clinical problems* (7th ed.). St. Louis: Mosby.

Linton, A. (2007). *Introduction to medical-surgical nursing* (4th ed.). Philadelphia: Saunders.

Monahan, F., Marek, J., Neighbors, M., & Green, C. (2007). *Phipps' medical-surgical nursing: Health and illness perspectives* (8th ed.). St. Louis: Mosby.

National Council of State Boards of Nursing (Eds.). (2008). *2008 Detailed Test Plan for the NCLEX-PN® Examination, National Council of State Boards of Nursing.* Chicago: Author.

National Council of State Boards of Nursing. *NCSBN home page.* www.ncsbn.org. Accessed June 29, 2008.

Perry, A., & Potter, P. (2006). *Clinical nursing skills & techniques* (6th ed.). St. Louis: Mosby.

Potter, P., & Perry, A. (2005). *Fundamentals of nursing* (6th ed.). St. Louis: Mosby.

Maternity Nursing

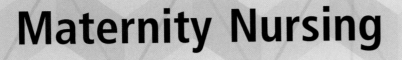

PYRAMID TERMS

amniotic fluid The straw-colored fluid that surrounds and protects the fetus. The fetus floats in the amniotic fluid, which serves as a cushion against injury from sudden blows or movements. It also helps maintain a constant body temperature for the fetus. The fetus modifies the amniotic fluid through the processes of swallowing, urinating, and movement through the respiratory tract.

ballottement The rebounding of the fetus against the examiner's finger on palpation. When the cervix is tapped, the fetus floats upward in the amniotic fluid. A rebound is felt by the examiner when the fetus falls back.

Chadwick's sign The violet coloration of the vaginal mucous membranes that is visible from about 4 weeks' gestation that is caused by increased vascularity. This is a probable sign of pregnancy.

delivery The actual event of birth. The expulsion or extraction of the neonate and the fetal membranes at birth.

fertilization The union of an ovum and sperm. Fertilization occurs within 12 hours of ovulation and within 2 to 3 days of insemination (i.e., the average duration of viability of the ovum and the sperm).

Goodell's sign The softening of the cervix. This occurs at the beginning of the second month of gestation and is a probable sign of pregnancy.

gravida A pregnant woman. The woman is called *gravida I* (or *primigravida*) during the first pregnancy, *gravida II* during the second, and so on.

Hegar's sign The compressibility and softening of the lower uterine segment. This occurs at about 6 weeks' gestation, and it is a probable sign of pregnancy.

implantation The embedding of the fertilized ovum in the uterine mucosa, which occurs 6 to 8 days after conception.

infant A baby who is born alive. Babies are considered infants from the time that they are 28 days old until the first birthday.

labor A coordinated sequence of rhythmic, involuntary uterine contractions that result in the effacement and dilation of cervix; this is followed by the expulsion of the products of conception.

lochia Vaginal discharge from the uterus that consists of blood from the vessels of the placental site, tissue debris from the decidua, and mucus. Lochia lasts for 2 to 6 weeks' postpartum, and it is differentiated by color: rubra, serosa, or alba.

Nägele's rule A way to determine the estimated date of birth that works on the premise that the woman has a 28-day menstrual cycle. Add 7 days to the first day of last menstrual period. Subtract 3 months from that date, and then add 1 year. Alternatively, add 7 days to the last menstrual period, and then count forward 9 months.

neonate A human offspring from the time of birth to day 28 of life; also called a *newborn*.

newborn A human offspring from the time of birth to day 28 of life; also called a *neonate*.

parity The number of pregnancies that have reached viability, regardless of whether the infants were alive or stillborn.

placenta The organ that provides for the exchange of nutrients and waste products between the fetus and the mother and that produces hormones to maintain pregnancy. It develops by the third month of gestation, and it is also called the *afterbirth*.

quickening The maternal perception of fetal movement, which usually appears around 16 to 20 weeks' gestation.

PYRAMID TO SUCCESS

The Pyramid to Success focuses on the physiological and psychosocial aspects related to the experience of pregnancy. The pyramid points begin with instructing the pregnant client with regard to measures that will promote a healthy environment for both the mother and fetus. Focus on the importance of antenatal follow-up care, nutrition, and the interventions for common discomforts that occur during pregnancy. Review the purpose of the commonly prescribed diagnostic tests and procedures during the antenatal period. Focus on disorders that can occur during pregnancy, particularly gestational hypertension and diabetes. Review the labor and delivery process and the immediate interventions when the mother or the fetal status is compromised (e.g., prolapsed cord, altered fetal heart rate). Review the fetal effects that result from the mother with acquired immunodeficiency syndrome or from the mother who abuses substances. Focus on the normal expectations of the postpartum period and the complications that can occur. The pyramid points also focus on the normal physical assessment findings of the newborn and the early identification of disorders of the newborn. The Integrated Processes addressed in this unit include Caring, the Clinical Problem-Solving Process (Nursing Process), Communication and Documentation, and Teaching and Learning.

▲ CLIENT NEEDS

Safe and Effective Care Environment

Collaborating with other members of the health care team

Establishing priorities of care

Handling infectious materials safely

Maintaining asepsis

Maintaining confidentiality

Obtaining informed consent for procedures

Providing continuity of care

Upholding parent rights

Using standard, transmission-based, and other precautions when delivering care

Health Promotion and Maintenance

Assessing growth and development

Assessing health and wellness

Discussing expected body-image changes

Identifying high-risk behaviors

Identifying lifestyle choices

Performing techniques of data collection

Providing antenatal, intrapartum, postpartum, and newborn care

Psychosocial Integrity

Considering cultural, spiritual, and religious influences regarding birth and motherhood

Discussing situational role changes

Ensuring therapeutic interactions within the family

Identifying available support systems

Identifying coping mechanisms

Physiological Integrity

Identifying at-risk clients during pregnancy

Instructing the client about prescribed diagnostic tests and procedures

Monitoring for expected outcomes and effects related to pharmacological and parenteral therapies

Monitoring for normal expectations during pregnancy

Monitoring the client during the labor and delivery process

Providing interventions for unexpected events during the pregnancy

Providing nonpharmacological and pharmacological comfort interventions during pregnancy

Teaching the client about nutrition during pregnancy and during the postpartum period

Teaching the client about the physiological changes that occur during pregnancy

REFERENCES

Chernecky, C., & Berger, B. (2008). *Laboratory tests and diagnostic procedures* (5th ed.). Philadelphia: Saunders.

Christensen, B., & Kockrow, E. (2006). *Foundations of nursing* (5th ed.). St. Louis: Mosby.

deWit, S. (2009). *Medical-surgical nursing: Concepts & practice*. St. Louis: Saunders.

Hill, S., & Howlett, H. (2005). *Success in practical/vocational nursing: From student to leader.* (5th ed.). Philadelphia: Saunders.

Hodgson, B., & Kizior, R. (2008). *Saunders nursing drug handbook 2008*. Philadelphia: Saunders.

Leifer, G. (2008). *Maternity nursing: An introductory text* (10th ed.). Philadelphia: Saunders.

Lilley, L., Harrington, S., & Snyder, J. (2007). *Pharmacology and the nursing process* (5th ed.). St. Louis: Mosby.

Linton, A. (2007). *Introduction to medical-surgical nursing* (4th ed.). Philadelphia: Saunders.

Lowdermilk, D., & Perry, S. (2007). *Maternity & women's health care* (9th ed.). St. Louis: Mosby.

Murray, S., & McKinney, E. (2006). *Foundations of maternal-newborn nursing* (4th ed.). Philadelphia: Saunders.

National Council of State Boards of Nursing (Eds.). (2008). *2008 Detailed Test Plan for the NCLEX-PN® Examination, National Council of State Boards of Nursing*. Chicago: Author.

National Council of State Boards of Nursing. *NCSBN home page*. www.ncsbn.org. Accessed June 30, 2008.

Nix, S. (2005). *Williams' basic nutrition and diet therapy* (11th ed.). St. Louis: Mosby.

Potter, P., & Perry, A. (2005). *Fundamentals of nursing* (6th ed.). St. Louis: Mosby.

Pagana, K., & Pagana, T. (2005). *Mosby's diagnostic and laboratory test reference* (7th ed.). St. Louis: Mosby.

Price, D., & Gwin, J. (2005). *Thompson's pediatric nursing* (9th ed.). Philadelphia: Saunders.

Female Reproductive System

I. FEMALE REPRODUCTIVE STRUCTURES
(Figure 20-1)
A. Ovaries
   1. Form and expel ova
   2. Primary source of estrogen and progesterone
B. Fallopian tubes
   1. Muscular tubes (oviducts) that are approximate to the ovaries and that connect into the uterus
   2. Provide transportation for the ova from the ovaries to the uterus
   3. Site for **fertilization**
C. Uterus
   1. Muscular organ shaped like an upside-down pear in which the fetus develops; a normal nulliparous uterus weighs about 2 oz and has a capacity of about 10 mL
   2. Organ from which menstruation occurs
   3. Serves for the reception, **implantation,** retention, and nutrition of the fertilized ovum and fetus
D. Cervix
   1. Protective entrance to the body of the uterus
   2. Internal os opens into the body of the uterine cavity
   3. Cervical canal is located between the internal os and the external os
   4. External os opens into the vagina
E. Vagina
   1. Mucous membrane–lined, fibromuscular channel through the muscles of the pelvic floor
   2. Known as the *birth canal*
   3. Passage between the cervical os and the external environment for the fetus and the menstrual flow

II. MENSTRUAL CYCLE (Table 20-1)
A. Menstrual cycle: The regularly recurring physiological changes in the endometrium that culminate in its shedding; may vary in duration, with average of approximately 28 days; ovarian and uterine changes occur

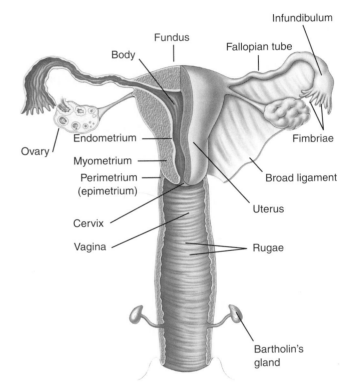

FIG. 20-1 Female reproductive organs. (From Herlihy, B., & Maebius, N. [2007]. *The human body in health and illness* [3rd ed.]. Philadelphia: Saunders.)

B. Ovarian hormones
   1. Include gonadotropin-releasing hormone, follicle-stimulating hormone, and luteinizing hormone
   2. Released by the hypothalamus and the anterior pituitary gland
   3. Produce changes in the ovaries
   4. Secretion of ovarian hormones leads to changes in the endometrium

III. FEMALE PELVIS AND MEASUREMENTS
A. True pelvis
   1. Lies below the pelvic brim (the lower, curved, bony canal)

TABLE 20-1	Menstrual Cycle

Ovarian Changes		
Hypothalamic-Pituitary Cycle	**Ovarian Cycle (Preovulatory Phase)**	**Ovarian Cycle (Luteal Phase)**
The hypothalamus, stimulated by the low blood levels of estrogen and progesterone that occur toward the end of the normal menstrual cycle, releases GnRH through the portal system to the anterior pituitary system	The follicle ruptures and releases an ovum into the peritoneal cavity	This cycle begins immediately after ovulation
GnRH stimulates the secretion of FSH by the anterior lobe of the pituitary gland		The body temperature drops and then rises by 0.5°-1° F around the time of ovulation
FSH stimulates the development of follicles and their production of estrogen		The corpus luteum is formed from follicle cells that remain in the ovary after ovulation
Estrogen produced by the follicle stimulates the increased secretion LH by the anterior lobe of the pituitary gland		The corpus luteum secretes estrogen and progesterone during the remaining 14 days of the cycle
Most follicles die, leaving one to mature into a large graafian follicle, which then begins to transform into a corpus luteum		The corpus luteum degenerates if the ovum is not fertilized, and the secretion of estrogen and progesterone declines
		Estrogen and progesterone inhibit the secretion of FSH and LH
		After the corpus luteum degenerates, the pituitary secretion of estrogen and progesterone decreases, and the ovarian cycle begins again

Uterine Changes			
Menstrual Phase	**Proliferative Phase**	**Secretory Phase**	**Ischemic Phase**
Consists of 4-6 days of bleeding as the endometrium breaks down and is shed as a result of the decreased amount of estrogen and progesterone	Estrogen stimulates the proliferation and growth of the endometrium	Lasts about 12 days	The corpus luteum regresses if fertilization and implantation do not occur
FSH rises, enabling the beginning of a new cycle	Lasts about 9 days	Follows ovulation	Rapid decrease in progesterone and estrogen
	As estrogen increases, it suppresses the secretion of FSH and increases the secretion of LH	Initiated in response to the increase in LH	Necrosis of the functional endometrium develops, and the functional layer separates from the basal layer
	LH stimulates ovulation and the development of the corpus luteum	The graafian follicle is replaced by the corpus luteum	Menstrual bleeding begins, marking day 1 of the next cycle
	Ovulation occurs between day 12 and day 16	The corpus luteum secretes progesterone and estrogen	
	Estrogen is high and progesterone is low	Progesterone prepares the endometrium for pregnancy should a fertilized ovum be implanted	

FSH, Follicle-stimulating hormone; *GnRH,* gonadotropin-releasing hormone; *LH,* luteinizing hormone.

2. Consists of the pelvic inlet, the mid pelvis, and the pelvic outlet
B. False pelvis
  1. Shallow portion above the pelvic brim
  2. Supports the abdominal viscera
C. Types of pelvis
  1. Gynecoid
    a. Normal female pelvis
    b. Transversely rounded or blunt
    c. Most favorable for successful **labor** and birth
  2. Android
    a. Wedge-shaped or angulated
    b. Resembles male pelvis
    c. Not favorable for **labor**
    d. Narrow pelvic planes can cause slow descent and mid-pelvis arrest
  3. Anthropoid
    a. Oval shape
    b. The outlet is adequate for **labor,** with a normal or moderately narrow pubic arch
  4. Platypelloid
    a. Flat shape with an oval inlet
    b. The transverse diameter is wide, but the anteroposterior diameter is short, thus making the outlet inadequate for **labor**
D. Pelvic inlet diameters
  1. Anteroposterior diameters
    a. Diagonal conjugate: Distance from the lower margin of the symphysis pubis to the sacral promontory
    b. True conjugate or conjugate vera: Distance from the upper margin of the symphysis pubis to the sacral promontory
    c. Obstetric conjugate: Smallest front-to-back distance through which the fetal head must pass when moving through the pelvic inlet
  2. Transverse diameter: Largest of the pelvic inlet diameters; located at right angles to the true conjugate
  3. Oblique (diagonal) diameter: Not clinically measurable
  4. Posterior sagittal diameter: Distance from the point where the anteroposterior and transverse diameters cross each other to the middle of the sacral promontory
E. Pelvic midplane diameters
  1. Transverse diameter (interspinous diameter)
  2. Midplane is normally the largest plane and has the longest diameter
F. Pelvic outlet diameters
  1. Transverse (intertuberous)
  2. Outlet presents the smallest plane of the pelvic canal

IV. **FERTILIZATION AND IMPLANTATION**
A. **Fertilization**
  1. Occurs in the upper region of the fallopian tubes

  2. Occurs within 12 hours of ovulation and within 2 to 3 days of insemination (the average duration of viability for the ovum and the sperm)
  3. Takes place when the sperm and ovum unite
  4. After **fertilization**, the membrane of the ovum undergoes changes that prevent the entry of other sperm
  5. Each reproductive cell carries 23 chromosomes
  6. Sperm carry an X or Y chromosome, and eggs carry an X chromosome; an XY combination results in a male child, and an XX combination results in a female
B. **Implantation**
  1. Zygote (fertilized ovum) is propelled toward the uterus
  2. Implants 6 to 8 days after **fertilization**
  3. Blastocyst (embryonic form) secretes chorionic gonadotropin to ensure that the corpus luteum remains viable; it secretes estrogen and progesterone for the first 2 to 3 months of gestation

V. **FETAL DEVELOPMENT** (Table 20-2)
A. Preembryonic period: First 2 weeks after conception
B. Embryonic stage: Begins on day 15 and continues through approximately the eighth week after conception
C. Fetal period: Begins the ninth week after conception and ends with birth

VI. **FETAL ENVIRONMENT**
A. Amnion
  1. Encloses the amniotic cavity
  2. Inner cell membrane that forms about the second week of embryonic development
  3. Forms a fluid-filled sac that surrounds the embryo and later the fetus
B. Chorion
  1. Outer membrane
  2. Becomes vascularized and forms the fetal part of the **placenta**
C. **Amniotic fluid**
  1. Consists of 800 to 1200 mL by term
  2. Surrounds, cushions, and protects the fetus and allows for fetal movement
  3. Maintains the body temperature of the fetus
  4. Consists largely of fetal urine and is therefore a measure of fetal kidney function
  5. The fetus modifies the **amniotic fluid** through the processes of swallowing, urinating, and movement through the respiratory tract.
D. **Placenta**
  1. Provides for the exchange of nutrients and waste products between the fetus and the mother
  2. Begins to form at **implantation**; structure completed by 12 weeks' gestation
  3. Dependent on maternal circulation
  4. Produces hormones to maintain pregnancy; assumes full responsibility for the production of these hormones by 12 weeks' gestation

TABLE 20-2   Fetal Development

Embryonic Stage	Fetal Period
Week 1 • Free-floating blastocyst **Weeks 2-3** • 2 mm in length • Groove formed along the middle of the back • Beginning of blood circulation • Heart is tubular in shape **Week 5** • 0.4-0.5 cm in length • 0.4 g in weight • Double heart chambers visible • Heart begins to beat; aortic arch and major veins completed • Body flexed and C-shaped; arm and leg buds present; head at right angle to body **Week 8** • 2.5-3 cm in length • 2 g in weight • Eyelids fuse • Circulatory system through umbilical cord well established • Testes and ovaries distinguishable; external genitalia sexless but beginning to differentiate • Every organ system present • Body fairly well formed; nose flat, eyes far apart; digits well formed; head elevating; tail almost disappeared; eyes, ears, nose, and mouth recognizable **Week 12** • 6-9 cm in length • 19 g in weight • Face well formed • Limbs long and slender • Kidneys able to secrete urine • Spontaneous movements occur • Heart tones detected by electronic devices between 10 and 12 weeks • Sex visually recognizable • Nails appearing; resembles a human; head erect but disproportionately large; skin pink and delicate	**Week 16** • 11.5-13.5 cm in length • 100 g in weight • Active movements are present • Fetal skin is transparent • Lanugo begins to develop • Skeletal ossification begins completion • Sex of fetus can be determined • Head still dominant; face looks human; eyes, ears, and nose approach typical appearance on gross examination; arm-to-leg ratio proportionate; scalp hair appears **Week 20** • 16-18.5 cm in length • 300 g in weight • Lanugo covers the entire body • Muscles developed • Enamel and dentin depositing • Heartbeat detected by fetoscope • Vernix caseosa appears; legs lengthen considerably; sebaceous glands appear **Week 24** • 23 cm in length • 600 g in weight • Hair on head well formed • Skin reddish and wrinkled • Reflex hand grasp • Vernix caseosa covers entire body • Has ability to hear **Week 28** • 27 cm in length • 1100 g in weight • Limbs are well flexed • Brain develops rapidly • Eyelids open and close; pupils capable of reacting to light • Lungs sufficiently developed to provide gas exchange; lecithin forming on alveolar surfaces • If born, neonate can breathe at this time **Weeks 30-31** • 31 cm in length • 1800-2100 g in weight • Bones are fully developed • Subcutaneous fat collected • Lecithin-to-sphingomyelin ratio switching to 1.2:1 • Skin pink and smooth • Has assumed birth position **Week 36** • 35 cm in length • 2200-2900 g in weight • Skin pink, body rounded • Less wrinkled • Lanugo disappearing • Lecithin-to-sphingomyelin ratio 2:1 or higher **Week 40** • 40 cm in length • 3200 g or more in weight • Skin pinkish and smooth • Lanugo present on upper arms and shoulders • Vernix caseosa decreases • Fingernails extend beyond fingertips • Sole (plantar) creases down to heel • Testes in scrotum • Labia majora well developed

5. Metabolic functions are respiration, nutrition, excretion, and storage

6. Large particles such as bacteria cannot pass through the **placenta**

7. In addition to nutrients, drugs, antibodies, and viruses can pass through the **placenta**

8. During the third trimester, the transfer of maternal immunoglobulin provides fetus passive immunity to certain diseases for the first few months after birth

9. By 8 weeks' gestation, genetic testing can be done (chorionic villus sampling)

VII. FETAL CIRCULATION (Figure 20-2)

A. Umbilical cord

1. Contains two arteries and one vein

2. Arteries carry deoxygenated blood and waste products from the fetus

3. Vein carries oxygenated blood and provides oxygen and nutrients to the fetus

B. Fetal heart rate

1. Depends on gestational age: 160 to 170 beats per minute during the first trimester, but slows with fetal growth to 120 to 160 beats per minute near or at term

2. Approximately twice the maternal heart rate

C. Fetal circulation bypass

1. Present as a result of nonfunctioning lungs

2. Bypasses must close after birth to allow blood to flow through the lungs and the liver

3. Ductus arteriosus connects the pulmonary artery to the aorta, bypassing the lungs

4. Ductus venosus connects the umbilical vein and the inferior vena cava, bypassing the liver

5. Foramen ovale is the opening between the right and left atria of heart, bypassing the lungs

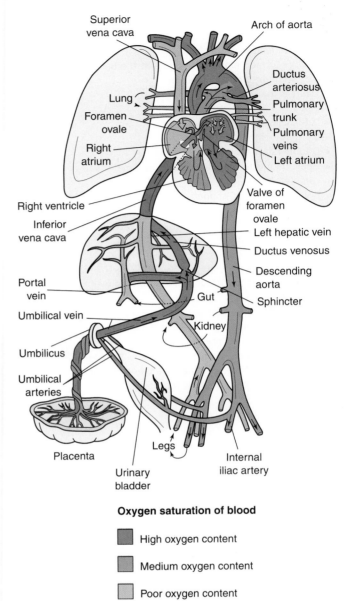

Oxygen saturation of blood

■ High oxygen content

■ Medium oxygen content

■ Poor oxygen content

FIG. 20-2 Schematic illustration of the fetal circulation. (From Lowdermilk, D., & Perry, S. [2007]. *Maternity & women's health care* [9th ed.]. St. Louis: Mosby.)

PRACTICE QUESTIONS

More questions on the companion CD!

192. A nurse is collecting data from a pregnant client when the client asks the nurse about the purpose of the fallopian tubes. The nurse responds to the client, knowing that the fallopian tubes:
   1. Are the organ of copulation
   2. Are where the fetus develops
   3. Are where fertilization occurs
   4. Secrete estrogen and progesterone

193. A nursing student is assigned to care for an adolescent female client in the health care clinic, and the instructor reviews the menstrual cycle with the student. The instructor determines that the student understands the process of the secretion of follicle-stimulating hormone (FSH) and luteinizing hormone (LH) if the student states:
   1. "FSH and LH are secreted by the adrenal glands."

   2. "FSH and LH are released from the anterior pituitary gland."
   3. "FSH and LH are secreted by the corpus luteum of the ovary."
   4. "FSH and LH stimulate the formation of milk during pregnancy."

194. A nurse working in a prenatal clinic reviews a client's chart and notes that the physician documents that the client has a gynecoid pelvis. The nurse understands that this type of pelvis is:
   1. Not favorable for labor
   2. Not normally a female pelvis type
   3. A wide pelvis with a short diameter
   4. The most favorable for labor and birth

195. A client asks the nurse about the purpose of the placenta. The nurse plans to respond to the client, knowing that the placenta:
    1. Cushions and protects the fetus
    2. Maintains the body temperature of the fetus
    3. Prevents antibodies and viruses from passing to the fetus
    4. Provides an exchange of nutrients and waste products between the mother and the fetus

196. A nurse is describing the process of fetal circulation to a client during a prenatal visit. The nurse tells the client that fetal circulation consists of:
    1. Two umbilical veins and one umbilical artery
    2. Two umbilical arteries and one umbilical vein
    3. Arteries that carry oxygenated blood to the fetus
    4. Veins that carry deoxygenated blood to the fetus

197. A nursing student is assigned to a client in labor. The nursing instructor asks the student to describe fetal circulation, specifically the ductus venosus. The instructor determines that the student understands the structure of the ductus venosus if the student states that it:
    1. Connects the pulmonary artery to the aorta
    2. Is an opening between the right and left atria
    3. Connects the umbilical vein to the inferior vena cava
    4. Connects the umbilical artery to the inferior vena cava

198. During a prenatal visit, the nurse checks the fetal heart rate (FHR) of a client in the third trimester of pregnancy. The nurse determines that the FHR is normal if which of the following heart rates is noted?
    1. 80 beats per minute
    2. 100 beats per minute
    3. 150 beats per minute
    4. 180 beats per minute

199. A nurse is teaching a pregnant woman about the physiological effects and hormone changes that occur during pregnancy. The woman asks the nurse about the purpose of estrogen. The nurse bases the response on which of the following purposes of estrogen?
    1. It maintains the uterine lining for implantation.
    2. It stimulates the metabolism of glucose, and it converts glucose to fat.
    3. It prevents the involution of the corpus luteum, and it maintains the production of progesterone until the placenta is formed.
    4. It stimulates uterine development to provide an environment for the fetus, and it stimulates the breasts to prepare for lactation.

200. A nursing student is asked to describe the size of the uterus in a nonpregnant client. Which of the following responses, if made by the student, indicates an understanding of the anatomy of this structure?
    1. "The uterus weighs about 2 ounces."
    2. "The uterus weighs about 2.2 pounds."
    3. "The uterus has a capacity of about 50 milliliters."
    4. "The uterus is round in shape and weighs approximately 1000 grams."

ALTERNATE ITEM FORMAT: MULTIPLE RESPONSE

201. A nursing instructor asks a nursing student to list the functions of the amniotic fluid. The student responds correctly by stating that which of the following are functions of amniotic fluid? Select all that apply.
    ☑ 1. Allows for fetal movement
    ☑ 2. Is a measure of kidney function
    ☑ 3. Surrounds, cushions, and protects the fetus
    ☑ 4. Maintains the body temperature of the fetus
    ☐ 5. Prevents large particles such as bacteria from passing to the fetus
    ☐ 6. Provides an exchange of nutrients and waste products between the mother and the fetus

ANSWERS

192. 3
Rationale: Each fallopian tube is a hollow muscular tube that transports a mature oocyte for final maturation and fertilization. Fertilization typically occurs near the boundary between the ampulla and the isthmus of the tube. Estrogen is a hormone that is produced by the ovarian follicles, the corpus luteum, the adrenal cortex, and the placenta during pregnancy. Progesterone is a hormone that is secreted by the corpus luteum of the ovary, the adrenal glands, and the placenta during pregnancy. The vagina is the organ of copulation, and the fetus develops in the uterus.
Test-Taking Strategy: Recalling the anatomy and physiology of the female reproductive system will direct you to the correct option. Remember that fertilization occurs in the fallopian tube. Review the female reproductive system if you had difficulty with this question.
Level of Cognitive Ability: Application
Client Needs: Physiological Integrity
Integrated Process: Nursing Process/Implementation
Content Area: Maternity/Antepartum
Reference: Leifer, G. (2008). *Maternity nursing: An introductory text* (10th ed., p. 30). Philadelphia: Saunders.

193. 2
Rationale: FSH and LH are released from the anterior pituitary gland in order to stimulate follicular growth and development, the growth of the graafian follicle, and the production of progesterone. Options 1, 3, and 4 are incorrect.

Test-Taking Strategy: Use the process of elimination. Option 4 can be eliminated, because the case of the question does not address pregnancy. Use your knowledge related to the menstrual cycle to select the correct option. Review the menstrual cycle if you had difficulty with this question.
Level of Cognitive Ability: Comprehension
Client Needs: Physiological Integrity
Integrated Process: Teaching and Learning
Content Area: Maternity/Antepartum
References: Leifer, G. (2008). *Maternity nursing: An introductory text* (10th ed., p. 22). Philadelphia: Saunders.
McKinney, E., James, S., Murray, S., & Ashwill, J. (2005). *Maternal-child nursing* (2nd ed., pp. 224-226). St. Louis: Saunders.

194. **4**
Rationale: A gynecoid pelvis is a normal female pelvis, and it is the most favorable for successful labor and birth. An android pelvis would not be favorable for labor because of the narrow pelvic planes. An anthropoid pelvis has an outlet that is adequate, with a normal or moderately narrow pubic arch. The platypelloid pelvis has a wide transverse diameter, but the anteroposterior diameter is short, thus making the outlet inadequate.
Test-Taking Strategy: Knowledge regarding pelvic types is required to answer this question. Remember that the gynecoid pelvis is the normal female pelvis. Review pelvic types if you had difficulty with this question.
Level of Cognitive Ability: Comprehension
Client Needs: Physiological Integrity
Integrated Process: Nursing Process/Data Collection
Content Area: Maternity/Antepartum
Reference: Leifer, G. (2008). *Maternity nursing: An introductory text* (10th ed., pp. 19-20). Philadelphia: Saunders.

195. **4**
Rationale: The placenta provides an exchange of nutrients and waste products between the mother and the fetus. The amniotic fluid surrounds, cushions, and protects the fetus, and it maintains the body temperature of the fetus.
Test-Taking Strategy: Knowledge regarding the purpose of the placenta and amniotic fluid is required to answer this question. Remember that the placenta provides nutrients. Review the structure and function of the placenta and the amniotic fluid if you had difficulty with this question.
Level of Cognitive Ability: Comprehension
Client Needs: Physiological Integrity
Integrated Process: Nursing Process/Planning
Content Area: Maternity/Antepartum
Reference: Leifer, G. (2008). *Maternity nursing: An introductory text* (10th ed., pp. 31-32). Philadelphia: Saunders.

196. **2**
Rationale: Blood pumped by the fetus' heart leaves the fetus through two umbilical arteries. After the blood is oxygenated, it is then returned by one umbilical vein. Arteries carry deoxygenated blood and waste products from the fetus, and veins carry oxygenated blood and provide oxygen and nutrients to the fetus.

Test-Taking Strategy: Recall the anatomy of fetal circulation to answer this question. Remember that there are three umbilical vessels within an umbilical cord (two arteries and one vein). Review the fetal circulation if you had difficulty with this question.
Level of Cognitive Ability: Application
Client Needs: Physiological Integrity
Integrated Process: Teaching and Learning
Content Area: Maternity/Antepartum
Reference: Leifer, G. (2008). *Maternity nursing: An introductory text* (10th ed., p. 34). Philadelphia: Saunders.

197. **3**
Rationale: The ductus venosus connects the umbilical vein to the inferior vena cava. The foramen ovale is a temporary opening between the right and left atria. The ductus arteriosus joins the aorta and the pulmonary artery.
Test-Taking Strategy: Recall the anatomy of the fetal circulation to answer this question. Remember that the ductus venosus connects the umbilical vein to the inferior vena cava. Review the fetal circulation if you had difficulty with this question.
Level of Cognitive Ability: Comprehension
Client Needs: Physiological Integrity
Integrated Process: Teaching and Learning
Content Area: Maternity/Antepartum
Reference: Leifer, G. (2008). *Maternity nursing: An introductory text* (10th ed., p. 34). Philadelphia: Saunders.

198. **3**
Rationale: Fetal heart rate depends on gestational age. It is normally 160 to 170 beats per minute during the first trimester, but it slows with fetal growth to 110 or 120 (low end) to 160 (high end) beats per minute near or at term.
Test-Taking Strategy: Note the strategic words "third trimester"; this will direct you to option 3. Review the fetal heart rate if you had difficulty with this question.
Level of Cognitive Ability: Comprehension
Client Needs: Physiological Integrity
Integrated Process: Nursing Process/Data Collection
Content Area: Maternity
Reference: Leifer, G. (2007). *Introduction to maternity and pediatric nursing* (5th ed., p.132). Philadelphia: Saunders.

199. **4**
Rationale: Estrogen stimulates uterine development to provide an environment for the fetus, and it stimulates the breasts to prepare for lactation. Progesterone maintains the uterine lining for implantation and relaxes all smooth muscle. Human placental lactogen stimulates the metabolism of glucose and converts the glucose to fat. Human chorionic gonadotropin prevents the involution of the corpus luteum and maintains the production of progesterone until the placenta is formed.
Test-Taking Strategy: Recalling the functions of various hormones related to pregnancy will direct you to the correct option. Remember that estrogen stimulates uterine development to provide an environment for the fetus and that it stimulates the breasts to prepare for lactation. Review these various hormones if you had difficulty with this question.

Level of Cognitive Ability: Application
Client Needs: Physiological Integrity
Integrated Process: Teaching and Learning
Content Area: Maternity/Antepartum
References: Leifer, G. (2007). *Introduction to maternity and pediatric nursing* (5th ed., p. 39). Philadelphia: Saunders.
McKinney, E., James, S., Murray, S., & Ashwill, J. (2005). *Maternal-child nursing* (2nd ed., p. 258). St. Louis: Saunders.

200. 1
Rationale: Before conception, the uterus is a small, pear-shaped organ that is contained entirely in the pelvic cavity. Before pregnancy, the uterus weighs approximately 60 g (2 oz), and it has a capacity of about 10 mL ($\frac{1}{3}$ oz). At the end of pregnancy, the uterus weighs approximately 1000 g (2.2 lb), and it has a capacity that is sufficient for the fetus, the placenta, and the amniotic fluid.
Test-Taking Strategy: Note the strategic word "nonpregnant." Visualizing each of the items identified in the options will direct you to the correct option. Review the anatomy of the uterus if you had difficulty with this question.
Level of Cognitive Ability: Comprehension
Client Needs: Physiological Integrity
Integrated Process: Teaching and Learning
Content Area: Maternity/Antepartum

Reference: Leifer, G. (2008). *Maternity nursing: An introductory text* (10th ed., p. 17). Philadelphia: Saunders.

ALTERNATE ITEM FORMAT: MULTIPLE RESPONSE

201. 1, 2, 3, 4
Rationale: The amniotic fluid surrounds, cushions, and protects the fetus. It allows the fetus to move freely, it maintains the body temperature of the fetus, and it helps to measure kidney function, because the amount of fluid is based on the amount of urination from the fetus. The placenta prevents large particles such as bacteria from passing to the fetus, and it provides an exchange of nutrients and waste products between the mother and the fetus.
Test-Taking Strategy: Focus on the subject of the question: the functions of the amniotic fluid. Visualizing the anatomical location of the amniotic fluid will direct you to the correct options. Review the function of the amniotic fluid if you had difficulty with this question.
Level of Cognitive Ability: Comprehension
Client Needs: Physiological Integrity
Integrated Process: Teaching and Learning
Content Area: Maternity/Antepartum
Reference: Wong, D., Perry, S., Hockenberry, M., Lowdermilk, D., & Wilson, D. (2006). *Maternal-child nursing care* (3rd ed., p. 197). St. Louis: Mosby.

REFERENCES

Leifer, G. (2008). *Maternity nursing: An introductory text* (10th ed.). Philadelphia: Saunders.
Leifer, G. (2007). *Introduction to maternity and pediatric nursing* (5th ed.). Philadelphia: Saunders.
Lowdermilk, D., & Perry, S. (2007). *Maternity & women's health care* (9th ed.). St. Louis: Mosby.

McKinney, E., James, S., Murray, S., & Ashwill, J. (2005). *Maternal-child nursing* (2nd ed.). St. Louis: Saunders.
Wong, D., Perry, S., Hockenberry, M., Lowdermilk, D., & Wilson, D. (2006). *Maternal-child nursing care* (3rd ed.). St. Louis: Mosby.

Obstetrical Assessment

I. GESTATION
A. Time from the **fertilization** of the ovum until the estimated date of birth
B. Lasts approximately 280 days or 40 weeks
C. First trimester lasts from week 1 through 13; second trimester last from weeks 14 through 26; third trimester last from weeks 27 through 40
D. **Nägele's rule** for estimating date of birth: To be accurate, the woman must have a regular 28-day menstrual cycle; the rule must be adjusted if woman's cycle is longer or shorter than 28 days (Box 21-1)

II. GRAVIDITY AND PARITY
A. Gravidity
  1. **Gravida**: A woman who is pregnant
  2. Gravidity: Number of pregnancies
  3. Nulligravida: A woman who has never been pregnant
  4. Primigravida: A woman who is pregnant for the first time
  5. Multigravida: A woman who has had two or more pregnancies
B. **Parity**
  1. **Parity**: The number of births (not the number of fetuses [e.g., twins]) carried past 20 weeks' gestation, whether or not the fetus was born alive
  2. Nullipara: A woman who has not had a birth at more than 20 weeks' gestation
  3. Primipara: A woman who has had one birth that occurred after 20 weeks' gestation
  4. Multipara: A woman who has had two or more pregnancies that resulted in viable offspring
C. Use of GTPAL: Pregnancy outcomes can be described with the GTPAL acronym (Box 21-2)
  1. G = Gravidity; number of pregnancies, including the present one
  2. T = Term births; number of children born at term (i.e., longer than 37 weeks' gestation)
  3. P = Preterm births; number of children born before 37 weeks' gestation
  4. A = Abortions or miscarriages; number of abortions/miscarriages (included in **gravida** if before 20 weeks' gestation; included in **parity** if past 20 weeks' gestation); note that a termination of the pregnancy after 20 weeks is referred to as a therapeutic termination
  5. L = Live births; number of live births or living children

III. PREGNANCY SIGNS
A. Presumptive signs
  1. Breast changes
  2. Amenorrhea
  3. Nausea and vomiting
  4. Urinary frequency
  5. Fatigue
  6. **Quickening**: First perception of fetal movement appearing usually in the sixteenth to twentieth week of gestation
B. Probable signs
  1. **Goodell's sign**: Softening of the cervix that occurs at the beginning of the second month of pregnancy
  2. **Chadwick's sign**: Violet coloration of the mucous membranes of the cervix, vagina, and vulva that occurs at about week 4
  3. **Hegar's sign**: Softening of the uterus that occurs at about week 6
  4. Positive result of pregnancy test (serum)
  5. Positive result of pregnancy test (urine)
  6. Braxton Hicks contractions: Irregular contractions that occur intermittently throughout pregnancy and that do not increase in intensity or duration or cause cervical dilation
  7. **Ballottement**: The rebounding of the fetus against the examiner's fingers on palpation
C. Positive signs
  1. Visualization of the fetus via radiography or ultrasound
  2. Fetal heart rate detected by ultrasound examination at 6 weeks' gestation; by electronic devices at 10 to 12 weeks' gestation, and by nonelectronic device (fetoscope) at 20 weeks' gestation
  3. Fetal movements palpated
  4. Fetal movements visible

BOX 21-1 **Nägele's Rule for Determining the Estimated Date of Birth**

Take the first day of the last menstrual period: September 12, 2009
- Add 7 days: September 19, 2009
- Subtract 3 months: June 19, 2009
- Add 1 year: June 19, 2010

Estimated date of birth: June 19, 2010

BOX 21-2 **GTPAL Acronym**

G = Gravidity
T = Term births
P = Preterm births
A = Abortions/miscarriages
L = Live births

Example: A woman is pregnant for the fourth time. She had one elective abortion during the first trimester, a daughter who was born at 40 weeks' gestation, and a son who was born at 36 weeks' gestation. Therefore, she is gravida (G) = 4; parity = 2; and term (T) = 1 (the daughter born at 40 weeks' gestation). She is also preterm (P) = 1 (the son born at 36 weeks' gestation); abortion (A) = 1 (the abortion is counted in the gravida, but it is not included in the parity, because it occurred before 20 weeks' gestation); and live births (L) = 2. Therefore, she would be considered GTPAL = 4, 1, 1, 1, 2.

IV. **FUNDAL HEIGHT** (Box 21-3)
A. Measured to evaluate the gestational age of the fetus (Fig. 21-1)
B. During the second and third trimesters (weeks 18 to 30), the fundal height in centimeters approximately equals the fetus's age in weeks, plus or minus 2 cm (Fig. 21-2)
C. At approximately 14 to 16 weeks, the fundus can be found above the symphysis pubis
D. At approximately 20 to 22 weeks, the fundus rises to the level of the umbilicus
E. At term, the fundus nearly reaches the xiphoid process
V. **MATERNAL RISK FACTORS**
A. TORCH infections
    1. Description: A group of organisms capable of crossing the **placenta** and adversely affecting the development of the fetus; infection may also occur during **delivery**
    2. Include *Toxoplasmosis; Other* infections, such as hepatitis and group B *Streptococcus; Rubella* (German measles); *Cytomegalovirus;* and *Herpes* and hepatitis A and B
    3. See Chapter 22 for information about these infections
B. Sexually transmitted infections
    1. Include chlamydia, syphilis, gonorrhea, condylomata acuminata (venereal warts),

BOX 21-3 **Measuring Fundal Height**

1. Place the client in a supine position.
2. Place the end of the tape measure at the level of the symphysis pubis.
3. Stretch the tape to the top of the uterine fundus.

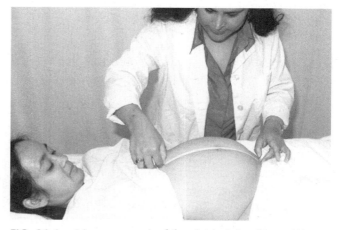

FIG. 21-1 Measurement of fundal height. (From Wong, D., Perry, S., Hockenberry, M., Lowdermilk, D., & Wilson, D. [2006]. *Maternal-child nursing care* [3rd ed.]. St. Louis: Mosby. Courtesy of Chris Rozales, San Francisco, CA.)

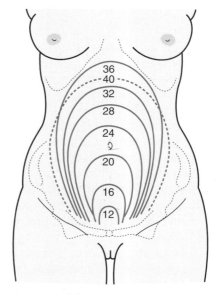

FIG. 21-2 Height of fundus by weeks of normal gestation with a single fetus. *Dashed line,* Height after lightening. (From Wong, D., Perry, S., Hockenberry, M., Lowdermilk, D., & Wilson, D. [2006]. *Maternal-child nursing care* [3rd ed.]. St. Louis: Mosby.)

bacterial vaginosis, vaginal candidiasis, and trichomoniasis
    2. See Chapter 22 for information about these infections
C. Substance abuse
    1. Many substances cross the **placenta**; therefore, no drugs, including over-the-counter

medications, should be taken unless prescribed by the physician

2. Substances commonly abused include alcohol, cocaine, crack, marijuana, amphetamines, barbiturates, heroin, and cigarettes

3. Substance abuse threatens normal fetal growth and the successful term completion of the pregnancy

4. Substance abuse places the pregnancy and the fetus/**newborn** at risk for bleeding, complications, miscarriage, stillbirth, prematurity, low birth weight, and sudden **infant** death syndrome

5. Physical signs of drug abuse may include dilated or contracted pupils, fatigue, track (needle) marks, skin abscesses, inflamed nasal mucosa, and inappropriate behavior by the mother

6. The consumption of alcohol during pregnancy may lead to fetal alcohol syndrome, congenital anomalies, and growth deficits; can also cause jitteriness and physical abnormalities

7. Smoking leads to low birth weights, a higher incidence of birth defects, and stillbirth

8. Neonatal abstinence syndrome can result as the **newborn** withdraws from the substance abused by the mother

D. Adolescent pregnancy

1. Factors that result in adolescent pregnancy include the early onset of menarche, changing sexual behaviors in this age group, problems with family development, poverty, and a lack of knowledge regarding reproduction and birth control

2. Major concerns related to adolescent pregnancy include poor nutritional status, emotional and behavioral difficulties, lack of support systems, increased risk of stillbirth, low birth weight, fetal mortality, cephalopelvic disproportion, and increased risks of maternal complications, such as hypertension, anemia, prolonged labor, and infections

3. The role of the nurse in reducing the risks and consequences of adolescent pregnancy is twofold

   a. To encourage early and continued prenatal care

   b. To refer the adolescent, if necessary, for appropriate assistance, which can help counter the effects of a negative socioeconomic environment

PRACTICE QUESTIONS

More questions on the companion CD!

202. A client arrives at the prenatal clinic for her first prenatal assessment. The client tells the nurse that the first day of her last menstrual period was October 20, 2010. Using Nägele's rule, the nurse determines the estimated date of birth to be:
   1. July 12, 2011
   2. July 27, 2011
   3. August 12, 2011
   4. August 27, 2011

203. A pregnant client asks the nurse in the clinic when she will be able to start feeling the fetus move. The nurse responds by telling the mother that fetal movements will be noted between:
   1. 6 and 8 weeks' gestation
   2. 8 and 10 weeks' gestation
   3. 10 and 12 weeks' gestation
   4. 16 and 20 weeks' gestation

204. A nurse is collecting data during the admission assessment of a client who is pregnant with twins. The client has a healthy 5-year-old child who was delivered at 38 weeks, and she tells the nurse that she does not have a history of any type of abortion or fetal demise. The nurse would document the GTPAL for this client as:
   1. G = 3, T = 2, P = 0, A = 0, L = 1
   2. G = 2, T = 1, P = 0, A = 0, L = 1
   3. G = 1, T = 1, P = 1, A = 0, L = 1
   4. G = 2, T = 0, P = 0, A = 0, L = 1

205. A nurse is collecting data during the admission assessment of a client who is pregnant with twins. The client also has a 5-year-old child. The nurse would document which gravida and para status on this client?
   1. Gravida I, para I
   2. Gravida II, para I
   3. Gravida II, para II
   4. Gravida III, para II

206. A nurse is reviewing the record of a client who has just been told that her pregnancy test is positive. The nurse notes that the physician has documented the presence of Goodell's sign. The nurse determines that this sign is indicative of:
   1. A softening of the cervix
   2. The presence of fetal movement
   3. The presence of human chorionic gonadotropin in the urine
   4. A soft blowing sound that corresponds with the maternal pulse that is heard while auscultating the uterus

207. A primipara is being evaluated in the clinic during her second trimester of pregnancy. Which of the following would indicate an abnormal physical finding that necessitates further testing?
   1. Quickening
   2. Braxton Hicks contractions
   3. Consistent increase in fundal height
   4. Fetal heart rate of 180 beats per minute

208. A nurse is collecting data from a pregnant client who is at 28 weeks' gestation. The nurse measures

the fundal height in centimeters and expects the findings to be which of the following?
1. 22 cm
2. 28 cm
3. 36 cm
4. 40 cm

209. A pregnant client is seen in the health care clinic for a regular prenatal visit. The client tells the nurse that she is experiencing irregular contractions. The nurse determines that the client is experiencing Braxton Hicks contractions. Based on this finding, which nursing action is appropriate?
1. Contact the physician.
2. Instruct the client to maintain bedrest for the remainder of the pregnancy.
3. Tell the client that these are common and that they may occur throughout the pregnancy.
4. Call the maternity unit, and inform them that the client will be admitted in a prelabor condition.

210. A nursing instructor asks a nursing student to describe the process of quickening. Which of the following statements, if made by the student, indicates an understanding of this term?

1. "It is the thinning of the lower uterine segment."
2. "It is the fetal movement that is felt by the mother."
3. "It is the irregular, painless contractions that occur throughout pregnancy."
4. "It is the soft blowing sound that can be heard when the uterus is auscultated."

ALTERNATE ITEM FORMAT: MULTIPLE RESPONSE

211. A nurse is collecting data from a client who suspects that she is pregnant. The nurse is checking the client for probable signs of pregnancy. Select all probable signs of pregnancy.
☐ 1. Ballottement
☐ 2. Chadwick's sign
☐ 3. Uterine enlargement
☐ 4. Braxton Hicks contractions
☐ 5. Outline of fetus via radiography or ultrasound
☐ 6. Fetal heart rate detected by a nonelectronic device

ANSWERS

202. 2
Rationale: The accurate use of Nägele's rule requires that the woman have a regular 28-day menstrual cycle. Add 7 days to the first day of the last menstrual period (LMP), subtract 3 months, and then add 1 year to that date. In this case, the first day of the LMP was October 20. If you add 7 days, you get October 27, 2010. When you subtract 3 months, you get July 27, 2010. Add 1 year to this, and you get the estimated date of birth: July 27, 2011.
Test-Taking Strategy: Follow Nägele's rule to answer this question. Read all of the options carefully and note the dates and years in the options before selecting an answer. Review Nägele's rule if you had difficulty with this question.
Level of Cognitive Ability: Comprehension
Client Needs: Health Promotion and Maintenance
Integrated Process: Nursing Process/Data Collection
Content Area: Maternity/Antepartum
Reference: Leifer, G. (2008). *Maternity nursing: An introductory text* (10th ed., p. 42). Philadelphia: Saunders.

203. 4
Rationale: Quickening is fetal movement that usually first occurs between 16 and 20 weeks' gestation. The expectant mother first notices subtle fetal movements during this time, and these gradually increase in intensity. Options 1, 2, and 3 are incorrect.
Test-Taking Strategy: Use the process of elimination and your knowledge regarding the occurrence of quickening. In this situation, it is best to select the option that indicates the greatest length of gestational time. Review the process of quickening if you had difficulty with this question.
Level of Cognitive Ability: Application
Client Needs: Health Promotion and Maintenance

Integrated Process: Teaching and Learning
Content Area: Maternity/Antepartum
Reference: Leifer, G. (2007). *Introduction to maternity and pediatric nursing* (5th ed., p. 49). Philadelphia: Saunders.

204. 2
Rationale: Pregnancy outcomes can be described with the GTPAL acronym: G = gravidity (number of pregnancies); T = term births (number born after 37 weeks); P = preterm births (number born before 37 weeks' gestation); A = abortions/miscarriages (number of abortions/miscarriages; included in gravida if before 20 weeks' gestation, and included in para if past 20 weeks' gestation); L = live births (number of live births or living children). Therefore, a woman who is pregnant with twins and who already has a child has a gravida of 2. Because the child was delivered at 38 weeks, the number of preterm births is 0, and the number of term births is 1. The number of abortions is 0, and the number of live births is 1. *Test-Taking Strategy:* Your knowledge and understanding of the GTPAL acronym will direct you to option 2. **Review the GTPAL method of describing pregnancy outcomes if you had difficulty answering this question.**
Level of Cognitive Ability: Application
Client Needs: Health Promotion and Maintenance
Integrated Process: Nursing Process/Data Collection
Content Area: Maternity/Antepartum
Reference: Leifer, G. (2008). *Maternity nursing: An introductory text* (10th ed., p. 42). Philadelphia: Saunders.

205. 2
Rationale: Gravida is a term that refers to a woman who is or who has been pregnant, regardless of the duration of the pregnancy. *Parity* is a term that means the number of births

after 20 weeks' gestation; it does not reflect the number of fetuses or infants. Options 1, 3, and 4 are incorrect on the basis of the above definitions.

Test-Taking Strategy: Knowledge of the terms *gravida* and *parity* is necessary to answer this question correctly. Remember that *gravida* refers to a woman who is or has been pregnant, regardless of the duration of the pregnancy. Parity means the number of births past 20 weeks' gestation. Review the definitions of these terms if you had difficulty with this question.

Level of Cognitive Ability: Application
Client Needs: Physiological Integrity
Integrated Process: Communication and Documentation
Content Area: Maternity/Antepartum
Reference: Leifer, G. (2007). *Introduction to maternity and pediatric nursing* (5th ed., p. 47). Philadelphia: Saunders.

206. 1
Rationale: During the early weeks of pregnancy, the cervix becomes softer as a result of pelvic vasoconstriction, which causes Goodell's sign. Cervical softening is noted by the examiner during a pelvic examination. A soft blowing sound that corresponds with the maternal pulse may be auscultated over the uterus; it is the result of blood circulating through the placenta. Human chorionic gonadotropin is noted in maternal urine with a positive urine pregnancy test. Goodell's sign does not indicate the presence of fetal movement.

Test-Taking Strategy: Use the process of elimination and your knowledge regarding the physiological findings of Goodell's sign to answer this question. Remember that Goodell's sign refers to a softening of the cervix. Review the changes in the cervix that occur during pregnancy if you had difficulty with this question.

Level of Cognitive Ability: Comprehension
Client Needs: Health Promotion and Maintenance
Integrated Process: Nursing Process/Data Collection
Content Area: Maternity/Antepartum
Reference: Leifer, G. (2008). *Maternity nursing: An introductory text* (10th ed., p. 43). Philadelphia: Saunders.

207. 4
Rationale: The fetal heart rate depends on the gestational age. It is 160 to 170 beats per minute during the first trimester, and it slows with fetal growth to approximately 120 to 160 beats per minute. Options 1, 2, and 3 are normal expected findings.

Test-Taking Strategy: Note the strategic words "indicate an abnormal physical finding." Recalling the normal fetal heart rate will direct you to option 4. Review the normal assessment findings of pregnancy if you had difficulty with this question.

Level of Cognitive Ability: Comprehension
Client Needs: Physiological Integrity
Integrated Process: Nursing Process/Data Collection
Content Area: Maternity/Antepartum
Reference: Leifer, G. (2007). *Introduction to maternity and pediatric nursing* (5th ed., p. 50). Philadelphia: Saunders.

208. 2
Rationale: During the second and third trimesters (18 to 30 weeks' gestation), the fundal height in centimeters approximately equals the fetus' age in weeks plus or minus 2 cm. At

14 to 16 weeks' gestation, the fundus can be located halfway between the symphysis pubis and the umbilicus. At 20 to 22 weeks' gestation, the fundus is at the umbilicus, and, at term, the fundus is at the xiphoid process.

Test-Taking Strategy: Use the process of elimination. Remember that, during the second and third trimesters, the fundal height in centimeters approximately equals the fetus' age in weeks plus or minus 2 cm. Review fundal height if you had difficulty with this question.

Level of Cognitive Ability: Comprehension
Client Needs: Health Promotion and Maintenance
Integrated Process: Nursing Process/Data Collection
Content Area: Maternity/Antepartum
References: Leifer, G. (2008). *Maternity nursing: An introductory text* (10th ed., p. 227). Philadelphia: Saunders.
Wong, D., Perry, S., Hockenberry, M., Lowdermilk, D., & Wilson, D. (2006). *Maternal-child nursing care* (3rd ed., pp. 239, 272-273). St. Louis: Mosby.

209. 3
Rationale: Braxton Hicks contractions are irregular, painless contractions that may occur intermittently throughout pregnancy. Because Braxton Hicks contractions may occur and are normal in some pregnant women during pregnancy, options 1, 2, and 4 are unnecessary and inappropriate actions.

Test-Taking Strategy: Use the process of elimination. Options 1 and 4 are comparable or alike and can thus be eliminated first. From the remaining options, knowing that Braxton Hicks contractions are common and that they can occur throughout pregnancy will assist with directing you to option 3. Review the physiology associated with Braxton Hicks contractions if you had difficulty with this question.

Level of Cognitive Ability: Application
Client Needs: Health Promotion and Maintenance
Integrated Process: Teaching and Learning
Content Area: Maternity/Antepartum
Reference: Leifer, G. (2008). *Maternity nursing: An introductory text* (10th ed., p. 47). Philadelphia: Saunders.

210. 2
Rationale: Quickening is fetal movement that appears usually at week 16 to 20, when the expectant mother first notices subtle fetal movements that gradually increase in intensity. A soft blowing sound that corresponds with the maternal pulse may be auscultated over the uterus; this is known as *uterine souffle.* This sound is the result of blood circulation to the placenta, and it corresponds with the maternal pulse. Braxton Hicks contractions are irregular, painless contractions that may occur throughout pregnancy. A thinning of the lower uterine segment occurs at about 6 weeks' gestation and is called *Hegar's sign.*

Test-Taking Strategy: Use the process of elimination and your knowledge regarding the term *quickening* to answer this question. Review quickening if you had difficulty with this question.

Level of Cognitive Ability: Comprehension
Client Needs: Health Promotion and Maintenance
Integrated Process: Teaching and Learning
Content Area: Maternity/Antepartum
Reference: Leifer, G. (2008). *Maternity nursing: An introductory text* (10th ed., pp. 43, 53). Philadelphia: Saunders.

ALTERNATE ITEM FORMAT: MULTIPLE RESPONSE

211. **1, 2, 3, 4**

Rationale: The probable signs of pregnancy include uterine enlargement, Hegar's sign (the softening and thinning of the lower uterine segment that occurs at about week 6), Goodell's sign (the softening of the cervix that occurs at the beginning of the second month of pregnancy), Chadwick's sign (the violet coloration of the mucous membranes of the cervix, vagina, and vulva that occurs at about week 4), ballottement (the rebounding of the fetus against the examiner's fingers on palpation), Braxton Hicks contractions, and a positive pregnancy test that measures for human chorionic gonadotropin. Positive signs of pregnancy include a fetal heart rate that is detected by an electronic device (Doppler transducer) at 10 to 12 weeks' gestation and by a nonelectronic device (fetoscope) at 20 weeks' gestation; active fetal movements that are palpable by the examiner; and an outline of the fetus via radiography or ultrasound.

Test-Taking Strategy: Focusing on the subject of the probable signs of pregnancy will assist you with answering this question. Remember that the detection of the fetal heart rate and of an outline of the fetus via radiography or ultrasound are positive signs of pregnancy. Review the probable signs of pregnancy if you had difficulty with this question.

Level of Cognitive Ability: Analysis
Client Needs: Health Promotion and Maintenance
Integrated Process: Nursing Process/Data Collection
Content Area: Maternity/Antepartum
Reference: Leifer, G. (2007). *Introduction to maternity and pediatric nursing* (5th ed., pp. 49-51). Philadelphia: Saunders.

REFERENCES

Leifer, G. (2007). *Introduction to maternity and pediatric nursing* (5th ed.). Philadelphia: Saunders.

Leifer, G. (2008). *Maternity nursing: An introductory text* (10th ed.). Philadelphia: Saunders.

Wong, D., Perry, S., Hockenberry, M., Lowdermilk, D., & Wilson, D. (2006). *Maternal-child nursing care* (3rd ed.). St. Louis: Mosby.

Prenatal Period and Risk Conditions

I. PHYSIOLOGICAL MATERNAL CHANGES

A. Cardiovascular system
   1. Circulating blood volume increases
   2. Heart is elevated upward and to the left because of displacement of the diaphragm as the uterus enlarges
   3. Pulse may increase about 10 beats per minute; blood pressure may slightly decline during the second trimester
   4. Increase in the body's demand for iron; physiological anemia may occur
   5. Sodium and water retention may occur, which can lead to weight gain

B. Respiratory system
   1. Oxygen consumption increases as a result of an increase in metabolic rate and tissue mass
   2. Diaphragm is elevated as a result of the enlarged uterus
   3. Respiratory rate remains unchanged
   4. Shortness of breath may be experienced

C. Gastrointestinal (GI) system
   1. Nausea and vomiting may occur as a result of the secretion of human chorionic gonadotropin (hCG), which subsides by the third month
   2. Increase in the body's nutritional requirements (i.e., vitamins, minerals, calories, protein, and iron)
   3. Constipation as a result of decreased GI motility or pressure of the uterus
   4. Changes in appetite, flatulence, and heartburn as a result of decreased GI motility and slow emptying of the stomach
   5. Alterations in taste and smell may occur
   6. Hemorrhoids as a result of increased venous pressure
   7. Altered gallbladder function that can lead to gallstone formation caused by an increase in progesterone

D. Renal system
   1. Frequency of urination occurs during the first and third trimesters as a result of the pressure of the enlarging uterus on the bladder, which causes decreased bladder capacity
   2. Decreased bladder tone is caused by hormonal changes
   3. Renal function increases
   4. Renal threshold for glucose may be reduced

E. Endocrine system: Basal metabolic rate rises

F. Reproductive system
   1. Uterus
      a. Uterus enlarges from 60 to 1000 g
      b. Irregular contractions occur
   2. Cervix
      a. Becomes shorter, more elastic, and larger in diameter
      b. Endocervical glands secrete a thick mucus plug, which is expelled from the canal when dilation begins
      c. Increased vascularization causes a softening and a violet discoloration (Chadwick's sign)
   3. Ovaries: Cease ovum production
   4. Vagina
      a. Hypertrophy and thickening of muscle occurs
      b. Increase in vaginal secretions occurs; secretions are usually thick, white, and acidic
   5. Breasts
      a. Breast size increases
      b. Increase in blood flow to the breasts; swelling, tingling, and tenderness are common
      c. Nipples become more pronounced and the areolae become darker, with an increase in ductal growth
      d. Colostrum may leak from the breasts

G. Skin
   1. A dark streak down the midline of the abdomen may appear (linea nigra; Figure 22-1)
   2. Chloasma (mask of pregnancy), which is a blotchy, brownish hyperpigmentation, may occur over the forehead, cheeks, and nose
   3. Reddish-purple stretch marks (striae) may occur on the abdomen, breasts, thighs, and upper arms

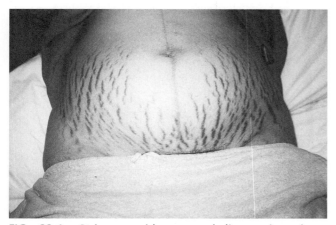

FIG. 22-1 Striae gravidarum and linea nigra in a dark-skinned person. (From Wong, D., Perry, S., Hockenberry, M., Lowdermilk, D., & Wilson, D. [2006]. *Maternal-child nursing care* [3rd ed.]. St. Louis: Mosby. Courtesy of Shannon Perry, Phoenix, AZ.)

H. Musculoskeletal system
   1. Postural changes occur as the increased weight of the uterus causes a forward pull of the bony pelvis
   2. Ligament laxity and the softening of connective tissue are seen throughout the body as a result of an increase in estrogen and relaxin

II. **PSYCHOLOGICAL MATERNAL CHANGES**
A. Ambivalence
   1. May occur even when the pregnancy is planned
   2. Mother may experience a dependence–independence conflict and ambivalence related to role changes, changes in body image, and fear of the unknown
   3. Partner may experience ambivalence related to assuming a new role, increased financial responsibilities, the mother's physical changes, and having to share attention with the child
B. Acceptance
   1. Factors that may be related to the acceptance of the pregnancy are the woman's readiness for the experience and her identification with the motherhood role
   2. Commonly occurs at 20 weeks, when **quickening** is likely to occur
C. Emotional lability
   1. Frequency in the change of emotional states or extremes in emotional states caused by hormone changes
   2. These emotional changes are common, but the mother may believe that these changes are abnormal
D. Body image changes: Perception of her image during pregnancy occurs gradually and may be either positive or negative; often influenced by her partner

E. Relationship with the fetus
   1. The woman may daydream to prepare for motherhood and think about the maternal qualities she would like to possess
   2. The woman first accepts the biological fact that she is pregnant
   3. The woman next accepts the growing fetus as distinct from herself and as a person to nurture
   4. Finally, the woman prepares realistically for the birth and parenting of the child

III. **DISCOMFORTS OF PREGNANCY**
A. Nausea and vomiting
   1. Occur during the first trimester
   2. Caused by elevated hCG levels and changes in carbohydrate metabolism
   3. Interventions
     a. Eating dry crackers before arising
     b. Avoiding brushing the teeth immediately after arising
     c. Eating small, frequent, low-fat meals during the day
     d. Drinking liquids between meals rather than at meals
     e. Avoiding fried foods and spicy foods
     f. Acupressure (some types may require a prescription)
     g. Herbal remedies, only if approved by a physician or nurse-midwife
B. Syncope
   1. Usually occurs during the first trimester; supine hypotension occurs, particularly during the second and third trimesters
   2. May be hormonally triggered or caused by increased blood volume, anemia, fatigue, sudden position changes, or lying supine
   3. Interventions
     a. Sitting with the feet elevated
     b. Changing positions slowly
     c. Changing to the lateral recumbent position to relieve the pressure of the uterus on the inferior vena cava
     d. Increasing fluid intake
C. Urinary urgency and frequency
   1. Usually occurs during the first and third trimesters
   2. Caused by the pressure of the uterus on the bladder
   3. Interventions
     a. Drinking 2 quarts of fluid during the day
     b. Limiting fluid intake during the evening
     c. Voiding at regular intervals
     d. Sleeping on the side at night
     e. Wearing perineal pads, if necessary
     f. Performing Kegel exercises
D. Breast tenderness and tingling
   1. Can occur from the first through the third trimesters

2. Caused by increased levels of estrogen and progesterone
3. Interventions
   a. Encouraging the use of a supportive bra with nonelastic straps
   b. Avoiding the use of soap on the nipples and areolae to prevent drying
E. Increased vaginal discharge
   1. Can occur from the first through the third trimesters
   2. Caused by hyperplasia of the vaginal mucosa and increased mucus production
   3. Interventions
      a. Wearing cotton underwear
      b. Avoiding douching
      c. Using proper cleansing and hygiene techniques
      d. Advising the client to consult the physician or nurse-midwife if infection is suspected
F. Nasal stuffiness or nosebleeds
   1. Occurs during the first through the third trimesters
   2. Occurs as a result of increased estrogen that causes swelling of the nasal tissues and dryness
   3. Interventions
      a. Encouraging the use of a humidifier
      b. Avoiding the use of nasal sprays or antihistamines
G. Fatigue
   1. Occurs usually during the first and third trimesters
   2. Is usually the result of hormonal changes
   3. Interventions
      a. Arranging frequent rest periods throughout the day
      b. Using correct body mechanics
      c. Engaging in regular exercise
      d. Performing muscle relaxation and strengthening exercises for the legs and hip joints
      e. Avoiding eating and drinking foods that contain stimulants throughout pregnancy
H. Heartburn
   1. Occurs during the second and third trimesters
   2. Results from increased progesterone levels, decreased GI motility, esophageal reflux, and the displacement of the stomach by the enlarging uterus
   3. Interventions
      a. Eating small, frequent meals and avoiding fatty and spicy food
      b. Sitting upright for 30 minutes after a meal
      c. Drinking milk between meals
      d. Performing tailor-sitting exercises (sitting cross-legged)
      e. Taking antacids only if recommended by the physician or the nurse-midwife

I. Ankle edema
   1. Usually occurs during the second and third trimesters
   2. Occurs as a result of vasodilation, venous stasis, and increased venous pressure below the uterus
   3. Interventions
      a. Elevating the legs during the day
      b. Sleeping on the left side
      c. Wearing supportive stockings
      d. Avoiding sitting or standing in one position for long periods
J. Varicose veins
   1. Usually occur during the second and third trimesters
   2. Occur because of weakening walls of the veins or valves and venous congestion
   3. Interventions
      a. Wearing support hose
      b. Elevating the feet when sitting
      c. Lying with the feet and hips elevated
      d. Avoiding long periods of standing or sitting
      e. Moving about while standing to improve circulation
      f. Avoiding leg crossing
      g. Avoiding constricting articles of clothing
K. Headaches
   1. Usually occur during the second and third trimesters
   2. Occur as a result of changes in blood volume and vascular tone
   3. Interventions
      a. Changing position slowly
      b. Applying a cool cloth to the forehead
      c. Eating a small snack
      d. Using acetaminophen (Tylenol) only if prescribed by the physician or nurse-midwife
L. Hemorrhoids
   1. Usually occur during the second and third trimesters
   2. Occur as a result of increased venous pressure and/or constipation
   3. Interventions
      a. Soaking in a warm sitz bath
      b. Sitting on a soft pillow
      c. Eating high-fiber foods and avoiding constipation
      d. Drinking sufficient fluids
      e. Increasing exercise, such as walking
      f. Applying ointments, suppositories, or compresses as prescribed by the physician or nurse-midwife
M. Constipation
   1. Usually occurs during the second and third trimesters
   2. Occurs as a result of decreased intestinal motility, the displacement of the intestines, and taking iron supplements

3. Interventions
    a. Eating high-fiber foods
    b. Drinking sufficient fluids
    c. Exercising regularly
    d. Avoiding laxatives and enemas unless their use is approved by the physician or nurse-midwife
N. Backache
    1. Usually occurs during the second and third trimesters
    2. Occurs as a result of the exaggerated lumbosacral curve, which is caused by the enlarged uterus
    3. Interventions
        a. Encouraging rest
        b. Using correct body mechanics and improving posture
        c. Wearing low-heeled shoes
        d. Performing pelvic rocking and abdominal breathing exercises
        e. Sleeping on a firm mattress
O. Leg cramps
    1. Usually occur during the second and third trimesters
    2. Occur as a result of an altered calcium–phosphorus balance, the pressure of the uterus on nerves, or fatigue
    3. Interventions
        a. Getting regular exercise, especially walking
        b. Dorsiflexing the foot of the affected leg
        c. Increasing calcium intake
P. Shortness of breath
    1. Can occur during the second and third trimesters
    2. Occurs as a result of pressure on the diaphragm
    3. Interventions
        a. Allowing frequent rest periods and avoiding overexertion
        b. Sleeping with the head elevated or on the side
        c. Performing tailor-sitting exercises

IV. LABORATORY TESTS/PRENATAL VISITS (Box 22-1)
A. Blood type and Rh factor
    1. ABO typing is performed to determine the woman's blood type
    2. Rh typing is done to determine the presence or absence of Rh antigen (Rh positive or Rh negative)
    3. If the client is Rh negative and has a negative antibody screen, the client will need repeat antibody screens and should receive Rh immune globulin at 28 weeks' gestation
B. Rubella titer
    1. If the client has a negative titer, this indicates susceptibility to the rubella virus; the client should receive the appropriate immunization postpartum
    2. The client must be using effective birth control at the time of the immunization; she must be counseled to not become pregnant for 1 to 3 months after immunization (as specified by the health care provider) and to avoid contact with anyone who is immunocompromised
    3. If the rubella vaccine is administered at the same time as the Rh immune globulin, it may not be effective
C. Hemoglobin and hematocrit levels
    1. Hemoglobin and hematocrit levels will drop during gestation as a result of increased plasma volume
    2. A decrease in the hemoglobin level below 10 g/dL or a decrease in the hematocrit level below 30 g/dL indicates anemia
D. Papanicolaou (Pap) smear: Done during the initial prenatal examination to screen for cervical neoplasia
E. Sexually transmitted infections (Table 22-1)

BOX 22-1 Prenatal Visits

- Every 4 weeks for the first 28 to 32 weeks' gestation
- Every 2 weeks from 32 to 36 weeks' gestation
- Every week from 36 to 40 weeks' gestation

TABLE 22-1 Monitoring for Sexually Transmitted Infections

Disease	Laboratory Test
Gonorrhea	A vaginal culture is performed during the initial prenatal examination to screen for gonorrhea; it may be repeated during the third trimester for high-risk clients.
Syphilis	A culture of lesions (if present) is performed during the initial prenatal examination to screen for syphilis. Diagnosis is dependent on the microscopic examination of primary and secondary lesion tissue and serology (Venereal Disease Research Laboratory or rapid plasma reagin test). The culture may be repeated during the third trimester for high-risk clients.
Herpes virus	A culture is indicated for clients with an infection-positive history and for those with active lesions. Testing is performed to determine the route of delivery; weekly cultures may be performed from 35 or 36 weeks' gestation until delivery.
Chlamydia	A vaginal culture is indicated if the client is in a high-risk group or if infants from previous pregnancies have developed neonatal conjunctivitis or pneumonia.

F. Sickle cell screening
 1. Indicated for clients who are at risk for sickle cell disease
 2. A positive test result may indicate a need for further screening
G. Tuberculin skin test
 1. The health care provider may prefer to perform this skin test after **delivery**
 2. A positive skin test indicates the need for a chest radiograph (using an abdominal lead shield) to rule out active disease; in a pregnant client, a chest radiograph will not be performed until after 20 weeks' gestation (i.e., after the fetal organs are formed)
 3. Those who convert to positive may be referred for treatment with medication after **delivery**
H. Hepatitis B surface antigen
 1. Recommended for all women because of the prevalence of the disease in the general population
 2. Vaccination for hepatitis B antigen may be specifically indicated for the following:
  a. Health care workers
  b. Clients born in Asia, Africa, Haiti, or the Pacific islands
  c. Clients with previously undiagnosed jaundice or chronic liver disease
  d. Intravenous (IV) drug abusers
  e. Clients with tattoos
  f. Clients with histories of blood transfusions
  g. Clients with histories of multiple episodes of sexually transmitted infections
  h. Clients who have been previously rejected as blood donors
  i. Clients with histories of dialysis or renal transplantation
  j. Clients from households having hepatitis B–infected members or hemodialysis clients
 3. See Chapter 46 for additional information about hepatitis
I. Urinalysis and urine culture
 1. A urine specimen for glucose and protein determinations should be obtained at every prenatal visit
 2. Glycosuria is a common result of decreased renal threshold that occurs during pregnancy
 3. If glycosuria persists, this may indicate diabetes mellitus
 4. White blood cells in the urine may indicate infection
 5. Ketonuria may result from insufficient food intake or vomiting
 6. Protein levels of 2+ to 4+ in the urine may indicate infection or gestational hypertension

V. DIAGNOSTIC TESTS
A. Ultrasonography
 1. Outlines and identifies fetal and maternal structures

 2. Helps confirm gestational age and estimated date of **delivery**
 3. May be done abdominally or transvaginally during pregnancy
 4. Interventions
  a. If an abdominal ultrasound is being performed, the woman may need to drink water to fill the bladder before the procedure to obtain a better image of the fetus
  b. If a transvaginal ultrasound is being performed, a lubricated probe is inserted into the vagina
  c. Inform the client that the test presents no known risks to the client or the fetus
B. Alpha-fetoprotein (AFP) screening
 1. Assesses the quantity of fetal serum proteins; if the AFP level is elevated, it is associated with open neural tube and abdominal wall defects
 2. Can detect spina bifida and Down syndrome
 3. Interventions
  a. Explain that the AFP level is determined by a single maternal blood sample that is drawn at 15 to 18 weeks' gestation
  b. If the level is elevated and the gestation is less than 18 weeks, a second sample is drawn
  c. Ultrasonography is performed if the AFP level is elevated to rule out fetal abnormalities and multiple gestations
C. Chorionic villus sampling (CVS)
 1. The physician aspirates a small sample of chorionic villus tissue at 8 to 12 weeks' gestation
 2. CVS is performed to detect genetic abnormalities
 3. Interventions
  a. Obtain informed consent
  b. Instruct the client to drink water to fill the bladder before the procedure to aid in positioning the uterus for catheter insertion
  c. Instruct the client to report bleeding, infection, or the leakage of fluid at the insertion site after the procedure
  d. Rh-negative women may be given Rho(D) immune globulin (RhoGAM), because CVS increases the risk of Rh sensitization
D. Kick counts (fetal movement counting)
 1. Mother sits quietly or lies down on her left side and counts fetal kicks for a period of time, as instructed
 2. Instruct the client to notify the physician or nurse-midwife if there are fewer than 10 kicks in a 12-hour period or as instructed by the physician or nurse-midwife
E. Amniocentesis
 1. Aspiration of **amniotic fluid** may be done at 16 weeks' gestation or thereafter

2. May reveal genetic disorders, metabolic defects, lung maturity, and sex
3. Risks
   a. Maternal hemorrhage
   b. Infection
   c. Rh isoimmunization
   d. Abruptio placentae
   e. **Amniotic fluid** emboli
   f. Premature rupture of the membranes
4. Interventions
   a. Obtain informed consent
   b. If less than 20 weeks' gestation, the woman must have a full bladder to support uterus; if more than 20 weeks' gestation, the woman must have an empty bladder to minimize the chance of puncture
   c. Prepare the client for ultrasonography, which is performed to locate the **placenta** and avoid puncture
   d. Obtain baseline vital signs and fetal heart rate; monitor every 15 minutes
   e. Position the client supine during the exam and on the left side after
   f. Instruct the client that if chills, fever, leakage of fluid at the needle-insertion site, decreased fetal movement, uterine contractions, or cramping occur, she is to notify the physician or nurse-midwife

F. Fern test
1. A microscopic slide test to determine the presence of **amniotic fluid** leakage
2. With the use of sterile technique, a specimen is obtained from the external os of the cervix and vaginal pool and examined on a slide under a microscope
3. A fernlike pattern that results from the salts of **amniotic fluid** indicates the presence of **amniotic fluid**
4. Interventions
   a. Place the client in the dorsal lithotomy position
   b. Instruct the client to cough; this causes the fluid to leak from the uterus if the membranes are ruptured

G. Nitrazine test
1. A Nitrazine test strip is used to detect the presence of **amniotic fluid** in vaginal secretions
2. Vaginal secretions have a pH of 4.5 to 5.5; they do not affect the yellow color of the Nitrazine strip or swab
3. **Amniotic fluid** has a pH of 7.0 to 7.5 and turns the yellow Nitrazine strip or swab a blue color
4. Interventions
   a. Place the client in the dorsal lithotomy position
   b. Touch the test tape to the fluid

BOX 22-2 **Nonstress Test**

Description
- Performed to assess placental function and oxygenation
- Determines fetal well-being
- Evaluates fetal heart rate (FHR) in response to fetal movement

Interventions
An external ultrasound transducer and tocodynamometer are applied to the mother, and a tracing of at least 20 minutes' duration is obtained so that the FHR and the uterine activity can be observed.
Obtain a baseline blood pressure reading, and monitor the blood pressure frequently.
Position the mother in the left lateral position to avoid vena cava compression.
The mother may be asked to press a button every time she feels fetal movement. The monitor records a mark at each point of fetal movement, and this is used as a reference point to assess FHR response.

Results
Reactive Nonstress Test (Normal, Negative)
"Reactive" indicates a healthy fetus.
The result requires two or more FHR accelerations of at least 15 beats per minute and lasting at least 15 seconds from the beginning of the acceleration to the end, in association with fetal movement, during a 20-minute period.
Nonreactive Nonstress Test (Abnormal)
No accelerations or accelerations of less than 15 beats per minute or lasting less than 15 seconds in duration during a 40-minute observation
Unsatisfactory
Cannot be interpreted because of the poor quality of the FHR tracing

---

   c. Assess the test tape for a blue-green, blue-gray, or deep blue color, which indicates that the membranes are probably ruptured
H. Nonstress test (Box 22-2)
I. Contraction stress test (Box 22-3)

VI. NUTRITION
A. General guidelines
1. A MyPyramid Web site (www.mypyramid.gov) designed specifically for pregnant and breast-feeding mothers provides unique, individualized nutrition guidance to meet the needs of the pregnant woman; the woman should be assisted with accessing this site and preparing a nutritional plan
2. The average expected weight gain during pregnancy is 25 to 35 pounds for women with a normal prepregnancy weight, depending on physician preference
3. An increase of about 300 calories per day is needed during pregnancy
4. Calorie needs are greater during the last two trimesters than in the first

BOX 22-3 **Contraction Stress Test**

Description
- Assesses placental oxygenation and function
- Determines fetal ability to tolerate labor
- Determines fetal well-being
- Fetus is exposed to the stressor of contractions to assess the adequacy of placental perfusion under simulated labor conditions
- Performed if the nonstress test is abnormal

Interventions
The external fetal monitor is applied to the mother, and a 20- to 30-minute baseline strip is recorded.

The uterus is stimulated to contract, either by the administration of a dilute dose of oxytocin (Pitocin) or by having the mother use nipple stimulation, until three palpable contractions with a duration of 40 seconds or more during a 10-minute period have been achieved.

Frequent maternal blood pressure readings are obtained, and the mother is monitored closely while increasing doses of oxytocin are given.

Results
Negative Contraction Stress Test
Represented by no late decelerations of the fetal heart rate (FHR)

Positive Contraction Stress Test (Abnormal)
Represented by late decelerations of the FHR with 50% or more of the contractions in the absence of hyperstimulation of the uterus

Equivocal
Contains decelerations but with less than 50% of the contractions, or uterine activity shows a hyperstimulated uterus

Unsatisfactory
Adequate uterine contractions cannot be achieved or the FHR tracing is not of sufficient quality for adequate interpretation

BOX 22-4 **Types of Vegetarian Diets**

Lacto-Ovo Vegetarian
Consumes eggs and dairy products, but excludes meat, poultry, and seafood

Lacto Vegetarian
Consumes dairy products, but excludes eggs, meat, poultry, and seafood

Vegan
Refrains from eating animal products

Pesco Vegetarian
Consumes seafood, but excludes meat, poultry, eggs, and dairy products

5. An increase of about 500 calories per day is needed during lactation
6. Encourage a diet high in folic acid and nutrient-dense foods, with prenatal supplements, as prescribed
7. A diet rich in folic acid is necessary for all women of childbearing age to prevent neural tube defects in the fetus during the first trimester of pregnancy
8. Encourage the consumption of at least 8 to 10 (8-oz) glasses of fluid each day, of which 4 to 6 glasses are water
9. Sodium is not restricted unless specifically ordered by the physician or nurse-midwife
10. Alcohol-containing beverages should not be consumed

B. Vegetarianism (Box 22-4)
  1. Ensure that the client eats a sufficient amount of varied foods to meet normal nutrient and energy needs
  2. Protein consumption can be increased by consuming a variety of vegetable protein sources that are based on whole grains, legumes, seeds, nuts, and vegetables combined to provide all essential amino acids
  3. Adequate energy intake is important to ensure that dietary protein is used for protein synthesis

C. Lactose intolerance
  1. Lactose consumed by an individual with lactose intolerance can cause abdominal distention, discomfort, nausea, vomiting, cramps, and loose stools
  2. Clients who experience lactose intolerance need to regularly incorporate sources of calcium (other than dairy products) into their dietary patterns
  3. Milk may be tolerated in cooked form (e.g., custards, fermented dairy products)
  4. Cheese and yogurt are sometimes tolerated
  5. Lactase, which is an enzyme, may be prescribed and taken before ingesting milk or milk products
  6. Lactase-treated milk and lactose-free products are also available commercially

D. Pica
  1. Definition: Eating nonfood substances such as dirt, clay, starch, and freezer frost
  2. The cause is unknown; cultural values, such as beliefs regarding a material's effect on the mother or fetus, may make pica a common practice
  3. Iron-deficiency anemia may occur as a result of pica

E. Cultural considerations: See Chapter 6 for information about cultural considerations and nutrition

VII. DANGER SIGNS OF PREGNANCY (Box 22-5)

VIII. ABORTION
A. Description: A pregnancy that ends before 20 weeks' gestation, either spontaneously or electively
B. Data collection
  1. Spontaneous vaginal bleeding with the passage of clots and tissue through the vagina

BOX 22-5	**Danger Signs of Pregnancy**

- Severe vomiting
- Chills
- Fever
- Burning on urination
- Diarrhea
- Abdominal cramping or vaginal bleeding
- Sudden discharge of fluid from the vagina before 37 weeks' gestation
- Severe backache or flank pain
- Change in fetal movements in pattern or amount
- Visual disturbances
- Swelling of the face or fingers or over the sacrum
- Headaches
- Epigastric or abdominal pain
- Muscular irritability or seizures
- Glycosuria or other signs of diabetes mellitus

Modified from Lowdermilk, D., & Perry, S. (2004). *Maternity & women's health care* (8th ed.). St. Louis: Mosby.

BOX 22-6	**Stages of Acquired Immunodeficiency Syndrome**

Stage 1
- Fever
- Myalgia
- Lymphadenopathy
- Headache

Stage 2
- Active infection but asymptomatic; may remain so for years
- May experience an outbreak of herpes zoster (shingles)
- May experience a transient thrombocytopenia

Stage 3
- Symptomatic
- Evidence of immune dysfunction
- All body systems can present with signs of immune dysfunction
- Integumentary and gynecological problems are common

Stage 4
- Advanced human immunodeficiency virus infection
- Vulnerable to common bacterial infections
- Development of opportunistic infections
- Serious immune compromise

  2. Low uterine cramping and contractions
  3. Hemorrhage and shock can occur
C. Interventions
  1. Maintain bedrest
  2. Monitor vital signs
  3. Monitor cramping and bleeding
  4. Count perineal pads to evaluate blood loss; save expelled tissues and clots
  5. Maintain IV fluids as prescribed; monitor for signs of shock
  6. Prepare the client for dilation and curettage, as prescribed, for incomplete abortion
  7. Rh immune globulin is given to appropriate Rh-negative women

IX. ACQUIRED IMMUNODEFICIENCY SYNDROME
A. Description
  1. The human immunodeficiency virus (HIV) is the causative factor of the development of acquired immunodeficiency syndrome
  2. Women infected with HIV virus may first demonstrate symptoms at the time of pregnancy or possibly develop life-threatening infections, because normal pregnancy involves some suppression of the maternal immune system
  3. Zidovudine (AZT) is recommended for the prevention of maternal–fetal HIV transmission; it is administered orally beginning after 14 weeks' gestation, intravenously during **labor,** and in the form of syrup to the **neonate** after birth for 6 weeks
B. Transmission
  1. Sexual exposure to genital secretions of an infected person
  2. Parenteral exposure to infected blood and tissue
  3. Perinatal exposure of an **infant** to infected maternal secretions through birth process or breast-feeding

C. Risks to the mother: The mother with HIV is managed as high risk because she is vulnerable to infections
D. Diagnosis (Box 22-6)
  1. Tests used to determine the presence of antibodies to HIV include enzyme-linked immunosorbent assay (ELISA), Western blot (WB), and indirect fluorescent antibody (IFA)
  2. A single reactive ELISA test result by itself cannot be used to diagnose HIV and should be repeated in duplicate with the same blood sample; if the result is repeatedly reactive, follow-up tests using WB or IFA should be performed
  3. A positive WB or IFA is considered confirmatory for HIV
  4. A positive ELISA that fails to be confirmed by WB or IFA should not be considered negative; repeat testing should take place in 3 to 6 months
  5. See Chapter 11 for additional laboratory tests
E. Interventions
  1. Prenatal period
    a. Prevention of opportunistic infections
    b. Avoid procedures that increase the risk of perinatal transmission, such as amniocentesis and fetal scalp sampling
  2. Intrapartum period
    a. If the fetus has not been exposed to HIV in utero, the highest risk exists during **delivery** through the birth canal

b. Avoid the use of scalp electrodes

c. Avoid episiotomy to decrease the amount of maternal blood in and around the birth canal

d. Avoid the administration of oxytocin (Pitocin), because oxytocin contractions can be strong, thus inducing vaginal tears or necessitating the need for an episiotomy

e. Place heavy absorbent pads under the mother's hips to absorb **amniotic fluid** and maternal blood

f. Minimize the **neonate's** exposure to maternal blood and body fluids; promptly remove the **neonate** from the mother's blood after **delivery**

g. Suction the **infant** promptly

h. Prepare to administer AZT intravenously, as prescribed, to the mother during **labor** and **delivery**

3. Postpartum period

a. Monitor for signs of infection

b. Place the mother in protective isolation if she is immunosuppressed

c. Restrict breast-feeding

d. Instruct the mother to monitor for signs of infection and to report any signs if they occur

F. The **neonate** and HIV

1. Description

a. **Neonates** born to HIV-positive clients may test positive, because the mother's positive antibodies may persist for as long as 18 months after birth; all **neonates** acquire maternal antibody to HIV infection, but not all acquire infection

b. The use of antiviral medication, the reduction of **neonate** exposure to maternal blood and body fluids, and the early identification of HIV during pregnancy reduce the risk of transmission to the **neonate**

2. Interventions

a. Bathe the **neonate** carefully before any invasive procedure, such as the administration of vitamin K, heel sticks, or venipunctures; the umbilical cord stump is cleaned meticulously every day until it is healed

b. The **neonate** can room with mother

c. Prepare to administer AZT to the **newborn infant,** as prescribed, for the first 6 weeks of life

d. All HIV-exposed **newborn infants** should be treated with medication to prevent infection with *Pneumocystis jiroveci*

e. Note that an HIV culture is recommended at the age of 1 month and after 4 months of age; **infants** at risk for HIV infection should

be seen by the physician at birth and at 1 week, 2 weeks, 1 month, 2 months, and 4 months of life

f. **Infants** at risk for HIV infection need to receive all recommended immunizations according to the regular schedule; no live-virus vaccines should be administered

g. The **neonate** may be asymptomatic for the first several years of life; he or she needs to be monitored for early signs of immunodeficiency

X. ANEMIA

A. Description

1. Develops as a result of iron deficiency

2. Predisposes the client to postpartum infection and hemorrhage

B. Data collection

1. Fatigue

2. Headache

3. Pallor

4. Tachycardia

5. Hemoglobin value usually less than 10 g/dL and hematocrit value usually less than 30%

C. Interventions

1. Monitor hemoglobin and hematocrit levels every 2 weeks

2. Administer and instruct the client about iron and folic acid supplements

3. Teach the client to monitor for signs and symptoms of infection

4. Prepare to administer injectable iron; may be prescribed for severe anemia

5. Prepare to administer transfusions if prescribed for severe anemia

6. Prepare for the administration of oxytocic medications during the postpartum period to prevent hemorrhage

XI. CARDIAC DISEASE

A. Description: Inability to cope with the added plasma volume and increased cardiac output

B. Data collection

1. Cough

2. Dyspnea and fatigue

3. Palpitations and tachycardia

4. Peripheral edema

5. Angina-type pain

6. Signs of pulmonary edema

7. Signs of respiratory infection

C. Interventions

1. Monitor vital signs, fetal heart rate, and condition of fetus

2. Plan activities and stress the need for sufficient rest

3. Encourage adequate nutrition to prevent anemia

4. Maintain bedrest for the client, as prescribed, during the last weeks of pregnancy

5. During **labor**
   a. Monitor vital signs frequently
   b. Place the client on a cardiac monitor and on an external fetal monitor
   c. Maintain bedrest with the mother lying on her side and her head and shoulders elevated
   d. Administer oxygen and pain medication, as prescribed
   e. Monitor for signs of heart failure

XII. CHORIOAMNIONITIS
A. Description
   1. A bacterial infection of the amniotic cavity; can result from the premature rupture of the membranes, vaginitis, amniocentesis, or intrauterine procedures
   2. May result in the development of postpartum endometritis
B. Data collection
   1. Uterine tenderness
   2. Elevated temperature
   3. Maternal or fetal tachycardia
   4. Foul odor to **amniotic fluid**
   5. Leukocytosis
C. Interventions
   1. Monitor maternal vital signs and fetal heart rate
   2. Monitor for uterine tenderness, contractions, and fetal activity
   3. Monitor the results of blood cultures; prepare for amniocentesis to obtain **amniotic fluid** for analysis
   4. Administer antibiotics, as prescribed, after cultures are obtained
   5. Oxytocic medications may be prescribed to increase uterine tone
   6. Obtain neonatal cultures after **delivery,** as prescribed

XIII. DIABETES MELLITUS
A. Description
   1. Pregnancy places demands on carbohydrate metabolism and causes insulin requirements to change
   2. Maternal glucose crosses the **placenta,** but insulin does not
   3. During the first trimester, maternal insulin needs decrease
   4. During the second and third trimesters, increases in placental hormones cause an insulin-resistant state that requires an increase in the client's insulin dose
   5. After placental **delivery,** placental hormone levels drop abruptly, and insulin requirements decrease
   6. The fetus produces its own insulin and pulls glucose from the mother, which predisposes the mother to hypoglycemic reactions

7. The **newborn infant** of a diabetic mother may be large in size but will have functions related to gestational age rather than size
8. The **newborn infant** of a diabetic mother is subject to hypoglycemia, hyperbilirubinemia, respiratory distress syndrome, hypocalcemia, and congenital anomalies

B. Gestational diabetes mellitus
   1. Occurs during pregnancy (during the second or third trimester) among clients not previously diagnosed as diabetic; occurs when the pancreas cannot respond to the demand for more insulin
   2. Pregnant women should be screened for gestational diabetes between 24 and 28 weeks' gestation
   3. An oral glucose tolerance test will be performed to confirm gestational diabetes mellitus
   4. Gestational diabetes frequently can be treated by diet alone; however, some clients may need insulin (oral hypoglycemic agents are never used during pregnancy)
   5. Most gestational diabetics convert to a euglycemic state after **delivery;** however, these individuals have an increased risk for developing diabetes mellitus during their lifetimes
C. Predisposing conditions for gestational diabetes
   1. Older than 35 years old
   2. Obese
   3. Multiple gestation
   4. Family history of diabetes mellitus
D. Data collection
   1. Excessive thirst
   2. Hunger
   3. Weight loss
   4. Blurred vision
   5. Frequent urination
   6. Recurrent urinary tract infections and vaginal yeast infections
   7. Glycosuria and ketonuria
   8. Signs of gestational hypertension
   9. Polyhydramnios
   10. Fetus may be large for gestational age
E. Interventions
   1. Include diet, insulin (if diet cannot control blood glucose levels), exercise, and blood glucose determinations to maintain blood glucose levels between 65 and 130 mg/dL
   2. Observe for signs of hyperglycemia, glycosuria, ketonuria, and hypoglycemia
   3. Monitor weight
   4. Increase calorie intake, as prescribed, with adequate insulin therapy so that glucose will move into the cells
   5. Assess for signs of maternal complications, such as preeclampsia (hypertension, proteinuria, and edema)

6. Monitor for signs of infection
7. Instruct the client to report burning and pain on urination, vaginal discharge or itching, or any other signs of infection to the health care provider
8. Assess the fetal status and monitor for signs of fetal compromise

▲ F. Interventions during **labor**
1. Monitor the fetal status continuously for signs of distress; if noted, prepare the client for immediate cesarean section
2. Carefully regulate insulin and provide IV glucose, as prescribed, because **labor** depletes glycogen

▲ G. Interventions during the postpartum period
1. Observe the client closely for a hypoglycemic reaction, because a precipitous drop in insulin requirements normally occurs; the client may not require insulin for the first 24 hours
2. Reregulate insulin needs, as prescribed, after the first day, according to blood glucose testing
3. Assess dietary needs on the basis of blood glucose and insulin requirements
4. Monitor for signs of infection or postpartum hemorrhage

XIV. DISSEMINATED INTRAVASCULAR COAGULATION

A. Description
1. A condition in the mother's body that results in an exaggerated clotting process, which increases the formation of clots in the microcirculation
2. The rapid and extensive formation of clots results in bleeding and the potential vascular occlusion of organs from thromboembolus formation

B. Predisposing conditions (Box 22-7)

C. Data collection
1. Uncontrolled bleeding
2. Bruising, purpura, petechiae, and ecchymosis
3. Hematuria, hematemesis, or vaginal bleeding
4. Signs of shock
5. Decreased fibrinogen level, platelet count, and hematocrit level
6. Increased prothrombin time, partial thromboplastin time, clotting time, and fibrin degradation products

---

BOX 22-7   **Predisposing Conditions for Disseminated Intravascular Coagulation**

- Abruptio placentae
- Amniotic fluid embolism
- Gestational hypertension
- Intrauterine fetal death
- Liver disease
- Sepsis

D. Interventions
1. Remove the underlying cause
2. Monitor vital signs; assess for bleeding and signs of shock
3. Prepare for oxygen therapy, volume replacement, blood-component therapy, and possibly heparin therapy
4. Monitor for complications associated with fluid and blood replacement and heparin therapy
5. Monitor the urine output, and maintain it at 30 mL/hr (renal failure is a complication of this condition)

XV. ECTOPIC PREGNANCY

A. Description: Pregnancy that occurs in a site other than a uterine site, with **implantation** usually occurring in the ampulla of the fallopian tube (Figure 22-2)

B. Data collection
1. Missed period
2. Abdominal pain
3. Vaginal spotting to bleeding that is dark red or brown
4. Rupture: Increased pain, referred shoulder pain, and signs of shock

C. Interventions
1. Obtain assessment data and vital signs
2. Monitor bleeding and initiate measures to prevent rupture and shock
3. Methotrexate (a folic acid antagonist) may be prescribed to inhibit cell division in the developing embryo
4. Prepare the client for laparotomy and the removal of the pregnancy and tube, if necessary, or repair of the tube
5. Administer antibiotics; Rh immune globulin is given to appropriate Rh-negative women

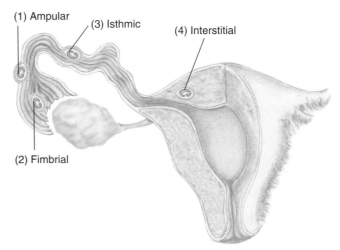

FIG. 22-2   Sites of tubal ectopic pregnancy. The numbers indicate the order of prevalence. (From Murray, S., & McKinney, E. [2006]. *Foundations of maternal-newborn nursing* [4th ed.]. Philadelphia: Saunders.)

XVI. ENDOMETRITIS

A. Description
   1. Infection of the lining of the uterus after **delivery**; caused by bacteria that invade the uterus at the placental site
   2. The infection may spread, involve the entire endometrium, and cause peritonitis, pelvic thrombophlebitis, or cellulitis

B. Data collection
   1. Chills and fever
   2. Increased pulse
   3. Decreased appetite
   4. Headache
   5. Backache
   6. Prolonged, severe afterpains
   7. Tender, large uterus
   8. Foul odor to **lochia** or reddish-brown **lochia**
   9. Ileus
   10. Elevated white blood cell count

C. Interventions
   1. Monitor vital signs
   2. Place the mother in Fowler's position to facilitate the drainage of **lochia**
   3. Provide a private room for the mother
   4. Inform the mother that it is not necessary to isolate the **newborn infant** from the mother
   5. Instruct the mother in proper handwashing techniques
   6. Initiate wound and skin precautions, as necessary
   7. Monitor intake and output (I&O), and encourage fluid intake
   8. IV antibiotics may be prescribed
   9. Administer comfort measures, such as back rubs, position changes, and pain medications, as prescribed
   10. Oxytocic medications may be prescribed to improve uterine tone

XVII. FETAL DEATH IN UTERO

A. Description
   1. Death of a fetus after 20 weeks' gestation and before birth
   2. Disseminated intravascular coagulation can develop if the dead fetus is retained in the uterus for 3 to 4 weeks or more

B. Data collection
   1. Absence of fetal movement
   2. Absence of fetal heart tones
   3. Maternal weight loss
   4. Lack of fetal growth or decrease in fundal height
   5. Lack of cardiac activity and other characteristics suggestive of fetal death noted on the ultrasound

C. Interventions
   1. Prepare for the **delivery** of the fetus
   2. Support the client's decision about **labor**, birth, and the postpartum period
   3. Facilitate the grieving process
   4. Allow the parents to hold the **infant** after birth
   5. Allow the parents to name the **infant**
   6. Accept such behaviors as anger and hostility from the parents
   7. Refer parents to an appropriate support group

XVIII. HEPATITIS B

A. Description
   1. The risks of prematurity, low birth weight, and neonatal death increases if the mother has hepatitis B infection
   2. It is transmitted through blood, saliva, vaginal secretions, semen, breast milk, and across the placental barrier

B. Interventions
   1. Minimize the risk for intrapartum ascending infections by limiting the number of vaginal examinations
   2. Remove the maternal blood from the **neonate** immediately after birth
   3. Suction the **neonate** immediately after birth
   4. Bathe the **neonate** before any invasive procedures
   5. Clean and dry the face and eyes of the **neonate** before instilling eye prophylaxis
   6. Infection of the **neonate** can be prevented by the administration of hepatitis B immune globulin and hepatitis B vaccine soon after birth
   7. Discourage the mother from kissing the **neonate** until the **neonate** has received the vaccine
   8. Support breast-feeding after neonatal treatment; breast-feeding is not contraindicated if the **neonate** has been vaccinated
   9. Inform the mother that the hepatitis B vaccine will be administered to the **neonate** and that the second dose will be administered at 1 month; the third dose is administered at 6 months

XIX. HEMATOMA

A. Description
   1. Occurs after the escape of blood into the tissues of the reproductive sac after the **delivery**
   2. Predisposing conditions include operative **delivery** with forceps or injury to a blood vessel

B. Data collection (Box 22-8)

BOX 22-8 **Hematoma: Data Collection Findings**

- Abnormal, severe pain
- Pressure in the perineal area (the client states that she feels like she has to have a bowel movement)
- Palpable, sensitive tumor in the perineal area, with discolored skin
- Inability to void
- Decreased hemoglobin and hematocrit levels
- Signs of shock, such as pallor, tachycardia, and hypotension, if significant blood loss has occurred

C. Interventions
1. Monitor vital signs
2. Monitor the client for abnormal pain, especially when forceps **delivery** has occurred
3. Apply ice to the hematoma site
4. Administer analgesics, as prescribed
5. Monitor I&O
6. Encourage fluids and voiding; prepare for urinary catheterization if the client is unable to void
7. Prepare to administer blood replacements, as prescribed
8. Monitor for signs of infection, such as increased temperature, pulse rate, and white blood cell count
9. Administer antibiotics, as prescribed, because infection is common after hematoma formation
10. Prepare for the incision and evacuation of the hematoma, if necessary

XX. HYDATIDIFORM MOLE

A. Description
1. Developmental anomaly of the **placenta** that changes chorionic villi into a mass of clear vesicles
2. Presents as an edematous, grapelike cluster that may be nonmalignant or that may develop into choriocarcinoma

B. Data collection
1. Fetal heart rate not detectable
2. Vaginal bleeding, which may occur as early as the fourth week or as late as the second trimester; it is usually bright red or dark brown in color, and it may be slight, profuse, or intermittent
3. Signs of gestational hypertension such as an elevated blood pressure, edema, and proteinuria, may be present before week 20
4. Fundal height is greater than expected for date
5. Elevated hCG levels
6. Ultrasound shows a characteristic snowstorm pattern

C. Interventions
1. Prepare the mother for uterine evacuation (before evacuation, diagnostic tests are done to detect metastatic disease)
2. Evacuation of the mole is done by vacuum aspiration; oxytocin (Pitocin) is administered after evacuation to contract the uterus
3. Tissue is sent to the laboratory for evaluation; follow-up is important to detect changes that are suggestive of malignancy
4. Monitor for postprocedure hemorrhage and infection
5. hCG levels are monitored every 1 to 2 weeks until normal prepregnancy levels are attained; the levels are then checked every 1 to 2 months for 1 year

6. Instruct parents regarding birth control measures so that pregnancy can be prevented during the 1-year follow-up

XXI. HYPEREMESIS GRAVIDARUM

A. Description: Intractable nausea and vomiting that persists beyond the first trimester and that causes disturbances in nutrition, electrolytes, and fluid balance

B. Data collection
1. Nausea is most pronounced on arising; however, it can occur at other times during the day
2. Persistent vomiting and weight loss
3. Signs of dehydration and electrolyte imbalances

C. Interventions
1. Measures to alleviate nausea, including medication therapy, are initiated; if this is unsuccessful and weight loss and electrolyte imbalances occur, the administration of IV fluid and electrolyte replacement or parenteral nutrition may be necessary
2. Monitor vital signs, intake, output, weight, and calorie count
3. Monitor the laboratory data and for signs of dehydration and electrolyte imbalances
4. Monitor the urine for ketones
5. Monitor the fetal heart rate, fetal activity, and fetal growth
6. Encourage the intake of small portions of food (low-fat, easily digestible carbohydrates, such as cereals, rice, and pasta)
7. Liquids should be taken between meals to avoid distending the stomach and triggering vomiting
8. Encourage the client to sit upright after meals

XXII. GESTATIONAL HYPERTENSION

A. Description and types (Table 22-2)
1. Hypertension can be mild or severe, leading to preeclampsia and then eclampsia (seizures)
2. Signs of preeclampsia are hypertension, generalized edema, and proteinuria

B. Data collection (Table 22-3)

C. Predisposing conditions
1. Primigravida
2. Age younger than 19 years or older than 40 years
3. Chronic renal disease
4. Chronic hypertension
5. Diabetes mellitus
6. Rh incompatibility
7. History of or family history of gestational hypertension (GH)

D. Complications of GH
1. Abruptio placentae
2. Disseminated intravascular coagulation
3. Thrombocytopenia
4. Placental insufficiency
5. Intrauterine growth restriction
6. Intrauterine fetal death

TABLE 22-2 **Classification of Hypertensive States of Pregnancy**

Type	Description
Gestational Hypertensive Disorders	
Gestational hypertension	Development of mild hypertension during pregnancy in previously normotensive woman without proteinuria or pathologic edema
Gestational proteinuria	Development of proteinuria after 20 weeks' gestation in a previously nonproteinuric woman without hypertension
Preeclampsia	Development of hypertension and proteinuria in a previously normotensive woman after 20 weeks' gestation or during the early postpartum period; in the presence of trophoblastic disease, it can develop before 20 weeks' gestation
Eclampsia	Development of convulsions or coma in a preeclamptic woman
Chronic Hypertensive Disorders	
Chronic hypertension	Hypertension and/or proteinuria in pregnant woman with chronic hypertension before 20 weeks' gestation and persistent 12 weeks after delivery
Superimposed preeclampsia or eclampsia	Development of preeclampsia or eclampsia in a woman with chronic hypertension before 20 weeks' gestation

Modified from Lowdermilk, D., & Perry, S. (2006). *Maternity nursing* (7th ed.). St. Louis: Mosby.

TABLE 22-3 **Mild Versus Severe Preeclampsia**

Parameter Evaluated	Mild	Severe
Systolic blood pressure	$\geq$140 but <160 mm Hg	$\geq$160 mm Hg (two readings, 6 hours apart, while on bedrest)
Diastolic blood pressure	$\geq$90 but <110 mm Hg	$\geq$110 mm Hg
Proteinuria (a 24-hour specimen is preferred to eliminate hour-to-hour variations)	$\geq$0.3 g but <2 g in a 24-hour specimen (1+ on a random dipstick test)	$\geq$5 g in a 24-hour specimen ($\geq$3+ on a random dipstick test)
Creatinine, serum (renal function)	Normal	Elevated (>1.2 mg/dL)
Platelets	Normal	Decreased (<100,000 cells/mm^3)
Liver enzymes (alanine aminotransferase or aspartate aminotransferase)	Normal or minimal increase in levels	Elevated levels
Urine output	Normal	Oliguria common, often <500 mL/day
Severe, unrelenting headache not attributable to other cause; mental confusion (cerebral edema)	Absent	Often present
Persistent right upper quadrant or epigastric pain or pain penetrating to the back (distention of the liver capsule); nausea and vomiting	Absent	May be present and often precedes seizure
Visual disturbances (spots or "sparkles," temporary blindness; photophobia)	Absent to minimal	Common
Pulmonary edema, heart failure, and cyanosis	Absent	May be present
Fetal growth restriction	Normal growth	Growth restriction and reduced amniotic fluid volume

Modified from Murray, S., & McKinney, E. (2006). *Foundations of maternal-newborn nursing* (4th ed.). St. Louis: Saunders.

E. Interventions for mild hypertension
1. Monitor blood pressure
2. Monitor fetal activity and fetal growth
3. Encourage frequent rest periods; instruct the client to lie in the lateral position
4. Administer antihypertensive medications, as prescribed; teach the client about the importance of the medications
5. Monitor I&O
6. Evaluate renal function through prescribed studies such as blood urea nitrogen, serum creatinine, and 24-hour urine levels for creatinine clearance and protein

F. Interventions for mild preeclampsia
1. Provide bedrest, and place the client in a lateral position
2. Monitor the blood pressure and weight
3. Monitor the neurological status, because changes can indicate cerebral hypoxia or impending seizure
4. Monitor the deep tendon reflexes and for the presence of clonus, because hyperreflexia

BOX 22-9 **Checking Reflexes**

Biceps Reflex
Position your thumb over the client's biceps tendon, and support the client's elbow with the palm of the hand.
Strike a downward blow over the thumb with the percussion hammer.
Normal Response: Flexion of the arm at the elbow

Patellar Reflex
Position the client with legs dangling over the edge of the examining table or lying on her back, with the legs slightly flexed.
Strike the patellar tendon just below the kneecap with the percussion hammer.
Normal Response: Extension or kicking out of the leg

Clonus Reflex
Position the client with the legs dangling over the edge of the examining table.
Support the leg with one hand, and sharply dorsiflex the client's foot with the other hand.
Maintain the dorsiflexed position for a few seconds; then release the foot.

Normal Response (Negative Clonus Response):
The foot will remain steady in the dorsiflexed position.
No rhythmic oscillations or jerking of the foot will be felt.
When released, the foot will drop to a plantarflexed position, with no oscillations.

Abnormal Response (Positive Clonus Response):
Rhythmic oscillations will occur when the foot is dorsiflexed.
Similar oscillations will be noted when the foot drops to the plantarflexed position.

Grading the Response
0 = Reflex absent
1+ = Reflex present but hypoactive
2+ = Normal reflex
3+ = Hyperactive reflex
4+ = Hyperactive reflex with clonus present

indicates increased central nervous system irritability (Box 22-9)
5. Provide adequate fluids
6. Monitor I&O; a urinary output of 30 mL/hr indicates adequate renal perfusion
7. Increase dietary protein and carbohydrates with no added salt
8. Administer medications, as prescribed, to lower the blood pressure; blood pressure should not be lowered drastically, because placental perfusion can be compromised
9. Monitor for HELLP syndrome: a laboratory diagnosis for severe preeclampsia characterized by hemolysis (H), elevated liver enzymes (EL), and low platelets (LP)
G. Interventions for severe preeclampsia
1. Maintain bedrest
2. Magnesium sulfate (use a controlled infusion device) may be prescribed to prevent seizures;

this may be continued for 24 to 48 hours postpartum
3. Monitor for signs of magnesium toxicity, including flushing, sweating, hypotension, depressed deep tendon reflexes, and central nervous system depression, including respiratory depression; keep antidote (calcium gluconate) at the client's bedside
4. Administer antihypertensives, as prescribed
5. Prepare for the induction of **labor**
H. Eclampsia
1. Data collection: Characterized by generalized seizures (Box 22-10)
2. Interventions
a. Maintain a patent airway and administer oxygen
b. Protect the client from injury
c. Monitor the fetal heart rate and contractions
d. Administer medications to control the seizures (magnesium sulfate may be prescribed)
e. Prepare for the delivery of the fetus after the stabilization of the client

XXIII. INCOMPETENT CERVIX
A. Description
1. Premature dilation of cervix, which occurs most often during the fourth or fifth month of pregnancy and is associated with structural or functional defects of the cervix
2. Treatment is surgical
B. Data collection
1. Vaginal bleeding
2. Fetal membranes visible through the cervix
C. Interventions
1. Provide bedrest, hydration, and tocolysis, as prescribed, to inhibit uterine contractions
2. Prepare for cervical cerclage (at 10 to 14 weeks' gestation), in which a band of fascia or nonabsorbable ribbon is placed around the cervix beneath the mucosa to constrict the internal os of the cervix
3. After cervical cerclage, the woman is told to refrain from intercourse and to avoid prolonged standing and heavy lifting
4. The cervical cerclage is removed at 37 weeks' gestation or left in place and a cesarean **delivery** is performed; if removed, the cerclage must be repeated with each successive pregnancy
5. After the procedure, monitor for contractions, rupture of the membranes, and signs of infection
6. Instruct the woman to report any postprocedure vaginal bleeding or increased uterine contractions immediately to the health care provider

XXIV. INFECTIONS
A. Toxoplasmosis
1. Caused by infection with the protozoan intracellular parasite *Toxoplasma gondii*

BOX 22-10 Eclampsia

An eclampsia seizure typically begins with twitching around the mouth. The body then becomes rigid in a state of tonic muscular contractions, which last 15 to 20 seconds. The facial muscles and then all of the body muscles alternatively contract and relax in rapid succession; this is the clonic phase, which may last about 1 minute. Respiration ceases during the seizure, because the diaphragm tends to remain fixed. Breathing resumes shortly after the seizure, and postictal sleep occurs.

2. Produces a rash and symptoms of acute, flu-like infection in the mother
3. Transmitted to the mother through raw meat or via the handling of the cat litter of infected cats
4. Organism is transmitted to the fetus across the **placenta**
5. Can cause spontaneous abortion

B. Rubella (German measles)
1. Extremely teratogenic during the first trimester
2. Transmitted to the fetus across the **placenta**
3. Causes congenital defects of the eyes, heart, ears, and brain
4. If not immune (titer of 1:8 or less), the mother should be vaccinated during the postpartum period; she must then wait 1 to 3 months (as specified by health care provider) before becoming pregnant again

C. Cytomegalovirus
1. Organism is transmitted through close personal contact or across the placenta to the fetus, or the fetus may be infected through the birth canal
2. The mother may be asymptomatic, and most **infants** are asymptomatic at birth
3. Diagnosis of neonatal infection is by urine; cytomegalovirus causes low birth weight, intrauterine growth retardation, enlarged liver and spleen, jaundice, mental retardation, blindness, hearing loss, and seizures
4. Antiviral medications may be prescribed for severe infections in the mother, but these medications are toxic and may only temporarily suppress the shedding of the virus

D. Genital herpes
1. Affects the external genitalia, vagina, and cervix
2. Causes draining, painful vesicles
3. Virus is usually transmitted to the fetus during birth through the infected vagina or via an ascending infection after the rupture of the membranes
4. No vaginal examinations are done in the presence of active vaginal herpetic lesions
5. Can cause death or severe neurological impairment in the **newborn**
6. **Delivery** of the fetus is usually by cesarean section if active lesions are present in the vagina;

delivery may be performed vaginally if the lesions are in the anal, perineal, or inner thigh area (strict precautions are necessary to protect the fetus during **delivery**)
7. Maintain contact precautions

E. Group B *Streptococcus* (GBS)
1. A leading cause of life-threatening perinatal infections
2. The gram-positive bacterium colonizes the rectum, **vagina,** cervix, and urethra of pregnant and nonpregnant women.
3. Meningitis, fasciitis, and intraabdominal abscess can occur in the pregnant client if she is infected at the time of birth
4. Transmission occurs during vaginal **delivery**
5. Early-onset **newborn** GBS occurs within the first week after birth, usually within 48 hours; it can include infections such as sepsis, pneumonia, or meningitis, and permanent neurological disability can result
6. Diagnosis of the mother is done via vaginal and rectal cultures between 35 and 37 weeks' gestation.
7. Antibiotics such as penicillin may be prescribed for the mother during **labor** and birth; IV antibiotics may be prescribed for infected infants

XXV. **MULTIPLE GESTATION**
A. Description
1. Results from the **fertilization** of two ova (fraternal or dizygotic) or a splitting of one of the fertilized ovum (identical or monozygotic)
2. Complications include spontaneous abortion, anemia, congenital anomalies, hyperemesis gravidarum, intrauterine growth restriction, GH, polyhydramnios, postpartum hemorrhage, premature rupture of membranes, and preterm **labor** and **delivery**

B. Data collection
1. Excessive fetal activity
2. Uterus large for gestational age
3. Palpation of three or four large fetal parts in the uterus
4. Auscultation of more than one fetal heart rate
5. Excessive weight gain

C. Interventions
1. Monitor vital signs
2. Monitor the fetal heart rates, fetal activity, and fetal growth
3. Monitor for cervical changes
4. Prepare the client for ultrasound, as prescribed
5. Monitor for anemia; administer supplemental vitamins, as prescribed
6. Monitor for preterm **labor** and treat it promptly
7. Prepare for cesarean section for abnormal presentations

8. Prepare to administer oxytocic medications after **delivery** to prevent postpartum hemorrhage from uterine overdistention

XXVI. PYELONEPHRITIS

A. Description
  1. Results from bacterial infections that extend upward from the bladder through the blood vessels and the lymphatics
  2. Frequently follows untreated urinary tract infections; associated with increased incidence of anemia, low birth weight, GH, premature **labor** and **delivery**, and premature rupture of the membranes

B. Data collection
  1. Flank pain
  2. Burning or painful urination
  3. Increased frequency of urination
  4. Chills, malaise, and nausea
  5. Increased temperature, pulse rate, and fetal heart rate
  6. Vomiting
  7. Uterine contractions
  8. Elevated white blood cell count

C. Interventions
  1. Monitor vital signs
  2. Monitor the fetal heart rate
  3. Monitor for uterine contractions
  4. Encourage fluids; monitor I&O
  5. Monitor renal function
  6. Administer antibiotics, as prescribed
  7. Administer antipyretics, such as acetaminophen (Tylenol), as prescribed
  8. Obtain urine cultures every 2 to 4 weeks after the resolution of infection

XXVII. SEXUALLY TRANSMITTED INFECTIONS

A. Chlamydia
  1. Description
    a. Common sexually transmitted pathogen associated with an increased risk of premature birth, stillbirth, neonatal conjunctivitis, and **newborn** chlamydial pneumonia
    b. In the nonpregnant state, can cause salpingitis, pelvic abscesses, chronic pelvic pain, and infertility
    c. Diagnostic test is a positive culture for *Chlamydia trachomatis*
  2. Data collection
    a. Usually asymptomatic
    b. Bleeding between periods or after coitus
    c. Mucoid or purulent cervical discharge
    d. Dysuria and pelvic pain
  3. Interventions
    a. Screen the client to determine whether the client is at high risk; instruct the client about the importance of rescreening, because reinfection can occur as the client nears term
    b. Ensure that the sexual partner is treated

B. Syphilis
  1. Description
    a. Chronic infectious disease caused by the organism *Treponema pallidum*
    b. Transmission is by intimate physical contact with syphilitic lesions, which are usually found on the skin or mucous membranes of the mouth and genitals
    c. Infection may cause abortion or premature **labor**; passed to the fetus after the fourth month of pregnancy as congenital syphilis
  2. Data collection (Box 22-11)
  3. Interventions
    a. Obtain a serum test (Venereal Disease Research Laboratory or rapid plasma reagin) for syphilis on the first prenatal visit; prepare to repeat the test at 36 weeks' gestation, because the disease may be acquired after the initial visit
    b. If the test result is positive, treatment with an antibiotic such as penicillin may be necessary
    c. Instruct the client that the treatment of her partner is necessary if infection is present

C. Gonorrhea
  1. Description
    a. Infection caused by *Neisseria gonorrhoeae*, which causes inflammation of the mucous membranes of the genital and urinary tracts
    b. Transmission of organism is by sexual intercourse
    c. Infection may be transmitted to the **newborn's** eyes during **delivery**, causing blindness (ophthalmia neonatorum)

BOX 22-11 Stages of Syphilis

Primary Stage
- Most infectious stage
- Appearance of ulcerative, painless lesions produced by spirochetes at the point of entry into the body

Secondary Stage
- Highly infectious stage
- Lesions appear about 3 weeks after the primary stage and may occur anywhere on the skin and mucous membranes
- Generalized lymphadenopathy occurs

Tertiary Stage
- Spirochetes enter the internal organs and cause permanent damage; symptoms may occur 10 to 30 years after the occurrence of an untreated primary lesion
- Disease invades the central nervous system, causing meningitis, ataxia, general paresis, and progressive mental deterioration
- Affects the aortic valve and the aorta

2. Data collection: Usually asymptomatic; vaginal discharge, urinary frequency, and lower abdominal pain are possible
3. Interventions
   a. Obtain a culture for gonorrhea on the first prenatal visit; prepare to repeat culture, because infection may occur during pregnancy
   b. Administer prophylactic antibiotics to the **newborn infant's** eyes, as prescribed
   c. Instruct the client that the treatment of her partner is necessary if infection is present

D. Condylomata acuminata (venereal warts)
1. Description
   a. Caused by human papillomavirus (HPV); affects the cervix, urethra, anus, penis, and scrotum
   b. Transmitted through sexual contact
2. Data collection
   a. Small to large wart-like growths on the genitals
   b. Cervical cell changes may be noted, because HPV is associated with cervical malignancies
3. Interventions
   a. Lesions are removed with the use of cytotoxic agents, cryotherapy, electrocautery, and laser
   b. Encourage a yearly Papanicolaou (Pap) smear
   c. Avoid sexual contact until the lesions are healed (condoms are used to reduce transmission)

E. Bacterial vaginosis
1. Description
   a. Caused by *Haemophilus vaginalis* or *Gardnerella*; transmitted via sexual contact
   b. Associated with premature **labor** and birth
2. Data collection
   a. Client complains of "fishy odor" to vaginal secretions and increased odor after intercourse
   b. Microscopic examination of vaginal secretions identifies the infection
3. Interventions
   a. Treatment with oral metronidazole (Flagyl) may be prescribed
   b. Sexual partner may need to be treated

F. Vaginal candidiasis
1. Description
   a. *Candida albicans* is the most common causative organism
   b. Predisposing factors include the use of antibiotics, diabetes mellitus, and obesity
   c. Diagnosis is by identifying the spores of *Candida albicans*
2. Data collection
   a. Vulvar and vaginal pruritus

b. White, lumpy, and cottage-cheese–like discharge from the **vagina**
3. Interventions
   a. An antifungal vaginal preparation such as miconazole (Monistat) may be prescribed
   b. For extensive irritation and swelling, sitz baths may be prescribed
   c. Sexual partner may need to be treated

G. Trichomoniasis
1. Description: Caused by *Trichomonas vaginalis*; transmitted via sexual contact
2. Data collection
   a. Yellowish to greenish, frothy, mucopurulent, copious, and malodorous vaginal discharge
   b. Inflammation of vulva, **vagina,** or both maybe present
3. Interventions
   a. Metronidazole (Flagyl) may be prescribed
   b. Sexual partner may need to be treated

XXVIII. TUBERCULOSIS
A. Description
1. A highly communicable disease caused by *Mycobacterium tuberculosis*
2. Transmitted by the airborne route
3. A multidrug-resistant strain can exist as a result of improper compliance or noncompliance with treatment programs and the development of mutations in the tubercle bacilli
B. Transmission
1. Transplacental transmission is rare
2. Can occur during birth through the aspiration of infected **amniotic fluid**
3. **Neonate** can become infected from contact with infected individuals
C. Risk to mother: Active disease during pregnancy has been associated with an increase in hypertensive disorders of pregnancy
D. Diagnosis
1. If a chest radiograph is required for the mother, it is obtained only after 20 weeks' gestation, and a lead shield for the abdomen is required
2. Skin testing is safe during pregnancy
E. Data collection
1. Maternal
   a. May be asymptomatic
   b. Fever and chills
   c. Night sweats
   d. Weight loss
   e. Fatigue
   f. Cough, hemoptysis, or green or yellow sputum
   g. Dyspnea
   h. Pleural pain
2. **Neonate**
   a. Fever
   b. Lethargy

c. Poor feeding
d. Failure to thrive
e. Respiratory distress
f. Hepatosplenomegaly
g. Meningitis
h. Disease may spread to all major organs

F. Interventions
   1. Pregnant client
      a. Administration of isoniazid (INH), pyrazinamide, and rifampin (Rifadin) daily for 9 months; ethambutol (Myambutol) is added if medication resistance is probable
      b. Pyridoxine (vitamin B6) should be administered along with INH to pregnant women to prevent fetal neurotoxicity caused by the INH
      c. Promote breast-feeding only if the mother is noninfectious
   2. **Newborn infant**
      a. Management focuses on preventing disease and treating early infection
      b. The **infant** is skin tested at birth and may be placed on INH therapy; the skin test is repeated in 3 to 4 months, and the INH may be stopped if the skin test results remain negative
      c. If the skin test result is positive, the **infant** should receive INH for at least 6 months
      d. If the mother's sputum is free of organisms, the **infant** does not need to be isolated from the mother while in the hospital

XXIX. URINARY TRACT INFECTION
A. Description: A urinary tract infection can occur during pregnancy; if untreated, the client can develop pyelonephritis.
B. Predisposing conditions
   1. History of urinary tract infections
   2. Sickle cell trait
   3. Poor hygiene
   4. Anemia
   5. Diabetes mellitus
   6. Pregnancy
C. Data collection
   1. Possibly asymptomatic during pregnancy
   2. Burning and pain on urination
   3. Increased frequency of urination
   4. Lower abdominal pain and costovertebral angle tenderness
   5. Fever
   6. Proteinuria, hematuria, bacteriuria, and white blood cells in urine
D. Interventions
   1. Monitor vital signs
   2. Monitor the fetal heart rate

3. Increase the fluid intake
4. Monitor the I&O
5. Monitor the urine for consistency and odor
6. Monitor for signs and symptoms of pyelonephritis (dip test the urine for increases in protein, glucose, and ketones with each prenatal visit)
7. Obtain urine for culture and sensitivity
8. Provide heat to the lower abdomen or back
9. Administer antibiotics, as prescribed
10. Instruct the client to complete the course of antibiotics, if prescribed
11. Instruct the client regarding the need to repeat the culture after treatment is completed

PRACTICE QUESTIONS

More questions on the companion CD!

212. A client is undergoing an amniocentesis at 16 weeks' gestation to detect the presence of biochemical or chromosomal abnormalities. The nurse instructs the client:
   1. That the bladder must be full during the exam
   2. That the bladder must be empty during the exam
   3. She will be given RhoGAM because she is Rh positive
   4. Not to eat or drink anything 4 to 6 hours before the exam

213. A client at 28 weeks' gestation is Rh negative and Coombs' antibody negative. The nurse determines that the client understands what the nurse has taught her about Rh sensitization when the client states:
   1. "I know I can never have another child."
   2. "I am glad I won't have to have these shots if I have another child."
   3. "I will have to have an injection once a month until the baby is born."
   4. "I will tell the nurse at the hospital that I had RhoGAM during pregnancy."

214. While assisting with the measurement of fundal height, the client at 36 weeks' gestation states that she is feeling lightheaded. On the basis of the nurse's knowledge of pregnancy, the nurse determines that this is most likely due to:
   1. A full bladder
   2. Emotional instability
   3. Insufficient iron intake
   4. Compression of the vena cava

215. A contraction stress test is scheduled for a client. The woman asks the nurse about the test. The most accurate description of the test includes which of the following?
   1. "Uterine contractions are stimulated by Leopold's maneuvers."

2. "An internal fetal monitor is attached, and you will walk on a treadmill until contractions begin."

3. "The uterus is stimulated to contract by either small amounts of oxytocin (Pitocin) or by nipple stimulation."

4. "Small amounts of oxytocin (Pitocin) are administered during internal fetal monitoring to stimulate uterine contractions."

216. A client at 38 weeks' gestation is admitted to the birthing center in early labor. The client is carrying twins, and one of the fetuses is in a breech presentation. The nurse assists with planning care for the client and identifies which of the following as the lowest priority for the care of this client?
    1. Measuring the fundal height
    2. Attaching electronic fetal monitoring
    3. Preparing the client for a possible cesarean section
    4. Gathering equipment for starting an intravenous line

217. A perinatal client is admitted to the obstetric unit during an exacerbation of a heart condition. When planning for the nutritional requirements of the client, the nurse would consult with the dietitian to ensure which of the following?
    1. A low-calorie diet to ensure the absence of weight gain
    2. A diet that is high in fluids and fiber to decrease constipation
    3. A diet that is low in fluids and fiber to decrease blood volume
    4. Unlimited sodium intake to increase the circulating blood volume

218. A nurse caring for a client with abruptio placentae is monitoring the client for signs of disseminated intravascular coagulopathy (DIC). The nurse would suspect DIC if he or she observes:
    1. Rapid clotting times
    2. Pain and swelling of the calf of one leg
    3. Laboratory values that indicate increased platelets
    4. Petechiae, oozing from injection sites, and hematuria

219. A nurse has a teaching session with a malnourished client regarding iron supplementation to prevent anemia during pregnancy. Which of the following statements, if made by the client, would indicate successful learning?
    1. "Iron supplements will give me diarrhea."
    2. "The iron is needed for the red blood cells."
    3. "Meat does not provide iron and should be avoided."
    4. "My body has all the iron it needs, and I don't need to take supplements."

220. During a prenatal visit, a nurse is explaining dietary management to a client with diabetes mellitus. The nurse determines that the teaching has been effective when the client states:
    1. "I can eat more sweets now, because I need more calories."
    2. "I need more fat in my diet so that the baby can gain enough weight."
    3. "I need to eat a high-protein, low-carbohydrate diet now to control my blood glucose."
    4. "I need to increase the fiber in my diet to control my blood glucose and prevent constipation."

221. A nurse is assigned to assist with caring for a client who is at risk for eclampsia. If the client progresses from preeclampsia to eclampsia, the nurse's first action should be to:
    1. Administer oxygen by face mask.
    2. Clear and maintain an open airway.
    3. Check the blood pressure and the fetal heart tones.
    4. Prepare for the administration of intravenous magnesium sulfate.

222. A client is in her second trimester of pregnancy. She complains of frequent low back pain and ankle edema at the end of the day. The nurse recommends which measure to help relieve both discomforts?
    1. Lie on the left side with the feet dorsiflexed.
    2. Soak the feet in hot water after performing 10 pelvic tilt exercises.
    3. Lie on the right side with the feet elevated on a pillow and a heating pad on the back.
    4. Lie on the floor with the legs elevated onto a couch or padded chair, with the hips and knees at a right angle.

223. A pregnant woman complains of being awakened frequently by leg cramps. The nurse reinforces instructions to the client's partner and tells the partner to:
    1. Dorsiflex the client's foot while flexing the knee.
    2. Plantarflex the client's foot while flexing the knee.
    3. Dorsiflex the client's foot while extending the knee.
    4. Plantarflex the client's foot while extending the knee.

224. A nurse is providing instructions to a pregnant client with heartburn regarding measures that will alleviate the discomfort. The nurse instructs the client to:
    1. Eliminate between-meal snacks.
    2. Drink decaffeinated coffee and tea.
    3. Lie down for 30 minutes after eating.
    4. Substitute salt in cooking for other spices.

225. A nurse is doing a 48-hour postpartum check on a client with mild gestational hypertension (GH). Which of the following data indicate that the GH is not resolving?
    1. Urinary output has increased.
    2. There is no evidence of dependent edema.
    3. The client complains of a headache and blurred vision.
    4. The blood pressure reading has returned to the prenatal baseline.

ALTERNATE ITEM FORMAT: MULTIPLE RESPONSE

226. A nurse is monitoring a pregnant client with gestational hypertension who is at risk for pre-eclampsia. The nurse checks the client for which classic signs of preeclampsia? Check all that apply.
    ☐ 1. Proteinuria
    ☑ 2. Hypertension
    ☐ 3. Low-grade fever
    ☑ 4. Generalized edema
    ☑ 5. Increased pulse rate
    ☐ 6. Increased respiratory rate

ANSWERS

212. **1**

Rationale: Before 20 weeks' gestation, the bladder must be kept full during amniocentesis to support the weight of the uterus. After 20 weeks' gestation, the bladder may be emptied to minimize the chance of puncturing the placenta or fetus. $Rh_0(D)$ immune globulin (RhoGAM) is administered to Rh-negative woman because of the risk of immunization from the fetal blood during the exam. There are no fluid or food restrictions. Monitoring the fetal heart tones and the vital signs throughout and after the exam is an important intervention.

Test-Taking Strategy: Focus on the strategic words "16 weeks' gestation." Remember that before 20 weeks' gestation, the bladder must be kept full to support the weight of the uterus. Review client instructions for amniocentesis if you had difficulty with this question.

Level of Cognitive Ability: Application
Client Needs: Physiological Integrity
Integrated Process: Nursing Process/Implementation
Content Area: Maternity/Antepartum
References: Chernecky, C., & Berger, B. (2008). *Laboratory tests and diagnostic procedures* (5th ed., p. 132). Philadelphia: Saunders.
Christensen, B., & Kockrow, E. (2006). *Foundations and adult health nursing* (5th ed., p. 486). St. Louis: Mosby.

213. **4**

Rationale: As described in the question, it is accepted practice to administer $Rh_0(D)$ immune globulin (RhoGAM) to a woman at 28 weeks' gestation, with a second injection within 72 hours of delivery. This prevents sensitization, which could jeopardize a future pregnancy. For subsequent pregnancies or abortions, the injections must be repeated, because the immunity is passive. Options 1, 2, and 3 are inaccurate information.

Test-Taking Strategy: Note the strategic words "that the client understands." Recalling the guidelines regarding the administration of RhoGAM will direct you to option 4. Review Rh sensitization if you had difficulty with this question.

Level of Cognitive Ability: Comprehension
Client Needs: Physiological Integrity
Integrated Process: Nursing Process/Evaluation
Content Area: Maternity/Antepartum
Reference: Leifer, G. (2007). *Introduction to maternity and pediatric nursing* (5th ed., p. 336). Philadelphia: Saunders.

214. **4**

Rationale: Compression of the inferior vena cava and aorta by the uterus may cause supine hypotension syndrome during pregnancy. Having the woman turn onto her left side or elevating the right buttock during fundal height measurement will prevent or correct the problem. Options 1, 2, and 3 are not the cause of the problem described in the question.

Test-Taking Strategy: Focus on the data in the question, and recall the complications associated with pregnancy. Use the ABCs—airway, breathing, and circulation—to direct you to option 4. Review the interventions for supine hypotension syndrome if you had difficulty with this question.

Level of Cognitive Ability: Comprehension
Client Needs: Physiological Integrity
Integrated Process: Nursing Process/Data Collection
Content Area: Maternity/Antepartum
Reference: Leifer, G. (2007). *Introduction to maternity and pediatric nursing* (5th ed., p. 52). Philadelphia: Saunders.

215. **3**

Rationale: A contraction stress test assesses placental oxygenation and function and determines the fetus' ability to tolerate labor as well as its well-being. The test is performed if the nonstress test result is abnormal. During the stress test, the fetus is exposed to the stressor of contractions to assess the adequacy of placental perfusion under simulated labor conditions. An external fetal monitor is applied to the mother, and a 20- to 30-minute baseline strip is recorded. The uterus is stimulated to contract, either by the administration of a dilute dose of oxytocin (Pitocin) or by having the mother use nipple stimulation, until three palpable contractions with a duration of 40 seconds or more during a 10-minute period have occurred. Frequent maternal blood pressure readings are performed, and the client is monitored closely while increasing doses of oxytocin are given.

Test-Taking Strategy: Knowledge regarding the contraction stress test is required to answer the question. Remember that during both the nonstress test and the contraction stress test, external monitoring is performed. Review the contraction stress test if you had difficulty with this question.

Level of Cognitive Ability: Application
Client Needs: Physiological Integrity
Integrated Process: Nursing Process/Implementation
Content Area: Maternity/Antepartum
Reference: Leifer, G. (2008). *Maternity nursing: An introductory text* (10th ed., p. 65). Philadelphia: Saunders.

216. **1**

Rationale: Option 1 is a low priority, because fundal height should be measured at each antepartal clinic visit; it is not a priority of care during the intrapartum period. Options 2, 3, and 4 are all high priorities. The twins should be monitored by dual electronic fetal monitoring, and any signs of distress should be reported. Many physicians choose to perform a cesarean birth if either of the twins is breech. The mother should have an intravenous line in place in case fluid or blood replacement is required.

Test-Taking Strategy: Note the strategic words "lowest priority." Use Maslow's Hierarchy of Needs theory and the ABCs—airway, breathing, and circulation—to prioritize and direct you to option 1. Review the care of the pregnant client with a breech presentation if you had difficulty with this question.

Level of Cognitive Ability: Application
Client Needs: Physiological Integrity
Integrated Process: Nursing Process/Planning
Content Area: Delegating/Prioritizing
Reference: Murray, S., & McKinney, E. (2006). *Foundations of maternal-newborn nursing* (4th ed., pp. 702-703). Philadelphia: Saunders.

217. **2**

Rationale: Constipation causes the client to use Valsalva's maneuver. This causes blood to rush to the heart and overload the cardiac system. The absence of weight gain is not recommended during pregnancy. Diets that are low in fluid and fiber cause a decrease in blood volume, which in turn deprives the fetus of nutrients. Too much sodium could cause an overload to the circulating blood volume and contribute to the cardiac condition.

Test-Taking Strategy: Use the process of elimination, and try to relate the situation to something with which you are familiar. Look for options that would apply to any heart condition, think about the needs of a pregnant client, and use the process of elimination. Review dietary measures for the client with cardiac disease if you had difficulty with this question.

Level of Cognitive Ability: Application
Client Needs: Physiological Integrity
Integrated Process: Nursing Process/Planning
Content Area: Maternity/Antepartum
References: Leifer, G. (2008). *Maternity nursing: An introductory text* (10th ed., p. 68). Philadelphia: Saunders.
Murray, S., & McKinney, E. (2006). *Foundations of maternal-newborn nursing* (4th ed., p. 674). Philadelphia: Saunders.

218. **4**

Rationale: DIC is a state of diffuse clotting in which clotting factors are consumed, which leads to widespread bleeding. Platelet counts are decreased, because they are consumed by the process. Coagulation studies show no clot formation (clotting times are thus prolonged), and fibrin plugs may clog the microvasculature diffusely rather than in an isolated area.

Test-Taking Strategy: Use the process of elimination. Eliminate option 2 on the basis of the knowledge that DIC is a widespread problem rather than a localized one. Eliminate options 1 and 3 next, because they are comparable

or alike. Review the signs related to DIC if you had difficulty with this question.

Level of Cognitive Ability: Comprehension
Client Needs: Physiological Integrity
Integrated Process: Nursing Process/Data Collection
Content Area: Maternity/Antepartum
Reference: Leifer, G. (2008). *Maternity nursing: An introductory text* (10th ed., p. 255). Philadelphia: Saunders.

219. **2**

Rationale: A nutritional supplement that is commonly needed during pregnancy is iron. Anemia of pregnancy is primarily caused by iron deficiency. Iron supplements usually cause constipation. Meats are an excellent source of iron. Iron for the fetus comes from the maternal serum.

Test-Taking Strategy: Use the process of elimination. Note the strategic word "malnourished." Eliminate options 3 and 4 because of the close-ended words "not" and "all." Knowledge regarding the effects of iron supplements will assist you with eliminating option 1. Review the relationship of nutrition to anemia if you had difficulty with this question.

Level of Cognitive Ability: Comprehension
Client Needs: Physiological Integrity
Integrated Process: Nursing Process/Evaluation
Content Area: Maternity/Antepartum.
References: Leifer, G. (2008). *Maternity nursing: An introductory text* (10th ed., pp. 264-265). Philadelphia: Saunders.
Leifer, G. (2007). *Introduction to maternity and pediatric nursing* (5th ed., pp. 103-104). Philadelphia: Saunders.

220. **4**

Rationale: An increase in calories is needed during pregnancy, but concentrated sugars should be avoided, because they may cause hyperglycemia. The fat intake should be 20% to 30% of the total calories. The client with diabetes needs about 50% to 60% of her caloric intake from carbohydrates and about 12% to 20% from protein. High-fiber foods will control blood glucose levels and prevent constipation.

Test-Taking Strategy: Note the strategic words "teaching has been effective." Use the process of elimination and your knowledge regarding diabetes mellitus and diet therapy to direct you to the correct option. Review the components of the diabetic diet if you had difficulty with this question.

Level of Cognitive Ability: Comprehension
Client Needs: Health Promotion and Maintenance
Integrated Process: Nursing Process/Evaluation
Content Area: Maternity/Antepartum
References: Leifer, G. (2008). *Maternity nursing: An introductory text* (10th ed., p. 268). Philadelphia: Saunders.
Lowdermilk, D., & Perry, A. (2007). *Maternity and woman's health care* (9th ed., p. 854) St. Louis: Mosby.

221. **2**

Rationale: The first actions are to maintain an open airway and to prevent injuries to the client. Options 1, 3, and 4 may be components of care, but they are not the first actions.

Test-Taking Strategy: Note the strategic word "first." Use the ABCs—airway, breathing, and circulation—to answer this question; airway is the first priority. Review the care of the client with eclampsia if you had difficulty with this question.

Level of Cognitive Ability: Application
Client Needs: Physiological Integrity
Integrated Process: Nursing Process/Implementation
Content Area: Delegating/Prioritizing
References: Lowdermilk, D., & Perry, A. (2007). *Maternity and woman's health care* (9th ed., p. 854) St. Louis: Mosby.
Murray, S., & McKinney, E. (2006). *Foundations of maternal-newborn nursing* (4th ed., p. 648). Philadelphia: Saunders.

222. 4
Rationale: The position described in option 4 will produce the posture of the pelvic tilt while countering gravity as the force that leads to the edema of the lower extremities. Although the other options may seem useful, options 2 and 3 identify heat, which should be prescribed by the physician. Option 1 will not relieve back pain and ankle edema.
Test-Taking Strategy: Use the process of elimination. Focus on the subject of the question—back pain and ankle edema. Eliminate options 2 and 3, because the application of heat needs to be prescribed by the physician. From the remaining options, focus on the subject to direct you to option 4. Review the measures that will reduce these discomforts if you had difficulty with this question.
Level of Cognitive Ability: Application
Client Needs: Physiological Integrity
Integrated Process: Nursing Process/Implementation
Content Area: Maternity/Antepartum
Reference: Leifer, G. (2007). *Introduction to maternity and pediatric nursing* (5th ed., p. 66). Philadelphia: Saunders.

223. 3
Rationale: Leg cramps often occur when the pregnant woman stretches her leg and plantarflexes her foot. Dorsiflexion of the foot while extending the knee stretches the gastrocnemius muscle, prevents the muscle from contracting, and halts the cramping.
Test-Taking Strategy: Use the process of elimination. Knowledge regarding the actions that will alleviate muscle cramps will assist you with answering the question. Visualize each of the descriptions in the options to help direct you to the correct option. Review the measures to alleviate muscle cramps if you had difficulty with this question.
Level of Cognitive Ability: Application
Client Needs: Health Promotion and Maintenance
Integrated Process: Teaching and Learning
Content Area: Maternity/Antepartum
Reference: Leifer, G. (2008). *Maternity nursing: An introductory text* (10th ed., p. 69). Philadelphia: Saunders.

224. 2
Rationale: Lying down after meals is likely to lead to the reflux of stomach contents. Spices tend to trigger heartburn. Salt leads to the retention of fluid. Eating smaller, more frequent portions is preferable to eating three large meals to control heartburn. Caffeine, like spices, may cause heartburn.
Test-Taking Strategy: Use the process of elimination, and recall those items that cause heartburn; this will direct you to option 2. Review the measures that alleviate heartburn if you had difficulty with this question.
Level of Cognitive Ability: Application
Client Needs: Health Promotion and Maintenance
Integrated Process: Teaching and Learning
Content Area: Maternity/Antepartum
References: Leifer, G. (2008). *Maternity nursing: An introductory text* (10th ed., pp. 50, 68). Philadelphia: Saunders.
Murray, S., McKinney, E., & Gorrie, T. (2006). *Foundations of maternal-newborn nursing* (4th ed., p. 148). Philadelphia: Saunders.

225. 3
Rationale: Options 1, 2, and 4 are all signs that the GH is being resolved. Option 3 is a symptom of the worsening of the GH.
Test-Taking Strategy: Note the strategic words "not resolving." Recalling the signs of worsening GH will direct you to the correct option. Review these signs if you had difficulty with this question.
Level of Cognitive Ability: Analysis
Client Needs: Physiological Integrity
Integrated Process: Nursing Process/Evaluation
Content Area: Maternity/Antepartum
Reference: Leifer, G. (2008). *Maternity nursing: An introductory text* (10th ed., p. 258). Philadelphia: Saunders.

ALTERNATE ITEM FORMAT: MULTIPLE RESPONSE

226. 1, 2, 4
Rationale: The three classic signs of preeclampsia are hypertension, generalized edema, and proteinuria. A low-grade fever, an increased pulse rate, and an increased respiratory rate are not associated with preeclampsia.
Test-Taking Strategy: Focus on the subject—the classic signs of preeclampsia. Thinking about the pathophysiology associated with this disorder will direct you to the correct options. Remember that the classic signs of preeclampsia are hypertension, generalized edema, and proteinuria. Review the signs of preeclampsia if you had difficulty with this question.
Level of Cognitive Ability: Application
Client Needs: Physiological Integrity
Integrated Process: Nursing Process/Data Collection
Content Area: Maternity/Antepartum
References: Leifer, G. (2008). *Maternity nursing: An introductory text* (10th ed., p. 258). Philadelphia: Saunders.
Wong, D., Perry, S., Hockenberry, M., Lowdermilk, D., & Wilson, D. (2006). *Maternal-child nursing care* (3rd ed., p. 277). St. Louis: Mosby.

REFERENCES

Chernecky, C., & Berger, B. (2008). *Laboratory tests and diagnostic procedures* (5th ed.). Philadelphia: Saunders.

Christensen, B., & Kockrow, E. (2006). *Foundations and adult health nursing* (5th ed.). St. Louis: Mosby.

Leifer, G. (2008). *Maternity nursing: An introductory text* (10th ed.). Philadelphia: Saunders.

Leifer, G. (2007). *Introduction to maternity and pediatric nursing* (5th ed.). Philadelphia: Saunders.

Lowdermilk, D., & Perry, A. (2007). *Maternity and woman's health care* (9th ed.). St. Louis: Mosby.

Murray, S., & McKinney, E. (2006). *Foundations of maternal-newborn nursing* (4th ed.). Philadelphia: Saunders.

Wong, D., Perry, S., Hockenberry, M., Lowdermilk, D., & Wilson, D. (2006). *Maternal-child nursing care* (3rd ed.). St. Louis: Mosby.

CHAPTER 23

Labor and Delivery and Associated Complications

I. THE PROCESS OF LABOR: "THE FOUR *P*'s" (Box 23-1)
A. Description
  1. **Labor**: A coordinated sequence of rhythmic involuntary uterine contractions
  2. **Delivery**: The actual event of birth
B. Four major factors—the four *P*'s—interact during normal childbirth; all four *P*'s are interrelated
C. Powers: Uterine and abdominal contractions
  1. The forces acting to expel the fetus and **placenta**
  2. Effacement: The shortening, thinning, and disappearance of the cervix during the first stage of labor
  3. Dilation: The enlargement of the cervical os and cervical canal during the first stage of labor
  4. Voluntary pushing efforts of the mother during the second stage
D. Passageway: Composed of the mother's rigid bony pelvis and the soft tissues of the cervix, pelvic floor, vagina, and introitus
E. Passenger: The fetus, membranes, and **placenta**
F. Attitude
  1. The relationship of the fetal body parts with one another
  2. The normal intrauterine attitude is flexion, in which the fetal back is rounded, the head is forward on the chest, and the arms and legs are flexed in against the body; the other attitude, extension, tends to present larger fetal diameters
G. Lie
  1. Relationship of the spine of the fetus to the spine of the mother
  2. Longitudinal or vertical: Fetal spine is parallel to the mother's spine; the fetus is in either a cephalic or breech presentation
  3. Transverse or horizontal: Fetal spine is at a right angle, or perpendicular, to the mother's spine; the presenting part is usually the shoulder, and **delivery** is by cesarean section
H. Presentation
  1. Portion of the fetus that enters the pelvis first
  2. Cephalic: The most common presentation; fetal head presents first
  3. Breech: Buttocks present first; **delivery** by cesarean section may be required, although it is often possible to deliver vaginally
  4. Shoulder: Fetus is in a transverse lie; the arm, back, abdomen, or side could present; if the fetus does not spontaneously rotate or if it is not possible to turn the fetus manually, a cesarean section may be performed
I. Presenting part: The specific fetal structure lying nearest to the cervix
J. Position: The relationship of the assigned area of the presenting part or landmark to the maternal pelvis (Box 23-2)
K. Station
  1. The measurement of the progress of descent in centimeters above or below the midplane from the presenting part to the ischial spine
  2. Station 0: At the ischial spine; the presenting part is "engaged" when it reaches 0 station
  3. Minus station: Above the ischial spine
  4. Plus station: Below the ischial spine
L. Psyche
  1. Mother may experience anxiety, fear, and/or pain
  2. Perception of pain affected by physiological, psychosocial, and environmental factors and the woman's previous experiences

II. MECHANISMS OF LABOR (Box 23-3)
A. Data collection
  1. Lightening or dropping: Fetus descends into the pelvis about 2 weeks before **delivery** for a primipara; the fetus may engage into the pelvis after **labor** commences for a multipara
  2. Braxton Hicks contractions increase
  3. Vaginal mucosa congested; vaginal mucus increases
  4. Appearance of bloody show (brownish or blood-tinged cervical mucus is passed)
  5. Cervix ripens and becomes soft and partly effaced; may begin to dilate
  6. Sudden burst of energy

BOX 23-1 The Four *P*'s

- Powers
- Passageway
- Passenger
- Psyche

BOX 23-2 Fetal Positions

- ROA: Right occiput anterior
- LOA: Left occiput anterior
- ROP: Right occiput posterior
- LOP: Left occiput posterior
- ROT: Right occiput transverse
- LOT: Left occiput transverse
- RMA: Right mentum anterior
- LMA: Left mentum anterior
- RMP: Right mentum posterior
- LSA: Left sacrum anterior
- LSP: Left sacrum posterior

    7. Loss of 1 to 3 pounds from water loss resulting from fluid shifts produced by changes in progesterone and estrogen levels

    8. Spontaneous rupture of the membranes

  B. True **labor** and false **labor** (Box 23-4)

▲ **III. LEOPOLD'S MANEUVERS**

  A. Description: A method of determining the presentation and position of the fetus; an aid for locating fetal heart sounds

  B. If the head is in the fundus, a hard, round, movable object is felt; the buttocks will feel soft and have an irregular shape, and they are more difficult to move

  C. The fetus' back, which is a smooth, hard surface, should be felt on one side of the abdomen

  D. Irregular knobs and lumps, which may be the hands, feet, elbows, and knees, will be felt on the opposite side of the abdomen

▲ **IV. BREATHING TECHNIQUES** (Box 23-5)

  A. Provide a focus during contractions, thus interfering with pain sensory transmission

  B. Promote relaxation and oxygenation

  C. Begin with simple breathing patterns and progress to more complex ones, as needed

▲ **V. FETAL MONITORING**

  A. Description

    1. Displays fetal heart rate (FHR) and uterine activity

    2. Monitors the uterine activity, frequency, and duration of contractions; only internal monitoring is capable of monitoring the intensity of contractions

    3. Monitors the FHR in relation to maternal contractions

    4. Baseline FHR is measured between contractions; the normal FHR at term is 120 to 160 beats per minute

BOX 23-3 Mechanisms of Labor

Engagement
Engagement is the mechanism by which the fetus nestles into the pelvis; it also is called *lightening* or *dropping*.

Descent
Descent is the process that the fetal head undergoes as it begins its journey through the pelvis. It is a continuous process from the time of engagement until birth, and it is assessed by the measurement called *station*.

Flexion
Flexion is the process of the fetal head's nodding forward toward the fetal chest.

Internal Rotation
The internal rotation of the fetus occurs most commonly from the occiput transverse position, which is assumed at engagement into the pelvis, to the occiput anterior position while continuously descending.

Extension
Extension enables the head to emerge when the fetus is in a cephalic position, and it begins after the head crowns. Extension is complete when the head passes under the symphysis pubis and occiput and the anterior fontanel, brow, face, and chin pass over the sacrum and coccyx and are over the perineum.

Restitution
Restitution is the realignment of the fetal head with the body after the head emerges.

External Rotation
The shoulders externally rotate after the head emerges and restitution occurs so that the shoulders are in the anteroposterior diameter of the pelvis.

Expulsion
Expulsion is the birth of the entire body.

BOX 23-4 True Labor and False Labor

True Labor
Contractions occur regularly; they become stronger, last longer, and occur closer together.
Cervical dilation and effacement are progressive.
The fetus usually becomes engaged in the pelvis and begins to descend.

False Labor
False labor does not produce dilation, effacement, or descent.
Contractions are irregular and without progression.
Walking has no effect on contractions and often relieves the condition.
For example, consider a woman who has been sleeping and who wakes up with contractions. If she gets up and moves around and her contractions become stronger and closer together, this is true labor. If the contractions go away when she does this, it is false labor.

B. External fetal monitoring
   1. Noninvasive; performed with the use of a toco-transducer or a Doppler ultrasonic transducer
   2. Leopold's maneuvers are performed to determine on which side the fetal back is located, and the ultrasound transducer is then placed over this area and fastened with a belt
   3. The tocotransducer is placed over the fundus of the **uterus,** where contractions feel the strongest, and fastened with a belt
   4. Allow the client to assume a comfortable position, avoiding vena cava compression (maternal supine hypotensive syndrome)
   5. The preferred maternal position is to have her lie on her side to increase perfusion
C. Internal fetal monitoring
   1. Invasive; requires rupturing the membranes and attaching an electrode to the presenting part of the fetus
   2. Mother must be dilated 2 to 3 cm before internal monitoring can be performed
D. Periodic patterns in the FHR
   1. Fetal bradycardia and tachycardia
      a. Bradycardia: FHR is less than 120 beats per minute for 10 minutes or longer; a later sign of fetal hypoxia
      b. Tachycardia: FHR is greater than 160 beats per minute for 10 minutes or longer; can be early sign of fetal hypoxia

---

BOX 23-5 **Breathing Techniques**

First-Stage Breathing
Cleansing Breath
- Each contraction begins and ends with a deep inspiration and expiration.
Slow-Paced Breathing
- A slow, deep breathing that promotes relaxation
- Used as long as possible during labor
Modified-Paced Breathing
- Used when slow-paced breathing is no longer effective
- Shallow, fast breathing
Pattern-Paced Breathing
- Sometimes called *pant-blow*
- After a certain number of breaths (modified-paced breathing), the woman exhales with a slight emphasis or blow and then begins the modified-paced breathing again.
Breathing to Prevent Pushing
- The woman blows repeatedly using short puffs when the urge to push is strong.
Second-Stage Breathing
Several variations of breathing can be used in the pushing stage of labor, and the woman may grunt, groan, sigh, or moan as she pushes. Prolonged breath-holding while pushing with a closed glottis may result in a decrease in cardiac output. Therefore, if breath-holding while pushing is used, the open glottis method (limiting breath-holding to less than 6 to 8 seconds) should be done.

c. Notify physician
d. Treatment based on cause: Change the position of the mother and administer oxygen; other interventions, as prescribed
2. Variability
   a. Fluctuations in the baseline FHR
   b. Absence of variability or undetected variability is considered nonreassuring
   c. Decreased variability can result from fetal hypoxemia, acidosis, or certain medications
   d. A temporary decrease in variability can occur when the fetus is in a sleep state (sleep states do not usually last more than 30 minutes)
3. Accelerations
   a. Brief, temporary increases in the FHR of at least 15 beats above the baseline and lasting at least 15 seconds, with the return to baseline less than 2 minutes from the beginning of the acceleration
   b. Usually a reassuring sign that reflects a responsive, nonacidotic fetus
   c. Usually occur with fetal movement or stimulation
   d. May occur with uterine contractions, vaginal examinations, mild cord compression, or when the fetus is in a breech presentation
4. Early decelerations
   a. Visually apparent gradual decrease in FHR and return to baseline in response to fetal head compression
   b. Occur during contractions as the fetal head is pressed against the woman's pelvis or soft tissues, such as the cervix
   c. FHR returns to baseline by the end of the contraction
   d. Not associated with fetal compromise; requires no intervention
5. Late decelerations
   a. Nonreassuring patterns that reflect impaired placental exchange or uteroplacental insufficiency
   b. Patterns look similar to early decelerations but begin well after the contraction begins and return to baseline after the contraction ends
   c. Degree of the fall in the heart rate from baseline is not related to the amount of uteroplacental insufficiency
   d. Interventions include improving placental blood flow and fetal oxygenation
6. Variable decelerations
   a. Variable decelerations are caused by conditions that restrict flow through the umbilical cord
   b. Variable decelerations do not have the uniform appearance of early and late decelerations

c. Their shape, duration, and degree of fall below baseline heart rate are variable; they fall and rise abruptly with the onset and relief of cord compression

d. Variable decelerations also may be nonperiodic, occurring at times that are unrelated to contractions

e. One considers the baseline rate and variability when evaluating variable decelerations.

f. Variable decelerations are significant when the FHR repeatedly decreases to less than 70 beats per minute and persists at that level for at least 60 seconds before returning to baseline

7. Hypertonic uterine activity

a. Checking uterine activity includes frequency, duration, intensity of contractions, and uterine resting tone

b. Uterus should relax between contractions for 60 seconds or more

c. In hypertonic uterine activity, reduced uterine blood flow and decreased fetal oxygen supply occur

8. Interventions for nonreassuring (altered) patterns (Box 23-6)

a. The registered nurse and physician are notified

b. Identify the cause (check for cord prolapse)

c. Change the mother's position (avoid the supine position for patterns associated with cord compression)

d. Administer oxygen by face mask at 8 to 10 L/minute

e. Oxytocin (Pitocin), if infusing, is discontinued, as prescribed

f. Intravenous (IV) fluids are increased, as prescribed

g. Prepare to obtain a fetal scalp pH monitor to determine a blood pH value

h. Prepare to initiate continuous electronic fetal monitoring with internal devices if not contraindicated

i. Prepare for cesarean **delivery**, if necessary

VI. **FOUR STAGES OF LABOR** (Table 23-1)

A. Stage 1, latent phase

1. Description/data collection

a. Cervical dilation of up to 3 cm

b. Uterine contractions every 5 to 30 minutes, 30 to 45 seconds in duration, and of mild to moderate intensity

c. Mother talkative; eager to be in **labor**; alert, happy, and excited, with mild anxiety

2. Interventions

a. Encourage the mother and partner to participate in care

b. Assist with comfort measures, changes of position, and ambulation; encourage effleurage, focusing, and relaxation techniques

c. Keep the mother and partner informed of progress

d. Offer fluids and ice chips

e. Encourage voiding every 1 to 2 hours and rest or sleep, if possible

B. Stage 1, active phase

1. Description/data collection

a. Cervical dilation of 4 to 7 cm

b. Uterine contractions every 3 to 5 minutes, 40 to 70 seconds in duration, and of moderate to strong intensity

c. Mother may experience feelings of helplessness; mood becomes seriously **labor** oriented, with concentration and energy needed for contractions

d. Mother becomes restless and anxious as contractions become stronger

---

BOX 23-6 Nonreassuring Patterns

- Tachycardia
- Bradycardia
- Diminished or absent variability
- Late decelerations
- Variable decelerations falling to less than 70 beats per minute for more than 60 seconds
- Prolonged decelerations
- Hypertonic uterine activity

TABLE 23-1 Four Stages of Labor

First Stage	Second Stage	Third Stage	Fourth Stage
Effacement and dilation of the cervix	Pushing stage	Separation of the placenta	Physical recovery
Divided into three stages: latent, active, and transition	Expulsion of the fetus	Expulsion of the placenta	1 to 4 hours after the expulsion of the placenta
Woman is sociable and excited in the latent phase, becoming more inwardly focused as labor intensifies	Woman has intense concentration on pushing with contractions; may doze between contractions	Woman is excited and relieved after baby's birth; usually very tired	Woman is tired but may find it difficult to rest because of excitement; eager to become acquainted with the newborn

2. Interventions
   a. Encourage the maintenance of effective breathing patterns; assist the woman to cope with contractions
   b. Provide a quiet environment
   c. Keep the mother and partner informed of progress
   d. Promote comfort with back rubs, sacral pressure, pillow support, frequent position changes, and oral care; fluids, food, and ice chips, as ordered; and ointment for dry lips
   e. Offer analgesics, as ordered
   f. Encourage voiding every 1 to 2 hours

C. Stage 1, transition phase
   1. Description/data collection
      a. Cervical dilation of 8 to 10 cm
      b. Uterine contractions every 2 to 3 minutes, 45 to 90 seconds in duration, and of strong intensity
      c. Mother becomes tired, restless, and irritable; may feel out of control and have nausea and vomiting
   2. Interventions
      a. Encourage rest between contractions
      b. Alert the woman to begin her breathing pattern before the contraction becomes too intense; remind, reassure, and encourage her to reestablish the breathing pattern and concentration as necessary; assist her with coping with contractions
      c. Keep the mother and partner informed of progress
      d. Provide privacy but also constant support
      e. Offer fluids, ice chips, and ointment for dry lips
      f. Encourage voiding every 1 to 2 hours
      g. Prompt panting respirations if woman begins to push prematurely

D. Interventions throughout stage 1
   a. Monitor maternal vital signs
   b. Monitor FHR via ultrasound, Doppler, fetoscope, or electronic fetal monitor
   c. Assess FHR before, during, and after a contraction, noting that the normal FHR is 120 to 160 beats per minute
   d. Monitor uterine contractions by palpation or monitor, and determine frequency, duration, and intensity
   e. Assist with monitoring the status of cervical dilation and effacement
   f. Assist with monitoring fetal station, presentation, and position by performing Leopold's maneuvers
   g. Assist with pelvic examinations and prepare for a Nitrazine or fern test to assess for the rupture of membranes

   h. Check the color of the **amniotic fluid** if the membranes have ruptured; meconium-stained fluid can indicate fetal distress

E. Stage 2
   1. Description/data collection
      a. Begins with complete cervical effacement and full dilation; ends with the baby's birth
      b. Progress of **labor** is measured by the descent of the fetal head through the birth canal (change in fetal station)
      c. Uterine contractions occur every 2 to 3 minutes and last 60 to 75 seconds, and the intensity is strong
      d. Increase in bloody show occurs
      e. Mother feels urge to bear down; assist the mother with pushing efforts
   2. Interventions
      a. Monitor maternal vital signs
      b. Check the FHR before, during, and after a contraction, noting that normal FHR is 120 to 160 beats per minute
      c. Monitor the uterine contractions with palpation or monitoring, determining the frequency, duration, and intensity
      d. Provide the mother with encouragement and praise, and provide for rest between contractions
      e. Keep the mother and partner informed of progress
      f. Maintain privacy
      g. Provide ice chips and ointment for dry lips
      h. Assist the mother into a position that promotes comfort and that assists with pushing efforts
      i. Monitor for signs of approaching birth, such as perineal bulging or visualization of the fetal head
      j. Prepare for birth

F. Stage 3
   1. Description
      a. Lasts from the birth of the baby until the **placenta** is expelled
      b. Contractions continue as placental separation and expulsion occur
      c. Birth of the **placenta** occurs 5 to 30 minutes after the birth of the baby
   2. Data collection
      a. Schultze mechanism: The center portion of the **placenta** separates first, and its shiny fetal surface emerges from the **vagina**
      b. Duncan mechanism: The margin of the **placenta** separates first, and the dull, red, rough maternal surface emerges from the **vagina**
      c. The surface of the **placenta** that appears first is of no clinical importance

3. Interventions
   a. Monitor maternal vital signs and uterine status
   b. After the birth of the **placenta,** the uterine fundus remains firm and is located approximately two fingerbreadths below the umbilicus
   c. Examine the **placenta** for cotyledons and membranes to verify that it is intact; examine the umbilical cord for the presence of one vein and two arteries
   d. Monitor the mother for a shivering reaction; provide warmth
   e. Promote parental–neonatal attachment

G. Stage 4
   1. Description: The period of time from 1 to 4 hours after **delivery**
   2. Data collection
      a. Blood pressure returns to prelabor level
      b. Pulse is slightly lower than during **labor**
      c. Fundus remains contracted, in the midline, and one to two fingerbreadths below the umbilicus
      d. **Lochia** is moderate to heavy for the first 2 hours; it is bright red and may contain small clots; flow should steadily decrease
   3. Interventions
      a. Maternal assessments are performed every 15 minutes for 1 hour, every 30 minutes for 1 hour, and hourly for 2 hours
      b. Provide warm blankets
      c. Apply ice packs to the perineum
      d. Massage the fundus, if needed; teach the mother to massage the fundus
      e. Provide breast-feeding support, as needed
      f. See Chapter 25 for information about caring for the **newborn**

VII. ANESTHESIA

A. Local anesthesia
   1. Used for blocking pain during episiotomy
   2. Administered just before the birth of the baby
   3. No effect on the fetus
B. Pudendal block
   1. Administered just before the birth of the baby
   2. Injection site at pudendal nerve through a transvaginal route
   3. Blocks perineal area for episiotomy
   4. Effect lasts about 30 minutes
   5. No effect on contractions or fetus
C. Lumbar epidural block
   1. Injection site in epidural space at L3-L4
   2. Administered after **labor** is established or just before a scheduled cesarean birth
   3. Relieves pain from contractions and numbs the vagina and perineum
   4. May cause hypotension, bladder distension, and a prolonged second stage.

5. Does not cause headache, because the dura mater is not penetrated
6. Monitor maternal blood pressure
7. Maintain the mother in a side-lying position or place a rolled blanket beneath the right hip to displace the uterus from the vena cava
8. IV fluids are administered, as prescribed
9. Increase fluids, as prescribed, if hypotension occurs

D. Subarachnoid (spinal) block
   1. Injection site in spinal subarachnoid space at L3-L5
   2. Acts quickly; may be administered just before birth
   3. Relieves uterine and perineal pain and numbs vagina, perineum, and lower extremities
   4. Usually causes maternal hypotension; may be marked
   5. May cause postpartum headache
   6. The mother must lie flat 8 to 12 hours after spinal injection
   7. IV fluids are administered, as prescribed
   8. Increase fluids, as prescribed, if hypotension occurs

E. General anesthesia
   1. Rarely used for uncomplicated vaginal birth; infrequently used for elective cesarean birth
   2. The mother is not awake
   3. Presents a danger of respiratory depression and vomiting

VIII. OBSTETRICAL PROCEDURES

A. Bishop score (Table 23-2)
   1. Used to determine maternal readiness for **labor** induction
   2. Evaluates cervical status and fetal position
   3. Indicated before the induction of **labor**
   4. The five factors are assigned a score of 0 to 3, and the total score is calculated
   5. A score of 6 or more indicates a readiness for labor induction
B. Induction
   1. The chemical or mechanical initiation of uterine contractions before their spontaneous

TABLE 23-2	Factors of the Bishop Score			
Score	0	1	2	3
Dilation of cervix	0	1-2 cm	3-4 cm	>5 cm
Effacement of cervix	0%-30%	40%-50%	60%-70%	>80%
Consistency of cervix	Firm	Medium	Soft	
Position of cervix	Posterior	Mid position	Anterior	
Station of presenting part	−3	−2	−1	+1, +2

onset for the purpose of bringing about the birth

2. Elective induction may be accomplished by oxytocin (Pitocin) infusion and/or amniotomy
3. Baseline tracing of uterine contractions and FHR is obtained
4. IV dosage of oxytocin may be increased, as prescribed, only after assessing contractions, FHR, and maternal blood pressure and pulse
5. The rate of oxytocin is not increased after the desired contraction pattern is obtained (i.e., contraction frequency of 2 to 3 minutes, duration of 60 seconds)
6. Oxytocin infusion is discontinued immediately, and the primary health care provider is notified if uterine hyperstimulation, nonreassuring FHR and pattern, or both occur

C. Amniotomy
1. Artificial rupture of membranes (AROM); performed by the health care provider to stimulate **labor**
2. The presenting part of the fetus should be engaged before this is performed
3. Increases risk of prolapsed cord and infection
4. Monitor FHR before and after AROM
5. Record time of AROM, FHR, and characteristics of fluid
6. Meconium-stained **amniotic fluid** may be associated with fetal distress
7. Bloody **amniotic fluid** may indicate abruptio placentae or fetal trauma
8. An unpleasant odor to the **amniotic fluid** is associated with infection
9. Polyhydramnios is associated with maternal diabetes and certain congenital disorders
10. Oligohydramnios is associated with intrauterine growth restriction and congenital disorders
11. Expect more variable decelerations after the rupture of the membranes as a result of cord compression during contractions
12. Limit client activity after AROM, if prescribed

D. External cephalic version (ECV)
1. External manipulation of the fetus from a breech or shoulder presentation into a vertex presentation
2. Indicated for an abnormal presentation that exists after 37 weeks' gestation
3. Attempted only in a **labor** and birth setting
4. Women who are Rh-negative should receive Rh immune globulin
5. Prepare for nonstress test to evaluate fetal well-being just before ECV
6. Ultrasound is used before attempting ECV to determine fetal position, rule out **placenta** previa, locate the umbilical cord, evaluate the adequacy of the maternal pelvis, and assess

the amount of **amniotic fluid,** the fetal age, and for the presence of anomalies

7. IV fluids and tocolytic therapy may be administered to relax the uterus and permit easier manipulation of the fetus
8. Accomplished by the exertion of gentle, constant pressure on the abdomen to direct the fetus into a cephalic presentation, if possible
9. Before, during, and after, monitor the FHR and pattern, the maternal vital signs, and the level of discomfort
10. Following the procedure
    a. Perform a nonstress test to evaluate fetal well-being
    b. Monitor for uterine activity, bleeding, ruptured membranes, and decreased fetal activity

E. Episiotomy
1. Incision made into the perineum to enlarge the vaginal outlet and facilitate **delivery**
2. Check episiotomy site routinely as part of postpartum assessment
3. Institute measures to relieve pain
4. Provide an ice pack during the first 24 hours
5. Instruct the client regarding the use of sitz baths
6. Apply analgesic spray or ointment, as prescribed
7. Provide perineal care with the use of clean technique
8. Instruct the client regarding the proper care of the incision
9. Instruct the client to dry the perineal area from front to back and to blot the area rather than wipe it
10. Instruct the client to shower rather than bathe in a tub
11. Apply a Peri-Pad without touching the inside surface of the pad
12. Report any bleeding or discharge to the physician

F. Forceps **delivery**
1. Two double-crossed, spoonlike articulated blades are used to assist in the **delivery** of the fetal head
2. Reassure the mother and explain the need for the forceps
3. Monitor the mother and fetus during **delivery**
4. Check the **neonate** and mother after **delivery** for any possible injury
5. Assist with the repair of any lacerations

G. Vacuum extraction
1. A cap-like suction device is applied to the fetal head to facilitate extraction
2. Suction is used to assist with the **delivery** of the fetal head
3. Traction is applied during uterine contractions until the descent of the fetal head is achieved

4. The suction device should not be kept in place any longer than 25 minutes
5. Monitor the FHR every 5 minutes if external fetal monitoring is not used
6. Check the **newborn** at birth and monitor him or her throughout the postpartum period for signs of cerebral trauma
7. Monitor for developing cephalhematoma
8. Caput succedaneum is normal and will resolve in 24 hours

H. Cesarean **delivery**
1. Birth of the fetus through a transabdominal incision of the uterus
2. Preoperative
   a. If planned, prepare the mother and partner
   b. If an emergency, quickly explain the need and procedure to the mother and partner
   c. Obtain informed consent
   d. Make sure that the preoperative diagnostic tests are done, including testing for the Rh factor
   e. Prepare the mother for the insertion of an IV line and a Foley catheter
   f. Prepare the abdomen, as prescribed
   g. Monitor the mother and fetus continuously for signs of **labor**
   h. Provide emotional support
   i. Administer preoperative medications, as prescribed
3. Postoperative
   a. Monitor the vital signs
   b. Provide pain relief
   c. Encourage turning, coughing, and deep breathing
   d. Encourage ambulation and measures to decrease the risk for deep vein thrombosis
   e. Monitor for signs of infection and bleeding
   f. Burning and pain on urination may indicate a bladder infection
   g. A tender uterus and foul-smelling **lochia** may indicate endometritis
   h. A productive cough or chills may indicate pneumonia
   i. A positive Homans' sign, pain, or edema of the extremity may indicate thrombophlebitis

IX. DYSTOCIA
A. Description
1. Difficult labor that is prolonged or more painful
2. Occurs as a result of problems caused by uterine contractions, the fetus, or the bones and tissues of the maternal pelvis
3. Contractions may be hypotonic or hypertonic
4. Fetus may be excessively large, malpositioned, or in an abnormal presentation
5. Dystocia can result in maternal dehydration, infection, fetal injury, or death

B. Data collection
1. Excessive abdominal pain
2. Abnormal contraction pattern
3. Fetal distress
4. Maternal or fetal tachycardia
5. Lack of progress of labor
C. Interventions
1. Check FHR; monitor for fetal distress
2. Monitor uterine contractions
3. Monitor the vital signs, paying special attention to maternal temperature and heart rate
4. Assist with pelvic examination, measurements, ultrasound, and other procedures
5. Prophylactic antibiotics may be prescribed to prevent infection
6. IV fluids may be prescribed
7. Monitor intake and output
8. Monitor for dehydration
9. Instruct the mother in breathing techniques and relaxation exercises
10. Fetal monitoring is needed if oxytocin (Pitocin) is prescribed
11. Monitor the color of the amniotic fluid
12. Provide rest and comfort as with a normal delivery, such as back rubs and position changes
13. Assess the mother's fatigue and pain; administer sedatives and pain medications, as prescribed
14. Monitor for prolapse of the cord after the rupture of the membranes

X. PROLAPSED CORD (Figure 23-1)
A. Description: The umbilical cord is displaced between the presenting part and the amnion, or it is protruding through the cervix, causing compression of the cord and compromising fetal circulation
B. Data collection
1. Mother has a feeling that something is coming through the **vagina**
2. Umbilical cord is visible or palpable
3. FHR is irregular and slow
4. Fetal heart monitor will show variable deceleration or bradycardia after the rupture of the membranes
5. If fetal hypoxia is severe, violent fetal activity may occur and then cease
C. Interventions (Box 23-7)

XI. PRECIPITOUS LABOR AND DELIVERY
A. Description: **Labor** that lasts less than 3 hours from the onset of contractions to birth
B. Interventions
1. Stay with the mother at all times
2. Provide emotional support and keep the mother calm
3. Encourage the mother to pant between contractions
4. Prepare for the rupturing of the membranes when the head crowns if they are not already ruptured

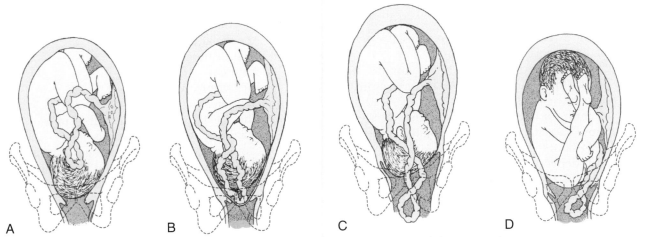

FIG. 23-1 Prolapse of the umbilical cord. Note the pressure of the presenting part on the umbilical cord; this endangers fetal circulation. **A,** Occult (hidden) prolapse of the cord. **B,** Complete prolapse of the cord. **C,** Cord presenting in front of the fetal head may be seen in the vagina. **D,** Frank breech presentation with prolapsed cord. (From Lowdermilk, D., & Perry, S. [2007]. *Maternity & women's health care* [9th ed.]. St. Louis: Mosby.)

BOX 23-7 **Interventions: Cord Prolapse**

Relieve cord pressure immediately.
Place the woman into an extreme Trendelenburg's position, a modified Sims' position, or a knee-chest position.
Elevate the fetal presenting part that is lying on the cord by applying finger pressure with a sterile gloved hand.
Do not attempt to push the cord into the uterus.
Monitor the fetal heart rate.
Assess the fetus for hypoxia.
Administer oxygen by face mask to the mother.
Prepare for emergency cesarean birth.

---

5. Do not try to keep the fetus from being delivered
6. If **delivery** is necessary before the arrival of the health care provider:
   a. Apply gentle pressure to fetal head upward toward the vagina to prevent damage to the fetal head and vaginal lacerations
   b. Support the **infant's** body during **delivery**
   c. Deliver the **infant** between contractions, checking for the cord around the neck
   d. Restitution is used to deliver the posterior shoulder
   e. Gentle downward pressure is used to move the anterior shoulder under the pubic symphysis
   f. Clear the **infant's** mouth
7. Dry and cover the **infant** to keep the body warm
8. Allow the **placenta** to separate naturally
9. Place the **infant** on the mother's abdomen or breast to induce uterine contractions

XII. PRETERM LABOR
A. Description
   1. Cervical changes and uterine contractions occurring between 20 and 37 weeks' gestation
   2. Cause is unknown but assumed to be multifactorial; may be associated with infection
B. Data collection
   1. Uterine contractions (painful or painless)
   2. Abdominal cramping (may be accompanied by diarrhea)
   3. Low back pain
   4. Pelvic pressure or heaviness
   5. Change in the character and amount of usual discharge; may be thicker or thinner, bloody, brown or colorless, or odorous
   6. Rupture of amniotic membranes
C. Interventions
   1. Focus is on stopping the **labor**: identify and treat infection, restrict activity, and ensure hydration
   2. Maintain bedrest, but recognize the potential for adverse effects of bedrest
   3. Monitor the fetal status
   4. Administer fluids
   5. Tocolytic medications may be prescribed to suppress **labor** (see Table 26-1 for a description of medications used to treat preterm **labor**)

XIII. PREMATURE RUPTURE OF THE MEMBRANES
A. Description
   1. The spontaneous rupture of the amniotic membrane before the onset of **labor**
   2. Gestational age usually determines the plan and intervention
   3. When the rupture of membranes is before term and **delivery** will be delayed, infection becomes a risk

Marginal   Partial   Total

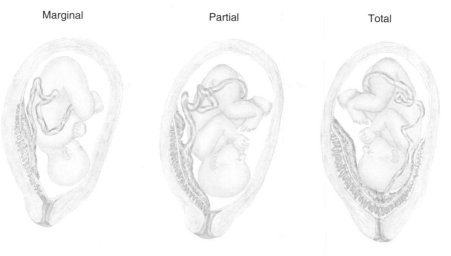

Placenta is implanted in lower uterus but its lower border is >3 cm from internal cervical os.

Lower border of placenta is within 3 cm of internal cervical os but does not fully cover it.

Placenta completely covers internal cervical os.

FIG. 23-2 The three classifications of placenta previa. (From Murray, S., & McKinney, E. [2006]. *Foundations of maternal-newborn nursing* [4th ed.]. Philadelphia: Saunders.)

B. Data collection
  1. Evidence of fluid pooling in the vaginal vault; Nitrazine test is positive
  2. Amount, color, consistency, and odor of fluid
  3. Vital signs; elevated temperature may indicate the presence of infection
  4. Fetal monitoring; tachycardia may indicate infection
C. Interventions
  1. Assist with tests to assess gestational age
  2. Monitor maternal and fetal status for signs of compromise or infection
  3. Administer antibiotics, as prescribed

XIV. **RUPTURE OF THE UTERUS**
A. Description
  1. Separation of the uterine tissue from the stress of **labor;** classified as complete or incomplete
  2. Complete: Extends through the entire uterine wall into the peritoneal cavity or the broad ligament
  3. Incomplete: Extends into the peritoneum but not into the peritoneal cavity or the broad ligament
  4. Manifestations vary with the extent of rupture; may be silent or dramatic; bleeding is usually internal
  5. Most frequent causes are the separation of the scar from a previous cesarean birth, uterine trauma (accidents, surgery), and a congenital uterine anomaly
  6. Occurrence is rare but very serious

B. Data collection
  1. Abdominal pain or tenderness
  2. Chest pain
  3. Contractions may stop or fail to progress
  4. Rigid abdomen
  5. Absent FHR
  6. Signs of maternal shock
  7. Fetus palpated outside of the uterus (complete rupture)
C. Interventions
  1. Prevention is the best treatment; assess risk factors
  2. Monitor for and assist with treating signs of shock (oxygen, IV fluids, and blood products may be prescribed)
  3. Prepare the client for cesarean section or hysterotomy with hysterectomy
  4. Provide emotional support for the mother and partner

XV. **PLACENTA PREVIA** (Figure 23-2)
A. Description
  1. The **placenta** is improperly implanted in the lower uterine segment near or over the internal cervical os
  2. Total: Internal os is entirely covered by the **placenta**
  3. Partial: Incomplete coverage of the internal os
  4. Marginal: Only an edge of the **placenta** extends to the internal os, but it may extend onto the os during the dilation of the cervix during **labor.**

5. Low-lying **placenta**: The **placenta** is implanted in the lower uterine segment but does not reach the os
6. Management depends on the classification of the previa and the gestational age of the fetus

B. Data collection
1. Sudden onset of painless, bright-red vaginal bleeding during the last half of pregnancy; suspect **placenta** previa whenever vaginal bleeding occurs after 24 weeks' gestation
2. Soft, relaxed, nontender uterus
3. Fundal height may be greater than expected for gestational age

C. Interventions
1. Monitor maternal vital signs, FHR, and fetal activity
2. Prepare for ultrasound to confirm diagnosis
3. Vaginal examination or any other action that would stimulate uterine activity is avoided
4. Maintain bedrest in a left lateral position
5. Monitor the amount of bleeding (treat signs of shock)
6. IV fluids, blood products, or tocolytic medications may be prescribed
7. If bleeding is heavy, a cesarean section may be performed
8. Prepare to administer Rh immune globulin if the mother is Rh-negative and has not been given the injection at 28 weeks' gestation

XVI. **ABRUPTIO PLACENTAE** (Figure 23-3)
A. Description
1. Premature separation of the **placenta** (the detachment of part or all of the **placenta** from its **implantation** site) after 20 weeks' gestation and before the birth of the baby
2. Classified according to type and severity

B. Data collection
1. Dark red vaginal bleeding; however, if the bleeding is high in the **uterus** or minimal, there can be an absence of visible blood
2. Uterine pain and/or tenderness
3. Uterine rigidity
4. Severe abdominal pain
5. Signs of fetal distress
6. Signs of maternal shock if bleeding is excessive

C. Interventions
1. Monitor maternal vital signs and FHR
2. Assess for excessive vaginal bleeding, abdominal pain, and an increase in fundal height
3. Maintain bedrest; administer oxygen, IV fluids, and blood products, as prescribed
4. Place the mother in Trendelenburg's position, if indicated, to decrease the pressure of the fetus on the **placenta** or in the lateral position with the head of the bed flat if signs of hypovolemic shock caused by blood loss occur
5. Monitor and report any uterine activity
6. Prepare for the **delivery** of the fetus as quickly as possible, with vaginal **delivery** preferable if the fetus is healthy and stable and the presenting part is in the pelvis; emergency cesarean section is performed if the fetus is alive but shows signs of distress
7. Monitor for signs of disseminated intravascular coagulopathy (DIC) during the postpartum period

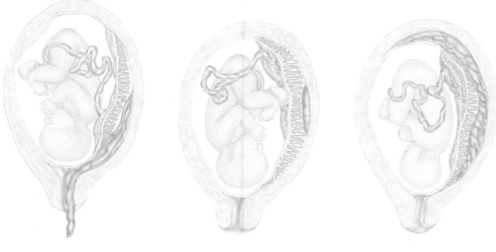

Marginal abruption with external bleeding   Partial abruption with concealed bleeding   Complete abruption with concealed bleeding

FIG. 23-3 Types of abruptio placentae. (From Murray, S., & McKinney, E. [2006]. *Foundations of maternal-newborn nursing* [4th ed.]. Philadelphia: Saunders.)

XVII. PLACENTAL ABNORMALITIES

A. Description: **Placenta** accreta is an abnormally adherent **placenta**; **placenta** increta occurs when the **placenta** penetrates the uterine muscle itself; **placenta** percreta occurs when the **placenta** goes all the way through the **uterus**

B. Data collection: May cause delayed hemorrhage immediately after birth because the **placenta** does not separate cleanly

C. Intervention
   1. Monitor for hemorrhage and shock
   2. Prepare the client for a hysterectomy if a large portion of the **placenta** is abnormally adherent

XVIII. UTERINE INVERSION

A. Description
   1. Uterus turns inside out; may be partial or complete
   2. Usually occurs during **delivery** or after the **delivery** of the **placenta**

B. Data collection
   1. A depression in the fundal area of the uterus is noted
   2. Interior of the uterus may be seen through the cervix or protruding through the vagina
   3. Severe pain
   4. Hemorrhage
   5. Signs of shock

C. Interventions
   1. Monitor for hemorrhage and signs of shock, and treat shock
   2. Prepare the client for a return of the uterus to the correct position via the vagina; if unsuccessful, laparotomy with replacement is done

XIX. AMNIOTIC FLUID EMBOLISM

A. Description
   1. Occurs when **amniotic fluid** containing particles of debris (e.g., vernix, hair, skin, cells, meconium) enters the maternal circulation and causes the release of endogenous mediators, thus obstructing maternal pulmonary vessels
   2. Causes respiratory distress and circulatory collapse; is usually fatal to the mother; if the mother survives, she is likely to have hemorrhage and DIC

B. Data collection
   1. Abrupt onset of respiratory distress and chest pain
   2. Cyanosis
   3. Seizures
   4. Heart failure and pulmonary edema
   5. Fetal bradycardia and distress if **delivery** has not occurred at the time of the embolism

C. Interventions
   1. Institute or assist with cardiopulmonary resuscitation

   2. Administer oxygen at 8 to 10 L/minute by face mask or resuscitation bag delivering 100% oxygen, as prescribed
   3. Prepare the client for intubation and mechanical ventilation
   4. Position the woman on her side
   5. IV fluids, blood products, and medications may be prescribed to correct coagulation failure and to maintain cardiac output and replace fluid losses
   6. Monitor the fetal status
   7. Prepare for emergency **delivery** after the woman is stabilized
   8. Provide emotional support to the woman, the partner, and the family

XX. SUPINE HYPOTENSIVE SYNDROME (VENA CAVA SYNDROME)

A. Description
   1. Occurs when the venous return to the heart is impaired by the weight of the uterus
   2. Results from the partial occlusion of the vena cava and the descending aorta and causes reduced cardiac return, cardiac output, and blood pressure

B. Data collection
   1. Faintness, lightheadedness, dizziness, and breathlessness
   2. Pallor, clammy (damp, cool) skin, and sweating
   3. Hypotension and tachycardia
   4. Nausea
   5. Fetal distress

C. Interventions
   1. Position the client on her side to shift the weight of the fetus off of the inferior vena cava until signs and symptoms subside and vital signs stabilize
   2. Monitor the vital signs and the FHR

XXI. FETAL DISTRESS

A. Description/data collection
   1. FHR of less than 120 or more than 160 beats per minute
   2. Meconium-stained **amniotic fluid**
   3. Fetal hyperactivity
   4. Progressive decrease in baseline variability
   5. Severe variable decelerations
   6. Late decelerations

B. Interventions depend on the cause of distress
   1. Place the mother in a lateral position; elevate her legs
   2. Administer oxygen at 8 to 10 L/minute via face mask, as prescribed
   3. Oxytocin (Pitocin) infusion is discontinued
   4. Monitor the maternal and fetal status
   5. Prepare for emergency cesarean section

XXII. INTRAUTERINE FETAL DEMISE

A. Data collection
   1. Loss of fetal movement

2. Absence of fetal heart tones
3. DIC screen (monitor for coagulation abnormalities, because DIC is a complication that is related to intrauterine fetal demise)
4. Low hemoglobin and hematocrit levels; low platelet count; prolonged bleeding and clotting times
5. Bleeding from puncture sites (could be indicative of DIC)

B. Interventions
1. Encourage the mother and her family to verbalize feelings
2. Allow the mother choices related to **labor** and **delivery**
3. Administer blood and blood products, as ordered, if DIC occurs

PRACTICE QUESTIONS

More questions on the companion CD!

227. A nurse is assigned to care for a client who is in early labor. When collecting data from the client, it is most important for the nurse to first determine which of the following?
1. Baseline fetal heart rate
2. Intensity of contractions
3. Maternal blood pressure
4. Frequency of contractions

228. Leopold's maneuvers will be performed on a pregnant client. The client asks the nurse about the procedure. The nurse responds, knowing that this procedure:
1. Measures the height of the maternal fundus
2. Determines the "lie" and "attitude" of the fetus
3. Is a systematic method for palpating the fetus through the maternal back
4. Is a sytematic method for palpating the fetus through the maternal abdominal wall

229. A nurse is caring for a client who is in labor. The nurse rechecks the client's blood pressure and notes that it has dropped. To decrease the incidence of supine hypotension, the nurse should encourage the client to remain in which position?
1. Squatting
2. Left lateral
3. Tailor sitting
4. Semi-Fowler's

230. After a precipitous delivery, a nurse notes that the new mother is passive and only touches her newborn infant briefly with her fingertips. The nurse would do which of the following to help the woman process what has happened?
1. Encourage the mother to breast-feed soon after birth.
2. Support the mother in her reaction to the newborn infant.

3. Tell the mother that it is important to hold the newborn infant.
4. Document a complete account of the mother's reaction in the birth record.

231. A primigravida's membranes rupture spontaneously. The nurse's first action is to:
1. Determine the fetal heart rate.
2. Prepare for immediate delivery.
3. Monitor the contraction pattern.
4. Note the amount, color, and odor of the amniotic fluid.

232. After a client vaginally delivers a viable newborn, the nurse sees the umbilical cord lengthen and observes a spurt of blood from the vagina. The nurse recognizes these findings as signs of:
1. Uterine atony
2. Placenta previa
3. Abruptio placentae
4. Placental separation

233. The nurse is assigned to assist with caring for a client who has been admitted to the labor unit. The client is 9 cm dilated and is experiencing precipitous labor. A priority nursing action is to:
1. Prepare for an oxytocin infusion.
2. Keep the client in a side-lying position.
3. Prepare the client for epidural anesthesia.
4. Encourage the client to start pushing with the contractions.

234. A client is admitted to the labor suite complaining of painless vaginal bleeding. The nurse assists with the examination of the client, knowing that a routine labor procedure that is contraindicated with this client's situation is:
1. Leopold's maneuvers
2. A manual pelvic examination
3. Hemoglobin and hematocrit evaluation
4. External electronic fetal heart rate monitoring

235. A nurse is assigned to assist with caring for a client with abruptio placentae who is experiencing vaginal bleeding. The nurse collects data from the client, knowing that abruptio placentae is accompanied by which additional finding?
1. Soft abdomen on palpation
2. Uterine tenderness on palpation
3. No complaints of abdominal pain
4. Lack of uterine irritability or tetanic contractions

236. A nurse is assigned to work in the delivery room and is assisting with caring for a client who has just delivered a newborn infant. The nurse is monitoring for signs of placental separation, knowing that which of the following indicates that the placenta has separated?
1. A change in the uterine contour
2. Sudden and sharp abdominal pain
3. A shortening of the umbilical cord

4. A decrease in blood loss from the introitus

237. A nurse is assisting with caring for a client with abruptio placenta. While caring for the client, the nurse notes that the client begins to develop signs of shock. The nurse would first:
   1. Monitor the urinary output.
   2. Monitor the maternal pulse.
   3. Turn the client onto her side.
   4. Monitor the maternal blood pressure.

238. A client who is being prepared for a cesarean delivery is brought to the delivery room. To maintain the optimal perfusion of oxygenated blood to the fetus, the nurse places the client in the:
   1. Prone position
   2. Semi-Fowler's position
   3. Trendelenburg's position
   4. Supine position with a wedge under the right hip

239. A woman in active labor has contractions every 2 to 3 minutes that last for 45 seconds. The fetal heart rate between contractions is 100 beats per minute. On the basis of these findings, the priority nursing intervention is to:
   1. Monitor the maternal vital signs.
   2. Notify the registered nurse (RN) immediately.
   3. Continue monitoring labor and the fetal heart rate.
   4. Encourage relaxation and breathing techniques between contractions.

240. A nurse is assigned to assist with caring for a client who is being admitted to the birthing center in early labor. On admission, the nurse would initially:
   1. Estimate the fetal size.
   2. Check pelvic adequacy.
   3. Administer an analgesic.
   4. Determine the maternal and fetal vital signs.

ALTERNATE ITEM FORMAT: MULTIPLE RESPONSE

241. A nurse is collecting data from a client who has been diagnosed with placenta previa. Choose the findings that the nurse would expect to note. Select all that apply.
   ☐ **1.** Uterine rigidity
   ☐ **2.** Uterine tenderness
   ☐ **3.** Severe abdominal pain
   ☑ **4.** Bright red vaginal bleeding
   ☑ **5.** Soft, relaxed, nontender uterus
   ☐ **6.** Fundal height may be greater than expected for gestational age

ANSWERS

227. 1
Rationale: The nurse should first determine the baseline fetal heart rate. Although options 2, 3, and 4 are components of the data collection process, the fetal heart rate is the priority.
Test-Taking Strategy: Note the strategic word "first." Use the ABCs—airway, breathing, and circulation—when selecting an answer. Fetal heart rate reflects the use of the ABCs. Review the care of the client in labor if you had difficulty with this question.
Level of Cognitive Ability: Application
Client Needs: Physiological Integrity
Integrated Process: Nursing Process/Implementation
Content Area: Delegating/Prioritizing
Reference: Leifer, G. (2008). *Maternity nursing: An introductory text* (10th ed., p. 114). Philadelphia: Saunders.

228. 4
Rationale: Leopold's maneuvers comprise a systematic method for palpating the fetus through the maternal abdominal wall. Options 1, 2, and 3 are incorrect.
Test-Taking Strategy: Knowledge of the purpose of and procedure for Leopold's maneuvers is required to answer this question. Visualizing this procedure will assist with directing you to option 4. Review Leopold's maneuvers if you had difficulty with this question.
Level of Cognitive Ability: Comprehension
Client Needs: Physiological Integrity
Integrated Process: Nursing Process/Implementation
Content Area: Maternity/Intrapartum
Reference: Leifer, G. (2008). *Maternity nursing: An introductory text* (10th ed., p. 125). Philadelphia: Saunders.

229. 2
Rationale: Pressure from the enlarged uterus on the aorta and the vena cava when the woman is supine can result in hypotension. This can be relieved by having the woman lie on her left side. Options 1, 3, and 4 are incorrect.
Test-Taking Strategy: Use the process of elimination and your knowledge of the anatomy of the pregnant uterus and the physiological response caused by pressure on the large abdominal vessels. Note that options 1, 3, and 4 are all comparable or alike in that the client would be upright. Review nursing measures for the hypotensive pregnant client if you had difficulty with this question.
Level of Cognitive Ability: Application
Client Needs: Physiological Integrity
Integrated Process: Nursing Process/Implementation
Content Area: Maternity/Intrapartum
Reference: Leifer, G. (2007). *Introduction to maternity and pediatric nursing* (5th ed., p. 52). Philadelphia: Saunders.

230. 2
Rationale: Women who have experienced precipitous labor and delivery often describe feelings of disbelief that their labor has progressed so rapidly. To assist the woman with understanding what has happened, it is best to support the mother in her reaction to the newborn infant. Options 1, 3, and 4 do not acknowledge the mother's feelings.
Test-Taking Strategy: Use therapeutic communication techniques. Option 2 is the only option that acknowledges the mother's feelings. Review the care of the mother after a precipitous birth if you had difficulty with this question.
Level of Cognitive Ability: Application
Client Needs: Psychosocial Integrity

Integrated Process: Caring
Content Area: Maternity/Intrapartum
Reference: Leifer, G. (2007). *Introduction to maternity and pediatric nursing* (5th ed., p. 192). Philadelphia: Saunders.

231. **1**
Rationale: When the membranes rupture, the nurse immediately assesses the fetal heart rate to detect changes associated with prolapse or the compression of the umbilical cord. Monitoring the contraction pattern and noting the amount, color, and odor of the amniotic fluid may be performed, but these would not be the first actions. There is no information in the question that indicates the need to prepare the client for immediate delivery.
Test-Taking Strategy: Note the strategic word "first." Use the ABCs—airway, breathing, and circulation. Fetal heart rate is associated with fetal breathing and circulation. Review the initial nursing interventions when the membranes rupture if you had difficulty with this question.
Level of Cognitive Ability: Application
Client Needs: Physiological Integrity
Integrated Process: Nursing Process/Implementation
Content Area: Maternity/Intrapartum
Reference: Leifer, G. (2008). *Maternity nursing: An introductory text* (10th ed., p. 288). Philadelphia: Saunders.

232. **4**
Rationale: As the placenta separates, it settles downward into the lower uterine segment, the umbilical cord lengthens, and a sudden trickle or spurt of blood appears. The clinical manifestations identified in the question are not related to options 1, 2, and 3.
Test-Taking Strategy: Use the process of elimination. Note that options 1, 2, and 3 are comparable or alike in that they represent complications associated with pregnancy. Option 4 indicates a normal finding after the vaginal delivery of the newborn. Review this stage of labor if you had difficulty with this question.
Level of Cognitive Ability: Comprehension
Client Needs: Physiological Integrity
Integrated Process: Nursing Process/Data Collection
Content Area: Maternity/Intrapartum
Reference: Leifer, G. (2008). *Maternity nursing: An introductory text* (10th ed., pp. 97-98). Philadelphia: Saunders.

233. **2**
Rationale: Priority care of this client includes the promotion of fetal oxygenation. Precipitous labor progresses quickly, with frequent contractions and short periods of relaxation between them. This does not allow for the maximal reperfusion of the placenta with oxygenated blood. A side-lying position can assist with providing blood flow to the uterus by preventing vena cava and abdominal aorta compression. Further stimulation with oxytocin is contraindicated. There may not be enough time to administer epidural anesthesia before delivery with such quick progression. Pushing with contractions is not indicated, especially with this type of labor. The controlled delivery of the fetus is essential to prevent maternal and fetal injury.
Test-Taking Strategy: Note the strategic words "precipitous" and "priority." Use the ABCs—airway, breathing, and circulation—and include the baby's needs as well as the mother's

needs. Option 2 will promote fetal oxygenation. Review the care of the client with precipitous labor if you had difficulty with this question.
Level of Cognitive Ability: Application
Client Needs: Physiological Integrity
Integrated Process: Nursing Process/Implementation
Content Area: Maternity/Intrapartum
Reference: Murray, S., & McKinney, E. (2006). *Foundations of maternal-newborn nursing* (4th ed., p. 706). Philadelphia: Saunders.

234. **2**
Rationale: Painless vaginal bleeding is a sign of possible placenta previa. Digital examination of the cervix can lead to maternal and fetal hemorrhage. Leopold's maneuvers can reveal a nonengaged presenting part or malpresentation, both of which often accompany placenta previa because of the placenta filling the lower uterine segment. Hemoglobin and hematocrit values help estimate the amount of blood loss. External electronic fetal monitoring is crucial for evaluating the status of the fetus, who is at risk for severe hypoxia. Options 1, 3, and 4 are procedures that would not place the client at further risk.
Test-Taking Strategy: Use the process of elimination, and note the strategic word "contraindicated." Option 2 is the only procedure that is invasive to the pregnancy and that endangers the physiological safety of the client and fetus. Review the care of the client with placenta previa if you had difficulty with this question.
Level of Cognitive Ability: Analysis
Client Needs: Physiological Integrity
Integrated Process: Nursing Process/Data Collection
Content Area: Maternity/Intrapartum
Reference: Leifer, G. (2007). *Introduction to maternity and pediatric nursing* (5th ed., pp. 87-89). Philadelphia: Saunders.

235. **2**
Rationale: Vaginal bleeding in a pregnant client is most often caused by placenta previa or a placental abruption. Uterine tenderness accompanies abruptio placentae, especially with a central abruption and trapped blood behind the placenta. The abdomen will feel hard and boardlike on palpation as the blood penetrates the myometrium and causes uterine irritability. A sustained tetanic contraction can occur if the client is in labor and the uterine muscle cannot relax.
Test-Taking Strategy: Note the subject of the question—abruptio placentae. It can be easy to confuse a placenta previa and abruption. Remember, the difference involves the presence of uterine pain and tenderness with an abruptio placentae as opposed to painless bleeding with a placenta previa. Options 1, 3, and 4 describe the absence of a sign or symptom of abruptio placentae, whereas option 2 is the only one that describes the presence of one. Review the signs of abruptio placentae if you had difficulty with this question.
Level of Cognitive Ability: Comprehension
Client Needs: Physiological Integrity
Integrated Process: Nursing Process/Data Collection
Content Area: Maternity/Intrapartum
Reference: Leifer, G. (2008). *Maternity nursing: An introductory text* (10th ed., p. 255). Philadelphia: Saunders.

236. 1

Rationale: Signs of placental separation include the lengthening of the umbilical cord, a sudden gush of dark blood from the introitus, a firmly contracted uterus, and the uterus changing from a discoid to a globular shape. The client may experience vaginal fullness but not sudden and sharp abdominal pain.

Test-Taking Strategy: Use the process of elimination. Thinking about what one would expect to occur when the placenta separates will assist you with eliminating options 3 and 4. Option 2 is eliminated because of the words "sudden and sharp." Review the signs of placental separation if you had difficulty with this question.

Level of Cognitive Ability: Comprehension
Client Needs: Physiological Integrity
Integrated Process: Nursing Process/Data Collection
Content Area: Maternity/Intrapartum
Reference: Leifer, G. (2008). *Maternity nursing: An introductory text* (10th ed., pp. 97-98). Philadelphia: Saunders.

237. 3

Rationale: With a client who is in shock, the nurse would want to increase perfusion to the placenta. A simple way to do this that requires no equipment is to turn the mother on her side. This would increase blood flow to the placenta by relieving pressure from the gravid uterus on the great vessels. The nurse would immediately contact the registered nurse, who would then contact the physician. The other options would follow quickly.

Test-Taking Strategy: Note the strategic word "first." Eliminate options 2 and 4, because they are comparable or alike. Recalling that positioning will affect the status of blood flow will assist with directing you to option 3 from the remaining options. Review the care of the client in shock if you had difficulty with this question.

Level of Cognitive Ability: Application
Client Needs: Physiological Integrity
Integrated Process: Nursing Process/Implementation
Content Area: Delegating/Prioritizing
References: McKinney, E., James, S., Murray, S., & Ashwill, J. (2005). *Maternal-child nursing* (2nd ed., p. 629). Philadelphia: Saunders.
Wong, D., Perry, S., Hockenberry, M., Lowdermilk, D., & Wilson, D. (2006). *Maternal-child nursing care* (3rd ed., p. 401). St. Louis: Mosby.

238. 4

Rationale: Vena cava and descending aorta compression by the pregnant uterus impede blood return from the lower trunk and extremities, thereby decreasing cardiac return, cardiac output, and blood flow to the uterus and subsequently to the fetus. The best position to prevent this would be side-lying, with the uterus displaced off of the abdominal vessels. Positioning for abdominal surgery necessitates a supine position; however, a wedge placed under the right hip provides for the displacement of the uterus. Trendelenburg's position places pressure from the pregnant uterus on the diaphragm and lungs, thus decreasing respiratory capacity and oxygenation. A semi-Fowler's or prone position is not practical for this type of abdominal surgery.

Test-Taking Strategy: Note the strategic words "maintain the optimal perfusion." Use the process of elimination, and

visualize each of the positions and their effect on the fetus. Review client positioning if you had difficulty with this question.

Level of Cognitive Ability: Application
Client Needs: Physiological Integrity
Integrated Process: Nursing Process/Implementation
Content Area: Maternity/Intrapartum
References: Leifer, G. (2007). *Introduction to maternity and pediatric nursing* (5th ed., p. 180). Philadelphia: Saunders.
Murray, S., & McKinney, E. (2006). *Foundations of maternal-newborn nursing* (4th ed., p. 382). Philadelphia: Saunders.

239. 2

Rationale: Fetal bradycardia between contractions may indicate the need for immediate medical management. The nurse would immediately contact the RN, who would then contact the physician. Options 1, 3, and 4 will delay necessary and immediate interventions.

Test-Taking Strategy: Use the ABCs—airway, breathing, and circulation. Note that the woman is in active labor and that the fetal heart rate is below normal. It is imperative that the circulation in the fetus be restored to normal limits. Review the care of the client in active labor if you had difficulty with this question.

Level of Cognitive Ability: Application
Client Needs: Physiological Integrity
Integrated Process: Nursing Process/Implementation
Content Area: Maternity/Intrapartum
Reference: Leifer, G. (2008). *Maternity nursing: An introductory text* (10th ed., p. 121). Philadelphia: Saunders.

240. 4

Rationale: To evaluate a woman's physical well-being, her temperature, pulse, respirations, and blood pressure (as well as the fetal heartbeat) are checked. Option 3 is incorrect, because it would be too premature for an analgesic; medication given too early tends to slow or stop labor contractions. Options 1 and 2 are incorrect; these assessments should be performed by the physician or nurse-midwife during prenatal visits.

Test-Taking Strategy: Note the strategic word "initially," and use the ABCs—airway, breathing, and circulation; this will direct you to option 4. Remember, measuring the vital signs is the priority. Review the care of the client in labor if you had difficulty with this question.

Level of Cognitive Ability: Application
Client Needs: Physiological Integrity
Integrated Process: Nursing Process/Implementation
Content Area: Maternity/Intrapartum
Reference: Leifer, G. (2008). *Maternity nursing: An introductory text* (10th ed., p. 113). Philadelphia: Saunders.

ALTERNATE ITEM FORMAT: MULTIPLE RESPONSE

241. 4, 5, 6

Rationale: Painless bright red vaginal bleeding during the second or third trimester of pregnancy is a sign of placenta previa. The client will have a soft, relaxed, nontender uterus, and the fundal height may be greater than expected for gestational age. In clients with abruptio placentae, severe abdominal pain is present. Uterine tenderness accompanies placental abruption. Additionally, with abruptio placentae, the abdomen will feel hard and boardlike on palpation as the blood penetrates the myometrium and causes uterine irritability.

Test-Taking Strategy: Remember that the difference between placenta previa and abruptio placentae involves the presence of uterine pain and tenderness with an abruption as opposed to painless bleeding with a previa. Review the signs of placenta previa and abruptio placentae if you had difficulty with this question.

Level of Cognitive Ability: Analysis
Client Needs: Physiological Integrity
Integrated Process: Nursing Process/Data Collection
Content Area: Maternity/Intrapartum
Reference: Leifer, G. (2008). *Maternity nursing: An introductory text* (10th ed., pp. 252-253). Philadelphia: Saunders.

REFERENCES

Leifer, G. (2008). *Maternity nursing: An introductory text* (10th ed.). Philadelphia: Saunders.

Leifer, G. (2007). *Introduction to maternity and pediatric nursing* (5th ed.). Philadelphia: Saunders.

Murray, S., & McKinney, E. (2006). *Foundations of maternal-newborn nursing* (4th ed.). Philadelphia: Saunders.

National Council of State Boards of Nursing (Eds.). (2008). *2008 Detailed Test Plan for the NCLEX-PN® Examination, National Council of State Boards of Nursing.* Chicago: Author.

National Council of State Boards of Nursing. *NCSBN home page.* www.ncsbn.org. Accessed July 4, 2008.

Wong, D., Perry, S., Hockenberry, M., Lowdermilk, D., & Wilson, D. (2006). *Maternal-child nursing care* (3rd ed.). St. Louis: Mosby.

The Postpartum Period and Associated Complications

I. POSTPARTUM
A. Description: Period when the reproductive tract returns to the normal, nonpregnant state
B. Postpartum period: Starts immediately after **delivery** and is usually completed by week 6 after **delivery**

II. PHYSIOLOGICAL MATERNAL CHANGES
A. Involution (Figure 24-1)
1. Description
a. The rapid decrease in the size of the uterus as it returns to the nonpregnant state
b. Clients who breast-feed may experience a more rapid involution
2. Data collection
a. Weight of the uterus decreases from 2 lbs to 2 oz in 6 weeks
b. Fundus steadily descends into the pelvis; the fundal height decreases about one finger-breadth (1 cm) per day
c. By 10 days postpartum, the uterus cannot be palpated abdominally
d. A flaccid fundus indicates uterine atony and should be massaged until firm
e. A tender fundus indicates an infection
B. **Lochia** (Figure 24-2)
1. Description: Discharge from the uterus that consists of blood from the vessels of the placental site and debris from the decidua
2. Data collection
a. Rubra: Bright red discharge that occurs from **delivery** day to day 3 postpartum
b. Serosa: Brownish-pink discharge that occurs from days 4 to 10 postpartum
c. Alba: White discharge that occurs from days 10 to 14 postpartum
d. Normally the discharge smells like normal menstrual flow
e. Discharge decreases daily in amount
f. Discharge increases with ambulation
g. Weigh the perineal pad before and after use and identify the amount of time between pad changes to determine the amount of lochial flow most accurately

C. Cervix: Cervical involution occurs; after 1 week, the muscle begins to regenerate
D. Vagina: Vaginal distentsion decreases, although muscle tone is never restored completely to the pregravid state
E. Ovarian function and menstruation
1. Ovarian function depends on the rapidity with which pituitary function is restored
2. Menstrual flow resumes within 8 weeks among non–breast-feeding mothers
3. Menstrual flow usually resumes within 3 to 4 months among breast-feeding mothers
4. Breast-feeding mothers may experience amenorrhea during the entire period of lactation
5. A woman may ovulate without menstruating, so breast-feeding should not be considered a form of birth control
F. Breasts
1. A decrease of estrogen and progesterone levels after **delivery** stimulates increased prolactin levels, which promote breast milk production
2. Breasts become distended with milk on the third day
3. Engorgement occurs within 48 to 72 hours among non–breast-feeding mothers; breast-feeding will relieve engorgement
4. The non–breast-feeding mother should avoid nipple stimulation; she can also apply a breast binder, wear a tight-fitting bra, apply ice packs, or take a mild analgesic to relieve the discomfort of engorgement
G. Urinary tract
1. May have urinary retention because of a loss of elasticity, tone, and sensation in the bladder from trauma, medications, anesthesia, and lack of privacy
2. Diuresis usually begins within the first 12 hours after **delivery**
H. Gastrointestinal tract
1. Women are usually very hungry after **delivery**
2. Constipation can occur
3. Hemorrhoids are common

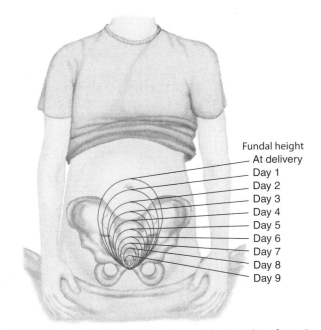

FIG. 24-1   Involution of the uterus. The height of uterine fundus decreases by approximately 1 cm/day. (From McKinney, E., James, S., Murray, S., & Ashwill, J. [2005]. *Maternal-child nursing* [2nd ed.]. Philadelphia: Saunders.)

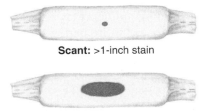

Scant: >1-inch stain

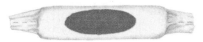

Light: 1- to 4-inch stain

Moderate: 4- to 6-inch stain

Large: Saturated in 1 hour

FIG. 24-2   Guidelines for assessing the amount of lochia on the perineal pad. (From McKinney, E., James, S., Murray, S., & Ashwill, J. [2005]. *Maternal-child nursing* [2nd ed.]. Philadelphia: Saunders.)

I. Vital signs (Table 24-1)
1. Temperature may be elevated during the first 24 hours as a result of dehydration
2. Bradycardia is common during the first week, with a range of 50 to 70 beats per minute
3. Blood pressure remains unchanged

III. POSTPARTUM INTERVENTIONS
A. Data collection
1. Monitor the vital signs

TABLE 24-1	Normal Postpartum Vital Signs
Vital Sign	**Description**
Temperature	May rise to 100.4° F as a result of the dehydrating effects of labor; any higher elevation may be caused by infection and must be reported
Pulse	May decrease to 50 beats per minute (normal puerperal bradycardia); a pulse rate of >100 beats per minute may indicate excessive blood loss or infection
Blood pressure	Should be normal; suspect hypovolemia if it decreases
Respirations	Rarely changes; if respirations increase significantly, suspect pulmonary embolism, uterine atony, or hemorrhage

2. Monitor the height, consistency, and location of the fundus (Figure 24-3)
3. Monitor the color, amount, and odor of the **lochia**
4. Check the breasts for engorgement
5. Monitor the perineum for swelling or discoloration; check the episiotomy for healing
6. Check the incisions or dressings of the cesarean birth client
7. Monitor the intake and output (I&O)
8. Monitor the bowel status
9. Encourage frequent voiding
10. Encourage ambulation
11. Rh$_0$(D) immune globulin (RhoGAM) is prescribed to be administered within 72 hours postpartum to the Rh-negative client who has given birth to an Rh-positive **neonate**
12. Monitor parent–**newborn** bonding
13. Monitor the mother's emotional status
B. Client teaching
1. Demonstrate **newborn** care skills as necessary
2. Provide the opportunity for the mother to bathe the **newborn**
3. Instruct the mother regarding feeding technique
4. Instruct the mother to avoid heavy lifting for at least 3 weeks
5. Instruct the mother to plan at least one rest period per day
6. Instruct the mother that contraception should begin after **delivery** or with the initiation of intercourse
7. Instruct the mother regarding the importance of follow-up care, which should be scheduled at 4 to 6 weeks postpartum
8. Instruct the mother to report immediately any signs of chills, fever, increased **lochia**, or depressed feelings to the physician

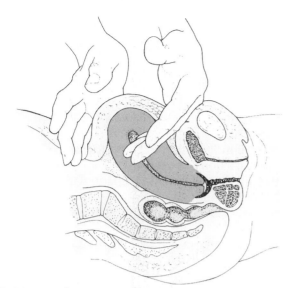

FIG. 24-3 Palpating the fundus of the uterus during the fourth stage of labor. Note that the upper hand is cupped over the fundus; the lower hand dips in above the symphysis pubis and supports the uterus while it is massaged gently. (From Lowdermilk, D., & Perry, S. [2006]. *Maternity nursing* [7th ed.]. St. Louis: Mosby.)

IV. POSTPARTUM DISCOMFORTS

A. Afterbirth pains
1. Occur as a result of contractions of the uterus
2. Are more common among multiparas, breast-feeding mothers, clients treated with oxytocin (Pitocin), and clients who had an overdistended uterus during pregnancy (e.g., those who carried twins)

B. Perineal discomfort
1. Apply ice packs to the perineum, as prescribed, during the first 24 hours to reduce swelling
2. After the first 24 hours, apply warmth by sitz baths, as prescribed

C. Episiotomy
1. Instruct the client to administer perineal care after each voiding
2. Encourage the use of analgesic spray, as prescribed
3. Administer analgesics, as prescribed, if comfort measures are unsuccessful

D. Breast discomfort from engorgement
1. Encourage the wearing of a support bra at all times, even while sleeping
2. Encourage the use of ice packs if the client is not breast-feeding
3. Encourage the use of warm soaks before feeding for the breast-feeding mother
4. Administer analgesics, as prescribed, if comfort measures are unsuccessful

E. Postpartum blues (Box 24-1)
1. The condition may be caused by physiological or emotional stress

---

2. The mother may feel upset and depressed at times
3. Verbalization should be encouraged
4. If unresolved, postpartum blues may progress to postpartum depression

V. NUTRITION

A. Discuss caloric intake for breast-feeding and non–breast-feeding mothers
B. Nutritional needs depend on prepregnancy weight, ideal weight for height, and whether the mother is breast-feeding
C. If the mother is breast-feeding, calorie needs increase by approximately 200 to 500 cal/day, and the mother may require increased fluids and the continuance of prenatal vitamins and minerals

VI. BREAST-FEEDING

A. Interventions
1. Put the baby to the mother's breast as soon as the mother's and baby's conditions are stable (on the **delivery** table, if possible)
2. Stay with the mother each time she nurses until she feels secure and confident with the baby and her feelings
3. Assess LATCH (L = latch achieved by **infant**; A = audible swallowing; T = type of nipple; C = comfort of mother; H = help given to mother with nursing)
4. Uterine cramping may occur during the first day after **delivery** while the mother is nursing, when oxytocin stimulation causes the uterus to contract

5. Use general hygiene and wash the breasts once daily
6. If engorgement occurs, have the mother breast-feed frequently, apply warm packs before feeding, apply ice packs after feedings, and massage the breasts
7. Do not use soap on the breasts, because it tends to remove natural oils, which increases the chance of cracked nipples
8. If cracked nipples develop, expose the nipples to air for 10 to 20 minutes after feeding, rotate the position of the baby for each feeding, and be sure that the baby is latched on to the areola and not just the nipple
9. Bra should be well-fitted and supportive
10. Breasts may leak between feedings or during coitus; place breast pad in bra
11. Calories should be increased by 200 to 500 cal/day, and the diet should include additional fluids; prenatal vitamins should be taken, as prescribed
12. Baby's stools will be light yellow, seedy, watery, and frequent
13. Medications should be avoided, unless prescribed
14. Gas-producing foods and caffeine should be avoided
15. Hormonal contraceptives may cause a decrease in the milk supply and are best avoided during the first 6 weeks after birth
16. Oral contraceptives that contain estrogen are not recommended for breast-feeding mothers; progestin-only birth control pills are less likely to interfere with the milk supply
17. Baby will develop his or her own feeding schedule

B. Breast-feeding procedure for mother (Box 24-2)
C. Engorgement
1. Breast-feed frequently
2. Apply warm packs before feeding
3. Apply ice packs between feedings

BOX 24-2   Breast-Feeding Procedure for Mother

Wash the hands and assume a comfortable position.
Start with the breast with which the last feeding ended.
Brush the newborn infant's lower lip with the nipple.
Tickle the lips to have the infant open the mouth wide.
Guide the nipple and the surrounding areola into the infant's mouth.
Listen for audible sucking and swallowing.
After the baby has nursed, release suction by depressing the infant's chin or inserting a clean finger into the infant's mouth.
Burp the infant after the first breast.
Repeat the procedure on the second breast until the infant stops nursing.
Burp the infant again.

D. Cracked nipples
1. Expose nipples to air for 10 to 20 minutes after feeding
2. Rotate the position of the baby for each feeding
3. Be sure that the baby is latched on to the areola and not just the nipple

VII. CYSTITIS
A. Description: Infection of the bladder
B. Data collection
1. Burning and pain on urination
2. Lower abdominal pain
3. Increased frequency of urination
4. Fever
5. Proteinuria, hematuria, bacteriuria, and white blood cells (WBCs) in the urine
C. Interventions
1. Palpate the bladder for distention
2. Palpate the fundus for position
3. Obtain a urine specimen for culture and sensitivity, if prescribed
4. Institute measures to assist the client with voiding
5. Encourage the frequent and complete emptying of the bladder
6. Encourage fluids to 3000 mL/day
7. Administer antibiotics, as prescribed, after the urine culture is obtained
8. Instruct the client in the methods of the prevention and treatment of cystitis

VIII. HEMATOMA
A. Description
1. Localized collection of blood into the tissues of the reproductive sac after **delivery**
2. Predisposing conditions include operative **delivery** with forceps or injury to a blood vessel
3. Can be a life-threatening condition
B. Data collection
1. Abnormal severe pain
2. Pressure in the perineal area
3. Sensitive, bulging mass in the perineal area with discolored skin
4. Inability to void
5. Decreased hemoglobin and hematocrit levels
6. Signs of shock (e.g., pallor, tachycardia, hypotension) if significant blood loss has occurred
C. Interventions
1. Monitor the vital signs
2. Monitor the client for abnormal pain, especially when a forceps **delivery** has occurred
3. Place ice on the hematoma site
4. Administer analgesics and antibiotics, as prescribed
5. Monitor the I&O; encourage fluids
6. Prepare for urinary catheterization if the client is unable to void
7. Monitor for signs of infection, such as increased temperature, pulse rate, and WBC count

8. Prepare the client for the incision and evacuation of the hematoma, if necessary

IX. HEMORRHAGE (Box 24-3)

A. Description: Bleeding of 500 mL or more after **delivery**

B. Data collection
1. Early
   a. Hemorrhage occurs during the first 24 hours after **delivery**
   b. Caused by uterine atony, lacerations, or the inversion of the uterus
2. Late
   a. Hemorrhage occurs more than 24 hours after **delivery**
   b. Caused by retained placental fragments

C. Interventions
1. Massage the fundus, taking care to not overmassage
2. The physician or health care provider is notified if hemorrhage occurs; monitor the vital signs and fundus every 5 to 15 minutes
3. Monitor and estimate blood loss by pad count
4. Maintain asepsis, because hemorrhage predisposes the mother to infection
5. Administer fluids, as prescribed, and monitor the I&O
6. Monitor the level of consciousness
7. Oxytocin (Pitocin) may be administered
8. Hemoglobin and hematocrit levels are monitored; blood transfusions may be administered

X. INFECTION

A. Description: Any infection of the reproductive organs that occurs within 28 days of **delivery** or abortion

B. Data collection
1. Fever and chills
2. Pelvic discomfort or pain
3. Vaginal discharge
4. Elevated WBC count

BOX 24-3 Postpartum Hemorrhage

Causes
- Uterine atony (poor muscle tone)
- Laceration of the vagina
- Cervix, perineum, or labia hematoma development
- Retained placental fragments

Predisposing Factors
- High parity
- Dystocia
- Prolonged labor
- Operative delivery (cesarean or forceps delivery, intrauterine manipulation)
- Overdistention of the uterus (polyhydramnios, multiple gestation, large neonate)
- Abruptio placentae
- Previous history of postpartum hemorrhage
- Infection
- Placenta previa

C. Interventions
1. Monitor the vital signs and temperature every 2 to 4 hours
2. Make the mother as comfortable as possible; position her for comfort and to promote drainage
3. Keep the mother warmed if she is chilled
4. Isolate the baby from the mother only if the mother can infect the baby
5. Provide a nutritious, high-calorie, high-protein diet
6. Encourage fluids to 3000 to 4000 mL/day, if not contraindicated
7. Encourage frequent voiding; monitor the I&O
8. Monitor culture results if cultures were prescribed
9. Administer antibiotics, as prescribed

XI. MASTITIS

A. Description
1. Inflammation of the breast as a result of infection
2. Primarily seen among breast-feeding mothers 2 to 3 weeks after **delivery** but may occur at any time during lactation

B. Data collection
1. Localized heat and swelling
2. Pain
3. Elevated temperature
4. Complaints of flu-like symptoms

C. Interventions
1. Instruct the mother in good handwashing and breast hygiene techniques
2. Apply heat or cold to the site, as prescribed
3. Maintain lactation among breast-feeding mothers
4. Encourage the manual expression of breast milk or the use of a breast pump every 4 hours
5. Encourage the mother to support the breasts with a supportive bra
6. Administer analgesics or antibiotics, as prescribed

XII. PULMONARY EMBOLISM

A. Description: The passage of a thrombus (often originates in one of the uterine or other pelvic veins) into the lungs, where it disrupts the circulation of blood

B. Data collection
1. Dyspnea, tachypnea, and tachycardia
2. Congested cough
3. Hemoptysis
4. Pleuritic chest pain
5. Feeling of impending doom

C. Interventions
1. Administer oxygen, as prescribed
2. Position the client with the head of the bed elevated to promote comfort
3. Monitor the vital signs frequently
4. Monitor the respiratory rate frequently

5. Monitor for signs of respiratory distress and hypoxemia, such as tachypnea, tachycardia, restlessness, cool and clammy skin, cyanosis, and the use of accessory muscles
6. Intravenous fluids may be prescribed
7. Anticoagulants may be prescribed

XIII. SUBINVOLUTION

A. Description: Incomplete involution or the failure of the uterus to return to its normal size and condition
B. Data collection
1. Uterine pain on palpation
2. Uterus is larger than expected
3. More vaginal bleeding than normal
C. Interventions
1. Monitor the vital signs
2. Monitor the uterus and fundus and for vaginal bleeding
3. Elevate the legs to promote venous return
4. Encourage frequent voiding
5. Monitor the hemoglobin and hematocrit levels
6. Methylergonovine maleate (Methergine) may be prescribed

XIV. THROMBOPHLEBITIS

A. Description
1. A condition in which a clot forms in a vessel wall as a result of the inflammation of the vessel wall
2. A partial obstruction of the vessel can occur
3. Increased blood-clotting factors during the postpartum period place the client at risk
B. Types
1. Superficial thrombophlebitis
2. Femoral thrombophlebitis
3. Pelvic thrombophlebitis
C. Data collection (Box 24-4)
D. Interventions
1. Assess the lower extremities for edema, tenderness, varices, and increased skin temperature

---

BOX 24-4   Data Collection: Types of Thrombophlebitis

Superficial
- Tenderness and pain in the affected lower extremity
- Warm and pinkish-red color over the thrombus area
- Palpable thrombus that feels bumpy and hard

Femoral
- Chills and fever
- Malaise
- Pain, stiffness, and swelling of the affected leg
- Shiny, white skin over the affected area
- Positive Homans' sign
- Diminished peripheral pulses

Pelvic
- Severe chills
- Dramatic body temperature changes
- Occurrence of pulmonary embolism may be the first sign

---

2. Maintain bedrest, if prescribed
3. Elevate the affected leg
4. Apply a bed cradle, and keep bedclothes off of the affected leg
5. Never massage the leg
6. Monitor for manifestations of pulmonary embolism
7. Superficial thrombophlebitis
   a. Provide rest
   b. Apply hot packs to the affected site, as prescribed
   c. Apply elastic stockings
   d. Administer analgesics, as prescribed
8. Femoral thrombophlebitis
   a. Provide bedrest
   b. Elevate the affected leg
   c. Apply moist heat continuously to the affected area, if prescribed, to alleviate discomfort
   d. Administer analgesics, as prescribed
   e. Administer antibiotics, if prescribed
   f. Intravenous heparin sodium may be prescribed to prevent further thrombus formation
9. Pelvic thrombophlebitis
   a. Provide bedrest
   b. Administer analgesics, as prescribed
   c. Administer antibiotics, if prescribed
   d. Intravenous heparin sodium may be prescribed to prevent further thrombus formation
E. Client teaching (Box 24-5)

XV. PERINATAL LOSS

A. Description
1. Perinatal loss is associated with miscarriage, neonatal death, stillbirth, and therapeutic abortion
2. Loss and grief may also coincide with the birth of a preterm **infant**, an **infant** who has suffered complications, or an **infant** with congenital anomalies; it may also occur within a family who is giving up a child for adoption
B. Interventions
1. Communicate therapeutically and actively listen, providing parents with time to grieve

---

BOX 24-5   Client Teaching for Thrombophlebitis

Avoid pressure behind the knees.
Avoid prolonged sitting.
Avoid constrictive clothing.
Avoid crossing the legs.
Never massage the leg.
Know how to apply support hose, if prescribed.
Understand the importance of anticoagulant therapy, if prescribed.
Understand the importance of follow-up with the health care provider.

2. Notify the hospital chaplain

3. Inform the parents about options such as seeing, holding, bathing, and/or dressing the deceased **infant,** visitation by other family members or friends, religious rituals, and funeral arrangements

4. Prepare a special memories box with keepsakes such as footprints, handprints, locks of hair, and pictures

5. Admit the mother to a private room; if possible, mark the door to the room with a special card (per agency procedure) that denotes to hospital staff that this family has experienced a loss

PRACTICE QUESTIONS

More questions on the companion CD!

242. A client received epidural anesthesia during labor and had a forceps delivery after pushing for 2 hours. At 6 hours postpartum, the client's systolic blood pressure (BP) dropped 20 points, the diastolic BP dropped 10 points, and her pulse is 120 beats per minute. The client is very anxious and restless. The nurse is told that the client has a vulvar hematoma. On the basis of this diagnosis, the nurse would plan to:
 1. Reassure the client.
 2. Apply perineal pressure.
 3. Monitor the fundal height.
 4. Prepare the client for surgery.

243. A nurse is assigned to care for a client after a cesarean section. To prevent thrombophlebitis, the nurse encourages the woman to:
 1. Ambulate frequently.
 2. Wear support stockings.
 3. Apply warm, moist packs to the legs.
 4. Remain on bedrest, with the legs elevated.

244. A postpartum client is getting ready for discharge. The nurse suspects that the client is in need of further teaching related to breast-feeding when she states:
 1. "I don't need birth control since I will be breast-feeding."
 2. "I need to increase my caloric intake by 500 calories a day."
 3. "I shouldn't use soap to wash my breasts since I will be breast-feeding."
 4. "Since I will not breast-feed, I will wear a supportive bra for 1 to 2 weeks."

245. A nurse is caring for a postpartum client with a diagnosis of thrombophlebitis. The client suddenly complains of chest pain and dyspnea. The nurse would initially check the:
 1. Vital signs
 2. Fundal height
 3. Presence of Homans' sign
 4. Level of consciousness (LOC)

246. A nurse suspects that a client has a pulmonary embolism. The most important nursing action is to:
 1. Monitor the vital signs.
 2. Elevate the head of the bed.
 3. Increase the intravenous flow rate.
 4. Administer oxygen by face mask, as prescribed.

247. A nurse notes that the 4-hour postpartum client has cool, clammy skin and that she is restless and excessively thirsty. The nurse immediately notifies the registered nurse and then:
 1. Checks the vital signs
 2. Begins fundal massage
 3. Encourages ambulation
 4. Encourages the client to drink fluids

248. A nurse is assisting with caring for a postpartum client who is experiencing uterine hemorrhage. When planning to meet the psychosocial needs of the client, the nurse would:
 1. Maintain strict bedrest.
 2. Monitor the vital signs every 2 hours.
 3. Perform firm fundal massage every 2 hours.
 4. Keep the client and her family members informed of her progress.

249. A nurse palpates the fundus and checks the character of the lochia of a postpartum client who is in the fourth stage of labor. The nurse expects the lochia to be:
 1. Red
 2. Pink
 3. White
 4. Serosanguineous

250. After episiotomy and the delivery of a newborn, the nurse performs a perineal check on the mother. The nurse notes a trickle of bright red blood coming from the perineum. The nurse checks the fundus and notes that it is firm. The nurse determines that:
 1. This is a normal expectation after episiotomy.
 2. The mother should be allowed bathroom privileges only.
 3. The bright red bleeding is abnormal and should be reported.
 4. The perineal assessment should be performed more frequently.

251. A nurse is assigned to care for a client during the postpartum period. The client asks the nurse what the term *involution* means. The nurse responds to the client, knowing that involution is:
 1. The inverted uterus returning to normal
 2. The gradual reversal of the uterine muscle into the abdominal cavity
 3. The descent of the uterus into the pelvic cavity, which occurs at a rate of 2 cm/day
 4. The progressive descent of the uterus into the pelvic cavity, which occurs at a rate of approximately 1 cm/day

252. A mother is breast-feeding her newborn baby and experiences breast engorgement. The nurse encourages the mother to do which of the following to provide relief of the engorgement?
1. Breast-feed only during the daytime hours.
2. Apply cold compresses to the breast before feeding.
3. Avoid the use of a bra while the breasts are engorged.
4. Massage the breasts before feeding to stimulate let-down.

253. After delivery, a nurse checks the height of the uterine fundus. The nurse expects that the position of the fundus would most likely be noted:
1. To the right of the abdomen
2. At the level of the umbilicus
3. Above the level of the umbilicus
4. One fingerbreadth above the symphysis pubis

254. A nurse is caring for a postpartum client. At 4 hours postpartum, the client's temperature is 102° F (38.9° C). The appropriate nursing action would be to:
1. Apply cool packs to the abdomen.
2. Continue to monitor the temperature.
3. Remove the blanket from the client's bed.
4. Notify the registered nurse, who will then contact the physician.

255. A nurse is assisting with planning care for a postpartum woman who has small vulvar hematomas. To assist with reducing the swelling, the nurse should:
1. Check the vital signs every 4 hours.
2. Measure the fundal height every 4 hours.
3. Prepare a heat pack for application to the area.
4. Prepare an ice pack for application to the area.

ALTERNATE ITEM FORMAT: MULTIPLE RESPONSE

256. A nurse is preparing a list of self-care instructions for a postpartum client who has been diagnosed with mastitis. Choose the instructions that would be included on the list. Select all that apply.
☐ 1. Wear a supportive bra.
☐ 2. Rest during the acute phase.
☐ 3. Maintain a fluid intake of at least 3000 mL.
☐ 4. Continue to breast-feed if the breasts are not too sore.
☐ 5. Take the prescribed antibiotics until the soreness subsides.
☐ 6. Avoid decompression of the breasts by breast-feeding or breast pump.

ANSWERS

242. **4**
Rationale: The information provided in the question indicates that the client is experiencing blood loss. Surgery would be indicated for this complication to stop the bleeding. Options 1, 2, and 3 would not assist with controlling the bleeding in this emergency situation.
Test-Taking Strategy: Focus on the information provided in the question. Note that the signs and symptoms in the question indicate the presence of bleeding; this should direct you to option 4. Review the nursing interventions related to vulvar hematomas if you had difficulty with this question.
Level of Cognitive Ability: Analysis
Client Needs: Physiological Integrity
Integrated Process: Nursing Process/Planning
Content Area: Maternity/Postpartum
Reference: Leifer, G. (2008). *Maternity nursing: An introductory text* (10th ed., p. 339). Philadelphia: Saunders.

243. **1**
Rationale: Stasis is believed to be a major predisposing factor for the development of thrombophlebitis. Because cesarean delivery poses a risk factor, the client should ambulate early and frequently to promote circulation and prevent stasis. Options 2, 3, and 4 are implemented if thrombophlebitis occurs.
Test-Taking Strategy: Focus on the subject of the question —the prevention of thrombophlebitis. Options 2, 3, and 4 are implemented if thrombophlebitis occurs.

Ambulating frequently (option 1) is a preventive measure. Review the content related to the prevention of thrombophlebitis during the postoperative period if you had difficulty with this question.
Level of Cognitive Ability: Application
Client Needs: Physiological Integrity
Integrated Process: Nursing Process/Implementation
Content Area: Maternity/Postpartum
Reference: Leifer, G. (2008). *Maternity nursing: An introductory text* (10th ed., p. 297). Philadelphia: Saunders.

244. **1**
Rationale: Amenorrhea may occur during breast-feeding, but the client can still ovulate without menstruating. The use of soap on the breasts is avoided because it tends to remove natural oils, which can lead to cracked nipples. The caloric intake should be increased by 200 to 500 cal/day, and the diet should include additional fluids and prenatal vitamins, as prescribed.
Test-Taking Strategy: Use the process of elimination. Recalling the physiology related to amenorrhea and ovulation during breast-feeding will direct you to the correct option. Review these concepts if you had difficulty answering this question.
Level of Cognitive Ability: Comprehension
Client Needs: Physiological Integrity
Integrated Process: Teaching and Learning
Content Area: Maternity/Postpartum
References: Leifer, G. (2008). *Maternity nursing: An introductory text* (10th ed., pp. 215-217). Philadelphia: Saunders.

Wong, D., Perry, S., Hockenberry, M., Lowdermilk, D., & Wilson, D. (2006). *Maternal-child nursing care* (3rd ed., p. 781). St. Louis: Mosby.

245. 1
Rationale: Pulmonary embolism is a complication of thrombophlebitis. Changes in the vital signs will be one of the first things to occur with pulmonary embolism, because pulmonary blood flow is compromised. LOC may change as the condition worsens; this would indicate hypoxia. Homans' sign is an indicator of thrombophlebitis. Fundal height is unrelated to the subject of the question.
Test-Taking Strategy: Note the strategic word "initially." Use the ABCs—airway, breathing, and circulation—to direct you to option 1. Review the complications of thrombophlebitis if you had difficulty with this question.
Level of Cognitive Ability: Application
Client Needs: Physiological Integrity
Integrated Process: Nursing Process/Data Collection
Content Area: Maternity/Postpartum
References: Leifer, G. (2008). *Maternity nursing: An introductory text* (10th ed., p. 231). Philadelphia: Saunders.
Murray, S., & McKinney, E. (2006). *Foundations of maternal-newborn nursing* (4th ed., pp. 745-746). Philadelphia: Saunders.

246. 4
Rationale: Because pulmonary circulation is compromised in the presence of an embolus, cardiorespiratory support is initiated by oxygen administration. Options 1 and 2 may be components of the plan of care, but they are not the most important actions. The nurse would not increase the intravenous rate without a physician's order to do so.
Test-Taking Strategy: Note the strategic words "most important," and use the ABCs—airway, breathing, and circulation. This will direct you to option 4. Review the care of the client in the event of a pulmonary embolism if you had difficulty with this question.
Level of Cognitive Ability: Application
Client Needs: Physiological Integrity
Integrated Process: Nursing Process/Implementation
Content Area: Maternity/Postpartum
Reference: Leifer, G. (2008). *Maternity nursing: An introductory text* (10th ed. p. 343). Philadelphia: Saunders.

247. 1
Rationale: Symptoms of hypovolemia include cool, clammy, and pale skin; feelings of anxiety and restlessness; and thirst. The nurse would check the vital signs. The nurse would not ambulate the client or encourage fluids until specific orders are given to do so. There is no information in the question to indicate the need for fundal massage.
Test-Taking Strategy: Focus on the symptoms in the question. Use the ABCs—airway, breathing, and circulation—to direct you to option 1. Review the nursing care of the client with hypovolemia if you had difficulty with this question.
Level of Cognitive Ability: Application
Client Needs: Physiological Integrity
Integrated Process: Nursing Process/Implementation
Content Area: Maternity/Postpartum

Reference: Leifer, G. (2008). *Maternity nursing: An introductory text* (10th ed., pp. 338-339). Philadelphia: Saunders.

248. 4
Rationale: Keeping the client and her family informed about her condition will help minimize fear and apprehension. Options 1, 2, and 3 identify physiological interventions.
Test-Taking Strategy: Use the process of elimination. Focus on the strategic words "meet the psychosocial needs." Option 4 is the only option that addresses psychosocial needs. Review the interventions that will meet the psychosocial needs of a client if you had difficulty with this question.
Level of Cognitive Ability: Application
Client Needs: Psychosocial Integrity
Integrated Process: Nursing Process/Implementation
Content Area: Maternity/Postpartum
Reference: Leifer, G. (2008). *Maternity nursing: An introductory text* (10th ed., pp. 341-342). Philadelphia: Saunders.

249. 1
Rationale: The color of the lochia during the fourth stage of labor is bright red, and this may last from 1 to 3 days. The color of the lochia then changes to a pinkish brown, which lasts for 4 to 10 days. Finally, the lochia changes to a creamy white color that lasts for approximately 10 to 14 days.
Test-Taking Strategy: Focus on the strategic words "fourth stage of labor"; this will direct you to option 1. Review the expected postpartum findings if you had difficulty with this question.
Level of Cognitive Ability: Comprehension
Client Needs: Physiological Integrity
Integrated Process: Nursing Process/Data Collection
Content Area: Maternity/Postpartum
Reference: Leifer, G. (2008). *Maternity nursing: An introductory text* (10th ed., p. 228). Philadelphia: Saunders.

250. 3
Rationale: Lochial flow should be distinguished from bleeding that originates from a laceration or an episiotomy, which is usually brighter red than lochia and presents as a continuous trickle of bleeding, even though the fundus of the uterus is firm. This bright red bleeding is abnormal and needs to be reported.
Test-Taking Strategy: Note the strategic words "bright red." This should be an indication that the flow is not normal. Review the lochial flow and the complications associated with episiotomy if you had difficulty with this question.
Level of Cognitive Ability: Analysis
Client Needs: Physiological Integrity
Integrated Process: Nursing Process/Data Collection
Content Area: Maternity/Postpartum
Reference: Leifer, G. (2008). *Maternity nursing: An introductory text* (10th ed., pp. 228-229). Philadelphia: Saunders.

251. 4
Rationale: Involution is the progressive descent of the uterus into the pelvic cavity. After birth, descent occurs at a rate of approximately one fingerbreadth or 1 cm per day.
Test-Taking Strategy: Use your knowledge of medical terminology to help you to define the word *involution*. This will assist with directing you to the correct option. Review the

process of involution if you had difficulty with this question.

Level of Cognitive Ability: Comprehension
Client Needs: Physiological Integrity
Integrated Process: Nursing Process/Implementation
Content Area: Maternity/Postpartum
References: Leifer, G. (2008). *Maternity nursing: An introductory text* (10th ed., p. 226). Philadelphia: Saunders.
McKinney, E., James, S., Murray, S., & Ashwill, J. (2005). *Maternal-child nursing* (2nd ed., p. 465). Philadelphia: Saunders.

252. 4
Rationale: Comfort measures for breast engorgement include massaging the breasts before feeding to stimulate let-down, wearing a supportive and well-fitting bra at all times, taking a warm shower or applying warm compresses just before feeding, and alternating breasts during feeding.
Test-Taking Strategy: Use the process of elimination to answer the question. Eliminate option 1 because of the close-ended word "only." From the remaining options, recalling the self-care measures that promote the comfort of the mother with breast engorgement will direct you to option 4. Review these measures if you had difficulty with this question.
Level of Cognitive Ability: Application
Client Needs: Health Promotion and Maintenance
Integrated Process: Nursing Process/Implementation
Content Area: Maternity/Postpartum
References: Leifer, G. (2007). *Introduction to maternity and pediatric nursing* (5th ed., p. 229). Philadelphia: Saunders.
McKinney, E., James, S., Murray, S., & Ashwill, J. (2005). *Maternal-child nursing* (2nd ed., pp. 587-588). Philadelphia: Saunders.

253. 2
Rationale: Immediately after delivery, the uterine fundus should be at the level of the umbilicus or one to three fingerbreadths below it and in the midline of the abdomen. If the fundus is above the umbilicus, this may indicate that there are blood clots in the uterus that need to be expelled by fundal massage. If the fundus is noted to the right of the abdomen, it may indicate a full bladder.
Test-Taking Strategy: Note the strategic words "after delivery." Remember that immediately after delivery, the uterine fundus should be at the level of the umbilicus or one to three fingerbreadths below it and in the midline of the abdomen. Review expected postdelivery findings if you had difficulty with this question.
Level of Cognitive Ability: Comprehension
Client Needs: Physiological Integrity
Integrated Process: Nursing Process/Data Collection
Content Area: Maternity/Postpartum
References: Leifer, G. (2008). *Maternity nursing: An introductory text* (10th ed., p. 227). Philadelphia: Saunders.
Lowdermilk, D., & Perry, A. (2007). *Maternity and woman's health care* (9th ed., p. 619) St. Louis: Mosby.

254. 4
Rationale: During the first 24 hours postpartum, the mother's temperature may be elevated as a result of dehydration. However, if the temperature is more than 2° F above normal, this may indicate infection, and the physician will need to be notified.
Test-Taking Strategy: Use the process of elimination. Focus on the strategic words "4 hours" and "102° F." Noting that this temperature is extreme as compared with the normal temperature will direct you to option 4. Review the expected postpartum findings if you had difficulty with this question.
Level of Cognitive Ability: Application
Client Needs: Physiological Integrity
Integrated Process: Nursing Process/Implementation
Content Area: Maternity/Postpartum
Reference: Leifer, G. (2008). *Maternity nursing: An introductory text* (10th ed., p. 244). Philadelphia: Saunders.

255. 4
Rationale: The application of ice will reduce the swelling caused by hematoma formation in the vulvar area. Options 1, 2, and 3 will not reduce swelling.
Test-Taking Strategy: Use the process of elimination. Focus on the subject of the question—the reduction of swelling. This will assist you with eliminating options 1 and 2. Recalling the principles related to heat and cold will direct you to option 4. Review the nursing care of the client with a hematoma if you had difficulty with this question.
Level of Cognitive Ability: Application
Client Needs: Physiological Integrity
Integrated Process: Nursing Process/Implementation
Content Area: Maternity/Postpartum
Reference: Leifer, G. (2008). *Maternity nursing: An introductory text* (10th ed., p. 339). Philadelphia: Saunders.

ALTERNATE ITEM FORMAT: MULTIPLE RESPONSE

256. 1, 2, 3, 4
Rationale: Mastitis is an infection of the lactating breast. Client instructions include resting during the acute phase, maintaining a fluid intake of at least 3000 mL per day, and taking analgesics to relieve discomfort. Antibiotics may be prescribed and are taken until the complete prescribed course is finished; they are not stopped when the soreness subsides. Additional supportive measures include the use of moist heat or ice packs and the wearing of a supportive bra. Continued decompression of the breast by breast-feeding or breast pump is important to empty the breast and to prevent the formation of an abscess.
Test-Taking Strategy: Think about the pathophysiology associated with mastitis. Recalling that supportive measures include rest, moist heat or ice packs, antibiotics, analgesics, increased fluid intake, breast support, and the decompression of the breasts will assist you with answering the question. Review the treatment of mastitis if you had difficulty with this question.
Level of Cognitive Ability: Application
Client Needs: Physiological Integrity
Integrated Process: Teaching and Learning
Content Area: Maternity/Postpartum
Reference: Leifer, G. (2008). *Maternity nursing: An introductory text* (10th ed., p. 345). Philadelphia: Saunders.

REFERENCES

Leifer, G. (2008). *Maternity nursing: An introductory text* (10th ed.). Philadelphia: Saunders.

Leifer, G. (2007). *Introduction to maternity and pediatric nursing* (5th ed.). Philadelphia: Saunders.

McKinney, E., James, S., Murray, S., & Ashwill, J. (2005). *Maternal-child nursing* (2nd ed.). Philadelphia: Saunders.

Murray, S., & McKinney, E. (2006). *Foundations of maternal-newborn nursing* (4th ed.). Philadelphia: Saunders.

National Council of State Boards of Nursing (Eds.) (2008). *2008 Detailed Test Plan for the NCLEX-PN® Examination, National Council of State Boards of Nursing.* Chicago: Author.

National Council of State Boards of Nursing. *NCSBN home page.* www.ncsbn.org. Accessed July 4, 2008.

Wong, D., Perry, S., Hockenberry, M., Lowdermilk, D., & Wilson, D. (2006). *Maternal-child nursing care* (3rd ed.). St. Louis: Mosby.

Care of the Newborn

I. INITIAL CARE OF THE NEWBORN

A. Data collection
1. Observe or assist with the initiation of respirations
2. Determine Apgar score
3. Note characteristics of cry
4. Monitor for nasal flaring, grunting, retractions, and abnormal respirations
5. Obtain vital signs
6. Observe for signs of hypothermia or hyperthermia
7. Check for gross anomalies

B. Interventions
1. Suction the mouth and then the nares with a bulb syringe
2. Dry the baby and stimulate crying by rubbing
3. Maintain temperature stability; wrap the baby in warm blankets and place a stockinette cap on the **newborn's** head
4. Keep the baby with the mother to facilitate bonding
5. Place the baby at mother's breast if breast-feeding is planned, or place the baby on mother's abdomen
6. Place the baby in a preheated warmer after initial parent–**infant** acquaintance process
7. Position the baby on his or her side with a rolled blanket at the back to facilitate the drainage of mucus
8. Ensure proper identification
9. Footprint the **newborn** and mother on an identification sheet, per agency policies and procedures
10. Place matching identification bracelets on the mother and the **newborn**

C. Apgar scoring system
1. Determine and record the Apgar score at 1 minute and at 5 minutes
2. Assess each of the five items to be scored, and assign a value of 0 (very poor) to 2 (excellent) for each item
3. Add the points assessed for each item to determine the **newborn's** total score
4. Five vital indicators (Table 25-1)
5. Interventions: Apgar score (Table 25-2)

II. INITIAL PHYSICAL EXAMINATION

A. General guidelines
1. Keep the **newborn** warm during the examination
2. Begin with general observations; then first perform the assessments that are the least disturbing to the **newborn**
3. Initiate nursing interventions for abnormal findings
4. Document all findings, especially abnormal ones

B. Vital signs
1. Heart rate: 100 to 160 beats per minute (apical); check for a full minute because of irregularities after birth, especially with crying
2. Respirations: 30 to 60 breaths per minute; check for a full minute
3. Axillary temperature: 96.8° to 99° F (36° to 37.2° C)
4. Blood pressure: Systolic, 60 to 80 mm Hg; diastolic 40 to 50 mm Hg

C. Body measurements
1. Length: 45 to 55 cm (18 to 22 inches)
2. Weight: 2500 to 4300 g (5.5 to 9.5 pounds)
3. Head circumference: 32 to 36.8 cm (12.6 to 14.4 inches)
4. Chest circumference: 30 to 33 cm (12 to 13 inches); should be equal to or 2 to 3 cm less than the head circumference

D. Head
1. 25% of the body length (cephalocaudal development)
2. Bones of the skull are not fused
3. Palpable sutures (connective tissue between the skull bones)
4. Fontanels: Unossified membranous tissue at the junction of the sutures (Table 25-3)
5. Molding: Asymmetry of the head as a result of pressure in the birth canal; disappears in about 72 hours

TABLE 25-1	The Five Vital Indicators of the Apgar Score			
Indicator	0 Points	1 Point		2 Points
Heart rate	Absent	Less than 100 beats/minute		More than 100 beats/minute
Respiratory rate	Absent	Slow, irregular, weak cry		Good, vigorous cry
Muscle tone	Flaccid, limp	Minimal flexion of the extremities		Good flexion, active motion
Reflex irritability	No response	Minimal response (grimace) to suction or the gentle slap on the soles		Responds promptly with a cry or active movement
Skin color	Pallor or cyanosis	Body skin color normal, extremities blue		Body and extremity skin color normal

TABLE 25-2	Apgar Score Interventions
Score	Intervention
8-10	No intervention except support the infant's spontaneous efforts
4-7	Gently stimulate Rub the infant's back Administer oxygen to the infant
0-3	Infant requires resuscitation

Note: The newborn's Apgar score obtained at 5 minutes of age reflects the efficacy of any resuscitation efforts.

TABLE 25-3	Fontanels	
Location	Characteristics	Closure
Anterior	Soft, flat, and diamond-shaped; 5 cm wide by 2-3 cm long	Closes between the ages of 12 and 18 months
Posterior	Triangular, 0.5-1 cm wide; located between the occipital and parietal bones	Closes between birth and the age of 2 or 3 months

6. Masses from birth trauma
   a. Caput succedaneum: Edema of the soft tissue over bone (crosses over suture line); subsides within a few days
   b. Cephalhematoma: Swelling caused by bleeding into an area between the bone and its periosteum (does not cross over suture line); usually absorbed within 6 weeks with no treatment
7. Head lag
   a. Common when pulling the **newborn** to a sitting position
   b. When prone, the **newborn** should be able to lift the head slightly and turn the head from side to side
E. Eyes
   1. Slate gray (light skin) or brown gray (dark skin)
   2. Symmetrical and clear
   3. Pupils are equal and round; react to light by accommodation
   4. Blink reflex present
   5. Eyes cross because of weak extraocular muscles
   6. Able to track and fixate momentarily
   7. Red reflex present
   8. Eyelids often edematous as a result of pressure during the birth process and the effects of eye medication
F. Ears
   1. Symmetrical
   2. Firm cartilage with recoil
   3. Pinna should be on or above a line drawn from the canthus of the eye
   4. Low-set ears associated with Down syndrome
G. Nose
   1. Flat, broad, and located in the center of the face

2. Obligatory nose breathing
3. Occasional sneezing to remove obstructions
H. Mouth
   1. Gums pink and moist
   2. Soft and hard palates intact
   3. Epstein's pearls (small, white cysts) may be present on the hard palate
   4. Uvula in midline
   5. Tongue symmetrical and moves freely, with a short frenulum
   6. Sucking and crying movements are symmetrical
   7. Able to swallow
   8. Gag reflex present
I. Neck
   1. Short and thick
   2. Head held in midline
   3. Trachea in midline
   4. Good range of motion with flexion and extension
J. Chest
   1. Appears circular because anteroposterior and lateral diameters are about equal
   2. Respirations appear diaphragmatic
   3. Bronchial sounds on auscultation
   4. Nipples prominent and often edematous
   5. Milky secretion (witch's milk) common
   6. Breast tissue present
   7. Palpate clavicles to check for fractures
K. Skin
   1. Pinkish red (light-skinned **newborn**) to pinkish brown or pinkish yellow (dark-skinned **newborn**)
   2. Vernix caseosa

3. Lanugo

4. Milia

5. Dry, peeling skin

6. Dark red color common among premature **newborns**

7. Cyanosis common with hypothermia, infection, and hypoglycemia and with cardiac, respiratory, or neurological abnormalities

8. Acrocyanosis (peripheral cyanosis) is normal during the first few hours after birth and if the **infant** becomes cold; results from the poor perfusion of blood to the periphery of the body

9. Check for ecchymosis and petechiae as a result of the trauma of birth

10. Check the skin turgor over the abdomen to determine hydration status

11. Observe for forceps marks

12. Harlequin sign
   a. Deep pink or red color develops over one side of the **newborn's** body while the other side remains pale or of normal color
   b. May indicate sepsis or a shunting of blood caused by a cardiac problem

13. Birthmarks (Table 25-4)

L. Abdomen

1. Umbilical cord
   a. Three vessels (two arteries and one vein) in the cord; if fewer than three vessels are noted, notify the physician
   b. Small, thin cord may be associated with poor fetal growth
   c. Check for intact cord, and ensure that clamp is secured
   d. Cord should be clamped for at least the first 24 hours after birth; clamp can be removed when the cord is dried and occluded
   e. Note any bleeding or drainage from the cord
   f. Hospital protocol and physician's preference determine the technique for cord care; an antibiotic ointment or triple dye may be prescribed, or cleansing with sterile water or soap and water
   g. If symptoms of infection (e.g., moistness, oozing, discharge, reddened base) occur, notify the physician and use antibiotic treatment, as prescribed

2. Gastrointestinal
   a. Monitor the cord for meconium staining
   b. Check for umbilical hernia
   c. Note abdominal depression associated with diaphragmatic hernia
   d. Check for abdominal distention associated with obstruction, mass, or sepsis
   e. Monitor the bowel sounds, which should occur within 1 to 2 hours after birth

3. Anus
   a. Anal opening is patent
   b. First stool (meconium) should pass within the first 24 hours

M. Genitals

1. Female
   a. Labia edematous and clitoris enlarged
   b. Smegma present (thick, white mucous discharge)
   c. Pseudomenstruation possible (blood-tinged mucus)

TABLE 25-4	Birthmarks			
Birthmark	**Characteristics**	**Location**	**Treatment**	**Length of Presence**
Telangiectatic nevi (stork bites)	Pale pink or red; flat, dilated capillaries Blanch easily More noticeable during crying periods	Eyelids, nose, lower occipital bone, and nape of neck	None	Usually disappear by the age of 2 years
Nevus flammeus (port-wine stain)	Capillary angioma directly below the epidermis Nonelevated; sharply demarcated; red to purple; dense areas of capillaries	Commonly appears on the face	May require surgery in the future	Only removed by surgery; does not fade with time
Nevus vasculosus (strawberry mark)	Capillary hemangioma Raised; clearly delineated; dark red with rough surface	Common in the head region	None	Disappears by the age of 7 to 9 years
Mongolian spots	Bluish-black pigmentation common among Asian and dark-skinned individuals	Lumbar dorsal area and buttocks	None	Gradually fade during the first and second years of life

d. Hymen tag may be visible

e. First voiding should occur within 24 hours

2. Male

a. Prepuce (foreskin) covers glans penis

b. Scrotum edematous

c. Meatus at tip of penis

d. Testes descended but may retract with cold

e. Check for hernia or hydrocele

f. First voiding should occur within 24 hours

N. Spine

1. Straight

2. Posture flexed

3. Supports head momentarily when prone

4. Arms and legs flexed

5. Chin flexed on upper chest

6. Sporadic movements that are well coordinated

7. A degree of hypotonicity or hypertonicity is indicative of central nervous system damage

O. Extremities

1. Flexed

2. Full range of motion and symmetrical movements

3. Fists clenched

4. Should be 10 fingers and 10 toes, all separate

5. Legs bowed

6. Major gluteal folds are even

7. Creases on soles of feet

8. Check for fractures (especially clavicle) or dislocations (hip)

9. Check for hip dysplasia; when thighs are rotated outward, no clicks should be heard

10. Pulses palpable (radial, brachial, and femoral)

11. Slight tremors are common but could be a sign of hypoglycemia or drug withdrawal

III. BODY SYSTEMS

A. Cardiovascular system

1. Keep the **newborn** warm

2. Take the apical heart rate for 1 full minute

3. Listen for murmurs

4. Palpate pulses

5. Check for cyanosis; blanch the skin on the trunk and extremities to assess circulation

6. Observe for cardiac distress when the **newborn** is feeding

B. Respiratory system

1. Position the **newborn** on his or her side

2. Suction as necessary: Use a bulb syringe for upper-airway suctioning (compress bulb before insertion) and a French catheter for deeper suctioning

3. Observe for respiratory distress and hypoxemia

a. Nasal flaring

b. Increasingly severe retractions

c. Grunting

d. Cyanosis

e. Bradycardia and periods of apnea that last more than 15 seconds

4. Administer oxygen via hood if necessary and as prescribed

C. Hepatic system

1. Normal or physiological jaundice appears after the first 24 hours in full-term **neonates** and after the first 48 hours in premature **neonates**; jaundice occurring before this time (pathological jaundice) may indicate the early hemolysis of red blood cells and must be reported to the physician

2. Physiological jaundice peaks about the fifth day of life (indirect bilirubin levels: 6 to 7 mg/dL)

3. Monitor the serum bilirubin levels

4. Feed early to stimulate intestinal activity and to keep the bilirubin level low

5. Prevent chilling, because hypothermia can cause acidosis, which interferes with bilirubin conjugation and excretion

6. The **newborn's** liver stores iron that was passed from the mother for 5 to 6 months

7. Glycogen storage occurs in the liver

8. The **neonate** is at risk for hemorrhagic disorders; coagulation factors synthesized in the liver are dependent on vitamin K, which is not synthesized until intestinal bacteria are present

9. Handle the **neonate** carefully and monitor for any bruising or bleeding episodes

10. Watch for meconium stool and subsequent stools

11. Administer one dose of vitamin K (AquaMEPHYTON; usually 0.5 to 1.0 mg intramuscularly, as prescribed) to the **neonate** in the lateral aspect of the middle third of the vastus lateralis muscle to prevent hemorrhagic disorders

12. Check the **newborn's** hemoglobin and blood glucose levels per facility protocol

D. Renal system

1. The immature kidneys cannot concentrate urine

2. A weight loss of 5% to 15% during the first week of life occurs as a result of voiding and limited intake

3. Weigh the **newborn** daily

4. Monitor intake and output (I&O); weigh diapers, if necessary

5. Measure the specific gravity of the urine, if necessary

6. Monitor for signs of dehydration (dry mucous membranes, sunken eyeballs, poor skin turgor, sunken fontanels)

E. Immune system

1. Passive immunity via the placenta (immunoglobulin G)

2. Passive immunity from the colostrum (immunoglobulin A)

3. Elevations in immunoglobulin M indicate infection in utero

4. Use aseptic technique when caring for the **newborn**
5. Observe standard precautions when handling the **newborn**
6. Ensure meticulous handwashing
7. Ensure that infection-free staff members care for the **newborn**
8. Monitor the **newborn's** temperature
9. Observe for any cracks or openings in the skin
10. Administer eye medication within 1 hour after birth to prevent ophthalmia neonatorum
    a. Eye prophylaxis may be delayed until an hour or so after birth so that eye contact and parent–**infant** attachment and bonding are facilitated
    b. Erythromycin (0.5%) and tetracycline (1%) ophthalmic ointment or drops are both bacteriostatic and bactericidal; they provide prophylaxis against infection by *Neisseria gonorrhoeae* and *Chlamydia trachomatis*
    c. Silver nitrate (1%) solution may be prescribed, but its use is minimal, because it does not protect against chlamydial infection, and it can cause chemical conjunctivitis
11. Provide cord care
    a. Umbilical clamp can be removed after 24 hours
    b. Teach the mother how to perform cord care
    c. Keep the cord clean and dry; wash with soap and water at least two or three times a day, during a bath, and/or with diaper changes
    d. Keep the diaper from covering the cord; fold the diaper below the cord
    e. Monitor the cord for odor, swelling, or discharge
    f. Sponge bathe the **newborn** until the cord falls off (within 2 weeks)
12. Provide circumcision care
    a. Apply petroleum jelly gauze to the penis, except when a Plastibell is used
    b. Remove the petroleum jelly gauze, if applied, after the first voiding after circumcision
    c. Observe for swelling, infection, or bleeding from the circumcision site
    d. Teach the mother how to care for the circumcision site
    e. Cleanse the penis after each voiding by squeezing warm water over it
    f. A milky covering over the glans penis is normal and should not be disrupted
    g. Monitor for urinary retention
13. Hepatitis B vaccination
    a. Usually administered within 12 hours of birth

b. Parental consent should be obtained before administration
c. Administer in the vastus lateralis injection site with a 25-gauge, ⅝-inch needle
d. After administration, record name, date and time of administration, amount, route, and site of injection on the **newborn's** chart

F. Metabolic system and gastrointestinal system
1. **Newborns** can digest simple carbohydrates, but they cannot digest fats as a result of their lack of lipase
2. Proteins may be only partially broken down, so they may serve as antigens and provoke an allergic reaction
3. The **newborn** has a small stomach capacity (about 90 mL) with rapid intestinal peristalsis (bowel emptying time is 2.5 to 3 hours)
4. Breast-feeding can usually begin immediately after birth; bottle-fed **newborns** may be offered a few milliliters of sterile water or 5% dextrose 1 to 4 hours after birth before a feeding with formula
5. Observe feeding reflexes, such as rooting, sucking, and swallowing
6. Assist the mother with breast-feeding or formula feeding
7. Burp the **newborn** during and after feeding
8. Monitor for regurgitation or vomiting
9. Position the **newborn** on his or her right side after a feeding
10. Observe for normal stool and the passage of meconium
    a. Meconium stool, which is greenish black with a thick, sticky, tar-like consistency, is usually passed within the first 24 hours of life
    b. Transitional stool, which is the second type of stool excreted by the **newborn,** is greenish brown and of looser consistency than meconium
    c. Seedy, yellow stools are noted in breast-fed **newborns**; pale yellow to light brown stools are seen in formula-fed **newborns**
11. **Newborn**: A screening test is performed (includes the test for phenylketonuria) before discharge after sufficient protein intake occurs; the **newborn** should be on formula or breast milk for a minimum of 24 hours before screening

G. Neurological system
1. The **newborn's** head size is proportionally larger than that of adults as a result of cephalocaudal development
2. Myelinization of the nerve fibers is incomplete, so primitive reflexes are present
3. Fontanels are open to allow for brain growth
4. Check for an abnormal head size and a bulging or depressed anterior fontanel

5. Measure and graph the head circumference in relation to the chest circumference and length
6. Monitor the **newborn's** movements, noting symmetry, posture, and abnormal movements
7. Observe for jitteriness, marked tremors, and seizures
8. Test the **newborn's** reflexes
9. Monitor for lethargy
10. Monitor the pitch of the cry

H. Thermal regulatory system
1. **Newborns** do not shiver to produce heat
2. **Newborns** have brown fat deposits that produce heat
3. Heat is dissipated through vasodilation
4. Prevent heat loss that results from evaporation by keeping the **newborn** dry and well-wrapped with a blanket
5. Prevent heat loss that results from radiation by keeping the **newborn** away from cold objects and outside walls
6. Prevent heat loss that results from convection by shielding the **newborn** from drafts
7. Prevent heat loss that results from conduction by performing all treatments on a warm, padded surface
8. Keep the temperature in the room warm
9. Take the **newborn's** axillary temperature every hour for the first 4 hours of life, every 4 hours for the remainder of the first 24 hours, and then every shift

I. Reflexes
1. Sucking and rooting
   a. Touch the **newborn's** lip, cheek, or the corner of the mouth with a nipple
   b. The **newborn** turns his or her head toward the nipple, opens the mouth, takes hold of the nipple, and sucks
   c. The rooting reflex usually disappears after 3 to 4 months but may persist for up to 1 year
2. Swallowing reflex
   a. Occurs spontaneously after sucking and obtaining fluids
   b. **Newborn** swallows in coordination with sucking without gagging, coughing, or vomiting
3. Tonic neck or fencing position
   a. While the **newborn** is falling asleep or sleeping, gently and quickly turn the head to one side
   b. As the **newborn** faces the left side, the left arm and leg extend outward while the right arm and leg flex
   c. When the head is turned to the right side, the right arm and leg extend outward while the left arm and leg flex
   d. Usually disappears within 3 to 4 months

4. Palmar–plantar grasp
   a. Place a finger in the palm of the **newborn's** hand, and then place a finger at the base of the toes
   b. The **newborn's** fingers curl around the examiner's fingers, and the **newborn's** toes curl downward
   c. Palmar response lessens within 3 to 4 months
   d. Plantar response lessens within 8 months
5. Moro reflex
   a. Hold the **newborn** in a semi-sitting position, and then allow the head and trunk to fall backward to at least a 30-degree angle
   b. The **newborn** symmetrically abducts and extends the arms
   c. The **newborn** fans the fingers out and forms a C with the thumb and the forefinger
   d. The **newborn** adducts the arms to an embracing position and returns to a relaxed flexion state
   e. Present at birth; a complete response may occur for up to 8 weeks
   f. A body jerk motion occurs from 8 to 18 weeks
   g. No response may be noted by 6 months as long as neurological maturation has not been delayed
   h. A persistent response lasting more than 6 months may indicate the occurrence of brain damage during pregnancy
6. Startle reflex
   a. The response is best elicited if the **newborn** is at least 24 hours old
   b. The examiner makes a loud noise or claps the hands to elicit the response
   c. The **newborn's** arms adduct while the elbows flex
   d. The hands stay clenched
   e. The reflex should disappear within 4 months
7. Pull to sit
   a. Pull the **newborn** up from the wrist while he or she is in the prone position
   b. The head will lag until the **newborn** is in an upright position; then the head will be level with the chest and shoulders momentarily before falling forward
   c. The head will then lift for a few minutes
   d. The response depends on the **newborn's** general muscle tone and condition as well as his or her maturity level
8. Babinski sign (plantar reflex)
   a. Beginning at the heel of the foot, gently stroke upward along the lateral aspect of the sole; the examiner then moves the finger along the ball of the foot

b. The **newborn's** toes hyperextend while the big toe dorsiflexes

c. Reflex disappears after the **newborn** is 1 year old

d. The absence of this reflex indicates the need for a neurological examination

9. Stepping or walking

a. Hold the **newborn** in a vertical position, allowing one foot to touch a table surface

b. The **newborn** simulates walking, alternately flexing and extending the feet

c. The reflex is usually present for 3 to 4 months

10. Crawling

a. Place the **newborn** on his or her abdomen

b. The **newborn** begins making crawling movements with the arms and legs

c. The reflex usually disappears after about 6 weeks

▲ IV. NEWBORN SAFETY

A. **Infant** identification

1. Information bracelets are applied to the mother and the **newborn** immediately after birth and before the mother and the **newborn** are separated

2. Include name, sex, date, time of birth, and identification numbers

B. **Infant** abduction

1. The mother is taught to check the identification of any person who comes to remove the baby from her room and other precautions to prevent **infant** abduction (Box 25-1)

2. Closed-circuit televisions, code-alert bands, or computer monitoring systems may be used on some units

3. The **newborn** is wheeled in a bassinette rather than carried in a staff member's arms

V. PARENT TEACHING

A. Formula feeding

1. Teach sterilization techniques if the water supply is from an area where the purification process of the water is questionable

2. Remind the mother not to heat the bottle of formula in a microwave oven

3. Inform the mother that formula is a sufficient diet for the first 4 to 6 months

4. Determine the mother's ability to burp the **newborn**

B. Breast-feeding

1. Monitor the **newborn's** ability to properly attach to the mother's breast and suck (Figure 25-1)

2. Teach the mother about engorgement

3. Teach the mother how to pump her breasts and how to store breast milk properly

4. Inform the mother that breast milk is a sufficient and superior diet for the first 4 to 6 months

5. Give the mother the phone numbers of local organizations that offer support to breast-feeding mothers

C. Bathing

1. Bathe the **newborn** in a warm room before feeding

2. Have all equipment for bathing available

3. Use a mild soap (not on the face)

4. Proceed from the cleanest area to the dirtiest area

5. Clean the eyes from the inner canthus outward

6. Special care should be taken to clean the groin, genital, underarms, and under the folds of the neck

BOX 25-1	Precautions to Prevent Infant Abductions

All personnel must wear identification that is easily visible at all times.

Teach the parents to only allow hospital staff with proper identification to take their infants from them.

Question anyone with a newborn near an exit or in an unusual part of the facility.

Never leave infants unattended.

Teach the parents that the infants must be observed at all times.

When the infant is in the mother's room, position the crib away from the doorway.

Suggest that the parents do not place announcements in the paper or signs in their yard that may alert an abductor that a new baby is in the home.

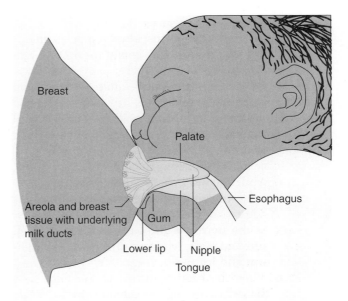

FIG. 25-1 Correct attachment (latch-on) of an infant at the breast. (From Lowdermilk, D., & Perry, S., [2006]. *Maternity nursing* [7th ed.] St. Louis: Mosby.)

7. Make bath time enjoyable for both the **newborn** and the mother

D. Clothing
   1. Determine diaper and clothing needs for the **newborn** with the mother
   2. Instruct the mother that the **newborn's** head should be covered during cold weather to prevent heat loss
   3. Instruct the mother to layer the **newborn's** clothing in cooler weather

E. Cord care: See cord care under Body Systems

F. Circumcision: See circumcision care under Body Systems

G. Uncircumcised **newborn**
   1. Inform the mother that the foreskin and glans are two similar layers of cells that separate from each other and that the separation process is normally complete by 3 years of age, but can remain adhered until puberty
   2. Instruct the mother to not pull back the foreskin but rather to allow for the natural separation to occur
   3. Inform the mother that, as the process of separation occurs, sterile sloughed cells build up between the layers of the foreskin and the glans; when retraction occurs, daily gentle washing of the glans with soap and water is sufficient to maintain adequate cleanliness

VI. PRETERM NEWBORN

A. Description
   1. A **neonate** born before 37 weeks' gestation
   2. The primary concern relates to the immaturity of all body systems

B. Data collection
   1. Respirations irregular with periods of apnea
   2. Body temperature is below normal
   3. Poor suck and swallow reflexes
   4. Bowel sounds are diminished
   5. Increased or decreased urinary output
   6. Extremities are thin, with minimal creasing on the soles and palms
   7. Extremities extend but do not maintain flexion
   8. Lanugo on the skin and in the hair on the **newborn's** head is present in woolly patches
   9. Skin is thin, with visible blood vessels and minimal subcutaneous fat pads
   10. Skin may appear jaundiced
   11. Testes are undescended in boys
   12. Labia are narrow in girls

C. Interventions
   1. Monitor the vital signs every 2 to 4 hours
   2. Maintain cardiopulmonary function
   3. Administer oxygen and humidification, as prescribed
   4. Monitor I&O and electrolyte balance
   5. Monitor the weight daily
   6. Maintain the **newborn** in a warming device

7. Position the **newborn** every 1 to 2 hours, and handle the **newborn** carefully
8. Avoid exposing the **newborn** to infections
9. Provide the **newborn** with appropriate stimulation, such as touch and cuddling

VII. POSTTERM NEWBORN

A. Description: A **neonate** born after 42 weeks' gestation

B. Data collection
   1. Hypoglycemia
   2. Parchment-like skin (dry and cracked) without lanugo
   3. Fingernails long and extended over the ends of the fingers
   4. Profuse scalp hair
   5. Long and thin body
   6. Extremities show wasting of fat and muscle
   7. Meconium staining may be present on nails and umbilical cord

C. Interventions
   1. Provide normal **newborn** care
   2. Monitor for hypoglycemia
   3. Maintain temperature
   4. Monitor for meconium aspiration

VIII. SMALL FOR GESTATIONAL AGE

A. Description: A **neonate** who is plotted at or below the 10th percentile on the intrauterine growth curve

B. Data collection
   1. Fetal distress
   2. Gestational age and physical maturity
   3. Lowered or elevated body temperature
   4. Physical abnormalities
   5. Hypoglycemia
   6. Signs of polycythemia
      a. Ruddy appearance
      b. Cyanosis
      c. Jaundice
   7. Signs of infection
   8. Signs of meconium aspiration

C. Interventions
   1. Maintain airway
   2. Maintain body temperature
   3. Observe for signs of respiratory distress
   4. Monitor for infection; initiate measures to prevent sepsis
   5. Monitor the blood glucose levels and for signs of hypoglycemia
   6. Initiate early feedings; monitor for signs of aspiration
   7. Provide stimulation, such as touch and cuddling

IX. LARGE FOR GESTATIONAL AGE

A. Description: A **neonate** who is plotted at or above the 90th percentile on the intrauterine growth curve

B. Data collection
   1. Gestational age
   2. Birth trauma or injury

3. Respiratory distress
4. Hypoglycemia
C. Interventions
1. Monitor the vital signs
2. Monitor the blood glucose levels and for signs of hypoglycemia
3. Initiate early feedings
4. Monitor for infection; initiate measures to prevent sepsis
5. Provide stimulation, such as touch and cuddling

X. RESPIRATORY DISTRESS SYNDROME
A. Description: A serious lung disorder caused by immaturity and the inability to produce surfactant that results in hypoxia and acidosis
B. Data collection
1. Tachypnea
2. Flaring nares
3. Expiratory grunting
4. Retractions
5. Decreased breath sounds
6. Apnea
7. Pallor and cyanosis
8. Hypothermia
9. Poor muscle tone
C. Interventions
1. Monitor the color, respiratory rate, and degree of effort when breathing
2. Support respirations, as prescribed
3. Monitor the arterial blood gases (ABGs) and the oxygen saturation levels (ABGs from umbilical artery)
4. Monitor the ABGs so that oxygen administered to the **newborn** is at the lowest possible concentration necessary to maintain adequate arterial oxygenation
5. Before discharge, schedule any premature **newborn** who has been given oxygen support for an eye examination to check for retinal damage
6. Suction every 2 hours or more often, as necessary
7. Position the **newborn** on his or her side or back, with the neck slightly extended
8. Prepare to administer surfactant replacement therapy (instilled into the endotracheal tube)
9. Administer respiratory therapy (percussion and vibration), as prescribed; use a padded small plastic cup or a small oxygen mask for percussion; use a padded electric toothbrush for vibration
10. Provide nutrition
11. Support bonding
12. Prepare parents for a short- to long-term period of oxygen dependency, if necessary
13. Encourage the mother to pump her breasts for future breast-feeding, if she so desires
14. Encourage as much parental participation in the **newborn's** care as the condition allows

XI. MECONIUM ASPIRATION SYNDROME
A. Description
1. Occurs in term or postterm **infants**
2. Fetal distress increases intestinal peristalsis, relaxing the anal sphincter and releasing meconium into the **amniotic fluid**
3. Aspiration can occur in utero or with the first breath
B. Data collection
1. Respiratory distress is present at birth; tachypnea, cyanosis, retractions, nasal flaring, grunting, crackles, and rhonchi may be present
2. The **infant's** nails, skin, and umbilical cord may be stained a yellow-green color
C. Interventions
1. Suctioning must be done immediately after the head is delivered before the first breath is taken; vocal cords should be viewed to see if the airway is clear before stimulation and crying
2. **Infants** with severe meconium aspiration syndrome may benefit from extracorporeal membrane oxygenation

XII. BRONCHOPULMONARY DYSPLASIA
A. Description
1. A chronic pulmonary condition that affects **infants** who have experienced respiratory failure or who have been oxygen dependent for more than 28 days
2. X-ray findings are abnormal and indicate areas of overinflation and atelectasis
3. **Neonate** may exhibit respiratory symptoms
B. Data collection
1. Tachypnea and tachycardia
2. Retractions, nasal flaring, and labored breathing
3. Crackles, decreased air movement, and occasional expiratory wheezing
C. Interventions
1. Oxygen therapy
2. Fluid restriction
3. Medications may include **surfactant**, diuretics, corticosteroids, and bronchodilators

XIII. TRANSIENT TACHYPNEA OF THE NEWBORN
A. Description
1. Respiratory condition that results from the incomplete evacuation of the fetal lung fluid in full-term **infants**
2. Usually disappears within 24 to 48 hours
B. Assessment
1. Tachypnea
2. Nasal flaring, expiratory grunting, and retractions
3. Wet lung sounds heard during auscultation
4. Cyanosis that responds to minimal oxygen
C. Interventions
1. Supportive care
2. Oxygen administration

XIV. INTRAVENTRICULAR HEMORRHAGE

A. Description
   1. Bleeding within the ventricles of the brain
   2. Risk factors include prematurity, respiratory distress syndrome, trauma, or asphyxia
B. Data collection
   1. Diminished or absent Moro reflex, lethargy, apnea, poor feeding, high-pitched and shrill cry, and seizure activity
C. Interventions: Treatment is supportive

XV. RETINOPATHY OF PREMATURITY

A. Description
   1. A vascular disorder that involves the gradual replacement of the retina by fibrous tissue and blood vessels
   2. Primarily caused by prematurity and the use of supplemental oxygen for more than 30 days
B. Data collection
   1. Leucoria (white tissue on the retrolental space), vitreous hemorrhage, miopia, strabismus, and cataracts (check for red reflex)
C. Interventions: Laser photocoagulation surgery

XVI. NECROTIZING ENTEROCOLITIS

A. Description
   1. An acute inflammatory disease of the gastrointestinal tract
   2. Usually occurs 4 to 10 days after birth in a term baby
B. Data collection: Increased abdominal girth, decreased or absent bowel sounds, loops of bowel seen through the abdominal wall, vomiting, bile-stained emesis, abdominal tenderness, and occult blood in the stools
C. Interventions
   1. Hold oral feedings
   2. Insert an oral gastric tube to decompress the abdomen
   3. Intravenous antibiotics
   4. Intravenous fluids to correct fluid, electrolyte, and acid–base imbalances
   5. Surgery, if indicated

XVII. HYPERBILIRUBINEMIA

A. Description
   1. At any serum bilirubin level, the appearance of jaundice during the first day of life indicates a pathological process
   2. Immediate attention is indicated when serum bilirubin levels are more than 12 mg/dL in the term **newborn**
   3. Therapy is aimed at preventing kernicterus, which results in permanent neurological damage as a result of the deposition of bilirubin in the brain cells
B. Data collection
   1. Jaundice
   2. Elevated serum bilirubin levels
   3. Enlarged liver
   4. Poor muscle tone
   5. Lethargy
   6. Poor sucking reflex
C. Interventions
   1. Monitor for the presence of jaundice
      a. Examine the **newborn's** skin color in natural light
      b. Press a finger over a bony prominence or the tip of the **newborn's** nose to press out capillary blood from the tissues
      c. Note that jaundice starts at the head first and then spreads to the chest, the abdomen, the arms and legs, and the hands and feet, which are the last to be jaundiced
   2. Keep the **newborn** well hydrated to maintain blood volume
   3. Facilitate early, frequent feeding to hasten the passage of meconium and to encourage the excretion of bilirubin
   4. Report any signs of jaundice during the first 24 hours and any abnormal signs and symptoms to the physician
   5. Prepare for phototherapy, and monitor the **newborn** closely during the treatment
D. Phototherapy
   1. Description
      a. Use of intense fluorescent lights to reduce serum bilirubin levels in the **newborn**
      b. Injury from treatment (e.g., eye damage, dehydration, sensory deprivation) can occur
   2. Interventions
      a. Expose as much of the **newborn's** skin as possible
      b. Cover the genital area, and monitor the genital area for skin irritation or breakdown
      c. Cover the **newborn's** eyes with shields or patches; make sure the eyelids are closed when shields or patches are applied
      d. Remove the shields or patches at least once per shift to inspect the eyes for infection or irritation and to allow for eye contact
      e. Measure the quantity of light every 8 hours
      f. Monitor the skin temperature closely
      g. Increase fluids to compensate for water loss
      h. Expect loose green stools and green urine
      i. Monitor the **newborn's** skin color with the fluorescent light turned off every 4 to 8 hours
      j. Monitor the skin for bronze baby syndrome, which is a grayish-brown discoloration of the skin
      k. Reposition the **newborn** every 2 hours
      l. Provide stimulation
      m. After treatment, continue monitoring for signs of hyperbilirubinemia, because rebound elevations are normal after therapy is discontinued

XVIII. ERYTHROBLASTOSIS FETALIS

A. Description
1. Destruction of the red blood cells that results from an antigen–antibody reaction
2. Characterized by hemolytic anemia or hyperbilirubinemia
3. Exchange of fetal and maternal blood takes place primarily when the placenta separates at birth
4. Rh antigens from the baby's blood enter the maternal bloodstream
5. The mother produces anti-Rh antibodies against the fetal blood cells
6. Antibodies are harmless to the mother but attach to the erythrocytes in the fetus and cause hemolysis
7. Sensitization is rare with the first pregnancy
8. ABO incompatibility is usually less severe

B. Data collection
1. Anemia
2. Jaundice that develops rapidly after birth and before 24 hours
3. Edema

C. Interventions
1. Administer $Rh_0(D)$ immune globulin (RhoGAM) to the mother during the first 72 hours after **delivery** if the Rh-negative mother delivers an Rh-positive fetus but remains unsensitized
2. Assist with exchange transfusion after birth or intrauterine transfusion, as prescribed
3. The baby's blood is replaced with Rh-negative blood to stop the destruction of the baby's red blood cells; the Rh-negative blood is gradually replaced with the baby's own blood
4. Reassure the mother that the **newborn** will suffer no untoward effects as a result of the condition

XIX. SEPSIS

A. Description: Generalized infection that results from the presence of bacteria in the blood

B. Data collection
1. Pallor
2. Tachypnea and tachycardia
3. Poor feeding
4. Abdominal distention
5. Temperature instability

C. Interventions
1. Monitor for periods of apnea or irregular respirations
2. If apnea is present, stimulate by gently rubbing the chest or foot
3. Administer oxygen, as prescribed
4. Monitor the vital signs
5. Maintain warmth in an isolette
6. Provide isolation, as necessary

7. Monitor for a fever
8. Monitor I&O and obtain daily weight
9. Monitor for diarrhea
10. Monitor feeding and sucking reflex, which may be poor
11. Monitor for jaundice
12. Monitor for irritability and lethargy
13. Administer antibiotics, as prescribed, and observe carefully for toxicity, because a **newborn's** liver and kidneys are immature

XX. TORCH SYNDROME

A. Description
1. Refers to infection of the fetus or **newborn**
2. Caused by one of the following:
   a. Toxoplasmosis
   b. Other infections
   c. Rubella
   d. Cytomegalovirus
   e. Herpes

B. Infections (Table 25-5)

XXI. SYPHILIS

A. Description
1. Sexually transmitted infection
2. Congenital syphilis can result in premature **delivery**, skin lesions, and abnormal skeletal development
3. The organism *Treponema pallidum*, a spirochete, can cross the placenta throughout pregnancy and infect the fetus, usually after 18 weeks' gestation
4. Risks include preterm birth, stillbirth, and low birth weight
5. Congenital effects are irreversible and may include central nervous system damage and hearing loss

B. Data collection
1. Hepatosplenomegaly
2. Joint swelling
3. Palmar rash
4. Anemia
5. Jaundice
6. Snuffles (syphilitic rhinitis)
7. Ascites
8. Pneumonitis
9. Cerebrospinal fluid changes

C. Interventions
1. Monitor the **newborn** for signs of syphilis
2. Monitor for palmar rash and snuffles
3. Prepare the **newborn** for serological testing, if prescribed
4. Administer antibiotic therapy, as prescribed
5. Use standard precautions and drainage and secretion precautions with suspected congenital syphilis
6. Wear gloves when handling the **neonate** until antibiotic therapy has been administered for 24 hours

TABLE 25-5 Infections Included in TORCH Syndrome

Infection	Characteristics
Toxoplasmosis	• Caused by a protozoal infection • Produces no serious effects in the mother • Can be transmitted to the fetus • Can result in severe physical and developmental abnormalities • Common carriers include cat feces and raw beef
Other infections	• Can include syphilis, gonorrhea, varicella, hepatitis B, and HIV
Rubella	• Systemic viral infection. • Causes congenital rubella syndrome, which includes congenital heart disease, cataracts, growth retardation, and pneumonia if the mother becomes infected within the first trimester • Deafness and some learning disabilities can occur if the mother becomes infected during the first trimester
Cytomegalovirus	• Viral infection that persists in the body indefinitely, with periods of reactivation without symptoms • Can infect the fetus or infant during delivery or after birth through breast milk, blood transfusions, or contact with infected secretions • May cause microcephaly, blindness, deafness, and mental and motor retardation.
Herpes simplex	• Sexually transmitted infection that is caused by a virus • Has periods of reactivation • Neonate commonly infected during delivery by direct contact with lesions in the genital tract • Can cause neurological impairment or death

7. Provide psychological support to the mother, and provide instructions regarding follow-up care of the **newborn**

XXII. ADDICTED NEWBORN
A. Description: A **newborn** who has become passively addicted to drugs that have passed through the placenta
B. Addicting drugs
1. Heroin
   a. The **newborn** may appear normal at birth, with a low birth weight
   b. Withdrawal occurs within 12 to 24 hours and may last 5 to 7 days
2. Methadone
   a. Withdrawal occurs within 1 to 2 days to 1 week or more, is most evident at 48 to 72 hours, and may last 6 days to 8 weeks
   b. The **newborn** appears very ill
   c. May develop jaundice as a result of prematurity
3. Cocaine
   a. Causes decreased interactive behavior
   b. Feeding problems are present
   c. Irregular sleep patterns and diarrhea occur
C. Data collection
1. Irritability
2. Tremors
3. Hyperactivity and hypertonicity
4. Respiratory distress
5. Vomiting
6. High-pitched cry
7. Sneezing
8. Fever
9. Diarrhea
10. Excessive sweating
11. Poor feeding
12. Extreme sucking of fists
13. Convulsions
D. Interventions
1. Monitor the respiratory and cardiac statuses frequently
2. Monitor the temperature and vital signs
3. Hold the **newborn** firm and close to the body during feeding and when giving care
4. Initiate seizure precautions (pad the sides of the crib)
5. Provide small frequent feedings and allow a longer period for feeding
6. Monitor the I&O
7. Administer intravenous hydration, as prescribed
8. Protect the **neonate's** skin from injury, which can be caused by constant rubbing from hyperactive jitters
9. Swaddle the **newborn**
10. Place the **newborn** in a quiet room and reduce stimulation
11. Allow the mother to ventilate feelings of anxiety and guilt
12. Refer the mother for treatment of her substance abuse problem

XXIII. FETAL ALCOHOL SYNDROME
A. Description
1. Caused by maternal alcohol use during pregnancy
2. Most serious cause of teratogenesis
3. Causes mental and physical retardation
B. Data collection
1. Facial changes
   a. Short palpebral fissures
   b. Hypoplastic philtrum

c. Short, upturned nose
d. Flat midface
e. Thin upper lip
f. Low nasal bridge
2. Abnormal palmar creases
3. Respiratory distress (apnea, cyanosis)
4. Congenital heart disorders
5. Irritability and hypersensitivity to stimuli
6. Tremors
7. Poor feeding
8. Seizures
C. Interventions
1. Monitor for respiratory distress
2. Position the **newborn** on his or her side to facilitate the drainage of secretions
3. Keep resuscitation equipment at the bedside
4. Monitor for hypoglycemia
5. Check the suck and swallow reflex
6. Administer small feedings and burp the baby well
7. Suction as necessary
8. Monitor the I&O
9. Monitor the weight and head circumference
10. Decrease environmental stimuli

▲ XXIV. **NEWBORN WITH ACQUIRED IMMUNODEFICIENCY SYNDROME**
A. Description
1. The fetus of a human immunodeficiency virus (HIV)-positive woman should be monitored closely throughout the pregnancy
2. Serial ultrasound screenings should be done during pregnancy to identify intrauterine growth restriction
3. Weekly nonstress testing after 32 weeks' gestation and biophysical profiles may be necessary during pregnancy
4. **Neonates** born to HIV-positive clients may test positive because the mother's positive antibodies may persist for as long as 18 months after birth
5. The use of antiviral medication, the reduction of **neonate** exposure to maternal blood and body fluids, and the early identification of HIV during pregnancy reduce the risk of transmission to the **newborn**
6. All **neonates** born to HIV-positive mothers acquire maternal antibody to HIV infection, but not all acquire the infection
7. The **neonate** may be asymptomatic for the first several years of life
B. Transmission
1. Across placental barrier
2. During **labor** and **delivery**
3. Via breast milk
C. Data collection
1. May have no outward signs for the first several months of life

2. Signs of immuno deficiency
3. Hepatomegaly
4. Splenomegaly
5. Lymphadenopathy
6. Impairment in growth and development
D. Interventions
1. Cleanse the **newborn's** skin carefully with soap, water, and alcohol before any invasive procedure, such as the administration of vitamin K, heel sticks, or venipunctures
2. Circumcisions are not done on **newborns** with HIV-positive mothers until the **newborn's** status is determined
3. **Newborn** can room with mother
4. All HIV-exposed **newborns** should be treated with medication to prevent infection by *Pneumocystis jiroveci*
5. Antiretroviral medication may be administered, as prescribed, for the first 6 weeks of life
6. Monitor for early signs of immunodeficiency, such as hepatomegaly, splenomegaly, lymphadenopathy, and impairment in growth and development
7. **Newborns** at risk for HIV infection should be seen by the physician at birth and at 1 week, 2 weeks, 1 month, and 2 months of life
8. Inform the mother that an HIV culture is recommended at the ages of 1 month and 4 months
E. Immunizations
1. **Newborns** at risk for HIV infection need to receive all recommended immunizations according to the regular schedule
2. Immunizations with live vaccines, such as measles–mumps–rubella, should not be done until the **newborn's, infant's,** or child's HIV status is confirmed
3. If a child is infected, live vaccine will not be given

XXV. **NEWBORN OF A DIABETIC MOTHER** ▲
A. Description
1. A **neonate** born to an insulin-dependent or gestational diabetic mother
2. High incidence of hypoglycemia, hyperbilirubinemia, respiratory distress syndrome, hypocalcemia, and congenital anomalies
B. Data collection
1. Excessive size and weight as a result of excess fat and glycogen in tissues
2. Edema or puffiness in the face and cheeks
3. Signs of hypoglycemia, such as twitching, difficulty feeding, lethargy, apnea, seizures, and cyanosis
4. Hyperbilirubinemia
5. Signs of respiratory distress, such as tachypnea, cyanosis, retractions, grunting, and nasal flaring

C. Interventions
1. Monitor for signs of respiratory distress
2. Monitor the bilirubin and blood glucose levels
3. Monitor the weight
4. Feed the **infant** soon after birth with glucose in water, breast milk, or formula, as prescribed
5. Administer intravenous glucose to treat hypoglycemia, if necessary and as prescribed
6. Monitor for edema
7. Monitor for apnea, tremors, and seizures

XXVI. HYPOGLYCEMIA

A. Description
1. Abnormally low levels of glucose in the blood (<40 mg/dL during the first 72 hours or <45 mg/dL after the first 3 days of life)
2. Normal blood glucose level is 40 to 60 mg/dL in a 1-day-old **neonate** and 50 to 90 mg/dL in a **neonate** who is more than 1 day old

B. Data collection
1. Increased respiratory rate
2. Twitching, nervousness, or tremors
3. Unstable temperature
4. Cyanosis

C. Interventions
1. Prevent low blood glucose with early feedings
2. Administer glucose orally or intravenously, as prescribed
3. Monitor the blood glucose levels, as prescribed
4. Monitor for feeding problems
5. Monitor for apneic periods
6. Monitor for shrill or intermittent cries
7. Evaluate lethargy and poor muscle tone

PRACTICE QUESTIONS

More questions on the companion CD!

257. A nurse administers erythromycin ointment (0.5%) to the newborn's eyes, and the mother asks the nurse why this is done. The nurse tells the client that this is routinely done to:
1. Prevent cataracts in the neonate born to a woman who is susceptible to rubella.
2. Protect the neonate's eyes from possible infections acquired while hospitalized.
3. Minimize the spread of microorganisms to the neonate from invasive procedures during labor.
4. Prevent ophthalmia neonatorum from occurring after delivery to a neonate born to a woman with an untreated gonococcal infection.

258. A client asks the nurse why her newborn baby needs an injection of vitamin K. The nurse makes which statement to the client?
1. "Your newborn needs vitamin K to develop immunity."

2. "The vitamin K will protect your newborn from becoming jaundiced."
3. "Newborns are deficient in vitamin K. This injection prevents your baby from abnormal bleeding."
4. "Newborns have sterile bowels. The vitamin K will colonize the bowel with the necessary bacteria."

259. A nurse is assigned to assist with caring for a neonate born to a mother with acquired immunodeficiency syndrome (AIDS). The nurse understands that which of the following should be included in the plan of care?
1. Monitor the neonate's vital signs routinely.
2. Maintain standard precautions at all times while caring for the neonate.
3. Instruct breast-feeding mothers regarding the treatment of their nipples with an antifungal cream.
4. Initiate a referral to evaluate for blindness, deafness, learning, or behavioral problems in the neonate.

260. A nurse in the newborn nursery receives a telephone call to prepare for the admission of an infant born at 43 weeks' gestation with Apgar scores of 1 and 4. When planning for the admission of this infant, the nurse's highest priority should be to:
1. Turn on the apnea and cardiorespiratory monitor.
2. Connect the resuscitation bag to the oxygen outlet.
3. Set up the intravenous line with 5% dextrose in water.
4. Set the radiant warmer control temperature at 36.5° C (97.6° F).

261. A nurse is caring for a postterm neonate immediately after admission to the nursery. The priority nursing action would be to monitor:
1. Urinary output
2. Blood glucose levels
3. Total bilirubin levels
4. Hemoglobin and hematocrit level

262. A nurse is reinforcing instructions to a new mother about cord care and how to monitor for infection. The nurse tells the mother that which of the following is a sign of infection?
1. A darkened drying stump
2. A moist cord with discharge
3. A purple stump that shows pinkness around the base
4. A purple stump that shows some moistness at the base

263. A nurse is reinforcing measures regarding the care of the newborn with a mother. To bathe the newborn, the mother should be taught to:
1. Begin with the eyes and face.

2. Start with the dirtiest area first.

3. Begin with the feet and work upward.

4. Only wash the diaper area, because this is the only part of the baby that gets soiled.

264. After birth, the nurse prevents hypothermia as a result of evaporation in the newborn by:
   1. Warming the crib pad
   2. Closing the doors of the room
   3. Drying the baby with a warm blanket
   4. Turning on the overhead radiant warmer

265. A nurse is planning to teach cord care to a new mother. The nurse plans to tell the mother that:
   1. Alcohol is the only agent used to clean the cord.
   2. It takes 21 days for the cord to dry up and fall off.
   3. Cord care is done only at birth to control bleeding.
   4. The process of keeping the cord clean and dry will decrease bacterial growth.

266. A male neonate has just been circumcised. The nurse would expect the surgical site to appear:
   1. Pink, without drainage
   2. Reddened, with a small amount of bloody drainage
   3. Reddened, with a small amount of yellow exudate on the glans
   4. Reddened, with a large amount of bloody drainage that requires a dressing change every 30 minutes

267. Preterm newborns are at the risk for developing respiratory distress syndrome (RDS). The nurse monitors for the clinical signs associated with RDS, knowing that these signs include:
   1. Tachypnea and retractions
   2. Acrocyanosis and grunting
   3. Hypotension and bradycardia
   4. The presence of a barrel chest with acrocyanosis

268. A nurse notes hypotonia, irritability, and a poor sucking reflex in a full-term newborn infant after admission to the nursery. The nurse suspects fetal alcohol syndrome (FAS) and is aware that which of the following additional signs would be consistent with FAS?
   1. A length of 19 inches
   2. Abnormal palmar creases

3. A birth weight of 6 pounds and 14 ounces

4. A head circumference that is appropriate for gestational age

269. A pregnant human immunodeficiency virus (HIV)-positive woman delivers a baby. The nurse provides guidance to help the client make decisions regarding newborn care. The nurse determines that additional guidance is needed if the woman states that she will:
   1. Be sure to wash her hands before feeding the newborn.
   2. Breast-feed, especially for the first 6 weeks postpartum.
   3. Be sure to wash her hands before and after bathroom use.
   4. Administer the prescribed antiviral medication to the newborn for the first 6 weeks after delivery.

270. A pregnant woman has a positive history of genital herpes, but she has not had lesions during her pregnancy. The nurse plans to provide which of the following information to the client?
   1. "You will be isolated from your newborn after delivery."
   2. "There is little risk to your neonate during your pregnancy, birth, and after delivery."
   3. "Vaginal deliveries can reduce neonatal infection risks, even if you have an active lesion at birth."
   4. "You will be evaluated at the time of delivery for herpetic genital tract lesions. If they are present, a cesarean delivery will be needed."

ALTERNATE ITEM FORMAT: MULTIPLE RESPONSE

271. The nurse is preparing to care for a newborn who is receiving phototherapy. Choose the measures that would be implemented. Select all that apply.
   ☐ 1. Avoid stimulation.
   ☐ 2. Decrease fluid intake.
   ☐ 3. Expose all of the newborn's skin.
   ☐ 4. Monitor the skin temperature closely.
   ☐ 5. Reposition the newborn every 2 hours.
   ☐ 6. Cover the newborn's eyes with shields or patches.

ANSWERS

257. **4**

Rationale: Erythromycin ophthalmic ointment 0.5% is used as a prophylactic treatment for ophthalmia neonatorum, which is caused by the bacteria *Neisseria gonorrhoeae*. The preventive treatment of gonorrhea is required by law. Options 1, 2, and 3 are not the purposes of administering this medication to the newborn infant.

Test-Taking Strategy: Use the process of elimination and your knowledge of the purpose of administering erythromycin ophthalmic ointment to the newborn infant. Remember that erythromycin ophthalmic ointment 0.5% is used as a prophylactic treatment of ophthalmia neonatorum in newborns. Review the initial care of the newborn infant if you had difficulty with this question.

Level of Cognitive Ability: Application

Clients Needs: Safe and Effective Care Environment
Integrated Process: Nursing Process/Implementation
Content Area: Maternity/Postpartum
References: Leifer, G. (2008). *Maternity nursing: An introductory text* (10th ed., p. 188). Philadelphia: Saunders.
Leifer, G. (2007). *Introduction to maternity and pediatric nursing* (5th ed., p. 151). Philadelphia: Saunders.

258. 3

Rationale: Vitamin K is necessary for the body to synthesize coagulation factors, and it is administered to the newborn infant to prevent abnormal bleeding. It promotes the liver's formation of the clotting factors II, VII, IX, and X. Newborn infants are deficient in vitamin K, because the bowel does not have the bacteria necessary for synthesizing this fat-soluble vitamin. The normal flora in the intestinal tract produces vitamin K, but the newborn's bowel does not support the normal production of vitamin K until bacteria have adequately colonized it. The bowel becomes colonized by bacteria as food is ingested. Vitamin K does not promote the development of immunity or prevent the infant from becoming jaundiced.

Test-Taking Strategy: Use the process of elimination. Because jaundice and immunity are not related to the action of vitamin K, eliminate options 1 and 2. From the remaining options, recall the action of vitamin K to direct you to option 3. Review the purpose of vitamin K injection if you had difficulty with this question.

Level of Cognitive Ability: Application
Client's Needs: Psychological Integrity
Integrated Process: Nursing Process/Implementation
Content Area: Maternity/Postpartum
Reference: Leifer, G. (2007). *Introduction to maternity and pediatric nursing* (5th ed., p. 151). Philadelphia: Saunders.

259. 2

Rationale: The neonate born to a mother with AIDS must be cared for with strict attention to standard precautions. This prevents the transmission of the infection from the neonate, if he or she is infected, to others, and it prevents the transmission of other infectious agents to the possibly immunocompromised neonate. A mother with AIDS should not breast-feed. Options 1 and 4 are not specifically associated with the care of a potentially AIDS-infected neonate.

Test-Taking Strategy: Use the process of elimination and your knowledge regarding the care of a neonate infant born to a woman with AIDS. Eliminate options 1 and 4 first, because they are not specifically associated with the care of a potentially infected neonate. Recalling that AIDS-infected mothers should not breast-feed will direct you to option 2. Review the care of a neonate born to a woman with AIDS if you had difficulty with this question.

Level of Cognitive Ability: Application
Client Needs: Safe and Effective Care Environment
Integrated Process: Nursing Process/Planning
Content Area: Maternity/Postpartum
Reference: Leifer, G. (2007). *Introduction to maternity and pediatric nursing* (5th ed., pp. 105, 718, 726-728). Philadelphia: Saunders.

260. 2

Rationale: The highest priority during the admission to the nursery of a newborn with low Apgar scores is airway support, which would involve preparing respiratory resuscitation equipment. The remaining options are also important, although they are of lower initial priority. The newborn infant will be placed on a cardiorespiratory monitor. Setting up an intravenous line with 5% dextrose in water would provide circulatory support. The radiant warmer will provide an external heat source, which is necessary to prevent further respiratory distress.

Test-Taking Strategy: Use the process of elimination, and note the strategic words "highest priority." This question asks you to prioritize care on the basis of information about a newborn infant's condition. Use the ABCs—airway, breathing, and circulation. A method of planning for airway support is to have the resuscitation bag connected to an oxygen source. Review the care of the newborn infant with low Apgar scores if you had difficulty with this question.

Level of Cognitive Ability: Application
Client Needs: Physiological Integrity
Integrated Process: Nursing Process/Planning
Content Area: Delegating/Prioritizing
References: Leifer, G. (2007). *Introduction to maternity and pediatric nursing* (5th ed., pp.150, 286). Philadelphia: Saunders.
Price, D., & Gwin, J. (2008). *Pediatric nursing: An introductory text* (10th ed., p. 50). St. Louis: Saunders.

261. 2

Rationale: The most common metabolic complication in the postterm newborn is hypoglycemia, which can produce central nervous system abnormalities and mental retardation if it is not corrected immediately. Urinary output, although important, is not the highest priority action. Hemoglobin and hematocrit levels are monitored, because the postterm neonate exhibits polycythemia; however, this also does not require immediate attention. The polycythemia contributes to increased bilirubin levels, usually beginning on the second day after delivery.

Test-Taking Strategy: Use the process of elimination, and note the strategic word "priority." Recalling that hypoglycemia is a primary concern in the postterm newborn will direct you to option 2. Review the care of the postterm newborn if you had difficulty with this question.

Level of Cognitive Ability: Application
Client Needs: Physiological Integrity
Integrated Process: Nursing Process/Data Collection
Content Area: Delegating/Prioritizing
References: Leifer, G. (2007). *Introduction to maternity and pediatric nursing* (5th ed., pp. 316-317). Philadelphia: Saunders.
Price, D., & Gwin, J. (2008). *Pediatric nursing: An introductory text* (10th ed., p. 73). St. Louis: Saunders.

262. 2

Rationale: Signs of infection of the umbilical cord are moistness, oozing, discharge, and a reddened base. If signs of infection occur, the health care provider is notified. Antibiotic treatment may be necessary.

Test-Taking Strategy: Use the process of elimination. Options 1 and 3 identify normal signs and are eliminated first. From the remaining options, noting the word "discharge" in option 2 will direct you to this option. Review the signs and symptoms of infection if you had difficulty with this question.
Level of Cognitive Ability: Application
Client Needs: Safe and Effective Care Environment
Integrated Process: Teaching and Learning
Content Area: Maternity/Postpartum
Reference: Leifer, G. (2007). *Introduction to maternity and pediatric nursing* (5th ed., pp. 218-219). Philadelphia: Saunders.

263. 1
Rationale: Bathing should start at the eyes and face, which are usually the cleanest areas. Next, the external ears and behind the ears are cleansed. The newborn's neck should be washed, because formula, breast milk, or lint will often accumulate in the folds of the neck. The hands and arms are then washed. The baby's legs are washed, with the diaper area being washed last.
Test-Taking Strategy: Use the basic techniques of bathing a client to answer the question. Remember, when bathing an adult or a baby, start with the cleanest part of the body and proceed to the dirtiest part. Options 2, 3, and 4 are incorrect. Review the techniques for bathing a newborn if you had difficulty with this question.
Level of Cognitive Ability: Application
Client Needs: Health Promotion and Maintenance
Integrated Process: Nursing Process/Implementation
Content Area: Maternity/Postpartum
Reference: Leifer, G. (2007). *Introduction to maternity and pediatric nursing* (5th ed., p. 294). Philadelphia: Saunders.

264. 3
Rationale: Evaporation occurs when moisture from the newborn's wet body surface dissipates heat along with moisture. By keeping the newborn dry (and by drying the wet newborn at birth), evaporation is prevented. Conduction occurs when the newborn is on a cold surface, such as a cold pad or mattress. Convection occurs as air moves across the newborn's skin from an open door and heat is transferred to the air. Radiation occurs when heat from the newborn radiates to a colder surface.
Test-Taking Strategy: Recalling the methods of preventing heat loss in a newborn and focusing on the subject of evaporation will direct you to option 3. Review the methods of heat loss if you had difficulty with this question.
Level of Cognitive Ability: Application
Client Needs: Physiological Integrity
Integrated Process: Nursing Process/Implementation
Content Area: Maternity/Postpartum
Reference: Price, D., & Gwin, J. (2008). *Pediatric nursing: An introductory text* (10th ed., p. 51). St. Louis: Saunders.

265. 4
Rationale: The cord should be kept clean and dry to decrease bacterial growth; this includes keeping the diaper folded below the cord to keep urine away from the cord. The cord should be cleansed two to three times a day. It usually falls off

within 7 to 14 days. Agents other than alcohol may be prescribed to clean the cord.
Test-Taking Strategy: Use the process of elimination. Eliminate options 1 and 3, noting the close-ended word "only." Recall that cord care is required until the cord dries up and falls off and that agents other than alcohol may be prescribed for cord care. Option 2 is incorrect, because the cord should fall off between 7 and 14 days after birth. Review the concepts of cord care if you had difficulty with this question.
Level of Cognitive Ability: Comprehension
Client Needs: Physiological Integrity
Integrated Process: Teaching and Learning
Content Area: Maternity/Postpartum
References: Leifer, G. (2007). *Introduction to maternity and pediatric nursing* (5th ed., p. 218). Philadelphia: Saunders.
Price, D., & Gwin, J. (2008). *Pediatric nursing: An introductory text* (10th ed., p. 68). St. Louis: Saunders.

266. 2
Rationale: The glans penis is normally dark red. After circumcision, a small amount of bloody drainage is expected. During the normal healing process, the glans becomes covered with a yellow exudate. If excessive bleeding is noted from the circumcision, the nurse applies gentle pressure to the site of bleeding with a sterile gauze pad. If the bleeding is not controlled, the physician is notified, because a blood vessel may need to be ligated.
Test-Taking Strategy: Use the process of elimination, and focus on the subject of the expected appearance. Remember that a small amount of bloody drainage is expected. Review the expected findings after circumcision if you had difficulty with this question.
Level of Cognitive Ability: Comprehension
Client Needs: Physiological Integrity
Integrated Process: Nursing Process/Data Collection
Content Area: Maternity/Postpartum
Reference: Leifer, G. (2007). *Introduction to maternity and pediatric nursing* (5th ed., pp. 290-291). Philadelphia: Saunders.

267. 1
Rationale: The newborn infant with RDS may present with clinical signs of cyanosis, tachypnea, apnea, nasal flaring, chest wall retractions, or audible grunts. Acrocyanosis is a bluish discoloration of the hands and feet that is associated with immature peripheral circulation, and it is not uncommon during the first few hours of life. Options 2, 3, and 4 do not indicate clinical signs of RDS.
Test-Taking Strategy: Use the process of elimination. Recalling that acrocyanosis may be a normal sign in a newborn infant will assist you with eliminating options 2 and 4. From the remaining options, it is necessary to be familiar with the signs of RDS. In addition, note the relationship between the diagnosis and the signs noted in option 1. Review the signs of RDS if you had difficulty with this question.
Level of Cognitive Ability: Analysis
Client Needs: Physiological Integrity
Integrated Process: Nursing Process/Data Collection
Content Area: Maternity/Postpartum

Reference: Price, D., & Gwin, J. (2008). *Pediatric nursing: An introductory text* (10th ed., p. 75). St. Louis: Saunders.

268. 2
Rationale: Features of newborn infants who are diagnosed with FAS include craniofacial abnormalities, intrauterine growth restriction, cardiac abnormalities, abnormal palmar creases, and respiratory distress. Options 1, 3, and 4 are normal findings in the full-term newborn infant.
Test-Taking Strategy: Use the process of elimination and your knowledge regarding the normal findings in the full-term newborn infant to answer this question. Note that options 1, 3, and 4 are comparable or alike and that they represent normal findings. Review the content related to normal newborn infant findings and FAS if you had difficulty with this question.
Level of Cognitive Ability: Analysis
Client Needs: Physiological Integrity
Integrated Process: Nursing Process/Data Collection
Content Area: Maternity/Postpartum
References: Leifer, G. (2007). *Introduction to maternity and pediatric nursing* (5th ed., pp. 108-109). Philadelphia: Saunders. Murray, S., & McKinney, E. (2006). *Foundations of maternal-newborn nursing* (4th ed., pp. 601-602). Philadelphia: Saunders.

269. 2
Rationale: The mode of perinatal transmission of HIV to the fetus or neonate of an HIV-positive woman can occur during the antenatal, intrapartal, or postpartum periods. HIV transmission can occur during breast-feeding; thus, HIV-positive clients need to bottle-feed their neonates. Antiviral medications will be prescribed for the neonate for the first 6 weeks of life. The principles related to handwashing need to be taught to the mother.
Test-Taking Strategy: Use the process of elimination, and note the strategic words "additional guidance is needed." These words indicate a negative event query and ask you to select an option that is an incorrect statement. Options 1 and 3 can be eliminated first, because they are comparable or alike. From the remaining options, recalling the modes of transmission of HIV from the mother to the newborn will direct you to option 2. Review these modes of HIV transmission if you had difficulty with this question.
Level of Cognitive Ability: Analysis
Clients Needs: Safe and Effective Care Environment
Integrated Process: Teaching and Learning
Content Area: Maternity/Postpartum
Reference: Leifer, G. (2007). *Introduction to maternity and pediatric nursing* (5th ed., p. 105). Philadelphia: Saunders.

270. 4
Rationale: If herpetic genital lesions are present at the time of delivery, a cesarean delivery will be necessary to reduce the risk of infecting the neonate. In the absence of herpetic genital lesions, a vaginal delivery may be indicated, unless there are other reasons for performing a cesarean delivery. Maternal isolation is not necessary, but potentially exposed neonates should be cultured on the day of delivery.
Test-Taking Strategy: Use the process of elimination. Focusing on the subject of a positive history of genital herpes and recalling the risks to the neonate will direct you to option 4. Review the methods of transmission of genital herpes to the neonate if you had difficulty with this question.
Level of Cognitive Ability: Application
Clients Needs: Safe and Effective Care Environment
Integrated Process: Nursing Process/Implementation
Content Area: Maternity/Antepartum
Reference: Leifer, G. (2007). *Introduction to maternity and pediatric nursing* (5th ed., p. 105). Philadelphia: Saunders.

ALTERNATE ITEM FORMAT: MULTIPLE RESPONSE
271. 4, 5, 6
Rationale: Phototherapy is the use of intense fluorescent lights to reduce serum bilirubin levels in the newborn. Injury from treatment (e.g., eye damage, dehydration, sensory deprivation) can occur. Interventions include exposing as much of the newborn's skin as possible; however, the genital area is covered. The newborn's eyes are also covered with shields or patches to ensure that the eyelids are closed. The shields or patches are removed at least once per shift to inspect the eyes for infection or irritation and to allow for eye contact. The nurse measures the quantity of light every 8 hours, monitors the skin temperature closely, and increases fluids to compensate for water loss. The newborn will have loose green stools and green-colored urine. The newborn's skin color is monitored with the fluorescent light turned off every 4 to 8 hours, and he or she is monitored for bronze baby syndrome, which is a grayish-brown discoloration of the skin. The newborn is repositioned every 2 hours, and stimulation is provided. After treatment, the newborn is monitored for signs of hyperbilirubinemia, because rebound elevations are normal after therapy is discontinued.
Test-Taking Strategy: Focus on the subject of phototherapy. Recalling that injury from treatment and sensory deprivation can occur will assist you with determining the correct interventions. Review the interventions for the newborn who is receiving phototherapy if you had difficulty with this question.
Level of Cognitive Ability: Application
Client Needs: Safe and Effective Care Environment
Integrated Process: Nursing Process/Implementation
Content Area: Maternity/Postpartum
Reference: Murray, S., & McKinney, E., (2006). *Foundations of maternal-newborn nursing* (4th ed., pp. 793-794). Philadelphia: Saunders.

REFERENCES

Leifer, G. (2008). *Maternity nursing: An introductory text* (10th ed.). Philadelphia: Saunders.

Leifer, G. (2007). *Introduction to maternity and pediatric nursing* (5th ed.). Philadelphia: Saunders.

Murray, S., & McKinney, E. (2006). *Foundations of maternal-newborn nursing* (4th ed.). Philadelphia: Saunders.

National Council of State Boards of Nursing (Eds.). (2008). *2008 Detailed Test Plan for the NCLEX-PN® Examination, National Council of State Boards of Nursing.* Chicago: Author.

National Council of State Boards of Nursing. *NCSBN home page.* www.ncsbn.org. Accessed July 7, 2008.

Price, D., & Gwin, J. (2008). *Pediatric nursing: An introductory text* (10th ed.). St. Louis: Saunders.

Maternity and Newborn Medications

CHAPTER

26

I. OXYTOCIC MEDICATION: OXYTOCIN (PITOCIN)

A. Description
1. Stimulates the smooth muscle of the **uterus** and induces the contraction of the myocardium
2. Promotes milk let-down
3. Routes of administration include intranasal, intramuscular, and intravenous (IV)
4. Minimal cervical change usually is noted until the active phase of **labor** is achieved

B. Uses
1. Induce or augment **labor**
2. Control postpartum bleeding
3. Promote milk let-down and facilitate breast-feeding (intranasal route)
4. Induce or complete an abortion

C. Adverse reactions and contraindications
1. Rare, but may include allergies, dysrhythmias, changes in blood pressure, uterine rupture, and water intoxication; intranasal administration may cause nasal vasoconstriction
2. May produce uterine hypertonicity that results in fetal or maternal injury
3. High doses may cause hypotension, with rebound hypertension
4. Postpartum hemorrhage can occur, because the uterus may become atonic when the medication wears off
5. Should not be used with a client who cannot deliver vaginally or one with hypertonic uterine contractions

D. Interventions
1. Monitor maternal vital signs every 15 minutes, especially blood pressure, heart rate, weight, intake and output, level of consciousness, and lung sounds
2. Monitor the frequency, duration, and force of contractions and the resting uterine tone every 15 minutes
3. Monitor the fetal heart rate every 15 minutes, and notify the registered nurse or health care provider if significant changes occur; an internal fetal scalp electrode should be used, if possible
4. Administered by IV infusion via an infusion monitoring device (Y setup or stopcock is used with normal saline in the primary line); dose being administered is carefully monitored
5. Do not leave the client unattended while the oxytocin is infusing
6. Administer oxygen, if prescribed
7. Monitor for hypertonic contractions
8. Notify the registered nurse or the health care provider if uterine hyperstimulation or a non-reassuring fetal heart rate occurs
9. The infusion will be stopped, the client will be turned on her side, the IV rate of normal saline will be increased, and oxygen will be administered via a face mask
10. Monitor for signs of water intoxication
11. Have emergency equipment available
12. Document the dose of the medication and the times that the medication was started, increased, maintained, and discontinued
13. Keep the family informed about the client's progress

II. MEDICATIONS USED TO MANAGE POSTPARTUM HEMORRHAGE (Box 26-1)

A. Ergot alkaloids
1. Description
   a. Ergonovine maleate (Ergotrate, ergometrine) and methylergonovine maleate (Methergine) are ergot alkaloids
   b. Directly stimulate uterine muscle, increase the force and frequency of contractions, and produce a firm tetanic contraction of the uterus
   c. Can produce arterial vasoconstriction and vasospasm of the coronary arteries
   d. Ergot alkaloids are not administered before the **delivery** of the **placenta**
2. Uses
   a. Postpartum hemorrhage
   b. Postabortal hemorrhage resulting from atony or involution

BOX 26-1	Medications Used to Manage Postpartum Bleeding

- Ergonovine maleate (Ergotrate, Ergometrine)
- Methylergonovine maleate (Methergine)
- Oxytocin (Pitocin)
- Prostaglandin F$_2\alpha$ (carboprost tromethamine, Hemabate)

BOX 26-2	Medications Used to Stop Preterm Labor Contractions

- Indomethacin
- Magnesium sulfate
- Nifedipine (Procardia, Adalat)
- Ritodrine hydrochloride
- Terbutaline (Brethine)

3. Adverse reactions and contraindications
   a. Can cause nausea, uterine cramping, bradycardia, dysrhythmias, myocardial infarction, and severe hypertension
   b. High doses associated with peripheral vasospasm or vasoconstriction, angina, miosis, confusion, respiratory depression, seizures, or unconsciousness; uterine tetany can occur
   c. Contraindicated during pregnancy and in clients with significant cardiovascular disease, peripheral vascular disease, or hypertension
4. Interventions
   a. Monitor maternal vital signs, weight, intake and output, level of consciousness, and lung sounds
   b. Monitor the client's blood pressure closely; the medication produces vasoconstriction, and, if a rise in blood pressure is noted, withhold the medication and notify the registered nurse or the health care provider.
   c. Monitor the uterine contractions for frequency, strength, and duration
   d. Assess for chest pain, headache, shortness of breath, itching, pale or cold hands or feet, nausea, diarrhea, and dizziness
   e. Notify the registered nurse or health care provider if chest pain occurs
   f. Assess the extremities for color, warmth, movement, and pain
   g. Assess vaginal bleeding
   h. Administer analgesics, as prescribed; they may be required, because the medication produces painful uterine contractions
B. Prostaglandin F$_2\alpha$ (carboprost tromethamine, Hemabate)
   1. Description: Contracts the uterus
   2. Uses: Postpartum hemorrhage
   3. Adverse reactions and contraindications
      a. Can cause headache, nausea, vomiting, and fever
      b. Contraindicated if the client has asthma
   4. Interventions
      a. Check the temperature every 1 to 2 hours
      b. Auscultate the breath sounds frequently

III. MEDICATIONS TO STOP PRETERM LABOR CONTRACTIONS
A. Description: Tocolytics are medications that produce uterine relaxation and suppress uterine activity in an attempt to prevent preterm birth (Box 26-2 and Table 26-1)
B. Uses: To prevent preterm birth
C. Adverse reactions and contraindications
   1. See Table 26-1 for a description of adverse reactions
   2. Maternal contraindications include severe preeclampsia and eclampsia, active vaginal bleeding, intrauterine infection, cardiac disease, or a medical or obstetric condition that contraindicates the continuation of pregnancy
   3. Fetal contraindications include estimated gestational age of more than 37 weeks, cervical dilation of more than 4 cm, fetal demise, lethal fetal anomaly, chorioamnionitis, acute fetal distress, or chronic intrauterine growth restriction
D. Interventions for the client who is receiving tocolytic therapy
   1. Position the client on her side to enhance placental perfusion and reduce pressure on the cervix
   2. Monitor maternal vital signs, fetal status, and **labor** status frequently, according to agency protocol
   3. Monitor for signs of adverse reactions to the medication
   4. Monitor daily weight and intake and output status; limit fluid intake, as prescribed
   5. Offer comfort measures, and provide psychosocial support to the client and family
   6. See Table 26-1 for interventions specific to each tocolytic medication
IV. PROSTAGLANDINS (Box 26-3)
A. Description
   1. Ripen the cervix, thus making it softer and causing it to begin to dilate and efface
   2. Stimulate uterine contractions
   3. Administered vaginally
B. Uses
   1. Preinduction cervical ripening (ripening of the cervix before the induction of **labor**)
   2. To induce **labor**
   3. To induce abortion (abortifacient agent)

TABLE 26-1	Medications Used for Preterm Labor	
Medication/Classification	**Adverse Reactions**	**Nursing Interventions**
Magnesium sulfate • Central nervous system depressant • Relaxes smooth muscle, including the uterus • Used to halt preterm labor contractions • Used for preeclamptic clients to prevent seizures	• Depressed respirations • Depressed deep tendon reflexes • Hypotension • Extreme muscle weakness • Flushing • Decreased urine output • Pulmonary edema • Serum magnesium levels ≥9 mg/dL	• Use controller pump for administration • Follow agency protocol for administration • Discontinue infusion and notify physician if adverse reactions occur • Monitor for respirations of <12 per minute and for urine output of <100 mL per 4 hours (25-30 mL/hr) • Monitor deep tendon reflexes • Monitor magnesium levels and report values outside therapeutic range (4-7.5 mEq/L or 5-8 mg/dL) • Keep calcium gluconate (antidote) at bedside
Ritodrine • β-Adrenergic agonist • Relaxes smooth muscles, inhibiting uterine activity and causing bronchodilation	• Shortness of breath, coughing, tachypnea, and pulmonary edema • Tachycardia, palpitations, chest pain, and hypotension • Fluid retention and decreased urine production • Tremors, dizziness, muscle cramps, and weakness • Headache • Hypokalemia, hyperglycemia, and hypocalcemia	• Discontinue infusion and notify physician if the following occur: maternal heart rate >120-140 beats per minute, dysrhythmias, chest pain, blood pressure <90/60 mm Hg, signs of pulmonary edema, or fetal heart rate >180 beats per minute • Ensure that a β-blocking agent such as propranolol (Inderal) is available to reverse adverse cardiovascular reactions
Terbutaline (Brethine) • β-Adrenergic agonist • Relaxes smooth muscles, inhibiting uterine activity and causing bronchodilation	• Similar to ritodrine but limited and less severe	• Monitor for adverse reactions and notify the physician if they occur • Teach the woman and family to monitor for adverse reactions and when to notify the physician
Nifedipine (Procardia, Adalat) • Calcium channel blocker • Relaxes smooth muscles, including the uterus, by blocking calcium entry	• Transient tachycardia • Palpitations • Hypotension • Dizziness, headache, and nervousness • Facial flushing • Fatigue and nausea	• Follow agency protocol for administration • Avoid use or use cautiously with magnesium sulfate, because severe hypotension can occur • Monitor for adverse reactions
Indomethacin • Prostaglandin inhibitor • Relaxes uterine smooth muscle	• Maternal: nausea and vomiting, dyspepsia, and dizziness • Fetal: premature closure of ductus arteriosus • Neonate: bronchopulmonary dysplasia, respiratory distress syndrome, intracranial pressure, necrotizing enterocolitis, and hyperbilirubinemia	• Used only when other methods fail and only if gestational age is <32 weeks • Not used in women with bleeding potential, peptic ulcer disease, or oligohydramnios • Follow agency protocol for administration • Prepare to determine amniotic fluid volume and the function of the ductus arteriosus before therapy and within 48 hours of discontinuing therapy

Modified from Wong, D., Hockenberry, M., Perry, S., Lowdermilk, D., & Wilson, D. (2006). *Maternal-child nursing care* (3rd ed.). St. Louis: Mosby.

BOX 26-3 **Prostaglandins**

- Prostaglandin E_1: Misoprostol (Cytotec)
- Prostaglandin E_2: Dinoprostone (Cervidil vaginal insert, Prepidil Gel)

BOX 26-4 **Contraindications to the Use of Prostaglandins**

- Active cardiac, hepatic, pulmonary, or renal disease
- Acute pelvic inflammatory disease
- Clients for whom vaginal delivery is not indicated
- Fetal malpresentation
- History of cesarean section or major uterine surgery
- History of difficult or traumatic labor
- Hypersensitivity to prostaglandins
- Maternal fever or infection
- Nonreassuring fetal heart rate pattern
- Placenta previa or unexplained vaginal bleeding
- Regular progressive uterine contractions
- Significant cephalopelvic disproportion

C. Adverse reactions and contraindications
1. Significant gastrointestinal side effects, including diarrhea, nausea, vomiting, and stomach cramps
2. Fever, chills, flushing, headache, and hypotension
3. Tachysystole (12 or more uterine contractions in 20 minutes without an alteration in the fetal heart rate pattern)
4. Hyperstimulation of the uterus
5. Fetal passage of meconium
6. Contraindications (Box 26-4)

D. Interventions
1. Monitor maternal vital signs, fetal heart rate pattern, and status of pregnancy, including indications of cervical ripening or the induction of **labor,** signs of **labor** or impending **labor,** and the Bishop score (see Chapter 23 for information about the Bishop score)
2. Monitor for adverse reactions to the medication
3. Have the client void before the administration of the medication, and then have her maintain a supine with a lateral tilt or a side-lying position for 30 to 40 minutes after administration
4. Follow agency protocol and instructions from the health care provider for the induction of **labor** if cervical ripening has occurred and **labor** has not begun

V. **MAGNESIUM SULFATE**
A. Description (see Table 26-1)
1. Central nervous system depressant and anticonvulsant
2. Causes smooth muscle relaxation
3. Antidote is calcium gluconate

B. Uses
1. To stop preterm **labor**
2. To prevent and control seizures in preeclamptic and eclamptic clients
C. Adverse reactions and contraindications
1. Can cause respiratory depression, depressed reflexes, flushing, hypotension, extreme muscle weakness, decreased urine output, pulmonary edema, and elevated serum magnesium levels.
2. Continuous IV infusion increases the risk of magnesium toxicity in the **neonate**
3. IV administration should not be used for 2 hours preceding **delivery**
4. Usually continued for the first 12 to 24 hours postpartum if it is used for preeclampsia
5. High doses can cause loss of deep tendon reflexes, heart block, respiratory paralysis, and cardiac arrest
6. Contraindicated in the client with heart block, myocardial damage, or renal failure
7. Used with caution in the client with severe renal impairment
D. Interventions
1. Monitor maternal vital signs, especially respirations, every 30 to 60 minutes
2. Notify the registered nurse or health care provider if respirations are less than 12 breaths per minute (indicating respiratory depression) or if any other adverse reactions occur
3. Assess renal function and electrocardiogram for cardiac function
4. Monitor magnesium levels for the target range of 4 to 7.5 mEq/L (5 to 8 mg/dL); if a rise in the magnesium level occurs, notify the registered nurse or health care provider
5. Administered by IV infusion via an infusion monitoring device such as a controller pump; dose being administered is carefully monitored; follow agency protocol for administration
6. Keep calcium gluconate on hand in case of a magnesium sulfate overdose, because calcium gluconate antagonizes the effect of magnesium sulfate
7. Deep tendon reflexes need to be monitored hourly for signs of developing toxicity
8. Patellar reflex or knee-jerk reflex is tested before the administration of repeat parenteral doses (used as an indicator of central nervous system depression; suppressed reflexes may be a sign of impending respiratory arrest; Table 26-2)
9. Patellar reflex must be present and respiratory rate must be more than 16 breaths per minute (or as designated by agency protocol) before each parenteral dose
10. Monitor intake and output hourly; output should be maintained at 30 mL per hour,

TABLE 26-2 **Assessing Deep Tendon Reflexes**

Grade	Deep Tendon Reflex Response
0	No response
1+	Sluggish or diminished
2+	Active or expected response
3+	More brisk than expected, slightly hyperactive
4+	Brisk, hyperactive, with intermittent or transient clonus

From Seidel, H., et al. (2003). *Mosby's guide to physical examination* (5th ed.). St. Louis: Mosby.

because the medication is eliminated through the kidneys

VI. OPIOID ANALGESICS
A. Used to relieve moderate to severe pain associated with **labor**
B. Administered by the intramuscular or IV route
C. Regular use of opioids during pregnancy may produce withdrawal symptoms in the **neonate** (i.e., irritability, excessive crying, tremors, hyperactive reflexes, fever, vomiting, diarrhea, yawning, sneezing, and seizures)
D. Antidote for opioids: Naloxone (Narcan)
E. Meperidine hydrochloride (Demerol)
   1. Can cause dizziness, nausea, vomiting, sedation, decreased blood pressure, decreased respirations, diaphoresis, flushed face, and decreased urination
   2. May be prescribed to be administered with promethazine (Phenergan) to prevent nausea
   3. High doses may result in respiratory depression, skeletal muscle flaccidity, cold and clammy skin, cyanosis, extreme somnolence progressing to convulsions, stupor, and coma
   4. Is used cautiously in clients delivering preterm **infants**
   5. Is not administered in early **labor,** because it may slow the **labor** process
   6. Is not administered in advanced **labor** (within 1 hour of **delivery**) if the **neonate** is to be delivered before the medication is removed adequately from the fetal circulation (may cause respiratory depression)
F. Morphine sulfate, fentanyl (Sublimaze): Can cause respiratory depression, fetal narcosis/distress, hypotension, and urinary retention
G. Butorphanol tartrate (Stadol), nalbuphine (Nubain)
   1. Cause less respiratory depression than the agonists (morphine)
   2. Use with caution in a client with preexisting opioid dependency, because withdrawal symptoms occur immediately
H. Interventions
   1. Obtain a drug history before administration (butorphanol tartrate [Stadol] is contraindicated if the client has a history of opioid dependency)

BOX 26-5 **Lung Surfactant Replacement Therapy**

- Beractant (Survanta)
- Colfosceril palmitate (Exosurf)

2. Monitor the vital signs, particularly the respiratory status; if respirations are 12 breaths per minute or fewer, withhold the medication and contact the health care provider
3. Monitor the fetal heart rate and characteristics of uterine contractions
4. Monitor for blood pressure changes (hypotension), and notify the registered nurse if they occur; maintain the client in a recumbent position
5. Record the client's response and level of pain relief
6. Monitor the bladder for distention/retention
7. Have antidote available
8. Have antidote naloxone (Narcan) available, especially if **delivery** is going to occur during peak drug absorption time

VII. BETAMETHASONE
A. Description: A corticosteroid that increases the production of **surfactant**
B. Uses: For a client in preterm **labor** between 28 and 32 weeks' gestation whose **labor** can be inhibited for 48 hours without jeopardizing the mother or fetus
C. Adverse reactions and contraindications
   1. May decrease mother's resistance to infection
   2. Pulmonary edema secondary to sodium and fluid retention
   3. Elevated blood glucose levels in the client with diabetes mellitus
D. Interventions
   1. Monitor maternal vital signs, lung sounds, and for edema
   2. Monitor the mother for signs of infection
   3. Monitor the white blood cell count
   4. Monitor the blood glucose levels

VIII. LUNG SURFACTANTS (Box 26-5)
A. Description
   1. Replenish surfactant and restore surface activity to the lungs
   2. Administered by the intratracheal route
B. Uses: To prevent or treat respiratory distress syndrome (hyaline membrane disease) in premature **infants**
C. Adverse reactions and contraindications
   1. Include transient bradycardia and oxygen desaturation
   2. Administered with caution to those at risk for circulatory overload
D. Interventions
   1. Surfactant is instilled through a catheter inserted into the **infant's** endotracheal tube;

avoid suctioning for at least 2 hours after administration

2. Monitor for bradycardia and decreased oxygen saturation during administration

3. Assess lung sounds for crackles and moist breath sounds

IX. RH$_0$(D) IMMUNE GLOBULIN (RHOGAM)

A. Description

1. Prevention of anti-Rh$_0$(D) antibody formation is most successful if the medication is administered twice: at 28 weeks' gestation and again within 72 hours after **delivery**

2. The immune globulin should also be administered within 72 hours after potential or actual exposure to Rh-positive blood; must be given with each subsequent exposure or potential exposure to Rh-positive blood

3. The immune globulin is of no benefit after the client has developed a positive antibody titer to the Rh antigen

B. Uses: To prevent isoimmunization in Rh-negative clients who are exposed or potentially exposed to Rh-positive red blood cells by transfusion, termination of pregnancy, amniocentesis, chorionic villus sampling, abdominal trauma, or bleeding during pregnancy or the birth process

C. Adverse reactions and contraindications

1. Elevated temperature

2. Tenderness at the injection site

3. Contraindicated for Rh-positive women

4. Contraindicated for clients with a history of systemic allergic reactions to preparations containing human immunoglobulins

5. Not administered to a **newborn infant**

D. Interventions

1. Administer to the mother by intramuscular injection at 28 weeks' gestation and within 72 hours after **delivery**

2. Never administered by the IV route

3. Monitor for temperature elevation

4. Monitor the injection site for tenderness

X. EYE PROPHYLAXIS FOR THE NEONATE

A. Description

1. Erythromycin (0.5% Ilotycin) and tetracycline (1%) ophthalmic ointment or drops are bacteriostatic and bactericidal and provide prophylaxis against infection by *Neisseria gonorrhoeae* and *Chlamydia trachomatis*

2. Silver nitrate (1%) solution may be prescribed, but its use is minimal, because it does not protect against chlamydial infection and can cause chemical conjunctivitis

3. Preventive treatment of gonorrhea is required by law

B. Uses: As a prophylactic measure to protect against *Neisseria gonorrhoeae* and *Chlamydia trachomatis*

C. Adverse reactions: Silver nitrate (1%) solution can cause chemical conjunctivitis

D. Interventions

1. Cleanse the **neonate's** eyes before instilling drops or ointment

2. Instill into each of the **neonate's** conjunctival sacs within 1 hour after **delivery**

3. Do not flush the eyes after instillation

XI. VITAMIN K (AQUAMEPHYTON)

A. Description

1. Vitamin K is necessary for aiding in the production of active prothrombin

2. **Newborns** are deficient in vitamin K for the first 5 to 8 days of life because of the lack of intestinal flora that are necessary to absorb vitamin K

B. Uses: For prophylaxis and to treat hemorrhagic disease of the **newborn**

C. Adverse reactions: Can cause hyperbilirubinemia in the **newborn**

D. Interventions

1. Protect the medication from light

2. Administer during the early neonatal period

3. Administer in the vastus lateralis muscle of the thigh

4. Monitor for bruising at the injection site and for bleeding from the cord

5. Monitor for jaundice

6. Monitor the bilirubin level, because the medication can cause hyperbilirubinemia in the **newborn**

XII. RUBELLA VACCINE

A. Description: Given subcutaneously before hospital discharge to nonimmune postpartum clients

B. Uses: Given if rubella titer is less than 1:8

C. Adverse reactions: Transient rash and hypersensitivity

D. Interventions

1. Do not give if the client or other family members are immunocompromised

2. Teach about contraception; the client should avoid pregnancy for 1 to 3 months (as prescribed by the health care provider) after immunization

XIII. HEPATITIS B VACCINE

A. Description: Given intramuscularly to the **newborn** before discharge

B. Use: Recommended for all **infants** to prevent hepatitis B

C. Adverse reactions: Rash, fever, erythema, and pain at the injection site

D. Interventions

1. Parental consent must be obtained

2. Administer in the middle third of the vastus lateralis intramuscularly

3. If the **infant** was born to a mother who is positive for hepatitis B surface antigen, hepatitis B

immune globulin should be given within 12 hours of birth in addition to the hepatitis B vaccine; the regularly scheduled hepatitis B virus vaccination schedule should then be followed

PRACTICE QUESTIONS

More questions on the companion CD!

272. Methylergonovine (Methergine) is prescribed for a woman to treat postpartum hemorrhage. Before the administration of methylergonovine, the priority nursing assessment is to check the:
    1. Uterine tone
    2. Blood pressure
    3. Amount of lochia
    4. Deep tendon reflexes

273. A nurse is caring for a client who is receiving oxytocin (Pitocin) to induce labor. The nurse discontinues the oxytocin infusion and notifies the registered nurse if which of the following is noted during the assessment of the client?
    1. Fatigue
    2. Drowsiness
    3. Uterine hyperstimulation
    4. Early decelerations of the fetal heart rate

274. A pregnant client is receiving magnesium sulfate for the management of preeclampsia. A nurse determines that the client is experiencing toxicity from the medication if which of the following is noted on assessment?
    1. Proteinuria of 3+
    2. Presence of deep tendon reflexes
    3. Serum magnesium level of 6 mEq/L
    4. Respirations of 10 breaths per minute

275. Epidural analgesia is administered to a woman for pain relief after a cesarean birth. The nurse assigned to care for the woman ensures that which medication is readily available if respiratory depression occurs?
    1. Betamethasone
    2. Morphine sulfate
    3. Naloxone (Narcan)
    4. Meperidine hydrochloride (Demerol)

276. $Rh_0(D)$ immune globulin (RhoGAM) is prescribed for a woman after the delivery of a newborn infant, and the nurse provides information to the woman about the purpose of the medication. The nurse determines that the woman understands the purpose of the medication if the woman states that it will protect her next baby from which of the following?
    1. Having Rh-positive blood
    2. Developing a rubella infection
    3. Developing physiological jaundice
    4. Being affected by Rh incompatibility

277. A woman with preeclampsia is receiving magnesium sulfate. The nurse assigned to care for the client determines that the magnesium sulfate therapy is effective if:
    1. Scotomas are present.
    2. Seizures do not occur.
    3. Ankle clonus is noted.
    4. The blood pressure decreases.

278. Methylergonovine (Methergine) is prescribed for a client with postpartum hemorrhage. Before administering the medication, a nurse contacts the health care provider who prescribed the medication if which of the following conditions is documented in the client's medical history?
    1. Hypotension
    2. Hypothyroidism
    3. Diabetes mellitus
    4. Peripheral vascular disease

279. A nursing instructor asks a nursing student to describe the procedure for administering erythromycin (0.5% Ilotycin) ointment to the eyes of a neonate. The instructor determines that the student needs to research this procedure further if the student states:
    1. "I will flush the eyes after instilling the ointment."
    2. "I will cleanse the neonate's eyes before instilling the ointment."
    3. "The administration of the eye ointment is within 1 hour after delivery."
    4. "I will instill the eye ointment into each of the neonate's conjunctival sacs."

280. A 31-week preterm labor client dilated to 4 centimeters has been started on magnesium sulfate. Her contractions have stopped. If the client's labor can be inhibited for the next 48 hours, what medication does the nurse anticipate will be prescribed?
    1. Betamethasone
    2. Nalbuphine (Nubain)
    3. Misoprostol (Cytotec)
    4. $Rh_0(D)$ immune globulin (RhoGAM)

ALTERNATE ITEM FORMAT: MUTIPLE RESPONSE

281. A nurse is monitoring a preterm labor client who is receiving magnesium sulfate intravenously. The nurse monitors for which adverse reactions of this medication? Select all that apply.
    ☑ 1. Flushing
    ☐ 2. Hypertension
    ☐ 3. Increased urine output
    ☑ 4. Depressed respirations
    ☑ 5. Extreme muscle weakness
    ☐ 6. Hyperactive deep tendon reflexes

ANSWERS

272. 2

Rationale: Methylergonovine, which is an ergot alkaloid, is an agent that is used to prevent or control postpartum hemorrhage by contracting the uterus. Methylergonovine causes continuous uterine contractions and may elevate the blood pressure. A priority assessment before the administration of the medication is to check the blood pressure. The physician should be notified if hypertension is present. Although options 1, 3, and 4 may be components of the postpartum assessment, option 2 is related specifically to the administration of this medication.

Test-Taking Strategy: Use the process of elimination. Eliminate options 1 and 3 first, because they are comparable or alike and related to one another. From the remaining options, use the ABCs—airway, breathing, and circulation. Obtaining the blood pressure is a method of assessing circulation. Review the adverse effects of methylergonovine if you had difficulty with this question.

Level of Cognitive Ability: Analysis
Client Needs: Physiological Integrity
Integrated Process: Nursing Process/Data Collection
Content Area: Maternity/Postpartum
References: Lilley, L., Harrington, S., & Snyder, J. (2005). *Pharmacology and the nursing process* (4th ed., p. 59). St. Louis: Mosby.
Murray, S., & McKinney, E., (2006). *Foundations of maternal-newborn nursing* (4th ed., p. 662). Philadelphia: Saunders.

273. 3

Rationale: Oxytocin stimulates uterine contractions, and it is one of the common pharmacological methods used to induce labor. An adverse reaction associated with the administration of the medication is the hyperstimulation of uterine contractions. Therefore, oxytocin infusion must be stopped when any signs of uterine hyperstimulation are present. Drowsiness and fatigue may be caused by the labor experience. Early decelerations of the fetal heart rate are a reassuring sign and do not indicate fetal distress.

Test-Taking Strategy: Use the process of elimination, and focus on the subject of an adverse reaction to oxytocin. Options 1 and 2 can be eliminated first. From the remaining options, recalling that early decelerations of the fetal heart rate are a reassuring sign will direct you to option 3. Review the nursing responsibilities associated with oxytocin if you had difficulty with this question.

Level of Cognitive Ability: Analysis
Client Needs: Physiological Integrity
Integrated Process: Nursing Process/Implementation
Content Area: Maternity/Intrapartum
References: Hodgson, B., & Kizior, R. (2007). *Saunders nursing drug handbook 2007* (p. 885). St. Louis: Saunders.
Wong, D., Hockenberry, M., Perry, S., Lowdermilk, D. & Wilson, D. (2006). *Maternal-child nursing care* (3rd ed., p. 567). St. Louis: Mosby.

274. 4

Rationale: Magnesium toxicity can occur as a result of magnesium sulfate therapy. Signs of magnesium sulfate toxicity relate to the central nervous system depressant effects of the medication and include respiratory depression, a loss of deep tendon reflexes, and a sudden drop in fetal heart rate, maternal heart rate, and blood pressure. Therapeutic serum levels of magnesium are 4 to 7.5 mEq/L. Proteinuria of 3+ is likely to be noted in a client with preeclampsia.

Test-Taking Strategy: Use the process of elimination. Eliminate option 2 first, because it is a normal finding. Next, eliminate option 3, knowing that the therapeutic serum level of magnesium is between 4 and 7.5 mEq/L. From the remaining options, recalling that proteinuria of 3+ would be noted in a client with preeclampsia will direct you to the correct option. Review the adverse effects of magnesium sulfate if you had difficulty with this question.

Level of Cognitive Ability: Analysis
Client Needs: Physiological Integrity
Integrated Process: Nursing Process/Data Collection
Content Area: Maternity/Intrapartum
References: Hodgson, B., & Kizior, R. (2007). *Saunders nursing drug handbook 2007* (pp. 717-720). St. Louis: Saunders.
McKinney, E., James, S., Murray, S., & Ashwill, J. (2005). *Maternal-child nursing* (2nd ed., pp. 640-641, 637). Philadelphia: Saunders.

275. 3

Rationale: Opioids are used for epidural analgesia. An adverse reaction of epidural analgesia is a delayed respiratory depression. Naloxone (Narcan) is a opioid antagonist, which reverses the effects of opioids and is given for respiratory depression. Morphine sulfate and meperidine hydrochloride are opioid analgesics. Betamethasone is a corticosteroid that is administered to enhance fetal lung maturity.

Test-Taking Strategy: Use the process of elimination, and focus on the subject of the question: the antidote for respiratory depression. Eliminate options 2 and 4 first, knowing that these medications are opioid analgesics. Next, eliminate option 1, knowing that this medication is a corticosteroid. Review the purposes and actions of these medications if you had difficulty with this question.

Level of Cognitive Ability: Application
Client Needs: Physiological Integrity
Integrated Process: Nursing Process/Planning
Content Area: Maternity/Postpartum
References: Lilley, L., Harrington, S., & Snyder, J. (2005). *Pharmacology and the nursing process* (4th ed., p. 154). St. Louis: Mosby.
Murray, S., & McKinney, E., (2006). *Foundations of maternal-newborn nursing* (4th ed., pp. 348, 351). Philadelphia: Saunders.

276. 4

Rationale: Rh incompatibility can occur when an Rh-negative mother becomes sensitized to the Rh antigen. Sensitization may develop when an Rh-negative woman becomes pregnant with a fetus who is Rh positive. During pregnancy and at delivery, some of the baby's Rh-positive blood can enter the maternal circulation, thus causing the woman's immune system to form antibodies against the Rh-positive blood. The administration of $Rh_0(D)$ immune globulin prevents the woman from developing antibodies against Rh-positive blood by providing passive antibody protection against the Rh antigen.

Test-Taking Strategy: Use the process of elimination. Options 2 and 3 can be eliminated first. From the remaining options, note the relationship between the name of the medication, $Rh_0(D)$ immune globulin, and the word "incompatibility" in the correct option. Review the purpose of $Rh_0(D)$ immune globulin if you had difficulty with this question.
Level of Cognitive Ability: Analysis
Client Needs: Physiological Integrity
Integrated Process: Teaching and Learning
Content Area: Maternity/Postpartum
References: Hodgson, B., & Kizior, R. (2007). *Saunders nursing drug handbook 2007* (pp. 1014-1016). St. Louis: Saunders.
Murray, S., & McKinney, E., (2006). *Foundations of maternal-newborn nursing* (4th ed., p. 411). Philadelphia: Saunders.

277. 2
Rationale: For a client with preeclampsia, the goal of care is directed at preventing eclampsia (seizures). Magnesium sulfate is an anticonvulsant rather than an antihypertensive agent. Although a decrease in blood pressure may be noted initially, this effect is usually transient. Ankle clonus indicates hyperreflexia and may precede the onset of eclampsia. Scotomas are areas of complete or partial blindness. Visual disturbances, such as scotomas, often precede an eclamptic seizure.
Test-Taking Strategy: Use the process of elimination. Knowing that magnesium sulfate is an anticonvulsant will direct you to option 2. Review magnesium sulfate if you had difficulty with this question.
Level of Cognitive Ability: Analysis
Client Needs: Physiological Integrity
Integrated Process: Nursing Process/Evaluation
Content Area: Maternity/Intrapartum
References: Lilley, L., Harrington, S., & Snyder, J. (2005). *Pharmacology and the nursing process* (4th ed., p. 906). St. Louis: Mosby.
McKinney, E., James, S., Murray, S., & Ashwill, J. (2005). *Maternal-child nursing* (2nd ed., p. 638). St. Louis: Saunders.

278. 4
Rationale: Methylergonovine is an ergot alkaloid that is used to treat postpartum hemorrhage. Ergot alkaloids are avoided in clients with significant cardiovascular disease, peripheral vascular disease, hypertension, eclampsia, or preeclampsia, because these conditions are worsened by the vasoconstrictive effects of the ergot alkaloids. Options 1, 2, and 3 are not contraindications related to the use of ergot alkaloids.
Test-Taking Strategy: Use the process of elimination. Recalling that ergot alkaloids produce vasoconstriction will direct you to option 4. Review the effects of ergot alkaloids and the associated contraindications if you had difficulty with this question.
Level of Cognitive Ability: Analysis
Client Needs: Physiological Integrity
Integrated Process: Nursing Process/Implementation
Content Area: Maternity/Postpartum
References: Hodgson, B., & Kizior, R. (2007). *Saunders nursing drug handbook 2007* (pp. 754-756). St. Louis: Saunders.
McKinney, E., James, S., Murray, S., & Ashwill, J. (2005). *Maternal-child nursing* (2nd ed., p. 704). St. Louis: Saunders.

279. 1
Rationale: Eye prophylaxis protects the neonate against *Neisseria gonorrhoeae* and *Chlamydia trachomatis*. The eyes are not flushed after the instillation of the medication, because the flush will wash away the administered medication. Options 2, 3, and 4 are correct statements regarding the procedure for administering eye medication to the neonate.
Test-Taking Strategy: Use the process of elimination, and note the strategic words "needs to research." These words indicate a negative event query and ask you to select an option that is an incorrect statement. Eliminate options 3 and 4 first, because they are comparable or alike. From the remaining options, visualize the effect of each. This will direct you to option 1. Review the procedure for administering eye medication to the neonate if you had difficulty with this question.
Level of Cognitive Ability: Analysis
Client Needs: Safe and Effective Care Environment
Integrated Process: Teaching and Learning
Content Area: Maternity/Postpartum
Reference: Murray, S., & McKinney, E. (2006). *Foundations of maternal-newborn nursing* (4th ed., p. 513). Philadelphia: Saunders.

280. 1
Rationale: Betamethasone, which is a glucocorticoid, is given to stimulate fetal lung maturation. It is used for clients in preterm labor between 28 and 32 weeks' gestation if the labor can be inhibited for 48 hours. Nalbuphine (Nubain) is an opioid analgesic. Misoprostol (Cytotec) is a prostaglandin that is given to ripen and soften the cervix and to stimulate uterine contractions. $Rh_0(D)$ immune globulin (RhoGAM) is given to RH-negative clients to prevent sensitization.
Test-Taking Strategy: Use the process of elimination. Noting the strategic words "31-week preterm labor client" and recalling that betamethasone is used to stimulate surfactant release will direct you to option 1. Review the purpose and actions of the medications in the options if you had difficulty with this question.
Level of Cognitive Ability: Analysis
Client Needs: Physiological Integrity
Integrated Process: Nursing Process/Planning
Content Area: Maternity/Intrapartum
Reference: Lowdermilk, D., & Perry, S. (2006). *Maternity nursing* (7th ed., p. 780). St. Louis: Mosby.

ALTERNATE ITEM FORMAT: MULTIPLE RESPONSE
281. 1, 4, 5
Rationale: Magnesium sulfate is a central nervous system depressant, and it relaxes smooth muscle, including the uterus. It is used to halt preterm labor contractions, and it is used for preeclamptic clients to prevent seizures. Adverse effects include flushing, depressed respirations, depressed deep tendon reflexes, hypotension, extreme muscle weakness, decreased urine output, pulmonary edema, and elevated serum magnesium levels.
Test-Taking Strategy: Focus on the subject of adverse effects of magnesium sulfate. Recalling that this medication is a central nervous system depressant will assist you with answering

correctly. Review the adverse effects of magnesium sulfate if you had difficulty with this question.
Level of Cognitive Ability: Analysis
Client Needs: Physiological Integrity

Integrated Process: Nursing Process/Data Collection
Content Area: Maternity/Intrapartum
Reference: Hodgson, B., & Kizior, R. (2007). *Saunders nursing drug book 2007* (pp. 717-720). St. Louis: Saunders.

REFERENCES

Hodgson, B., & Kizior, R. (2007). *Saunders nursing drug handbook 2007* St. Louis: Saunders.

Kee, J., Hayes, E., & McCuistion, L. (2006). *Pharmacology: A nursing process approach* (5th ed.). St. Louis: Saunders.

Lilley, L., Harrington, S., & Snyder, J. (2005). *Pharmacology and the nursing process* (4th ed.). St. Louis: Mosby.

Lowdermilk, D., & Perry, S. (2006). *Maternity nursing* (7th ed.). St. Louis: Mosby.

Lowdermilk, D., & Perry, S. (2004). *Maternity and women's health care* (8th ed.). St. Louis: Mosby.

McKinney, E., James, S., Murray, S., & Ashwill, J. (2005). *Maternal-child nursing* (2nd ed.). St. Louis: Saunders.

Murray, S., & McKinney, E. (2006). *Foundations of maternal-newborn nursing* (4th ed.). Philadelphia: Saunders.

National Council of State Boards of Nursing (Eds.). (2008). *2008 Detailed Test Plan for the NCLEX-PN® Examination, National Council of State Boards of Nursing.* Chicago: Author.

National Council of State Boards of Nursing. *NSCBN home page.* www.ncsbn.org. Accessed July 9, 2008.

Wong, D., Hockenberry, M., Perry, S., Lowdermilk, D., & Wilson, D. (2006). *Maternal-child nursing care* (3rd ed.). St. Louis: Mosby.

Growth and Development Across the Life Span

PYRAMID TERMS

abuse The willful infliction of pain, injury, mental anguish, or unreasonable confinement. Abuse can include verbal assaults, the demand to perform demeaning tasks, theft, or the mismanagement of personal belongings. Abuse can be physical, emotional, or sexual.

accommodation The ability to change a schema (an individual's cognitive structure or framework of thought) to introduce new ideas, objects, or experiences.

aging The biopsychosocial process of change that occurs between birth and death.

assimilation The ability to incorporate new ideas, objects, and experiences into the framework of one's thoughts.

conscious All experiences that are within an individual's awareness and that the individual is able to control.

dementia An organic syndrome that is identified by a gradual and progressive deterioration in intellectual functioning. Long- and short-term memory loss occurs with impairments in judgment, abstract thinking, problem-solving ability, and behavior; these result in a self-care deficit. A common type of dementia is Alzheimer's disease.

depression A mood disorder that can be identified by feelings of sadness, hopelessness, and worthlessness and a decreased interest in activities.

ego One's "sense of self." The ego provides functions such as problem solving, the mobilization of defense mechanisms, reality testing, and the capability of functioning independently; it is the mediator between the id and the superego.

exploitation The illegal or improper use of an individual's resources.

gerontology The study of the process of aging.

id The source of all primitive drives and instincts; the id is thought of as the reservoir of all psychic energy.

neglect The lack of providing the services necessary for physical or mental health, including a failure to prevent injury.

polypharmacy The taking of multiple prescription and/or over-the-counter medications together.

self-neglect The choice to avoid medical care or other services that could improve one's optimal function. Unless an individual has been declared legally incompetent, he or she has the right to refuse care.

subconscious The experiences, thoughts, feelings, and desires that may not be in immediate awareness of an individual but that can be recalled to consciousness. The subconscious helps to repress unpleasant thoughts or feelings; it is often called the *preconscious*.

superego The moral component of the personality that includes the internalization of the values, ideals, and moral standards of society.

unconscious Memories, feelings, thoughts, and wishes that are repressed and that are not available to the conscious mind.

PYRAMID TO SUCCESS

Normal growth and development proceed in an orderly, systematic, and predictable pattern that provides a basis for identifying and assessing an individual's abilities. Understanding the path of growth and development across the life span assists the nurse with identifying appropriate and expected human behavior. The Pyramid to Success focuses on Sigmund Freud's theory of psychosexual development, Jean Piaget's theory of cognitive development, Erik Erikson's psychosocial theory, and Lawrence Kohlberg's theory of moral development. Growth and development concepts focus on the aging process and on physical characteristics, nutritional behaviors, skills, play, and specific safety measures that are relevant to a particular age group that will ensure a safe and hazard-free environment. When a question is presented on the NCLEX-PN, if an age is identified in the question, note the age, and think about the associated growth and developmental concepts. The Integrated Processes addressed in this unit include Caring, Communication and Documentation, the Clinical Problem-Solving Process (Nursing Process), and Teaching and Learning.

▲ CLIENT NEEDS

Safe and Effective Care Environment

Acting as a client advocate
Consulting with members of the health care team
Establishing priorities
Maintaining confidentiality
Preventing accidents
Providing care in accordance with ethical and legal standards
Respecting client and family needs on the basis of their preferences
Upholding client's rights

Health Promotion and Maintenance

Identifying changes that occur as a result of the aging process
Providing client and family education
Identifying developmental stages and transitions
Identifying expected body image changes
Monitoring growth and development
Respecting health care beliefs and preferences
Discussing lifestyle choices

Psychosocial Integrity

Assessing for abuse and neglect
Monitoring for adjustment to potential deteriorations in physical and mental health and well-being in the older client
Monitoring for changes in and adjustment to role functioning in the older client (i.e., threats to independent functioning)
Identifying coping mechanisms
Considering grief and loss issues with the older client
Identifying the loss of the quantity and quality of relationships with the older client
Monitoring for sensory and perceptual alterations
Identifying support systems
Providing resources for the client and family

Physiological Integrity

Monitoring for alterations in body systems and the related risks of the aging process
Providing basic care and comfort needs
Identifying health care preferences
Providing interventions that are compatible with the client's age; cultural, religious, and health care beliefs; education level; and language
Identifying practices or restrictions related to procedures and treatments
Providing care with the use of a nonjudgmental approach
Administering medications safely

REFERENCES

Burke, M., & Laramie, J. (2004). *Primary care of the older adults: A multidisciplinary approach* (2nd ed.). St. Louis: Mosby.

Ebersole, P., Hess, P., & Luggan, A. (2004). *Toward healthy aging: Human needs and nursing response* (6th ed.). St. Louis: Mosby.

Hockenberry, M., Wilson, D., & Winkelstein, M. (2005). *Wong's essentials of pediatric nursing* (7th ed.). St. Louis: Mosby.

Ignatavicius, D., & Workman, M. (2006). *Medical-surgical nursing: Critical thinking for collaborative care* (5th ed.). Philadelphia: Saunders.

Leifer, G. (2007). *Introduction to maternity and pediatric nursing* (5th ed.). Philadelphia: Saunders.

Meiner, S., & Leuckenotte, A. (2006). *Gerontologic nursing* (3rd ed.). St. Louis: Mosby.

Murray, S., & McKinney, E. (2006). *Foundations of maternal-newborn nursing* (4th ed.). Philadelphia: Saunders.

National Council of State Boards of Nursing (Eds.). (2008). *2008 Detailed Test Plan for the NCLEX-PN® Examination, National Council of State Boards of Nursing.* Chicago: Author.

National Council of State Boards of Nursing. *NCSBN home page.* www.ncsbn.org. Accessed July 9, 2008.

Potter, P., & Perry, A. (2005). *Fundamentals of nursing* (6th ed.). St. Louis: Mosby.

Price, D., & Gwin, J. (2008). *Pediatric nursing: An introductory text* (10th ed.). St. Louis: Saunders.

Stuart, G., & Laraia, M. (2005). *Principles and practice of psychiatric nursing* (8th ed.). St. Louis: Mosby.

Varcarolis, E., Carson, V., & Shoemaker, N. (2006). *Foundations of psychiatric mental health nursing: A clinical approach* (5th ed.). Philadelphia: Saunders.

Wold, G. (2008). *Basic geriatric nursing* (4th ed.). St. Louis: Mosby.

Wong, D., Hockenberry, M., Perry, S., Lowdermilk, D., & Wilson, D. (2006). *Maternal-child nursing care* (3rd ed.). St. Louis: Mosby.

Theories of Growth and Development

I. PSYCHOSOCIAL DEVELOPMENT AND ERIK ERIKSON
A. The theory
1. Describes the human life cycle as a series of eight **ego** developmental stages from birth to death
2. Each stage presents a psychosocial crisis, the goal of which is to integrate physical, maturational, and societal demands
3. Focuses on psychosocial tasks that are accomplished throughout the life cycle
4. The **ego** is separate and liberated from the **id**, developing across the course of the complete life cycle
5. **Ego** development is influenced by familial, social, and developmental factors
B. Psychosocial development
1. A lifelong series of conflicts affected by social and cultural factors
2. Each conflict must be resolved for the child or adult to progress emotionally
3. Unsuccessful resolution leaves the individual emotionally handicapped
C. Stages of psychosocial development (Table 27-1)

II. COGNITIVE DEVELOPMENT AND JEAN PIAGET
A. The theory
1. Defines cognitive acts as the ways in which the mind organizes and adapts to its environment
2. Schema: Refers to an individual's cognitive structure or framework of thought
3. Schemata
   a. Categories that an individual forms in his or her mind to organize and understand the world
   b. A young child has only a few schemata with which to understand the world; gradually these are increased
   c. Adults use a wide variety of schemata to understand the world
4. **Assimilation**
   a. The ability to incorporate new ideas, objects, and experiences into the framework of one's thoughts
   b. The growing child will perceive and give meaning to new information according to what is already known and understood
5. **Accommodation**
   a. The ability to change a schema to introduce new ideas, objects, or experiences
   b. Changes the mental structure so that new experiences can be added
B. Stages of cognitive development
1. Sensorimotor stage
   a. 0 to 2 years
   b. Development proceeds from reflex activity to imagining and solving problems through the senses and movement
2. Preoperational stage
   a. 2 to 7 years
   b. Learning to think in terms of past, present, and future
   c. The child moves from knowing the world through sensation and movement to prelogical thinking and finding solutions to problems
3. Concrete operational
   a. 7 to 11 years
   b. Able to classify, order, and sort facts
   c. The child moves from prelogical thought to solving concrete problems through logic
4. Formal operations
   a. 11 years to adulthood
   b. Able to think abstractly and logically
   c. Logical thinking is expanded to include solving abstract and concrete problems

III. MORAL DEVELOPMENT AND LAWRENCE KOHLBERG
A. Moral development
1. A complicated process involving the acceptance of the values and rules of society in a way that shapes behavior
2. Classified into a series of levels and behaviors
B. Levels of moral development (Box 27-1)

TABLE 27-1 Erik Erikson's Stages of Psychosocial Development

Age	Psychosocial Crisis	Task
Infancy (birth to 18 months)	Trust vs. mistrust	Attachment to the mother
Resolution of Crisis		
Trust in other people; faith and hope about the environment and the future		
Unsuccessful Resolution of Crisis		
General difficulties relating to others effectively; suspicion; trust/fear conflict; fear of the future		

Age	Psychosocial Crisis	Task
Early childhood (18 months to 3 years)	Autonomy vs. shame and doubt	Gaining some basic control over the self and the environment
Resolution of Crisis		
Sense of self-control and adequacy; will power		
Unsuccessful Resolution of Crisis		
Independence/fear conflict; severe feelings of self-doubt		

Age	Psychosocial Crisis	Task
Late childhood (3-6 years)	Initiative vs. guilt	Becoming purposeful and directive
Resolution of Crisis		
Ability to initiate one's own activities; sense of purpose		
Unsuccessful Resolution of Crisis		
Aggression/fear conflict; sense of inadequacy or guilt		

Age	Psychosocial Crisis	Task
School age (6-12 years)	Industry vs. inferiority	Developing social, physical, and learning skills
Resolution of Crisis		
Competence; ability to learn and work		
Unsuccessful Resolution of Crisis		
Sense of inferiority; difficulty learning and working		

Age	Psychosocial Crisis	Task
Adolescence (12-20 years)	Identity vs. role confusion	Developing a sense of identity
Resolution of Crisis		
Sense of personal identity		
Unsuccessful Resolution of Crisis		
Confusion about who one is; identity submerged in relationships or group memberships		

Age	Psychosocial Crisis	Task
Early adulthood (20-35 years)	Intimacy vs. isolation	Establishing intimate bonds of love and friendship
Resolution of Crisis		
Ability to love deeply and commit oneself		
Unsuccessful Resolution of Crisis		
Emotional isolation; egocentricity		

Age	Psychosocial Crisis	Task
Middle adulthood (35-65 years)	Generativity vs. stagnation	Fulfilling life goals that involve family, career, and society
Resolution of Crisis		
Ability to give and care for others		
Unsuccessful Resolution of Crisis		
Self-absorption; inability to grow as a person		

Age	Psychosocial Crisis	Task
Later (65 years to death)	Integrity vs. despair	Looking back over one's life and accepting its meaning
Resolution of Crisis		
Sense of integrity and fulfillment		
Unsuccessful Resolution of Crisis		
Dissatisfaction with life		

Modified from Varcarolis, E. (2006). *Foundations of psychiatric mental health nursing* (5th ed.). Philadelphia: Saunders.

BOX 27-1   **Moral Development and Lawrence Kohlberg**

Level One: Preconventional Morality
Stage 0 (Birth-2 years): Egocentric Judgment
The infant has no awareness of right or wrong.
Stage 1 (2-3 years): Punishment-Obedience Orientation
At this stage, children cannot reason as mature members of society.
Children view the world in a selfish way, with no real understanding of right or wrong.
The child obeys rules and demonstrates acceptable behavior to avoid punishment and displeasing those who are in power and because he or she fears punishment from a superior force, such as a parent.
A toddler typically is at the first substage of the preconventional stage; this involves a punishment-obedience orientation in which the toddler makes judgments on the basis of avoiding punishment or obtaining a reward.
Physical punishment and withholding privileges tend to give the toddler a negative view of morals.
Withdrawing love and affection as punishment leads to feelings of guilt in the toddler.
Appropriate discipline includes providing simple explanations of why certain behaviors are not acceptable, praising appropriate behavior, and using distractions when the toddler is headed for danger.
Stage 2 (4-7 years): Instrumental Relativist Orientation
The child conforms to rules to obtain rewards or to have favors returned.
The child's moral standards are those of others, and the child observes them to avoid punishment or obtain rewards.
A preschooler is in the preconventional stage of moral development.
During this stage, the conscience emerges, and the emphasis is on external control.
Level Two: Conventional Morality
The child conforms to rules to please others.
The child has an increased awareness of others' feelings.
A concern for social order begins to emerge.
A child views good behavior as that of which those in authority will approve.
If the behavior is not acceptable, the child feels guilty.
Stage 3 (7-10 years): Good Boy–Nice Girl Orientation
Conformity occurs to avoid disapproval or dislike by others.

This stage involves living up to what is expected by individuals close to the child or what individuals generally expect of others in their roles as son, brother, friend, and so on.
Being good is important and is interpreted as having good motives and showing concern about others.
It also means maintaining mutual relationships with the use of such characteristics as trust, loyalty, respect, and gratitude.
Stage 4 (10-12 years): Law and Order Orientation
The child has more concern with society as a whole.
The emphasis is on obeying laws to maintain social order.
Moral reasoning develops as the child shifts the focus of living to society.
The school-age child is at the conventional level of the role-conformity stage and has an increased desire to please others.
The child observes and to some extent internalizes the standards of others.
The child wants to be considered "good" by those individuals whose opinions matter to him or her.
Level Three: Postconventional Morality
The individual focuses on individual rights and principles of conscience.
The focus is a concern regarding what is best for all.
Stage 5 (12 years and older): Social Contract and Legalistic Orientation
The adolescent is aware that people hold a variety of values and opinions and that most values and rules are relative to the group.
The adolescent in this stage gives as well as takes and does not expect to get something without paying for it.
Stage 6: Universal Ethical Principles Orientation
Conformity is based on universal principles of justice and occurs to avoid self-condemnation.
This stage involves following self-chosen ethical principles.
The development of the postconventional level of morality occurs in the adolescent at about the age of 13 years; it is marked by the development of an individual conscience and a defined set of moral values.
The adolescent can now acknowledge a conflict between two socially accepted standards and try to decide between them.
The control of conduct is now internal, both in standards observed and in reasoning about right and wrong.

IV. **PSYCHOSEXUAL DEVELOPMENT**
   AND SIGMUND FREUD
A. Components of the theory (Box 27-2)
   1. Levels of awareness
   2. Agencies of the mind (**id, ego, superego**)
   3. Concept of anxiety and defense mechanisms
   4. Psychosexual stages of development
B. Levels of awareness
   1. **Conscious** level of awareness
      a. The **conscious** mind is logical and regulated by the reality principle
      b. Includes all experiences that are within an individual's awareness and that the individual is able to control

BOX 27-2   **Psychosexual Development and Sigmund Freud: Components of the Theory**

- Levels of awareness
- Agencies of the mind: id, ego, and superego
- Concept of anxiety and defense mechanisms
- Psychosexual stages of development

      c. Includes all information that is easily remembered and immediately available to an individual

2. Preconscious level of awareness
   a. Also called the *subconscious*
   b. Includes experiences, thoughts, feelings, or desires that might not be in an individual's immediate awareness but that can be recalled to consciousness
   c. Can help repress unpleasant thoughts or feelings and examine and censor certain wishes and thinking
3. **Unconscious** level of awareness
   a. Not logical; governed by the pleasure principle, which refers to seeking immediate tension reduction
   b. Memories, feelings, thoughts, and wishes are repressed and not available to the **conscious** mind
   c. These repressed memories, thoughts, or feelings, if made prematurely **conscious**, can cause anxiety
C. Agencies of the mind
   1. Id, **ego**, and **superego**
      a. The three systems of personality
      b. The psychological processes that follow different operating principles
      c. In a mature and well-adjusted personality, they work together as a team under the leadership of the **ego**
   2. The **id**
      a. Source of all drives
      b. Present at birth
      c. Includes genetic inheritance, reflexes, capacities to respond, instincts, basic drives, needs, and wishes that motivate an individual
      d. Operates according to the pleasure principle
      e. The **id** does not tolerate uncomfortable states and seeks to discharge tension and return to a more comfortable, constant level of energy
      f. The **id** acts immediately in an impulsive, irrational way; pays no attention to the consequences of its actions; and therefore often behaves in ways that are harmful to the self and others
      g. The primary process is a psychological activity in which the **id** attempts to reduce tension
      h. The primary process can include hallucinating or forming an image of the object that will satisfy needs and remove tension
      i. The primary process by itself is not capable of reducing tension; therefore, a secondary psychological process must develop if the individual is to survive; when this occurs, the structure of the second system of the personality, the **ego**, begins to take form
   3. The **ego**
      a. The functions of the **ego** include reality testing and problem solving

b. Begins its development during the fourth or fifth month of life
c. The **ego** emerges out of the **id** and acts as an intermediary between the **id** and the external world
d. Emerges because the needs, wishes, and demands of the **id** require appropriate exchanges with the outside world of reality
e. Distinguishes between things in the mind and things in the external world
f. Reality testing is a function of the **ego**, and the **ego** uses realistic thinking
g. The **ego** follows the reality principle and operates by means of the secondary process of realistic thinking
h. The aim of the reality principle is to satisfy the **id's** impulses in the external world with an object that is suitable; the reality principle determines whether an experience is true or false and whether it has external existence
i. The **ego** devises a plan and tests the plan by some kind of action to see if it will work
4. The **superego**
   a. A necessary part of socialization that develops during the phallic stage of 3 to 6 years of age
   b. It develops from the interactions with one's parents during the extended period of childhood dependency
   c. It includes the internalization of the values, ideals, and moral standards of society
   d. The child internalizes the moral standards of the parents and society
   e. The **superego** consists of the conscience and the **ego** ideal
   f. The conscience refers to the capacity for self-evaluation and criticism
   g. When moral codes are violated, the conscience punishes the individual by instilling guilt
   h. What parents approve of and what they reward the child for doing become incorporated as the **ego** ideal by the mechanism of introjection
   i. The **superego** strives for perfection rather than pleasure and represents the ideal rather than the real
   j. Living up to one's **ego** ideal results in the individual feeling proud and increases self-esteem
D. Anxiety and defense mechanisms
   1. The **ego** develops defenses or defense mechanisms to fight off anxiety
   2. Defense mechanisms operate on an **unconscious** level (except for suppression), so the individual is not aware of their operation

BOX 27-3 **Freud's Psychosexual Stages of Development**

Oral Stage (Birth-1 year)
During this stage, the infant is concerned with his or her own gratification.

The infant is all id, operating on the pleasure principle and striving for the immediate gratification of his or her needs.

When the infant experiences the gratification of basic needs, a sense of trust and security begins.

The ego begins to emerge as the infant begins to see him- or herself as separate from the mother; this marks the beginning of the development of a sense of self.

Anal Stage (1-3 years)
Toilet training occurs during this period, and the child gains pleasure from both the elimination and retention of feces.

The conflict of this stage is between demands from society and parents and the sensations of pleasure associated with the anus.

The child begins to gain a sense of control over instinctive drives and learns to delay immediate gratification to gain a future goal.

Phallic Stage (3-6 years)
The child experiences both pleasurable and conflicting feelings associated with the genital organs.

The pleasures of masturbation and the fantasy life of children set the stage for the Oedipus complex.

The child's unconscious sexual attraction to and wish to possess the parent of the opposite sex, the hostility toward and desire to remove the parent of the same sex, and the subsequent guilt regarding these wishes comprise the conflict that the child faces.

The conflict is resolved when the child identifies with the parent of the same sex.

The emergence of the superego is both the solution to and the result of these intense impulses.

Latency Stage (6-12 years)
During this stage, there is a tapering off of conscious biological and sexual urges.

The sexual impulses are channeled and elevated into a more culturally accepted level of activity.

The growth of ego functions and the ability to care about and relate to others outside of the home are the tasks of this stage of development.

Genital Stage (12 years and beyond)
This emerges at adolescence with the onset of puberty, when the genital organs mature.

The individual gains gratification from his or her own body.

During this stage, the individual develops satisfying sexual and emotional relationships with members of the opposite sex.

The individual plans life goals and gains a strong sense of personal identity.

---

3. Defense mechanisms deny, falsify, or distort reality to make it less threatening

4. An individual cannot survive without defense mechanisms; however, if they become too extreme in distorting reality, then interference in healthy adjustment and personal growth may occur

E. Psychosexual stages of development (Box 27-3)

▲ 1. Human development proceeds through a series of stages from infancy to adulthood

2. Each stage is characterized by the inborn tendency of all individuals to reduce tension and seek pleasure

▲ 3. Each stage is associated with a particular conflict that must be resolved before the child can move successfully to the next stage

▲ 4. Experiences during the early stages determine an individual's adjustment patterns and the personality traits that the individual has as an adult

PRACTICE QUESTIONS

More questions on the companion CD!

282. A nursing instructor asks a nursing student about Kohlberg's theory of moral development. The instructor determines that the student needs to further research this theory if the student states

that a component of the theory includes which of the following?

1. Individuals move through all six stages in a sequential fashion.
2. Moral development progresses in relationship to cognitive development.
3. A person's ability to make moral judgments develops over a period of time.
4. It provides a framework for understanding how individuals determine a moral code to guide their behavior.

283. The mother of an 8-year-old child tells the nurse that she is concerned about the child because the child seems to be more attentive to friends than anything else. The appropriate nursing response would be which of the following?

1. "You need to be concerned."
2. "You need to monitor the child's behavior closely."
3. "At this age, the child is developing his or her own personality."
4. "You need to provide more praise to the child to stop this behavior."

284. A mother of a 4-year-old child tells the nurse that she is concerned because the child has been masturbating. The appropriate response by the nurse is which of the following?

1. "This is a normal behavior at this age."

2. "Children usually begin this behavior at the age of 8 years."
3. "This is not normal behavior. The child should be brought to the mental health clinic."
4. "The child is very young to begin this behavior and should be brought to the mental health clinic."

285. A nurse is providing instructions to a new mother regarding the psychosocial development of the infant. Using Erikson's psychosocial development theory, the nurse would instruct the mother to:
1. Allow the infant to signal a need.
2. Anticipate all of the needs of the infant.
3. Attend to the crying infant immediately.
4. Avoid the infant during the first 10 minutes of crying.

286. The mother of a 3-year-old tells the nurse that the child is constantly rebelling and having temper tantrums. The appropriate instruction to the mother is to:
1. Set limits on the child's behavior.
2. Ignore the child when this behavior occurs.
3. Allow the behavior, because this is normal at this age period.
4. Punish the child every time the child says "no" to change the behavior.

287. A nurse who is employed in long-term care facility is caring for a 70-year-old woman. The client reminisces about past life experiences in a positive way. The nurse interprets this behavior as:
1. A mental status alteration
2. A normal psychosocial response
3. Requiring a psychiatric consultation
4. A sensory deficit requiring social activities

288. A nursing instructor asks a nursing student to present a clinical conference to peers regarding Freud's psychosexual stages of development, specifically the anal stage. The nursing student prepares for the conference knowing that which of the following appropriately relates to this stage of development?
1. This stage is associated with toilet training.
2. This stage is characterized by the gratification of the self.

3. This stage is characterized by a tapering off of conscious biological and sexual urges.
4. This stage is associated with pleasurable and conflicting feelings about the genital organs.

289. A nursing instructor asks a nursing student to describe the formal operations stage of Piaget's cognitive developmental theory. The appropriate response by the nursing student is:
1. "The child has the ability to think abstractly."
2. "The child develops logical thought patterns."
3. "The child begins to understand the environment."
4. "The child has difficulty separating fantasy from reality."

290. According to Kohlberg's theory of moral development, at the preconventional level, moral development is thought to be motivated by which of the following?
1. Peer pressure
2. Social pressures
3. The parents' behavior
4. Punishment and reward

ALTERNATE ITEM FORMAT: MULTIPLE RESPONSE

291. Which of the following are components of Kohlberg's theory of moral development? Select all that apply.
☐ 1. Individuals move through all six stages in a sequential fashion.
☐ 2. Moral development progresses in relationship to cognitive development.
☐ 3. A person's ability to make moral judgments develops over a period of time.
☐ 4. The theory provides a framework for understanding how individuals determine a moral code to guide their behavior.
☐ 5. In stage 1 (punishment-obedience orientation), children are expected to reason as mature members of society.
☐ 6. In stage 2 (instrumental relativist orientation), the child conforms to rules to obtain rewards or to have favors returned.

ANSWERS

282. **1**
Rationale: Kohlberg's theory states that individuals move through the six stages of development in a sequential fashion but that not everyone reaches stages 5 or 6 as part of their development of personal morality. Options 2, 3, and 4 are correct statements regarding Kohlberg's theory.
Test-Taking Strategy: Note the strategic words "needs to further research." These words indicate a negative event query and ask you to select an option that is an incorrect statement. Also, note the close-ended word "all" in option 1. Review Kohlberg's theory if you had difficulty with this question.

Level of Cognitive Ability: Comprehension
Client Needs: Psychosocial Integrity
Integrated Process: Teaching and Learning
Content Area: Fundamental Skills
Reference: Price, D., & Gwin, J. (2008). *Pediatric nursing: An introductory text* (10th ed., p. 178). St. Louis: Saunders.

283. **3**
Rationale: According to Erikson, from the ages of 7 to 12 years, the child begins to move toward receiving support from peers and friends and away from that of parents. The child also begins to develop special interests that reflect his or

her own developing personality instead of those of the parents.

Test-Taking Strategy: Use Erikson's psychosocial development theory related to school-age children to assist with eliminating options 1 and 2. Eliminate option 4 next, because, although praising the child for accomplishments is important at this age, the behavior that the child is exhibiting is normal. Review Erikson's psychosocial development theory if you had difficulty with this question.

Level of Cognitive Ability: Application
Client Needs: Psychosocial Integrity
Integrated Process: Caring
Content Area: Child Health
Reference: Price, D., & Gwin, J. (2008). *Pediatric nursing: An introductory text* (10th ed., p. 21). St. Louis: Saunders.

284. 1

Rationale: According to Freud's psychosexual stages of development, the child is in the phallic stage between the ages of 3 and 6 years. At this time, the child devotes much energy to examining his or her genitalia, masturbating, and expressing interest in sexual concerns.

Test-Taking Strategy: Use the process of elimination. Eliminate options 3 and 4, because they are comparable or alike. From the remaining options, use Freud's psychosexual stages of development to direct you to option 1. Review Freud's psychosexual stages of development if you had difficulty with this question.

Level of Cognitive Ability: Application
Client Needs: Psychosocial Integrity
Integrated Process: Nursing Process/Implementation
Content Area: Child Health
Reference: Leifer, G. (2007). *Introduction to maternity and pediatric nursing* (5th ed., p. 361). Philadelphia: Saunders.

285. 1

Rationale: According to Erikson, the caregiver should not try to anticipate the infant's needs at all times but rather must allow the infant to signal his or her needs. If an infant is not allowed to signal a need, he or she will not learn how to control the environment. Erikson believed that a delayed or prolonged response to an infant's signal would inhibit the development of trust and lead to the mistrust of others.

Test-Taking Strategy: Use the process of elimination. Eliminate options 3 and 4 first because of the words "immediately" and "avoid." Additionally, option 2 can be eliminated because of the close-ended word "all." Review Erikson's psychosocial development theory if you had difficulty with this question.

Level of Cognitive Ability: Application
Client Needs: Psychosocial Integrity
Integrated Process: Teaching and Learning
Content Area: Child Health
Reference: Leifer, G. (2007). *Introduction to maternity and pediatric nursing* (5th ed., p. 361). Philadelphia: Saunders.

286. 1

Rationale: According to Erikson, the child focuses on independence between the ages of 1 and 3 years. Gaining independence often means that the child has to rebel against the parents' wishes. Saying things like "no" and "mine" and having temper tantrums are common during this period of development. Being consistent and setting limits on the child's behavior are necessary elements.

Test-Taking Strategy: Use the process of elimination. Options 2 and 3 can be eliminated first, because they are comparable or alike. Eliminate option 4 next, because this action is likely to produce a negative response during this normal developmental pattern. Review the psychosocial development of the toddler according to Erikson if you had difficulty with this question.

Level of Cognitive Ability: Application
Client Needs: Psychosocial Integrity
Integrated Process: Nursing Process/Implementation
Content Area: Child Health
Reference: Leifer, G. (2007). *Introduction to maternity and pediatric nursing* (5th ed., p. 361). Philadelphia: Saunders.

287. 2

Rationale: According to Erikson, the later years of life are from 65 years of age until death. The adult reminisces about past life experiences, often viewing them in a positive way. The adult needs to feel good about his or her accomplishments, to see successes in his or her life, and to feel that he or she has made a contribution to society.

Test-Taking Strategy: Use your knowledge regarding Erikson's theory of psychosocial development of late adulthood to answer the question. Note that options 1, 3, and 4 are comparable or alike; this will direct you to option 2. Review Erikson's theory of psychosocial development if you had difficulty with this question.

Level of Cognitive Ability: Comprehension
Client Needs: Psychosocial Integrity
Integrated Process: Nursing Process/Data Collection
Content Area: Fundamental Skills
Reference: Wold, G. (2008). *Basic geriatric nursing* (4th ed., pp. 191-192). St. Louis: Mosby.

288. 1

Rationale: Toilet training generally occurs during this period. According to Freud, the child gains pleasure from both the elimination and retention of feces. Option 2 relates to the oral stage. Option 3 relates to the latency period. Option 4 relates to the phallic stage.

Test-Taking Strategy: Use the process of elimination. Note the relationship between the words "anal" in the question and "toilet training" in the correct option. Review Freud's psychosocial stages of development if you had difficulty with this question.

Level of Cognitive Ability: Comprehension
Client Needs: Psychosocial Integrity
Integrated Process: Nursing Process/Planning
Content Area: Child Health
Reference: Price, D., & Gwin, J. (2008). *Pediatric nursing: An introductory text* (10th ed., pp. 21, 178). St. Louis: Saunders.

289. 1

Rationale: In the formal operations stage, the child has the abilities to think abstractly and to solve problems. Option 2 identifies the concrete operations stage. Option 3 identifies the sensorimotor stage. Option 4 identifies the preoperational stage.

Test-Taking Strategy: Knowledge regarding the characteristics of Piaget's cognitive developmental theory is required to answer this question. Remember, in the formal operations stage, the child has the abilities to think abstractly and to solve problems. Review Piaget's cognitive developmental theory if you had difficulty with this question.
Level of Cognitive Ability: Comprehension
Client Needs: Psychosocial Integrity
Integrated Process: Teaching and Learning
Content Area: Child Health
Reference: Leifer, G. (2007). *Introduction to maternity and pediatric nursing* (5th ed., p. 361). Philadelphia: Saunders.

290. 4
Rationale: In the preconventional stage, morals are thought to be motivated by punishment and reward. If the child is obedient and not punished, then he or she is being moral. The child sees actions as either good or bad. If the child's actions are good, then the child is praised. If the child's actions are bad, then the child is punished.
Test-Taking Strategy: Use the process of elimination. Eliminate options 1 and 2, because they are comparable or alike. Knowledge that the preconventional stage occurs between the ages of 2 and 7 years will assist with directing you to option 4. Review Kohlberg's theory of moral development if you had difficulty with this question.
Level of Cognitive Ability: Comprehension
Client Needs: Psychosocial Integrity
Integrated Process: Nursing Process/Data Collection
Content Area: Child Health
Reference: Price, D., & Gwin, J. (2008). *Pediatric nursing: An introductory text* (10th ed., p. 21). St. Louis: Saunders.

ALTERNATE ITEM FORMAT: MULTIPLE RESPONSE

291. 2, 3, 4, 6
Rationale: Kohlberg's theory states that individuals move through the six stages of development in a sequential fashion but that not everyone reaches stages 5 and 6 during his or her development of personal morality. The theory provides a framework for understanding how individuals determine a moral code to guide their behavior. It also states that moral development progresses in relationship to cognitive development and that a person's ability to make moral judgments develops over a period of time. In stage 1 (ages 2-3 years; punishment-obedience orientation), children cannot reason as mature members of society. In stage 2 (ages 4-7 years; instrumental relativist orientation), the child conforms to rules to obtain rewards or to have favors returned.
Test-Taking Strategy: Read each option carefully. Recalling the ages associated with each stage and that the theory provides a framework for understanding how individuals determine a moral code to guide their behavior will assist you with answering the question. Review Kohlberg's theory if you had difficulty with this question.
Level of Cognitive Ability: Comprehension
Client Needs: Psychosocial Integrity
Integrated Process: Nursing Process/Planning
Content Area: Fundamental Skills
Reference: Hockenberry, M., Wilson, D., & Winkelstein, M. (2005). *Wong's essentials of pediatric nursing* (7th ed., pp. 89-90). St. Louis: Mosby.

REFERENCES

Hockenberry, M., Wilson, D., & Winkelstein, M. (2005). *Wong's essentials of pediatric nursing* (7th ed.). St. Louis: Mosby.
Leifer, G. (2007). *Introduction to maternity and pediatric nursing* (5th ed.). Philadelphia: Saunders.
National Council of State Boards of Nursing (Eds.). (2008). *2008 Detailed Test Plan for the NCLEX-PN® Examination, National Council of State Boards of Nursing.* Chicago: Author.

National Council of State Boards of Nursing. *NCSBN home page.* www.ncsbn.org. Accessed July 9, 2008.
Price, D., & Gwin, J. (2008). *Pediatric nursing: An introductory text* (10th ed.). St. Louis: Saunders.
Wold, G. (2008). *Basic geriatric nursing* (4th ed.). St. Louis: Mosby.

Developmental Stages

▲ I. THE HOSPITALIZED INFANT AND TODDLER
A. Separation anxiety
   1. Protest
      a. Cries, screams, searches for a parent; avoids and rejects contact with strangers
      b. Verbal attacks on others
      c. Physical fighting; kicks, fights, hits, and pinches
   2. Despair
      a. Withdrawn, depressed, and uninterested in the environment
      b. Loss of newly learned skills
   3. Detachment
      a. Rather uncommon; sometimes called denial
      b. Superficially, the toddler appears to have adjusted to the loss
      c. During this phase, the toddler again becomes more interested in the environment, plays with others, and seems to form new relationships; this behavior is a form of resignation and is not a sign of contentment
      d. The toddler detaches from the parents in an effort to escape the emotional pain of desiring the parent's presence
      e. The toddler copes by forming shallow relationships with others, becoming increasingly self-centered, and attaching primary importance to material objects
      f. This is the most serious phase, because the reversal of the potential adverse effects is less likely to occur after detachment is established; in most situations, the temporary separation imposed by hospitalization does not cause such prolonged parental absence that the toddler enters into detachment
B. Fear of injury and pain: Affected by previous experiences, separation from parents, and preparation for the experience
▲ C. Loss of control
   1. Hospitalization with its own set of rituals and routines can severely disrupt the life of a toddler
   2. The lack of control is often exhibited in behaviors related to feeding, toileting, playing, and bedtime
   3. The toddler may demonstrate regression
D. Interventions ▲
   1. Provide swaddling and soft talking to the infant
   2. Provide opportunities for sucking and oral stimulation for the infant using a pacifier if the infant is not to receive anything by mouth
   3. Provide stimulation for the infant, if appropriate, with the use of objects of contrasting colors and textures
   4. Provide routines and rituals that are as close as possible to what the toddler is used to at home
   5. Provide as many choices to the toddler as possible to provide some control
   6. Approach the toddler with a positive attitude
   7. Allow the toddler to express feelings of protest
   8. Encourage the toddler to talk about his or her parents or others in his or her life
   9. Accept regressive behavior without ridiculing the toddler
   10. Provide the toddler with favorite and comforting objects
   11. Allow the toddler as much mobility as possible
   12. Anticipate temper tantrums from the toddler, and maintain a safe environment for physical acting out
   13. Employ pain-reduction techniques, as appropriate
II. THE HOSPITALIZED PRESCHOOLER ▲
A. Separation anxiety
   1. Generally less obvious and less serious than that seen in the toddler
   2. As stress increases, the preschooler's ability to separate from the parents decreases
   3. Protest
      a. Less direct and aggressive than that seen in the toddler
      b. May displace feelings onto others
   4. Despair
      a. Similar to the toddler

b. Quietly withdrawn, depressed, and uninterested in the environment
c. Loss of newly learned skills
d. The preschooler becomes generally uncooperative, refusing to eat or take medication
e. The preschooler repeatedly asks when the parents will be visiting
5. Detachment: Similar to that of the toddler

B. Fear of injury and pain
1. The preschooler has a general lack of understanding of body integrity
2. Fears invasive procedures and mutilation
3. Imagines things to be much worse than they are
4. Preschoolers believe that they are ill because of something they did or thought

C. Loss of control
1. Likes familiar routines and rituals; may show regression if not allowed to maintain some control
2. Has attained a good deal of independence and self-care at home; may expect that to continue in the hospital

D. Interventions
1. Provide a safe and secure environment
2. Take time for communication
3. Allow the preschooler to express anger
4. Acknowledge fears and anxieties
5. Accept regressive behavior; assist the preschooler with moving from regressive to appropriate behaviors according to age
6. Encourage rooming in or leave a favorite toy
7. Allow mobility, and provide play and diversional activities
8. Place the preschooler with other children of the same age, if possible
9. Encourage the preschooler to be independent
10. Explain procedures simply, on the preschooler's level
11. Avoid intrusive procedures, when possible
12. Allow for the wearing of underpants

III. THE HOSPITALIZED SCHOOL-AGE CHILD
A. Separation anxiety
1. Accustomed to periods of separation from the parents, but, as stressors are added, the separation becomes more difficult
2. More concerned with missing school and the fear that friends will forget him or her
3. Usually do not see the stage of behavior of protest, despair, and detachment with school-age children

B. Fear of injury and pain
1. Fear bodily injury and pain
2. Fear of illness itself, disability, death, and intrusive procedures in genital areas
3. Uncomfortable with any type of sexual examination

4. Groans, whines, holds rigidly still, and communicates about pain

C. Loss of control
1. Is usually highly social, independent, and involved with activities
2. Seeks information and asks relevant questions about tests, procedures, and the illness
3. Associates his or her actions with the cause of the illness
4. May feel helpless and dependent if physical limitations occur

D. Interventions
1. Encourage rooming in
2. Focus on the school-age child's abilities and needs
3. Encourage the school-age child to become involved with his or her own care
4. Accept regression but encourage independence
5. Provide choices to the school-age child
6. Allow for the expression of feelings, both verbally and nonverbally
7. Acknowledge fears and concerns and allow for discussion
8. Explain all procedures with the use of body diagrams or outlines
9. Provide privacy
10. Avoid intrusive procedures, if possible
11. Allow the school-age child to wear underpants
12. Involve the school-age child in activities that are appropriate to his or her developmental level and illness
13. Encourage the school-age child to contact friends
14. Provide for educational needs
15. Employ appropriate interventions to relieve pain

IV. THE HOSPITALIZED ADOLESCENT
A. Separation anxiety
1. Not sure whether they want their parents with them when they are hospitalized
2. Separation from friends is a source of anxiety
3. Become upset if friends go on with their lives and exclude them

B. Fear of injury and pain
1. Fear of being different from others and their peers
2. May give the impression that they are not afraid although they are terrified
3. Become guarded when any areas related to sexual development are examined

C. Loss of control
1. Behaviors exhibited include anger, withdrawal, and uncooperativeness
2. Seek help and then reject it

D. Interventions
1. Encourage questions about appearance and the effects of the illness on the future

2. Explore feelings about the hospital and the significance that the illness might have with regard to relationships
3. Encourage the adolescent to wear his or her own clothes and to perform normal grooming
4. Allow favorite foods to be brought in to the hospital, if possible
5. Provide privacy
6. Use body diagrams to prepare for procedures
7. Introduce to other adolescents in the nursing unit
8. Encourage the maintenance of contact with peer groups
9. Provide for educational needs
10. Identify the formation of future plans
11. Help develop positive coping mechanisms

V. COMMUNICATION APPROACHES
A. General guidelines
  1. Allow the child to feel comfortable with the nurse
  2. Communicate with the use of objects
  3. Allow the child to express fears and concerns
  4. Speak clearly and in a quiet, unhurried voice
  5. Offer choices, when possible
  6. Be honest with the child
  7. Set limits with the child, as appropriate
B. Infant
  1. Infants respond to the nonverbal communication behaviors of adults, such as holding, rocking, patting, and touching
  2. Use a slow approach; allow the infant to get to know the nurse
  3. Use a calm, soft, soothing voice
  4. Be responsive to cries
  5. Talk and read to infants
  6. Allow security objects such as blankets and pacifiers, if the infant uses them
C. Toddler
  1. Approach the toddler cautiously
  2. Remember that toddlers accept the verbal communications of others literally
  3. Learn the toddler's words for common items and use them in conversations
  4. Use short, concrete terms
  5. Prepare the toddler for procedures immediately before the event
  6. Repeat explanations and descriptions
  7. Use play for demonstrations
  8. Use visual aids such as picture books, puppets, and dolls
  9. Allow the toddler to handle the equipment or instruments; explain what the equipment or instrument does and how it feels
  10. Encourage the use of comfort objects
D. Preschooler
  1. Seek opportunities to offer choices
  2. Speak in simple sentences

3. Be concise; limit the length of explanations
4. Allow for the asking of questions
5. Describe the procedures as they are about to be performed
6. Use play to explain procedures and activities
7. Allow the handling of equipment or instruments, which will ease fear and help answer questions
E. School-age child
  1. Establish limits
  2. Provide reassurance to help with alleviating fears and anxieties
  3. Engage in conversations that encourage thinking
  4. Use medical play techniques
  5. Use photographs, books, dolls, and videos to explain procedures
  6. Explain in clear terms
  7. Allow time for composure and privacy
F. Adolescent
  1. Remember that the adolescent may be preoccupied with body image
  2. Encourage and support independence
  3. Provide privacy
  4. Use photographs, books, and videos to explain procedures
  5. Engage in conversations about the adolescent's interests
  6. Avoid becoming too abstract, too detailed, and too technical
  7. Avoid responding to less-than-desirable social behaviors by prying, confrontation, or judgmental attitudes

VI. DEVELOPMENTAL CHARACTERISTICS
A. Infant
  1. Physical
     a. Height increases by $^3/_4$ inch per month
     b. Weight is doubled at 5 to 6 months and tripled at 12 months
     c. At birth, head circumference is 2 to 3 cm greater than chest circumference
     d. By 1 to 2 years of age, head circumference and chest circumference are equal
     e. Anterior fontanel (soft and flat in a normal infant) closes at 12 to 18 months
     f. Posterior fontanel (soft and flat in a normal infant) closes by 2 to 3 months
     g. Has 10 upper and 10 lower deciduous teeth by the age of 2½ years
     h. Lower central incisors present by 6 to 8 months
     i. Sleeps most of the time
  2. Vital signs (Box 28-1)
  3. Nutrition
     a. The infant may breast-feed or bottle-feed, depending on the mother's choice
     b. Iron stores from birth are depleted by 4 months

Newborn
Temperature: Axillary, 97.7° to 99.5° F
Apical rate: 120 to 140 beats per minute (100 sleeping, 180 crying)
Respirations: 30 to 60 breaths per minute (average, 40 breaths per minute)
Blood pressure: 73/55 mm Hg
1-Year-Old Infant
Temperature: Axillary, 96.8° to 99° F
Apical rate: 90 to 130 beats per minute
Respirations: 20 to 40 breaths per minute
Blood pressure: 90/56 mm Hg

c. Human milk is the best food for infants less than 6 months old
d. Infants should remain on human milk or iron-fortified formula for the first year of life
e. Whole milk should not be introduced to infants until after 1 year of age
f. Skim and low-fat milk should not be given, because the essential fatty acids are inadequate and the solute concentration of protein and electrolytes is too high
g. Fluoride supplementation may be needed at about 6 months of age, depending on the infant's intake of fluoridated tap water
h. Solid foods are introduced at 5 to 6 months old; introduce solid foods one at a time, usually at intervals of 4 to 5 days, to identify food allergens
i. The sequence of introduction of solid foods is as follows: rice cereal; fruits and vegetables, starting with yellow and then green; meats; and then egg yolks, avoiding egg whites (introduce egg whites toward the end of the first year); cheese may be used as a substitute for meat and as a finger food
j. Avoid solid foods that place the infant at risk for choking, such as nuts, foods with seeds, raisins, popcorn, grapes, and pieces of hot dog
k. Avoid microwaving baby bottles and baby food
l. Never mix food and/or medications with formula
m. To prevent botulism, avoid adding honey to formula, water, or other fluids
n. Offer fruit juice from a cup (12 to 13 months) rather than a bottle to prevent nursing (bottle-mouth) caries
4. Skills (Box 28-2)
5. Play
a. Solitary

| BOX 28-2 | Infant Skills |

2 to 3 Months
- Smiles
- Turns head from side to side
- Cries
- Follows objects
- Holds head in midline

4 to 5 Months
- Grasps objects
- Switches objects from hand to hand
- Rolls over for the first time
- Enjoys social interaction
- Begins to show memory
- Aware of unfamiliar surroundings

6 to 7 Months
- Creeps
- Sits with support
- Imitates
- Exhibits fear of strangers
- Holds arms out
- Frequent mood swings
- Waves bye-bye

8 to 9 Months
- Sits steadily unsupported
- Crawls
- May stand while holding on to something
- Begins to stand without help

10 to 11 Months
- Can change from a prone to a sitting position
- Walks while holding onto furniture
- Stands securely
- Entertains self for periods of time

12 to 13 Months
- Walks with one hand held
- Can take a few steps without falling

14 to 15 Months
- Walks alone
- Can crawl up stairs
- Shows emotions such as anger and affection
- Will explore away from his or her mother in familiar surroundings

b. Birth to 3 months: Verbal, visual, and tactile stimuli
c. 4 to 6 months: Initiates actions and recognizes new experiences
d. 6 to 12 months: Aware of self, imitates, and repeats pleasurable actions
e. Enjoys soft stuffed animals, crib mobiles with contrasting colors, squeeze toys, rattles, musical toys, water toys during the bath, large picture books, and push toys after he or she begins to walk
6. Safety
a. Baby-proof the home
b. An infant should ride in a car in a semi-reclined, rear-facing position in an infant-only seat or a convertible seat until he or

she weighs at least 20 lbs and is at least 1 year old; convertible seats can be used as rear-facing seats for infants and then converted to a forward-facing position when the child is old enough and big enough to do so safely

c. Infants are placed in the back seat of the car in their safety seats; they could be seriously injured if the air bag is released in the passenger side of the front seat of the car, because rear-facing safety seats extend close to the dashboard

d. Guard the infant when he or she is on a bed or changing table

e. Use gates to protect the infant from stairs

f. Never shake an infant

g. Be sure that bath water is not hot; do not leave infant unattended in the bath

h. Do not hold the infant while drinking or working near hot liquids

i. Cool vaporizers should be used rather than steam vaporizers to prevent burn injuries

j. Avoid offering food that is round and similar in size to the airway to prevent choking

k. Be sure that toys have no small pieces

l. Hanging toys or mobiles over the crib should be well out of reach to prevent strangulation

m. Avoid placing large toys in the crib; an older infant may use them as steps to climb out

n. Cribs should be positioned away from curtains and blind cords

o. Cover electrical outlets

p. Remove hazardous objects from low, reachable places

q. Remove chemicals, medications, poisons, and plants from the infant's reach

r. Keep the poison control number available

s. The mother is instructed to contact the poison control center immediately in the event of a poisoning

B. Toddler
  1. Physical
    a. Height and weight increase in a steplike fashion that reflects growth spurts and lags
    b. The head circumference increases about 1 inch between the ages of 1 and 2 years; thereafter, head circumference increases about ½ inch per year until the age of 5 years
    c. Anterior fontanel closes between ages 12 and 18 months
    d. Weight gain is slower than in infancy; by 2 years old, the average weight is 27 pounds
    e. Normal height changes include a growth of about 3 inches per year; the average height of a toddler is 34 inches at 2 years old
    f. Lordosis (pot belly) is evident

> **BOX 28-3** **Toddler's Vital Signs**
>
> *Temperature:* Axillary, 97.5° to 98.6° F
> *Apical rate:* 80 to 120 beats per minute
> *Respirations:* 20 to 30 breaths per minute
> *Blood pressure:* Average, 92/55 mm Hg

g. The toddler should see a dentist soon after the first teeth erupt, usually around 1 year old; fluoride supplements may be necessary if the water is not fluoridated

h. A toddler should never be allowed to fall asleep with a bottle containing milk, juice, soda, or sweetened water because of the risk of nursing (bottle-mouth) caries

i. A toddler typically sleeps through the night; he or she has one daytime nap, which is usually discontinued at about the age of 3 years

j. A consistent bedtime ritual helps prepare the toddler for sleep

k. Security objects at bedtime may assist with sleep

2. Vital signs (Box 28-3)
3. Nutrition
  a. Most toddlers prefer to feed themselves
  b. The toddler generally does best by eating several small nutritious meals each day rather than three large meals
  c. Offer a limited number of foods at any one time
  d. Offer finger foods; avoid concentrated sweets and empty calories
  e. Toddlers are at risk for the aspiration of small foods that are not easily chewed, such as nuts, foods with seeds, raisins, popcorn, grapes, and pieces of hot dog
  f. Physiological anorexia is normal as a result of the alternating periods of fast and slow growth
  g. Sit the toddler in a high chair at the family table for meals
  h. Allow sufficient time to eat, but remove food when the toddler begins playing with it
  i. The toddler drinks well from a cup that is held with both hands
  j. Avoid using food as a reward or punishment
4. Skills
  a. The toddler begins to walk with one hand held by the age of 12 to 13 months
  b. Runs by the age of 2 years; walks backward and hops on one foot by the age of 3 years
  c. The toddler usually cannot alternate feet when climbing stairs

BOX 28-4 **Signs of Readiness for Toilet Training**

- Able to stay dry for 2 hours
- Waking dry from a nap
- Able to sit, squat, and walk
- Able to remove clothing
- Recognizes urge to defecate or urinate
- Expresses willingness to please parent
- Able to sit on toilet for 5 to 10 minutes without fussing or getting off

    d. The toddler begins to master fine motor skills for building, undressing, and drawing lines

    e. The young toddler often uses the word "no," even when he or she means "yes," to assert independence

    f. Begins to use short sentences and has a vocabulary of about 300 words by the age of 2 years

    g. Tends to ask many "why" questions

5. Bowel and bladder control

    a. Signs that a toddler is ready for toilet training (Box 28-4)

    b. Bowel control develops before bladder control

    c. By the age of 3 years, the toddler achieves fairly good bowel and bladder control

    d. The toddler may stay dry during the day but may need a diaper at night until about the age of 4 years

6. Play

    a. The major socializing mechanism is parallel play; therapeutic play can begin at this age

    b. The toddler has a short attention span that causes him or her to change toys often

    c. Explores the body parts of self and others

    d. Typical toys include push-pull toys, blocks, sand, finger paints, bubbles, large balls, crayons, trucks, dolls, containers, Play-Doh, toy telephones, cloth books, and wooden puzzles

7. Safety

    a. Toddlers are eager to explore the world around them

    b. The toddler should be supervised when at play

    c. The toddler can be placed in an upright forward-facing position in a car safety seat (convertible restraint); the transition point for switching to a forward-facing position is defined by the manufacturer of the car seat but is generally at a body weight of at least 20 lbs and an age of 1 year

    d. Convertible restraints (car safety seats) are used until the child weighs at least 40 lbs

    e. Booster seats are used for children who are shorter than 4 feet and 9 inches tall and who weigh more than 40 lbs (typically between 4 and 8 years old); the booster seat is used until the child is able to sit against the back of the seat with the feet hanging down and the legs bent at the knees

    f. Children should use specially designed car restraints until they weigh at least 60 lbs or are 8 years old

    g. Lock car doors

    h. Use back burners on the stove to prepare a meal, and turn pot handles inward and toward the middle of the stove

    i. Keep dangling cords from small appliances away from the toddler

    j. Place inaccessible locks on windows and doors, and keep furniture away from windows

    k. Secure screens on all windows

    l. Place gates at stairways

    m. Do not allow the toddler to sleep or play in an upper bunk bed

    n. Never leave the toddler alone near a bathtub, pail of water, swimming pool, or any other body of water

    o. Keep toilet lids closed

    p. Keep all medicines, poisons, household plants, and toxic products high and locked out of reach

    q. Keep the poison control number available

    r. The mother is instructed to contact the poison control center immediately in the event of a poisoning

C. Preschooler

  1. Physical

    a. Grows 2½ to 3 inches per year

    b. Average height is 37 inches at age 3, 40½ inches at age 4, and 43 inches at age 5

    c. Gains 5 pounds per year; average weight of 32 pounds at age 5

    d. Requires about 12 hours of sleep each day

    e. A security object and a nightlight help with sleeping

    f. At the beginning of the preschool period, the eruption of the deciduous (primary) teeth is complete

    g. Regular dental care is essential, and the preschooler requires assistance with the brushing and flossing of teeth; fluoride supplements may be necessary if the water is not fluoridated

  2. Vital signs (Box 28-5)

  3. Nutrition

    a. Exhibits food fads and strong taste preferences

    b. By 5 years old, tends to focus on social aspects of eating, table conversations, manners, and willingness to try new foods

BOX 28-5 Preschooler's Vital Signs

Temperature: Axillary, 97.5° to 98.6° F
Apical rate: 70 to 110 beats per minute
Respirations: 16 to 22 breaths per minute
Blood pressure: Average, 95/57 mm Hg

4. Skills
   a. Has good posture
   b. Develops fine motor coordination
   c. Can hop, skip, and run more smoothly
   d. Athletic abilities begin to develop
   e. Demonstrates increased balancing skills
   f. Alternates feet when climbing stairs
   g. Can tie shoelaces
   h. May talk continuously and ask many "why" questions
   i. Vocabulary increases to about 900 words by age 3 and to about 2100 words by age 5
   j. By age 3, usually talks in three- or four-word sentences and speaks in short phrases
   k. By age 4, uses five- or six-word sentences; by age 5, speaks in longer sentences that contain all parts of speech
   l. Can be readily understood by others and can clearly understand what others are saying
5. Bowel and bladder control
   a. By age 4, the preschooler has daytime control of bowel and bladder but may experience bed-wetting accidents at night
   b. By age 5, the preschooler achieves both bowel and bladder control, although accidents may occur in stressful situations
6. Play
   a. Cooperative
   b. Imaginary playmates
   c. Likes to build and create things; play is simple and imaginative
   d. Understands sharing and is able to interact with peers
   e. Requires regular socialization with children of same age
   f. Play activities include a large space for running and jumping
   g. Likes dress-up clothes, paints, paper, and crayons for creative expression
   h. Swimming and sports aid with growth and development
   i. Puzzles and toys aid with fine motor development
7. Safety
   a. Preschoolers are active and inquisitive
   b. Because of their magical thinking, they may believe that daring feats seen in cartoons are possible and may attempt them
   c. Can learn simple safety practices, because they can follow simple and verbal directions, and their attention span is lengthened
   d. After the child has outgrown the convertible restraint car safety seat (weight of more than 40 lbs), then he or she should be placed and restrained in a booster seat.
   e. Booster seats are used for children who are shorter than 4 feet and 9 inches tall and who weigh more than 40 lbs (typically between 4 and 8 years old); the booster seat is used until the child is able to sit against the back of the seat with the feet hanging down and the legs bent at the knees
   f. Children should use specially designed car restraints until they weigh at least 60 lbs or are 8 years old
   g. Teach the preschooler basic safety rules to ensure safety when playing in a playground near swings and ladders
   h. Never allow the preschooler to play with matches or lighters
   i. The preschooler should be taught what to do in the event of a fire or if his or her clothes catch fire; fire drills should be practiced with the preschooler
   j. Guns should be stored unloaded and secured under lock and key; the preschooler should be taught to leave an area immediately if a gun is seen and to tell an adult
   k. The preschooler should be taught never to point a toy gun at another person
   l. Teach the preschooler that if another person touches his or her body in an inappropriate way, to tell an adult
   m. Teach the preschooler to avoid speaking to strangers and to never accept a ride, toys, or gifts from a stranger
   n. Teach the preschooler his or her full name, address, parents' names, and telephone number
   o. Teach the preschooler how to dial 911 in an emergency situation
   p. Keep the poison control number available
   q. The mother is instructed to contact the poison control center immediately in the event of a poisoning
D. School-age child
   1. Physical
      a. Girls usually grow faster than boys
      b. Growth of about 2 inches per year between the ages of 6 and 12 years
      c. Height ranges from 45 inches at age 6 to 59 inches at age 12
      d. Weight gain of 4½ to 6½ pounds per year

e. Average weight of 46 pounds at age 6 and 88 pounds at age 12
f. The first permanent (secondary) teeth erupt around age 6, and the deciduous teeth are gradually lost
g. Regular dentist visits are necessary, and the school-age child needs to be supervised during the brushing and flossing of teeth; fluoride supplements may be necessary if the water is not fluoridated
h. For school-age children with primary and permanent dentition, the best toothbrush is one with soft nylon bristles and an overall length of about 6 inches
i. Sleep requirements range from 10 to 12 hours per night
2. Vital signs (Box 28-6)
3. Nutrition
   a. Increased growth needs
   b. Balanced diet from foods in MyPyramid (http://www.mypyramid.gov)
   c. May still be a picky eater but is willing to try new foods
4. Skills
   a. Refinement of fine motor skills
   b. Continued development of gross motor skills
   c. Increase in strength and endurance
5. Play
   a. Play is more competitive
   b. Rules and rituals are important aspects of play and games
   c. Enjoys drawing, collecting items, dolls, pets, guessing games, board games, listening to the radio, television, reading, videos, and computer games
   d. Participates in team sports
   e. Participates in secret clubs, peer-group activities, and scout organizations
6. Safety
   a. Experiences less fear during play activities; frequently imitates real life with the use of tools and household items
   b. School-age children are ready to transition from booster seats when the adult seat belts fit correctly (i.e., the shoulder belt fits across the chest and shoulder, the lap belt fits across the thighs, and the child is tall enough to sit comfortably against the seat back with the knees bent, without slouching,

for the length of the trip); this typically occurs when the child is at least 4 feet and 9 inches tall and is between 8 and 12 years old
   c. Car safety belts should be worn across the thighs; the shoulder belt is used only if it does not cross over the child's neck and face
   d. Major causes of injuries include bicycles, skateboards, and team sports as the child increases motor abilities and independence
   e. Children should always wear a helmet when riding a bike or using inline skates or skateboards
   f. Teach the school-age child water safety rules
   g. Instruct the school-age child to avoid teasing or playing roughly with animals
   h. Never allow the school-age child to play with matches or lighters
   i. The school-age child should be taught what to do in the event of a fire or if clothes catch fire; fire drills should be practiced with the school-age child
   j. Guns should be stored unloaded and secured under lock and key; the school-age child should be taught to leave an area immediately if a gun is seen and to tell an adult
   k. Teach the school-age child that if another person touches his or her body in an inappropriate way, to tell an adult
   l. Teach the school-age child to avoid speaking to strangers and to never accept a ride, toys, or gifts from a stranger
   m. Teach the school-age child traffic safety rules
   n. Teach the school-age child how to dial 911 in an emergency situation
   o. Keep the poison control number available
   p. The mother is instructed to contact the poison control center immediately in the event of a poisoning
E. Adolescent
1. Physical
   a. Puberty: The maturational, hormonal, and growth process that occurs when the reproductive organs begin to function and the secondary sex characteristics develop
   b. Body mass increases to adult size
   c. Sebaceous and sweat glands become active and fully functional
   d. Body hair distribution occurs
   e. Increase in height, weight, breast development, and pelvic girth in girls
   f. Menstrual periods occur about 2½ years after the onset of puberty
   g. In boys, an increase in height, weight, muscle mass, and penis and testicle size occurs

---

BOX 28-6 **School-Age Child's Vital Signs**

Temperature: Oral, 97.5° to 98.6° F
Apical rate: 60 to 100 beats per minute
Respirations: 16 to 20 breaths per minute
Blood pressure: Average, 107/64 mm Hg

h. Voice deepens in boys

i. Normal weight gain during puberty: Girls gain 15 to 55 pounds and boys gain 15 to 65 pounds

j. Careful brushing and care of the teeth are important, and many adolescents need to wear braces

k. Sleep patterns include a tendency to stay up late; therefore, in an attempt to catch up on missed sleep, adolescents sleep late whenever possible; an overall average of 8 hours per night is recommended

2. Vital signs (Box 28-7)

3. Nutrition

a. Teaching about the food guide MyPyramid is important

b. Typically eat whenever they have a break in activities

c. Calcium, zinc, iron, folic acid, and protein are especially important nutritional needs

d. Tend to snack on empty calories

e. Body image is very important

4. Skills

a. Gross and fine motor skills are well developed

b. Strength and endurance increase

5. Play

a. Games and athletics are the most common forms of play

b. Competition and strict rules are important

c. Enjoy activities such as sports, videos, movies, reading, parties, dancing, hobbies, computer games, music, and experimenting, such as with makeup, hairstyles, tattoos, and piercings

d. Friends are important; adolescents like to gather in small groups

6. Safety

a. Risk takers

b. Have a natural urge to experiment and be independent

c. Instruct adolescents regarding the dangers related to drugs, alcohol, cigarettes, caffeine, suntanning, and motor vehicles of any type

d. Help them to recognize that there are choices when difficult or potentially dangerous situations arise

e. Advocate the use of seat belts

f. Instruct them regarding the consequences of the injuries that motor vehicle crashes can cause

g. Instruct them regarding water safety; emphasize that they should enter the water feet first, as opposed to diving, especially when the depth of the water is unknown

h. Instruct them about the dangers associated with guns, violence, and gangs

i. Instruct them about the complications associated with body piercing, tattooing, and suntanning

j. Discuss issues such as date rape, sexual relationships, and the transmission of sexually transmitted infections

F. Early adulthood

1. Description: Period between the late teens and the mid to late 30s

2. Physical changes

a. Has completed physical growth by the age of 20 years

b. Quite active

c. Severe illnesses are less common than those seen among older age groups

d. Tend to ignore physical symptoms and postpone seeking health care

e. Lifestyle habits such as smoking, stress, lack of exercise, poor personal hygiene, and family history of disease increase the risk of future illness

3. Cognitive changes

a. Rational thinking habits

b. Conceptual, problem-solving, and motor skills increase

c. Identifying preferred occupational areas

4. Psychosocial changes

a. Separate from their families of origin

b. Give much attention to occupational and social pursuits to improve socioeconomic status

c. Make decisions regarding career, marriage, and parenthood

d. Need to adapt to new situations

5. Sexuality

a. Have the emotional maturity to develop mature sexual relationships

b. At risk for sexually transmitted infections

G. Middle adulthood

1. Description: Period between the mid to late 30s and the mid 60s

2. Physical changes

a. Occur between the ages of 40 and 65 years

b. Individual becomes aware that changes in reproductive and physical abilities signify the beginning of another stage in life

c. Menopause occurs in women; climacteric occurs in men

BOX 28-7 **Adolescent's Vital Signs**

Temperature: Oral, 97.5° to 98.6° F
Apical rate: 55 to 90 beats per minute
Respirations: 12 to 20 breaths per minute
Blood pressure: Average, 121/70 mm Hg

d. Physiological changes often have an impact on self-concept and body image

e. Physiological concerns include stress, level of wellness, and the formation of positive health habits

3. Cognitive changes
   a. May be interested in learning new skills
   b. May become involved with educational or vocational programs for entering the job market or for changing careers

4. Psychosocial changes
   a. May include expected events, such as children moving away from home (postparental family stage), or unexpected events, such as the death of a close friend
   b. Time and financial demands decrease as children move away from home and the couple faces redefining their relationship
   c. May become grandparents
   d. Achieving generativity

5. Sexuality
   a. Many couples renew their relationships and find increased marital and sexual satisfaction
   b. The onset of menopause and climacteric may affect sexual health
   c. Stress, health, and medications can affect sexuality

PRACTICE QUESTIONS

More questions on the companion CD!

292. The mother of a 16-year-old child tells the nurse that she is concerned because the child sleeps until noon every weekend and whenever there is a day off from school. Which of the following is the appropriate nursing response?
    1. "Adolescents love to sleep late in the morning."
    2. "The child shouldn't be staying up so late at night."
    3. "If the child eats properly, that shouldn't be happening."
    4. "The child should have a blood test to check for anemia."

293. A 16-year-old child is admitted to the hospital for acute appendicitis, and an appendectomy is performed. Which of the following interventions is most appropriate to facilitate normal growth and development?
    1. Encourage the child to rest and read.
    2. Encourage the parents to room in with the child.
    3. Allow the family to bring in favorite computer games.
    4. Allow the child to participate in activities with other individuals in the same age group when the condition permits.

294. A 2-year-old child is treated in the emergency department for a burn to the chest and abdomen. The child sustained the burn from grabbing a cup of hot coffee that was left on the kitchen counter. The nurse reinforces safety principles with the parents before discharge. Which statement, if made by the parents, indicates an understanding of the measures required to provide safety in the home?
    1. "We will be sure not to leave hot liquids unattended."
    2. "I guess my children need to understand what the word 'hot' means."
    3. "We will be sure that the children stay in their rooms when we work in the kitchen."
    4. "We will install a safety gate as soon as we get home so that the children can't get into the kitchen."

295. The mother of a 4-year-old child expresses concern because her hospitalized child has started sucking his thumb. The mother states that this behavior began 2 days after hospital admission. Which of the following is the appropriate nursing response?
    1. "It is best to ignore the behavior."
    2. "Your child is acting like a baby."
    3. "The doctor will need to be notified."
    4. "A 4-year-old is too old for this type of behavior."

296. The mother of a toddler asks a nurse when it is safe to place the car safety seat in a face-forward position. Which of the following is the best nursing response?
    1. When the toddler weighs 20 lbs and is 1 year old
    2. When the weight of the toddler is more than 40 lbs
    3. The seat should not be placed in a face-forward position unless there are safety locks in the car.
    4. The seat should never be placed in a face-forward position because of the risk of the child unbuckling the harness.

297. The parents of a 2-year-old arrive at the hospital to visit the child. The child is in the play room and ignores the parents during the visit. This behavior in a 2-year-old child indicates:
    1. A normal pattern
    2. That the child is withdrawn
    3. That the child has adjusted to the hospitalized setting
    4. That the child is more interested in playing with other children

298. Which of the following is the most appropriate toy to provide to a 3-year-old child?
    1. A puzzle
    2. A wagon
    3. A golf set
    4. A farm set

299. A nurse is assigned to monitor a 3-month-old infant for increased intracranial pressure. On palpation of the fontanels, the nurse notes that the anterior fontanel has not closed and that it is soft and flat. Which of the following actions should the nurse take?
   1. Increase oral fluids.
   2. Document the findings.
   3. Notify the registered nurse.
   4. Elevate the head of the bed to 90 degrees.
300. A nurse is caring for a 5-year-old child who has been placed in traction after a fracture of the femur. Which of the following is the most appropriate activity for this child?
   1. A radio
   2. Finger paints
   3. A sports video
   4. Large picture books

ALTERNATE ITEM FORMAT: MULTIPLE RESPONSE

301. Select the interventions that are appropriate for the care of an infant. Select all that apply.
   ☐ **1.** Provide swaddling.
   ☐ **2.** Talk in a loud voice.
   ☐ **3.** Provide the infant with a bottle of juice at naptime.
   ☐ **4.** Hang mobiles with black-and-white contrast designs.
   ☐ **5.** Caress the infant while bathing or during diaper changes.
   ☐ **6.** Allow the infant to cry for at least 10 minutes before responding.

ANSWERS

292. 1
Rationale: The sleep patterns of the adolescent vary according to individual needs. Adolescents love to sleep late in the morning, but they should be encouraged to be responsible for waking themselves, particularly in time to get ready for school. Options 2, 3, and 4 are incorrect.
Test-Taking Strategy: Use the process of elimination. Options 2 and 3 can be eliminated first, because they are inappropriate responses. From the remaining options, there is no indication that a physiological alteration is present; therefore, option 1 is most appropriate. Review adolescent sleep patterns if you had difficulty with this question.
Level of Cognitive Ability: Application
Client Needs: Physiological Integrity
Integrated Process: Nursing Process/Implementation
Content Area: Child Health
Reference: Price, D., & Gwin, J. (2008). *Pediatric nursing: An introductory text* (10th ed., p. 335). St. Louis: Saunders.

293. 4
Rationale: Adolescents often are not sure whether they want their parents with them when they are hospitalized. Because of the importance of the peer group, separation from friends is a source of anxiety. Ideally, the peer group will support the ill friend. Options 1, 2, and 3 isolate the child from the peer group.
Test-Taking Strategy: Consider the psychosocial needs of the adolescent when answering the question. Options 1, 2, and 3 are comparable or alike in that they isolate the child from their own peer group. Review the psychosocial needs of the adolescent if you had difficulty with this question.
Level of Cognitive Ability: Application
Client Needs: Psychosocial Integrity
Integrated Process: Nursing Process/Implementation
Content Area: Child Health
Reference: Price, D., & Gwin, J. (2008). *Pediatric nursing: An introductory text* (10th ed., p. 313). St. Louis: Saunders.

294. 1
Rationale: Toddlers, with their increased mobility and developing motor skills, can reach hot water, open fires, or hot objects placed on counters and stoves above their eye level. Parents should be encouraged to remain in the kitchen when preparing a meal and reminded to use the back burners on the stove; pot handles should be turned inward and toward the middle of the stove. Hot liquids should never be left unattended, and the toddler should always be supervised. Options 2, 3, and 4 do not reflect an adequate understanding of the principles of safety.
Test-Taking Strategy: Use the process of elimination. Option 2 can be easily eliminated. Options 3 and 4 are comparable or alike in that they isolate the child from the environment. Review safety principles for the toddler if you had difficulty with question.
Level of Cognitive Ability: Comprehension
Client Needs: Safe and Effective Care Environment
Integrated Process: Nursing Process/Evaluation
Content Area: Child Health
Reference: Price, D., & Gwin, J. (2008). *Pediatric nursing: An introductory text* (10th ed., p. 190). St. Louis: Saunders.

295. 1
Rationale: In the hospitalized preschooler, it is best to accept regression if it occurs, because it is most often caused by the stress of the hospitalization. Parents may be overly concerned about regression and should be told that their child may continue the behavior at home. There is no need to call the physician. Options 2 and 4 are inappropriate.
Test-Taking Strategy: Use the process of elimination. Options 2, 3, and 4 will cause additional stress and concern in the parent. Review the psychosocial issues related to the hospitalized preschool child if you had difficulty with this question.
Level of Cognitive Ability: Application
Client Needs: Psychosocial Integrity
Integrated Process: Nursing Process/Implementation
Content Area: Child Health

Reference: Price, D., & Gwin, J. (2008). *Pediatric nursing: An introductory text* (10th ed., p. 30). St. Louis: Saunders.

296. 1
Rationale: The transition point for switching to the forward-facing position is defined by the manufacturer of the convertible car safety seat, but it is generally at a body weight of 9 kg (20 lbs) and an age of 1 year. Convertible car safety seats are used until the child weighs at least 40 lbs. Options 2, 3, and 4 are incorrect.
Test-Taking Strategy: Use the process of elimination, and focus on the subject of the question. Eliminate options 3 and 4 first because of the close-ended words "not" and "never." From the remaining options, use your knowledge regarding car safety and the toddler to answer the question. Review these safety principles if you had difficulty with this question.
Level of Cognitive Ability: Application
Client Needs: Safe and Effective Care Environment
Integrated Process: Teaching and Learning
Content Area: Child Health
References: American Academy of Pediatrics. *Car safety seats: A guide for families 2008.* www.aap.org/family/carseatguide.htm. Accessed July 13, 2008.
McKinney, E., James, S., Murray, S., & Ashwill, J. (2005). *Maternal-child nursing* (2nd ed., p. 97). Philadelpha: Saunders.

297. 1
Rationale: The toddler is particularly vulnerable to separation. A toddler often shows anger at being left by ignoring the parent or by pretending to be more interested in play than in going home. The parents of hospitalized toddlers are frequently distressed by such behavior. The toddler normally engages in parallel play and plays alongside (but not with) other children. Options 2, 3, and 4 are incorrect.
Test-Taking Strategy: Use the concepts of growth and development. Option 3 can be easily eliminated first. There is no information in the question to support option 2. From the remaining options, knowledge regarding separation anxiety in the toddler will direct you to option 1. Review these concepts if you had difficulty with this question.
Level of Cognitive Ability: Comprehension
Client Needs: Psychosocial Integrity
Integrated Process: Nursing Process/Data Collection
Content Area: Child Health
Reference: Price, D., & Gwin, J. (2008). *Pediatric nursing: An introductory text* (10th ed., pp. 24-25). St. Louis: Saunders.

298. 2
Rationale: Toys for the toddler must be strong, safe, and too large to swallow or place in the ear or nose. Toddlers need supervision at all times. Push-pull toys, large balls, large crayons, trucks, and dolls are some appropriate toys. A puzzle with large pieces only may be appropriate. A farm set and a golf set may contain items that the child could swallow.
Test-Taking Strategy: Use the process of elimination. Options 3 and 4 can be easily eliminated, because they contain items that could be swallowed by the child. From the remaining options, the most appropriate toy is a wagon. Remember that large and strong toys are safest for the toddler.

Review safety measures for the toddler if you had difficulty with this question.
Level of Cognitive Ability: Comprehension
Client Needs: Safe and Effective Care Environment
Integrated Process: Nursing Process/Implementation
Content Area: Child Health
Reference: Price, D., & Gwin, J. (2008). *Pediatric nursing: An introductory text* (10th ed., p. 188). St. Louis: Saunders.

299. 2
Rationale: The anterior fontanel is diamond shaped and located on the top of the head. It should be soft and flat in a normal infant, and it normally closes by 12 to 18 months of age. The posterior fontanel closes by 2 to 3 months of age. Therefore, because the findings are normal, the nurse would document the findings.
Test-Taking Strategy: Use the process of elimination. Note the strategic words "soft and flat." These should provide you with the clue that this is a normal finding. A bulging or tense fontanel may result from crying or increased intracranial pressure. Review normal findings in the infant if you had difficulty with this question.
Level of Cognitive Ability: Application
Client Needs: Physiological Integrity
Integrated Process: Nursing Process/Implementation
Content Area: Child Health
Reference: Price, D., & Gwin, J. (2008). *Pediatric nursing: An introductory text* (10th ed., pp. 53-54). St. Louis: Saunders.

300. 2
Rationale: In the preschooler, play is simple and imaginative, and it includes activities such as dressing up, finger paints, clay, pasting, and simple board and card games. Large picture books are most appropriate for the infant. A radio and a sports video are most appropriate for the adolescent.
Test-Taking Strategy: Note the age of the child, and think about the age-related activity that would be appropriate. Eliminate options 1 and 3, knowing that they are most appropriate for the adolescent. From the remaining options, the word "large" in option 4 should provide you with the clue that this activity would be more appropriate for a child who is less than 5 years old. Review the appropriate activities for a preschooler if you had difficulty with this question.
Level of Cognitive Ability: Application
Client Needs: Psychosocial Integrity
Integrated Process: Nursing Process/Implementation
Content Area: Child Health
Reference: Price, D., & Gwin, J. (2008). *Pediatric nursing: An introductory text* (10th ed., p. 210). St. Louis: Saunders.

ALTERNATE ITEM FORMAT: MULTIPLE RESPONSE
301. 1, 4, 5
Rationale: Holding, caressing, and swaddling provide warmth and tactile stimulation for the infant. To provide auditory stimulation, the nurse should talk to the infant in a soft voice and should instruct the mother to do so also. Additional interventions include playing a music box, radio, or television or having a ticking clock or metronome nearby. Hanging a bright, shiny object within 20 to 25 cm of the

infant's face in the midline and hanging mobiles with contrasting colors (e.g., black and white) provide visual stimulation. Crying is an infant's way of communicating; therefore, the nurse would respond to the infant's crying. The mother is taught to do so also. An infant or child should never be allowed to fall asleep with a bottle containing milk, juice, soda, or sweetened water because of the risk of nursing (bottle-mouth) caries.

Test-Taking Strategy: Focus on the subject of the care of the infant. Noting the word "loud" in option 2 and the words "at least 10 minutes before responding" in option 6 will assist

you with eliminating these interventions. Recalling the concerns related to dental caries will assist you with eliminating option 3. Review the guidelines related to the care of an infant if you had difficulty with this question.

Level of Cognitive Ability: Application
Client Needs: Psychosocial Integrity
Integrated Process: Nursing Process/Implementation
Content Area: Child Health
Reference: Hockenberry, M., Wilson, D., & Winkelstein, M. (2005). *Wong's essentials of pediatric nursing* (7th ed., p. 408). St. Louis: Mosby.

REFERENCES

American Academy of Pediatrics. *Car safety seats: A guide for families 2008.* www.aap.org/family/carseatguide.htm. Accessed July 13, 2008.

Hockenberry, M., Wilson, D., & Winkelstein, M. (2005). *Wong's essentials of pediatric nursing* (7th ed.). St. Louis: Mosby.

McKinney, E., James, S., Murray, S., & Ashwill, J. (2005). *Maternal-child nursing* (2nd ed.). St. Louis: Saunders.

Leifer, G. (2005). *Maternity nursing* (9th ed.). Philadelphia: Saunders.

Lowdermilk, D., & Perry, S. (2003). *Maternity nursing* (6th ed.). St. Louis: Mosby.

National Council of State Boards of Nursing (Eds.) (2008). *2008 Detailed Test Plan for the NCLEX-PN® Examination, National Council of State Boards of Nursing.* Chicago: Author.

National Council of State Boards of Nursing. *NCSBN home page.* www.ncsbn.org. Accessed July 13, 2008.

Price, D., & Gwin, J (2008). *Pediatric nursing: An introductory text* (10th ed.). St. Louis: Saunders.

Care of the Older Client

I. PHYSIOLOGICAL CHANGES
  A. Integumentary system
    1. Loss of pigment in hair and skin
    2. Wrinkling of the skin
    3. Thinning of the epidermis; easy bruising and tearing of the skin
    4. Decreased skin turgor, elasticity, and subcutaneous fat
    5. Increased nail thickness and decreased nail growth
    6. Decreased perspiration
    7. Dry, itchy, and scaly skin
    8. Seborrheic dermatitis and keratosis formation
  B. Neurological system
    1. Slowed reflexes
    2. Slight tremors and difficulty with fine motor movement
    3. Loss of balance
    4. An increased incidence of awakening after sleep onset
    5. Increased susceptibility to hypothermia and hyperthermia
    6. Short-term memory may decline
    7. Long-term memory usually maintained
  C. Musculoskeletal system
    1. Muscle mass and strength decrease; muscles atrophy
    2. Decreased mobility, range of motion, flexibility, coordination, and stability
    3. Change of gait, with a shortened step and a wider base
    4. Posture and stature changes that cause a decrease in height (Figure 29-1)
    5. Increased brittleness of the bones
    6. Joint capsule component deterioration
    7. Kyphosis of the dorsal spine
  D. Cardiovascular system
    1. Diminished energy and endurance, with lowered tolerance to exercise
    2. Decreased compliance of the heart muscle; heart valves become thicker and more rigid
    3. Decreased cardiac output; decreased efficiency of blood return to the heart
    4. Decreased resting heart rate
    5. Weak peripheral pulses
    6. Increased blood pressure but susceptible to postural hypotension
  E. Respiratory system
    1. Decreased stretch and compliance of the chest wall
    2. Decreased strength and function of the respiratory muscles
    3. Decreased size and number of alveoli
    4. Increased rate of respirations (generally 16 to 25 breaths per minute)
    5. Decreased depth of respirations and oxygen intake
    6. Decreased ability to cough and expectorate sputum
  F. Hematological system
    1. Hemoglobin and hematocrit levels average toward the low end of normal
    2. Prone to increased blood clotting
  G. Immune system
    1. Lymphocyte counts tend to be low
    2. Decreased resistance to infection and disease
  H. Gastrointestinal system
    1. Decreased need for calories
    2. Decreased appetite, thirst, and oral intake
    3. Decreased lean body mass
    4. Digestive disturbances
    5. Decreased stomach-emptying time
    6. Decreased absorption of carbohydrates, proteins, fats, and vitamins
    7. Increased tendency toward constipation
    8. Increased susceptibility to dehydration
    9. Tooth loss
    10. Difficulty with chewing and swallowing food
  I. Endocrine system
    1. Decreased secretion of hormones, with specific changes related to each hormone function
    2. Decreased metabolic rate
    3. Decreased glucose tolerance, with resistance to insulin in the peripheral tissues
  J. Renal system
    1. Decreased kidney size, function, and ability to concentrate urine

2. Decreased glomerular filtration rate
3. Decreased capacity of the bladder
4. Increased residual urine; increased incidence of infection and incontinence
5. Impaired medication excretion

K. Reproductive system
1. Decreased testosterone production and size of testes
2. Changes in the prostate gland that lead to urinary problems
3. Decreased secretion of hormones, with the cessation of menses
4. Vaginal changes, including decreased muscle tone and lubrication
5. Impotence or sexual dysfunction for both sexes; sexual function varies and depends on general physical condition, mental health status, and medications

L. Special senses
1. Decreased visual acuity
2. Decreased accommodation in eyes, which requires increased time for adjustment to changes in light
3. Decreased peripheral vision and increased sensitivity to glare
4. Presbyopia and cataract formation

5. Possible loss of hearing ability; low-pitched tones more easily heard
6. Inability to discern taste of food
7. Decreased smell acuity
8. Changes in touch sensation
9. Decreased pain awareness

II. **PSYCHOSOCIAL CONCERNS**
A. Adjustment to deterioration in physical and mental health and well-being
B. Threat to independent functioning; fear of becoming a burden to loved ones
C. Adjustment to retirement and loss of income
D. Loss of skills and competencies developed early in life
E. Coping with changes in role function and social life
F. Diminished quantity and quality of relationships; coping with loss
G. Dependence on governmental and social systems
H. Access to social support systems
I. Costs of health care and medications

III. **MENTAL HEALTH CONCERNS** (Box 29-1)
A. Isolation: Client is alone and desires contact with others but is unable to make that contact
B. Grief: Reaction to the client's perception of loss, including physical, psychological, social, and spiritual aspects
C. **Depression**: The increased dependency that older adults may experience can lead to hopelessness, helplessness, a lowered sense of self-control, and decreased self-esteem and self-worth; these changes can interfere with daily functioning and lead to **depression**
D. Suicide: All suicide threats from an older client should be taken seriously

IV. **PAIN**
A. Description
1. Pain can occur from numerous causes and most often occurs from degenerative changes in the musculoskeletal system
2. The failure to alleviate pain in the older client can lead to functional limitations that affect the client's ability to function independently
B. Data collection
1. Agitation
2. Moaning
3. Crying
4. Restlessness
5. Verbal reporting of pain

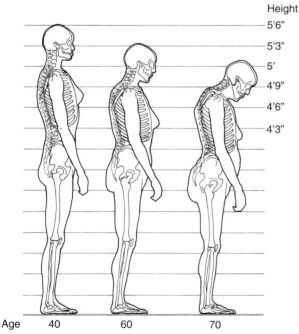

FIG. 29-1 A normal spine at 40 years of age and osteoporotic changes at 60 and 70 years of age. These changes can cause a loss of as much as 6 inches in height and can result in a malformation called dowager's hump *(far right)* in the upper thoracic vertebrae. (From Ignatavicius, D., & Workman, M. [2006]. *Medical surgical nursing: Critical thinking for collaborative care* [5th ed.]. Philadelphia: Saunders.)

| BOX 29-1 | **Mental Health Concerns** |

- Isolation
- Grief
- Depression
- Suicide

C. Interventions
1. Monitor the client for signs of pain
2. Identify the pattern of pain
3. Identify the precipitating factor(s) of the pain
4. Monitor the impact of the pain on the client's activities of daily living
5. Provide pain relief through measures such as distraction, relaxation, massage, and biofeedback
6. Administer pain medications, as prescribed; instruct the client in their use
7. Evaluate the effects of pain-reducing measures

V. INFECTION

A. Confusion is a common sign of infection in the older adult, especially of infection of the urinary tract
B. Carefully monitor the older adult with an infection because of the diminished and altered immune response seen in these patients
C. Nonspecific symptoms may indicate illness or infection (Box 29-2)

VI. MEDICATIONS

A. Major problems with prescription medications include adverse affects, interactions, errors, noncompliance, and cost
B. Determine the use of over-the-counter medications
C. **Polypharmacy**
1. Routinely monitor the number of prescription and nonprescription medications used and determine if any can be eliminated or combined
2. Keep the use of medications to a minimum
3. Overprescribing medications leads to increased problems with more side effects, increased interaction among medications, the replication of medication treatment, diminished quality of life, and pointless costs.
D. Medication dosages normally are prescribed at one third to one half of the normal adult doses
E. Closely monitor the client for adverse effects and response to therapy because of the increased risk for medication toxicity

---

BOX 29-2 **Nonspecific Symptoms That May Indicate Illness or Infection**

- Apathy
- Anorexia
- Changes in functional status
- Confusion
- Dyspnea
- Falling
- Fatigue
- Incontinence
- Self-neglect
- Shortness of breath
- Tachypnea
- Vital sign changes

F. Note that a common sign of an adverse reaction in the older client in an acute change in mental status
G. Assess for medication interactions in the client who is taking multiple medications
H. Advise the client to use one pharmacy and to notify the consulting physicians of the medications taken
I. Administration of medications
1. Place the client in a sitting position when administering medication
2. Check for mouth dryness, because medication may stick and dissolve in the mouth
3. Administer liquid preparations if the client has difficulty swallowing tablets
4. Crush tablets, if necessary, and give with textured food (e.g., nectar, applesauce) if not contraindicated
5. Do not crush enteric-coated tablets; do not open capsules
6. If administering a suppository, do not insert the suppository immediately after removing it from the refrigerator
7. A suppository may take longer to dissolve because of a decreased body core temperature
8. When administering parenteral medication, monitor the site, because it may ooze medication or bleed as a result of decreased tissue elasticity
9. Do not use an immobile limb for administering parenteral medication
10. Monitor client compliance with the taking of prescribed medications
11. Monitor the client for safety with regard to correctly taking medications, including an assessment of the client's ability to read the instructions and to discriminate among the pills and their colorations
12. Use a medication cassette to facilitate the proper administration of medication

VII. ABUSE OF THE OLDER ADULT

A. **Abuse** involves physical, emotional, or sexual **abuse** and also can involve **neglect** or economic **exploitation**
B. Categories of mistreatment of the older client
1. Domestic mistreatment takes place in the home of the older adult and is usually carried out by a family member or a significant other; this can include physical maltreatment, **neglect**, or abandonment
2. Institutional mistreatment takes place when an older adult experiences **abuse** when hospitalized or living in another type of facility other than the home
3. **Self-neglect** is the lack of caring for oneself by a mentally competent individual who is cognitively competent but who engages in actions that negatively affect his or her personal safety

C. Individuals who are at most risk for **abuse** include those who are dependent because of their immobility or altered mental status.

D. Factors that contribute to **abuse** and **neglect** include longstanding family violence, caregiver stress, and the individual's increasing dependence on others

E. Abusers tend to be male, engage in substance **abuse,** and have a mental illness or **dementia**; in addition, they tend to depend on the older client for financial assistance or other resources

F. Victims may attempt to dismiss injuries as accidental, and abusers may prevent victims from receiving proper medical care to avoid discovery

G. Victims often are socially isolated by their abusers

H. For additional information about **abuse** of the older client, see Chapter 65

PRACTICE QUESTIONS

More questions on the companion CD!

302. The nurse is providing medication instructions to an older client who is taking digoxin (Lanoxin) on a daily basis. The nurse bears in mind that which age-related body changes could place the client at risk for digitalis toxicity?
    1. Decreased cough efficiency and vital capacity
    2. Decreased salivation and gastrointestinal motility
    3. Decreased muscle strength and loss of bone density
    4. Decreased lean body mass and glomerular filtration rate

303. A nurse who is employed in a long-term care facility is caring for an older male client. Which of the following nursing actions would contribute to encouraging autonomy in the client?
    1. Planning his meals
    2. Decorating his room
    3. Scheduling his barber appointments
    4. Allowing him to choose his social activities

304. A nurse is caring for an older female client whose husband died 6 months ago. Which behavior by the client indicates ineffective coping?
    1. Neglecting her personal grooming
    2. Looking at old snapshots of her family
    3. Participating in a senior citizens' program
    4. Visiting her husband's grave once a month

305. The nurse is preparing to communicate with an older client who is hearing impaired. The appropriate initial nursing action is to:
    1. Stand in front of the client.
    2. Exaggerate the lip movements.
    3. Obtain a sign-language interpreter.
    4. Pantomime and write the client notes.

306. The nurse is assigned to care for an older client with hearing loss. The nurse plans care, knowing that older clients:
    1. Are often distracted
    2. Have middle-ear changes
    3. Respond to low-pitched tones
    4. Develop moist cerumen production

307. The nurse is attending an educational session, and the topic is the abuse of the older client. The nurse understands that which type of client is commonly a victim of abuse?
    1. A 75-year-old man with moderate hypertension
    2. A 68-year-old man with newly diagnosed cataracts
    3. A 90-year-old woman with advanced Parkinson's disease
    4. A 70-year-old woman with early diagnosed Lyme disease

308. A nurse is assigned to care for an older client. To reduce the risk of aspiration during meals, the nurse positions the client:
    1. Upright in a chair
    2. On the left side in bed
    3. On the right side in bed
    4. In a low Fowler's position, with the legs elevated

309. A nurse who volunteers at a senior citizens' center is planning activities for the members who attend the center. Which activity would best promote the health and maintenance of these senior citizens?
    1. Gardening every day for an hour
    2. Sculpting once a week for 40 minutes
    3. Cycling three times a week for 20 minutes
    4. Walking three to five times a week for 30 minutes

310. A nurse is working with older clients in a long-term care facility. Which of the following activities performed by the nurse fosters reminiscence among these clients?
    1. Having storytelling hours
    2. Setting up pet therapy sessions
    3. Displaying calendars and clocks
    4. Encouraging client participation in a pottery class

311. A nurse is teaching an older client about measures to prevent constipation. Which statement, if made by the client, indicates that further teaching about bowel elimination is necessary?
    1. "I walk 1 to 2 miles per day."
    2. "I need to decrease fiber in my diet."
    3. "I have a bowel movement every other day."
    4. "I drink six to eight glasses of water per day."

312. The nurse is collecting data from an older client who is having difficulty sleeping at night. Which statement, if made by the client, indicates that teaching about promoting sleep is necessary?

1. "I swim three times a week."
2. "I have stopped smoking cigars."
3. "I drink hot chocolate before bedtime."
4. "I read for 40 minutes before bedtime."

313. The nurse observes that an older male client is confined by his daughter-in-law to his room. When the nurse suggests that he walk to the den and join the family, he says, "I'm in everyone's way, and my son needs me to stay here." The most important action for the nurse to take is to:
   1. Say to the son, "Confining your father to his room is inhumane."
   2. Say nothing; it is best for the nurse to remain neutral and to wait to be asked for help.
   3. Suggest to the client and daughter-in-law that they consider a nursing home for the client.
   4. Suggest appropriate resources to the client and daughter-in-law, such as respite care and a senior citizens' center.

314. The nurse provides medication instructions to an older hypertensive client who is taking 20 mg of lisinopril (Prinivil, Zestril) orally daily. Which statement, if made by the client, indicates that further teaching is necessary?
   1. "I can skip a dose once a week."

2. "I need to change my position slowly."
3. "I take the pill after breakfast each day."
4. "If I get a bad headache, I should call my doctor immediately."

315. The nurse is caring for an older client who is on bedrest. The nurse plans which intervention to prevent respiratory complications?
   1. Decreasing oral fluid intake
   2. Monitoring the vital signs every shift
   3. Changing the client's position every 2 hours
   4. Instructing the client to bear down every hour and to hold his or her breath

ALTERNATE ITEM FORMAT: MULTIPLE RESPONSE

316. Select all of the normal age-related physiological changes.
   ☐ 1. Increased heart rate
   ☐ 2. Decline in visual acuity
   ☐ 3. Decreased respiratory rate
   ☐ 4. Decline in long-term memory
   ☐ 5. Increased susceptibility to urinary tract infections
   ☐ 6. Increased incidence of awakening after sleep onset

ANSWERS

302. 4

Rationale: The older client is at risk for medication toxicity because of decreased lean body mass and an age-associated decreased glomerular filtration rate. Although options 1, 2, and 3 identify age-related changes that occur in the older client, they are not specifically associated with this risk.

Test-Taking Strategy: Use the process of elimination, and focus on the subject of an age-related body change that could place the client at risk for medication toxicity. Note that option 4 is the only option that addresses renal excretion. Review the physiological changes associated with aging if you had difficulty with this question.

Level of Cognitive Ability: Comprehension
Client Needs: Physiological Integrity
Integrated Process: Teaching and Learning
Content Area: Fundamental Skills
Reference: Wold, G. (2008). *Basic geriatric nursing* (4th ed., p. 117). St. Louis: Mosby.

303. 4

Rationale: Autonomy is the personal freedom to direct one's own life as long as it does not impinge on the rights of others. An autonomous person is capable of rational thought. This individual can identify problems, search for alternatives, and choose solutions that allow for continued personal freedom as long as the rights and property of others are not harmed. The loss of autonomy—and, therefore, independence—is a very real fear among older clients. Option 4 is the only option that allows the client to be a decision maker.

Test-Taking Strategy: Use the process of elimination, and focus on the subject of encouraging autonomy. Recalling the definition of autonomy will direct you to the correct option. Remember that to promote independence in clients, it is essential to give the client choices. Review the concept of autonomy if you had difficulty with this question.

Level of Cognitive Ability: Application
Client Needs: Safe and Effective Care Environment
Integrated Process: Caring
Content Area: Fundamental Skills
Reference: Linton, A. (2007). *Introduction to medical-surgical nursing* (4th ed., pp. 24, 27). Philadelphia: Saunders.

304. 1

Rationale: Coping mechanisms are behaviors that are used to decreased stress and anxiety. In response to a death, ineffective coping is manifested by an extreme behavior that in some instances may be harmful to the individual, either physically, psychologically, or both. Option 1 is indicative of a behavior that identifies an ineffective coping behavior as part of the grieving process.

Test-Taking Strategy: Use the process of elimination, and note the subject of an ineffective coping behavior. Eliminate options 2, 3, and 4, because they are comparable or alike and are positive activities that the individual is engaging in to get on with her life. Review the coping mechanisms for dealing with grief and loss if you had difficulty with this question.

Level of Cognitive Ability: Analysis
Client Needs: Mental Health
Integrated Process: Nursing Process/Data Collection

Content Area: Fundamental Skills
Reference: Wold, G. (2008). *Basic geriatric nursing* (4th ed., p. 212). St. Louis: Mosby.

305. 1
Rationale: The nurse would ensure that the hearing-impaired client can see the nurse when the nurse is speaking by providing adequate lighting and by standing in front of the client. The nurse should enunciate words clearly but not exaggerate lip movements. If the client is profoundly hearing impaired and uses signing, a sign-language interpreter should be obtained. If a client cannot understand by reading lips, the nurse would try using gestures, pantomiming, or writing notes.
Test-Taking Strategy: Note the strategic words "initial nursing action." To communicate effectively with a hearing-impaired client, the nurse first makes sure that the client can see him or her. Review the nursing interventions for the hearing-impaired client if you had difficulty with this question.
Level of Cognitive Ability: Application
Client Needs: Psychosocial Integrity
Integrated Process: Nursing Process/Implementation
Content Area: Fundamental Skills
Reference: Wold, G. (2008). *Basic geriatric nursing* (4th ed., p. 93). St. Louis: Mosby.

306. 3
Rationale: Presbycusis refers to the age-related, irreversible, degenerative changes of the inner ear that lead to decreased hearing acuity. As a result of these changes, the older client has a decreased response to high-frequency sounds. Low-pitched tones of voice are more easily heard and interpreted by the older client. Options 1, 2, and 4 are not accurate.
Test-Taking Strategy: Use the process of elimination. Recalling that the client with a hearing loss responds better to low-pitched tones will direct you to option 3. Review the characteristics associated with presbycusis and hearing loss if you had difficulty with this question.
Level of Cognitive Ability: Application
Client Needs: Physiological Integrity
Integrated Process: Nursing Process/Planning
Content Area: Adult Health/Ear
Reference: Wold, G. (2008). *Basic geriatric nursing* (4th ed., pp. 64, 165-166). St. Louis: Mosby.

307. 3
Rationale: Elder abuse is widespread and occurs among all subgroups of the population. It includes physical and psychological abuse, the misuse of property, and the violation of rights. The typical abuse victim is a woman of advanced age with few social contacts and at least one physical or mental impairment that limits her ability to perform activities of daily living. In addition, the client usually lives alone or with the abuser and depends on the abuser for care.
Test-Taking Strategy: Use the process of elimination. Read each option carefully, and identify the client who is most defenseless as a result of the disease process. Review the characteristics of elder abuse if you had difficulty with this question.
Level of Cognitive Ability: Comprehension
Client Needs: Psychosocial Integrity

Integrated Process: Nursing Process/Data Collection
Content Area: Mental Health
Reference: Fortinash, K., & Holoday Worret, P. (2008). *Psychiatric mental health nursing* (4th ed., p. 502). St. Louis: Mosby.

308. 1
Rationale: It is preferable to get clients out of bed and sitting in a chair for meals. This position facilitates chewing and swallowing and prevents the reflux of stomach contents and aspiration. Options 2, 3, and 4 do not identify positions that will reduce the risk of aspiration.
Test-Taking Strategy: Use the process of elimination. Focus on the subject of the question—reducing the risk of aspiration. This should direct you to option 1. Review the measures that will prevent aspiration if you had difficulty with this question.
Level of Cognitive Ability: Application
Client Needs: Safe and Effective Care Environment
Integrated Process: Nursing Process/Implementation
Content Area: Fundamental Skills
Reference: Wold, G. (2008). *Basic geriatric nursing* (4th ed., p.263). St. Louis: Mosby.

309. 4
Rationale: Exercise and activity are essential for health promotion and maintenance in the older adult and for achieving an optimal level of functioning. Approximately half of the physical deterioration of the older client is caused by disuse rather than by the aging process or disease. One of the best exercises for an older adult is walking, with the goal of progressing to 30-minute sessions three to five times each week. Swimming and dancing are also beneficial.
Test-Taking Strategy: Use the process of elimination, and note the strategic word "best." Options 1, 2, and 3, although possible, are not the best activities. Remember that walking is one of the best forms of exercise. Review health promotion activities for the older client if you had difficulty with this question.
Level of Cognitive Ability: Application
Client Needs: Health Promotion and Maintenance
Integrated Process: Nursing Process/Planning
Content Area: Fundamental Skills
Reference: Wold, G. (2008). *Basic geriatric nursing* (4th ed., pp. 302-304). St. Louis: Mosby.

310. 1
Rationale: Clients who like to retell stories or to describe past events need to be provided with the opportunity to do so. This phenomenon is called life review or reminiscence. In a sense, it is a way for the elder client to relive and restructure life experiences, and it is a part of achieving ego identity. Option 3 indicates reality orientation techniques. Options 2 and 4 indicate socialization and physical activity.
Test-Taking Strategy: Use the process of elimination. Focusing on the strategic word "reminiscence" and recalling its definition will direct you to option 1. Review this form of activity if you had difficulty with this question.
Level of Cognitive Ability: Application
Client Needs: Psychosocial Integrity
Integrated Process: Caring

Content Area: Mental Health
Reference: Wold, G. (2008). *Basic geriatric nursing* (4th ed., p. 192). St. Louis: Mosby.

311. 2
Rationale: Adequate dietary fiber is an important factor for improving bowel function. Dietary fiber increases fecal weight and water content and accelerates the transit of the fecal mass through the gastrointestinal tract. The retention of water by the fiber has the ability to soften stools and promote regularity. Fluid intake and exercise also facilitate bowel elimination.
Test-Taking Strategy: Note the strategic words "further teaching about bowel elimination is necessary." These words indicate a negative event query and ask you to select an option that is an incorrect statement. Use the process of elimination and basic principles related to preventing constipation. Review these basic principles if you had difficulty with this question.
Level of Cognitive Ability: Comprehension
Client Needs: Physiological Integrity
Integrated Process: Teaching and Learning
Content Area: Fundamental Skills
Reference: Wold, G. (2008). *Basic geriatric nursing* (4th ed., pp. 288-290). St. Louis: Mosby.

312. 3
Rationale: Many nonpharmacological sleep aids can be used to influence sleep. The client should avoid caffeinated beverages and stimulants (e.g., tea, cola, chocolate) and foods that contain tyrosine (e.g., cheddar cheese). The client should exercise regularly, because exercise promotes sleep by burning off tension that accumulates during the day. A 20- to 30-minute walk, swim, or bicycle ride three time a week is helpful. Smoking and alcohol should be avoided. The client should avoid large meals, peanuts, beans, fruit and raw vegetables that produce gas, and snacks that are high in fat and difficult to digest.
Test-Taking Strategy: Focus on the subject of teaching being necessary. Options 1, 2, and 4 are positive statements that indicate that the client understands the methods of promoting sleep. Review the factors that can interfere with sleep if you had difficulty with this question.
Level of Cognitive Ability: Comprehension
Client Needs: Physiological Integrity
Integrated Process: Teaching and Learning
Content Area: Fundamental Skills
Reference: Wold, G. (2008). *Basic geriatric nursing* (4th ed., p. 330). St. Louis: Mosby.

313. 4
Rationale: Assisting clients and families with becoming aware of available community support systems is a role and responsibility of the nurse. Option 3 involves suggesting committing the client to a nursing home and is a premature action on the nurse's part. Although the data provided tell the nurse that this client requires nursing care, the nurse does not know the extent of nursing care required. Observing that the client has begun to be confined to his room makes it necessary for the nurse to intervene legally and ethically, so option 2 is not appropriate and is passive in terms of advocacy. Option 1 is incorrect and judgmental.

Test-Taking Strategy: Use the process of elimination. Note the strategic words "most important action." Using the principles related to the ethical and legal responsibilities of the nurse and your knowledge of the nurse's role will direct you to option 4. Review these principles if you had difficulty with this question.
Level of Cognitive Ability: Application
Client Needs: Safe and Effective Care Environment
Integrated Process: Nursing Process/Implementation
Content Area: Fundamental Skills
Reference: Wold, G. (2008). *Basic geriatric nursing* (4th ed., pp. 25, 177). St. Louis: Mosby.

314. 1
Rationale: Lisinopril is an antihypertensive angiotensin-converting enzyme inhibitor. The usual dosage range is 20 to 40 mg per day. Adverse effects include headache, dizziness, fatigue, orthostatic hypotension, tachycardia, and angioedema. Specific client teaching points include taking one pill a day, not stopping the medication without consulting the physician, and monitoring for side effects and adverse reactions. The client should notify the physician if side effects occur.
Test-Taking Strategy: Use the process of elimination. Note the strategic words "further teaching is necessary." Basic principles related to the administration of prescribed medications will direct you to option 1. Review the teaching points related to medication administration if you had difficulty with this question.
Level of Cognitive Ability: Analysis
Client Needs: Physiological Integrity
Integrated Process: Teaching and Learning
Content Area: Pharmacology
Reference: Hodgson, B., & Kizior, R. (2008). *Saunders nursing drug handbook 2008* (pp. 695-697). Philadelphia: Saunders.

315. 3
Rationale: Frequent position changes help mobilize lung secretions and prevent pooling. This is the only intervention identified in the options that will prevent respiratory complications. The nurse should assess the client's vital signs every 4 hours to identify an elevated temperature, which may suggest infection. The nurse would encourage fluid intake to thin secretions and thus enable the client to expectorate more easily. It is important to encourage coughing and deep breathing to mobilize lung secretions. The client should be instructed to avoid Valsalva's maneuver or any activity that involves holding the breath.
Test-Taking Strategy: Use the process of elimination. Note the strategic words "prevent respiratory complications." Changing the position of the immobilized client every 2 hours will help prevent the pooling of lung secretions. The other options do not assist the client with improving ventilatory efforts or preventing respiratory complications. Review the nursing interventions to prevent respiratory complications in the client who is immobilized if you had difficulty with this question.
Level of Cognitive Ability: Application
Client Needs: Physiological Integrity
Integrated Process: Nursing Process/Planning
Content Area: Fundamental Skills

Reference: Linton, A. (2007). *Introduction to medical-surgical nursing* (4th ed., p. 314). Philadelphia: Saunders.

ALTERNATE FORMAT QUESTION: MULTIPLE RESPONSE

316. **2, 5, 6**
Rationale: Anatomical changes to the eye affect the individual's visual ability, which leads to potential problems with activities of daily living. Light adaptation and visual fields are reduced. Respiratory rates are generally higher among older adults, ranging from 16 to 25 breaths per minute. The heart rate decreases, and the heart valves thicken. Age-related changes that affect the urinary tract increase an older client's susceptibility to urinary tract infections. Short-term memory may decline with age, but long-term memory is usually maintained. Changes in sleep patterns are consistent, age-related changes. Older persons experience an increased incidence of awakening after sleep onset.
Test-Taking Strategy: Knowledge regarding normal age-related changes is needed to answer this question. Read each characteristic carefully, and think about the physiological changes that occur with aging to select the correct items. Review normal age-related changes if you had difficulty with this question.
Level of Cognitive Ability: Analysis
Client Needs: Health Promotion and Maintenance
Integrated Process: Nursing Process/Data Collection
Content Area: Fundamental Skills
Reference: Meiner, S., & Lueckenotte, A. (2006). *Gerontologic nursing* (3rd ed, pp. 27-30). St. Louis: Mosby.

REFERENCES

Fortinash, K., & Holoday Worret, P. (2008). *Psychiatric mental health nursing* (4th ed.). St. Louis: Mosby.

Hodgson, B., & Kizior, R. (2008). *Saunders nursing drug handbook 2008.* Philadelphia: Saunders.

Jarvis, C. (2008). *Physical examination & health assessment* (5th ed.). Philadelphia: Saunders.

Linton, A. (2007). *Introduction to medical-surgical nursing* (4th ed.). Philadelphia: Saunders.

Meiner, S., & Lueckenotte, A. (2006). *Gerontologic nursing* (3rd ed.). St. Louis: Mosby.

National Council of State Boards of Nursing (Eds.). (2008). *2008 Detailed Test Plan for the NCLEX-PN® Examination, National Council of State Boards of Nursing.* Chicago: Author.

National Council of State Boards of Nursing. *NCSBN home page.* www.ncsbn.org. Accessed July 13, 2008.

Wold, G. (2008). *Basic geriatric nursing* (4th ed.). St. Louis: Mosby.

Pediatric Nursing

PYRAMID TERMS

abuse The nonaccidental physical injury or the nonaccidental act of omission of care by a parent or a person responsible for a child; includes neglect as well as physical, sexual, and emotional maltreatment.

active immunity A form of long-term acquired antibody protection that develops either naturally after an initial infection or by exposure to antigens or artificially after a vaccination.

atresia The congenital absence or closure of a body orifice.

attenuated vaccines Vaccines derived from microorganisms or viruses with virulence that has been weakened as a result of passage through another host.

cephalocaudal Characterized by growth and development that proceeds from head to toe.

crackles Audible high-pitched crackling or popping sounds heard during lung auscultation that result from fluid in the airways and that are not cleared by coughing; formerly called rales.

chronological age The age in years.

cyanosis The bluish color that is seen in tissues, nail beds, and mucous membranes when tissues are deprived of adequate amounts of oxygen.

developmental age The age based on functional behavior and the ability to adapt to the environment; developmental age does not necessarily correspond with chronological age.

encopresis Fecal incontinence after the age of 4 years.

functional age The age equivalent at which a child actually is able to perform specific self-care or related tasks.

growth Measurable physical and physiological body changes that occur over time.

grunting The sound made by forced expiration, which is the body's attempt to improve oxygenation when hypoxemia is present.

hereditary The transmission of genetic characteristics from parent to offspring.

inactivated vaccines Vaccines that contain killed microorganisms.

nasal flaring A widening of the nares to enable an infant or child to take in more oxygen; a serious indicator of air hunger.

passive immunity A form of acquired immunity that occurs artificially through injection or that is acquired naturally as a result of antibody transfer through the placenta to a fetus or through colostrum to an infant; this type of immunity is not permanent.

prodromal Pertaining to early symptoms that mark the onset of a disease.

puberty The period of time during which the adolescent experiences a growth spurt, develops secondary sex characteristics, and achieves reproductive maturity.

regression Behavior that is more appropriate for an earlier stage of development and that is often used to cope with stress or anxiety.

regurgitation An abnormal backward flow of body fluid.

retraction An abnormal movement of the chest wall during inspiration in which the skin appears to be drawn in between the ribs and above and/or below the clavicle and scapula; this condition indicates respiratory difficulty.

shunt The movement of blood or body fluid through an abnormal anatomical or surgically created opening.

stenosis The narrowing or constriction of an opening.

stridor A shrill, harsh sound heard during inspiration, expiration, or both that is produced by the flow of air through a narrowed segment of the respiratory tract.

vaccine A suspension of attenuated or killed microorganisms that is administered to induce active immunity to an infectious disease.

wheezing A high-pitched musical whistling sound that is heard with or without a stethoscope as air is compressed through narrowed or obstructed airways as a result of swelling, secretions, or tumors.

PYRAMID TO SUCCESS

The pyramid points focus on growth and development; safety and the age-appropriate measures for ensuring a safe and hazard-free environment for the child; and acute disorders that can occur in children. Focus on specific feeding techniques, positioning techniques, and interventions that will provide and maintain adequate airway, breathing, and circulation patterns in the child. On the NCLEX-PN, be alert to the age of the child if the age is presented in the question. The Integrated Processes addressed in this unit include Caring, the Clinical Problem-Solving Process (Nursing Process), Communication and Documentation, and Teaching and Learning.

▲ CLIENT NEEDS

Safe and Effective Care Environment

Considering issues related to informed consent for minors

Ensuring environmental and personal safety related to the developmental age of the child

Establishing priorities

Instituting measures related to the spread and control of infectious agents, particularly communicable diseases

Maintaining confidentiality

Preventing accidents

Providing continuity of care

Providing protective measures

Protecting the child and other contacts to prevent illness

Upholding parent's and child's rights

Health Promotion and Maintenance

Considering concepts of family systems when planning care

Ensuring that immunization schedules are up to date

Focusing on developmental stages when planning care

Preventing disease in the pediatric population

Providing health-promotion programs for the pediatric client

Providing instructions to the child and parents regarding care at home

Psychosocial Integrity

Assessing for child abuse and neglect

Communicating with the pediatric client

Considering cultural, religious, and spiritual beliefs when planning care

Considering end-of-life issues, grief, and loss in the pediatric population

Identifying family and support systems for the child

Providing play therapies

Physiological Integrity

Following medication administration procedures

Following nutritional guidelines for the pediatric population

Identifying comfort measures that are appropriate for the child

Maintaining sensitivity during intrusive procedures that are required for the pediatric client

Managing childhood illnesses

Monitoring elimination patterns

Monitoring for age-appropriate normal body structure and function

Monitoring for infectious diseases of the pediatric client

Monitoring for potential alterations in body systems as a result of disease

Monitoring for responses to treatments

Providing for consistent rest and sleep patterns

Responding to medical emergencies

REFERENCES

deWit, S. (2005). *Fundamental concepts and skills for nursing* (2nd ed.). Philadelphia: Saunders.

Hockenberry, M., & Wilson, D. (2007). *Nursing care of infants and children* (8th ed.). St. Louis: Mosby.

Leifer, G. (2007). *Introduction to maternity and pediatric nursing* (5th ed.). Philadelphia: Saunders.

Malarkey, L., & McMorrow, M. (2005). *Nursing guide to laboratory and diagnostic tests*. Philadelphia: Saunders.

Merenstein, G.B., & Gardner, S.A. (2007). *Handbook of neonatal intensive care* (6th ed.). St. Louis: Mosby.

National Council of State Boards of Nursing (Eds.). (2008). *2008 Detailed Test Plan for the NCLEX-PN® Examination, National Council of State Boards of Nursing*. Chicago: Author.

National Council of State Boards of Nursing. *NCSBN home page*. www.ncsbn.org. Accessed July 16, 2008.

Pagana, K., & Pagana, T. (2005). *Mosby's diagnostic and laboratory test reference* (7th ed.). St. Louis: Mosby.

Potter, P., & Perry, A. (2005). *Fundamentals of nursing* (6th ed.). St. Louis: Mosby.

Price, D., & Gwin, J. (2008). *Pediatric nursing: an introductory text* (10th ed.). St. Louis: Saunders.

Skidmore-Roth, L. (2005). *Mosby's drug guide for nurses* (6th ed.). St. Louis: Mosby.

Stuart, G., & Laraia, M. (2005). *Principles and practice of psychiatric nursing* (8th ed.). St. Louis: Mosby.

Wong, D., Perry, S., Hockenberry, M., Lowdermilk, D., & Wilson, D. (2006). *Maternal-child nursing care* (3rd ed.). St. Louis: Mosby.

Neurological, Cognitive, and Psychosocial Disorders

▲ **I. HEAD INJURY**

A. Description

    1. Head injury is the pathological result of any mechanical force to the skull, scalp, meninges, or brain

        a. Open head injury occurs when there is a fracture of the skull or a penetration of the skull by an object

        b. Closed head injury is the result of blunt trauma; it is more serious as a result of the chance of increased intracranial pressure (ICP) in a "closed" vault

    2. Manifestations depend on the type of injury and the subsequent amount of increased ICP

▲ B. Data collection (increased ICP)

    1. Early signs

        a. Headache

        b. Visual disturbances; diplopia

        c. Nausea and vomiting

        d. Dizziness or vertigo

        e. Slight change in vital signs

        f. Change in pupillary response and equality

        g. Sunsetting eyes (sclera is visible above the iris)

        h. Slight change in level of consciousness

        i. Infant: Bulging fontanel; wide sutures, increased head circumference; dilated scalp veins; high-pitched cry

        j. Child: Headache, nausea, vomiting, ataxia, nystagmus

    2. Late signs

        a. Significant decrease in level of consciousness

        b. Bradycardia

        c. Decorticate posturing: Adduction of the arms at the shoulders, the arms being flexed on the chest with the wrists flexed and the hands fisted, and the lower extremities being extended and adducted; seen with severe dysfunction of the cerebral cortex (Figure 30-1)

        d. Decerebrate posturing: Rigid extension and pronation of the arms and the legs; a sign of dysfunction at the level of the midbrain (see Figure 30-1)

        e. Fixed and dilated pupils

C. Interventions

    1. Monitor the airway

    2. Assess injuries; immobilize the neck if a cervical injury is suspected

    3. Monitor the vital signs and the neurological function

    4. Monitor for decreased responsiveness to pain (this is a significant sign of an altered level of consciousness)

    5. Initiate seizure precautions (Box 30-1)

    6. Maintain a nothing-by-mouth status or provide clear liquids, if prescribed, until it is determined that vomiting will not occur

    7. Administer oxygen and intravenous (IV) fluids, as prescribed

    8. Monitor IV fluids carefully to avoid aggravating any cerebral edema and to minimize the possibility of overhydration

    9. Elevate the head of the bed 15 to 30 degrees, if not contraindicated, to facilitate venous drainage

    10. Position the child so that the head is maintained in the midline to avoid jugular vein compression, which can increase ICP

    11. Assess the wound dressings for the presence of drainage; monitor for nose or ear drainage, which could indicate the leakage of cerebrospinal fluid (CSF); drainage that is positive for glucose (as tested with reagent strips) indicates the leakage of CSF from a skull fracture

    12. Administer tepid sponge baths or place the child on a hypothermia blanket if hyperthermia occurs

    13. Avoid suctioning through the nares because of the possibility of the catheter entering the brain through a fracture and placing the child at high risk for a secondary infection

    14. Administer acetaminophen (Tylenol) for headache, anticonvulsants for seizures, antibiotics if a laceration is present, an osmotic diuretic

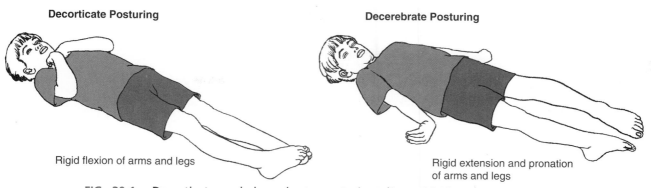

Decorticate Posturing

Rigid flexion of arms and legs

Decerebrate Posturing

Rigid extension and pronation of arms and legs

FIG. 30-1 Decorticate and decerebrate posturing. (From McKinney, E., James, S., Murray, S., & Ashwill, J. [2005]. *Maternal-child nursing* [2nd ed.]. Philadelphia: Saunders.)

BOX 30-1 Seizure Precautions

Raise the side rails when the child is sleeping or resting.
Pad the side rails and other hard objects.
Place a waterproof mattress or pad in the bed or crib.
Instruct the child to wear or carry medical identification.
Instruct the child regarding precautions to take during potentially hazardous activities.
Instruct the child to swim with a companion.
Instruct the child to use a protective helmet and padding during bicycle riding, skateboarding, and inline skating.
Alert caregivers to the need for any special precautions.

BOX 30-2 Signs of Brainstem Involvement

- Deep, rapid, or intermittent and gasping respirations
- Wide fluctuations or noticeable slowing of the pulse
- Widening pulse pressure or extreme fluctuations in blood pressure

(Mannitol) to reduce cerebral edema, corticosteroids such as dexamethasone (Decadron) to reduce brain edema, and tetanus toxoid, as appropriate and as prescribed

15. Withhold sedating medications during the acute phase of the injury so that changes in levels of consciousness can be assessed
16. Monitor for signs of brainstem involvement (Box 30-2)
17. Monitor for signs of epidural hematoma, such as asymmetric pupils (one dilated, unreactive pupil), which can be a neurosurgical emergency that may require the evacuation of the hematoma
18. Keep stimuli to a minimum; attempt to minimize crying in the infant

II. NEAR DROWNING
A. Description
   1. Survival of at least 24 hours after submersion in a fluid medium

BOX 30-3 Types of Hydrocephalus

Communicating
Hydrocephalus occurs as a result of impaired absorption within the subarachnoid space.
Interference of the cerebrospinal fluid within the ventricular system does not occur.
Noncommunicating
The obstruction of cerebrospinal fluid flow within the ventricular system occurs.

   2. Hypoxia is the primary problem, because it results in global cell damage; cerebral cells sustain irreversible damage after 4 to 6 minutes of submersion
B. Interventions
   1. Monitor the respiratory status, because respiratory compromise and cerebral edema may occur 24 hours after the incident
   2. Monitor for aspiration pneumonia
   3. If the child has had a severe cerebral insult, endotracheal intubation and mechanical ventilation may be required
   4. Teach the parents to provide adequate supervision of infants and small children around water to prevent accidents

III. HYDROCEPHALUS
A. Description
   1. An imbalance of CSF absorption and production caused by malformations, tumors, hemorrhage, infections, or trauma
   2. Results in head enlargement and increased ICP
B. Types (Box 30-3)
C. Data collection
   1. Infant
      a. Increased head circumference
      b. Thin, widely separated bones of the head that produce a cracked-pot sound (Macewen's sign) on percussion
      c. Anterior fontanel that is tense, bulging, and nonpulsating
      d. Dilated scalp veins

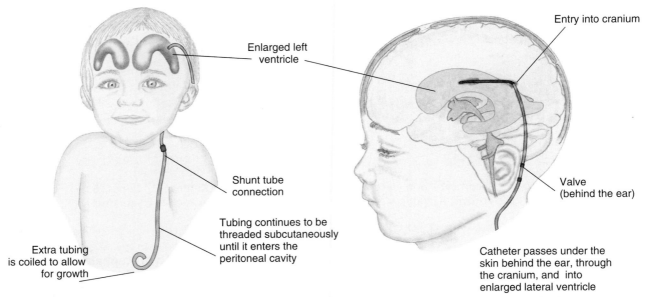

FIG. 30-2 Ventriculoperitoneal shunt. (From McKinney, E., James, S., Murray, S., & Ashwill, J. [2005]. *Maternal-child nursing* [2nd ed.]. Philadelphia: Saunders.)

e. Frontal bossing

f. Sunsetting eyes

2. Child

a. Behavior changes (e.g., irritability, lethargy)

b. Headache on awakening

c. Nausea and vomiting

d. Ataxia

e. Nystagmus

3. Late signs: A high, shrill cry and seizures

D. Surgical interventions

1. The goal of surgical treatment is to prevent further CSF accumulation by bypassing the blockage and draining the fluid from the ventricles to a location where it may be reabsorbed

2. In a ventriculoperitoneal **shunt,** the CSF drains into the peritoneal cavity from the lateral ventricle (Figure 30-2)

3. In an atrioventricular **shunt,** the CSF drains into the right atrium of the heart from the lateral ventricle, bypassing the obstruction; this is used for older children and children with pathological conditions of the abdomen

E. Interventions preoperatively

1. Monitor intake and output (I&O); administer small frequent feedings as tolerated until a preoperative nothing-by-mouth status is prescribed

2. Reposition the head frequently and use an eggcrate mattress under the head to prevent pressure sores

3. Prepare the child and family for diagnostic procedures and surgery

F. Interventions postoperatively

1. Monitor the vital signs and the neurological signs

2. Position the child on the unoperated side to prevent pressure on the **shunt** valve

3. Keep the child flat, as prescribed, to avoid the rapid reduction of intracranial fluid

4. Observe for increased ICP; if increased ICP occurs, elevate the head of the bed to 15 to 30 degrees to enhance gravity flow through the **shunt**

5. Monitor for signs of infection; assess dressings for drainage

6. Measure the head circumference

7. Monitor I&O

8. Provide comfort measures; administer medications, as prescribed, which may include diuretics, antibiotics, or anticonvulsants

9. Instruct the parents regarding how to recognize **shunt** infection or malfunction

10. In an infant, irritability, lethargy, and feeding poorly may indicate **shunt** malfunction or infection

11. In a toddler, headache and a lack of appetite are the earliest common signs of **shunt** malfunction

12. In older children, the most valuable indicator of **shunt** malfunction is an alteration in the child's level of consciousness

IV. **SPINA BIFIDA**

A. Description

1. A central nervous system defect that results from the failure of the neural tube to close during embryonic development

2. Associated deficits may include sensorimotor disturbance, dislocated hips, talipes equinovarus (clubfoot), and hydrocephalus

3. Defect closure is performed immediately after birth

B. Types
1. Spina bifida occulta
   a. Posterior vertebral arches fail to close in the lumbosacral area
   b. Spinal cord remains intact and usually is not visible
   c. Meninges are not exposed on the skin surface
   d. Neurological deficits are not usually present
2. Spina bifida cystica
   a. Protrusion of the spinal cord and/or its meninges occurs
   b. Defect results in the incomplete closure of the vertebral and neural tubes, which results in a saclike protrusion in the lumbar or sacral area with varying degrees of nervous tissue involvement
   c. Defect can include meningocele, myelomeningocele, lipomeningocele, and lipomeningomyelocele
3. Meningocele
   a. Protrusion involves meninges and a saclike cyst that contains CSF in the midline of the back, usually in the lumbosacral area
   b. Spinal cord is not involved
   c. Neurological deficits are usually not present
4. Myelomeningocele
   a. Protrusion of the meninges, CSF, nerve roots, and a portion of the spinal cord occurs
   b. The sac (defect) is covered by a thin membrane that is prone to leakage or rupture
   c. Neurological deficits are evident
C. Data collection
   1. Depends on the spinal cord involvement
   2. Visible spinal defect
   3. Flaccid paralysis of the legs
   4. Altered bladder and bowel function
   5. Hip and joint deformities
   6. Hydrocephalus
D. Interventions
   1. Evaluate the sac and measure the lesion
   2. Perform a neurological assessment
   3. Monitor for increased ICP, which may indicate developing hydrocephalus
   4. Measure the head circumference; assess the anterior fontanel for fullness
   5. Protect the sac; cover with a sterile, moist (normal saline), nonadherent dressing to maintain the moisture of the sac and its contents; change the dressing every 2 to 4 hours, as prescribed
   6. Place the child in a prone position to minimize tension on the sac and the risk of trauma; the head is turned to one side for feeding
   7. Change the dressing that covers the sac whenever it becomes soiled to reduce the risk of infection; diapering may be contraindicated until the defect has been repaired
   8. Use aseptic technique to prevent infection
   9. Assess the sac for redness, clear or purulent drainage, abrasions, irritation, and signs of infection
   10. Early signs of infection include elevated axillary temperature, irritability, lethargy, and nuchal rigidity
   11. Assess for physical impairments such as hip and joint deformities
   12. Prepare the child and family for surgery
   13. Administer antibiotics preoperatively, as prescribed, to prevent infection
   14. Teach the parents and eventually the child about long-term home care
       a. Positioning, feeding, skin care, and range-of-motion exercises
       b. Performing clean intermittent catheterization technique
       c. Administering propantheline (Pro-Banthine), as prescribed, to improve continence
       d. Implementing a bowel program that includes a high-fiber diet, increased fluids, and suppositories, as needed
       e. The child is at high risk for a latex allergy

V. REYE'S SYNDROME
A. Description
   1. An acute encephalopathy that follows a viral illness and that is characterized pathologically by cerebral edema and fatty changes in the liver
   2. The exact cause is not clear
   3. The administration of aspirin is not recommended for children with varicella or influenza because of its association with Reye's syndrome
   4. Acetaminophen (Tylenol) is considered the medication of choice for pediatric clients
   5. The goals of treatment are to maintain effective cerebral perfusion and to control increasing ICP
B. Data collection
   1. History of systemic viral illness 4 to 7 days before the onset of symptoms
   2. Malaise
   3. Nausea and vomiting
   4. Progressive neurological deterioration
C. Interventions
   1. Assess the neurological status
   2. Monitor for an altered level of consciousness and signs of increased ICP
   3. Monitor I&O
   4. Provide rest; decrease stimulation in the environment
   5. Monitor for signs of bleeding and impaired coagulation (e.g., a prolonged bleeding time)
   6. Monitor the liver function studies

▲ **VI. MENINGITIS**

A. Description

1. Meningitis is an infectious process of the central nervous system that is caused by bacteria and viruses that may be acquired as a primary disease or as a result of complications of neurosurgery, trauma, infection of the sinuses or ears, or systemic infections

2. The diagnosis of bacterial meningitis is made by testing CSF obtained by lumbar puncture; the fluid of a child with meningitis is cloudy with increased pressure, increased white blood cell count, elevated protein, and decreased glucose

3. Bacterial meningitis (*Haemophilus influenzae* type B, *Streptococcus pneumoniae*, or *Neisseria meningitidis*) occurs in epidemic form and can be transmitted by droplets from nasopharyngeal secretions

4. Viral meningitis is associated with viruses such as mumps, paramyxovirus, herpesvirus, and enterovirus

▲ B. Data collection

1. Signs and symptoms vary, depending on the type, the age of the child, and the duration of the preceding illness; there is no one classic sign or symptom

2. Fever, chills, and headache

3. Vomiting and diarrhea

4. Poor feeding or anorexia

5. Nuchal rigidity

6. Poor or high-pitched cry

7. Altered level of consciousness (e.g., lethargy, irritability)

8. Bulging anterior fontanel in the infant

9. Positive Kernig's sign (the inability to extend the leg when the thigh is flexed anteriorly at the hip) and Brudzinski's sign (neck flexion causes adduction and flexion movements of the lower extremities) in children and adolescents

10. Muscle or joint pain

11. Petechial or purpuric rashes (meningococcal infection)

▲ C. Interventions

1. Provide isolation and maintain it for at least 24 hours after antibiotics are initiated

2. Administer antibiotics and antipyretics, as prescribed

3. Perform a neurological assessment and monitor for seizures; assess for the complication of inappropriate antidiuretic hormone secretion, which causes fluid retention (cerebral edema) and dilutional hyponatremia

4. Assess for changes in the level of consciousness and irritability

5. Monitor I&O

6. Assess the nutritional status

7. Determine the close contacts of the child with meningitis, because those contacts will require prophylactic treatment

8. Meningococcal **vaccine** is recommended to protect against meningitis; see Chapter 38 for information about vaccines

VII. SEIZURE DISORDERS ▲

A. Description

1. Sudden, transient alterations in brain function that result from excessive levels of electrical activity in the brain

2. Classified as generalized, partial, or unclassified, depending on the area of the brain involved

3. Types of generalized seizures
   a. Tonic-clonic (grand mal); consciousness is lost
   b. Absence (petit mal); momentary loss of consciousness, posture is maintained; minor face, eye, and hand movements

4. Partial seizures arise from a specific area in the brain and cause limited symptoms; examples include focal and psychomotor seizures

B. Data collection ▲

1. Obtain information from the parents about the time of onset, precipitating events, and behavior before and after the seizure

2. Determine the child's history related to seizures

3. Aura (a warning sign of impending seizure)

4. Apnea and **cyanosis**

5. Postseizure: Disoriented and sleepy

6. Absence seizures: Occur between 4 and 12 years of age and last 5 to 10 seconds; child appears inattentive

C. Seizure precautions (see Box 30-1) ▲

D. Interventions (Box 30-4)

E. Anticonvulsant medications (see Chapter 57 for information about medications)

VIII. CEREBRAL PALSY

A. Description

1. A disorder characterized by impaired movement and posture resulting from an abnormality in the extrapyramidal or pyramidal motor system

2. The most common clinical type is spastic cerebral palsy, which represents an upper motor neuron type of muscle weakness

3. Less common types are athetoid, ataxic, and mixed

B. Data collection

1. Extreme irritability and crying

2. Feeding difficulties

3. Stiff and rigid arms or legs

4. Delayed developmental milestones

5. Abnormal motor performance

6. Alterations of muscle tone

7. Abnormal posturing (e.g., opisthotonic [exaggerated arching of the back]) ▲

BOX 30-4 **Emergency Treatment for Seizures**

Ensure airway patency.

Have suction equipment and oxygen available.

Time the seizure episode.

If the child is standing or sitting, ease the child down to the floor and place him or her in a side-lying position.

Place a pillow or folded blanket under the child's head; if no bedding is available, place your own hands under the child's head, or place the child's head in your own lap.

Loosen restrictive clothing.

Remove eyeglasses from the child, if present.

Clear the area of any hazards or hard objects.

Allow the seizure to proceed and end without interference.

If vomiting occurs, turn the child to one side as a unit.

Do not restrain the child, place anything in the child's mouth, or give any food or liquids to the child.

Prepare to administer medications, as prescribed.

Remain with the child until the child fully recovers.

Observe for incontinence, which may have occurred during the seizure.

Document the occurrence.

---

8. Persistence of primitive infantile reflexes (e.g., Moro, tonic neck) after 6 months
9. Seizures

C. Interventions
1. The goal of management is early recognition and intervention to maximize the child's abilities
2. A multidisciplinary team approach is implemented to meet the many needs of the child
3. Therapeutic management includes physical therapy, occupational therapy, speech therapy, education, and recreation
4. Assess the child's developmental level and intelligence
5. Encourage early intervention and participation in school programs
6. Prepare for the use of mobilizing devices to help prevent or reduce deformities
7. Encourage communication and interaction with the child on his or her developmental level rather than his or her **chronological age** level
8. Provide a safe environment by removing sharp objects, using a protective helmet if the child falls frequently, and implementing seizure precautions, if necessary
9. Provide safe and appropriate toys for the child's age and developmental level
10. Position the child upright after meals.
11. Administer medications, as prescribed, to decrease spasticity

12. Surgical interventions are reserved for the child who does not respond to more conservative measures or for the child whose spasticity causes progressive deformity.
13. Intrathecal baclofen (Lioresal) may be used to provide relief of spasticity

IX. **MENTAL RETARDATION**
A. Description
1. In mental retardation, the child manifests subaverage intellectual functioning along with deficits in adaptive skills
2. Down syndrome is a congenital condition that results in moderate to severe retardation and has been linked to an extra group G chromosome (chromosome 21/trisomy 21)

B. Data collection
1. Deficits in cognitive skills and level of adaptive functioning
2. Delays in fine and gross motor skills
3. Speech delays
4. Decreased spontaneous activity
5. Nonresponsiveness
6. Irritability
7. Poor eye contact during feeding

C. Interventions
1. Medical strategies are focused at correcting structural deformities and treating associated behaviors
2. Implement community and educational services with the use of a multidisciplinary approach
3. Promote care skills as much as possible
4. Assist with communication and socialization skills
5. Facilitate appropriate playtime
6. Initiate safety precautions, as necessary
7. Assist the family with decisions regarding care
8. Provide information regarding support services and community agencies

X. **AUTISM**
A. Description
1. A severe mental disorder that begins during infancy or toddlerhood
2. Apparent to the parents before the child is 3 years old
3. Characterized by impairments in reciprocal social interaction and in verbal and nonverbal communication
4. Cause is unknown; prognosis may be poor
5. Diagnosis is established on the basis of symptoms and with the use of specialized autism assessment tools
6. Also called infantile autism

B. Data collection
1. The child experiences a disturbance in the rate and appearance of physical, social, and language skills

2. The child experiences abnormal responses of body sensations

3. The child has abnormal ways of relating to persons, objects, and events; he or she is self-absorbed and unable to relate to others

4. The child has no delusions, hallucinations, or incoherence; the facies is intelligent and responsive

5. The child may play happily alone for hours but have temper tantrums if interrupted

6. Language disturbance often includes the repetition of previously heard speech (echolalia) and the reversal of the pronouns "I" and "you"

7. If the child can talk, he or she uses speech not for communication but to repeat words or phrases meaninglessly

8. The child may develop an unusual attachment to a significant object and display frequent rocking, spinning, twirling, or other bizarre behaviors

C. Interventions

1. Determine the child's routines, habits, and preferences, and maintain consistency as much as possible

2. Determine the specific ways in which the child communicates

3. Facilitate communication with the use of picture boards

4. Evaluate the child for safety

5. Implement safety precautions, as necessary, for self-injurious behaviors such as head banging

6. Monitor for stress and anxiety

7. Avoid placing demands on the child

8. Initiate referrals to special programs, as required

9. Provide support to the parents

XI. ATTENTION DEFICIT HYPERACTIVITY DISORDER

A. Description

1. A developmental disorder that is characterized by inappropriate degrees of inattention, overactivity, and impulsivity

2. One of the most common reasons for the referral of children to mental health services

3. Childhood problems include lowered intellectual development, some minor physical abnormalities, sleep disturbances, behavioral or emotional disorders, and difficulty with social relationships

4. Diagnosis is established on the basis of self-reports, parent and teacher reports, and psychological assessments

B. Data collection

1. Fidgets with hands or feet or squirms in a seat

2. Easily distracted by external or internal stimuli

3. Difficulty with following through on instructions

4. Poor attention span

5. Shifts from one uncompleted activity to another

6. Talks excessively

7. Interrupts or intrudes on others

8. Engages in physically dangerous activities without considering the possible consequences

C. Interventions

1. Provide environmental and physical safety measures

2. Enhance capabilities and self-esteem

3. Encourage support groups for the parents

4. Administer prescribed medication; some commonly prescribed medications include methylphenidate hydrochloride (Ritalin), pemoline (Cylert), and dextroamphetamine sulfate (Dexedrine).

5. Instruct the child and parents regarding medication administration

6. Inform the child and parents that positive effects of the medication may be seen within 1 to 2 weeks if taken as prescribed

XII. CHILD ABUSE

A. Description: Child **abuse** involves emotional or physical **abuse** or neglect as well as sexual exploitation or molestation by caretakers or other individuals

B. Data collection

1. Physical **abuse**
   a. Unexplained bruises, burns, or fractures
   b. Bald spots on the scalp
   c. Apprehensive child
   d. Extreme aggressiveness or withdrawal
   e. Fear of parents
   f. Lack of crying (older infant, toddler, or young preschool child) when approached by a stranger

2. Physical neglect
   a. Inadequate weight gain
   b. Poor hygiene
   c. Consistent hunger
   d. Inconsistent school attendance
   e. Constant fatigue
   f. Reports of a lack of child supervision
   g. Delinquency

3. Emotional **abuse**
   a. Speech disorders
   b. Habit disorders, such as sucking, biting, and rocking
   c. Psychoneurotic reactions
   d. **Learning** disorders
   e. Suicide attempts

4. Sexual **abuse**
   a. Difficulty walking or sitting
   b. Torn, stained, or bloody underclothing
   c. Pain, swelling, or itching of the genitals
   d. Bruises, bleeding, or lacerations in the genital or anal area

e. Unwillingness to change clothes or to participate in gym activities

f. Poor peer relations

5. Shaken baby syndrome: Intracranial (usually subdural hemorrhage) trauma that is caused by violent shaking of a child who is less than 1 year old

a. Ophthalmoscopic assessment reveals retinal hemorrhages; external signs of trauma are usually absent

b. Can cause intracranial hemorrhage that leads to cerebral edema and death

c. Full bulging fontanelles and a head circumference greater than expected would be noted

C. Interventions

1. Support the child during a thorough physical assessment

2. Assess injuries

3. Report a case of suspected **abuse**; nurses are legally required to report all cases of suspected **abuse** to the appropriate local or state agency

4. Place the child in an environment that is safe, thereby preventing further injury

5. Document in an objective manner information related to the suspected **abuse**

6. Assess the parents' strengths and weaknesses, normal coping mechanisms, and the presence or absence of support systems

7. Assist the family with identifying stressors, support systems, and resources

8. Refer the family to appropriate support groups

9. If shaken baby syndrome is suspected, monitor the infant's level of consciousness

XIII. CHILD ABDUCTION

A. Description

1. Child abduction is the kidnapping of a child (or baby) by an older person

a. A stranger removes a child for criminal or mischievous purposes

b. A stranger removes a child (usually a baby) to bring up as that person's own child

c. A parent removes or retains a child from the other parent's care (often during the course of or after divorce proceedings)

2. Around the preschool age, parents are less able to provide the constant protection that they once did

B. Interventions

1. Instruct the parents to teach the child basic guidelines about personal safety, including the following:

a. Do not go anywhere alone

b. Always tell an adult where he or she is going and when he or she will return

c. Say "no" if he or she feels uncomfortable with a situation

d. Do not give directions to a stranger

e. Do not talk with strangers or get into their cars

f. Do not help anyone look for a lost dog or cat

g. Do not accept candy from a stranger.

h. If lost in a store, do not wander around looking for the parent; go at once to a clerk or guard

2. Children need to learn their full name, address, and parents' names

3. Watch for posttraumatic stress disorder in any child who has experienced an abduction

PRACTICE QUESTIONS

More questions on the companion CD!

317. A nurse is collecting data about a child who has been admitted to the hospital with a diagnosis of seizures. The nurse checks for causes of the seizure activity by:

1. Testing the child's urine for specific gravity

2. Asking the child what happens during a seizure

3. Obtaining a family history of psychiatric illness

4. Obtaining a history regarding factors that may precipitate seizure activity

318. A child has a basilar skull fracture. Which of the following physician orders should the nurse question?

1. Restrict fluid intake.

2. Insert an indwelling urinary catheter.

3. Keep an intravenous (IV) line patent.

4. Suction via the nasotracheal route as needed.

319. Which of the following laboratory results would verify the diagnosis of bacterial meningitis?

1. Clear cerebrospinal fluid with high protein and low glucose levels

2. Cloudy cerebrospinal fluid with low protein and low glucose levels

3. Cloudy cerebrospinal fluid with high protein and low glucose levels

4. Decreased pressure and cloudy cerebrospinal fluid with a high protein level

320. A child has been diagnosed with meningococcal meningitis. Which of the following isolation techniques is appropriate?

1. Enteric precautions

2. Neutropenic precautions

3. No precautions are required as long as antibiotics have been started.

4. Isolation precautions for at least 24 hours after the initiation of antibiotics

321. Which of the following represents a primary characteristic of autism?

1. Normal social play

2. Consistent imitation of others' actions

3. Lack of social interaction and awareness
4. Normal verbal and nonverbal communication

322. Which assessment finding would indicate the possibility of the sexual abuse of a child?
1. Poor hygiene
2. Fear of the parents
3. Bald spots on the scalp
4. Swelling of the genitals

323. A nurse is assisting with data collection from an infant who has been diagnosed with hydrocephalus. If the infant's level of consciousness diminishes, a priority nursing intervention is:
1. Taking the apical pulse
2. Taking the blood pressure
3. Testing the urine for protein
4. Palpating the anterior fontanel

324. A mother arrives at the emergency department with her 5-year-old child and states that the child fell off a bunk bed. A head injury is suspected, and a nurse is assessing the child continuously for signs of increased intracranial pressure (ICP). Which of the following is a late sign of increased ICP in this child?
1. Nausea
2. Bradycardia
3. Bulging fontanel
4. Dilated scalp veins

325. A child has been diagnosed with Reye's syndrome. The nurse understands that the major symptom associated with Reye's syndrome is:
1. Persistent vomiting
2. Protein in the urine
3. Symptoms of hyperglycemia
4. A history of a *Staphylococcus* infection

326. The nurse assists with preparing a nursing care plan for a child who has Reye's syndrome. Which of the following is the priority nursing intervention?
1. Monitoring the output
2. Checking for hearing loss
3. Changing the body position every 2 hours

4. Providing a quiet atmosphere with dimmed lights

327. Which of the following is indicative of a potential complication associated with a tonic-clonic seizure?
1. High-pitched cry
2. Blanched toenails
3. Blood on the pillow
4. Migraine headaches

328. A nurse is initiating seizure precautions. Which of the following items should the nurse place at the bedside?
1. Oxygen with a nasal cannula
2. A suction apparatus and oxygen
3. An airway and a tracheotomy set
4. An emergency cart and an oxygen mask

329. A nurse is providing instructions to an adolescent who has a history of seizures and who is taking an anticonvulsant medication. Which of the following statements indicates that the client understands the instructions?
1. "I will never be able to drive a car."
2. "My anticonvulsant medication will clear up my skin."
3. "I can't drink alcohol while I am taking my medication."
4. "If I forget my morning medication, I can take two pills at bedtime."

ALTERNATE ITEM FORMAT: MULTIPLE RESPONSE

330. A nurse is developing a plan of care for a child who is at risk for seizures. Select all of the interventions that apply if the child has a seizure.
☐ 1. Time the seizure.
☐ 2. Restrain the child.
☐ 3. Stay with the child.
☐ 4. Place the child in a prone position.
☐ 5. Move furniture away from the child.
☐ 6. Insert a padded tongue blade into the child's mouth.

ANSWERS

317. 4
Rationale: Fever and infections increase the body's metabolic rate; this can cause seizure activity among children who are less than 5 years old. Dehydration and electrolyte imbalance can also contribute to the occurrence of a seizure. Falls can cause head injuries, which would increase intracranial pressure or cerebral edema. Some medications could cause seizures. Specific gravity would not be a reliable test, because it varies, depending on the existing condition. Psychiatric illness has no impact on seizure occurrence or cause. Children do not remember what happened during the seizure itself.
Test-Taking Strategy: Use the process of elimination, and focus on the subject of the cause of the seizure

activity. Note the relationship between the subject and option 4. Review the precipitating factors associated with seizures if you had difficulty with this question.
Level of Cognitive Ability: Application
Client Needs: Physiological Integrity
Integrated Process: Nursing Process/Data Collection
Content Area: Child Health
Reference: Price, D., & Gwin, J. (2008). *Pediatric nursing: An introductory text* (10th ed., p. 252). St. Louis: Saunders.

318. 4
Rationale: Nasotracheal suctioning is contraindicated in a child with a basilar skull fracture. Because of the nature of the injury, the suction catheter may be introduced into

the brain. The child may require a urinary catheter for the accurate monitoring of intake and output. Fluids are restricted to prevent fluid overload. An IV line is maintained to administer fluids or medications, if necessary.

Test-Taking Strategy: Use the process of elimination, and note the strategic words "should the nurse question." Note that options 1, 2, and 3 are comparable or alike in that they all address the issue of fluid intake or output. Review the care of the child with a basilar skull fracture if you had difficulty with this question.

Level of Cognitive Ability: Analysis
Client Needs: Safe and Effective Care Environment
Integrated Process: Nursing Process/Implementation
Content Area: Child Health
Reference: Wong, D., Perry, S., Hockenberry, M., Lowdermilk, D., & Wilson, D. (2006). *Maternal child nursing care* (3rd ed., p. 1678). St. Louis: Mosby.

319. 3
Rationale: A diagnosis of meningitis is made by testing the cerebrospinal fluid (CSF) obtained by lumbar puncture. In the case of bacterial meningitis, findings usually include increased pressure, cloudy CSF, a high protein level, and a low glucose level.

Test-Taking Strategy: Use the process of elimination and your knowledge regarding the diagnostic findings in clients with meningitis. Eliminate options 1 and 4 first, because clear CSF and decreased pressure are not likely to be found if an infectious process such as meningitis is suspected. From this point, recalling that a high protein level indicates a possible diagnosis of meningitis will direct you to option 3. Review the findings in clients with meningitis if you had difficulty with this question.

Level of Cognitive Ability: Comprehension
Client Needs: Physiological Integrity
Integrated Process: Nursing Process/Data Collection
Content Area: Child Health
References: Hockenberry, M., & Wilson, D. (2007). *Nursing care of infants and children* (8th ed., p. 1646). St. Louis: Mosby. Pagana, K., & Pagana, T. (2005). *Mosby's diagnostic and laboratory test reference* (7th ed., pp. 603-606). St. Louis: Mosby.

320. 4
Rationale: Meningococcal meningitis is transmitted primarily by droplet infection. Isolation is begun and maintained for at least 24 hours after antibiotics are given. Options 1, 2, and 3 are incorrect.

Test-Taking Strategy: Use the process of elimination, and eliminate options 1 and 2 first. Both enteric and neutropenic precautions are unrelated to the mode of transmission of meningococcal meningitis. Recalling that it takes approximately 24 hours for antibiotics to reach a therapeutic blood level will assist with directing you to option 4 from the remaining options. Review the mode of transmission of meningococcal meningitis if you had difficulty with this question.

Level of Cognitive Ability: Application
Client Needs: Safe and Effective Care Environment
Integrated Process: Nursing Process/Planning
Content Area: Child Health
Reference: Leifer, G. (2007). *Introduction to maternity and pediatric nursing* (5th ed., p. 531). Philadelphia: Saunders.

321. 3
Rationale: Autism is a severe developmental disorder that begins during infancy or toddlerhood. The primary characteristic is a lack of social interaction and awareness. Social behaviors in autism include a lack of or an abnormal imitation of others' actions and a lack of or abnormal social play. Additional characteristics include a lack of or impaired verbal communication and markedly abnormal nonverbal communication.

Test-Taking Strategy: Use the process of elimination. Eliminate options 1 and 4 first, because they address normal behaviors. From the remaining options, recalling that the autistic child lacks social interaction and awareness will direct you to option 3. Review the characteristics associated with autism if you had difficulty with this question.

Level of Cognitive Ability: Comprehension
Client Needs: Psychosocial Integrity
Integrated Process: Nursing Process/Data Collection
Content Area: Child Health
Reference: Leifer, G. (2007). *Introduction to maternity and pediatric nursing* (5th ed., p. 732). Philadelphia: Saunders.

322. 4
Rationale: The most likely findings among children who have been sexually abused include difficulty walking or sitting; torn, stained, or bloody underclothing; pain, swelling, or itching of the genitals; and bruises, bleeding, or lacerations in the genital or anal area. Poor hygiene may be indicative of physical neglect. Bald spots on the scalp and fear of the parents are most likely associated with physical abuse.

Test-Taking Strategy: Use the process of elimination. Note the strategic words "sexual abuse." The only option that specifically addresses a finding related to sexual abuse is option 4. Review the findings in a child who is suspected of being abused if you had difficulty with this question.

Level of Cognitive Ability: Comprehension
Client Needs: Physiological Integrity
Integrated Process: Nursing Process/Data Collection
Content Area: Child Health
Reference: Price, D., & Gwin, J. (2008). *Pediatric nursing: An introductory text* (10th ed., p. 173). St. Louis: Elsevier.

323. 4
Rationale: A full or bulging anterior fontanel indicates an increase in cerebrospinal fluid collection in the cerebral ventricle. Proteinuria, apical pulse, and blood pressure changes are not specifically associated with increasing cerebrospinal fluid in the brain tissue in an infant.

Test-Taking Strategy: Use the principles associated with excessive fluid buildup in the cranial cavity, and note that the question addresses an infant. Additionally, correlate "hydrocephalus" in the question with "anterior fontanel" in option 4. Review the symptoms associated with hydrocephalus if you had difficulty with this question.

Level of Cognitive Ability: Application
Client Needs: Physiological Integrity
Integrated Process: Nursing Process/Data Collection
Content Area: Child Health
Reference: Price, D., & Gwin, J. (2008). *Pediatric nursing: An introductory text* (10th ed., pp. 110-111). St. Louis: Saunders.

324. 2
Rationale: Late signs of increased ICP include a significant decrease in the level of consciousness, bradycardia, and fixed and dilated pupils. A bulging fontanel and dilated scalp veins are early signs of increased ICP and would be noted in an infant rather than in a 5-year-old child. Nausea is an early sign of increased ICP.
Test-Taking Strategy: Use the process of elimination, and note the age of the child and the strategic word "late." Options 3 and 4 can be eliminated first, because these signs would be noted in an infant rather than a 5-year-old child. Focusing on the strategic word "late" will direct you to option 2. Review the early and late signs of increased ICP in an infant and in a child if you had difficulty with this question.
Level of Cognitive Ability: Analysis
Client Needs: Physiological Integrity
Integrated Process: Nursing Process/Data Collection
Content Area: Child Health
Reference: Price, D., & Gwin, J. (2008). *Pediatric nursing: An introductory text* (10th ed., p. 212). St. Louis: Saunders.

325. 1
Rationale: Persistent vomiting is a major symptom that is associated with increased intracranial pressure (ICP). Options 2, 3, and 4 are incorrect. Protein is not present in the urine. Reye's syndrome is related to a history of viral infections, and hypoglycemia is a symptom of this disease.
Test-Taking Strategy: Note the strategic words "major symptom." Recalling that increased ICP is an associated characteristic will direct you to option 1. Review the symptoms of Reye's syndrome and the signs of increased ICP if you had difficulty with this question.
Level of Cognitive Ability: Comprehension
Client Needs: Physiological Integrity
Integrated Process: Nursing Process/Data Collection
Content Area: Child Health
Reference: Price, D., & Gwin, J. (2008). *Pediatric nursing: An introductory text* (10th ed., p. 318). St. Louis: Saunders.

326. 4
Rationale: The major elements of care are to maintain effective cerebral perfusion and to control intracranial pressure. Decreasing stimuli in the environment would decrease the stress on the cerebral tissue and the neuron responses. Cerebral edema is a progressive part of this disease process. Hearing loss and output are not affected. Changing the body position every 2 hours would not affect the cerebral edema and intracranial pressure directly. The child should be in a head-elevated position to decrease the progression of the cerebral edema and to promote the drainage of cerebrospinal fluid.
Test-Taking Strategy: Focus on the pathophysiology associated with Reye's syndrome to answer the question. Recalling the effects of environmental stimuli, the responses of the brain cells to stimuli, and how cerebral edema can result will direct you to option 4. Review the symptoms of Reye's syndrome and the signs of increased intracranial pressure if you had difficulty with this question.
Level of Cognitive Ability: Application
Client Needs: Physiological Integrity
Integrated Process: Nursing Process/Planning

Content Area: Child Health
References: Leifer, G. (2007). *Introduction to maternity and pediatric nursing* (5th ed., pp. 527-529). Philadelphia: Saunders. Wong, D., Perry, S., Hockenberry, M., Lowdermilk, D., & Wilson, D. (2006). *Maternal-child nursing care* (3rd ed., p. 1702). St. Louis: Mosby.

327. 3
Rationale: The complications associated with seizures include airway compromise, extremity and teeth injuries, and tongue lacerations. Night seizures can cause the child to bite down on the tongue. Cyanosis can occur during the tonic-clonic part of the seizure activity, but blanching does not occur. Migraine headaches are not common in children with seizures. Seizures do not cause a high-pitched cry unless a tumor or intracranial pressure is the cause of the seizure diagnosis.
Test-Taking Strategy: Use your knowledge of tonic-clonic activity and of the involuntary tightening of all of the body muscles that occurs during seizure activity when answering this question. Recall that the tongue can easily get caught by the child's teeth when the seizure activity occurs; this causes injury, swelling, and bleeding of the tongue tissue. Review the complications associated with seizures if you had difficulty with this question.
Level of Cognitive Ability: Analysis
Client Needs: Physiological Integrity
Integrated Process: Nursing Process/Data Collection
Content Area: Child Health
Reference: Price, D., & Gwin, J. (2008). *Pediatric nursing: An introductory text* (10th ed., pp. 252-254). St. Louis: Saunders.

328. 2
Rationale: Seizures cause a tightening of all body muscles that is followed by tremors. An obstructed airway and increased oral secretions are the major complications during and after the seizure. Suctioning and oxygen is helpful to prevent choking and cyanosis. Option 3 is incorrect, because inserting a tracheostomy is not done. Option 4 is incorrect, because an emergency cart would not be left at the bedside; however, it would be available in the treatment room or on the nursing unit.
Test-Taking Strategy: Use the process of elimination. Recalling that seizures produce excessive oral secretions and airway obstruction will direct you to option 2. Review the plan of care associated with seizure precautions if you had difficulty with this question.
Level of Cognitive Ability: Application
Client Needs: Safe and Effective Care Environment
Integrated Process: Nursing Process/Implementation
Content Area: Child Health
References: Price, D., & Gwin, J. (2008). *Pediatric nursing: An introductory text* (10th ed., p. 254). St. Louis: Saunders.

329. 3
Rationale: Alcohol will lower the seizure threshold and should be avoided. Adolescents can obtain a driver's license in most states when they have been seizure free for 1 year. Anticonvulsants cause acne and oily skin; therefore, a dermatologist may need to be consulted. If an anticonvulsant medication is missed, the physician should be notified.

Test-Taking Strategy: Use the process of elimination, and note the strategic words "indicates that the client understands." Using general principles related to medication instructions will direct you to option 3. Review the teaching points related to anticonvulsant medications if you had difficulty with this question.
Level of Cognitive Ability: Comprehension
Client Needs: Physiological Integrity
Integrated Process: Nursing Process/Evaluation
Content Area: Pharmacology
Reference: Price, D., & Gwin, J. (2008). *Pediatric nursing: An introductory text* (10th ed., p. 256). St. Louis: Saunders.

ALTERNATE ITEM FORMAT: MULTIPLE RESPONSE

330. **1, 3, 5**
Rationale: During a seizure, the child is placed on his or her side in a lateral position. This type of positioning will prevent aspiration, because saliva will drain out of the corner of the child's mouth. The child is not restrained, because this could cause injury. The nurse would loosen clothing around the child's neck and ensure a patent airway. Nothing is placed into the child's mouth during a seizure, because this action may cause injury to the child's mouth, gums, or teeth. The nurse would stay with the child to reduce the risk of injury and to allow for the observation and timing of the seizure.
Test-Taking Strategy: Visualize this clinical situation. Recalling that airway patency and safety are the priorities will assist you with determining the appropriate interventions. Review the care of the child who is experiencing a seizure if you had difficulty with this question.
Level of Cognitive Ability: Application
Client Needs: Physiological Integrity
Integrated Process: Nursing Process/Implementation
Content Area: Child Health
Reference: Price, D., & Gwin, J. (2008). *Pediatric nursing: An introductory text* (10th ed., p. 254). St. Louis: Saunders.

REFERENCES

Hockenberry, M., & Wilson, D. (2007). *Nursing care of infants and children* (8th ed.). St. Louis: Mosby.
Leifer, G. (2007). *Introduction to maternity and pediatric nursing* (5th ed.). Philadelphia: Saunders.
National Council of State Boards of Nursing (Eds.). (2008). *2008 Detailed Test Plan for the NCLEX-PN® Examination, National Council of State Boards of Nursing.* Chicago: Author.
National Council of State Boards of Nursing. *NCSBN home page.* www.ncsbn.org. Accessed July 15, 2008.
Price, D., & Gwin, J. (2008). *Pediatric nursing: An introductory text* (10th ed.). St. Louis: Saunders.
Pagana, K., & Pagana, T. (2005). *Mosby's diagnostic and laboratory test reference* (7th ed.). St. Louis: Mosby.
Wong, D., Perry, S., Hockenberry, M., Lowdermilk, D., & Wilson, D. (2006). *Maternal-child nursing care* (3rd ed.). St. Louis: Mosby.

Eye, Ear, Throat, and Respiratory Disorders

CHAPTER 31

I. STRABISMUS

A. Description
1. Called squint or lazy eye
2. A condition in which the eyes are not aligned as a result of a lack of coordination of the extraocular muscles
3. Most often results from a muscle imbalance or the paralysis of the extraocular muscles, but it may also result from conditions such as a brain tumor, hydrocephalus, retinoblastoma, or infection
4. Normal in the young infant but should not be present after about 4 months

B. Data collection
1. Amblyopia may coexist
2. Permanent loss of vision if not treated early
3. Loss of binocular vision
4. Impairment of depth perception
5. Frequent headaches
6. Squints or tilts head to see

C. Interventions
1. Corrective lenses to improve eye alignment
2. Instruct the parents regarding patching (occlusion therapy) of the "good" eye to strengthen the weak eye; may also use atropine drops to "fog" the strong eye to strengthen the weak eye
3. Prepare for botulinum toxin (Botox) injection into the eye muscle, which produces temporary paralysis and allows muscles opposite the paralyzed muscle to straighten the eye
4. Inform the parents that the injection of botulinum toxin wears off in about 2 months and that, if it is successful, correction will occur
5. Prepare for surgery to realign the weak muscles, as prescribed, if nonsurgical interventions are unsuccessful
6. Instruct the parents about the need for follow-up visits

II. CONJUNCTIVITIS

A. Description
1. Inflammation of the conjunctiva; also known as pinkeye
2. Usually caused by allergy, infection, or trauma
3. Bacterial or viral conjunctivitis is extremely contagious (usually for 10 to 14 days from the day of onset)
4. Chlamydial conjunctivitis is rare among older children; if diagnosed in a child who is not sexually active, he or she should be assessed for possible sexual **abuse**

B. Data collection
1. Itching, burning, or scratchy eyelids
2. Redness of the conjunctiva and sclera
3. Edema
4. Mucoid or purulent discharge; may vary in coloration from white to yellowish or greenish; may cause morning crusting and difficulty with opening the eyes first thing in the morning

C. Interventions
1. Instruct the child in infection control measures such as good handwashing and not sharing towels and washcloths
2. Administer antibiotic or antiviral eyedrops or ointment, as prescribed, if infection is present
3. Administer antihistamines, as prescribed, if an allergy is present
4. Instruct the child and parents in the administration of the prescribed medications
5. Instruct the parents that the child should be kept home from school or day care until antibiotics and/or antibiotic eyedrops have been administered for 24 hours and until the eyes are no longer red and no longer have discharge
6. Instruct the child and parents in the use of cool compresses to lessen irritation and in the wearing of dark glasses for photophobia (eye irrigation with sterile saline may be performed until the discharge is gone)
7. Instruct the child to avoid rubbing the eye to prevent injury
8. Instruct the child who is wearing contact lenses to discontinue wearing them until treatment is complete; new lenses need to be obtained to eliminate the chance of reinfection

9. Instruct the adolescent that the eye makeup they are currently using should be discarded and replaced with new makeup to prevent reinfection

III. OTITIS MEDIA
A. Description
1. Infection of the middle ear that occurs as a result of a blocked Eustachian tube, which prevents normal drainage
2. A complication of an acute respiratory infection; passive smoking exposure increases the risk of otitis media
3. Infants and children are more prone to otitis media, because their Eustachian tubes are shorter, wider, and straighter
B. Data collection
1. Fever, irritability, and restlessness
2. Loss of appetite
3. Rolling of head from side to side; pulling on or rubbing the ear
4. Earache or pain
5. Signs of hearing loss
6. Purulent ear drainage
7. Red, opaque, bulging, or retracting tympanic membrane
C. Interventions
1. Instruct the parents in the administration of analgesics or antipyretics such as acetaminophen (Tylenol) to decrease fever and pain
2. Encourage fluids, as tolerated
3. Teach the parents to feed the infant in an upright position
4. Instruct the child to avoid chewing during the acute period, because chewing increases pain; soft foods should be provided
5. Provide local heat, and have the child lie with the affected ear down
6. Instruct the parents in the appropriate procedure to clean the drainage from the ear with a soft cloth or wicks
7. Instruct the parents in the administration of prescribed antibiotics, emphasizing that the 10- to 14-day period is necessary to eradicate infective organisms
8. Instruct the parents that screening for hearing loss may be necessary
9. Instruct the parents about the procedure for administering ear medications if antibiotic eardrops are prescribed (Box 31-1)

BOX 31-1 Administering Ear Medications

For a child who is younger than 3 years old, pull the pinna down and back.
For a child who is older than 3 years old, pull the pinna up and back.

D. Myringotomy
1. The insertion of tympanoplasty tubes into the middle ear to equalize pressure and keep the ear aerated
2. The tubes may stay in place for weeks, months, or years to allow for external ventilation of the middle-ear space
3. The most common complications include the early extrusion of the tube(s) and the failure of the eardrum to heal after the tube has fallen out
4. Interventions postoperatively
a. Instruct the parents and child to keep the ears dry
b. Earplugs should be worn during bathing, shampooing, and swimming
c. Diving and submerging under water are not encouraged

IV. TONSILLECTOMY AND ADENOIDECTOMY
A. Description
1. Tonsillitis refers to inflammation and infection of the tonsils (Figure 31-1)
2. Adenoiditis refers to inflammation and infection of the adenoids
B. Data collection
1. Persistent or recurrent sore throat
2. Enlarged bright red tonsils that may be covered with white exudate
3. Difficulty swallowing
4. Mouth breathing and an unpleasant mouth odor
5. Fever
6. Cough

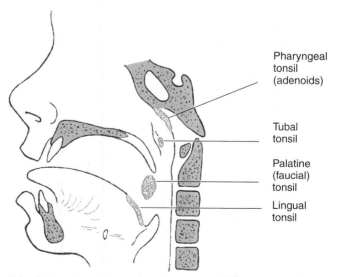

FIG. 31-1 Location of various tonsillar masses. (From Hockenberry, M., & Wilson, D. [2007]. *Wong's nursing care of infants and children* [8th ed.]. St. Louis: Mosby.)

7. Enlarged adenoids may cause a nasal quality of speech, mouth breathing, hearing difficulty, snoring, or obstructive sleep apnea

C. Interventions preoperatively
1. Monitor for signs of active infection
2. Monitor bleeding and clotting studies, because the throat is very vascular
3. Prepare the child for a sore throat postoperatively, and inform the child that he or she will need to drink liquids
4. Check for any loose teeth to decrease the risk of aspiration during surgery

D. Interventions postoperatively
1. Position the child prone or side lying to facilitate drainage
2. Have suction equipment available, but do not suction unless there is an airway obstruction
3. Monitor for signs of hemorrhage (e.g., frequent swallowing); if hemorrhage occurs, turn the child to the side and notify the physician
4. Discourage coughing and clearing of the throat
5. Provide clear, cool, noncitrus, and noncarbonated fluids
6. Avoid milk products initially, because they will coat the throat
7. Avoid red and purple liquids, which will simulate the appearance of blood if the child vomits
8. Do not give the child any straws, forks, or sharp objects that can be put into the mouth
9. Administer acetaminophen (Tylenol) for sore throat, as prescribed
10. Instruct the parents to notify the physician if bleeding, a persistent earache, or fever occurs
11. Instruct the parents to keep the child away from crowds until healing has occurred

V. EPISTAXIS (NOSEBLEEDS)
A. Description
1. The nose, especially the septum, is a highly vascular structure, and bleeding usually results from direct trauma, foreign bodies, nose picking, and mucosal inflammation
2. Recurrent epistaxis and severe bleeding may indicate underlying disease

B. Interventions
1. Have the child sit up and lean forward (not lying down)
2. Apply continuous pressure to the nose with the thumb and forefinger for at least 10 minutes
3. Insert cotton or wadded tissue into each nostril; apply ice or a cold cloth to bridge of nose if bleeding persists
4. Keep the child calm and quiet
5. If bleeding cannot be controlled, packing or cauterization of the bleeding vessel may be prescribed

VI. EPIGLOTTITIS
A. Description
1. A bacterial form of croup
2. An inflammation of the epiglottis, which may be caused by *Haemophilus influenzae* type B or *Streptococcus pneumoniae*
3. Occurs most frequently among children who are 2 to 5 years old
4. Onset is abrupt; occurs most often in the winter
5. Considered an emergency situation

B. Data collection
1. High fever
2. Sore, red, and inflamed throat
3. Absence of spontaneous cough
4. Drooling
5. Difficulty swallowing
6. Muffled voice
7. Inspiratory **stridor**
8. Agitation
9. Tripod positioning; while supporting the body with the hands and arms, the child leans forward, thrusts the chin forward, and opens the mouth in an attempt to widen the airway

C. Interventions
1. Maintain a patent airway; epiglottitis may progress to complete airway obstruction in a very short time period
2. Avoid agitating or frightening the child; may consider having the parents or caregiver remain nearby to reassure the child
3. Check the respiratory status and breath sounds; note **nasal flaring,** sternal **retractions,** and the presence of inspiratory **stridor** (Figure 31-2)
4. Check the temperature by the axillary route rather than the oral route

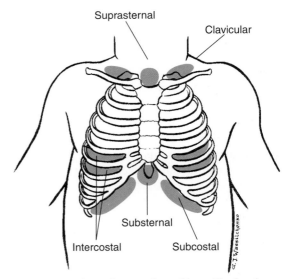

FIG. 31-2   Location of retractions. (From Hockenberry, M., & Wilson, D. [2007]. *Wong's nursing care of infants and children* [8th ed.]. St. Louis: Mosby.)

5. To prevent spasm of the epiglottis and airway occlusion, no attempts should be made to visualize the posterior pharynx or to obtain a throat culture
6. Prepare the child for lateral neck films to confirm the diagnosis
7. Maintain nothing by mouth status
8. Do not leave the child unattended
9. Do not force the child to lie down
10. Do not restrain the child
11. Administer intravenous (IV) fluids and antibiotics, as prescribed
12. Administer analgesics and antipyretics (acetaminophen [Tylenol]) per rectum to reduce fever and throat pain, as prescribed
13. Provide cool-mist oxygen therapy, as prescribed
14. Provide high humidification to cool the airway and decrease swelling
15. Have resuscitation equipment available, and prepare for endotracheal intubation or tracheotomy for severe respiratory distress
16. Immediate intubation is required when impending airway obstruction threatens; this is considered a medical emergency; intubation should be performed in the operating department; intubation may be required for several days until the epiglottic swelling resolves
17. Ensure that the child is up to date with his or her immunization schedule, including the *Haemophilus influenzae* type b conjugate **vaccine**

VII. LARYNGOTRACHEOBRONCHITIS (CROUP)

A. Description (Figure 31-3)
  1. Inflammation of larynx, trachea, and bronchi
  2. Most common type of croup; may be viral or bacterial
  3. Has a gradual onset and may be preceded by an upper respiratory infection
B. Data collection (Box 31-2)

C. Interventions
  1. Maintain a patent airway
  2. Monitor the respiratory status, and check for **nasal flaring**, sternal **retraction,** and inspiratory **stridor**
  3. Monitor for pallor or **cyanosis**
  4. Elevate the head of the bed and provide bedrest
  5. Provide humidified oxygen via a cool-mist tent for the hospitalized child
  6. Instruct the parents to use a cool-air vaporizer or humidifier at home; other measures include having the child breathe in the cool night air or the air from an open freezer and taking the child to a cool basement or garage
  7. Provide and encourage fluid intake; IV fluids may be prescribed to maintain hydration status if the child is unable to take oral fluids
  8. Administer acetaminophen (Tylenol), as prescribed, to reduce fever
  9. Avoid cough syrups and cold medicines, which may dry and thicken secretions
  10. Administer bronchodilators, if prescribed, to relax smooth muscle and relieve **stridor**
  11. Administer corticosteroids, if prescribed, for their anti-inflammatory effects
  12. Administer nebulized epinephrine (racemic epinephrine), as prescribed, for children with severe disease, **stridor** at rest, **retractions,** or difficulty breathing

---

BOX 31-2 **Progression of Symptoms in Laryngotracheobronchitis**

Stage I
- Low-grade fever
- Fear
- Seal bark and brassy cough
- Inspiratory stridor
- Irritability and restlessness

Stage II
- Continuous respiratory stridor
- Retractions
- Use of accessory muscles
- Crackles and wheezing
- Labored respirations

Stage III
- Restlessness
- Anxiety
- Pallor
- Diaphoresis
- Tachypnea
- Signs of anoxia and hypercapnia

Stage IV
- Intermittent cyanosis that progresses to permanent cyanosis
- Apneic episodes that progress to cessation of breathing

Modified from Hockenberry, M., & Wilson, D. (2007). *Wong's nursing care of infants and children* (8th ed.). St. Louis: Mosby.

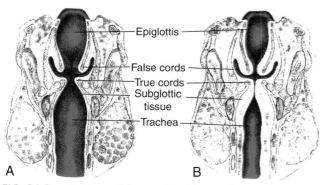

FIG. 31-3 **A,** Normal larynx. **B,** Obstruction and narrowing resulting from edema of croup. (From Hockenberry, M., & Wilson, D. [2007]. *Wong's nursing care of infants and children* [8th ed.]. St. Louis: Mosby.)

13. Administer antibiotics, as prescribed, noting that they are not indicated unless a bacterial infection is present
14. Have resuscitation equipment available
15. Provide appropriate reassurance and education to the parents or caregivers

VIII. **BRONCHITIS**
A. Description: Infection of the major bronchi; may be referred to as tracheobronchitis
B. Data collection
   1. Fever
   2. Dry, hacking, and nonproductive cough that is worse at night and that becomes productive in 2 to 3 days
C. Interventions: Primarily supportive
   1. Monitor for respiratory distress
   2. Monitor with pulse oximetry
   3. Apnea may occur, particularly in those infants who were born preterm
   4. Provide respiratory support, as needed
   5. Provide cool, humidified air
   6. Monitor for signs of dehydration, such as a sunken fontanel, poor skin turgor, and decreased and concentrated urinary output
   7. Increase fluid intake
   8. Administer acetaminophen (Tylenol) for fever, as prescribed
   9. Antibiotics are generally not necessary unless there is a superimposed bacterial infection
   10. Recurrent episodes of bronchitis could indicate the presence of asthma

IX. **BRONCHIOLITIS/RESPIRATORY SYNCYTIAL VIRUS**
A. Description
   1. An inflammation of the bronchioles that causes a thick production of mucus, which occludes the bronchiole tubes and the small bronchi
   2. Respiratory syncytial virus (RSV) is a common cause of bronchiolitis
   3. RSV, although not airborne, is highly communicable and usually transferred by direct contact with respiratory secretions
   4. Occurs primarily from the late fall to the early spring
   5. Rare among children who are more than 2 years old, with a peak incidence at approximately 6 months old
B. Data collection (Box 31-3)
C. Interventions
   1. Maintain a patent airway
   2. Position the child at a 30- to 40-degree angle with the neck slightly extended to maintain an open airway and to decrease pressure on the diaphragm
   3. Provide cool, humidified oxygen
   4. Encourage fluids; IV fluids may be necessary until the acute stage has passed

---

BOX 31-3 | **Data Collection: Respiratory Syncytial Virus**

Initial Manifestations
- Rhinorrhea
- Pharyngitis
- Coughing
- Wheezing
- Intermittent fever

Manifestations as the Disease Progresses
- Increased coughing and wheezing
- Signs of air hunger
- Tachypnea and retractions
- Periods of cyanosis

Manifestations in Severe Illness
- Tachypnea greater than 70 breaths per minute
- Decreased breath sounds and poor air exchange
- Listlessness
- Apneic episodes

Modified from Hockenberry, M., & Wilson, D. (2007). *Wong's nursing care of infants and children* (8th ed.). St. Louis: Mosby.

BOX 31-4 **Administering Ribavirin (Virazole)**

Ribavirin is administered via aerosol by hood, tent, or mask or through ventilator tubing.
Pregnant health care providers should not care for a child who is receiving ribavirin.
The nurse who is wearing contact lenses should wear goggles when coming in contact with ribavirin, because the mist may dissolve soft lenses.

BOX 31-5 | **Respiratory Syncytial Virus Immune Globulin**

- Used prophylactically to prevent respiratory syncytial virus in high-risk infants
- Not administered to infants or children with congenital heart disease

   5. Monitor for signs of dehydration
   6. Provide support and appropriate information to the family
D. The child with RSV
   1. Isolate the child in a single room or place him or her in a room with another child with RSV
   2. Maintain good handwashing procedures
   3. Ensure that nurses caring for these children do not care for other high-risk children
   4. Wear gowns when the soiling of clothing may occur during care
   5. Administer ribavirin (Virazole), an antiviral respiratory medication, if prescribed (Box 31-4)
   6. Prepare for the administration of RSV immune globulin (RSV-IG or RespiGam) or palivizumab (Synagis) (Box 31-5)

> **BOX 31-6   Types of Pneumonia**
> - Viral pneumonia
> - Primary atypical pneumonia *(Mycoplasma pneumoniae)*
> - Bacterial pneumonia
> - Aspiration pneumonia

X. PNEUMONIA

A. Description (Box 31-6)
1. Inflammation of the alveoli caused by a virus, a mycoplasmal agent, bacteria, or the aspiration of a foreign substance
2. The causative agent is usually introduced into the lungs through inhalation or from the bloodstream
3. Viral pneumonia occurs more frequently than bacterial pneumonia and is often associated with a viral upper respiratory infection
4. Primary atypical pneumonia *(Mycoplasma pneumoniae)* is the most common cause of pneumonia in children between the ages of 5 and 12 years; it occurs primarily during the fall and winter months and is more prevalent in crowded living conditions
5. Bacterial pneumonia is often a serious infection; hospitalization is indicated when pleural effusion or empyema accompanies the disease and is mandatory for children with staphylococcal pneumonia
6. Aspiration pneumonia occurs when food, secretions, liquids, or other materials enter the lung and cause inflammation and a chemical pneumonitis; classic symptoms include an increasing cough or fever with foul-smelling sputum, deteriorating results on chest x-rays, and other signs of airway involvement

B. Viral pneumonia
1. Data collection
   a. Mild fever, slight cough, and malaise to high fever, severe cough, and prostration
   b. Nonproductive or productive cough of small amounts of whitish sputum
   c. Wheezes or fine **crackles**
2. Interventions
   a. Administer oxygen with cool mist, as prescribed
   b. Increase fluid intake
   c. Administer antipyretics for fever, as prescribed
   d. Administer chest physiotherapy and postural drainage, as prescribed
   e. Antimicrobial therapy is reserved for children in whom the presence of infection is demonstrated by cultures

C. Primary atypical pneumonia
1. Data collection
   a. Fever, chills, anorexia, headache, malaise, and muscle pain
   b. Rhinitis, sore throat, and dry, hacking cough
   c. Cough is nonproductive initially and then produces seromucoid sputum, which becomes mucopurulent or blood streaked
2. Interventions: Symptomatic

D. Bacterial pneumonia
1. Data collection
   a. Acute onset, fever, and toxic appearance
   b. Infant: Irritability, lethargy, poor feeding, abrupt fever (may be accompanied by seizures), and respiratory distress (air hunger, tachypnea, and circumoral **cyanosis**)
   c. Older child: Headache, chills, abdominal pain, chest pain, and meningeal symptoms (meningism)
   d. Hacking, nonproductive cough
   e. Diminished breath sounds or scattered **crackles**
   f. As the infection resolves, coarse **crackles** and **wheezing** are heard; the cough becomes productive with purulent sputum
2. Interventions
   a. Antimicrobial therapy is initiated as soon as the diagnosis is suspected
   b. Administer humidified oxygen via hood, mist tent, or nasal cannula for respiratory distress, as prescribed, and monitor the child's oxygen saturation (Table 31-1)
   c. Place the child in a mist tent, as prescribed; cool humidification moistens the airways and assists with temperature reduction
   d. Suction the infant to maintain a patent airway if he or she is unable to handle secretions
   e. Administer chest physiotherapy and postural drainage every 4 hours, as prescribed
   f. Promote bedrest to conserve energy
   g. Encourage the child to lie on the affected side (if pneumonia is unilateral) to splint the chest and to reduce the discomfort caused by pleural rubbing
   h. Provide liberal fluid intake (administer cautiously to prevent aspiration); IV fluids may be necessary
   i. Administer antipyretics for fever, as prescribed; monitor the temperature frequently because of the risk for febrile seizures
   j. Institute isolation precautions with pneumococcal or staphylococcal pneumonia, according to agency policy
   k. Administer antitussives, as prescribed, before rest times and meals if the cough is disturbing

TABLE 31-1	Advantages and Disadvantages of Various Oxygen-Delivery Systems	
Systems	Advantages	Disadvantages
Oxygen mask	Various sizes available Delivers higher O_2 concentration than cannula Able to provide a predictable concentration of oxygen (with Venturi mask) whether child breathes through nose or mouth	Skin irritation Fear of suffocation Accumulation of moisture on face Possibility of aspiration of vomitus Difficulty with controlling O_2 concentrations
Nasal cannula	Provides low to moderate O_2 concentration (22%-40%) Child able to eat and talk while receiving O_2 Possibility of more complete observation of child because nose and mouth remain unobstructed	Must have patent nasal passages May cause abdominal distention, discomfort, or vomiting Difficulty controlling O_2 concentration if child breathes through mouth Inability to provide mist, if desired
Oxygen tent	Provides of lower O_2 concentrations (F_{IO_2} up to 0.3-0.5) Child able to receive desired inspired O_2 concentrations, even while eating	Necessity for proper fit around bed to prevent the leakage of gas Cool and wet tent environment Poor access to child; inspired O_2 levels fall when the tent is entered
Oxygen hood	Provides of high O_2 concentrations (F_{IO_2} up to 1.00) Free access to child's chest for assessment	High-humidity environment Need to remove child for feeding and care

O_2, Oxygen; F_{IO_2}, fraction of inspired oxygen.
Modified from Hockenberry, M., & Wilson, D. (2007). *Wong's nursing care of infants and children* (8th ed.). St. Louis: Mosby.

l. Continuous closed-chest drainage may be instituted if purulent fluid is present; this is usually noted with staphylococcal infections

m. Fluid accumulation in the pleural cavity may be removed by thoracentesis; thoracentesis also provides a means for obtaining fluid for culture and for instilling antibiotics directly into the pleural cavity

XI. ASTHMA

A. Description
  1. A chronic inflammatory disease of the airways
  2. Asthma is commonly caused by physical and chemical irritants such as foods, pollens, dust mites, cockroaches, smoke, animal dander, temperature changes, respiratory infection, activity, and stress
  3. The allergic reaction in the airways can cause an immediate reaction involving obstruction, and it can precipitate a late bronchial obstructive reaction several hours after the initial exposure
  4. Mast cell release of histamine leads to a bronchoconstrictive process
  5. A common symptom is coughing in the absence of respiratory infection, especially at night
  6. Status asthmaticus
    a. Child displays respiratory distress despite vigorous treatment measures
    b. This is a medical emergency that can result in respiratory failure and death if left untreated

B. Data collection
  1. Child has episodes of **wheezing**, breathlessness, dyspnea, chest tightness, and cough, particularly at night and/or in the early morning

  2. Child may present with **prodromal** itching localized at the front of the neck or over the upper part of the back
  3. Exacerbations include episodes of progressively worsening shortness of breath, cough, **wheezing,** chest tightness, decreases in expiratory airflow secondary to bronchospasm, mucosal edema, and mucus plugging; air is trapped behind occluded or narrow airways, and hypoxemia can occur
  4. Asthmatic episode
    a. The episode begins with irritability, restlessness, headache, feeling tired, and/or chest tightness
    b. Respiratory symptoms include a hacking, irritable, nonproductive cough caused by bronchial edema
    c. Accumulated secretions stimulate the cough; the cough becomes rattling, and there is production of frothy, clear, gelatinous sputum
    d. Child experiences **retractions**
    e. Hyperresonance on percussion of the chest is noted
    f. Breath sounds are coarse and loud, with **crackles,** coarse rhonchi, and inspiratory and expiratory **wheezing;** expiration is prolonged
    g. Exercise-induced bronchospasm: Cough, shortness of breath, chest pain or tightness, **wheezing,** and endurance problems occur during exercise
    h. Severe spasm or obstruction: Breath sounds and **crackles** may become inaudible, and the cough is ineffective (represents a lack of air movement)

BOX 31-7 Interventions in the Event of an Acute Asthma Attack

Assess airway patency.
Administer humidified oxygen by nasal prongs or face mask.
Administer quick-relief (rescue) medications.
Continuously monitor respiratory status, pulse oximetry, and color; be alert to decreased wheezing or a silent chest, which may signal the inability to move air.
Prepare to initiate an intravenous line, and prepare to correct dehydration, acidosis, or electrolyte imbalances.
Prepare the child for a chest radiograph.
Prepare to obtain samples for determining arterial blood gas and serum electrolyte levels.

BOX 31-8 Quick-Relief (Rescue) Medications

- Short-acting β_2-agonists
- Anticholinergics (for the relief of acute bronchospasm)
- Systemic corticosteroids (for their anti-inflammatory action to treat reversible airflow obstruction)

BOX 31-9 Long-Term Control (Preventer) Medications

- Corticosteroids
- Antiallergic medications
- Nonsteroidal anti-inflammatory drugs
- Long-acting β_2-agonists
- Leukotriene modifiers (to prevent bronchospasm and inflammatory cell infiltration)
- Long-acting bronchodilators

---

i. Ventilatory failure and asphyxia: Shortness of breath, with air movement in the chest restricted to the point of absent breath sounds accompanied by a sudden rise in the respiratory rate
j. Child may be pale or flushed, and the lips may have a deep, dark red color that may progress to **cyanosis** observed in the nail beds and skin, especially around the mouth
k. Restlessness, apprehension, and diaphoresis occur
l. Younger children assume the tripod sitting position; older children sit upright with the shoulders in a hunched-over position, with the hands on the bed or a chair and the arms braced to facilitate the use of the accessory muscles of breathing; the child refuses to lie down
m. Child speaks in short, broken phrases

C. Interventions: Acute episode (Box 31-7)
D. Medications
1. Quick-relief (rescue) medications to treat symptoms and exacerbations (Box 31-8)
2. Long-term control (preventer) medications to achieve and maintain control of inflammation (Box 31-9)
3. Nebulizers, metered-dose inhalers, or peak expiratory flowmeters may be used to administer medications; if the child has difficulty using the metered-dose inhaler, medication can be administered by nebulization (i.e., the medication is mixed with saline and then nebulized with compressed air by a machine)
E. Chest physiotherapy
1. Chest physiotherapy includes clapping, vibration, postural drainage, suctioning, and breathing exercises
2. Chest physiotherapy is not recommended during an acute exacerbation

F. Allergen control
1. Prevention and reduction of exposure to airborne and environmental allergens
2. Skin testing to identify allergens; immunotherapy (hyposensitization) is not recommended for allergens that can be eliminated effectively
G. Home-care measures
1. Instruct the family regarding measures to eliminate allergens
2. Avoid extremes of environmental temperature; in cold temperatures, instruct the child to breathe through the nose rather than the mouth and to cover the nose and mouth with a scarf
3. Avoid exposure to individuals with respiratory infections
4. Instruct the child and family regarding how to recognize the early symptoms of an asthma attack
5. Teach the child and family how to administer medications, as prescribed
6. Instruct the child and family regarding use of a nebulizer, a metered-dose inhaler, or a peak expiratory flowmeter
7. Instruct the child and family regarding the importance of home monitoring of the peak expiratory flow rate; a decrease in the expiratory flow rate may indicate an impending infection or exacerbation
8. Instruct the child with regard to the cleaning of the devices used for inhaled medications; oral candidiasis can occur with the use of aerosolized steroids
9. Encourage adequate rest and sleep and a well-balanced diet
10. Instruct the child regarding the importance of adequate fluid intake to liquefy secretions
11. Assist with the development of an exercise program for the child

12. Instruct the child regarding the procedures for respiratory treatments and exercises, as prescribed
13. Encourage the child to cough effectively
14. Encourage the parents to keep the child's immunizations up to date; annual influenza vaccinations may also be recommended
15. Inform other health care providers and school personnel of the child's asthma condition
16. Allow the child to take control of self-care measures on the basis of age appropriateness

XII. TUBERCULOSIS
A. Description
1. A contagious disease caused by *Mycobacterium tuberculosis*, which is an acid-fast bacillus
2. Multidrug-resistant strains of *M. tuberculosis* occur as a result of client or family noncompliance with therapeutic regimens
3. The route of transmission of *M. tuberculosis* is via the inhalation of droplets from an individual with active tuberculosis (TB)
4. Most children are infected by a family member or by another individual with whom they have frequent contact (e.g., a babysitter)

B. Data collection
1. May be asymptomatic or develop symptoms such as malaise, fever, cough, weight loss, anorexia, and lymphadenopathy
2. Specific symptoms related to the site of infection (e.g., lungs, brain, bone) may be present
3. Chest x-rays must be obtained and interpreted

C. Mantoux test (Box 31-10)
1. Will produce a positive reaction 2 to 10 weeks after the initial infection
2. Determines whether the child has been infected and has developed a sensitivity to the protein of the tubercle bacillus; a positive reaction does not confirm the presence of active disease
3. After the child reacts positively, he or she will always react positively; a positive reaction in a previously negative child indicates that the child has been infected since the last test
4. Measles **vaccine** may cause a false-negative reaction

D. Sputum culture
1. A definitive diagnosis is made by demonstrating the presence of mycobacteria in a culture
2. Because an infant or young child often swallows sputum rather than expectorates, gastric washings (the aspiration of lavaged contents from the fasting stomach) may be performed to obtain a specimen; the specimen is obtained in the early morning, before breakfast

E. Interventions
1. Medications
   a. Include isoniazid (INH), rifampin (Rifadin), and pyrazinamide

---

> ### BOX 31-10 Mantoux Test Results
>
> Induration that measures 15 mm or more is considered to be a positive reaction in children 4 years old or older who do not have any risk factors.
> Induration that measures 10 mm or more is considered to be a positive reaction in children younger than 4 years old and in those with chronic illness or who are at high risk for exposure to tuberculosis.
> Induration that measures 5 mm or more is considered to be positive for those in the highest-risk groups, such as children with immunosuppressive conditions or human immunodeficiency virus infection.

---

   b. A 9-month course of INH may be prescribed to prevent a latent infection from progressing to clinically active TB and to prevent initial infection in children in high-risk situations; a 12-month course may be prescribed for the child with human immunodeficiency virus infection
   c. Recommendations for the child with clinically active TB may include INH, rifampin, and pyrazinamide daily for 2 months followed by INH and rifampin twice weekly for 4 months
2. Place children with infectious disease on airborne precautions until medications have been initiated, sputum cultures demonstrate a diminished number of organisms, and cough is improving
3. Wear a mask if the child is coughing and does not reliably cover his or her mouth
4. Maintain airborne precautions (mask) with family members until they are demonstrated to not have infectious TB
5. Stress the importance of adequate rest and diet
6. Instruct the child and family regarding measures to prevent the transmission of TB
7. Instruct the child and family about the importance of strict adherence to the treatment program; to ensure compliance, directly observed therapy may be recommended
8. Family members should be assessed for possible infection and subsequently treated
9. Identified cases of TB should be reported to the local health department

XIII. CYSTIC FIBROSIS (Figure 31-4)
A. Description
1. A chronic multisystem disorder and autosomal-recessive trait disorder that is characterized by exocrine gland dysfunction
2. The mucus produced by the exocrine glands is abnormally thick, which causes the obstruction of the small passageways of the affected organs

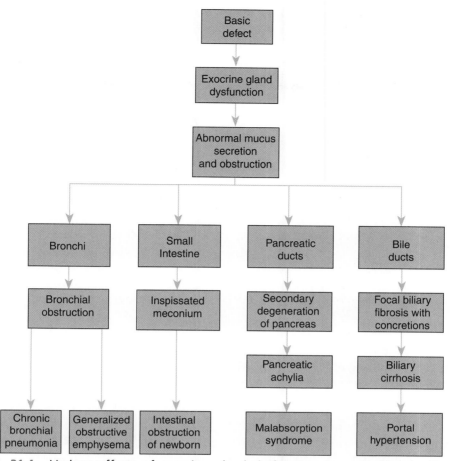

FIG. 31-4 Various effects of exocrine gland dysfunction in cystic fibrosis. (From Hockenberry, M., & Wilson, D. [2007]. *Wong's nursing care of infants and children* [8th ed.]. St. Louis: Mosby.)

3. The most common symptoms are pancreatic enzyme deficiency caused by duct blockage, progressive chronic lung disease associated with infection, and sweat-gland dysfunction that results in increased sodium and chloride sweat concentrations

4. An increase in sodium and chloride in both sweat and saliva forms the basis for the most reliable diagnostic test, which is the sweat chloride test

B. Respiratory system
  1. Symptoms are produced by the stagnation of mucus in the airway, which leads to bacterial colonization and the destruction of lung tissue
  2. Emphysema and atelectasis occur as the airways become increasingly obstructed
  3. Chronic hypoxemia causes the contraction and hypertrophy of the muscle fibers in the pulmonary arteries and arterioles, thus leading to pulmonary hypertension and eventual cor pulmonale
  4. Pneumothorax from ruptured bullae and hemoptysis from the erosion of the bronchial wall through an artery occur as the disease progresses
  5. **Wheezing** and dry, nonproductive cough
  6. Dyspnea
  7. **Cyanosis**
  8. Clubbing of the fingers and toes (Figure 31-5)
  9. Repeated episodes of bronchitis and pneumonia

C. Gastrointestinal system
  1. Meconium ileus in the neonate
  2. Intestinal obstruction (distal intestinal obstructive syndrome) caused by thick intestinal secretions; signs include pain, abdominal distention, nausea, and vomiting
  3. Steatorrhea (frothy, foul-smelling stools)
  4. Deficiency of the fat-soluble vitamins A, D, E, and K, which causes easy bruising and anemia
  5. Malnutrition and failure to thrive; demonstration of hypoalbuminemia from the diminished absorption of protein, which results in generalized edema
  6. Rectal prolapse can occur as a result of the large, bulky stools and a lack of supportive fat pads around the rectum

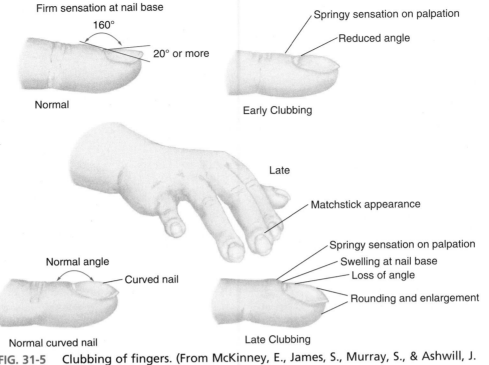

FIG. 31-5 Clubbing of fingers. (From McKinney, E., James, S., Murray, S., & Ashwill, J. [2005]. *Maternal-child nursing* [2nd ed.]. Philadelphia: Saunders.)

D. Integumentary system
1. Abnormally high concentrations of sodium and chloride in the sweat
2. Parents report that the infant tastes "salty" when kissed
3. Dehydration and electrolyte imbalances, especially during hyperthermic conditions

E. Reproductive system
1. Delayed **puberty** in females
2. Fertility can be inhibited by highly viscous cervical secretions, which act as a plug and block sperm entry
3. Males are usually sterile as a result of the blockage of the vas deferens by abnormal secretions or by the failure of the normal development of duct structures

F. Diagnostic tests
1. Quantitative sweat chloride test (Box 31-11)
2. Chest x-ray reveals atelectasis and obstructive emphysema
3. Pulmonary function tests provide evidence of abnormal small airway function
4. Stool fat and/or enzyme analysis: A 72-hour stool sample is collected to check the fat and/ or enzyme (trypsin) content (food intake is recorded during the collection)

G. Interventions
1. Respiratory system
a. Goals of treatment include preventing and treating pulmonary infection by improving

---

BOX 31-11 **Quantitative Sweat Chloride Test**

The production of sweat is stimulated (via pilocarpine iontophoresis), the sweat is collected, and the sweat electrolytes are measured; a minimum of 50 mg of sweat is needed.
Normally, the chloride concentration of sweat is less than 40 mEq/L.
A chloride concentration of greater than 60 mEq/L is a positive test result.
Chloride concentrations of 40 to 60 mEq/L are highly suggestive of cystic fibrosis and necessitate a repeat test.

---

aeration, removing secretions, and administering antimicrobial medications
b. Chest physiotherapy (CPT; percussion and postural drainage) on awakening and in the evening (more frequently during pulmonary infection)
c. CPT should not be performed before or immediately after a meal
d. Bronchodilator medications by aerosol to open the bronchi for easier expectoration (administered before CPT when the child has reactive airway disease or is **wheezing**)
e. Use of a Flutter Mucus Clearance Device (a small, hand-held plastic pipe with a stainless steel ball on the inside), which facilitates the removal of mucus; store this device away from small children, because, if the device

separates, the steel ball poses a choking hazard

f. Use of a ThAIRapy Vest device, which provides high-frequency chest wall oscillations to help loosen secretions

g. Administration of medications as prescribed to decrease the viscosity of mucus

h. Instruct the parents not to give cough suppressants, because they will inhibit the expectoration of secretions and promote infection

i. Teach the child forced expiratory technique (huffing) to mobilize secretions

j. Develop a physical exercise program with the aim of establishing a good habitual breathing pattern

k. Administer antibiotics, as prescribed; they may be prescribed prophylactically or when pulmonary symptoms develop

l. Aerosolized antibiotics may be prescribed and are administered after CPT is performed; IV antibiotics may be prescribed and administered at home through a central venous access device

m. Administer oxygen, as prescribed, during acute episodes; monitor closely for oxygen narcosis

n. Monitor for hemoptysis; more than 300 mL in 24 hours for the older child (less for a younger child) needs to be treated immediately

o. Hemoptysis may be controlled by bedrest, cough suppressants, antibiotics, and vitamin K; if hemoptysis persists, the site of bleeding may be cauterized or embolized

p. Lung transplantation is a final therapeutic option for the child with end-stage disorder

2. Gastrointestinal system

a. The goal of treatment of pancreatic insufficiency is to replace pancreatic enzymes; the enzymes are administered with meals and snacks (or within 30 minutes of eating meals and snacks) to ensure that digestive enzymes are mixed with food in the duodenum

b. The amount of pancreatic enzymes administered is adjusted to achieve normal **growth** and a decrease in the number of stools to two or three per day

c. Enteric-coated pancreatic enzymes should not be crushed or chewed

d. Pancreatic enzymes should not be given if the child is to receive nothing by mouth

e. Encourage a well-balanced, high-protein, high-calorie diet; multivitamins and vitamins A, D, E, and K are also administered

f. Monitor the child's weight and for failure to thrive

g. Monitor the child for constipation and intestinal obstruction

h. Ensure adequate salt intake and fluids that provide an adequate supply of electrolytes during extremely hot weather or if the child has a fever

H. Home care

1. Instruct the parents about the prescribed treatment measures and their importance

2. Instruct the parents to be sure that the child's immunizations are up to date

3. Inform the parents that the child should be vaccinated yearly for influenza; pneumococcus vaccine may also be prescribed

4. Inform the parents about the Cystic Fibrosis Foundation

XIV. SUDDEN INFANT DEATH SYNDROME

A. Description

1. Unexpected death of an apparently healthy infant who is less than 1 year old for which a thorough autopsy fails to demonstrate an adequate cause of death

2. Cause may be related to a brainstem abnormality in the neurological regulation of cardiorespiratory control

3. Most frequently occurs during the winter months

4. Death usually occurs during a sleep period but not necessarily at night

5. Most frequently affects infants who are 2 to 4 months old

6. Incidence is higher among males

7. Incidence is higher among Native Americans, blacks, and Hispanics

8. High-risk behaviors
   a. Prone position
   b. Use of soft bedding
   c. Overheating (thermal stress)
   d. Possibly sleeping with an adult

B. Data collection

1. Child is apneic, blue, and lifeless

2. Frothy, blood-tinged fluid is in the nose and mouth

3. Child may be found in any position but is typically found in a disheveled bed with blankets over the head and huddled in a corner

4. Child may appear to have been clutching bedding

5. Diaper may be wet and full of stool

C. Prevention

1. Infants should be placed in the supine position for sleep

2. Soft, moldable mattresses and bedding, such as pillows and quilts, should not be used for bedding

3. Stuffed animals should be removed from the crib while the infant is sleeping

4. Discourage bed sharing (sleeping with an adult)

5. Avoid overheating during sleep

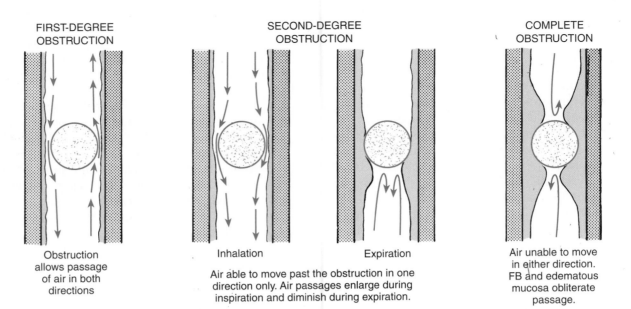

FIRST-DEGREE OBSTRUCTION

Obstruction allows passage of air in both directions

SECOND-DEGREE OBSTRUCTION

Inhalation

Expiration

Air able to move past the obstruction in one direction only. Air passages enlarge during inspiration and diminish during expiration.

COMPLETE OBSTRUCTION

Air unable to move in either direction. FB and edematous mucosa obliterate passage.

FIG. 31-6 Manifestations of airway obstruction by foreign body (FB). (From Hockenberry, M., & Wilson, D. [2007]. *Wong's nursing care of infants and children* [8th ed.]. St. Louis: Mosby.)

XV. FOREIGN-BODY ASPIRATION

A. Description (Figure 31-6)
1. Swallowing and aspirating a foreign body (or bodies) into the air passages
2. Most inhaled foreign bodies lodge in the mainstem or lobar bronchus
3. The most common offending foods are round in shape and include hot dogs, candy, peanuts, and grapes

B. Data collection
1. Initially, choking, gagging, coughing, and retractions are general findings
2. If the condition worsens, **cyanosis** may occur
3. Laryngotracheal obstruction leads to dyspnea, **stridor,** cough, and hoarseness
4. Bronchial obstruction produces paroxysmal cough, **wheezing,** asymmetrical breath sounds, and dyspnea
5. If any obstruction progresses, unconsciousness and asphyxiation may occur
6. Partial obstructions may occur without symptoms
7. The distressed child cannot speak, becomes cyanotic, and collapses

C. Interventions: See Chapter 16 for information about the removal of a foreign body in the airway

D. Prevention
1. Keep small objects out of reach of small children
2. Keep rubber balloons out of reach of small children
3. Avoid giving small children small, round-shaped food items

4. Provide parent, day care provider, and babysitter education

PRACTICE QUESTIONS

More questions on the companion CD!

331. The appropriate child position after a tonsillectomy is which of the following?
 1. Supine position
 2. Side-lying position
 3. High Fowler's position
 4. Trendelenburg's position

332. After a tonsillectomy, the child begins to vomit bright red blood. The initial nursing action would be to:
 1. Turn the child to the side.
 2. Notify the registered nurse (RN).
 3. Administer the prescribed antiemetic.
 4. Maintain nothing-by-mouth (NPO) status.

333. After a tonsillectomy, which of the following fluid or food items would be appropriate to offer to the child?
 1. Yellow Jell-O
 2. Cold ginger ale
 3. Vanilla pudding
 4. Cool cherry Kool-Aid

334. A nurse reinforces instructions to the mother of a child with croup about the measures to take if an acute spasmodic episode occurs. Which statement by the mother indicates the need for further instruction?

1. "I will place a steam vaporizer in my child's room."
2. "I will take my child out into the cool, humid night air."
3. "I will place a cool-mist humidifier in my child's room."
4. "I will place my child in a closed bathroom and allow my child to inhale steam from the running water."

335. A nurse reinforces instructions to the mother of a child who has been hospitalized with croup. Which of the following statements, if made by the mother, would indicate the need for further instruction?
1. "I will give my child cough syrup if a cough develops."
2. "Sips of warm fluid will help if my child develops a croup attack."
3. "I will give acetaminophen (Tylenol) if my child develops a fever."
4. "I will be sure that my child drinks at least three to four glasses of fluids every day."

336. A nurse who is working in the emergency department is caring for a child who has been diagnosed with epiglottitis. Indications that the child may be experiencing airway obstruction include which of the following?
1. Nasal flaring and bradycardia
2. The child thrusts the chin forward and opens the mouth
3. A low-grade fever and complaints of a sore throat
4. The child leans backward, supporting him- or herself with the hands and arms

337. A nurse is caring for a hospitalized infant with bronchiolitis. Diagnostic tests have confirmed respiratory syncytial virus (RSV). On the basis of this finding, which of the following would be the appropriate nursing action?
1. Initiate strict enteric precautions.
2. Wear a mask when caring for the child.
3. Plan to move the infant to a room with another child with RSV.
4. Leave the infant in the present room, because RSV is not contagious.

338. A nurse is instructing the mother of a child with cystic fibrosis (CF) about the appropriate dietary measures. Which type of diet will be included in the instructions?
1. A low-calorie, low-fat diet
2. A high-calorie, low-protein diet
3. A low-calorie, restricted-fat diet
4. A high-calorie, high-protein diet

339. A nurse reviews the results of a Mantoux test performed on a 3-year-old child. The results indicate an area of induration that measures 10 mm. The nurse would interpret these results as:
1. Positive
2. Negative
3. Inconclusive
4. Definitive, requiring a repeat test

340. Isoniazid (INH) is prescribed for a 2-year-old child with a positive Mantoux test. The mother of the child asks the nurse how long the child will need to take the medication. The appropriate response is:
1. 6 months
2. 9 months
3. 15 months
4. 18 months

341. A day-care nurse is observing a 2-year-old child and suspects that the child may have strabismus. Which of the following observations may be indicative of this condition?
1. The child has difficulty hearing.
2. The child does not respond when spoken to.
3. The child consistently tilts his or her head to see.
4. The child consistently turns his or her head to see.

342. A nurse has provided instructions to the mother of a child who has been diagnosed with bacterial conjunctivitis. Which of the following, if stated by the mother, would indicate the need for further instructions?
1. "I need to wash my hands frequently."
2. "I need to clean the eye, as prescribed."
3. "It is OK to share towels and washcloths."
4. "I need to give the eyedrops, as prescribed."

343. A nurse is assigned to care for a child after a myringotomy with the insertion of tympanostomy tubes. The nurse notes a small amount of reddish drainage from the child's ear after the surgery. On the basis of this finding, the nurse takes which action?
1. Documents the findings
2. Notifies the registered nurse immediately
3. Changes the ear tubes so that they do not become blocked
4. Checks the ear drainage for the presence of cerebrospinal fluid

344. A nurse prepares a teaching plan regarding the administration of eardrops for the parents of a 2-year-old child. Which of the following would be included in the plan?
1. Wear gloves when administering the eardrops.
2. Pull the ear up and back before instilling the eardrops.
3. Pull the earlobe down and back before instilling the eardrops.
4. Hold the child in a sitting position when administering the eardrops.

ALTERNATE ITEM FORMAT: MULTIPLE RESPONSE

345. A nurse is preparing for the admission of an infant with a diagnosis of bronchiolitis caused by the respiratory syncytial virus (RSV). Choose the interventions that would be included in the plan of care. Select all that apply.
    ☑ **1.** Place the infant in a private room.
    ☑ **2.** Place the infant in a room near the nurses' station.
    ☐ **3.** Ensure that the infant's head is in a flexed position.
    ☐ **4.** Wear a mask at all times when in contact with the infant.
    ☐ **5.** Place the child in a tent that delivers warm, humidified air.
    ☐ **6.** Position the infant side lying, with the head lower than the chest.

ANSWERS

331. **2**
Rationale: The child should be placed in a prone or side-lying position after tonsillectomy to facilitate drainage. Options 1, 3, and 4 will not achieve this goal.
Test-Taking Strategy: Visualize each of the positions described in the options. Keeping in mind that the goal is to facilitate drainage will direct you to option 2. Review positioning procedures after tonsillectomy if you had difficulty with this question.
Level of Cognitive Ability: Application
Client Needs: Physiological Integrity
Integrated Process: Nursing Process/Implementation
Content Area: Child Health
Reference: Price, D., & Gwin, J. (2008). *Pediatric nursing: An introductory text* (10th ed., p. 249). St. Louis: Saunders.

332. **1**
Rationale: After a tonsillectomy, if bleeding occurs, the child is turned to the side, and the RN is then notified; the RN will then contact the physician. An NPO status would be maintained, and an antiemetic may be prescribed; however, the initial nursing action would be to turn the child to the side.
Test-Taking Strategy: Note the strategic word "initial." Although all of the options may be appropriate, to maintain physiological integrity, the initial action is to turn the child to the side. Review the care to the child after tonsillectomy if you had difficulty with this question.
Level of Cognitive Ability: Application
Client Needs: Physiological Integrity
Integrated Process: Nursing Process/Implementation
Content Area: Child Health
Reference: Hockenberry, M., Wilson, D., & Winkelstein, M. (2005). *Wong's essentials of pediatric nursing* (7th ed., pp. 796-797). St. Louis: Mosby.

333. **1**
Rationale: After a tonsillectomy, clear, cool liquids should be administered. Citrus, carbonated, and extremely hot or cold liquids need to be avoided, because they may irritate the throat. Red liquids need to be avoided, because they give the appearance of blood if the child vomits. Milk and milk products (pudding) are avoided, because they coat the throat and cause the child to clear the throat, thus increasing the risk of bleeding.
Test-Taking Strategy: Use the process of elimination. Remember that avoiding foods and fluids that may irritate the throat or cause bleeding is the concern; this will assist you with eliminating options 2 and 3. The word "cherry" in option 4 should be the clue that this is not an appropriate food item. Review the dietary measures after tonsillectomy if you had difficulty with this question.
Level of Cognitive Ability: Application
Client Needs: Physiological Integrity
Integrated Process: Nursing Process/Implementation
Content Area: Child Health
Reference: Leifer, G. (2007). *Introduction to maternity and pediatric nursing* (5th ed., p. 581). Philadelphia: Saunders.

334. **1**
Rationale: Steam from warm running water in a closed bathroom and cool mist from a bedside humidifier are effective for reducing mucosal edema. Cool-mist humidifiers are recommended as compared with steam vaporizers, which present a danger of scalding burns. Taking the child out into the cool, humid night air may also relieve mucosal swelling. Remember, however, that a cold mist may precipitate bronchospasm.
Test-Taking Strategy: Note the strategic words "need for further instruction." Focus on the subjects of reducing mucosal edema and providing a safe environment. Option 1 is the option that would provide an unsafe environment for the child. Review the management of acute spasmodic croup if you had difficulty with this question.
Level of Cognitive Ability: Comprehension
Client Needs: Safe and Effective Care Environment
Integrated Process: Teaching and Learning
Content Area: Child Health
Reference: Leifer, G. (2007). *Introduction to maternity and pediatric nursing* (5th ed., p. 576). Philadelphia: Saunders.

335. **1**
Rationale: Cough syrups and cold medicines are not to be given, because they may dry and thicken secretions. Adequate hydration of 500 to 1000 mL of fluids daily is important for thinning secretions. Acetaminophen is used if a fever develops. Sips of warm fluids during a croup attack help to relax the vocal cords and thin the mucus.
Test-Taking Strategy: Note the strategic words "the need for further instruction." These words indicate a negative event query and ask you to select an option that is an incorrect statement. Knowledge of the pathophysiology related to croup will assist you with eliminating options 3 and 4 first. Recalling that warm fluids can relax membranes and thin secretions will direct you to option 1 from the remaining options. Review the effects of cough medicines if you had difficulty with this question.

Level of Cognitive Ability: Comprehension
Client Needs: Physiological Integrity
Integrated Process: Teaching and Learning
Content Area: Child Health
References: Hockenberry, M., & Wilson, D. (2007). *Wong's nursing care of infants and children* (8th ed., p. 1337). St. Louis: Mosby.
Price, D., & Gwin, J. (2008). *Pediatric nursing: An introductory text* (10th ed., p. 198). St. Louis: Saunders.

336. **2**
Rationale: Clinical manifestations that are suggestive of airway obstruction include tripod positioning (leaning forward supported by the hands and arms with the chin thrust out and the mouth open), nasal flaring, tachycardia, a high fever, and a sore throat.
Test-Taking Strategy: Use the process of elimination. Eliminate option 1 first, because tachycardia rather than bradycardia will occur in a child who is experiencing respiratory distress. Eliminate option 3 next, knowing that a high fever occurs with epiglottitis. From the remaining options, visualize the descriptions given in each, and determine which position would best assist a child who is experiencing respiratory distress. Review the tripod position if you had difficulty with this question.
Level of Cognitive Ability: Comprehension
Client Needs: Physiological Integrity
Integrated Process: Nursing Process/Data Collection
Content Area: Child Health
Reference: Leifer, G. (2007). *Introduction to maternity and pediatric nursing* (5th ed., pp. 514-515, 576). Philadelphia: Saunders.

337. **3**
Rationale: RSV is a highly communicable disorder, but it is not transmitted via the airborne route. It is usually transferred by the hands, and meticulous handwashing is necessary to decrease the spread of organisms. The infant with RSV is isolated in a single room or placed in a room with another child with RSV. Enteric precautions are not necessary; however, the nurse should wear a gown when the soiling of clothing may occur.
Test-Taking Strategy: Knowledge regarding the transmission of RSV will direct you to option 3. Remember that RSV is usually transferred by the hands and that meticulous handwashing is necessary to decrease the spread of organisms. Review the care of the child with RSV if you had difficulty with this question.
Level of Cognitive Ability: Application
Client Needs: Safe and Effective Care Environment
Integrated Process: Nursing Process/Implementation
Content Area: Child Health
Reference: Leifer, G. (2007). *Introduction to maternity and pediatric nursing* (5th ed., p. 577). Philadelphia: Saunders.

338. **4**
Rationale: Children with CF are managed with a high-calorie, high-protein diet. Pancreatic enzyme replacement therapy is undertaken, and fat-soluble vitamin supplements are administered. Fats are not restricted unless steatorrhea cannot be controlled by increased levels of pancreatic enzymes.
Test-Taking Strategy: Use the process of elimination. Eliminate options 1 and 3 first because of the word "low-

calorie." From the remaining options, recalling the appropriate diet for the child with CF will direct you to option 4. Review the treatment measures for CF if you had difficulty with this question.
Level of Cognitive Ability: Application
Client Needs: Physiological Integrity
Integrated Process: Nursing Process/Implementation
Content Area: Child Health
Reference: Price, D., & Gwin, J. (2008). *Pediatric nursing: An introductory text* (10th ed., p. 154). St. Louis: Elsevier.

339. **1**
Rationale: An induration that measures 10 mm or more is considered to be a positive result for children who are younger than 4 years old and for those with chronic illness or with a high risk for environmental exposure to tuberculosis. A reaction of 5 mm or more is considered to be a positive result for those in the highest-risk groups.
Test-Taking Strategy: Use the process of elimination and your knowledge regarding a positive Mantoux test in children to answer this question. Option 4 can be easily eliminated first. Note the child's age in the question to determine the correct option from the remaining three options. Review the analysis of the Mantoux test for children if you had difficulty with this question.
Level of Cognitive Ability: Analysis
Client Needs: Physiological Integrity
Integrated Process: Nursing Process/Data Collection
Content Area: Child Health
References: Chernecky, C., & Berger, B. (2008). *Laboratory tests and diagnostic procedures* (5th ed., pp. 758-759). Philadelphia: Saunders.
Hockenberry, M., Wilson, D., & Winkelstein, M. (2005). *Wong's essentials of pediatric nursing* (7th ed., pp. 808-809). St. Louis: Mosby.

340. **2**
Rationale: INH is given to prevent tuberculosis (TB) infection from progressing to active disease. A chest x-ray film is obtained before the initiation of preventive therapy. In infants and children, the recommended duration of INH therapy is 9 months. For children with human immunodeficiency virus infection, a minimum of 12 months is recommended.
Test-Taking Strategy: Knowledge regarding treatment with INH in a 2-year-old child is required to answer this question. Remember that in infants and children, the recommended duration of INH therapy is 9 months. Review the recommended treatment plans for a child with TB if you had difficulty with this question.
Level of Cognitive Ability: Application
Client Needs: Safe and Effective Care Environment*Integrated Process:* Nursing Process/Implementation
Content Area: Child Health
References: Leifer, G. (2007). *Introduction to maternity and pediatric nursing* (5th ed., p. 715). Philadelphia: Saunders.
Price, D., & Gwin, J. (2008). *Pediatric nursing: An introductory text* (10th ed., pp. 91-92). St. Louis: Saunders.

341. **3**
Rationale: The nurse may suspect strabismus in a child when the child complains of frequent headaches, squints, or tilts the

head to see. Options 1, 2, and 4 are not indicative of this condition.

Test-Taking Strategy: Use the process of elimination. Begin by eliminating options 1 and 2, because they are comparable or alike and refer to hearing. From the remaining options, recalling the signs of strabismus will direct you to option 3. Review these signs if you had difficulty with this question.

Level of Cognitive Ability: Comprehension
Client Needs: Physiological Integrity
Integrated Process: Nursing Process/Data Collection
Content Area: Child Health
Reference: Price, D., & Gwin, J. (2008). *Pediatric nursing: An introductory text* (10th ed., p. 241). St. Louis: Saunders.

342. 3
Rationale: Bacterial conjunctivitis is highly contagious, and infection control measures should be taught; these include frequent handwashing and not sharing towels and washcloths. Options 2 and 4 are correct treatment measures.

Test-Taking Strategy: Note the strategic words "indicate the need for further instructions." These words indicate a negative event query and ask you to select an option that is an incorrect statement. Recalling that bacterial conjunctivitis is highly contagious will direct you to option 3. Review the infection control measures for bacterial conjunctivitis if you had difficulty with this question.

Level of Cognitive Ability: Comprehension
Client Needs: Safe and Effective Care Environment
Integrated Process: Teaching and Learning
Content Area: Child Health
Reference: Hockenberry, M., & Wilson, D. (2007). *Wong's nursing care of infants and children* (8th ed., p. 677). St. Louis: Mosby.

343. 1
Rationale: After a myringotomy with the insertion of tympanostomy tubes, the child is monitored for ear drainage. A small amount of reddish drainage is normal during the first few days after surgery. However, any heavy bleeding or bleeding that occurs after 3 days should be reported. The nurse would document the findings. Options 2, 3, and 4 are not necessary.

Test-Taking Strategy: Use the process of elimination. Note the strategic words "small amount." Considering both the anatomical location of the surgery and these strategic words will direct you to the correct option. Review postoperative findings after a myringotomy with the insertion of tympanostomy tubes if you had difficulty with this question.

Level of Cognitive Ability: Application
Client Needs: Physiological Integrity
Integrated Process: Nursing Process/Implementation
Content Area: Child Health
References: Hockenberry, M., & Wilson, D. (2007). *Wong's nursing care of infants and children* (8th ed., p. 1327). St. Louis: Mosby.

McKinney, E., James, S., Murray, S., & Ashwill, J. (2005). *Maternal-child nursing* (2nd ed., p. 1199). Philadelphia: Saunders.

344. 3
Rationale: When administering eardrops to a child who is less than 3 years old, the ear should be pulled down and back. For children who are more than 3 years old, the ear is pulled up and back. Gloves do not need to be worn by the parents, but handwashing needs to be performed before and after the procedure. The child should be in a side-lying position with the affected ear facing upward to facilitate the flow of medication down the ear canal by gravity.

Test-Taking Strategy: Use the process of elimination. Visualizing this procedure will assist you with eliminating options 1 and 4 first. From the remaining options, recalling the anatomy of the child's ear canal will direct you to option 3. Review the administration of eardrops if you had difficulty with this question.

Level of Cognitive Ability: Application
Client Needs: Health Promotion and Maintenance
Integrated Process: Teaching and Learning
Content Area: Child Health
Reference: Price, D., & Gwin, J. (2008). *Pediatric nursing: An introductory text* (10th ed., p. 384). St. Louis: Saunders.

ALTERNATE ITEM FORMAT: MULTIPLE RESPONSE

345. 1, 2
Rationale: The infant with RSV should be isolated in a private room or in a room with another child with RSV. The infant should be placed in a room near the nurses' station for easy observation. The infant should be positioned with the head and chest at a 30- to 40-degree angle and the neck slightly extended to maintain an open airway and to decrease pressure on the diaphragm. Cool, humidified oxygen is delivered to relieve dyspnea, hypoxemia, and insensible water loss from tachypnea. Contact precautions (wearing gloves and a gown) reduce the nosocomial transmission of RSV.

Test-Taking Strategy: Recalling the mode of transmission of RSV will assist you with determining that the infant needs to be placed in a private room or in a room with another child with RSV and that contact precautions need to be maintained. Recalling the reasons to maintain a patent airway (edema and the accumulation of mucus obstruct the bronchioles) will assist you with determining that the infant needs to be observed closely, that the infant's head should be elevated, and that the infant should receive cool, humidified oxygen. Review the care of the child with bronchiolitis and RSV if you had difficulty with this question.

Level of Cognitive Ability: Application
Client Needs: Physiological Integrity
Integrated Process: Nursing Process/Planning
Content Area: Child Health
Reference: Leifer, G. (2007). *Introduction to maternity and pediatric nursing* (5th ed., pp. 577-578). Philadelphia: Saunders.

REFERENCES

Chernecky, C., & Berger, B. (2008). *Laboratory tests and diagnostic procedures* (5th ed.). Philadelphia: Saunders.

Hockenberry, M., Wilson, D., & Winkelstein, M. (2005). *Wong's essentials of pediatric nursing* (7th ed.). St. Louis: Mosby.

Hockenberry, M., & Wilson, D. (2007). *Wong's nursing care of infants and children* (8th ed.). St. Louis: Mosby.

Leifer, G. (2007). *Introduction to maternity and pediatric nursing* (5th ed.). Philadelphia: Saunders.

McKinney, E., James, S., Murray, S., & Ashwill, J. (2005). *Maternal-child nursing* (2nd ed.). Philadelphia: Saunders.

National Council of State Boards of Nursing (Eds.). (2008). *2008 Detailed Test Plan for the NCLEX-PN® Examination, National Council of State Boards of Nursing*. Chicago: Author.

National Council of State Boards of Nursing. *NCSBN home page.* www.ncsbn.org. Accessed July 17, 2008.

Price, D., & Gwin, J. (2008). *Pediatric nursing: An introductory text* (10th ed.). St. Louis: Saunders.

Cardiovascular Disorders

▲ I. CONGESTIVE HEART FAILURE

A. Description

1. The inability of the heart to pump sufficiently to meet the metabolic needs of the body
2. In infants and children, inadequate cardiac output is most commonly caused by congenital heart defects that produce an excessive volume or pressure load on the myocardium
3. In infants and children, a combination of both left- and right-sided heart failure is usually present (Box 32-1)
4. The goals of treatment are to improve cardiac function, remove accumulated fluid and sodium, decrease cardiac demands, improve tissue oxygenation, and decrease oxygen consumption

▲ B. Data collection of early signs

1. Tachycardia, especially during rest and slight exertion
2. Tachypnea and **wheezing**
3. Profuse scalp sweating, especially in infants
4. Diaphoresis, especially with feeding
5. Fatigue and irritability
6. Sudden weight gain related to excess fluid retention
7. Failure to thrive or poor weight gain related to the inability to meet metabolic needs

▲ C. Interventions

1. Monitor the vital signs closely and for the early signs of congestive heart failure (CHF)
2. Monitor for respiratory distress (count respirations for 1 full minute)
3. Monitor the apical pulse (count the pulse for 1 full minute) and for dysrhythmias
4. Monitor for signs of infection, particularly respiratory infection
5. Monitor intake and output (I&O); weigh diapers
6. Monitor daily weight to assess for fluid retention; a weight gain of 0.5 kg (1 pound) in 1 day is a result of the accumulation of fluid
7. Monitor for facial or peripheral edema, auscultate lung sounds, and report abnormal findings

8. Elevate the head of the bed (semi-Fowler's position)
9. Maintain a neutral thermal environment to prevent cold stress in infants
10. Provide rest; decrease environmental stimuli
11. Administer cool, humidified oxygen, as prescribed; use an oxygen hood for young infants and a nasal cannula or face tent for older infants and children
12. Organize nursing activities to allow for uninterrupted sleep
13. Maintain adequate nutritional status
14. Feed the infant when he or she is hungry, accommodating the infant's sleep and wake patterns; the infant should be well rested before feeding (avoid overfeeding, which will contribute to worsening CHF)
15. Provide small, frequent feedings, which will be less tiring
16. Administer sedation, as prescribed, during the acute stage to promote rest
17. Administer digoxin (Lanoxin), as prescribed; monitor digoxin levels and for signs of digoxin toxicity, especially bradycardia and vomiting
18. Count the apical heart rate for 1 minute before administering digoxin
19. Check regarding the parameters for withholding digoxin; generally, digoxin is withheld if the pulse is less than 90 beats per minute in infants and young children and less than 70 beats per minute in older children
20. Note that infants rarely receive more than 1 mL (50 mcg or 0.05 mg) of digoxin (Lanoxin) in one dose
21. Angiotensin-converting enzyme (ACE) inhibitors such as captopril (Capoten) or enalapril (Vasotec) may be prescribed
22. Monitor for hypotension, renal dysfunction, and cough when ACE inhibitors are administered
23. Administer diuretics, as prescribed; monitor for hypokalemia with furosemide (Lasix) and with thiazide diuretics

BOX 32-1 Signs and Symptoms of Congestive Heart Failure

Left-Sided Failure
- Crackles and wheezes
- Cough
- Dyspnea
- Grunting (infants)
- Head bobbing (infants)
- Nasal flaring
- Orthopnea
- Periods of cyanosis
- Retractions
- Tachypnea

Right-Sided Failure
- Ascites
- Hepatosplenomegaly
- Jugular vein distention
- Oliguria
- Peripheral edema, especially dependent and periorbital edema
- Weight gain

BOX 32-2 Home-Care Instructions for Administering Digoxin (Lanoxin)

Administer the medication as prescribed.
Administer the medication 1 hour before or 2 hours after feedings.
Use a calendar to mark off the dose that has been administered.
Do not mix the medication with food or fluid.
If a dose is missed and more than 4 hours have elapsed, withhold the dose, and give the next dose at the scheduled time; if less than 4 hours have elapsed, administer the missed dose.
If the child vomits, do not administer a second dose.
If more than two consecutive doses have been missed, notify the physician; do not increase or double the dose to make up for missed doses.
If the child has teeth, give him or her water after the medication; if possible, brush the child's teeth to prevent tooth decay from the sweetened liquid.
If the child becomes ill, notify the physician.
Keep the medication in a locked cabinet.
Call the poison control center immediately if accidental overdose occurs.

24. Administer potassium supplements and provide dietary sources of potassium, as prescribed
25. Monitor the serum electrolytes, particularly the potassium level
26. Restrict fluid, as prescribed, during the acute stage; monitor for dehydration
27. Check the physician's orders regarding sodium restriction; note that most infant formulas have slightly more sodium than breast milk
28. Instruct the parents regarding the diagnosis and administration of medications (Box 32-2)
29. Instruct the parents in cardiopulmonary resuscitation
30. Provide the parents and caregivers with support, appropriate information, and resources

BOX 32-3 Defects With Increased Pulmonary Blood Flow

- Atrial septal defect
- Ventricular septal defect
- Atrioventricular canal defect
- Patent ductus arteriosus

BOX 32-4 Signs and Symptoms of Decreased Cardiac Output

- Decreased peripheral pulses
- Exercise intolerance
- Feeding difficulties
- Hypotension
- Irritability, restlessness, and lethargy
- Oliguria
- Pale, cool extremities
- Tachycardia

II. **DEFECTS WITH INCREASED PULMONARY BLOOD FLOW** (Box 32-3)
A. Description
  1. Intracardiac communications along the septum or an abnormal connection between the great arteries allow blood to flow from the high-pressure left side of the heart to the low-pressure right side of the heart (left-to-right **shunt**)
  2. The infant typically demonstrates signs and symptoms of CHF
B. Atrial septal defect (ASD)
  1. An abnormal opening between the atria that causes an increased flow of oxygenated blood into the right side of the heart
  2. Right atrial and ventricular enlargement occur
  3. Infants may be asymptomatic or may develop CHF
  4. Signs and symptoms of decreased cardiac output may be present (Box 32-4)
  5. Nonsurgical treatment: May be closed with the use of devices during a cardiac catheterization
  6. Surgical treatment: Open repair with cardiopulmonary bypass is usually performed before the child reaches school age
C. Ventricular septal defect (VSD)
  1. An abnormal opening between the right and left ventricles (frequently associated with other congenital defects)
  2. Many VSDs close spontaneously during the first year of life in children who have small or moderate defects
  3. A characteristic murmur is present; CHF is common

4. Nonsurgical treatment: Device closure during cardiac catheterization may be possible
5. Surgical treatment: Open repair with cardiopulmonary bypass
6. Educate parents and caregivers regarding the use of antibiotic prophylaxis for dental care or minor surgical procedures to prevent bacterial endocarditis

D. Atrioventricular canal defect
1. Incomplete fusion of the endocardial cushions
2. Most common cardiac defect in children with Down syndrome
3. A characteristic murmur is present
4. The infant usually has mild to moderate CHF; mild **cyanosis** increases with crying
5. Surgical treatment: Can include either pulmonary artery banding for infants with severe symptoms (palliative) or complete repair via cardiopulmonary bypass

E. Patent ductus arteriosus (PDA)
1. Failure of the fetal ductus arteriosus (i.e., the artery that connects the aorta and the pulmonary artery) to close within the first weeks of life
2. A characteristic machine-like murmur is present; the infant may be asymptomatic, or he or she may show signs of CHF
3. A widened pulse pressure and bounding pulses are present
4. Medical management: Indomethacin (prostaglandin inhibitor) may be administered to close a patent ductus in premature infants and some newborns
5. Other therapy: The defect may be closed during cardiac catheterization or may require surgical management

III. **OBSTRUCTIVE DEFECTS** (Box 32-5)
A. Description
1. Blood exiting the heart meets an area of anatomic narrowing (**stenosis**), thus causing obstruction of the blood flow
2. The location of narrowing is usually near the valve of the obstructive defect
3. Infants and children exhibit signs of CHF
4. Children with mild obstruction may be asymptomatic

B. Coarctation of the aorta
1. Localized narrowing of the aortic arch or descending aorta, frequently near the insertion of the ductus arteriosus
2. Collateral circulation develops during fetal life to maintain flow from the ascending to the descending aorta
3. Signs of CHF in infants
4. High blood pressure and bounding pulses in the arms, weak or absent femoral pulses, and cool lower extremities may be present

---

BOX 32-5 **Obstructive Defects**

- Coarctation of the aorta
- Aortic stenosis
- Pulmonary stenosis

---

5. Children may experience headaches, dizziness, fainting, and epistaxis as a result of hypertension
6. Treatment: Surgical treatment to remove the narrowed portions of the vessels and subsequent anastomosis of the ends or balloon angioplasty; however, restenosis can occur, or surgical treatment may be necessary

C. Aortic **stenosis**
1. Narrowing or stricture of the aortic valve that causes resistance to blood flow in the left ventricle, decreased cardiac output, left ventricular hypertrophy, and pulmonary vascular congestion
2. A characteristic murmur is present
3. Infants with severe defects demonstrate signs of decreased cardiac output with faint pulses, hypotension, tachycardia, and poor feeding
4. Children show signs of exercise intolerance, chest pain, and dizziness when standing for long periods
5. Treatment: Balloon angioplasty during cardiac catheterization to dilate the narrowed valve may be performed, or surgery may be necessary

D. Pulmonary **stenosis** (PS)
1. Narrowing at the entrance to the pulmonary artery
2. Resistance to blood flow causes right ventricular hypertrophy and decreased pulmonary blood flow; the right ventricle may be hypoplastic
3. Pulmonary **atresia** is the extreme form of PS (i.e., total fusion of the commissures and no blood flows to the lungs)
4. A characteristic murmur is present
5. May be asymptomatic; mild **cyanosis** or CHF occurs
6. Newborns with severe narrowing will be cyanotic
7. If PS is severe, CHF occurs
8. Treatment: Balloon angioplasty during cardiac catheterization to dilate the narrowed valve may be performed, or surgery may be necessary

IV. **DEFECTS WITH DECREASED PULMONARY BLOOD FLOW** (Box 32-6)
A. Description
1. Obstructed pulmonary blood flow and an anatomic defect (ASD or VSD) between the right and left sides of the heart
2. Pressure on the right side of the heart increases, exceeding left-sided pressure, which allows

| BOX 32-6 | Defects With Decreased Pulmonary Blood Flow |

- Tetralogy of Fallot
- Tricuspid atresia

| BOX 32-7 | Mixed Defects |

- Transposition of the great arteries or transposition of the great vessels
- Total anomalous pulmonary venous connection
- Truncus arteriosus
- Hypoplastic left heart syndrome

desaturated blood to **shunt** right to left; this causes desaturation in the left side of the heart and in the systemic circulation

3. Typically, hypoxemia and **cyanosis** appear

B. Tetralogy of Fallot
1. Includes four defects: VSD, PS, overriding aorta, and right ventricular hypertrophy
2. If pulmonary vascular resistance is higher than systemic resistance, the **shunt** is from right to left; if systemic resistance is higher than pulmonary resistance, the **shunt** is from left to right
3. Infants
    a. May be acutely cyanotic at birth or may have mild **cyanosis** that progresses over the first year of life as the pulmonic **stenosis** worsens
    b. A characteristic murmur is present
    c. Acute episodes of **cyanosis** and hypoxia (hypercyanotic spells), called blue spells or tet spells, occur when the infant's oxygen requirements exceed the blood supply (usually during crying or after feeding); the infant's knees may be brought to his or her chest and oxygen administered to relieve a tet spell
4. Children: With increasing **cyanosis,** there may be clubbing of the fingers, squatting after learning to walk (increases systemic vascular resistance to ward off cyanotic spells), easy fatigability and dyspnea on exertion, and poor **growth**
5. Surgical treatment may include a palliative **shunt** or complete repair

C. Tricuspid **atresia**
1. Failure of the tricuspid valve to develop
2. There is no communication from the right atrium to the right ventricle
3. Blood flows through an ASD or a patent foramen ovale to the left side of the heart and through a VSD to the right ventricle and out to the lungs
4. Often associated with pulmonic **stenosis** and the transposition of the great arteries
5. A complete mixing of unoxygenated and oxygenated blood in the left side of the heart occurs, which results in systemic desaturation, pulmonary obstruction, and decreased pulmonary blood flow
6. **Cyanosis,** tachycardia, fatigability with feeding, and dyspnea are seen in the newborn
7. Poor **growth** and development

8. Older children exhibit signs of chronic hypoxemia and clubbing
9. Surgical treatment is necessary; for the neonate whose pulmonary blood flow depends on the patency of the ductus arteriosus, a continuous infusion of prostaglandin E_1 is initiated until surgery

V. **MIXED DEFECTS** (Box 32-7)
A. Description
1. Fully saturated systemic blood flow mixes with the desaturated blood flow, which causes a desaturation of the systemic blood flow
2. Pulmonary congestion occurs and cardiac output decreases
3. Signs of CHF; symptoms depend on the degree of desaturation

B. Transposition of the great arteries or transposition of the great vessels
1. The pulmonary artery leaves the left ventricle, and the aorta exits from the right ventricle
2. No communication between the systemic and pulmonary circulations
3. Infants with minimal communication are severely cyanotic and depressed at birth
4. Infants with large septal defects or a patent ductus arteriosus may be less severely cyanotic but may have symptoms of CHF
5. Cardiomegaly is evident a few weeks after birth
6. Treatment includes balloon atrial septostomy during cardiac catheterization; surgery may be required

C. Total anomalous pulmonary venous connection
1. Failure of the pulmonary veins to join the left atrium
2. Results in mixed blood being returned to the right atrium and shunted from the right to the left through an ASD
3. The right side of the heart hypertrophies, whereas the left side of the heart may remain small
4. CHF develops
5. **Cyanosis** worsens with pulmonary vein obstruction; after obstruction occurs, the infant's condition deteriorates rapidly
6. Surgical treatment is necessary

D. Truncus arteriosus
1. The failure of normal septation and the division of the embryonic bulbar trunk into the

pulmonary artery and the aorta, which results in a single vessel that overrides both ventricles

2. Blood from both ventricles mixes in the common great artery, thus causing desaturation and hypoxemia
3. A characteristic murmur is present
4. The infant exhibits moderate to severe CHF, variable **cyanosis,** poor **growth,** and activity intolerance
5. Surgical treatment is necessary

E. Hypoplastic left heart syndrome
1. The underdevelopment of the left side of the heart that results in a hypoplastic left ventricle and aortic **atresia**
2. Mild **cyanosis** and signs of CHF occur until the ductus arteriosus closes; progressive deterioration with **cyanosis** and decreased cardiac output then occurs, which lead to cardiovascular collapse
3. Fatal during the first few months of life without intervention
4. Surgical treatment is necessary

▲ VI. INTERVENTIONS: CARDIOVASCULAR DEFECTS
A. Monitor for signs of a defect in the infant or child
B. Monitor the vital signs closely
C. Monitor the respiratory status for the presence of **nasal flaring** and the use of accessory muscles; the physician is notified if any changes occur
D. Breath sounds are auscultated for **crackles,** wheezes, or rhonchi
E. If respiratory effort is increased, place the child in reverse Trendelenburg's position (elevate the head and upper body) to decrease the work of breathing
F. Administer humidified oxygen, as prescribed
G. Endotracheal tube and ventilator care may be necessary; restrain the hands of an intubated child
H. Monitor for hypercyanotic spells (Box 32-8)
I. Monitor for signs of CHF, such as fluid retention in the hands, feet, chest, and around the eyes
J. Monitor the peripheral pulses
K. Monitor the I&O and notify the physician if a decrease in urine output occurs
L. Monitor the urine output, weighing diapers as necessary
M. Obtain a daily weight
N. Maintain fluid restriction, if prescribed

BOX 32-8 **Treatment for Hypercyanotic Spells**

Place the infant in a knee-chest position.
Administer 100% oxygen by face mask.
Administer morphine sulfate, as prescribed.
Administer intravenous fluids, as prescribed.

O. Provide adequate nutrition (high-calorie requirements), as prescribed
P. Administer medications, as prescribed
Q. Keep the child as stress-free as possible; plan interventions to allow for maximal rest for the child
R. Prepare the parents and child, if appropriate, for surgery
S. Allow the parents and child to verbalize their feelings and concerns regarding the disorder
T. Familiarize the parents and child with hospital procedures and equipment

VII. CARDIAC CATHETERIZATION
A. Description
1. The most invasive diagnostic procedure used to determine cardiac defects
2. Provides information about the oxygenation saturation of the blood in the great vessels and heart chambers
3. May be diagnostic, interventional, or electrophysiologic in purpose
4. Risks include hemorrhage from the entry site, clot formation and subsequent blockage distally, and transient dysrhythmias

B. Preprocedure nursing interventions
1. Assess for the accurate height and weight, because it assists with the selection of the correct catheter size
2. Obtain a history of the presence of allergic reactions to iodine
3. Assess for symptoms of infection, including diaper rash
4. Assess and mark bilateral pulses (e.g., dorsalis pedis, posterior tibial)
5. Assess the baseline oxygen saturation
6. Familiarize the parents and child with hospital procedures and equipment
7. Educate the parents and child, if he or she is of an appropriate age, about the procedure
8. Allow the parents and child to verbalize their feelings and concerns regarding the procedure and the disorder

C. Postprocedure nursing interventions
1. Monitor findings on the cardiac monitor and the oxygen saturation for up to 4 hours after the procedure
2. Assess the pulses below the catheter site for equality and symmetry
3. Assess the temperature and color of the affected extremity, and report coolness, which may indicate arterial obstruction
4. Monitor the vital signs frequently, per the physician's orders
5. Assess the pressure dressing for intactness and signs of hemorrhage
6. Assess for signs of bleeding under the extremity on the bedsheets

7. If bleeding is present, apply continuous direct pressure above the entry site, and report it immediately

8. Immobilize the affected extremity for at least 4 to 6 hours for a venous entry site and for 6 to 8 hours for an arterial entry site

9. Hydrate the child via the oral route, the intravenous route, or both, as prescribed

10. Administer acetaminophen (Tylenol) or ibuprofen (Advil, Motrin) for pain or discomfort, as prescribed

11. Prepare the parents and child, if appropriate, for surgery

▲ D. Discharge teaching for the child and parents

1. Remove the dressing on the day after the procedure and cover it with a Band-Aid for 2 to 3 days

2. Keep the site clean and dry

3. Have the child avoid tub baths for 2 to 3 days

4. Observe for redness, edema, drainage, bleeding, and fever, and report any of these signs immediately

5. Avoid strenuous activity, if applicable (the child may return to school, if appropriate)

6. Provide a diet as tolerated

7. Administer acetaminophen (Tylenol) or ibuprofen (Advil, Motrin) for pain, discomfort, or fever

8. Stress the importance of keeping follow-up appointments with the primary care provider

VIII. CARDIAC SURGERY

A. Postoperative interventions

1. Monitor the vital signs, per protocol

2. Monitor the temperature; notify the physician if a fever occurs

3. Monitor for signs of sepsis, such as fever, chills, diaphoresis, lethargy, and altered levels of consciousness

4. Monitor for increased oxygen requirements and poor perfusion

5. Maintain aseptic technique

6. Assist with monitoring lines, tubes, or catheters that are in place; remove them promptly, as prescribed, when they are no longer needed to prevent infection

7. Monitor for signs of discomfort, such as irritability; changes in heart rate, respiratory rate, and blood pressure; and the inability to sleep

8. Administer pain medications, as prescribed, and note their effectiveness

9. Administer antibiotics and antipyretics, as prescribed

10. Encourage rest periods

11. Facilitate parent–child contact as soon as possible

▲ B. Postoperative home care (Box 32-9)

IX. RHEUMATIC FEVER

A. Description

1. An inflammatory autoimmune disease that affects the connective tissues of the heart, joints, subcutaneous tissues, and/or blood vessels of the central nervous system

2. The most serious complication is rheumatic heart disease, which affects the cardiac valves

3. Presents 2 to 6 weeks after an untreated or partially treated group A β-hemolytic streptococcal infection of the upper respiratory tract

4. Jones criteria are used to determine the diagnosis

B. Data collection (Figure 32-1)

1. Low-grade fever that spikes in the late afternoon

2. Elevated antistreptolysin O titer

3. Elevated sedimentation rate

4. Elevated C-reactive protein

5. Aschoff's bodies (lesions) in the heart, blood vessels, brain, and serous surfaces of the joints and pleurae

6. A macular erythematous rash, primarily on the trunk and extremities

C. Interventions

1. Monitor the vital signs

2. Control joint pain and inflammation with massage and alternating hot and cold applications, as prescribed

3. Provide bedrest during the acute febrile phase

4. Limit physical exercise in the child with carditis

5. Administer antibiotics, as prescribed

BOX 32-9 **Home Care After Cardiac Surgery**

Omit outside play for several weeks.

Avoid activities in which the child could fall (e.g., bike riding) for 2 to 4 weeks.

Avoid crowds for 2 weeks after discharge.

Follow a no-salt added diet, if prescribed.

Do not add new foods to the infant's eating schedule.

Do not place creams, lotions, or powders on the incision until it is completely healed.

The child may return to school the third week after discharge, starting with half days.

The child should have no physical education for 2 months.

Instruct the parents to discipline the child normally.

Instruct the parents about the importance of the 2-week follow-up appointment.

Avoid immunizations, invasive procedures, and dental visits for 2 months.

Advise the parents regarding the importance of a dental visit every 6 months after the age of 3 years and to inform the dentist of the cardiac problem so that antibiotics can be prescribed, if necessary.

Instruct the parents to call the physician if the child displays coughing, tachypnea, cyanosis, vomiting, diarrhea, anorexia, pain, or fever or if any swelling, redness, or drainage occurs at the site of the incision.

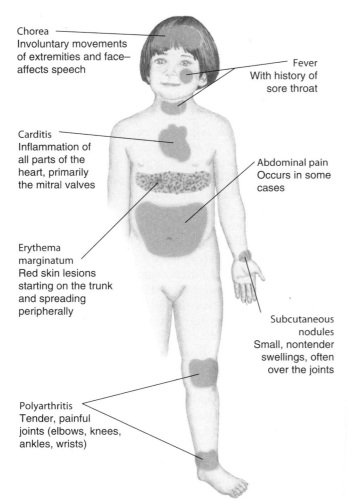

Chorea
Involuntary movements
of extremities and face–
affects speech

Fever
With history of
sore throat

Carditis
Inflammation of
all parts of the
heart, primarily
the mitral valves

Abdominal pain
Occurs in some
cases

Erythema
marginatum
Red skin lesions
starting on the trunk
and spreading
peripherally

Subcutaneous
nodules
Small, nontender
swellings, often
over the joints

Polyarthritis
Tender, painful
joints (elbows, knees,
ankles, wrists)

FIG. 32-1 Clinical manifestations of rheumatic fever. (From McKinney, E., James, S., Murray, S., & Ashwill, J. [2005]. *Maternal-child nursing* [2nd ed.]. Philadelphia: Saunders.)

6. Administer salicylates and anti-inflammatory agents, as prescribed (these medications should not be instituted before the diagnosis is confirmed, because they mask polyarthritis)
7. Initiate seizure precautions if the child is experiencing chorea
8. Instruct the parents about the importance of follow-up and the need for antibiotic prophylaxis for dental work, infection, and invasive procedures
9. Advise the child to tell the parents if anyone in school develops a streptococcal throat infection

X. KAWASAKI DISEASE
A. Description
1. Also called mucocutaneous lymph node syndrome; it is an acute systemic inflammatory illness
2. The cause is unknown but may be associated with an infection by an organism or toxin
3. Cardiac involvement is the most serious complication; aneurysms can develop

BOX 32-10 **Parent Education for Kawasaki Disease**

Follow-up care is essential to recovery.
The signs and symptoms of Kawasaki disease include the following:
• Irritability may last for up to 2 months after the onset of symptoms.
• Peeling of the hands and feet may occur.
• Pain in the joints may persist for several weeks.
• Stiffness in the morning, after naps, and in cold temperatures may occur.
Record the temperature (fever is expected) until the child has been afebrile for several days.
Notify the physician if the temperature is 101° F or higher.
Administer salicylates, such as acetylsalicylic acid (aspirin), as prescribed.
Monitor for signs of aspirin toxicity, including tinnitus, headache, vertigo, and bruising.
Do not administer aspirin or aspirin-containing products (ibuprofen [Advil, Motrin]) if the child has been exposed to chickenpox or influenza.
Monitor for signs and symptoms of bleeding, including epistaxis, hemoptysis, hematemesis, hematuria, melena (blood in the stool), and bruises on the body.
Monitor for signs and symptoms of cardiac complications, including chest pain or tightness (older children), cool and pale extremities, abdominal pain, nausea, vomiting, irritability, restlessness, and uncontrollable crying.
The child should avoid contact sports (if age appropriate) if he or she is taking aspirin or anticoagulants.
Avoid the administration of measles/mumps/rubella or varicella vaccines to the child for 11 months after intravenous immunoglobulin therapy, if appropriate.

B. Data collection
1. Acute stage (weeks 1 to 2)
a. Fever that may be present as long as 5 days
b. Conjunctival hyperemia
c. Red throat
d. Swollen hands, rash, and enlargement of the cervical lymph nodes
e. Irritability
2. Subacute stage (weeks 2 to 4)
a. Cracking lips and fissures
b. Desquamation of the skin on the tips of the fingers and toes
c. Joint pain
d. Cardiac manifestations
e. Thrombocytosis
f. Persistent irritability
3. Convalescent stage: Child appears normal but signs of inflammation may be present; generally the child returns to normal within 6 to 8 weeks
C. Interventions
1. Monitor the temperature frequently

2. Monitor the heart sounds and rhythm
3. Monitor the extremities for edema, redness, and desquamation
4. Examine the eyes for conjunctivitis
5. Monitor the mucous membranes for inflammation
6. Monitor the dietary and fluid intake (I&O)
7. Administer soft foods and liquids that are neither too hot nor too cold
8. Weigh the child daily
9. Provide passive range-of-motion exercises to facilitate joint movement
10. Administer acetylsalicylic acid (aspirin), as prescribed, for its antipyretic and antiplatelet effects
11. Intravenous immune globulin may be prescribed to reduce the duration of fever and the incidence of coronary artery lesions and aneurysms
12. Parent education (Box 32-10)

PRACTICE QUESTIONS

More questions on the companion CD!

346. A nurse reviews the record of a child who was just seen by a physician. The physician has documented a diagnosis of suspected aortic stenosis. Which clinical manifestation that is specifically found in children with this disorder should the nurse anticipate?
1. Pallor
2. Hyperactivity
3. Exercise intolerance
4. Gastrointestinal disturbances

347. A nurse has reinforced home-care instructions to the mother of a child who is being discharged after cardiac surgery. Which statement, if made by the mother, indicates the need for further instructions?
1. "A balance of rest and exercise is important."
2. "I can apply lotion or powder to the incision if it is itchy."
3. "Activities during which the child could fall need to be avoided for 2 to 4 weeks."
4. "Large crowds of people need to be avoided for at least 2 weeks after this surgery."

348. A nurse is told that a child with rheumatic fever (RF) will be arriving to the nursing unit for admission. Which question should the nurse ask the family to elicit information specific to the development of RF?
1. "Has the child complained of back pain?"
2. "Has the child complained of headaches?"
3. "Has the child had any nausea or vomiting?"
4. "Did the child have a sore throat or an unexplained fever within the past 2 months?"

349. Acetylsalicylic acid (aspirin) is prescribed for a child with rheumatic fever (RF). The nurse would question this order if the child had documented evidence of which condition?
1. Arthralgia
2. Joint pain
3. Facial edema
4. A viral infection

350. A nurse assists with admitting a child with a diagnosis of acute-stage Kawasaki disease. When obtaining the child's medical history, which clinical manifestation is likely to be reported?
1. Cracked lips
2. A normal appearance
3. Conjunctival hyperemia
4. Desquamation of the skin

351. A nurse caring for an infant with congenital heart disease is monitoring the infant closely for signs of congestive heart failure (CHF). The nurse looks for which early sign of CHF?
1. Pallor
2. Cough
3. Tachycardia
4. Slow and shallow breathing

352. A physician has prescribed oxygen as needed for a 10-year-old child with congestive heart failure (CHF). In which situation would the nurse administer the oxygen to the child?
1. When the child is sleeping
2. When changing the child's diapers
3. When the mother is holding the child
4. When drawing blood for the measurement of electrolyte levels

353. A nurse is monitoring the daily weight of an infant with congestive heart failure (CHF). Which of the following alerts the nurse to suspect fluid accumulation and thus to the need to notify the registered nurse?
1. Bradypnea
2. Diaphoresis
3. Decreased blood pressure (BP)
4. A weight gain of 1 pound in 1 day

354. A nurse provides home-care instructions to the parents of a child with congestive heart failure regarding the procedure for the administration of digoxin (Lanoxin). Which statement, if made by a parent, indicates the need for further instruction?
1. "I will not mix the medication with food."
2. "If more than one dose is missed, I will call the physician."
3. "I will take my child's pulse before administering the medication."
4. "If my child vomits after medication administration, I will repeat the dose."

ALTERNATE ITEM FORMAT: MULTIPLE RESPONSE

355. A nurse is caring for an infant with a diagnosis of tetralogy of Fallot. The infant suddenly becomes cyanotic, and the nurse recognizes that the infant is experiencing a hypercyanotic spell. Choose the interventions that the nurse should perform. Select all that apply.

☐ **1.** Call a code blue.
☐ **2.** Notify the registered nurse.
☐ **3.** Place the infant in a prone position.
☐ **4.** Prepare to administer morphine sulfate.
☐ **5.** Prepare to administer intravenous fluids.
☐ **6.** Prepare to administer 100% oxygen by face mask.

ANSWERS

346. **3**

Rationale: The child with aortic stenosis shows signs of exercise intolerance, chest pain, and dizziness when standing for long periods. Pallor may be noted, but it is not specific to this type of disorder alone. Options 2 and 4 are not related to this disorder.
Test-Taking Strategy: Use the process of elimination, and focus on the disorder. Options 2 and 4 can be eliminated first, because they are not associated with a cardiac disorder. From the remaining options, noting the word "specifically" in the query of the question will direct you to option 3. Review the manifestations associated with aortic stenosis if you had difficulty with this question.
Level of Cognitive Ability: Comprehension
Client Needs: Physiological Integrity
Integrated Process: Nursing Process/Data Collection
Content Area: Child Health
Reference: Hockenberry, M., & Wilson, D. (2007). *Nursing care of infants and children* (8th ed., pp. 1464-1465). St. Louis: Mosby.

347. **2**

Rationale: The mother should be instructed that lotions and powders should not be applied to the incision site. Options 1, 3, and 4 are accurate instructions regarding home care after cardiac surgery.
Test-Taking Strategy: Note the strategic words "indicates the need for further instructions." These words indicate a negative event query and ask you to select an option that is an incorrect statement. Using the general principles related to postoperative incisional site care will direct you to option 2. Review the home-care instructions after cardiac surgery if you had difficulty with this question.
Level of Cognitive Ability: Comprehension
Client Needs: Health Promotion and Maintenance
Integrated Process: Teaching and Learning
Content Area: Child Health
References: Hockenberry, M., Wilson, D., & Winkelstein, M. (2005). *Wong's essentials of pediatric nursing* (7th ed., pp. 921-922). St. Louis: Mosby.
Price, D., & Gwin, J. (2005). *Thompson's pediatric nursing* (9th ed., p. 95). Philadelphia: Saunders.

348. **4**

Rationale: RF characteristically presents 2 to 6 weeks after an untreated or partially treated group A β-hemolytic streptococcal infection of the upper respiratory tract. Initially, the nurse determines if the child has had a sore throat or an unexplained fever within the past 2 months. Options 1, 2, and 3 are unrelated to RF.

Test-Taking Strategy: Use the process of elimination. Note the similarity between rheumatic "fever" in the question and the word "fever" in the correct option. Review the causes of RF if you had difficulty with this question.
Level of Cognitive Ability: Application
Client Needs: Physiological Integrity
Integrated Process: Nursing Process/Data Collection
Content Area: Child Health
Reference: Leifer, G. (2007). *Introduction to maternity and pediatric nursing* (5th ed., p. 603). Philadelphia: Saunders.

349. **4**

Rationale: Anti-inflammatory agents, including aspirin, may be prescribed for the child with RF. Aspirin should not be given to a child who has chickenpox or other viral infections such as influenza because of the risk of Reyes syndrome. Options 1 and 2 are clinical manifestations of RF. Facial edema may be associated with the development of a cardiac complication.
Test-Taking Strategy: Use the process of elimination. Options 1 and 2 can be eliminated first, because they are comparable or alike. Recalling that facial edema may indicate a cardiac complication will assist you with eliminating this option. Review the contraindications related to the use of aspirin if you had difficulty with this question.
Level of Cognitive Ability: Application
Client Needs: Safe and Effective Care Environment
Integrated Process: Nursing Process/Implementation
Content Area: Child Health
Reference: Price, D., & Gwin, J. (2008). *Pediatric nursing: An introductory text* (10th ed., pp. 311-312). St. Louis: Saunders.

350. **3**

Rationale: During the acute stage of Kawasaki disease, the child presents with fever, conjunctival hyperemia, a red throat, swollen hands, a rash, and enlargement of the cervical lymph nodes. During the subacute stage, cracking lips and fissures, desquamation of the skin on the tips of the fingers and toes, joint pain, cardiac manifestations, and thrombocytosis occur. During the convalescent stage, the child appears normal, but signs of inflammation may be present.
Test-Taking Strategy: Use the process of elimination. Noting the strategic words "acute-stage" in the question will assist with directing you to option 3. Review the clinical manifestations associated with each stage of Kawasaki disease if you had difficulty with this question.
Level of Cognitive Ability: ComprehensionClient Needs: Physiological Integrity
Integrated Process: Nursing Process/Data Collection
Content Area: Child Health
Reference: Leifer, G. (2007). *Introduction to maternity and pediatric nursing* (5th ed., pp. 606-607). Philadelphia: Saunders.

351. **3**

Rationale: The early signs of CHF include tachycardia, tachypnea, profuse scalp sweating, fatigue, irritability, sudden weight gain, and respiratory distress. A cough may occur with CHF as a result of mucosal swelling and irritation, but it is not an early sign. Pallor may be noted in the infant with CHF, but it is also not an early sign.

Test-Taking Strategy: Use the process of elimination and note the strategic word "early." Think about the physiology and the effects on the heart when fluid overload occurs. These concepts will assist with directing you to option 3. Review the early signs of CHF in an infant if you had difficulty with this question.

Level of Cognitive Ability: Application
Client Needs: Physiological Integrity
Integrated Process: Nursing Process/Data Collection
Content Area: Child Health
Reference: Price, D., & Gwin, J. (2008). *Pediatric nursing: An introductory text* (10th ed., p. 97). St. Louis: Saunders.

352. **4**

Rationale: Oxygen administration may be ordered for stressful periods, especially during bouts of crying or invasive procedures. Drawing blood is an invasive procedure that would likely cause the child to cry.

Test-Taking Strategy: Use the process of elimination. Read the options and recall the situations that would place stress and an increased workload on the heart. This concept should direct you to option 4. Review care of the child with CHF if you had difficulty with this question.

Level of Cognitive Ability: Application
Client Needs: Physiological Integrity
Integrated Process: Nursing Process/Implementation
Content Area: Child Health
Reference: Leifer, G. (2007). *Introduction to maternity and pediatric nursing* (5th ed., p. 602). Philadelphia: Saunders.

353. **4**

Rationale: A weight gain of 0.5 kg (1 pound) in 1 day is a result of the accumulation of fluid. The nurse should monitor the urine output, monitor for evidence of facial or peripheral edema, check the lung sounds, and report the weight gain. Tachypnea and an increased BP would occur with fluid accumulation. Diaphoresis is a sign of CHF, but it is not specific to fluid accumulation, and it usually occurs with exertional activities.

Test-Taking Strategy: Use the process of elimination, and focus on the subject of fluid accumulation. Note the relationship between "fluid accumulation" in the question and "weight gain" in the correct option. Review the indications of fluid accumulation in the infant with CHF if you had difficulty with this question.

Level of Cognitive Ability: Comprehension
Client Needs: Physiological Integrity
Integrated Process: Nursing Process/Data Collection
Content Area: Child Health
Reference: Price, D., & Gwin, J. (2008). *Pediatric nursing: An introductory text* (10th ed., p. 97). St. Louis: Saunders.

354. **4**

Rationale: The parents need to be instructed that, if the child vomits after the digoxin is administered, they are not to repeat the dose. Options 1, 2, and 3 are accurate instructions regarding the administration of this medication. Additionally, the parents should be instructed that if a dose is missed and it is not noticed until 4 hours later, the dose should not be administered.

Test-Taking Strategy: Note the strategic words "need for further instruction." These words indicate a negative event query and ask you to select an option that is an incorrect statement. Principles related to the administration of medication to children will assist you with eliminating option 1. General knowledge regarding digoxin administration will assist you with eliminating option 3. From the remaining options, select option 4 over option 2, because, if the child vomits, it would be difficult to determine whether the medication was absorbed by the body. Review home-care instructions regarding the administration of digoxin if you had difficulty with this question.

Level of Cognitive Ability: Comprehension
Client Needs: Physiological Integrity
Integrated Process: Teaching and Learning
Content Area: Child Health
Reference: Price, D., & Gwin, J. (2008). *Pediatric nursing: An introductory text* (10th ed., pp. 99-100). St. Louis: Saunders.

ALTERNATE ITEM FORMAT: MULTIPLE RESPONSE

355. **2, 4, 5, 6**

Rationale: Hypercyanotic episodes often occur among infants with tetralogy of Fallot, and they may occur among infants whose heart defect includes the obstruction of pulmonary blood flow and communication between the ventricles. If a hypercyanotic episode occurs, the infant is placed in a knee-chest position immediately. The registered nurse is notified, who will then contact the physician. The knee-chest position improves systemic arterial oxygen saturation by decreasing venous return so that smaller amounts of highly saturated blood reach the heart. Toddlers and children squat to get into this position and relieve chronic hypoxia. There is no reason to call a code blue unless respirations cease. Additional interventions include administering 100% oxygen by face mask, morphine sulfate, and intravenous fluids, as prescribed.

Test-Taking Strategy: Focus on the infant's diagnosis. Review the nursing interventions when a hypercyanotic episode occurs in an infant if you had difficulty with this question.

Level of Cognitive Ability: Application
Client Needs: Physiological Integrity
Integrated Process: Nursing Process/Implementation
Content Area: Child Health
Reference: Price, D., & Gwin, J. (2008). *Pediatric nursing: An introductory text* (10th ed., pp. 95-97). St. Louis: Saunders.

REFERENCES

Hockenberry, M., & Wilson, D. (2007). *Nursing care of infants and children* (8th ed.). St. Louis: Mosby.

Hockenberry, M., Wilson, D., & Winkelstein, M. (2005). *Wong's essentials of pediatric nursing* (7th ed.). St. Louis: Mosby.

Leifer, G. (2007). *Introduction to maternity and pediatric nursing* (5th ed.). Philadelphia: Saunders.

National Council of State Boards of Nursing (Eds.). (2008). *2008 Detailed Test Plan for the NCLEX-PN® Examination, National Council of State Boards of Nursing*. Chicago: Author.

National Council of State Boards of Nursing. *NCSBN home page*. www.ncsbn.org. Accessed July 20, 2008.

Price, D., & Gwin, J. (2008). *Pediatric nursing: An introductory text* (10th ed.). St. Louis: Saunders.

Price, D., & Gwin, J. (2005). *Pediatric nursing: An introductory text* (9th ed.). Philadelphia: Saunders.

Metabolic, Endocrine, and Gastrointestinal Disorders

I. FEVER
A. Description
1. A rectal temperature of more than 38° C
2. A child's temperature can vary depending on activity, emotional stress, the type of clothing that the child is wearing, and the temperature of the environment
3. Data collection findings associated with the fever provide important indications of its seriousness

B. Data collection
1. Temperature elevation
2. Flushed skin
3. Diaphoresis
4. Chills
5. Restlessness or lethargy

C. Interventions
1. Monitor the vital signs
2. Administer a sponge bath with lukewarm water for 20 to 30 minutes
3. Administer antipyretics such as acetaminophen (Tylenol), as prescribed
4. Do not administer aspirin (acetylsalicylic acid) because of the risk of Reye's syndrome
5. Retake the temperature 30 to 60 minutes after the antipyretic is administered
6. Provide adequate fluid intake, as tolerated and as prescribed
7. Monitor for dehydration and fluid and electrolyte imbalance
8. Instruct the parents regarding how to take the child's temperature, how to safely medicate the child, and when it is necessary to call the physician

II. VOMITING
A. Description
1. The major concerns when a child is vomiting are the risk of dehydration, the loss of fluid and electrolytes, and the development of metabolic alkalosis
2. Additional concerns include aspiration, atelectasis, and the development of pneumonia

B. Data collection
1. Signs of aspiration
2. Character of vomitus
3. Pain and abdominal cramping
4. Dehydration
5. Fluid and electrolyte imbalances
6. Metabolic alkalosis

C. Interventions
1. Maintain a patent airway
2. Position the child on his or her side to prevent aspiration
3. Monitor the vital signs
4. Monitor the character, amount, and frequency of vomiting
5. Note the force of the vomiting, because projectile vomiting is indicative of pyloric **stenosis** or increased intracranial pressure
6. Monitor the intake and output (I&O) and for signs of dehydration
7. Monitor the electrolyte levels
8. Provide oral rehydration therapy, as tolerated and as prescribed; start feeding slowly, with small amounts of fluid at frequent intervals (intravenous [IV] fluids may need to be prescribed)
9. Monitor for diarrhea or abdominal pain
10. Tell the parents to contact the physician when signs of dehydration, blood in the vomitus, forceful vomiting, or abdominal pain is present

III. DIARRHEA
A. Description: The major concerns when a child is having diarrhea are the risk of dehydration, the loss of fluid and electrolytes, and the development of metabolic acidosis

B. Data collection
1. Character of stools
2. Pain and abdominal cramping
3. Dehydration
4. Fluid and electrolyte imbalances
5. Metabolic acidosis

C. Interventions
1. Monitor the vital signs

2. Monitor the character, amount, and frequency of diarrhea
3. Monitor the skin integrity
4. Monitor the I&O and for signs of dehydration
5. Monitor the electrolyte levels
6. For mild to moderate dehydration, prepare to provide oral rehydration therapy; avoid carbonated beverages and those that contain high amounts of sugar
7. For severe dehydration, prepare to maintain nothing-by-mouth (NPO) status to place the bowel at rest; provide fluid and electrolyte replacement with IV fluids, as prescribed; if potassium is prescribed intravenously, monitor the urine output
8. Prepare to reintroduce a normal diet after rehydration is achieved
9. Provide enteric isolation, as required
10. Instruct the parents in good handwashing technique

IV. DEHYDRATION (Box 33-1)

A. Description
1. Dehydration is a common fluid and electrolyte imbalance in infants and children
2. Infants and children are more vulnerable to fluid volume deficit, because a greater amount of their body water is in the extracellular fluid compartment
3. In infants and children, the organs that conserve water are immature, thus placing them at risk for fluid volume deficit
4. The causes can include decreased fluid intake, diaphoresis, vomiting, diarrhea, diabetic ketoacidosis, and extensive burns or other serious injuries

B. Data collection
1. Tachycardia
2. Dry skin and mucous membranes
3. Sunken periorbital areas and fontanels
4. Decreased urine output and increased urine specific gravity
5. Changes in the level of consciousness and responses to stimuli
6. Signs of circulatory failure, such as coolness and mottling of the extremities
7. Loss of skin elasticity and turgor
8. Delayed capillary filling time
9. Weight loss
10. Decreased blood pressure; this is a late sign in infants and children, and they can lose up to 25% of their circulating blood volume before their blood pressure is affected
11. Thirst
12. Absence of tears

C. Interventions
1. Monitor the vital signs
2. Monitor for signs of dehydration

BOX 33-1 **Types of Dehydration**

Isotonic Dehydration
Electrolyte and water deficits occur in approximately balanced proportions.
Hypertonic Dehydration
Water loss exceeds electrolyte loss.
Hypotonic Dehydration
Electrolyte loss exceeds water loss.

---

3. Monitor the weight and for weight changes, including fluid gains and losses
4. Monitor the I&O and the urine for specific gravity
5. Monitor the level of consciousness
6. Monitor the skin turgor and mucous membranes for dryness
7. Provide oral rehydration therapy with solutions, as prescribed, if the child is able to take fluids orally
8. IV fluids and electrolyte replacements may be prescribed if the child is unable to take sufficient fluids orally
9. Introduce a regular diet, as prescribed and as tolerated, when the child is rehydrated
10. Provide instructions to the parents regarding the types and amounts of fluid to encourage, the signs of dehydration, and when to notify the physician

V. PHENYLKETONURIA

A. Description
1. A genetic disorder that results in central nervous system damage from toxic levels of phenylalanine in the blood; children with this condition lack the hepatic enzyme that converts phenylalanine to tyrosine
2. An autosomal-recessive disorder that occurs with equal frequency in males and females; primarily seen in Caucasians and Asians
3. Characterized by blood phenylalanine levels greater than 8 mg/dL (a normal level is less than 2 mg/dL 2 to 5 days after birth)
4. Early detection and treatment are essential for positive outcomes; irreversible brain damage can occur within the first few weeks of life if phenylketonuria (PKU) is undetected or untreated
5. All 50 states require routine screening of all newborn infants for PKU

B. Data collection
1. In all children:
   a. Digestive problems and vomiting
   b. Seizures
   c. Musty or mousy odor of the urine
   d. Mental retardation
2. In older children:
   a. Eczema

b. Hypertonia (increased muscle tone and more active muscle tendon reflexes)

c. Hypopigmentation of the hair, skin, and irises (occurs mainly in blond, blue-eyed children as a result of a lack of tyrosine, which is a necessary component of melanin)

d. Hyperactive behavior

3. Untreated children

a. Microcephaly

b. Prominent cheek and upper jaw bones

c. Widely spaced teeth and poor development of tooth enamel

d. Poor physical **growth**

C. Interventions

1. Screening of newborn infants for PKU: the infant should have begun formula or breast-feeding before specimen collection

2. If initial screening is positive, a repeat test is performed and further diagnostic evaluation is required to verify the diagnosis

3. Infants are rescreened by 14 days of age if the initial screening was done before 48 hours of age

4. If PKU is diagnosed:

a. Phenylalanine intake is restricted for life; high-protein foods (meats and dairy products) and aspartame are avoided, because they contain large amounts of phenylalanine

b. Monitor the physical, neurological, and intellectual development

c. Stress the importance of follow-up treatment and the need for periodic blood levels

d. Encourage the parents to express their feelings about the diagnosis and the risk of PKU in future children

VI. DIABETES MELLITUS

A. Description (Figure 33-1)

1. Type 1 diabetes mellitus is characterized by the destruction of the pancreatic beta cells, which produce insulin; this results in absolute insulin deficiency

2. Type 2 diabetes mellitus usually arises as a result of insulin resistance, in which the body fails to use insulin properly, in combination with relative (rather than absolute) insulin deficiency

3. Complete insulin deficiency requires the use of exogenous insulin to promote appropriate glucose use and to prevent complications related to elevated blood glucose levels, such as hyperglycemia, diabetic ketoacidosis, and death

4. Diagnosis is based on the presence of classic symptoms and an elevated blood glucose level (a normal blood glucose level is between 70 and 110 mg/dL)

5. Children may be admitted directly to the pediatric intensive care unit because of the manifestations of diabetic ketoacidosis, which may be

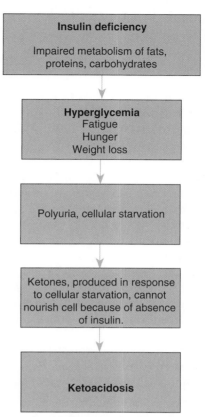

FIG. 33-1 Insulin deficiency leading to ketoacidosis. (From McKinney, E., James, S., Murray, S., & Ashwill, J. [2005]. *Maternal-child nursing* (2nd ed.). Philadelphia: Saunders.)

the initial occurrence when they are diagnosed with diabetes mellitus

B. Data collection

1. Polyuria, polydipsia, and polyphagia

2. Hyperglycemia

3. Weight loss

4. Unexplained fatigue or lethargy

5. Headaches

6. Stomachaches

7. Occasional enuresis in a previously toilet-trained child

8. Vaginitis in adolescent girls (caused by *Candida*, which thrives in hyperglycemic tissues)

9. Fruity odor to the breath

10. Dehydration

11. Blurred vision

12. Slow wound healing

13. Changes in the level of consciousness

C. Long-term effects

1. Failure to grow at a normal rate

2. Delayed maturation

3. Recurrent infections

4. Neuropathy

5. Cardiovascular disease

6. Retinal microvascular disease

7. Renal microvascular disease

D. Complications
1. Hypoglycemia
2. Hyperglycemia
3. Diabetic ketoacidosis
4. Coma
5. Hypokalemia
6. Hyperkalemia
7. Microvascular changes
8. Cardiovascular changes

E. Diet
1. Normal, healthy nutrition is encouraged; the total number of calories is individualized on the basis of the child's age and **growth** expectations
2. As prescribed by the physician, the child may be instructed to follow the food exchange from the American Diabetic Association diet or the dietary guidelines for Americans (MyPyramid) issued by the U.S. Departments of Agriculture and Health and Human Services
3. Dietary intake should include three meals per day, eaten at consistent intervals, plus a mid-afternoon carbohydrate snack and a bedtime snack that is high in protein; a consistent intake of carbohydrates at each meal and snack is needed
4. Tell the child and the parents that the child should carry a source of glucose (e.g., glucose tablets) with him or her at all times to treat hypoglycemia if it occurs
5. Incorporate the diet into the individual child's needs, likes, dislikes, lifestyle, and cultural and socioeconomic patterns
6. Allow the child to participate in making food choices to provide a sense of control

F. Exercise
1. Instruct the child regarding dietary adjustments to consider when exercising
2. Extra food needs to be consumed for increased activity (usually 10 g to 15 g of carbohydrates for every 30 to 45 minutes of activity)
3. Instruct the child to check the blood glucose level before exercising
4. Plan an appropriate exercise regimen with the child, and incorporate the child's developmental stage

G. Insulin
1. Diluted insulin may be required for some infants to provide small-enough doses to avoid hypoglycemia; diluted insulin should be clearly labeled to avoid dosage errors
2. A laboratory evaluation of the glycosylated hemoglobin level should be performed every 3 months
3. Illness, infection, and stress increase the need for insulin; insulin should not be withheld in these situations, because hyperglycemia and ketoacidosis can result
4. When the child is NPO for a special procedure, verify with the physician the need to withhold the morning insulin and when food, fluids, and insulin are to be given
5. Instruct the child and parents regarding the administration of the insulin
6. Instruct the child and parents regarding how to recognize the symptoms of hypoglycemia and hyperglycemia
7. Instruct the parents in the administration of intramuscular or subcutaneous glucagon if the child has a hypoglycemic reaction and is unable to consume sugar-containing items orally
8. Instruct the child and parents to always have a spare bottle of insulin available
9. Advise the parents to obtain a Medic-Alert bracelet that indicates the type and daily insulin dosage that has been prescribed for the child

H. Blood glucose monitoring
1. Results provide information needed to maintain good glycemic control
2. More accurate than urine testing
3. Requires that the child prick him- or herself several times a day, as prescribed (Box 33-2)
4. Instruct the child and parents in the proper procedure for obtaining the blood glucose level
5. Inform the child and parents that the procedure must be performed precisely to obtain accurate results
6. Stress the importance of handwashing before and after performing the procedure to prevent infection
7. Stress the importance of following the manufacturer's instructions for the blood glucose monitoring device

---

BOX 33-2 | **Lessening the Pain of Blood Glucose Monitoring**

Hold the finger under warm water for a few seconds before puncture; this enhances blood flow to the finger.

Use the ring finger or thumb to obtain a blood sample, because blood flows more easily to these areas.

Puncture the finger just to the side of the finger pad, because there are more blood vessels and fewer nerve endings in this area.

Press the lancet device lightly against the skin to prevent a deep puncture.

Use glucose monitors that require very small blood samples for measurement.

Apply an anesthetic cream (e.g., lidocaine/prilocaine cream) to the site before puncture.

Modified from Hockenberry, M., Wilson, D., & Winkelstein, M. (2005). *Wong's essentials of pediatric nursing* (7th ed.). St. Louis: Mosby.

8. Instruct the child and parents to calibrate the monitor as instructed by the manufacturer
9. Instruct the child and parents to check the expiration date on the test strips used for blood glucose monitoring
10. Instruct the child and parents that, if the blood glucose results do not seem reasonable, to reread the instructions, reassess the technique, check the expiration date of the test strips, and perform the procedure again to verify the results

I. Urine testing
1. Instruct the parents and child in the procedure for testing the urine for ketones and glucose
2. Teach the child that the second voided urine specimen is the most accurate
3. The presence of ketones may indicate impending ketoacidosis
4. Urine glucose testing is not recommended as the only means of monitoring control for the child who is taking insulin, because it is a less-reliable indicator as compared with blood glucose monitoring

J. Hypoglycemia
1. Description
   a. A blood glucose level less than 70 mg/dL
   b. Occurs as a result of too much insulin, not enough food, or excessive activity
2. Interventions (Boxes 33-3 and 33-4)

K. Hyperglycemia
1. Description: Elevated blood glucose level more than 200 mg/dL
2. Interventions (Box 33-5)
3. Sick-day rules (Box 33-6)

L. Diabetic ketoacidosis (see Figure 33-1)
1. Description
   a. A complication of diabetes mellitus that develops when a severe insulin deficiency occurs
   b. A life-threatening condition
   c. Hyperglycemia that progresses to metabolic acidosis occurs
   d. Develops over a period of several hours to days
   e. The blood glucose level is more than 300 mg/dL, and urine and serum ketones are positive
2. Interventions
   a. Restore the circulating volume and protect against cerebral, coronary, or renal hypoperfusion

---

BOX 33-4 **Food Items to Treat Hypoglycemia**

- Half a cup of orange juice or a sugar-sweetened carbonated beverage
- One small box of raisins
- Three or four hard candies (e.g., LifeSavers)
- Two to four sugar cubes
- One candy bar
- 1 tsp of honey
- Two or three glucose tablets

BOX 33-5 **Interventions for Hyperglycemia**

Instruct the parents to notify the physician when any of the following occur:
- The blood glucose results are higher than the target range (usually >200 mg/dL).
- Moderate or high ketonuria is present.
- The child is unable to take food or fluids.
- Illness persists.

BOX 33-3 **Interventions for Hypoglycemia**

If possible, confirm the hypoglycemia with a blood glucose reading.
Administer glucose immediately; the rapid-releasing glucose is followed by a complex carbohydrate and protein, such as a slice of bread or a peanut butter cracker.
Give the child an extra snack if the next meal is not planned for more than 30 minutes or if activity is planned.
If the child becomes unconscious, squeeze cake frosting or glucose paste onto the gums and retest the blood glucose level if the child does not improve within 15 to 20 minutes; if the reading remains low, administer additional glucose.
If the child remains unconscious, it may be necessary to administer glucagon.
In the hospital setting, prepare to administer intravenous dextrose.

BOX 33-6 **Sick-Day Rules for the Diabetic Child**

Always give insulin, even if the child does not have an appetite, or contact the physician for specific instructions.
Test the blood glucose level at least every 4 hours.
Test for urinary ketones with each voiding.
Notify the physician if moderate or large amounts of urinary ketones are present.
Follow the child's usual meal plan.
Encourage the consumption of calorie-free liquids to help with clearing ketones.
Encourage rest, especially if urinary ketones are present.
Notify the physician if vomiting; a fruity odor to the breath; deep, rapid respirations; a decreasing level of consciousness; or persistent hyperglycemia occurs.

b. Dehydration is corrected with IV infusions of 0.9% or 0.45% saline, as prescribed

c. Hyperglycemia is corrected with IV regular insulin administration, as prescribed

d. Monitor the vital signs, urine output, and mental status closely

e. Correct acidosis and electrolyte imbalances

f. Administer oxygen, as prescribed

g. Monitor the blood glucose level frequently

h. Monitor the potassium level closely, because, when the child receives insulin to lower the blood glucose level, the serum potassium level will decrease as the acidosis improves, and potassium replacement may be required

i. Monitor the child closely for signs of fluid overload

j. IV dextrose is added, as prescribed, when the blood glucose reaches an appropriate level

k. Treat the cause of hyperglycemia

VII. CLEFT LIP AND CLEFT PALATE (Figure 33-2)

A. Description

1. A congenital anomaly that occurs as a result of the failure of soft tissue or a bony structure to fuse during embryonic development; occurs more frequently among males

2. Involves abnormal openings in the lip or palate that may occur unilaterally or bilaterally and that are readily apparent at birth

3. Causes include genetic, **hereditary**, and environmental factors; exposure to radiation or rubella virus; chromosome abnormalities; and teratogenic factors

4. Closure of a cleft lip defect precedes that of the palate and is usually performed between 6 and 12 weeks of age, when weight gain is established and the infant is free of infection

5. Cleft palate repair is performed sometime between 12 and 18 months of age to allow for the palatal changes that take place with normal **growth**; a cleft palate is closed before the child develops faulty speech habits; the goals of treatment are improved feeding, improved speech, improved dental development, and the development of a positive self-image

B. Data collection

1. Cleft lip can range from a slight notch to a complete separation from the floor of the nose

2. Cleft palate can include nasal distortion, midline or bilateral cleft, and variable extension from the uvula and the soft and hard palate

C. Interventions

1. Check the ability to suck, swallow, handle normal secretions, and breathe without distress

2. Monitor the fluid and calorie intake daily, and monitor the weight

3. Breast-feeding is encouraged; this promotes bonding, and many infants actually feed better

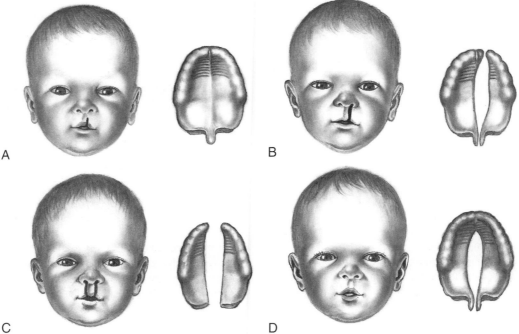

A

B

C

D

FIG. 33-2   Variations in clefts of lip and palate at birth. **A,** Notch in vermilion border. **B,** Unilateral cleft lip and palate. **C,** Bilateral cleft lip and palate. **D,** Cleft palate. (From Hockenberry, M. J. [2005]. *Wong's essentials of pediatric nursing* [7th ed.]. St. Louis: Mosby.)

with the breast than the bottle; if it is not possible to breast-feed, encourage the mother to express her breast milk and to feed this to her infant with a bottle
4. Modify feeding techniques, as necessary; plan to use specialized feeding techniques, obturators, nipples, and feeders
5. Hold the child in an upright position, and direct the formula to the side and back of the mouth to prevent aspiration; feed the infant small amounts gradually, and burp him or her frequently
6. Position the infant on his or her side after feeding
7. Keep suction equipment and a bulb syringe at the bedside
8. Teach the parents the ESSR (Enlarge, Stimulate sucking, Swallow, Rest) method of feeding (Box 33-7)
9. Encourage the parents to describe their feelings about the deformity
D. Postoperative interventions
   1. Cleft lip repair
      a. A lip-protector device may be taped securely to the cheeks to prevent trauma to the suture line
      b. Position the child on the side lateral to the repair or on the back; avoid the prone position to prevent the rubbing of the surgical site on the mattress
      c. After feeding, cleanse the suture line of formula or serosanguineous drainage with a cotton-tipped swab dipped in saline; apply antibiotic ointment, if prescribed
      d. Provide appropriate pain relief
      e. Encourage the parents to hold the child to promote bonding and nurturing
   2. Cleft palate repair
      a. The child is allowed to lie on the abdomen
      b. Avoid crying episodes in the infant or child
      c. Feedings are resumed by bottle, breast, or cup
      d. It is important to keep the mouth clean; feedings may be followed by a little water, and the physician may prescribe a mild antiseptic mouthwash.
      e. Oral packing may be secured to the palate and removed in 2 to 3 days

---

BOX 33-7 **ESSR Method of Feeding**

Enlarge the nipple.
Stimulate the suck reflex.
Swallow.
Rest to allow the child to finish swallowing what has been placed in the mouth.

---

      f. Do not allow the child to brush his or her teeth
      g. Instruct the parents to avoid offering hard food items to the child (e.g., toast, cookies)
   3. Soft elbow or jacket restraints may be used (check agency policies and procedures) to keep the child from touching the repair site; remove the restraints at least every 2 hours to assess the skin integrity and to allow for exercising of the arms
   4. Avoid contact with sharp objects near the surgical site
   5. Avoid the use of oral suction and the placing of objects such as tongue depressors, thermometers, straws, spoons, forks, and pacifiers in the mouth
   6. Provide analgesics for pain, as prescribed
   7. Instruct the parents in feeding techniques and in the care of the surgical site
   8. Instruct the parents to monitor for signs of infection at the surgical site, such as redness, swelling, or drainage
   9. Encourage the parents to hold the child to provide for emotional and nurturing needs
   10. Assist with initiating appropriate referrals for speech impairment or language-based learning difficulties

VIII. ESOPHAGEAL ATRESIA AND TRACHEOESOPHAGEAL FISTULA
(Figure 33-3)
A. Description
   1. The esophagus terminates before it reaches the stomach, a fistula is present that forms an unnatural connection with the trachea, or both
   2. The condition causes oral intake to enter the lungs or a large amount of air to enter the stomach; choking, coughing, and severe abdominal distention can occur
   3. Aspiration pneumonia and severe respiratory distress will develop, and death will occur without surgical intervention
   4. Treatment includes maintenance of a patent airway, prevention of pneumonia, gastric or blind-pouch decompression, supportive therapy, and surgical repair
B. Data collection
   1. Frothy saliva in the mouth and nose; drooling
   2. Coughing, choking during feedings, and unexplained **cyanosis** as a result of respiratory distress (also called "the 3 Cs")
   3. **Regurgitation** and vomiting
   4. Abdominal distention
   5. Inability to pass a small-gauge (e.g., No. 5 French) orogastric feeding tube via the mouth into the stomach

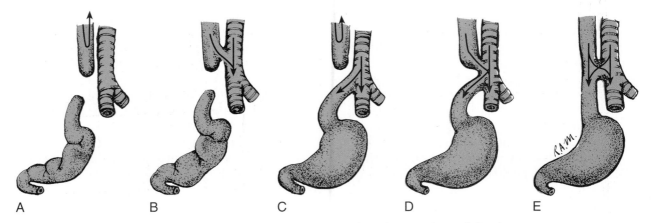

FIG. 33-3 Congenital atresia of esophagus and tracheoesophageal fistula. **A,** Upper and lower segments of esophagus end in blind sac (occurring in 5% to 8% of such infants). **B,** Upper segment of esophagus ends in atresia and connects to trachea by fistulous tract (occurring rarely). **C,** Upper segment of esophagus ends in blind pouch; lower segment connects with trachea by small fistulous tract (occurring in 80% to 95% of such infants). **D,** Both segments of esophagus connect by fistulous tracts to trachea (occurring in less than 1% of such infants). Infant may aspirate with first feeding. **E,** Esophagus is continuous but connects by fistulous tract to trachea; known as H-type. (From Hockenberry, M., & Wilson, D. [2007]. *Wong's nursing care of infants and children* [8th ed.]. St. Louis: Mosby.)

C. Preoperative interventions
  1. The infant may be placed in an incubator or radiant warmer, and humidified oxygen is administered; intubation and mechanical ventilation may be necessary if respiratory distress occurs
  2. Maintain NPO status
  3. Maintain IV fluids, as prescribed
  4. Suction accumulated secretions from the mouth and pharynx
  5. A double-lumen catheter is placed into the upper esophageal pouch and attached to intermittent or continuous low suction to keep the pouch empty of secretions; it is irrigated with normal saline, as prescribed, to prevent clogging
  6. Maintain the infant in an upright position to facilitate drainage and to prevent the aspiration of gastric secretions
  7. A gastrostomy tube may be placed and is left open so that air entering the stomach through the fistula can escape, thus minimizing the danger of **regurgitation**
  8. Administer broad-spectrum antibiotics, as prescribed, because of the high risk for aspiration pneumonia

D. Postoperative interventions
  1. Monitor the respiratory status
  2. Maintain IV fluids, antibiotics, and parenteral nutrition, as prescribed
  3. Monitor the I&O and weight daily
  4. Inspect the surgical site
  5. Provide care to the chest tube, if placed
  6. Monitor for signs of pain
  7. Monitor for dehydration and possible fluid overload
  8. Monitor for anastomotic leaks as evidenced by purulent chest drainage, increased temperature, and an increased white blood cell count
  9. The double-lumen catheter is attached to low suction
  10. If a gastrostomy tube is present, it is attached to gravity drainage until the infant can tolerate feedings (usually postoperative day 5 to 7)
  11. Before oral feedings and the removal of the chest tube, a barium swallow is performed to verify the integrity of the esophageal anastomosis
  12. Before feeding, the gastrostomy tube is elevated and secured above the level of the stomach to allow gastric secretions to pass to the duodenum and swallowed air to escape through the open gastrostomy tube
  13. Feedings through the gastrostomy tube may be prescribed until the anastomosis is healed
  14. Oral feedings are begun with sterile water and followed by frequent small, feedings of formula
  15. The gastrostomy tube may be removed before discharge or maintained for supplemental feedings at home
  16. If the infant is awaiting esophageal replacement, a cervical esophagostomy may be performed
  17. Check the cervical esophagostomy site for redness, breakdown, or exudate (continued discharge or saliva can cause skin breakdown); remove drainage frequently, and apply a protective ointment, a barrier dressing, and/or a collection device

18. If the infant is awaiting esophageal replacement, nonnutritive sucking is provided by a pacifier; infants who remain NPO for extended periods and who have not received oral stimulation frequently have difficulty eating by mouth after surgery and may develop oral hypersensitivity and food aversion

19. Reinforce instructions to the parents regarding the techniques of suctioning, gastrostomy tube care and feedings, and skin site care, as appropriate

20. Instruct the parents to identify behaviors that indicate the need for suctioning, signs of respiratory distress, and signs of a constricted esophagus (e.g., poor feeding, dysphagia, drooling, regurgitating undigested food)

IX. GASTROESOPHAGEAL REFLUX

A. Description
1. The backflow of gastric contents into the esophagus as a result of relaxation or incompetence of the lower esophageal or cardiac sphincter
2. Complications include esophagitis (pain), esophageal strictures, aspiration of the gastric contents, and aspiration pneumonia
3. Most infants with this condition have mild problems that improve within several months and that require minimal interventions
4. Treatment (Box 33-8)

B. Data collection
1. Passive **regurgitation** or nonbilious emesis
2. Poor weight gain and failure to thrive
3. Hematemesis and melena
4. Irritability
5. Heartburn (in older children)
6. Anemia from blood loss

C. Interventions
1. Monitor the amount and characteristics of the emesis
2. Monitor the relationship of the vomiting to the times of feedings and infant activity
3. Monitor the breath sounds before and after feedings
4. Place suction equipment at the bedside
5. Monitor the I&O
6. Monitor for signs and symptoms of dehydration
7. Maintain the IV fluids, as prescribed

D. Positioning
1. Maintain the positioning of the infant at a 30-degree angle after feeding; appropriate positioning may be accomplished with the use of slings and the elevation of the head with pillow wedges or blankets under the mattress
2. For infants, maintain a nonprone position during sleep to reduce the incidence of sudden infant death syndrome; a prone position is only acceptable while the infant is awake

---

BOX 33-8	Treatment for Gastroesophageal Reflux

- Diet
- Positioning
- Medications
- Surgery (performed when severe complications occur)

---

3. Position a child who is more than 1 year old on his or her the left side, with the head of the bed elevated

E. Diet
1. Provide small, frequent, high-calorie feedings to decrease the amount of **regurgitation**; nasogastric tube feedings are indicated if severe **regurgitation** and poor **growth** are present
2. For infants, thicken formula by adding 1 Tbs of rice cereal per 6 oz of formula and cross-cut the nipple; monitor for coughing during feeding
3. Breast-feeding may continue, and the mother may provide more frequent feeding times or express milk for thickening with rice cereal
4. Burp the infant frequently when feeding, and handle the infant minimally after feedings
5. For toddlers, feed solids first, followed by liquids
6. The parents are instructed to avoid feeding the child fatty foods, chocolate, tomato products, carbonated liquids, fruit juices, citrus products, and spicy foods
7. Avoid vigorous play after feeding, and avoid feeding just before bedtime
8. Eliminate all tobacco exposure

F. Medications
1. Administer antacids and histamine receptor antagonists, as prescribed, to reduce the amount of acid present in gastric secretions and to prevent esophagitis
2. Administer prokinetic agents to accelerate gastric emptying and decrease reflux
3. Administer acetaminophen (Tylenol), as prescribed, to relieve reflux pain

G. Surgery
1. If surgery is prescribed, it will require a procedure known as fundoplication, in which a wrap to the stomach fundus is made around the distal esophagus; this restores the competence of the lower esophageal sphincter
2. A gastrostomy may be performed at the same time as the fundoplication for decompression of the stomach postoperatively
3. Fundoplication may be combined with pyloroplasty for children with gastroesophageal reflux who also have delayed gastric emptying

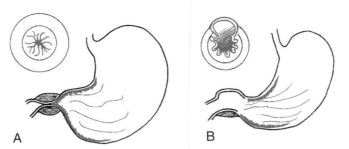

FIG. 33-4 Hypertrophic pyloric stenosis. **A,** Enlarged muscular tumor nearly obliterates pyloric channel. **B,** Longitudinal surgical division of muscle down to submucosa establishes adequate passageway. (From Hockenberry, M., & Wilson, D. [2007]. *Wong's nursing care of infants and children* [8th ed.]. St. Louis: Mosby.)

4. Postoperative care is similar to that for other types of abdominal surgery
5. Instruct the parents about potential postoperative problems, such as bloating symptoms or discomfort after consuming large, solid meals

X. HYPERTROPHIC PYLORIC STENOSIS
   (Figure 33-4)
A. Description
   1. Hypertrophy of the circular muscles of the pylorus causes the narrowing of the pyloric canal between the stomach and the duodenum
   2. Usually develops during the first few weeks of life and causes projectile vomiting, dehydration, metabolic alkalosis, and failure to thrive
   3. Predominantly seen among males
B. Data collection
   1. Vomiting that progresses from mild **regurgitation** to forceful and projectile that usually occurs after a feeding
   2. Vomitus contains gastric contents, such as milk or formula; may contain mucus, may be blood-tinged, and does not usually contain bile
   3. Hunger and irritability
   4. Peristaltic waves visible from left to right across the epigastrium during or immediately after a feeding
   5. Olive-shaped mass in the epigastrium just right of the umbilicus
   6. Dehydration and malnutrition
   7. Electrolyte imbalances
   8. Metabolic alkalosis
C. Interventions
   1. Monitor the vital signs
   2. Monitor the I&O and weight
   3. Monitor for signs of dehydration and electrolyte imbalances
   4. Prepare the child and parents for pyloromyotomy, if prescribed
D. Pyloromyotomy
   1. Description: An incision through the muscle fibers of the pylorus; may be performed by laparoscopy

2. Interventions preoperatively
   a. Monitor the hydration status by checking the daily weights, I&O, and urine for specific gravity
   b. Correct fluid and electrolyte imbalances; IV fluids may be prescribed for rehydration
   c. Maintain NPO status
   d. Monitor the number and character of stools
   e. Maintain the patency of the nasogastric (NG) tube that is placed for stomach decompression
3. Postoperative interventions
   a. Monitor the I&O
   b. Maintain IV fluids until the infant is taking and retaining adequate amounts by mouth
   c. Begin small, frequent feedings of glucose, water, or electrolyte solution 4 to 6 hours postoperatively, as prescribed; advance the diet to formula 24 hours postoperatively, as prescribed
   d. Gradually increase the amount of feedings and the interval between them until a full feeding schedule is reinstated, usually by 48 hours postoperatively
   e. Feed the infant slowly and burp him or her frequently; handle the infant minimally after feedings
   f. Monitor for abdominal distention
   g. Monitor the surgical wound for signs of infection
   h. Instruct the parents about wound care and feeding

XI. LACTOSE INTOLERANCE
A. Description: The inability to tolerate lactose as a result of an absence or deficiency of lactase, which is an enzyme found in the secretions of the small intestine that is required for the digestion of lactose
B. Data collection (Box 33-9)
C. Interventions
   1. Eliminate the offending dairy product or administer an enzyme replacement
   2. Provide information to parents about enzyme tablets (Lactaid, Lactrase, Dairy Ease) that

BOX 33-9 **Data Collection Findings: Lactose Intolerance**

- Symptoms occur after the ingestion of milk products
- Diarrhea
- Abdominal distention
- Crampy abdominal pain
- Excessive flatus

BOX 33-10 **Celiac Crisis**

- Precipitated by infection, fasting, and the ingestion of gluten
- Can lead to electrolyte imbalance, rapid dehydration, and severe acidosis
- Causes profuse, watery diarrhea and vomiting

BOX 33-11 **Basics of a Gluten-Free Diet**

Foods That Are Allowed
- Meats such as beef, pork, and poultry
- Fish
- Eggs, milk, and dairy products
- Vegetables and fruits
- Grains, rice, corn, gluten-free wheat flour, puffed rice, cornflakes, cornmeal, and precooked, gluten-free cereals

Foods That Are Prohibited
- Commercially prepared ice cream
- Malted milk
- Prepared puddings
- Grains, including anything made from wheat, rye, oats, or barley, such as breads, rolls, cookies, cakes, crackers, cereal, spaghetti, macaroni noodles, beer, and ale

predigest the lactose in milk or that supplement the body's own lactase

3. For infants, soy-based formula can be substituted for cow's milk formula or human milk
4. Provide calcium and vitamin D supplements to prevent deficiency
5. Limit milk consumption to one glass at a time
6. If milk is consumed, it should be taken when other foods are consumed rather than by itself
7. Encourage the consumption of hard cheese, cottage cheese, or yogurt (which contains inactive lactase enzyme) rather than milk
8. Encourage the consumption of small amounts of dairy foods daily to help colonic bacteria adapt to ingested lactose
9. Instruct the parents about the importance of calcium and vitamin D supplements
10. Instruct the parents about the foods that contain lactose, including hidden sources

XII. CELIAC DISEASE
A. Description
1. Also known as gluten enteropathy or tropical sprue
2. Malabsorption and intolerance to gluten, which is the protein component of wheat, barley, rye, and oats
3. Results in the accumulation of the amino acid glutamine, which is toxic to intestinal mucosal cells
4. Intestinal villi atrophy, which affects the absorption of ingested nutrients
5. Symptoms of the disorder occur most often between the ages of 1 and 5 years; there is usually an interval of several months between the introduction of gluten into the diet and the onset of symptoms
6. Children at higher risk for the development of celiac disease are those with first-degree relatives with the disease, those with Down syndrome, and those with diabetes mellitus
7. Strict dietary avoidance of gluten minimizes the risk of developing malignant lymphoma of the small intestine and other gastrointestinal (GI) malignancies
B. Data collection
1. Acute or insidious diarrhea; stools are watery and pale with an offensive odor
2. Anorexia

3. Abdominal pain and distention
4. Muscle wasting, particularly in the buttocks and extremities
5. Vomiting
6. Anemia
7. Irritability
C. Celiac crisis (Box 33-10)
D. Interventions
1. Gluten-free diet and the substitution of corn, rice, and millet as grain sources
2. Lifelong elimination of gluten sources such as wheat, rye, oats, and barley
3. Mineral and vitamin supplements, including iron, folic acid, and fat-soluble supplements A, D, E, and K
4. Teach the parents about a gluten-free diet and to read food labels carefully for hidden sources of gluten (Box 33-11)
5. Instruct the parents regarding measures to prevent celiac crisis
6. Inform the parents about the Celiac Sprue Association/United States of America

XIII. APPENDICITIS
A. Description
1. Inflammation of the appendix
2. When the appendix becomes inflamed or infected, perforation may occur within a matter of hours, which leads to peritonitis and sepsis
3. Treatment is the surgical removal of the appendix before perforation occurs

B. Data collection
1. Pain in periumbilical area that descends to the right lower quadrant
2. Abdominal pain that is most intense at McBurney's point
3. Referred pain that indicates the presence of peritoneal irritation
4. Rebound tenderness and abdominal rigidity
5. Elevated white blood cell count
6. Side-lying position with abdominal guarding (legs flexed)
7. Difficulty walking and pain in the right hip
8. Low-grade fever
9. Anorexia, nausea, and vomiting after the pain develops
10. Diarrhea
C. Peritonitis
1. Data collection
   a. Results from a perforated appendix
   b. Increased fever
   c. Sudden relief of pain after the perforation, followed by a subsequent increase in pain accompanied by guarding of the right abdomen
   d. Progressive abdominal distention
   e. Tachycardia, tachypnea, shallow breathing, and hypotension
   f. Pallor
   g. Chills
   h. Restlessness and irritability
D. Appendectomy
1. Description: Surgical removal of the appendix
2. Preoperative interventions
   a. Maintain NPO status
   b. IV fluids and electrolytes may be prescribed to prevent dehydration and to correct electrolyte imbalances
   c. Monitor for signs of a ruptured appendix and peritonitis
   d. Antibiotics may be prescribed
   e. Monitor for changes in the level of pain
   f. Monitor the bowel sounds
   g. Position the child in a right side-lying or low to semi-Fowler's position to promote comfort
   h. Apply ice packs to the abdomen for 20 to 30 minutes every hour, if prescribed
   i. Avoid the application of heat to the abdomen
   j. Avoid the administration of laxatives or enemas
3. Postoperative interventions
   a. Monitor the temperature for signs of infection
   b. Maintain NPO status until bowel function has returned; advance the diet gradually, as tolerated and as prescribed, when bowel sounds return

c. Monitor the incision for signs of infection, such as redness, swelling, drainage, and pain
d. If perforation of the appendix occurred, expect a drain (Penrose drain) to be inserted; alternatively, the incision may be left open to heal from the inside out
e. Expect that drainage from the drain may be profuse for the first 12 hours
f. Position the client in right side-lying or low to semi-Fowler's position with the legs flexed to facilitate drainage
g. Change the dressing, as prescribed, and record the type and amount of drainage
h. Perform wound irrigations, if prescribed
i. Maintain NG tube suction and the patency of the tube, if present
j. Administer antibiotics and analgesics, as prescribed

XIV. HIRSCHSPRUNG'S DISEASE (Figure 33-5)
A. Description
1. A congenital anomaly that is also known as congenital aganglionosis or megacolon
2. Occurs as the result of an absence or agenesis of ganglion cells in the rectum and upward in the colon
3. Results in mechanical obstruction from inadequate motility in an intestinal segment
4. May be a familial congenital defect or associated with other anomalies, such as Down syndrome and genital urinary abnormalities; predominantly seen among males
5. A rectal biopsy demonstrates histologic evidence of the absence of ganglionic cells
6. The most serious complication is enterocolitis; signs include fever, severe prostration, GI bleeding, and explosive, watery diarrhea
7. Treatment for mild or moderate disease is based on relieving the chronic constipation with stool

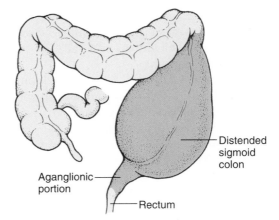

FIG. 33-5 Hirschsprung's disease. (From Wong, D., Perry, S., & Hockenberry, M. [2002]. *Maternal-child nursing care* [2nd ed.]. St. Louis: Mosby.)

softeners and rectal irrigations; however, most children require surgery

8. Treatment for moderate to severe disease involves a two-step surgical procedure
9. Initially, during the neonatal period, a temporary colostomy is created to relieve obstruction and to allow the normally innervated, dilated bowel to return to its normal size
10. A complete surgical repair is performed when the child weighs approximately 9 kg (20 pounds) via a pull-through procedure to excise portions of the bowel; at this time, the colostomy is closed

B. Data collection
1. Newborn infants
   a. Failure to pass meconium stool
   b. Refusal to suck
   c. Abdominal distention
   d. Bile-stained vomitus
2. Children
   a. Failure to gain weight and delayed **growth**
   b. Abdominal distention
   c. Vomiting
   d. Constipation alternating with diarrhea
   e. Ribbon-like and foul-smelling stools

C. Nonsurgical interventions
1. Dietary management
2. Stool softeners
3. Daily rectal irrigations with normal saline to promote adequate elimination and prevent obstruction

D. Surgical management: Preoperative interventions
1. Monitor the bowel function and administer bowel preparations, as prescribed
2. Maintain NPO status
3. Monitor hydration and fluid and electrolyte status; IV fluids may be prescribed for hydration
4. Antibiotics may be prescribed to clear the bowel of bacteria
5. Monitor I&O and weight
6. Measure the abdominal girth
7. Avoid taking rectal temperatures
8. Monitor for respiratory distress associated with abdominal distention

E. Postoperative interventions
1. Monitor the vital signs, and avoid taking rectal temperatures
2. Measure the abdominal girth
3. Check the surgical site for redness, swelling, and drainage
4. Check the stoma for bleeding or skin breakdown; the stoma should be pink and moist
5. Check the anal area for the presence of stool, redness, or discharge
6. Maintain NPO status until bowel sounds return or flatus is passed; bowel sounds usually return within 48 to 72 hours

7. Maintain the NG tube to allow for intermittent suction until peristalsis returns
8. Maintain the IV fluids until the child tolerates appropriate oral intake; begin the diet with clear liquids, advancing to a regular diet, as tolerated and as prescribed
9. Monitor for dehydration and fluid overload
10. Monitor I&O and weight
11. Monitor the pain level and provide comfort measures, as required
12. Provide the parents with instructions regarding colostomy care and skin care
13. Teach the parents about the appropriate diet and the need for adequate fluid intake
14. Provide the parents and caregivers with appropriate information and resources

XV. INTUSSUSCEPTION (Figure 33-6)
A. Description
1. The telescoping of one portion of the bowel into another portion of the bowel
2. Results in an obstruction of the passage of intestinal contents

B. Data collection
1. Colicky abdominal pain that causes the child to scream and draw his or her knees to the abdomen
2. Vomiting of gastric contents
3. Bile-stained fecal emesis
4. Currant jelly–like stools that contain blood and mucus
5. Hypoactive or hyperactive bowel sounds

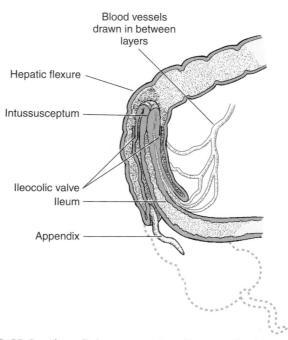

FIG. 33-6 Ileocolic intussusception. (From Hockenberry, M., & Wilson, D. [2007]. *Wong's nursing care of infants and children* [8th ed.]. St. Louis: Mosby.)

6. Tender and distended abdomen, possibly with a palpable sausage-shaped mass in the upper right quadrant

C. Interventions

1. Monitor for signs of perforation and shock as evidenced by fever, increased heart rate, changes in the level of consciousness or blood pressure, and respiratory distress; report these immediately
2. Prepare for hydrostatic reduction, if prescribed; this is not performed if signs of perforation or shock occur
   a. Antibiotics, IV fluids, and NG decompression may be prescribed
   b. Monitor for the passage of normal, brown stool, which indicates that the intussusception has reduced itself
3. After hydrostatic reduction:
   a. Monitor for the return of normal bowel sounds, the passage of barium, and the characteristics of stool
   b. Administer clear fluids, and advance the diet gradually, as prescribed
4. If surgery is required, postoperative care is similar to what occurs after any abdominal surgery
5. Provide the family with support and appropriate information and resources

XVI. ABDOMINAL WALL DEFECTS

A. Omphalocele

1. Occurs when there is a herniation of the abdominal contents through the umbilical ring (hernia of the umbilical cord), usually with an intact peritoneal sac
2. The protrusion is covered by a translucent sac that may contain bowel or other abdominal organs
3. Commonly associated with chromosomal abnormalities (trisomies 13, 18, and 21) and with cardiac, musculoskeletal, gastrointestinal, and genitourinary anomalies
4. Rupture of the sac results in the evisceration of the abdominal contents; gastric decompression is essential to prevent visceral distention
5. Immediately after birth, the sac is covered with sterile gauze soaked in normal saline to prevent the drying of the abdominal contents; a layer of plastic wrap is placed over the gauze to provide additional protection against heat and moisture loss
6. Monitor the vital signs every 2 to 4 hours; temperature is particularly important, because the infant can lose heat through the sac
7. Preoperatively: Maintain NPO status; IV fluids will be prescribed to maintain hydration and electrolyte balance; monitor for signs of infection, and handle the infant carefully to prevent the rupture of the sac

8. Primary reduction is possible with small or moderate defects; large defects may require a staged closure and frequent manual reductions
9. Postoperatively: Control pain, prevent infection, maintain fluid and electrolyte balance, and ensure adequate nutrition

B. Gastroschisis

1. Occurs when the herniation of the intestine is lateral (usually on the right) to the umbilical ring
2. There is no membrane covering the exposed bowel
3. The exposed bowel is loosely covered in saline-soaked pads, and the abdomen is wrapped in a plastic drape; wrapping around the exposed bowel is contraindicated, because, if the exposed bowel expands, the wrapping could cause pressure and necrosis
4. Gastric decompression is essential to prevent visceral distention
5. Preoperatively: Care is similar to that for omphalocele; surgery is performed within several hours after birth, because there is no membrane covering the sac
6. Postoperatively: Most infants have a prolonged ileus and require mechanical ventilation and parenteral nutrition; otherwise, care is similar to that for omphalocele

XVII. UMBILICAL HERNIA, INGUINAL HERNIA, OR HYDROCELE

A. Description

1. A hernia is a protrusion of the bowel through an abnormal opening in the abdominal wall
2. In children, a hernia most commonly occurs at the umbilicus and through the inguinal canal
3. A hydrocele is the presence of abdominal fluid in the scrotal sac

B. Data collection

1. Umbilical hernia: A soft swelling or protrusion around the umbilicus that is usually reducible with the finger
2. Inguinal hernia
   a. Painless inguinal swelling that is reducible
   b. Swelling may disappear during periods of rest and is most noticeable when the infant cries or coughs
3. Incarcerated hernia
   a. The descended portion of bowel becomes tightly caught in the hernial sac, thus compromising the blood supply
   b. This is a medical emergency that requires surgical repair
   c. Irritability
   d. Tenderness at site
   e. Anorexia
   f. Abdominal distention

g. Difficulty defecating

h. May lead to complete intestinal obstruction and gangrene

4. Noncommunicating hydrocele
   a. Occurs when residual peritoneal fluid is trapped with no communication with the peritoneal cavity
   b. Usually disappears by the age of 1 year

5. Communicating hydrocele
   a. Associated with a hernia that remains open from the scrotum to the abdominal cavity
   b. Data collection findings include a bulge in the inguinal area or the scrotum that increases with crying or straining and that decreases when the child is at rest

C. Postoperative interventions (hernia)
   1. Monitor the vital signs
   2. Monitor for wound infection
   3. Monitor for redness or drainage
   4. Monitor the I&O and hydration status
   5. Advance the diet, as tolerated and as prescribed
   6. Administer analgesics, as prescribed

D. Postoperative interventions (hydrocele)
   1. Provide ice bags and a scrotal support to relieve pain and swelling
   2. Instruct the child and parents to avoid tub bathing until the incision heals
   3. Instruct the child and parents to avoid strenuous physical activities

XVIII. CONSTIPATION AND ENCOPRESIS

A. Description
   1. Constipation is the infrequent and difficult passage of dry, hard stools
   2. **Encopresis** is fecal incontinence; children with this condition often complain that the soiling is involuntary and occurs without warning
   3. If the child does not have a neurological or anatomic disorder, **encopresis** is usually the result of fecal impaction and an enlarged rectum caused by chronic constipation

B. Data collection
   1. Constipation
      a. Abdominal pain and cramping without distention
      b. Palpable, movable fecal masses
      c. Normal or decreased bowel sounds
      d. Malaise and headache
      e. Anorexia, nausea, and vomiting
   2. **Encopresis**
      a. Evidence of soiling of clothing
      b. Scratching or rubbing of the anal area
      c. Fecal odor
      d. Social withdrawal

C. Interventions
   1. Simple constipation may resolve with the use of only dietary changes or methods to change the habit of retention

2. Severe **encopresis** may require that interventions be continued for a period of 3 to 6 months

3. Overcoming withholding
   a. Administer enemas, as prescribed, until the impaction is cleared
   b. Monitor for hypernatremia or hyperphosphatemia when administering repeated enemas
   c. Administer a stool softener or laxative, as prescribed
   d. If mineral oil is prescribed, administer it chilled or mixed with cold drinks to disguise the taste

4. Dietary changes
   a. Increase the water and fiber intake (Box 33-12)
   b. Decrease the sugar and milk intake
   c. Plan to administer fat-soluble vitamins while mineral oil is being used, because the oil can interfere with vitamin absorption in the small intestine

5. Changing the retention habit: Encourage the child sit on the toilet for 5 to 10 minutes approximately 20 to 30 minutes after breakfast and dinner to assist with defecation

XIX. IRRITABLE BOWEL SYNDROME

A. Description
   1. Occurs as a result of increased motility, which can lead to spasm and pain
   2. Diagnosis is based on the elimination of pathology

BOX 33-12 **High-Fiber Foods**

Bread and Grains
- Whole-grain bread or rolls
- Whole-grain cereals
- Bran
- Pancakes, waffles, and muffins with fruit or bran
- Unrefined (brown) rice

Vegetables
- Raw vegetables, especially broccoli, cabbage, carrots, cauliflower, celery, lettuce, and spinach
- Cooked vegetables, such as those listed previously, as well as asparagus, beans, brussels sprouts, corn, potatoes, rhubarb, squash, string beans, and turnips

Fruits
- Prunes, raisins, and other dried fruits
- Raw fruits, especially those with skins or seeds, other than bananas and avocados

Miscellaneous
- Legumes (beans), popcorn, nuts, and seeds
- High-fiber snack bars

Modified from Hockenberry, M., & Wilson, D. (2007) *Wong's nursing care of infants and children* (8th ed.) St. Louis: Mosby.

3. Self-limiting, intermittent problem with no definitive treatment
4. Stress and emotional factors may contribute to its occurrence

B. Data collection
1. Diffuse abdominal pain unrelated to meals or activity
2. Alternating constipation and diarrhea with the presence of undigested food and mucus in the stool

C. Interventions
1. Reassure the parents that the problem is self-limiting and intermittent and that it will resolve
2. Encourage the maintenance of a healthy, well-balanced, moderate-fiber diet
3. Avoid foods that may increase gastric distress, such as spicy foods
4. Encourage health-promotion activities, such as exercise and school activities
5. Inform the parents about psychosocial resources, if required

XX. IMPERFORATE ANUS

A. Description: The incomplete development or absence of the anus in its normal position in the perineum
B. Data collection (Box 33-13)
C. Preoperative interventions
1. Determine the patency of the anus
2. A low imperforate anus or the presence of a fistula on the perineum can be repaired with dilation and anoplasty; a high imperforate anus will require an initial colostomy with a formal repair at 3 to 6 months of age
3. Monitor for the presence of stool in the urine and vagina; report this immediately
D. Postoperative interventions
1. Monitor the skin for signs of infection
2. Place the child in a side-lying position with the legs flexed or in a prone position to keep the hips elevated to reduce edema and pressure on the surgical site
3. Keep the anal surgical incision clean and dry, and monitor for redness, swelling, or drainage
4. Maintain NPO status and the NG tube, if one has been placed
5. Maintain IV fluids until GI motility returns
6. Provide colostomy care, if prescribed
7. A fresh colostomy stoma will be red and edematous, but this should decrease with time

---

BOX 33-13 **Data Collection Findings: Imperforate Anus**

- Failure to pass meconium stool
- Absence or stenosis of the anal rectal canal
- Presence of an anal membrane
- External fistula to the perineum

---

8. Instruct the parents to perform anal dilation, if prescribed, to achieve and maintain bowel patency
9. Instruct the parents to use only the dilators supplied by the physician and a water-soluble lubricant and to insert the dilator no more than 1 to 2 cm into the anus to prevent damage to the mucosa

XXI. HEPATITIS

A. This section contains specific information regarding hepatitis as it relates to infants and children; refer to Chapters 22 and 46 for additional information about hepatitis
B. Description: An acute or chronic inflammation of the liver that may be caused by a virus, a medication reaction, or another disease process
C. Hepatitis A virus (HAV)
1. Highest incidence occurs among preschool or school-age children who are less than 15 years old
2. Many affected children are asymptomatic, but mild nausea, vomiting, and diarrhea may occur
3. Infected children who are asymptomatic can still spread HAV to others
D. Hepatitis B virus (HBV)
1. Most HBV in children is acquired perinatally
2. Newborn infants are at risk if the mother is infected with HBV or was a carrier of HBV during pregnancy
3. Possible routes of maternal-fetal (infant) transmission include the leakage of the virus across the placenta late in pregnancy or during labor, the ingestion of amniotic fluid or maternal blood, and breast-feeding, especially if the mother has cracked nipples
4. The severity in the infant varies from no liver disease to fulminant (severe, acute course) or chronic, active disease
5. In children and adolescents, HBV occurs in specific high-risk groups, including the following:
   a. Children with hemophilia or other disorders who have received multiple blood transfusions
   b. Children or adolescents who are involved in drug **abuse**
   c. Institutionalized children
   d. Preschool-age children in endemic areas
   e. Children who may be involved with heterosexual activity or sexual activity with homosexual males
6. HBV infection can cause a carrier state and lead to eventual cirrhosis or hepatocellular carcinoma during adulthood
E. Hepatitis C virus (HCV)
1. Transmission is primarily by the parenteral route

2. Some children may be asymptomatic, but HCV often becomes a chronic condition, and it can cause cirrhosis and hepatocellular carcinoma

F. Hepatitis D virus
   1. Occurs among children who are already infected with HBV
   2. Both acute and chronic forms tend to be more severe than HBV and can lead to cirrhosis

G. Hepatitis E virus
   1. Uncommon among children
   2. Is not a chronic condition, does not cause chronic liver disease, and has no carrier state

H. Hepatitis G virus
   1. Blood-borne and similar to HCV
   2. High-risk groups include transfusion recipients, IV drug users, and individuals infected with HCV
   3. Individuals are often asymptomatic, and most infections are chronic

I. Data collection (Box 33-14)

J. Diagnostic evaluation: See Chapter 11 for the laboratory studies that are used to diagnose hepatitis

K. Prevention
   1. Proper handwashing and standard precautions can prevent the spread of viral hepatitis
   2. Prophylactic use of standard immune globulin to prevent HAV in situations of preexposure (e.g., anticipated travel to areas where HAV is prevalent) or within 2 weeks of exposure
   3. Hepatitis B immune globulin is effective for preventing infection after one-time exposures (e.g., accidental needle punctures or other contact of contaminated material with mucous membranes); it should be given to newborns whose mothers are positive for hepatitis B surface antigen or within 72 hours of exposure
   4. HAV **vaccine** is recommended for children 2 years and older who reside in communities

with high endemic rates and for preexposure prophylaxis

   5. HBV **vaccine**: See Chapter 38 for an immunization schedule for this **vaccine**

L. Interventions
   1. Strict handwashing
   2. Hospitalization is required in the event of coagulopathy or fulminant hepatitis
   3. Standard precautions are followed during hospitalization
   4. A hospitalized child is not usually isolated in a separate room unless he or she is fecally incontinent and items are likely to become contaminated with feces
   5. Children are discouraged from sharing toys
   6. Instruct the child and parents regarding good handwashing techniques
   7. Instruct the parents to thoroughly disinfect diaper-changing surfaces using ¼ cup of bleach in 1 gallon of water
   8. Maintain comfort and provide adequate rest and sleep
   9. Provide a low-fat, balanced diet
   10. Provide enteric precautions for at least 1 week after the onset of jaundice with HAV
   11. Inform the parents that because HAV is not infectious within 1 week of the onset of jaundice, the child may return to school at that time if he or she feels well enough
   12. Inform the parents that jaundice may get worse before it resolves
   13. Caution the parents about administering any medications to the child (remember that the liver is unable to detoxify and excrete medications)
   14. Instruct the parents regarding the signs that indicate the worsening of the child's condition, such as changes in the neurological status, bleeding, and fluid retention

XXII. INGESTION OF POISONS

A. Lead poisoning
   1. Description: Excessive accumulation of lead in the blood
   2. Early detection is essential for a good outcomes
   3. Causes
      a. The pathway for exposure may be food, air, or water
      b. Dust and soil contaminated with lead may be a source of exposure
      c. Lead enters the child's body through ingestion or inhalation or through placental transmission to an unborn child when the mother is exposed; the most common route is ingestion either from hand-to-mouth behavior from contaminated objects or from eating loose paint chips or other items that may contain lead

---

BOX 33-14 **Data Collection Findings: Hepatitis**

Prodromal or Anicteric Phase
- Lasts 5 to 7 days
- Absence of jaundice
- Anorexia, malaise, lethargy, and easy fatigability
- Fever (especially among adolescents)
- Nausea and vomiting
- Epigastric or right upper quadrant abdominal pain
- Arthralgia and skin rashes (more likely with hepatitis B virus)
- Hepatomegaly

Icteric Phase
- Jaundice, which is best assessed in the sclera, nail beds, and mucous membranes
- Dark urine and pale stools
- Pruritus

d. When lead enters the body, it affects the erythrocytes, bones, teeth, organs, and tissues, including the brain and nervous system; the most serious consequences are the effects on the central nervous system

4. Universal screening
   a. Recommended in high-risk areas at the age of 1 to 2 years; children at high risk should be screened earlier
   b. Any child between the ages of 3 and 6 years who has not been screened should be tested

5. Targeted screening
   a. Acceptable in low-risk areas
   b. At the age of 1 to 2 years (or a child between the ages of 3 and 6 years who has not been screened) may be targeted for screening if determined to be at risk

6. Blood lead level test: Used for screening and diagnosis (Table 33-1)

7. Erythrocyte protoporphyrin test
   a. An indicator of anemia
   b. Normal value for a child is 35 mcg/100 mL of whole blood or less

8. Chelation therapy
   a. Removes lead from the circulating blood and from some organs and tissues
   b. Does not counteract any effects of the lead

TABLE 33-1 Blood Lead Levels

Level	Intervention
Less than 10 mcg/dL	Reassess or rescreen in 1 year or sooner if exposure status changes.
10 to 14 mcg/dL	Provide family lead education, follow-up testing, and social service referral, if necessary.
15 to 19 mcg/dL	Provide family lead education, follow-up testing, and social service referral, if necessary; during follow-up testing, initiate actions for a blood lead level of greater than 20 mcg/dL.
20 to 69 mcg/dL	A blood lead level greater than 20 mcg/dL is considered acute; provide coordination of care, clinical management including treatment, environmental investigation, and lead-hazard control; the child must not remain in a lead-hazardous environment if resolution is necessary.
70 mcg/dL or greater	Medical treatment is provided immediately, including coordination of care, clinical management, environmental investigation, and lead-hazard control.

c. Medications: Dimercaprol (BAL in Oil); calcium disodium edetate (CaNa$_2$EDTA); succimer (Chemet)
d. Dimercaprol (BAL in Oil) is contraindicated for children with an allergy to peanuts, because the medication is prepared in a peanut-oil solution
e. Ensure adequate urinary output before administering medications
f. Provide adequate hydration, and monitor kidney function for nephrotoxicity when the medication is given, because it is excreted via the kidneys
g. Monitoring the progress of the lead levels is essential
h. Provide instructions to the parents regarding safety from lead hazards, medication administration, and the need for follow-up
i. Confirm that the child will be discharged to a home without lead hazards

B. Acetaminophen (Tylenol) poisoning
   1. Description
      a. The seriousness of the ingestion is determined by the amount ingested and the length of time before intervention
      b. A toxic dose is 150 mg/kg or higher in children
   2. Data collection
      a. First 2 to 4 hours: Malaise, nausea, vomiting, sweating, pallor, and weakness
      b. Latent period: 24 to 36 hours; child improves
      c. Hepatic involvement: May last up to 7 days and be permanent; right upper quadrant pain, jaundice, confusion, stupor, elevated liver enzymes and bilirubin levels, and prolonged prothrombin time
   3. Interventions
      a. Vomiting may be induced or gastric lavage may be performed
      b. Administer antidote: N-acetylcysteine
      c. Dilute antidote in juice or soda because of its offensive odor
      d. Loading dose is followed by maintenance doses
      e. Monitor the liver enzymes

C. Acetylsalicylic acid (aspirin) poisoning
   1. Description
      a. May be caused by acute ingestion or chronic ingestion
      b. Acute: Severe toxicity occurs with 300 to 500 mg/kg
      c. Chronic: More than 100 mg/kg/day for 2 days or more; can be more serious than acute ingestion
   2. Data collection
      a. GI effects: Nausea, vomiting, and thirst from dehydration

b. Central nervous system effects: Hyperpnea, confusion, tinnitus, convulsions, coma, respiratory failure, and circulatory collapse

c. Renal effects: Oliguria

d. Hematopoietic effects: Bleeding tendencies

e. Metabolic effects: Diaphoresis, fever, hyponatremia, hypokalemia, dehydration, and hypoglycemia

3. Interventions

a. Activated charcoal may be prescribed to decrease the absorption of salicylate (this is important during early stages)

b. IV fluids, sodium bicarbonate, electrolytes, or volume expanders may be prescribed

c. Vitamin K may be given for bleeding tendencies, as prescribed

d. Glucose may be prescribed to treat hypoglycemia

e. Prepare the child for dialysis, as prescribed, if he or she is unresponsive to the therapy

XXIII. INTESTINAL PARASITES

A. Description: Common infections in children are giardiasis and pinworms

1. Giardiasis is caused by a protozoa, and it is prevalent among children in crowded environments, such as classrooms and day-care centers

2. Pinworms (enterobiasis) are universally present in temperate climate zones and easily transmitted in crowded environments

B. Data collection

1. Giardiasis

a. Diarrhea and vomiting

b. Anorexia

c. Failure to thrive

d. Abdominal cramps with intermittent loose stools and constipation

e. Steatorrhea

f. Resolves in 4 to 6 weeks spontaneously

g. Stool specimens from 3 or more collections are used for diagnosis

2. Pinworms

a. Intense perianal itching

b. Irritability and restlessness

c. Poor sleeping

d. Bed-wetting

C. Interventions

1. Giardiasis

a. Administer metronidazole (Flagyl), as prescribed

b. Performance of meticulous handwashing by caregivers

c. Provide education to the family and caregivers regarding sanitary practices

2. Pinworms

a. Perform a visual inspection of the anus with a flashlight 2 to 3 hours after sleep

b. The tape test is the most common diagnostic test

c. Educate the family and caregivers regarding the tape test: A loop of Scotch Tape is placed firmly against the child's perianal area; it is removed in the morning, placed in a glass jar or a plastic bag, and transported to the primary care provider for analysis

d. Mebendazole (Vermox) may be prescribed for children who are older than 2 years old

e. Piperazine phosphate may be prescribed for children who are younger than 2 years old

f. The medication regimen may be repeated in 2 weeks to prevent reinfection

g. All members of the family are treated for the infection

h. Teach the family and caregivers about the importance of meticulous handwashing and to wash all clothes and bed linens in hot water

PRACTICE QUESTIONS

More questions on the companion CD!

356. A nurse reviews the record of a 3-week-old infant and notes that the physician has documented a diagnosis of suspected Hirschsprung's disease. The nurse understands that which of the following symptoms led the mother to seek health care for the infant?
1. Diarrhea
2. Projectile vomiting
3. The regurgitation of feedings
4. Foul-smelling, ribbon-like stools

357. A nurse is caring for a child with a diagnosis of intussusception. Which of the following symptoms would the nurse expect to note in this child?
1. Watery diarrhea
2. Ribbon-like stools
3. Profuse projectile vomiting
4. Blood and mucus in the stools

358. A child with a diagnosis of a hernia has been scheduled for a surgical repair in 2 weeks. The nurse reinforces instructions to the parents about the signs of possible hernial strangulation. The nurse tells the parents that which of the following signs would require physician notification by the parents?
1. Fever
2. Diarrhea
3. Vomiting
4. Constipation

359. A nurse reinforces home-care instructions to the parents of a child with hepatitis regarding the care of the child and the prevention of the

transmission of the virus. Which statement by a parent indicates a need for further instruction?
1. "Frequent handwashing is important."
2. "I need to provide a well-balanced, high-fat diet to my child."
3. "I need to clean contaminated household surfaces with bleach."
4. "Diapers should not be changed near any surfaces that are used to prepare food."

360. A nursing instructor asks a nursing student about phenylketonuria (PKU). Which statement, if made by the student, indicates an understanding of this disorder?
1. "PKU is an autosomal-dominant disorder."
2. "PKU primarily affects the gastrointestinal system."
3. "Treatment of PKU includes the dietary restriction of tyramine."
4. "All 50 states require routine screening of all newborns for PKU."

361. A school-age child with type 1 diabetes mellitus has soccer practice three afternoons a week. The nurse reinforces instructions regarding how to prevent hypoglycemia during practice. The nurse tells the child to:
1. Drink a half a cup of orange juice before soccer practice.
2. Eat twice the amount that is normally eaten at lunchtime.
3. Take half of the amount of prescribed insulin on practice days.
4. Take the prescribed insulin at noontime rather than in the morning.

362. A mother of a 6-year-old child with type 1 diabetes mellitus calls the clinic nurse and tells the nurse that the child has been sick. The mother reports that she checked the child's urine and it showed positive ketones. Which of the following would the nurse instruct the mother to do?
1. Hold the next dose of insulin.
2. Come to the clinic immediately.
3. Administer an additional dose of regular insulin.
4. Encourage the child to drink calorie-free liquids.

363. A nurse is caring for an 18-month-old child who has been vomiting. The appropriate position in which to place the child during naps and sleep time is:
1. A supine position
2. A side-lying position
3. Prone, with the head elevated
4. Prone, with the face turned to the side

364. A nurse is monitoring for signs of dehydration in a 1-year-old child who has been hospitalized for diarrhea and prepares to take the child's

temperature. Which method of temperature measurement would be avoided?
1. Rectal
2. Axillary
3. Electronic
4. Tympanic

365. An infant returns to the nursing unit after the surgical repair of a cleft lip located on the right side of the lip. The best position in which to place this infant at this time is:
1. A prone position
2. A supine position
3. On his or her left side
4. On his or her right side

366. A nurse reviews the record of an infant who is seen in the clinic. The nurse notes that a diagnosis of esophageal atresia with tracheoesophageal fistula (TEF) is suspected. The nurse expects to note which most likely clinical manifestation of this condition in the medical record?
1. Incessant crying
2. Coughing at nighttime
3. Choking with feedings
4. Severe projectile vomiting

367. A nurse is reviewing the record of a child with a diagnosis of pyloric stenosis. Which data would the nurse expect to note as having been documented in the child's record?
1. Watery diarrhea
2. Projectile vomiting
3. Increased urine output
4. Vomiting large amounts of bile

368. A nurse reinforces instructions to the mother about dietary measures for a 5-year-old child with lactose intolerance. The nurse tells the mother that which of the following supplements will be required as a result of the need to avoid lactose in the diet?
1. Fats
2. Zinc
3. Protein
4. Calcium

369. A nurse reinforces home-care instructions to the parents of a child with celiac disease. Which of the following food items would the nurse advise the parents to include in the child's diet?
1. Rice
2. Oatmeal
3. Rye toast
4. Wheat bread

ALTERNATE ITEM FORMAT: MULTIPLE RESPONSE

370. A nurse is assigned to care for a child who is scheduled for an appendectomy. Select the

orders that the nurse anticipates will be prescribed.

☐ **1.** Administer a Fleet enema.
☐ **2.** Initiate an intravenous line.
☐ **3.** Maintain nothing-by-mouth status.
☐ **4.** Administer intravenous antibiotics.
☑ **5.** Administer preoperative medications.
☐ **6.** Place a heating pad on the abdomen to decrease pain.

ANSWERS

356. 4

Rationale: Chronic constipation that begins during the first month of life and that results in foul-smelling, ribbon-like or pellet-like stools is a clinical manifestation of Hirschsprung's disease. The delayed passage or absence of meconium stool during the neonatal period is the cardinal sign. Bowel obstruction (especially during the neonatal period), abdominal pain and distention, and failure to thrive are also clinical manifestations. Options 1, 2, and 3 are incorrect.

Test-Taking Strategy: Knowledge regarding the clinical manifestations associated with Hirschsprung's disease is required to answer this question. Remember that foul-smelling, ribbon-like or pellet-like stools are a clinical manifestation of this disorder. Review the manifestations of Hirschsprung's disease if you had difficulty with this question.

Level of Cognitive Ability: Comprehension
Client Needs: Physiological Integrity
Integrated Process: Nursing Process/Data Collection
Content Area: Child Health
Reference: Price, D., & Gwin, J. (2008). *Pediatric nursing: An introductory text* (10th ed., p. 162). St. Louis: Saunders.

357. 4

Rationale: The child with intussusception classically presents with severe abdominal pain that is crampy and intermittent and that causes the child to draw in his or her knees to the chest. Vomiting may be present, but it is not projectile. Bright red blood and mucus are passed through the rectum and commonly described as currant jelly–like stools. Ribbon-like stools are not a manifestation of this disorder.

Test-Taking Strategy: Knowledge related to the clinical manifestations associated with intussusception is required to answer this question. Recalling that a classic manifestation is currant jelly–like stools will assist in directing you to option 4. Review intussusception if you had difficulty with this question.

Level of Cognitive Ability: Comprehension
Client Needs: Physiological Integrity
Integrated Process: Nursing Process/Data Collection
Content Area: Child Health
Reference: Price, D., & Gwin, J. (2008). *Pediatric nursing: An introductory text* (10th ed., pp. 160-161). St. Louis: Saunders.

358. 3

Rationale: The parents of a child with a hernia need to be instructed about the signs of strangulation. These signs include vomiting, pain, and an irreducible mass. The parents should be instructed to contact the physician immediately if strangulation is suspected.

Test-Taking Strategy: Use the definition of the word "strangulation" to help answer this question; this will assist you with eliminating options 1 and 2. From the remaining options, knowledge regarding the signs of strangulation will assist you with answering the question. Review the signs of strangulation if you had difficulty with this question.

Level of Cognitive Ability: Application
Client Needs: Physiological Integrity
Integrated Process: Teaching and Learning
Content Area: Child Health
References: Leifer, G. (2007). *Introduction to maternity and pediatric nursing* (5th ed., p. 640). Philadelphia: Saunders.
Price, D., & Gwin, J. (2008). *Pediatric nursing: An introductory text* (10th ed., p. 156). St. Louis: Saunders.

359. 2

Rationale: The child with hepatitis should consume a well-balanced, low-fat diet to allow the liver to rest. Options 1, 3, and 4 are components of the home-care instructions to the family of a child with hepatitis.

Test-Taking Strategy: Note the strategic words "need for further instruction." These words indicate a negative event query and ask you to select an option that is an incorrect statement. Options 1, 3, and 4 can be eliminated by remembering the basic principles related to standard precautions. Review the home-care instructions for the parents of a child with hepatitis if you had difficulty with this question.

Level of Cognitive Ability: Comprehension
Client Needs: Safe and Effective Care Environment
Integrated Process: Teaching and Learning
Content Area: Child Health
Reference: Price, D., & Gwin, J. (2008). *Pediatric nursing: An introductory text* (10th ed., p. 265). St. Louis: Saunders.

360. 4

Rationale: PKU is an autosomal-recessive disorder. Treatment includes the dietary restriction of phenylalanine intake. PKU is a genetic disorder that results in central nervous system (CNS) damage from toxic levels of phenylalanine in the blood.

Test-Taking Strategy: Use the process of elimination. Recalling that PKU is a recessive disorder will assist you with eliminating option 1. Reading option 3 carefully will direct you to eliminate it, because tyramine is restricted among clients taking monoamine oxidase inhibitors rather than among those with PKU. Recalling that PKU affects the CNS will direct you to option 4. Review the characteristics associated with PKU if you had difficulty with this question.

Level of Cognitive Ability: Comprehension
Client Needs: Physiological Integrity
Integrated Process: Teaching and Learning
Content Area: Child Health
References: Hockenberry, M., Wilson, D., & Winkelstein, M. (2005). *Wong's essentials of pediatric nursing* (7th ed., pp. 742, 864). St. Louis: Mosby.
Leifer, G. (2007). *Introduction to maternity and pediatric nursing* (5th ed., p. 332). Philadelphia: Saunders.

361. 1

Rationale: An extra snack of 10 g to 15 g of carbohydrates eaten before activities and for every 30 to 45 minutes of activity will prevent hypoglycemia. A half cup of orange juice will

provide the needed carbohydrates. The child or parents should not be instructed to adjust the amount or time of insulin administration, and meal amounts should not be doubled.
Test-Taking Strategy: Use the process of elimination. Options 3 and 4 can be eliminated first, because insulin dosages and times should not be adjusted. From the remaining options, recalling the manifestations and treatment associated with hypoglycemia will direct you to option 1. Review the prevention of hypoglycemia if you had difficulty with this question.
Level of Cognitive Ability: Application
Client Needs: Health Promotion and Maintenance
Integrated Process: Teaching and Learning
Content Area: Child Health
Reference: Price, D., & Gwin, J. (2008). *Pediatric nursing: An introductory text* (10th ed., pp. 298, 300). St. Louis.

362. **4**
Rationale: When the child is sick, the mother should test for urinary ketones with each voiding. If ketones are present, liquids are essential to help with clearing them. The child should be encouraged to drink calorie-free liquids. It is not necessary to bring the child to the clinic immediately, and insulin doses should not be adjusted or changed.
Test-Taking Strategy: Use the process of elimination. Eliminate options 1 and 3 first, because insulin doses should not be adjusted or changed. From the remaining options, note the words "positive ketones." This finding does not require immediate physician referral. Review the home-care instructions for the sick diabetic child if you had difficulty with this question.
Level of Cognitive Ability: Application
Client Needs: Health Promotion and Maintenance
Integrated Process: Nursing Process/Implementation
Content Area: Child Health
References: Hockenberry, M., Wilson, D., & Winkelstein, M. (2005). *Wong's essentials of pediatric nursing* (7th ed., p.1083). St. Louis: Mosby.
McKinney, E., James, S., Murray, S., & Ashwill, J. (2005). *Maternal-child nursing* (2nd ed., p. 1478). Philadelphia: Saunders.

363. **2**
Rationale: The vomiting child should be placed in an upright or side-lying position to prevent aspiration. Options 1, 3, and 4 will place the child at risk for aspiration if vomiting occurs.
Test-Taking Strategy: Use the process of elimination. Eliminate options 3 and 4 first, because they are comparable or alike. In additional, these positions would place the child at risk for aspiration if vomiting occurred. Visualize the remaining two positions. Option 1 is also inappropriate and would cause aspiration. Review the appropriate positioning for the child who has been vomiting if you had difficulty with this question.
Level of Cognitive Ability: Application
Client Needs: Physiological Integrity
Integrated Process: Nursing Process/Implementation
Content Area: Child Health
Reference: Wong, D., Perry, S., Hockenberry, M., Lowdermilk, D., & Wilson, D. (2006). *Maternal-child nursing care* (3rd ed., p. 1507). St. Louis: Mosby.

364. **1**
Rationale: Rectal temperature measurements should be avoided if diarrhea is present. The use of a rectal thermometer can stimulate peristalsis and cause more diarrhea. Axillary or tympanic measurements of temperature would be acceptable. Most measurements are performed via electronic devices.
Test-Taking Strategy: Use the process of elimination, and note the strategic word "avoided." Eliminate option 3 first, because most methods of temperature measurement are performed with the use of an electronic device. Next, note the diagnosis stated in the question; this should direct you to option 1. Review the interventions for the child with diarrhea if you had difficulty with this question.
Level of Cognitive Ability: Application
Client Needs: Physiological Integrity
Integrated Process: Nursing Process/Implementation
Content Area: Child Health
References: Hockenberry, M., & Wilson, D. (2007). *Nursing care of infants and children* (8th ed., p. 1190). St. Louis: Mosby.
McKinney, E., James, S., Murray, S., & Ashwill, J. (2005). *Maternal-child nursing* (2nd ed., p. 1093). Philadelphia: Saunders.

365. **3**
Rationale: After the repair of a cleft lip, the infant should be positioned on the side opposite to the repair to prevent contact of the suture lines with the bed linens. In this case, it is best to place the infant on his or her left side rather than supine immediately after surgery to prevent the risk of aspiration if the infant vomits.
Test-Taking Strategy: Use the process of elimination. Consider the anatomical location of the surgical site and the strategic words "right side." You should be easily directed to the correct option with the use of these concepts. Review postoperative positioning techniques if you had difficulty with this question.
Level of Cognitive Ability: Application
Client Needs: Physiological Integrity
Integrated Process: Nursing Process/Implementation
Content Area: Child Health
References: Leifer, G. (2007). *Introduction to maternity and pediatric nursing* (5th ed., p. 326). Philadelphia: Saunders.
Price, D., & Gwin, J. (2008). *Pediatric nursing: An introductory text* (10th ed., p. 102). St. Louis: Saunders.

366. **3**
Rationale: Any child who exhibits the "3 Cs"—coughing and choking during feedings and unexplained cyanosis—should be suspected of having TEF. Options 1, 2, and 4 are not specifically associated with TEF.
Test-Taking Strategy: Use the process of elimination, and focus on the diagnosis. Recalling the "3 Cs" associated with TEF will direct you to the correct option. Review the clinical manifestations associated with TEF if you had difficulty with this question
Level of Cognitive Ability: Comprehension
Client Needs: Physiological Integrity
Integrated Process: Nursing Process/Data Collection
Content Area: Child Health
Reference: Leifer, G. (2007). *Introduction to maternity and pediatric nursing* (5th ed., p. 635). Philadelphia: Saunders.

367. 2

Rationale: Clinical manifestations of pyloric stenosis include projectile, nonbilious vomiting; irritability; hunger and crying; constipation; and signs of dehydration, including a decrease in urine output.

Test-Taking Strategy: Use the process of elimination. Considering the anatomical location of this disorder and its potential effects will assist you with eliminating options 1 and 3. Recalling that a major clinical manifestation is projectile, nonbilious vomiting will direct you to option 2. Review the clinical manifestations of pyloric stenosis if you had difficulty with this question.

Level of Cognitive Ability: Comprehension
Client Needs: Physiological Integrity
Integrated Process: Nursing Process/Data Collection
Content Area: Child Health
Reference: Leifer, G. (2007). *Introduction to maternity and pediatric nursing* (5th ed., p. 636). Philadelphia: Saunders.

368. 4

Rationale: Lactose intolerance is the inability to tolerate lactose, which is the sugar that is found in dairy products. Removing milk from the diet can provide relief from symptoms. Additional dietary changes may be required to provide adequate sources of calcium and, if the child is an infant, protein and calories.

Test-Taking Strategy: Knowledge that lactose is the sugar that is found in dairy products will easily direct you to option 4, because dairy products are major sources of calcium. Review the dietary management of lactose intolerance if you had difficulty with this question.

Level of Cognitive Ability: Application
Client Needs: Health Promotion and Maintenance
Integrated Process: Nursing Process/Implementation
Content Area: Child Health
Reference: Hockenberry, M., & Wilson, D. (2007). *Nursing care of infants and children* (8th ed., p. 586). St. Louis: Mosby.

369. 1

Rationale: Dietary management is the mainstay of treatment for celiac disease. All wheat, rye, barley, and oats should be eliminated from the diet and replaced with corn and rice.

Vitamin supplements, especially fat-soluble vitamins and folate, may be required during the early period of treatment to correct deficiencies. These restrictions are likely to be lifelong, although small amounts of grains may be tolerated after the ulcerations have healed.

Test-Taking Strategy: Use the process of elimination and your knowledge regarding the dietary management of celiac disease to answer this question. Recalling that corn and rice are substitute food replacements among clients with this disease will direct you to option 1. Review the dietary management of this disorder if you had difficulty with this question.

Level of Cognitive Ability: Application
Client Needs: Health Promotion and Maintenance
Integrated Process: Teaching and Learning
Content Area: Child Health
Reference: Price, D., & Gwin, J. (2008). *Pediatric nursing: An introductory text* (10th ed., pp. 249-250). St. Louis: Elsevier.

ALTERNATE ITEM FORMAT: MULTIPLE RESPONSE

370. 2, 3, 4, 5

Rationale: During the preoperative period, enemas or laxatives should not be administered. In addition, heat should not be applied to the abdomen. Any of these interventions can cause the rupture of the appendix and resultant peritonitis. Intravenous fluids would be started, and the child would receive nothing by mouth while awaiting surgery. Antibiotics are usually administered because of the risk of perforation. Preoperative medications are administered as prescribed.

Test-Taking Strategy: Consider the anatomical location of appendicitis, and think about the concern of rupture among clients with this disorder. This will assist you with determining the correct interventions. Review the preoperative care of the child with appendicitis if you had difficulty with this question.

Level of Cognitive Ability: Analysis
Client Needs: Physiological Integrity
Integrated Process: Nursing Process/Analysis
Content Area: Child Health
Reference: Hockenberry, M., & Wilson, D. (2007). *Nursing care of infants and children* (8th ed., p. 1405). St. Louis: Mosby.

REFERENCES

Hockenberry, M., & Wilson, D. (2007). *Nursing care of infants and children* (8th ed.). St. Louis: Mosby.

Hockenberry, M., Wilson, D., & Winkelstein, M. (2005). *Wong's essentials of pediatric nursing* (7th ed.). St. Louis: Mosby.

Leifer, G. (2007). *Introduction to maternity and pediatric nursing* (5th ed.). Philadelphia: Saunders.

McKinney, E., James, S., Murray, S., & Ashwill, J. (2005). *Maternal-child nursing* (2nd ed.). Philadelphia: Saunders.

National Council of State Boards of Nursing (Eds.). (2008). *2008 Detailed Test Plan for the NCLEX-PN® Examination, National Council of State Boards of Nursing.* Chicago: Author.

National Council of State Boards of Nursing. *NCSBN home page.* www.ncsbn.org. Accessed July 24, 2008.

Price, D., & Gwin, J. (2008). *Pediatric nursing: An introductory text* (10th ed.). St. Louis: Saunders.

Wong, D., Perry, S., Hockenberry, M., Lowdermilk, D., & Wilson, D. (2006). *Maternal-child nursing care* (3rd ed.). St. Louis: Mosby.

Renal and Urinary Disorders

I. GLOMERULONEPHRITIS

A. Description
1. Made up of a variety of disorders that may occur as a primary disease process or as a result of another disease process
2. Results in proliferative and inflammatory changes within the glomerular structure
3. Destruction, inflammation, and sclerosis of the glomeruli of both kidneys occur
4. Inflammation of the glomeruli results from an antigen–antibody reaction produced by an infection elsewhere in the body
5. Loss of kidney function develops

B. Causes
1. Immunological diseases
2. Autoimmune diseases
3. Antecedent group A β-hemolytic streptococcal infection of the pharynx or skin
4. History of pharyngitis or tonsillitis 2 to 3 weeks before the onset of symptoms

C. Types (Box 34-1)

D. Complications
1. Renal failure
2. Hypertensive encephalopathy
3. Pulmonary edema
4. Heart failure

E. Data collection
1. Periorbital and facial edema that is more prominent in the morning
2. Anorexia
3. Decreased urinary output
4. Cloudy, smoky, brown-colored urine (hematuria)
5. Pallor, irritability, and lethargy
6. In the older child, headaches, abdominal or flank pain, and dysuria
7. Hypertension
8. Proteinuria that produces a persistent and excessive foam in the urine
9. Azotemia
10. Increased blood urea nitrogen and creatinine levels
11. Increased antistreptolysin O titer (used to diagnose disorders caused by streptococcal infections)

F. Interventions
1. Monitor the vital signs, weight, intake and output (I&O), and characteristics of the urine
2. Limit activity; provide safety measures
3. Provide foods with high-quality nutrients
   a. Restrictions depend on the stage and severity of the disease, especially the extent of the edema
   b. In uncomplicated cases, a regular diet is permitted, but sodium is restricted to a "no-added salt" diet
   c. Moderate sodium restriction is prescribed for the child with hypertension or edema
   d. Foods high in potassium are restricted during periods of oliguria
   e. Protein is restricted if the child has severe azotemia as a result of prolonged oliguria
4. Monitor for complications (i.e., renal failure, hypertensive encephalopathy, seizures, pulmonary edema, and heart failure)
5. Administer diuretics (if significant edema and fluid overload are present), antihypertensives (for hypertension), and antibiotics (to the child with evidence of persistent streptococcal infections), as prescribed
6. Initiate seizure precautions and administer anticonvulsants, as prescribed, for seizures associated with hypertensive encephalopathy
7. Instruct the parents to report signs of bloody urine, headache, or edema
8. Instruct the parents that the child needs to obtain appropriate and adequate treatment for infections, specifically for sore throats, upper respiratory infections, and skin infections

II. NEPHROTIC SYNDROME

A. Description
1. A kidney disorder characterized by massive proteinuria, hypoalbuminemia (hypoproteinemia), and edema

BOX 34-1 Types of Glomerulonephritis

Acute: Occurs 2 to 3 weeks after a streptococcal infection

Chronic: Can occur after the acute phase or slowly over time

BOX 34-2 Findings in Nephrotic Syndrome

The child gains weight.

Periorbital and facial edema are most prominent in the morning.

Leg, ankle, labial, or scrotal edema occurs.

Urine output decreases, and the urine is dark and frothy.

Ascites (fluid in the abdominal cavity) is present.

Blood pressure is normal or slightly decreased.

Lethargy, anorexia, and pallor occur.

Massive proteinuria is seen.

Decreased serum protein (hypoproteinemia) and elevated serum lipid levels occur.

---

2. The primary objectives of therapeutic management are to reduce the excretion of urinary protein and to maintain protein-free urine

▲ B. Data collection (Box 34-2)

▲ C. Interventions
1. Monitor the vital signs, I&O, and daily weights
2. Monitor the urine for specific gravity, albumin, and protein
3. Monitor for edema
4. Nutrition: A regular diet without added salt is prescribed if the child is in remission; sodium is restricted during periods of massive edema
5. Corticosteroid therapy: Prescribed as soon as the diagnosis has been determined; monitor the child closely for signs of infection (Box 34-3)
6. Immunosuppressant therapy may be prescribed to reduce the relapse rate and to induce long-term remission; this may be administered in conjunction with the corticosteroid
7. Diuretics may be prescribed to reduce edema
8. Plasma expanders such as salt-poor human albumin may be prescribed for the severely edematous child
9. Instruct the parents about testing the urine for albumin, medication administration, the side effects of the medications, and the general care of the child
10. Instruct the parents regarding the signs of infection and the need to avoid contact with other children who may be infectious
11. Provide appropriate information and support to the child and family

III. CRYPTORCHIDISM

A. Description: Occurs when one or both testes fail to descend through the inguinal canal and into the scrotal sac

▲ B. Data collection: Testes not palpable or easily guided into the scrotum

C. Interventions
1. Monitor during the first 12 months of life to determine whether spontaneous descent occurs
2. After the age of 1 year, medical or surgical treatment may be instituted
3. Human chorionic gonadotropin, a pituitary hormone that stimulates the production of testosterone, may be prescribed

---

BOX 34-3 Adverse Reactions to Corticosteroid Therapy

- Impaired wound healing
- Hyperglycemia
- Skin fragility
- Abnormal fat deposition
- Emotional lability
- Hirsutism
- Moon face
- Osteoporosis

---

4. Surgical correction, if needed, is performed by orchiopexy before the child's second birthday (preferably between 1 and 2 years of age) if the testes do not descend spontaneously
5. Monitor for bleeding and infection postoperatively
6. Instruct the parents regarding postoperative home-care measures, including preventing infection, pain control, and activity restrictions
7. Provide an opportunity for parental counseling if the parents are concerned about the future fertility of the child
8. There is an increased incidence of testicular tumors among these children as they reach adulthood; parents should be instructed to teach their growing child the importance of testicular self-examination

IV. EPISPADIAS AND HYPOSPADIAS (Figure 34-1)

A. Description: Congenital defects that involve the abnormal placement of the urethral orifice of the penis

B. Data collection
1. Epispadias: Urethral orifice is located on the dorsal surface of the penis; often occurs with exstrophy of the bladder
2. Hypospadias: Urethral orifice is located below the glans penis, along the ventral surface

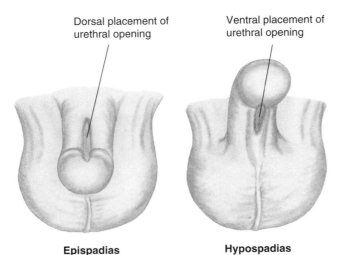

Dorsal placement of urethral opening

Ventral placement of urethral opening

Epispadias

Hypospadias

FIG. 34-1 Possible locations of the urethral meatus in the child with epispadias and hypospadias. (From Price, D., & Gwin, J. [2005]. *Thompson's pediatric nursing: An introductory text* [9th ed.]. Philadelphia: Saunders.)

C. Surgical interventions
  1. Performed before the age of toilet training, preferably between 16 and 18 months of age
  2. The child should not be circumcised, because the foreskin may be used in surgical reconstruction
D. Postoperative interventions
  1. The child will have a pressure dressing and may have some type of urinary diversion or a urinary stent (used to maintain the patency of the urethral opening) while the healing of the meatus occurs
  2. Monitor the vital signs
  3. Encourage fluid intake to maintain adequate urine output and to maintain the patency of the stent
  4. Monitor the I&O and the urine for cloudiness or a foul odor
  5. Notify the registered nurse if there is no urinary drainage for 1 hour, because this may indicate kinks in the system or obstruction by sediment
  6. Provide pain medication (acetaminophen [Tylenol]) or medication to relieve bladder spasms (anticholinergic), as prescribed
  7. Administer antibiotics, as prescribed
  8. Instruct the parents regarding the care of the urinary diversion or stent, if present
  9. Instruct the parents to avoid giving the child a tub bath until the stent, if present, is removed
  10. Instruct the parents about fluid intake, medication administration, the signs and symptoms of infection, and the need for physician follow-up for dressing removal approximately 4 days after surgery

V. BLADDER EXSTROPHY
A. Description
  1. A congenital anomaly characterized by the extrusion of the urinary bladder to the outside of the body through a defect in the lower abdominal wall
  2. Cause is unknown
  3. Treatment requires surgical management and occurs in a series of staged reconstructions
  4. Initial surgery for the closure of the abdominal defect should occur within the first few days of life
  5. Goals of subsequent surgeries are to reconstruct the bladder and genitalia and to enable the child to achieve urinary continence
B. Data collection
  1. Exposed bladder mucosa
  2. Widened symphysis pubis
  3. Defects of the external genitalia
C. Interventions
  1. Monitor the urinary output
  2. Monitor for signs of urinary tract or wound infection
  3. Maintain the integrity of the exposed bladder mucosa
  4. Prevent the bladder tissue from drying while allowing for the drainage of urine until surgical closure is performed
    a. The bladder is covered with sterile, nonadherent, clear plastic wrap or a sterile thin film dressing without adhesive
    b. Petroleum jelly is avoided, because it tends to dry out, adhere to the bladder mucosa, and damage the delicate tissues when the dressing is removed
  5. Monitor the laboratory values and urinalysis to assess for renal function
  6. Administer antibiotics, as prescribed
  7. Provide emotional support to the parents, and encourage the verbalization of their fears and concerns

VI. ENURESIS
A. Description
  1. The child is unable to control bladder function even though he or she has reached an age at which the control of voiding is expected
  2. By the age of 5 years, most children are aware of bladder fullness and are able to control voiding
B. Primary nocturnal enuresis
  1. Bed-wetting in a child who has never been dry for extended periods
  2. Common among children; most children will eventually outgrow bed-wetting without therapeutic intervention

3. The child is not able to sense a full bladder and does not awaken to void
4. The child may have delayed maturation of the central nervous system

C. Secondary or acquired enuresis
1. The onset of wetting after a period of established urinary continence
2. May occur during nighttime sleep (nocturnal), only during the waking hours (diurnal), or during both day and nighttime
3. The child may complain of dysuria, urgency, or frequency
4. The child should be assessed for urinary tract infections

D. Data collection
1. Normal voiding pattern
2. History of bed-wetting with no extended period of dryness in a child who is older than 5 years

E. Interventions
1. Obtain urinalysis and urine culture, as prescribed, to rule out infection or existing disorder
2. Assist the family with identifying a treatment plan that will best fit their needs
3. Limit fluid intake at night, and encourage the child to void just before going to bed
4. Involve the child in caring for the wet sheets and changing the bed to assist the child with taking ownership of the problem
5. Provide reward systems, as appropriate, for the child
6. Incorporate behavioral and motivational conditioning techniques
7. Pharmacologic therapy for an overactive bladder may be indicated
8. Encourage follow-up to determine the effectiveness of the treatment

VII. HEMOLYTIC-UREMIC SYNDROME

A. Description
1. Thought to be associated with bacterial toxins, chemicals, and viruses that cause acute renal failure in children
2. Occurs primarily among infants and small children between the ages of 6 months and 5 years
3. Clinical features include acquired hemolytic anemia, thrombocytopenia, renal injury, and central nervous system symptoms

B. Data collection
1. Triad of anemia, thrombocytopenia, and renal failure is diagnostic (Box 34-4)
2. Proteinuria, hematuria, and the presence of urinary casts
3. Blood urea nitrogen and serum creatinine levels are elevated; hemoglobin and hematocrit levels are decreased

BOX 34-4 Manifestations of Hemolytic-Uremic Syndrome
- Vomiting
- Irritability
- Lethargy
- Marked pallor
- Hemorrhagic manifestations, such as bruising, petechiae, jaundice, and bloody diarrhea
- Oliguria or anuria
- Central nervous system involvement, including seizures, stupor, and coma

C. Interventions
1. Hemodialysis or peritoneal dialysis may be prescribed if the child is anuric
   a. Hemodialysis requires venous access (arteriovenous **shunt**, fistula, or graft), and treatment is usually 3 to 8 hours in length (3 times per week); peritoneal dialysis requires the surgical placement of an abdominal catheter (the correction of fluid and electrolyte imbalance is slower than hemodialysis)
   b. Dialysate solution is prescribed to meet the child's electrolyte needs
2. Strict monitoring of fluid balance is necessary; fluid restrictions may be prescribed if the child is anuric
3. Institute measures to prevent infection
4. Provide adequate nutrition

PRACTICE QUESTIONS

More questions on the companion CD!

371. A nurse is assigned to care for a child who is suspected of having glomerulonephritis. The nurse reviews the child's record and notes that which finding is associated with the diagnosis of glomerulonephritis?
1. Hypotension
2. Red-brown urine
3. Low urinary specific gravity
4. A low blood urea nitrogen (BUN) level

372. A nurse is reviewing the health record of a child who has been recently diagnosed with glomerulonephritis. Which finding noted in the child's record is associated with the diagnosis of glomerulonephritis?
1. The child fell off a bike and onto the handlebars.
2. The child has had nausea and vomiting for the last 24 hours.
3. The child had urticaria and itching for 1 week before diagnosis.

4. The child had a streptococcal throat infection 2 weeks before diagnosis.

373. A nurse is planning care for a child with hemolytic-uremic syndrome (HUS). The child has been anuric and will be receiving peritoneal dialysis treatment. The nurse plans to:
   1. Restrict fluids, as prescribed.
   2. Administer analgesics, as prescribed.
   3. Care for the arteriovenous (AV) shunt.
   4. Encourage the intake of foods that are high in potassium.

374. A nurse is assisting with performing an admission assessment on a 2-year-old child who has been diagnosed with nephrotic syndrome. The nurse collects data knowing that a common characteristic associated with nephrotic syndrome is:
   1. Hypotension
   2. Generalized edema
   3. Increased urinary output
   4. Frank, bright red blood in the urine

375. The child with cryptorchidism is being discharged after orchiopexy, which was performed on an outpatient basis. The nurse informs the parents about which priority care measure?
   1. Measuring intake and output
   2. Administering anticholinergics
   3. Preventing infection at the surgical site
   4. Applying cold, wet compresses to the surgical site

376. A nurse is reinforcing discharge instructions to the mother of a 2-year-old child who has had an orchiopexy to correct cryptorchidism. Which of the following statements, if made by the mother of the child, indicates that further teaching is necessary?
   1. "I'll check his temperature."
   2. "I'll give him medication so he'll be comfortable."
   3. "I'll let him decide when to return to his play activities."
   4. "I'll check his voiding to be sure there are no problems."

377. A nurse collects a urine specimen preoperatively from a child with epispadias who is scheduled for surgical repair. The nurse reviews the child's record for the laboratory results of the urine test

and would most likely expect to note which of the following?
   1. Hematuria
   2. Bacteriuria
   3. Glucosuria
   4. Proteinuria

378. An 18-month-old child is being discharged after surgical repair of hypospadias. Which postoperative nursing care measure should the nurse stress to the parents as they prepare to take this child home?
   1. Leave diapers off to allow the site to heal.
   2. Avoid tub baths until the stent has been removed.
   3. Encourage toilet training to ensure that the flow of urine is normal.
   4. Restrict the fluid intake to reduce urinary output for the first few days.

379. The parents of a newborn have been told that their child was born with bladder exstrophy, and the parents ask the nurse about this condition. The nurse bases the response on knowledge that this condition is:
   1. A hereditary disorder that occurs in every other generation
   2. Caused by the use of medications taken by the mother during pregnancy
   3. A condition in which the urinary bladder is abnormally located in the pelvic cavity
   4. An extrusion of the urinary bladder to the outside of the body through a defect in the lower abdominal wall

ALTERNATE ITEM FORMAT: MULTIPLE RESPONSE

380. A child is admitted to the hospital with a probable diagnosis of nephrotic syndrome. Which findings would the nurse expect to observe?
   ☑ 1. Pallor
   ☐ 2. Edema
   ☐ 3. Anorexia
   ☑ 4. Proteinuria
   ☐ 5. Weight loss
   ☐ 6. Decreased serum lipids

ANSWERS

371. **2**

Rationale: Gross hematuria resulting in dark, smoky, cola-colored or red-brown urine is a classic symptom of glomerulonephritis, and hypertension is also common. BUN levels may be elevated. A mid to high urinary specific gravity is associated with glomerulonephritis.

Test-Taking Strategy: Use the process of elimination. Eliminate options 1 and 3 first, because hypertension and a high specific gravity are likely to occur with this kidney

disorder. Recalling that BUN levels elevate among clients with this condition will assist with directing you to option 2. Review the clinical manifestations associated with glomerulonephritis if you had difficulty with this question.

Level of Cognitive Ability: Comprehension
Client Needs: Physiological Integrity
Integrated Process: Nursing Process/Data Collection
Content Area: Child Health
Reference: Price, D., & Gwin, J. (2008). *Pediatric nursing: An introductory text* (10th ed., p. 258). St. Louis: Saunders.

372. 4

Rationale: Group A β-hemolytic streptococcal infection is a cause of glomerulonephritis. The child often becomes ill with streptococcal infection of the upper respiratory tract and then develops symptoms of acute poststreptococcal glomerulonephritis after an interval of 1 to 2 weeks. The data presented in options 1, 2, and 3 are unrelated to a diagnosis of glomerulonephritis.

Test-Taking Strategy: Use your knowledge regarding the causes of glomerulonephritis and the process of elimination to answer the question. Option 1 relates to a kidney injury. Options 2 and 3 are not related to the diagnosis of glomerulonephritis. Review the causes of glomerulonephritis if you had difficulty with this question.

Level of Cognitive Ability: Comprehension
Client Needs: Physiological Integrity
Integrated Process: Nursing Process/Data Collection
Content Area: Child Health
References: Leifer, G. (2007). *Introduction to maternity and pediatric nursing* (5th ed., pp. 668-669). Philadelphia: Saunders.
Price, D., & Gwin, J. (2008). *Pediatric nursing: An introductory text* (10th ed., pp. 257-258). St. Louis: Saunders.

373. 1

Rationale: HUS is thought to be associated with bacterial toxins, chemicals, and viruses that cause acute renal failure in children. Clinical features of the disease include acquired hemolytic anemia, thrombocytopenia, renal injury, and central nervous system symptoms. A child with HUS who is undergoing peritoneal dialysis for the treatment of anuria will be on fluid restrictions. Pain is not associated with HUS, and potassium would be restricted rather than encouraged if the child was anuric. Peritoneal dialysis does not require an AV shunt (only hemodialysis does).

Test-Taking Strategy: Focus on the child's diagnosis, and recall your knowledge of the care of a client with acute renal failure. Also focus on the data in the question. Noting the word "peritoneal" will assist you with eliminating option 3. From the remaining options, remember that because the child is anuric, fluids will be restricted. Review the care of the child with HUS if you had difficulty with this question.

Level of Cognitive Ability: Analysis
Client Needs: Physiological Integrity
Integrated Processes: Nursing Process/Planning
Content Area: Child Health
References: Hockenberry, M., & Wilson, D. (2007). *Nursing care of infants and children* (8th ed., pp. 1252-1253). St. Louis: Mosby.
Wong, D., Perry, S., Hockenberry, M., Lowdermilk, D., & Wilson, D. (2006). *Maternal-child nursing care* (3rd ed., p. 1658). St. Louis: Mosby.

374. 2

Rationale: Nephrotic syndrome is defined as massive proteinuria, hypoalbuminemia, and edema. The urine is dark, foamy, and frothy, but microscopic hematuria may be present; frank, bright red blood in the urine does not occur. Urine output is decreased, and the blood pressure is normal or slightly decreased.

Test-Taking Strategy: Use the process of elimination. Eliminate option 3 first, because urine output is likely to be decreased in a client with a renal disorder. From the remaining options, associate edema with nephrotic syndrome, because this will be helpful to you if you encounter a similar question. Review the characteristics of nephrotic syndrome if you had difficulty with this question.

Level of Cognitive Ability: Comprehension
Client Needs: Physiological Integrity
Integrated Process: Nursing Process/Data Collection
Content Area: Child Health
Reference: Price, D., & Gwin, J. (2008). *Pediatric nursing: An introductory text* (10th ed., p. 259). St. Louis: Saunders.

375. 3

Rationale: The most common complications associated with orchiopexy are bleeding and infection. The parents are instructed in postoperative home-care measures, including the prevention of infection, pain control, and activity restrictions. Anticholinergics are prescribed for the relief of bladder spasms; they are not necessary after orchiopexy. The measurement of intake and output is not required. Cold, wet compresses are not prescribed; the moisture from a wet compress presents a potential for infection.

Test-Taking Strategy: Note the strategic word "priority" in the question. Use Maslow's Hierarchy of Needs theory to answer the question. Of the options presented, the potential for infection is the physiological priority. Review the home-care instructions after orchiopexy if you had difficulty with this question.

Level of Cognitive Ability: Application
Client Needs: Physiological Integrity
Integrated Process: Teaching and Learning
Content Area: Child Health
Reference: Leifer, G. (2007). *Introduction to maternity and pediatric nursing* (5th ed., p. 672). Philadelphia: Saunders.
Price, D., & Gwin, J. (2008). *Pediatric nursing: An introductory text* (10th ed., pp. 167-168). St. Louis: Saunders.

376. 3

Rationale: All vigorous activities should be restricted for 2 weeks after surgery to promote healing and prevent injury; this will prevent dislodging of the suture, which is internal. Normally 2-year-old children will want to be very active; therefore, allowing the child to decide when to return to his play activities may prevent healing and cause injury. The parents should be taught to monitor the child's temperature; to provide analgesics, as needed; and to monitor the urine output.

Test-Taking Strategy: Note the strategic words "further teaching is necessary." These words indicate a negative event query and ask you to select an option that is an incorrect statement. Option 1 is an important action for recognizing signs of infection. Option 2 is appropriate for keeping pain to a minimum. Option 4 monitors the voiding pattern, which is also important after this type of surgery. Review the discharge instructions after the surgical correction of cryptorchidism if you had difficulty with this question.

Level of Cognitive Ability: Comprehension
Client Needs: Health Promotion and Maintenance
Integrated Process: Teaching and Learning*Content Area:* Child Health
Reference: Leifer, G. (2007). *Introduction to maternity and pediatric nursing* (5th ed., p. 672). Philadelphia: Saunders.

377. 2

Rationale: Epispadias is a congenital defect that involves the abnormal placement of the urethral orifice of the penis. Among clients with this condition, the urethral opening is located anywhere on the dorsum of the penis. This anatomical characteristic leads to the easy access of bacterial entry into the urine. Options 1, 3, and 4 are not characteristically noted with this condition.

Test-Taking Strategy: Use your knowledge regarding the anatomical characteristics of epispadias and the process of elimination to answer the question. Options 1, 3, and 4 do not relate to the potential for infection, which can be present with this condition. Review the diagnostic findings associated with epispadias if you had difficulty with this question.

Level of Cognitive Ability: Comprehension
Client Needs: Physiological Integrity
Integrated Process: Nursing Process/Data Collection
Content Area: Child Health
Reference: Hockenberry, M., Wilson, D., & Winkelstein, M. (2005). *Wong's essentials of pediatric nursing* (7th ed., p. 989). St. Louis: Mosby.

378. 2

Rationale: After hypospadias repair, the parents are instructed to avoid giving the child a tub bath until the stent has been removed to prevent infection. Diapers are placed on the child to prevent the contamination of the surgical site. Fluids should be encouraged to maintain hydration. Toilet training should not be an issue during this stressful period.

Test-Taking Strategy: Use the process of elimination. Option 3 is eliminated first, because toilet training should not be initiated during times of stress, such as after surgery. Eliminate option 1, because this action can cause the contamination of the surgical site. Option 4 is inappropriate, because fluids should be encouraged rather than restricted. Review the postoperative care after the surgical repair of hypospadias if you had difficulty with this question.

Level of Cognitive Ability: Application
Client Needs: Health Promotion and Maintenance
Integrated Process: Teaching and Learning
Content Area: Child Health
Reference: Price, D., & Gwin, J. (2008). *Pediatric nursing: An introductory text* (10th ed., p. 168). St. Louis: Saunders.

379. 4

Rationale: Bladder exstrophy is a congenital anomaly that is characterized by the extrusion of the urinary bladder to the outside of the body through a defect in the lower abdominal wall. The cause in unknown, and there is a higher incidence among males. Options 1, 2, and 3 are not characteristics of this disorder.

Test Taking Strategy: Use the process of elimination. If you are unfamiliar with this condition, note the relationship of the word "exstrophy" in the name of the disorder with the word "extrusion" in the correct option; this should remind you that this condition is located external to the body. Review the characteristics of bladder exstrophy if you had difficulty with this question.

Level of Cognitive Ability: Comprehension
Client Needs: Physiological Integrity
Integrated Process: Nursing Process/Implementation
Content Area: Child Health
Reference: Leifer, G. (2007). *Introduction to maternity and pediatric nursing* (5th ed., p. 663). Philadelphia: Saunders.

ALTERNATE ITEM FORMAT: MULTIPLE RESPONSE

380. 1, 2, 3, 4

Rationale: Nephrotic syndrome is a kidney disorder that is characterized by massive proteinuria, hypoalbuminemia, edema, elevated serum lipids, anorexia, and pallor. The urine volume is decreased, and the urine is dark and frothy in appearance. The child with this condition gains weight.

Test-Taking Strategy: Note the child's diagnosis and think about the definition of nephrotic syndrome and its associated characteristics to answer the question. Review the clinical manifestations associated with nephrotic syndrome if you had difficulty with this question.

Level of Cognitive Ability: Analysis
Client Needs: Physiological Integrity
Integrated Process: Nursing Process/Data Collection
Content Area: Child Health
References: McKinney, E., James, S., Murray, S., & Ashwill, J. (2005). *Maternal-child nursing* (2nd ed., p. 1175). Philadelphia: Saunders.
Price, D., & Gwin, J. (2008). *Pediatric nursing: An introductory text* (10th ed., pp. 258-260). Philadelphia: Saunders.

REFERENCES

Hockenberry, M., Wilson, D., & Winkelstein, M. (2005). *Wong's essentials of pediatric nursing* (7th ed.). St. Louis: Mosby.

Hockenberry, M., & Wilson, D. (2007). *Nursing care of infants and children* (8th ed.). St. Louis: Mosby.

Leifer, G. (2007). *Introduction to maternity and pediatric nursing* (5th ed.). Philadelphia: Saunders.

McKinney, E., James, S., Murray, S., & Ashwill, J. (2005). *Maternal-child nursing* (2nd ed.). Philadelphia: Saunders.

Merenstein, G.B., & Gardner, S.L, (2007). *Handbook of neonatal care* (6th ed.). St. Louis: Mosby.

National Council of State Boards of Nursing (Eds.). (2008). *2008 Detailed Test Plan for the NCLEX-PN® Examination, National Council of State Boards of Nursing*. Chicago: Author.

National Council of State Boards of Nursing. *NCSBN home page.* www.ncsbn.org. Accessed July 23, 2008.

Price, D., & Gwin, J. (2008). *Pediatric nursing: An introductory text* (10th ed.). St. Louis: Saunders.

Wong, D., Perry, S., Hockenberry, M., Lowdermilk, D., & Wilson, D. (2006). *Maternal-child nursing care* (3rd ed.). St. Louis: Mosby.

Integumentary Disorders

I. ATOPIC DERMATITIS (ECZEMA)

A. Description
   1. A superficial inflammatory process that primarily involves the epidermis and that is characterized by pruritic lesions
   2. The major goals of management are to relieve pruritus, hydrate the skin, reduce inflammation, and prevent or control secondary infections
   3. May be associated with a higher risk for the development of asthma and allergic rhinitis.

B. Forms of eczema (Box 35-1)

C. Data collection (Box 35-2)

D. Interventions
   1. Avoid exposure to skin irritants such as soaps, detergents, fabric softeners, diaper wipes, and powder
   2. Improve skin hydration
   3. Apply cool, wet compresses or colloidal oatmeal baths to soothe the skin
   4. Administer antihistamines and topical corticosteroids, as prescribed; corticosteroids are applied in a thin layer and rubbed into the area thoroughly
   5. Prevent or minimize scratching; keep the nails short and clean, and place gloves or cotton socks over the hands
   6. Eliminate conditions that increase itching, such as heat, woolen clothes or blankets, rough fabrics, and furry stuffed animals
   7. Instruct the parents to wash the child's clothing in a mild detergent and to rinse it thoroughly; putting the clothes through a second complete wash cycle without detergent will minimize the amount of residue remaining on the fabric
   8. Instruct the parents in the measures to prevent skin infections
   9. Instruct the parents to monitor the lesions for signs of infection (i.e., honey-colored crusts with surrounding erythema)

II. IMPETIGO

A. Description
   1. A highly contagious bacterial infection of the skin caused by β-hemolytic streptococci, *Staphylococcus aureus*, or both
   2. The most common sites of infection are the face, around the mouth, the hands, the neck, and the extremities
   3. The lesions begin as a vesicle or pustule that is surrounded by edema and redness, usually at a site that has been injured; this progresses to an exudative and crusting stage
   4. After the crusting of the lesions, the initially serous vesicular fluid becomes cloudy, and the vesicle ruptures, leaving a honey-colored crust that covers an ulcerated base

B. Data collection
   1. Lesions that may be red, edematous, draining, or crusting
   2. Pruritus and burning
   3. Secondary lymph node involvement

C. Interventions
   1. Contact isolation; use standard precautions and implement agency-specific isolation procedures for the hospitalized child
   2. Allow lesions to dry by air exposure
   3. Assist the child with daily bathing with antibacterial soap (e.g., pHisoHex), as prescribed
   4. Apply warm compresses to lesions two or three times per day, as prescribed, to remove crusts and to allow healing
   5. Apply and instruct the parents in the use of antibiotic ointments; the infection is still communicable for 48 hours beyond initiation of antibiotic treatment
   6. Administer oral antibiotics, which may be prescribed if there is no response to topical antibiotic treatment
   7. Apply and instruct the parents in the use of emollients, as prescribed, to prevent skin cracking

BOX 35-1 Forms of Eczema

Infantile
Usually begins at 2 to 6 months of age; generally undergoes spontaneous remission by 3 years of age
Childhood
May follow the infantile form; occurs at 2 to 3 years of age
Preadolescent and Adolescent
Begins at about 12 years of age; may continue into the early adult years or indefinitely

BOX 35-2 Data Collection Findings: Atopic Dermatitis

- Primary feature: Pruritus
Acute
- Erythematous patches, papules, or plaques
- Excoriations as a result of scratching
Chronic
- Thickening of the skin
- Fissures
- Alopecia as a result of scratching

Modified from Burg, F. D., Ingelfinger, J. R., Posin, R. A., & Gershon, A. A. (2006). *Current pediatric therapy* (18th ed.). Philadelphia: Saunders.

8. Instruct the parents in the methods of preventing the spread of the infection, especially careful handwashing
9. Inform the parents that the child needs to use separate towels, linens, and dishes
10. Inform the parents that all linens and clothing should be washed separately with detergent in hot water

III. PEDICULOSIS CAPITIS (LICE)
A. Description
   1. An infestation of the hair and scalp with lice
   2. The most common sites of involvement are the occipital area, behind the ears, at the nape of the neck, and, occasionally, the eyebrows and eyelashes; nits in the eyelashes and eyebrows are usually from pubic lice and may be a sign of sexual **abuse** in children; this would require further screening
   3. The female louse lays her eggs (nits) on the hair shaft, close to the scalp; the incubation period is 8 to 10 days
   4. Head lice live and reproduce only on humans and are transmitted by direct and indirect contact, such as the sharing of brushes, hats, towels, and bedding
   5. All contacts of the infested child should be examined
B. Data collection (Box 35-3)
C. Interventions (Table 35-1)
   1. Use a pediculicide shampoo; the hair is towel dried, the nits are removed with a

BOX 35-3 Data Collection Findings: Pediculosis Capitis

Intense pruritus is present.
Adult lice are difficult to see and appear as small gray specks; they may crawl very fast.
Nits are visible and firmly attached to the hair shaft near the scalp; they appear as tiny silver or gray specks that resemble dandruff.

   fine-toothed comb, and the treatment is repeated in 7 days
   2. Instruct the parents in the use of shampoo and rinse, as prescribed
   3. Instruct the parents that bedding and clothing used by the child should be changed daily, laundered in hot water with detergent, and dried in a hot dryer for 20 minutes
   4. Instruct the parents that nonessential bedding and clothing can be stored in a tightly sealed bag for 10 to 14 days and then washed
   5. Instruct the parents to seal toys that cannot be washed or dry cleaned in a plastic bag for 2 weeks
   6. Instruct the parents that hairbrushes or combs should be discarded or soaked in hot water (54.4° C [130° F]) for 15 minutes
   7. Instruct the parents that furniture and carpets need to be vacuumed frequently
   8. Teach the child not to share clothing, headwear, or brushes and combs

IV. SCABIES
A. Description (see Chapter 40 for additional information about scabies)
   1. A parasitic skin disorder caused by an infestation of *Sarcoptes scabiei* (itch mite)
   2. Endemic among schoolchildren and institutionalized populations as a result of close personal contact
   3. Incubation period
      a. Female mite burrows into the epidermis, lays eggs, and dies in the burrow after 4 to 5 weeks
      b. The eggs hatch in 3 to 5 days, and the larvae migrate to the skin to mature and complete their life cycle
   4. Infectious period: During the course of the infestation
   5. Transmission: By close personal contact with an infected person
B. Data collection (Box 35-4)
C. Interventions (Table 35-2)
   1. Instruct the parents in the application of the scabicide
   2. Application should be preceded by a warm soap-and-water bath
   3. Household members and contacts of the infected child need to be treated at the same time

TABLE 35-1 **Treatment of Pediculosis Capitis***

Generic Name (Trade Name)	Route of Administration	Instructions	Formulation	Side Effects	Strength	Comments
Permethrin (Nix), OTC	Topical	Apply to dry scalp for 5-10 minutes, then rinse; repeat in 1 week	Crème rinse	Irritant or allergic contact dermatitis	1%	Favorable safety profile; evidence of increasing resistance
Pyrethrins and piperonyl butoxide (RID, A-200, R and C, Pronto, Clear Lice), OTC	Topical	Apply to dry scalp for 5-10 minutes, then rinse; repeat in 1 week	Shampoo, mousse, or gel	Irritant or allergic contact dermatitis		
Lindane (Kwell), Rx	Topical	Apply to dry scalp for 5-10 minutes, then rinse; repeat in 1 week	Shampoo	Irritant or allergic contact dermatitis; risk of neurotoxicity and seizures	1%	Less ovicidal than permethrin; do not use with children <2 years old; use with caution with children with extensive dermatitis, seizure disorders, or HIV/AIDS
Malathion (Ovide), Rx	Topical	Apply to dry scalp for 8-12 hours, then rinse; repeat in 1 week	Lotion	Irritant or allergic contact dermatitis	0.5%	Highly ovicidal; flammable (avoid open flames or electric heat sources); odor

AIDS, Acquired immunodeficiency syndrome; *HIV*, human immunodeficiency virus; *OTC*, over the counter; *Rx*, prescription.
*All pediculicidal agents cause the death of the head louse.
Modified from Burg, F. D., Ingelfinger, J. R., Posin, R. A., & Gershon, A. A. (2006). *Current pediatric therapy* (18th ed.). Philadelphia: Saunders.

BOX 35-4 **Data Collection Findings: Scabies**

- Intense pruritus, especially at night
- Burrows (fine, grayish-red lines that may be difficult to see) on the skin

4. Instruct the parents about the importance of frequent handwashing
5. Instruct the parents that all clothing, bedding, and pillowcases used by the child need to be changed daily, washed in hot water with detergent, dried in a hot dryer, and ironed before reuse
6. Instruct the parents that nonwashable toys and other items should be sealed in plastic bags for 4 days

V. TINEA (RINGWORM)
A. Description
  1. Known as tinea capitis (scalp), tinea corporis (body), tinea pedis (feet), and tinea cruris (groin)
  2. A fungal infection spread by direct contact
B. Data collection
  1. Papules and dry scales
  2. Itching

C. Interventions
  1. Provide meticulous skin care
  2. Apply antifungal ointments, as prescribed
  3. Administer oral antifungal medications, as prescribed
VI. THE BURNED CHILD
A. Pediatric differences (see Chapter 40 for additional information about burns)
  1. Very young children who have been severely burned have a higher mortality rate than older children and adults with comparable burns
  2. The majority of childhood burns occur in the home, especially the kitchen and bathroom; most are preventable.
  3. Burns in children of all ages may be related to child **abuse** and should be thoroughly evaluated
  4. Young children are susceptible to burn injury because of their less acute perception of danger; they are likely to respond less quickly or properly to a dangerous fire situation
  5. Lower burn temperatures and shorter exposure to heat can cause a more severe burn in a child than an adult because a child's skin is thinner

TABLE 35-2	Treatment of Scabies*						
Generic Name (Trade Name)	Route of Administration	Instructions	Formulation	Side Effects	Strength	Comments	
Permethrin (Elimite, Acticin), Rx	Topical	Apply to whole body from neck down†; wash off after 8-14 hours; optional reapplication in 1 week	Cream	Irritant or allergic contact dermatitis; may temporarily worsen erythema or itching.	5%	First-line treatment; FDA approved down to 2 months of age; 96% cure rate after single application	
Lindane (Kwell), Rx	Topical	Apply to whole body from neck down†; wash off after 8-12 hours; repeat in 1 week	Lotion	Irritant or allergic contact dermatitis; risk of neurotoxicity or seizures	1%	Do not use with children <2 years old; use with caution with children with extensive dermatitis, seizure disorders, or HIV/AIDS	
Crotamiton (Eurax), Rx	Topical	Apply to whole body from neck down for 2-5 days; bathe every 24 hours	Lotion or cream	Irritant dermatitis or allergic contact dermatitis	10%	High failure rate	
Precipitated sulfur in petrolatum compounded, Rx	Topical	Apply nightly for 3 nights; wash off 24 hours after each application	Ointment	Allergic reaction; skin irritation	6%-10%	Some authors claim this is the treatment of choice for pregnant women and neonates; foul odor; messy; stains fabric	
Ivermectin (Stromectol), Rx	PO; 200 µg/kg; two doses spaced 2 weeks apart		Tablet: 3 mg or 6 mg	Nausea, vomiting, abdominal pain, drowsiness		Not FDA-approved for treating scabies; not approved for children <5 years old or weighing <15 kg	

AIDS, Acquired immunodeficiency syndrome; *FDA,* U.S. Food and Drug Administration; *HIV,* human immunodeficiency virus; *PO,* orally; *Rx,* prescription.
*All scabicide compounds listed are toxic to the *Sarcoptes scabiei* mite.
†In children ≤2 years old, also apply to scalp and face, but avoid the eyes, nose, and mouth.
Modified from Burg, F. D., Ingelfinger, J. R., Posin, R. A., & Gershon, A. A. (2006). *Current pediatric therapy* (18th ed.). Philadelphia: Saunders.

6. Severely burned children are at an increased risk for fluid and heat loss, dehydration, and metabolic acidosis as compared with adults
7. The higher proportion of body fluid to mass in children increases the risk of cardiovascular problems
8. Burns involving more than 10% of the total body surface area (TBSA) require some form of fluid resuscitation
9. Infants and children are at increased risk for protein and calorie deficiency, because they have a smaller muscle mass and less body fat than adults
10. Scarring is more severe in a child
11. An immature immune system presents an increased risk of infection among infants and young children
12. A delay in **growth** may occur after a burn
B. Extent of burn injury
  1. Burn size is expressed as a percentage of the TBSA that is burned
  2. The rule of nines, which is used for an adult with a burn injury, gives an inaccurate assessment in children; a modified rule of nines or the Lund-Browder classification may be used in a child
C. Treatment (Figure 35-1)

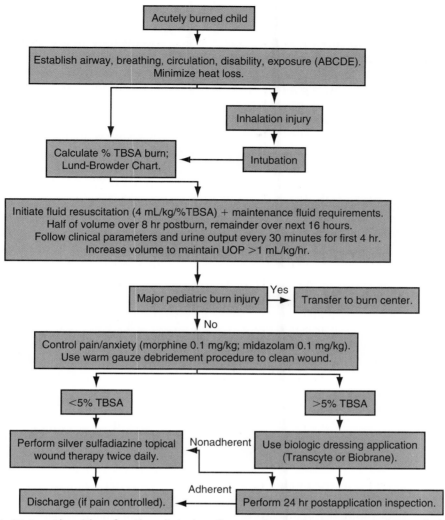

FIG. 35-1 Algorithm for the clinical pathway of care for an acutely burned child. (From Burg, F. D., Ingelfinger, J. R., Posin, R. A., & Gershon, A. A. [2006]. *Current pediatric therapy* (18th ed.]. Philadelphia: Saunders.)

PRACTICE QUESTIONS

More questions on the companion CD!

381. A school nurse prepares a list of home-care instructions for the parents of school children who have been diagnosed with pediculosis capitis (head lice). Which is included in the list?
    1. Use anti-lice sprays on all bedding and furniture.
    2. Boil combs and brushes in hot water for 2 hours.
    3. Take all bedding and linens to the cleaners to be dry cleaned.
    4. Vacuum floors, play areas, and furniture to remove any hairs that may carry live nits.
382. A mother of a 3-year-old child tells the nurse that the child has been continuously scratching the skin and has developed a rash. On assessment, which finding indicates that the child may have scabies?
    1. Fine, grayish-red lines
    2. Purple-colored lesions
    3. Thick, honey-colored crusts
    4. Clusters of fluid-filled vesicles
383. Permethrin 5% (Elimite) is prescribed for a 4-year-old child with a diagnosis of scabies. The nurse instructs the mother regarding the use of this treatment. Which instruction is appropriate?
    1. Apply the lotion and leave it on for 4 hours.
    2. Apply the lotion to the hair, the face, and the entire body.
    3. The child should wear no clothing while the lotion is in place.
    4. Apply the lotion to cool, dry skin at least half an hour after bathing.
384. A nurse is providing home-care instructions to an adolescent who has been diagnosed with tinea

pedis. Which statement by the adolescent indicates the need for further instruction?

1. "I need to wear clean socks."
2. "I need to wear shoes that are well ventilated."
3. "I should wear plastic shoes as much as possible."
4. "I need to dry my feet carefully, especially between the toes."

385. A corticosteroid cream is prescribed by a physician for a child with atopic dermatitis (eczema). The nurse teaches the mother how to apply the cream. Which instruction is appropriate?

1. Apply the cream over the entire body.
2. Apply a thick layer of cream in affected areas only.
3. Avoid cleansing the area before applying the cream.
4. Apply a thin layer of cream, and rub it into the area thoroughly.

386. A nurse assists with providing an instructional session to parents regarding impetigo. Which statement by a parent indicates the need for further instruction?

1. "It is extremely contagious."
2. "It is most common during humid weather."
3. "Lesions are most often located on the arms and chest."
4. "It begins in an area of broken skin, such as an insect bite."

387. A nurse provides instructions to the mother of a child with impetigo regarding the application of antibiotic ointment. The mother asks the nurse when the child can return to school. Which response by the nurse is accurate?

1. Ten days after using the antibiotic ointment
2. One week after using the antibiotic ointment
3. Forty-eight hours after using the antibiotic ointment
4. Twenty-four hours after using the antibiotic ointment

388. A nurse provides instructions regarding the use of permethrin 1% (Nix) to the parents of a child who has been diagnosed with pediculosis captits (head lice). Which statement by a parent indicates the need for further instruction?

1. "The hair should not be shampooed for 24 hours after treatment."
2. "The medication can be obtained over the counter in a local pharmacy."
3. "The medication is applied to the hair after shampooing and left on for 24 hours."
4. "The medication is applied to the hair after shampooing, left on for 5 to 10 minutes, and then rinsed out."

ALTERNATE ITEM FORMAT: MULTIPLE RESPONSE

389. Which of the following are characteristics of scabies? Select all that apply.

☐ 1. It is caused by a fungal infection.
☐ 2. It appears as burrows or fine, grayish-red lines.
☐ 3. It is transmitted by close personal contact with an infected person.
☐ 4. It is endemic among schoolchildren and institutionalized populations.
☐ 5. Meticulous skin care and the application of antifungal cream are components of treatment.
☐ 6. Household members and contacts of the infected child need to be treated at the same time that the child is being treated.

ANSWERS

381. **4**

Rationale: Anti-lice sprays are unnecessary. Additionally, they should never be used on a child. Bedding and linens should be washed with hot water and dried on a hot setting. Items that cannot be washed should be dry cleaned or sealed in plastic bags in a warm place for 3 weeks. Combs and brushes should be boiled or soaked in anti-lice shampoo or hot water for 15 minutes. Thorough home cleaning is necessary to remove any remaining lice or nits.

Test-Taking Strategy: Use the process of elimination. Eliminate option 1, knowing that anti-lice sprays should not be used. Knowing that bedding and linens can be washed will eliminate option 3. The time for boiling in option 2 is rather lengthy; therefore, eliminate this option. Review the home-care instructions for the child with pediculosis capitis if you had difficulty with this question.

Level of Cognitive Ability: Application
Client Needs: Safe and Effective Care Environment
Integrated Process: Teaching and Learning

Content Area: Child Health
References: Hockenberry, M., & Wilson, D. (2007). *Nursing care of infants and children* (8th ed., p. 773). St. Louis: Mosby. Price, D., & Gwin, J. (2008). *Pediatric nursing: An introductory text* (10th ed., p. 292). St. Louis: Saunders.

382. **1**

Rationale: Scabies appears as burrows or fine, grayish-red lines. They may be difficult to see if they are obscured by excoriation and inflammation. Purple-colored lesions may be indicative of various disorders, including systemic conditions. Clusters of fluid-filled vesicles are seen in clients with herpesvirus. Thick, honey-colored crusts are characteristic of impetigo.

Test-Taking Strategy: Use the process of elimination. Recalling that scabies infestation produces burrows will direct you to option 1. Review the characteristics of scabies if you had difficulty with this question.

Level of Cognitive Ability: Comprehension
Client Needs: Physiological Integrity
Integrated Process: Nursing Process/Data Collection
Content Area: Child Health
Reference: Hockenberry, M., & Wilson, D. (2007). *Nursing care of infants and children* (8th ed., pp. 271-272). St. Louis: Mosby.

383. 4
Rationale: Permethrin is applied from the neck downward, with care taken to ensure that the soles of the feet, the areas behind the ears, and the areas under the toenails and fingernails are covered. The lotion should be kept on for 8 to 14 hours, and then the child should be given a bath. The lotion should not be applied for at least 30 minutes after bathing, and it should be applied only to cool, dry skin. The child should be clothed during treatment.
Test-Taking Strategy: Use the process of elimination. Reading options 2 and 3 carefully will assist you with eliminating these options. From the remaining options, recalling the treatment time for this medication will direct you to option 4. Review permethrin treatment if you had difficulty with this question.
Level of Cognitive Ability: Application
Client Needs: Physiological Integrity
Integrated Process: Teaching and Learning
Content Area: Child Health
Reference: Hockenberry, M., & Wilson, D. (2007). *Nursing care of infants and children* (8th ed., pp. 771-772). St. Louis: Mosby.

384. 3
Rationale: Plastic shoes retain heat and should be avoided, because this condition is aggravated by heat and moisture. Options 1, 2, and 4 are appropriate measures for the treatment of this condition.
Test-Taking Strategy: Use the process of elimination. Note the strategic words "need for further instruction." These words indicate a negative event query and ask you to select an option that is an incorrect statement. Recalling that heat and moisture aggravate the condition will direct you to option 3. Review the measures used to treat tinea pedis if you had difficulty with this question.
Level of Cognitive Ability: Comprehension
Client Needs: Physiological Integrity
Integrated Process: Teaching and Learning
Content Area: Child Health
Reference: Leifer, G. (2007). *Introduction to maternity and pediatric nursing* (5th ed., p. 685). Philadelphia: Saunders.

385. 4
Rationale: Corticosteroid cream should be applied sparingly and rubbed into the area thoroughly. The affected area should be cleansed gently before application. The cream should not be applied over extensive areas. Systemic absorption is more likely to occur with extensive application.
Test-Taking Strategy: Use the process of elimination. Eliminate option 1, because the cream should only be applied to the area that is affected. Eliminate option 2 because of the words "thick" and "only." Eliminate option 3, because it does not make sense to avoid cleansing an affected area. Review the procedure for the application of corticosteriod cream if you had difficulty with this question.
Level of Cognitive Ability: Application

Client Needs: Physiological Integrity
Integrated Process: Teaching and Learning
Content Area: Child Health
Reference: Skidmore-Roth, L. (2008). *2008 Mosby's nursing drug reference* (21st ed., p. 1106). St. Louis: Mosby.

386. 3
Rationale: Impetigo is most common during the hot and humid summer months. It begins in an area of broken skin, such as an insect bite. It may be caused by *Staphylococcus aureus*, group A β-hemolytic streptococci, or a combination of these bacteria. It is extremely contagious. Lesions are usually located around the mouth and nose, but they may be present on the extremities.
Test-Taking Strategy: Use the process of elimination, and note the strategic words "indicates the need for further instruction." These words indicate a negative event query and ask you to select an option that is an incorrect statement. Recalling that the lesions are most commonly located around the mouth and nose will direct you to option 3. Review impetigo if you had difficulty with this question.
Level of Cognitive Ability: Comprehension
Client Needs: Health Promotion and Maintenance
Integrated Process: Teaching and Learning
Content Area: Child Health
Reference: Price, D., & Gwin, J. (2008). *Pediatric nursing: An introductory text* (10th ed., pp. 138, 140). St. Louis: Saunders.

387. 3
Rationale: The child should not attend school for 24 to 48 hours after the initiation of systemic antibiotics or for 48 hours after the use of the antibiotic ointment. The school should be notified of the diagnosis. Therefore, options 1, 2, and 4 are incorrect.
Test-Taking Strategy: Use your knowledge related to the administration of antibiotics to answer the question. Eliminate options 1 and 2 first, because the time frames are closely related and rather lengthy. Note the key strategic word "ointment" in the question; this should assist with directing you to option 3. Review the treatment measures for impetigo if you had difficulty with this question.
Level of Cognitive Ability: Application
Client Needs: Safe and Effective Care Environment
Integrated Process: Nursing Process/Implementation
Content Area: Child Health
Reference: McKinney, E., James, S., Murray, S., & Ashwill, J. (2005). *Maternal-child nursing* (2nd ed., p. 366). Philadelphia: Saunders.

388. 3
Rationale: Permethrin 1% is an over-the-counter anti-lice product that kills both lice and eggs with one application and that has residual activity for 10 days. It is applied to dried hair after shampooing and left for 5 to 10 minutes before it is rinsed out. The hair should not be shampooed for 24 hours after the treatment.
Test-Taking Strategy: Use the process of elimination, and note the strategic words "need for further instruction." These words indicate a negative event query and ask you to select an option that is an incorrect statement. Recalling the treatment uses of

this medication will direct you to option 3. Review permethrin 1% treatment if you had difficulty with this question.
Level of Cognitive Ability: Comprehension
Client Needs: Safe and Effective Care Environment
Integrated Process: Teaching and Learning
Content Area: Child Health
References: Lehne, R. (2007). *Pharmacology for nursing care* (6th ed., p. 1141). Philadelphia: Saunders.
Leifer, G. (2007). *Introduction to maternity and pediatric nursing* (5th ed., p. 685). Philadelphia: Saunders.

ALTERNATE ITEM FORMAT: MULTIPLE RESPONSE

389. **2, 3, 4, 6**
Rationale: Scabies appears as burrows or fine, grayish-red lines. It is not caused by a fungal infection, and it is treated with the application of a topical scabicide. It is transmitted by close personal contact with an infected person, and it is endemic among schoolchildren and institutionalized populations. Household members and contacts of the infected child need to be treated at the same time that the child is being treated.
Test-Taking Strategy: Focus on the pathophysiology and transmission of scabies. Recalling that scabies is not associated with a fungal infection will assist you with eliminating options 1 and 5. Review the characteristics of scabies if you had difficulty with this question.
Level of Cognitive Ability: Comprehension
Client Needs: Physiological Integrity
Integrated Process: Nursing Process/Data Collection
Content Area: Child Health
Reference: Hockenberry, M., & Wilson, D. (2007). *Nursing care of infants and children* (8th ed., pp. 271-272). St. Louis: Mosby.

REFERENCES

Burg, F.D., Ingelfinger, J.R., Posin, R.A., & Gershon, A.A. (2006). *Current pediatric therapy* (18th ed.). Philadelphia: Saunders.

Hockenberry, M., & Wilson, D. (2007). *Nursing care of infants and children* (8th ed.). St. Louis: Mosby.

Lehne, R. (2007). *Pharmacology for nursing care* (6th ed.). Philadelphia: Saunders.

Leifer, G. (2007). *Introduction to maternity and pediatric nursing* (5th ed.). Philadelphia: Saunders.

McKinney, E., James, S., Murray, S., & Ashwill, J. (2005). *Maternal-child nursing* (2nd ed.). Philadelphia: Saunders.

National Council of State Boards of Nursing (Eds.). (2008). *2008 Detailed Test Plan for the NCLEX-PN® Examination,* National Council of State Boards of Nursing. Chicago: Author.

National Council of State Boards of Nursing. NCSBN home page. www.ncsbn.org. Accessed July 25, 2008.

Price, D., & Gwin, J. (2008). *Pediatric nursing: An introductory text* (10th ed.). Philadelphia: Saunders.

Skidmore-Roth, L (2008). *2008 Mosby's nursing drug reference* (21st ed.). St. Louis: Mosby.

Musculoskeletal Disorders

I. DYSPLASIA OF THE HIP

A. Description
1. A condition in which the head of the femur is improperly seated in the acetabulum (hip socket) of the pelvis
2. Can range from very mild to severe dislocation
3. Can be congenital or develop after birth

B. Data collection (Figure 36-1)
1. Neonates: Laxity of the ligaments around the hip, which allows the femoral head to be displaced from the acetabulum with manipulation
2. Infants beyond the newborn period
   a. Asymmetry of the gluteal and thigh skin folds when the child is placed prone and the legs are extended against the examining table
   b. Limited range of motion of the affected hip
   c. Asymmetrical abduction of the affected hip when the child is placed supine with the knees and hips flexed
   d. Apparent short femur on the affected side
3. Positive Barlow or Ortolani maneuver; these tests should be performed gently on a relaxed child
4. The walking child: Minimal to pronounced variations in gait with lurching toward the affected side; positive Trendelenburg's sign

C. Interventions
1. During the neonatal period, splinting of the hips with a Pavlik harness to maintain flexion, abduction and, external rotation (Figure 36-2)
2. After the neonatal period, traction and/or surgery to release muscles and tendons
3. After surgery, positioning and immobilization in a spica cast until healing is achieved; then an abduction splint is used
4. Operative reduction may be required in the older child
5. Instruct the parents regarding the proper care of a Pavlik harness or spica cast

II. CONGENITAL CLUBFOOT

A. Description
1. A congenital malformation of the lower extremities

2. The defect may be unilateral or bilateral
3. These defects are rigid and cannot be manipulated into a neutral position
4. Long-term interval follow-up is required until the child reaches skeletal maturity

B. Data collection: The foot is plantarflexed with an inverted heel and an adducted forefoot

C. Interventions
1. Treatment begins as soon after birth as possible
2. Serial manipulation and casting are performed weekly, and, if correction is not achieved in 3 to 6 months, surgery is indicated
3. Monitor for pain
4. Monitor the neurovascular status of the toes
5. Instruct the parents with regard to cast care and the signs of neurovascular impairment that require physician notification

III. IDIOPATHIC SCOLIOSIS

A. Description
1. A three-dimensional spinal deformity that usually involves lateral curvature, spinal rotation that results in rib asymmetry, and hypokyphosis of the thorax
2. Usually diagnosed during the preadolescent **growth** spurt; screenings are important at times when **growth** spurts occur
3. Surgical (spinal fusion and placement of an instrumentation system) and nonsurgical (bracing) interventions are used; the type of treatment depends on the location and degree of the curvature, the age of the child, the amount of **growth** that is still anticipated, and any underlying disease processes
4. Long-term monitoring is essential to detect any progression of the curve

B. Data collection
1. Asymmetry of the ribs and flanks is noted when the child bends forward at the waist and hangs the arms down toward the feet (Adams' test)
2. Hip height, rib positioning, and shoulder height are asymmetrical (this can be noted when standing behind the undressed child); a leg-length discrepancy is also apparent

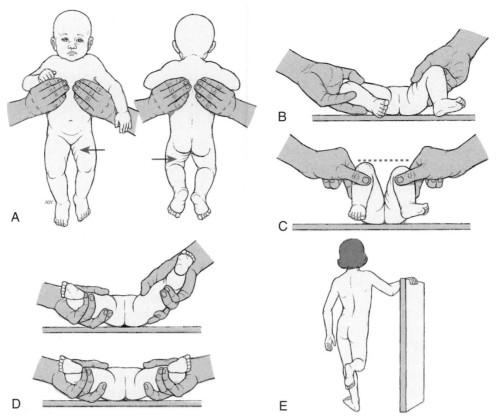

FIG. 36-1 Signs of developmental dysplasia of the hip. **A,** Asymmetry of gluteal and thigh folds. **B,** Limited hip abduction, as seen in flexion. **C,** Apparent shortening of the femur, as indicated by the level of the knees in flexion. **D,** Ortolani click (if infant is under 4 weeks of age). **E,** Positive Trendelenburg's sign of gait (if child is weight bearing) (Hockenberry, M. Wilson, D., & Wilkelstein, M. [2005]. *Wong's essentials of pediatric nursing* [7th ed.]. St. Louis: Mosby.)

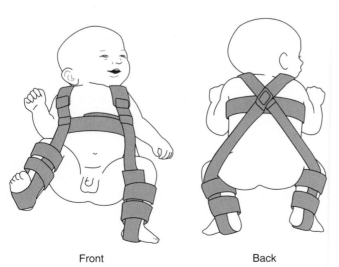

Front   Back

FIG. 36-2 Child in Pavlik harness. (From Hockenberry, M. Wilson, D., & Winkelstein, M. [2005]. *Wong's essentials of pediatric nursing* [7th ed.]. St. Louis: Mosby.)

3. Radiographs are performed to confirm the diagnosis

C. Interventions
   1. Monitor the progression of the curvatures
   2. Prepare the child and parents for the use of a brace, if prescribed; the potential for altered role performance, body-image disturbance, fear, anger, and isolation exists
   3. Prepare the child and parents for surgery (spinal fusion and the placement of internal instrumentation systems), if prescribed

D. Braces
   1. Braces are not curative, but they may slow the progression of the curvature to allow for skeletal **growth** and maturity
   2. Braces usually are prescribed to be worn from 16 to 23 hours a day
   3. Inspect the skin for signs of redness or breakdown
   4. Keep the skin clean and dry, and avoid lotions and powders
   5. Advise the child to wear soft, nonirritating clothing under the brace

6. Instruct the child and parents in the prescribed exercises, which help to maintain and strengthen the spinal and abdominal muscles during treatment
7. Encourage verbalization about body image and other psychosocial issues

E. Postoperative interventions
1. Maintain proper alignment; avoid twisting movements
2. Logroll the child when turning him or her to maintain alignment
3. Assess the extremities for neurovascular status
4. Encourage coughing, deep breathing, and the use of incentive spirometry
5. Assess for pain and administer analgesics, as prescribed
6. Monitor for incontinence
7. Monitor for signs and symptoms of infection
8. Monitor for superior mesenteric artery syndrome, which is caused by mechanical changes in the position of the child's abdominal contents during surgery, and notify the physician if it occurs; symptoms include emesis and abdominal distention similar to that which occurs with intestinal obstruction or paralytic ileus
9. Instruct the child and parents regarding activity restrictions
10. Instruct the child how to roll from a side-lying position to a sitting position, and assist with ambulation
11. Prepare the child for the use of a molded plastic orthosis (brace) jacket to provide external stability of the spine when resuming activities
12. Use extreme sensitivity and consider body-image disturbance when formulating a nursing care plan

IV. JUVENILE IDIOPATHIC RHEUMATOID ARTHRITIS
A. Description
1. An autoimmune inflammatory disease that affects the joints and other tissues (e.g., articular cartilage) and that most often occurs in girls
2. Treatment is supportive (there is no cure) and directed toward preserving joint function, controlling inflammation, minimizing deformity, and reducing the impact that the disease may have on the development of the child
3. Treatment includes medications, physical and occupational therapies, and child and family education
4. Surgical intervention may be implemented if the child has problems with joint contractures and the unequal **growth** of extremities.

B. Data collection (Box 36-1)
1. There are no definitive tests to diagnose the condition

BOX 36-1 **Data Collection: Juvenile Idiopathic Arthritis**

Stiffness, swelling, and limited motion occur in the affected joints.
The affected joints are warm to the touch, tender, and painful.
Joint stiffness is present on arising in the morning and after inactivity.
Uveitis (the inflammation of structures in the uveal tract) can occur and cause blindness.

---

2. Certain laboratory tests (e.g., an elevated erythrocyte sedimentation rate, the presence of leukocytosis) may support evidence of the disease
3. Radiographs may show soft tissue swelling and joint space widening as a result of increased synovial fluid in the joint

C. Interventions
1. Facilitate social and emotional development
2. Instruct the parents and child in the administration of medications; medications may be given alone or in combination and are prescribed in a steplike fashion that is dependent on the disease's response to each level (Box 36-2).
3. Assist the child with range-of-motion exercises; instruct the child and parents with regard to prescribed exercises
4. Encourage the normal performance of activities of daily living
5. Instruct the parents and child in the use of hot and cold packs, splinting, and positioning the affected joint in a neutral position during painful episodes
6. Encourage and support prescribed physical and occupational therapy
7. Instruct the child and parents in the importance of preventive eye care and the reporting of visual disturbances
8. Assess the child's and family's perceptions regarding the chronic illness; plan to discuss the nature of a chronic illness and the grief associated with the new recognition of life alterations that result from the chronic progression of the disorder

V. FRACTURES
A. Description
1. A break in the continuity of the bone as a result of trauma, twisting, or bone decalcification
2. Fractures in children usually result from increased mobility and inadequate or immature motor and cognitive skills
3. Fractures in children may result from trauma, bone diseases, or **abuse**
4. Fractures in infancy are generally rare and warrant further investigation to rule out the possibility of child **abuse**

BOX 36-2 **Medications Used to Treat Juvenile Idiopathic Arthritis**

Nonsteroidal Anti-inflammatory Drugs
- First medications used
- May cause gastrointestinal irritation and bruising

Methotrexate
- Used if NSAIDs are ineffective
- Complete blood cell counts and liver function studies are monitored closely

Corticosteroids
- Potent immunosuppressives that are used to treat life-threatening complications, incapacitating arthritis, and uveitis
- Administered at the lowest effective dose for the briefest period and discontinued on a tapering schedule
- Prolonged use can cause Cushing's syndrome, osteoporosis, increased infection risk, glucose intolerance, cataracts, and growth suppression

Tumor Necrosis Factor Receptor Inhibitors
Etanercept (Enbrel)
Infliximab (Remicade)
- Adverse effects include an allergic reaction at the injection site, increased risk for infection, demyelinating disease, and pancytopenia

Slower-Acting Antirheumatic Drugs (SAARDs)
- May require months to be effective
- Usually prescribed in combination with NSAIDs
- Category includes medications such as sulfasalazine (Azulfidine), hydroxychloroquine (Plaquenil), gold sodium thiomalate (Myochrysine), and D-penicillamine

BOX 36-3 **Initial Care of a Fracture**

Assess the extent of injury, and immobilize the affected extremity.
Observe for the "5 Ps": **P**ain, **P**ulselessness, **P**allor, **P**aresthesia, and **P**aralysis.
Monitor for compartment syndrome.
If a compound fracture exists, splint the extremity to minimize further soft tissue damage, and cover the wound with a sterile dressing.

  a. Used to stabilize a fractured femur before surgery
  b. Similar to Buck's traction but provides a double pull with the use of a knee sling
  c. Traction pulls at the knee and the foot
 2. Balanced suspension
  a. Used with skin or skeletal traction
  b. Used to approximate fractures of the femur, tibia, or fibula
  c. Produced by a counterforce other than the child
  d. Types include a Thomas ring splint with a Pearson attachment, a Steinmann pin, and Kirschner wires
  e. Protect the skin from breakdown
  f. Provide pin care if pins are used with the skeletal traction
 3. 90-degree–90-degree traction
  a. The lower leg is supported by a boot cast or a calf sling
  b. A skeletal Steinmann pin or Kirschner wire is placed in the distal fragment of the femur, which results in a 90-degree angle at both the hip and the knee
 4. Interventions
  a. Maintain the correct amount of weight, as ordered
  b. Ensure that the weights hang freely; they must not be resting on the floor or bed
  c. Check the ropes for fraying, and be sure that they are placed appropriately on the pulleys
  d. Monitor the neurovascular status of the involved extremity frequently
  e. Monitor for signs and symptoms of immobilization (e.g., constipation, skin breakdown) and of disuse syndrome of the unaffected extremities
  f. Monitor for sensory deprivation; provide therapeutic and diversional play
  g. Provide diet modifications, as needed; ensure adequate hydration
  h. Encourage the child to be as active as possible and to participate in his or her own care
  i. Keep in mind the child's developmental level; some regression may occur

  B. Data collection
   1. Pain or tenderness over the involved area
   2. Loss of function
   3. Obvious deformity
   4. Crepitation
   5. Ecchymosis
   6. Edema
   7. Muscle spasm
  C. Initial care of a fracture (Box 36-3)
  D. Interventions
   1. Reduction
    a. Restoring the bone to proper alignment
    b. Closed reduction: Accomplished by the manual alignment of the fragments and followed by immobilization
    c. Open reduction: Requires the surgical insertion of internal fixation devices (e.g., rods, wires, pins) that help maintain alignment while healing occurs
   2. Retention: The application of traction or a cast to maintain alignment until healing occurs
  E. Traction
   1. Russell's skin traction

▲ F. Casts
  1. Description
     a. Made of plaster or fiberglass to provide for the immobilization of bones and joints after a fracture or injury
     b. Fractures of the hip or the knee may require a spica cast
  2. Interventions
     a. Examine the cast for pressure areas
     b. Monitor the extremity for circulatory impairment, such as pain, swelling, discoloration, tingling, numbness, coolness, or diminished pulse
     c. Notify the physician if circulatory impairment occurs
     d. Prepare for bivalving or cutting the cast if circulatory impairment occurs
     e. Instruct the child to not stick objects down the cast
     f. Teach the child to keep the cast clean and dry if he or she is not wearing a waterproof cast.
     g. Instruct the child in isometric exercises to prevent muscle atrophy

PRACTICE QUESTIONS

More questions on the companion CD!

390. A nurse is providing instructions to the parents of a child with scoliosis regarding the use of a brace. Which statement by a parent indicates the need for further instruction?
  1. "I need to have my child wear a soft fabric under the brace."
  2. "I will apply lotion under the brace to prevent skin breakdown."
  3. "I need to encourage my child to perform the prescribed exercises."
  4. "I need to avoid applying powder under the brace, because it will cake."

391. The mother of a child with juvenile idiopathic arthritis calls the nurse because the child is experiencing a painful exacerbation of the disease. The mother asks the nurse if the child should perform range-of-motion (ROM) exercises at this time. The nurse makes which response to the mother?
  1. "Avoid all exercise during painful periods."
  2. "The ROM exercises must be performed every day."
  3. "Have the child perform simple isometric exercises during this time."
  4. "Administer additional pain medication before performing the ROM exercises."

392. A 4-year-old child sustains a fall at home and is brought to the emergency department by the mother. After an x-ray, it is determined that the child has a fractured arm, and a plaster cast is applied. The nurse provides instructions to the mother regarding cast care for the child. Which statement by the mother indicates the need for further instructions?
  1. "The cast may feel warm as it dries."
  2. "I can use lotion or powder around the cast edges to relieve itching."
  3. "A small amount of white shoe polish can touch up a soiled white cast."
  4. "If the cast becomes wet, a blow-dryer set on the cool setting may be used to dry it."

393. A nurse is preparing to perform a neurovascular check for tissue perfusion in the child with an arm cast. Which of the following is the priority when performing this procedure?
  1. Taking the temperature
  2. Taking the blood pressure
  3. Checking the apical heart rate
  4. Checking the peripheral pulse in the affected arm

394. A nurse is performing a neurovascular check on a child with a cast applied to the lower leg. The child complains of tingling in the toes distal to the fracture site. Which action should be taken by the nurse?
  1. Elevate the extremity.
  2. Document the findings.
  3. Notify the registered nurse (RN).
  4. Ambulate the child with crutches.

395. A nurse is assisting a physician during the examination of an infant with hip dysplasia. The physician performs the Ortolani maneuver. Which best describes the action/purpose of the Ortolani maneuver?
  1. Determining the extent of range of motion
  2. Checking for asymmetry on the affected side
  3. Pushing the unstable femoral head out of the acetabulum
  4. Reducing the dislocated femoral head back into the acetabulum

396. A nurse provides information to the mother of a 2-week-old infant who was diagnosed with clubfoot at the time of birth. Which statement by the mother indicates the need for further instruction regarding this disorder?
  1. "Treatment needs to be started as soon as possible."
  2. "I realize my child will require follow-up care until full grown."
  3. "I need to bring my child back to the clinic in 1 month for a new cast."
  4. "I need to come to the clinic every week with my child for the casting."

397. A nurse is assigned to care for a child after a spinal fusion for the treatment of scoliosis. The child complains of abdominal discomfort and begins to have episodes of vomiting. On assessment,

the nurse notes abdominal distention. Which action should the nurse take?
1. Administer an antiemetic.
2. Increase the intravenous fluids.
3. Notify the registered nurse (RN).
4. Place the child in a side-lying Sims' position.

398. A nurse is assigned to care for a child who is in skeletal traction. The nurse avoids which of the following when caring for the child?
1. Keeping the weights hanging freely
2. Ensuring that the ropes are in the pulleys
3. Placing the bed linens on the traction ropes
4. Ensuring that the weights are out of the child's reach

ALTERNATE ITEM FORMAT: MULTIPLE RESPONSE

399. A nurse prepares a list of home-care instructions for the parents of a child who has a plaster cast applied to the left forearm. Choose the instructions that would be included on the list. Select all that apply.
☐ 1. Use the fingertips to lift the cast while it is drying.
☑ 2. Keep small toys and sharp objects away from the cast.
☑ 3. Contact the physician if the child complains of numbness or tingling in the extremity.
☐ 4. Use a padded ruler or another padded object to scratch the skin under the cast if it itches.
☐ 5. Place a heating pad on the lower end of the cast and over the fingers if the fingers feel cold.
☑ 6. Elevate the extremity on pillows for the first 24 to 48 hours after casting to prevent swelling.

ANSWERS

390. 2
Rationale: The use of both lotions or powders should be avoided, because they can become sticky or cake under the brace, thus causing irritation. Options 1, 3, and 4 are appropriate statements regarding the care of a child with a brace.
Test-Taking Strategy: Use the process of elimination, and note the strategic words "need for further instruction." These words indicate a negative event query and ask you to select an option that is an incorrect statement. Recalling that lotions and powders need to be avoided will direct you to option 2. Review the home-care instructions for a child in a brace if you had difficulty with this question.
Level of Cognitive Ability: Comprehension
Client Needs: Health Promotion and Maintenance
Integrated Process: Teaching and Learning
Content Area: Child Health
Reference: Price, D., & Gwin, J. (2008). *Pediatric nursing: An introductory text* (10th ed., p. 348). St. Louis: Saunders.

391. 3
Rationale: During painful episodes, hot or cold packs, splinting, and positioning the affected joint in a neutral position help to reduce the pain. Although resting the extremity is appropriate, it is important to begin simple isometric or tensing exercises as soon as the child is able. These exercises do not involve joint movement.
Test-Taking Strategy: Use the process of elimination. Eliminate options 1, 2, and 4 because of the words "all," "must," and "additional," respectively, in each these options. Review pain management and care during exacerbations of juvenile idiopathic arthritis if you had difficulty with this question.
Level of Cognitive Ability: Application
Client Needs: Physiological Integrity
Integrated Process: Nursing Process/Implementation
Content Area: Child Health

Reference: Price, D., & Gwin, J. (2008). *Pediatric nursing: An introductory text* (10th ed., p. 317). St. Louis: Saunders.

392. 2
Rationale: The mother needs to be instructed to note use lotion or powders on the skin around the cast edges or inside the cast, because they can become sticky or caked and cause skin irritation. Options 1, 3, and 4 are appropriate instructions.
Test-Taking Strategy: Use the process of elimination, and note the strategic words "indicates the need for further instructions." These words indicate a negative event query and ask you to select an option that is an incorrect statement. Recalling the principles related to routine cast care should direct you to option 2. Review home-care instructions regarding cast care if you had difficulty with this question.
Level of Cognitive Ability: Comprehension
Client Needs: Health Promotion and Maintenance
Integrated Process: Teaching and Learning
Content Area: Child Health
Reference: Wong, D., Perry, S., Hockenberry, M., Lowdermilk, D., & Wilson, D. (2006). *Maternal-child nursing care* (3rd ed., p. 1811). St. Louis: Mosby.

393. 4
Rationale: The neurovascular check for tissue perfusion is performed on the toes or fingers distal to an injury or cast and includes peripheral pulse, color, capillary refill time, warmth, motion, and sensation. Options 1, 2, and 3 may be components of care, but they are not the priority in this situation.
Test-Taking Strategy: Use the process of elimination, and note the strategic word "priority." Option 4 is the only option that addresses a neurovascular check. Review the components of a neurovascular check if you had difficulty with this question.
Level of Cognitive Ability: Application
Client Needs: Physiological Integrity

Integrated Process: Nursing Process/Data Collection
Content Area: Delegating/Prioritizing
Reference: Leifer, G. (2007). *Introduction to maternity and pediatric nursing* (5th ed., p. 556). Philadelphia: Saunders.

394. **3**
Rationale: Reduced sensation to touch or complaints of numbness or tingling at a site distal to the fracture may indicate poor tissue perfusion. This finding should be reported to the RN. Options 1, 2, and 4 are inappropriate and would delay the required and immediate interventions.
Test-Taking Strategy: Use the process of elimination, and recall the signs of circulatory compromise. Noting the child's complaint will assist with directing you to option 3. Review the complications associated with a cast if you had difficulty with this question.
Level of Cognitive Ability: Application
Client Needs: Physiological Integrity
Integrated Process: Nursing Process/Implementation
Content Area: Child Health
Reference: Leifer, G. (2007). *Introduction to maternity and pediatric nursing* (5th ed., p. 556). Philadelphia: Saunders.

395. **4**
Rationale: When performing the Barlow maneuver, the examiner pushes the unstable femoral head out of the acetabulum. With the Ortolani maneuver, the examiner reduces the dislocated femoral head back into the acetabulum. A positive Ortolani maneuver is a palpable clink as the femoral head moves over the acetabular ring. Options 1 and 2 are data-collection techniques for the identification of the clinical manifestations of hip dysplasia, but they do not describe the Ortolani maneuver.
Test-Taking Strategy: Use the process of elimination. Eliminate options 1 and 2 first, because they are data-collection techniques. From the remaining options, it is necessary to know the action/purpose of the Ortolani maneuver. Review the Ortolani maneuver if you had difficulty with this question.
Level of Cognitive Ability: Comprehension
Client Needs: Physiological Integrity
Integrated Process: Nursing Process/Data Collection
Content Area: Child Health
Reference: Hockenberry, M., & Wilson, D. (2007). *Nursing care of infants and children* (8th ed., pp. 452-454). St. Louis: Mosby.

396. **3**
Rationale: The treatment for clubfoot is started as soon as possible after birth. Serial manipulation and casting are performed at least weekly. If sufficient correction is not achieved within 3 to 6 months, surgery is usually indicated. Because clubfoot can recur, all children with the condition require long-term interval follow-up until they reach skeletal maturity to ensure an optimal outcome.
Test-Taking Strategy: Use the process of elimination, and focus on the subject of the treatment plan for clubfoot. Note the strategic words "indicates the need for further instruction" to assist you with eliminating options 1 and 2. Recalling that serial manipulations and casting are required weekly will direct you to option 3. Review the treatment procedures for clubfoot if you had difficulty with this question.

Level of Cognitive Ability: Comprehension
Client Needs: Physiological Integrity
Integrated Process: Teaching and Learning
Content Area: Child Health
Reference: Price, D., & Gwin, J. (2008). *Pediatric nursing: An introductory text* (10th ed., p. 106). St. Louis: Saunders.

397. **3**
Rationale: A complication after the surgical treatment of scoliosis is superior mesenteric artery syndrome. This disorder is caused by mechanical changes in the position of the child's abdominal contents that result from the lengthening of the child's body. It results in a syndrome of emesis and abdominal distention that is similar to that which occurs with intestinal obstruction or paralytic ileus. Postoperative vomiting among children with body casts or among those who have undergone spinal fusion warrants attention because of the possibility of superior mesenteric artery syndrome.
Test-Taking Strategy: Use the process of elimination. Eliminate option 2 first, because it should not be implemented without a prescribed order. Eliminate option 4 next, because this child requires logrolling, and the Sims' position may cause injury after surgery. From the remaining options, note the signs and symptoms in the question; these should alert you that the RN needs to be notified. Review superior mesenteric artery syndrome if you had difficulty with this question.
Level of Cognitive Ability: Application
Client Needs: Physiological Integrity
Integrated Process: Nursing Process/Implementation
Content Area: Child Health
References: McKinney, E., James, S., Murray, S., & Ashwill, J. (2005). *Maternal-child nursing* (2nd ed., p. 1402). Philadelphia: Saunders.
Price, D., & Gwin, J. (2008). *Pediatric nursing: An introductory text* (10th ed., p. 347). St. Louis: Saunders.

398. **3**
Rationale: Bed linens should not be placed on the traction ropes because of the risk of disrupting the traction apparatus. Options 1, 2, and 4 are appropriate measures when caring for a child who is in skeletal traction.
Test-Taking Strategy: Note the strategic word "avoids." This word indicates a negative event query and asks you to select an option that is an incorrect intervention. Use the process of elimination and your knowledge regarding the care of the child in traction to direct you to option 3. Review the nursing measures for the child in traction if you had difficulty with this question.
Level of Cognitive Ability: Application
Client Needs: Physiological Integrity
Integrated Process: Nursing Process/Implementation
Content Area: Child Health
Reference: Leifer, G. (2007). *Introduction to maternity and pediatric nursing* (5th ed., p. 553). Philadelphia: Saunders.

ALTERNATE ITEM FORMAT: MULTIPLE RESPONSE

399. **2, 3, 6**
Rationale: While the cast is drying, the palms of the hands are used to lift the cast. If the fingertips are used, indentations in

the cast could occur and cause constant pressure on the underlying skin. Small toys and sharp objects are kept away from the cast, and no objects (including padded objects) are placed inside of the cast because of the risk of altered skin integrity. The extremity is elevated to prevent swelling, and the physician is notified immediately if any signs of neurovascular impairment develop. A heating pad is not applied to the cast or fingers. Cold fingers could indicate neurovascular impairment, and the physician should be notified.

Test-Taking Strategy: Use of the ABCs—airway, breathing, and circulation—and safety principles related to the care of a child with a cast will assist you with answering the question. Review these general principles if you had difficulty with this question.

Level of Cognitive Ability: Application
Client Needs: Physiological Integrity
Integrated Process: Teaching and Learning
Content Area: Child Health
References: McKinney, E., James, S., Murray, S., & Ashwill, J. (2005). *Maternal-child nursing* (2nd ed., p. 1411). Philadelphia: Elsevier.
Wong, D., Perry, S., Hockenberry, M., Lowdermilk, D., & Wilson, D. (2006). *Maternal-child nursing care* (3rd ed., p. 1811). St. Louis: Mosby.

REFERENCES

Hockenberry, M., & Wilson, D. (2007). *Nursing care of infants and children* (8th ed.). St. Louis: Mosby.

Leifer, G. (2007). *Introduction to maternity and pediatric nursing* (5th ed.). Philadelphia: Saunders.

McKinney, E., James, S., Murray, S., & Ashwill, J. (2005). *Maternal-child nursing* (2nd ed.). Philadelphia: Saunders.

National Council of State Boards of Nursing (Eds.). (2008). *2008 Detailed Test Plan for the NCLEX-PN® Examination, National Council of State Boards of Nursing.* Chicago: Author.

National Council of State Boards of Nursing. *NCSBN home page.* www.ncsbn.org. Accessed July 25, 2008.

Price, D., & Gwin, J. (2008). *Pediatric nursing: An introductory text* (10th ed.). St. Louis: Saunders.

Wong, D., Perry, S., Hockenberry, M., Lowdermilk, D., & Wilson, D. (2006). *Maternal-child nursing care* (3rd ed.). St. Louis: Mosby.

Hematological and Oncological Disorders

I. SICKLE CELL DISEASE
A. Description (Figure 37-1)
   1. One of a group of diseases that are collectively called hemoglobinopathies in which hemoglobin (Hgb) A is partly or completely replaced by abnormal sickle hemoglobin (HgbS)
   2. Caused by the inheritance of a gene for a structurally abnormal portion of the Hgb chain
   3. HgbS is sensitive to changes in the oxygen content of the red blood cell (RBC)
   4. Insufficient oxygen causes the cells to assume a sickle shape, and the cells become rigid and clumped together, thus obstructing capillary blood flow; this can cause a stroke
   5. Situations that precipitate sickling include fever and emotional or physical stress; any condition that increases the body's need for oxygen or that alters the transport of oxygen can result in sickle cell crisis
   6. Risk factors include having parents who are heterozygous for HgbS and being black
   7. The sickling response is reversible under conditions of adequate oxygenation and hydration; after repeated sickling, the cell becomes permanently sickled
   8. The clinical manifestations are primarily the result of obstruction caused by sickled RBCs and increased RBC destruction
   9. Sickle cell crises are acute exacerbations of the disease, which vary markedly in severity and frequency; these include vaso-occlusive crisis, splenic sequestration, and aplastic crisis
   10. Care focuses on the prevention (preventing exposure to infection and maintaining normal hydration) and treatment (oxygen, hydration, pain management, and bedrest) of the crisis
B. Sickle cell crisis: Data collection (Box 37-1)
C. Interventions
   1. Maintain adequate hydration and blood flow with intravenous (IV) normal saline, as prescribed, and with oral fluids
   2. Administer oxygen, as prescribed, to increase tissue perfusion; blood transfusions may also be prescribed
   3. Assess pain; maintain effective pain management with the administration of analgesics, as prescribed; the administration of meperidine (Demerol) is avoided because of the risk of normeperidine-induced seizures as a result of central nervous system toxicity
   4. Assist the child with assuming a comfortable position so that the child keeps the extremities extended to promote venous return; elevate the head of the bed no more than 30 degrees, avoid putting strain on painful joints, and do not raise the knee gatch of the bed
   5. Encourage the consumption of a high-calorie, high-protein diet with folic acid supplementation
   6. Administer antibiotics, as prescribed, to prevent infection
   7. Monitor for signs of increasing anemia and shock (i.e., mental status changes, pallor, and vital sign changes)
   8. Instruct the child and parents about the early signs and symptoms of crisis and the measures to prevent and alleviate a painful vaso-occlusive crisis
   9. Provide the parents with appropriate genetic counseling information and resources
   10. Emphasize the need to maintain strict adherence to immunization schedules

II. IRON DEFICIENCY ANEMIA
A. Description
   1. Iron stores are depleted, which results in a decreased supply of iron for the manufacture of hemoglobin in RBCs
   2. Commonly results from blood loss, increased metabolic demands, syndromes of gastrointestinal (GI) malabsorption, and dietary inadequacy
   3. Iron deficiency is associated with potentially irreversible developmental delays, behavioral disturbances, and learning impairments

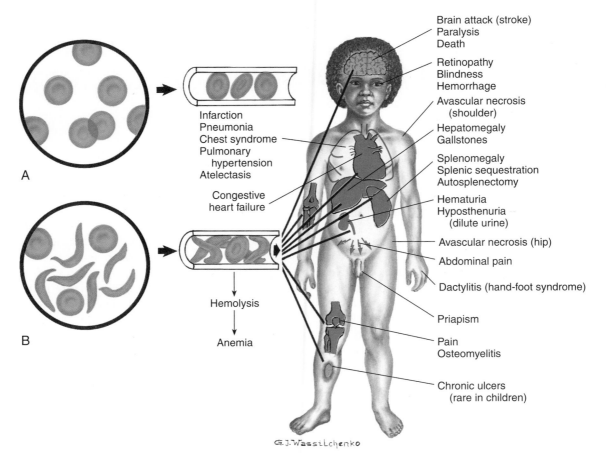

FIG. 37-1   Differences between **(A)** normal red blood cells and **(B)** sickled red blood cells in circulation with related complications. (From Hockenberry, M., & Wilson, D. [2007]. *Wong's nursing care of infants and children* [8th ed.]. St. Louis: Mosby.)

BOX 37-1   Sickle Cell Crisis

Vaso-Occlusive Crisis

The crisis is caused by ischemia, infarction, and the stasis of blood with clumping of the cells in the microcirculation.

Manifestations include fever; painful swelling of the hands, feet, and joints; and abdominal pain.

Splenic Sequestration

This is caused by the pooling and clumping of blood in the spleen (hypersplenism).

Manifestations include profound anemia, hypovolemia, and shock.

Aplastic Crisis

This is caused by the diminished production and increased destruction of red blood cells, which is triggered by viral infection or the depletion of folic acid.

Manifestations include profound anemia and pallor.

B. Data collection
   1. Pallor
   2. Weakness and fatigue
   3. Irritability
C. Interventions
   1. Increase oral intake of iron

2. Instruct the child and parents regarding food choices that are high in iron (Box 37-2)
3. Teach the parents how to administer the iron supplements
   a. Give them between meals for maximum absorption
   b. Give them with a multivitamin or fruit juice, because vitamin C increases absorption (fruit juice should be avoided among children who are less than 1 year old to prevent the introduction of allergens)
   c. Do not give them with milk or antacids, because these decrease absorption
   d. Teach the child and parents that liquid iron preparations stain the teeth and should be taken through a straw
   e. Instruct the child and parents about the side effects of iron supplements (i.e., black stools, constipation, and foul aftertaste)
4. Promote the universal screening of infants in communities with low incomes, recent immigration, and known risk factors

---

BOX 37-2 **Iron-Rich Foods**

- Breads and cereals
- Dark green, leafy vegetables
- Dried fruits
- Egg yolks
- Iron-enriched infant formula and cereal
- Kidney beans
- Legumes
- Liver
- Meats
- Molasses
- Nuts
- Potatoes
- Prune juice
- Raisins
- Seeds
- Shellfish
- Tofu
- Whole grains

BOX 37-3 **Hemophilia**

- *Hemophilia A* (classic hemophilia): Results from a deficiency of factor VIII
- *Hemophilia B* (Christmas disease): Results from a deficiency of factor IX

III. APLASTIC ANEMIA

A. Description
   1. A deficiency of circulating erythrocytes that results from the arrested development of RBCs within the bone marrow
   2. There are several possible causes, including chronic exposure to myelotoxic agents, viruses, infection, autoimmune disorders, and allergic states
   3. The definitive diagnosis is determined by bone marrow aspiration, which demonstrates the conversion of red bone marrow to yellow fatty bone marrow
   4. Therapeutic management focuses on restoring function to the bone marrow and involves immunosuppressive therapy and bone marrow transplantation (BMT); BMT is the treatment of choice if a suitable donor exists, and the preferable donor is a matched sibling

B. Data collection
   1. Pancytopenia (a deficiency of erythrocytes, leukocytes, and thrombocytes)
   2. Petechiae, purpura, bleeding, pallor, weakness, tachycardia, and fatigue

C. Interventions
   1. Prepare the child for BMT, if planned
   2. Immunosuppressive medications: Antilymphocyte globulin or antithymocyte globulin may be prescribed to suppress the autoimmune response
   3. Colony-stimulating factors may be prescribed to enhance bone marrow production
   4. Corticosteroids and cyclosporine (Sandimmune) may be prescribed
   5. Blood or platelet transfusions may be prescribed
   6. Advise the parents to obtain a Medic-Alert bracelet for the child

IV. HEMOPHILIA

A. Description (Box 37-3)
   1. Refers to a group of bleeding disorders resulting from a deficiency of specific coagulation proteins
   2. Is transmitted as an X-linked recessive disorder most frequently by the union of an unaffected male with a trait-carrier female; however, it can result from the union between an affected male and a normal female or a carrier female, leading to offspring such as an affected son, affected daughter, carrier daughter, or normal son.
   3. The primary treatment is the replacement of the missing clotting factor; additional medications, such as those to relieve pain, may be prescribed depending on the source of bleeding

B. Data collection
   1. Abnormal bleeding in response to trauma or surgery; this condition is often diagnosed during the newborn period after circumcision or vitamin K injection
   2. Joint bleeding that causes pain, tenderness, swelling, and a limited range of motion
   3. Tendency to bruise easily
   4. Prolonged partial thromboplastin time
   5. Results of tests that measure platelet function are normal; results of tests that measure clotting factor function may be abnormal

C. Interventions
   1. Monitor for bleeding and maintain bleeding precautions
   2. Factor VIII concentrate or DDAVP may be prescribed
   3. Monitor for joint pain; immobilize the affected extremity if joint pain occurs
   4. Monitor the neurological status; the child with this condition is at risk for intracranial hemorrhage
   5. Monitor the urine for hematuria
   6. Control bleeding by immobilization, elevation, and the application of ice; in addition, apply pressure (15 minutes) for superficial bleeding
   7. Instruct the child and parents about the signs of internal bleeding
   8. Instruct the parents regarding how to control the bleeding
   9. Instruct the parents regarding activities for the child, emphasizing the avoidance of contact sports
   10. Instruct the child to wear protective devices such as helmets and knee and elbow pads

when participating in sports such as bicycling and skating

11. Instruct the parents to obtain a Medic-Alert bracelet for the child

V. VON WILLEBRAND'S DISEASE

A. Description
1. A **hereditary** bleeding disorder characterized by a deficiency of or a defect in the protein called von Willebrand's factor (vWF)
2. The disorder causes platelets to adhere to damaged endothelium; the vWF protein also serves as a carrier protein for factor VIII
3. It is characterized by an increased tendency to bleed from the mucous membranes

B. Data collection
1. Epistaxis
2. Gum bleeding
3. Easy bruising
4. Excessive menstrual bleeding

C. Interventions
1. Treatment and care are similar to those measures implemented for hemophilia, including the administration of clotting factors
2. Provide emotional support to the child and parents, especially if the child is experiencing an episode of bleeding.

VI. β-THALASSEMIA

A. Description (Box 37-4)
1. An autosomal-recessive disorder characterized by the reduced production of a globin chain in the synthesis of hemoglobin
2. The incidence is highest among individuals of Mediterranean descent
3. Treatment is supportive; the goal of therapy is to maintain normal hemoglobin levels by the administration of blood transfusions
4. BMT may be offered as an alternative therapy
5. A splenectomy may be performed in a child with severe splenomegaly who demonstrates increased transfusion requirements; this treatment assists with relieving abdominal pressure and may increase the life span of supplemental red blood cells

B. Data collection
1. Frontal bossing
2. Maxillary prominence
3. Wide-set eyes with a flattened nose
4. Greenish-yellow skin tone
5. Hepatosplenomegaly
6. Severe anemia
7. Microcytic, hypochromic RBCs

C. Interventions
1. Blood transfusions may be prescribed
2. Monitor for iron overload, and administer chelation therapy with deferoxamine (Desferal), as prescribed, to treat iron overload and to prevent organ damage from the elevated levels

BOX 37-4 Types of β-Thalassemia

- *Thalassemia minor:* Asymptomatic, silent-carrier case
- *Thalassemia trait:* Produces a mild microcytic anemia
- *Thalassemia intermedia:* Manifested as splenomegaly and moderate to severe anemia
- *Thalassemia major:* Results in severe anemia that requires transfusion support to sustain life (also known as Cooley's anemia)

TABLE 37-1 Classification of Leukemia

Acute Lymphocytic Leukemia	Acute Myelogenous Leukemia
Mostly lymphoblasts present in bone marrow	Mostly myeloblasts present in bone marrow
Age of onset is younger than 15 years	Age of onset is between 15 and 39 years

of iron caused by the multiple transfusion therapy
3. If the child has had a splenectomy, instruct the parents to report any signs of infection because of the risk of sepsis
4. Provide resources for genetic counseling

VII. LEUKEMIA (Table 37-1)

A. Description
1. Malignant exacerbation in the number of leukocytes, usually at an immature stage, in the bone marrow
2. Affects the bone marrow, thus causing anemia from decreased erythrocytes, infection from neutropenia, and bleeding from decreased platelet production
3. The cause is unknown and appears to involve the gene damage of cells, thus leading to the transformation of cells from a normal state to a malignant state
4. Risk factors include genetic, viral, immunological, and environmental factors and exposure to radiation, chemicals, and medications
5. Acute lymphocytic leukemia is the most frequent type of cancer in children; the peak onset is from the ages of 2 to 6 years
6. More common among boys than girls after 1 year of age
7. Treatment involves the use of chemotherapeutic agents with or without cranial radiation
8. The phases of treatment include the following: induction, which achieves a complete remission or disappearance of leukemic cells; intensification or consolidation therapy, which further decreases the tumor burden; central nervous system prophylactic therapy, which prevents leukemic cells from invading the central nervous system; and

maintenance, which serves to maintain the remission phase

9. BMT may also be performed to treat some children with leukemia

B. Data collection
1. Infiltration of the bone marrow causes fever, pallor, fatigue, anorexia, hemorrhage (usually petechiae), and bone and joint pain; pathological fractures can occur as a result of bone marrow invasion with leukemic cells
2. Signs of infection as a result of neutropenia
3. Hepatosplenomegaly and lymphadenopathy
4. Normal, elevated, or low white blood cell count
5. Decreased hemoglobin and hematocrit levels
6. Decreased platelet count
7. Positive bone marrow biopsy identifying leukemic blast (immature) phase cells
8. Signs of increased intracranial pressure, such as severe headache, vomiting, papilledema, irritability, lethargy, and, eventually, coma, as a result of central nervous system involvement
9. Signs of cranial nerve (cranial nerve VII [the facial nerve] is most commonly affected) or spinal nerve involvement; clinical manifestations relate to the area involved
10. Clinical manifestations that indicate the invasion of leukemic cells in the kidneys, testes, prostate, ovaries, GI tract, and lungs

C. Infection (Box 37-5)
1. A major cause of death in the immunosuppressed child
2. Most common sites of infection are the skin (any break in the skin is a potential site of infection), respiratory tract, and GI tract

D. Bleeding (Box 37-6)
1. Children with platelet counts less than 20,000/mm^3 may need a platelet transfusion
2. For children with severe blood loss, packed red blood cells may be prescribed

E. Fatigue and nutrition
1. Assist the child with selecting a well-balanced diet
2. Provide small meals that require little chewing
3. Assist the child with self-care and mobility activities
4. Allow for adequate rest periods during care
5. Do not perform activities unless they are essential

F. Chemotherapy
1. Monitor for severe bone marrow suppression; during the period of greatest bone marrow suppression (the nadir), blood counts will be extremely low
2. Monitor for infection and bleeding
3. Protect the child from life-threatening infections
4. Monitor for nausea, vomiting, and diarrhea
5. Administer antiemetics, as prescribed
6. Monitor for signs of dehydration
7. Monitor for signs of hemorrhagic cystitis

BOX 37-5 Protecting the Child from Infection

Initiate protective isolation procedures.

Maintain frequent and thorough handwashing.

Maintain the child in a private room with high-efficiency particulate air filtration or laminar airflow system, if possible.

Be sure that the child's room is cleaned daily.

Use strict aseptic technique for all nursing procedures.

Limit the number of caregivers entering the child's room, and ensure that anyone entering the child's room is wearing a mask.

Keep supplies for the child separate from supplies for other children.

Reduce exposure to environmental organisms by eliminating raw fruits and vegetables and fresh flowers and by not leaving standing water in the child's room.

Assist the child with daily bathing with the use of antimicrobial soap.

Assist the child with performing oral hygiene frequently.

Monitor for signs and symptoms of infection.

Monitor the temperature, pulse, and blood pressure.

Change wound dressings daily, and inspect wounds for redness, swelling, or drainage.

Monitor the urine for color and cloudiness.

Monitor the skin and oral mucous membranes for signs of infection.

Check the lung sounds.

Encourage the child to cough and deep breathe.

Monitor the white blood cell and the neutrophil count.

Notify the physician if signs of infection are present; prepare to obtain specimens for the culture of open lesions, urine, and sputum.

Initiate a bowel program to prevent constipation and rectal trauma.

Avoid invasive procedures, such as injections, rectal temperatures, and urinary catheterization.

Administer antibiotic, antifungal, and antiviral medication, as prescribed.

Administer granulocyte colony-stimulating factor, as prescribed.

Instruct the parents to keep the child away from crowds and those with infections.

Instruct the parents that the child should not receive immunization with a live virus.

Keep any child with chickenpox or any child who has been exposed to the virus away from the child with leukemia.

Instruct the parents to inform the teacher that they should be notified immediately if a case of chickenpox occurs in another child at school.

---

8. Monitor for signs of peripheral neuropathy
9. Check the oral mucous membranes for mucositis; administer frequent mouth rinses (normal saline with or without sodium bicarbonate solution) to promote healing if mucositis occurs
10. Instruct the parents regarding the signs and symptoms to monitor after chemotherapy and when to notify the physician

BOX 37-6 **Protecting the Child From Bleeding**

Examine the child for signs and symptoms of bleeding.
Handle the child gently.
Measure the abdominal girth, which can indicate internal hemorrhage.
Instruct the child to use a soft toothbrush and to avoid dental floss.
Provide soft foods that are cool to warm in temperature.
Avoid injections, if possible, to prevent trauma to the skin and bleeding.
Apply firm and gentle pressure to a needle-stick site for at least 10 minutes.
Pad side rails and sharp corners of the bed and other furniture.
Discourage the child from engaging in activities that involve the use of sharp objects.
Instruct the child to avoid constrictive or tight clothing.
Use caution when taking the blood pressure to prevent skin injury.
Instruct the child to avoid blowing his or her nose.
Avoid rectal suppositories, enemas, and rectal thermometers.
Examine all body fluids and excrement for the presence of blood.
Count the number of pads or tampons used if the female adolescent is menstruating.
Instruct the child regarding the signs and symptoms of bleeding.
Instruct the parents to avoid administering nonsteroidal anti-inflammatory drugs and products that contain aspirin to the child.

11. Inform the parents that hair loss may occur from chemotherapy; the hair will regrow in 3 to 6 months and may be a slightly different color or texture
12. Instruct the parents about the care of a central venous access device, as necessary
13. Listen to the child and family, and encourage them to verbalize their feelings and express their concerns
14. Introduce the family to other families of children with cancer
15. Consult social services and chaplains, as necessary

VIII. HODGKIN'S DISEASE (Box 37-7)
A. Description
    1. A malignancy of the lymph nodes that originates in a single lymph node or a single chain of nodes
    2. It predictably metastasizes to non-nodal or extra-lymphatic sites, especially the spleen, liver, bone marrow, lungs, and mediastinum (Figure 37-2)
    3. Characterized by the presence of Reed-Sternberg cells in the lymph nodes
    4. Possible causes include viral infections and previous exposure to alkylating chemical agents

BOX 37-7 **Staging of Hodgkin's Disease**

Stage I
Involvement of a single lymph node region or only one extralymphatic organ or site, such as the liver, kidneys, lungs, or intestines
Stage II
Involvement of two or more lymph node regions on the same side of the diaphragm or one additional extralymphatic organ or site on the same side of the diaphragm
Stage III
Involvement of lymph node regions on both sides of the diaphragm or one extralymphatic organ or site, the spleen, or both
Stage IV
Diffuse or disseminated involvement of one or more extralymphatic organs, with or without associated lymph node involvement

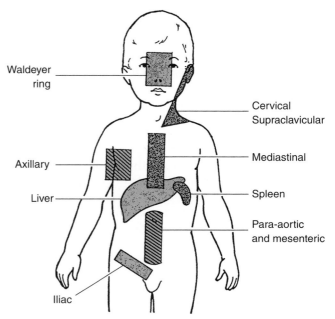

FIG. 37-2 Main areas of lymphadenopathy and organ involvement in Hodgkin's disease. (From Hockenberry, M., Wilson, D., & Winklestein, M. [2005]. *Wong's essentials of pediatric nursing* [7th ed.]. St. Louis: Mosby.)

    5. The prognosis is dependent on the stage of disease; it is excellent in children with localized disease
    6. The primary treatment modalities are radiation and chemotherapy; each may be used alone or in combination, depending on the clinical staging of the disease
    7. BMT may be a consideration for treatment
B. Data collection
    1. Painless enlargement of the lymph nodes
    2. Enlarged, firm, nontender, movable nodes in the supraclavicular area; in children, the

sentinel node located near the left clavicle may be the first enlarged node

3. Nonproductive cough as a result of mediastinal lymphadenopathy
4. Abdominal pain as a result of enlarged retroperitoneal nodes
5. Advanced lymph node and extralymphatic involvement may cause systemic symptoms, such as low-grade and/or intermittent fever, anorexia, nausea, weight loss, night sweats, and pruritus
6. Positive biopsy of a lymph node (presence of Reed-Sternberg cells) and positive bone marrow biopsy
7. Computed tomography scan of the liver, spleen, and bone marrow to detect metastasis

C. Interventions
1. For stages 1 and 2 without mediastinal node involvement, the treatment of choice is extensive external radiation of the involved lymph node regions
2. With more extensive disease, radiation in combination with multiagent chemotherapy is used
3. Monitor for drug-induced pancytopenia, which increases the risk for infection, bleeding, and anemia
4. Protect the child from infection
5. Provide a safe, hazard-free environment
6. Monitor for side effects related to chemotherapy or radiation; the most common complication of radiation of the neck area is hypothyroidism
7. Monitor for nausea and vomiting; administer antiemetics, as prescribed
8. Monitor for skin irritation and breakdown as a result of radiation therapy

IX. NEPHROBLASTOMA (WILMS' TUMOR)
A. Description
1. A tumor of the kidney that may present unilaterally and localized or bilaterally, sometimes with metastasis to other organs
2. The peak incidence is at 3 years of age
3. Associated with a genetic inheritance and with several congenital anomalies
4. Therapeutic management includes a combination treatment of surgery (partial to total nephrectomy) and chemotherapy with or without radiation, depending on the clinical stage and histologic pattern

B. Data collection
1. A swelling or mass within the abdomen; the mass is characteristically firm, nontender, confined to one side, and deep within the flank
2. Abdominal pain
3. Urinary retention and/or hematuria
4. Anemia secondary to hemorrhage within the tumor

5. Pallor, anorexia, and lethargy that occur as a result of anemia
6. Hypertension that is caused by the secretion of excess amounts of renin by the tumor
7. Weight loss and fever
8. Symptoms of lung involvement, such as dyspnea, shortness of breath, and pain in the chest, if metastasis has occurred

C. Preoperative interventions
1. Monitor the vital signs, particularly the blood pressure
2. Place a sign at the bedside that reads as follows: "Do not palpate abdomen"
3. Avoid the palpation of the abdomen
4. Measure the abdominal girth

D. Postoperative interventions
1. Monitor the temperature and blood pressure closely
2. Monitor for signs of hemorrhage and infection
3. Monitor strict intake and output closely
4. Monitor for abdominal distention, bowel sounds, and other signs of GI activity because of the risk for intestinal obstruction

X. NEUROBLASTOMA
A. Description
1. An embryonal tumor found in children that arises from the neural crest
2. The primary site is in the abdomen, because the tumor arises from the adrenal gland or from the retroperitoneal sympathetic chain; it may also occur in the head, neck, chest, or pelvis
3. Most presenting signs are caused by the tumor compressing adjacent normal tissue and organs
4. Diagnostic evaluation is aimed at locating the primary site of the tumor
5. The prognosis is poor because of the frequency of invasiveness of the tumor and because, in most cases, the diagnosis is not made until after metastasis has occurred
6. Surgery is performed to remove as much of the tumor as possible and to obtain samples for biopsy; in stages 1 and 2, complete surgical removal of the tumor is the treatment of choice
7. Surgery is usually limited to biopsy in stages 3 and 4 because of the extensive metastasis
8. Radiation is commonly used with stage 3 disease and provides palliation for metastatic lesions in the bones, lungs, liver, or brain
9. Chemotherapy is the mainstay of treatment for extensive local or disseminated disease

B. Data collection: Signs and symptoms depend on the location of the primary tumor
1. Firm, nontender, irregular mass in the abdomen that crosses the midline
2. Urinary frequency or retention from the compression of the kidney, ureter, or bladder

3. Lymphadenopathy, especially in the cervical and supraclavicular area
4. Bone pain if skeletal involvement occurs
5. Supraorbital ecchymosis (raccoon eyes), periorbital edema, and exophthalmos as a result of the invasion of retrobulbar soft tissue
6. Pallor, weakness, irritability, anorexia, fever, limping, anemia, and weight loss
7. Signs of respiratory impairment (thoracic lesion)
8. Signs of neurological impairment (intracranial lesion)
9. Paralysis from the compression of the spinal cord

C. Preoperative interventions
1. Monitor for signs and symptoms related to the location of the tumor
2. Provide emotional support to the child and parents

D. Postoperative interventions
1. Monitor for postoperative complications related to the location (organ) of the surgery
2. Monitor for complications related to chemotherapy or radiation, if prescribed
3. Provide support for the parents, and encourage them to express their feelings; many parents suffer from guilt for not having recognized signs in the child earlier
4. Refer the parents to appropriate community services

XI. OSTEOGENIC SARCOMA

A. Description
1. The most common bone cancer in children
2. Usually found in the metaphysis of the long bones, especially in the lower extremities, with most tumors occurring in the femur
3. Peak age of incidence is between 10 and 25 years
4. Symptoms during the earliest stage are almost always attributed to extremity injury or normal growing pains
5. Treatment may include surgical resection to save a limb or to remove affected tissue, or amputation
6. Chemotherapy plays a vital role in treatment and may be employed both before and after surgery
7. Metastasis may occur, with the lungs being the most frequent site;

B. Data collection
1. Localized pain at the affected site (may be severe or dull) that may be attributed to trauma or the vague complaint of "growing pains"; pain is often relieved by a flexed position
2. Palpable mass
3. Limping if weight-bearing limb is affected
4. Progressively limited range of motion; child curtails physical activity

5. Child may be unable to hold heavy objects
6. Pathological fractures at the tumor site

C. Interventions
1. Prepare the child and family for prescribed treatment modalities, which may include surgical resection to remove affected tissue, amputation, and chemotherapy
2. Provide honesty and support to the child and family
3. Prepare for prosthetic fitting, as necessary
4. Assist the child with dealing with self-image problems

XII. BRAIN TUMORS

A. Description
1. An infratentorial (below the tentorium cerebelli) tumor is located in the posterior third of the brain (primarily in the cerebellum or brainstem) and accounts for the frequency of symptoms that result from increased intracranial pressure (ICP)
2. A supratentorial tumor is located within the anterior two thirds of the brain, mainly the cerebrum
3. The signs and symptoms of a brain tumor depend on its anatomical location and size and, to some extent, on the age of the child
4. Therapeutic management includes surgery, radiation, and chemotherapy; the treatment of choice is the total removal of the tumor without residual neurological damage

B. Data collection
1. Headache that is worse on awakening and that improves during the day
2. Vomiting that is unrelated to feeding or eating
3. Behavioral changes
4. Lethargy or hyperactivity
5. Clumsiness; awkward gait or difficulty walking
6. Seizures
7. Infant may display failure to thrive, bulging fontanels, and increased head circumference

C. Preoperative interventions
1. Monitor the neurological status
2. Institute safety measures
3. Monitor the weight and nutritional status
4. Initiate seizure precautions
5. The child's head will be shaved (provide a favorite cap or hat for the child)
6. Prepare the child as much as possible; tell the child that he or she will wake up with a large head dressing

D. Postoperative interventions
1. Monitor for signs of increased ICP or hemorrhage; check the back of the head dressing for the posterior pooling of blood
2. Monitor the neurological and motor function and the level of consciousness

BOX 37-8 **Positioning After Craniotomy**

Check the physician's order for positioning, including the degree of neck flexion.

If a large tumor was removed, the child is not placed on the operative side, because the brain may suddenly shift into the cavity.

After an infratentorial procedure, the child is usually positioned flat or on either side.

After a supratentorial procedure, the head is usually elevated above the level of the heart to facilitate the drainage of cerebrospinal fluid and to decrease excessive blood flow to the brain to prevent hemorrhage.

Never place the child in Trendelenburg's position, because it increases the intracranial pressure and the risk of hemorrhage.

3. Monitor the temperature closely, because it may be elevated as a result of hypothalamus or brainstem involvement during surgery; maintain a cooling blanket by the bedside

4. Monitor for signs of respiratory infection

5. Monitor for signs of meningitis (opisthotonos, Kernig's and Brudzinski's signs)

6. Monitor the pupillary response; sluggish, dilated, or unequal pupils are reported immediately, because they may indicate increased ICP and potential brainstem herniation

7. Monitor for colorless drainage on the dressing or from the ears or nose; this is indicative of cerebrospinal fluid and should be reported immediately

8. Check the physician's order for positioning, including the degree of neck flexion (Box 37-8)

9. Monitor IV fluids closely to prevent volume overload or extravasation

10. Promote measures that prevent vomiting; vomiting increases ICP and the risk for incisional rupture

11. Provide a quiet environment

12. Administer analgesics, as prescribed

13. Provide emotional support to the child and parents, and promote maximum functioning in the child

14. Educate the family regarding appropriate follow-up and the potential need for rehabilitation

PRACTICE QUESTIONS

More questions on the companion CD!

400. A nurse instructs the mother of a child with sickle cell disease regarding the precipitating factors related to pain crisis. Which of the following, if identified by the mother as a precipitating factor, indicates the need for further instructions?
1. Stress
2. Trauma
3. Infection
4. Fluid overload

401. Oral iron supplements are prescribed for a 6-year-old child with iron deficiency anemia. The nurse instructs the mother to administer the iron with which best food item?
1. Milk
2. Water
3. Apple juice
4. Orange juice

402. A nurse who is caring for a child with aplastic anemia reviews the laboratory results and notes a white blood cell (WBC) count of 6000/μL and a platelet count of 27,000/mm³. Which nursing intervention should be incorporated into the plan of care?
1. Encourage naps.
2. Encourage a diet high in iron.
3. Encourage quiet play activities.
4. Maintain strict isolation precautions.

403. A nurse reinforces home-care instructions to the parents of a 3-year-old child who has been hospitalized with hemophilia. Which statement by a parent indicates the need for further instructions?
1. "I will supervise my child closely."
2. "I will pad the corners of the furniture."
3. "I will remove household items that can easily fall over."
4. "I will avoid immunizations and dental hygiene treatments for my child."

404. A nurse provides instruction to the parents of a child with leukemia regarding measures related to monitoring for infection. Which statement by the parents indicates the need for further instructions?
1. "I need to use proper handwashing techniques."
2. "I need to take my child's rectal temperature daily."
3. "I need to inspect my child's skin daily for redness."
4. "I need to inspect my child's mouth daily for lesions."

405. A nurse is reviewing the health record of a 14-year-old child who is suspected of having Hodgkin's disease. Which of the following is most characteristic of this disease?
1. Fever and malaise
2. Anorexia and weight loss
3. Painful, enlarged inguinal lymph nodes
4. Painless, firm, and movable adenopathy in the cervical area

406. A 4-year-old child is hospitalized with a suspected diagnosis of Wilms' tumor. The nurse assists with developing a plan of care. The nurse questions which intervention that is written in the plan of care?
    1. Palpating the abdomen for a mass
    2. Checking the urine for the presence of hematuria
    3. Monitoring the temperature for the presence of a kidney infection
    4. Monitoring the blood pressure for the presence of hypertension

407. A nursing instructor asks a student nurse to describe osteogenic sarcoma. Which statement by the student indicates the need to further research the disease?
    1. "The femur is the most common site of this sarcoma."
    2. "The child does not experience pain at the primary tumor site."
    3. "If a weight-bearing limb is affected, then limping is a clinical manifestation."
    4. "The symptoms of the disease during the early stage are almost always attributed to normal growing pains."

408. A nurse is monitoring for bleeding in a child after surgery for the removal of a brain tumor. The nurse checks the head dressing for the presence of blood and notes a colorless drainage on the back of the dressing. Which nursing action is appropriate?
    1. Reinforce the dressing.
    2. Notify the registered nurse (RN).
    3. Document the findings and continue to monitor.
    4. Circle the area of drainage and continue to monitor.

ALTERNATE ITEM FORMAT: MULTIPLE RESPONSE

409. A nurse is reviewing a physician's orders for a child with sickle cell anemia who was admitted to the hospital for the treatment of vaso-occlusive crisis. Which orders documented in the child's record should the nurse question?
    ☐ 1. Restrict fluid intake.
    ☐ 2. Position for comfort.
    ☐ 3. Avoid strain on painful joints.
    ☐ 4. Apply nasal oxygen at 2 L per minute.
    ☐ 5. Provide a high-calorie, high-protein diet.
    ☐ 6. Administer meperidine (Demerol) 25 mg IV every 4 hours for pain.

ANSWERS

400. **4**
Rationale: Pain crisis may be precipitated by infection, dehydration, hypoxia, trauma, or general stress. The mother of a child with sickle cell disease should encourage a fluid intake of 1.5 to 2 times the daily requirement to prevent dehydration.
Test-Taking Strategy: Note the strategic words "need for further instructions." These words indicate a negative event query and ask you to select an option that is an incorrect statement. Recalling that fluid administration is a main component of the treatment of sickle cell disease to prevent dehydration and pain crisis will direct you to option 4. Review the precipitating factors of pain crisis if you had difficulty with this question.
Level of Cognitive Ability: Comprehension
Client Needs: Health Promotion and Maintenance
Integrated Process: Teaching and Learning
Content Area: Child Health
Reference: Leifer, G. (2007). *Introduction to maternity and pediatric nursing* (5th ed., p. 616). Philadelphia: Saunders.

401. **4**
Rationale: Vitamin C increases the absorption of iron by the body. The mother should be instructed to administer the medication with a citrus fruit or a juice that is high in vitamin C.
Test-Taking Strategy: Use the process of elimination. Recalling that vitamin C increases the absorption of iron will assist you with eliminating options 1 and 2. From the remaining options, select option 4, because this food item contains the highest amount of vitamin C. Review the procedure for administering oral iron if you had difficulty with this question.
Level of Cognitive Ability: Application
Client Needs: Physiological Integrity
Integrated Process: Teaching and Learning
Content Area: Pharmacology
Reference: Leifer, G. (2007). *Introduction to maternity and pediatric nursing* (5th ed., p. 612). Philadelphia: Saunders.

402. **3**
Rationale: Precautionary measures to prevent bleeding should be taken when a child has a low platelet count. These include no injections, no rectal temperatures, the use of a soft toothbrush, and abstinence from contact sports or activities that could cause an injury. Strict isolation would be required if the WBC count was low. Options 1 and 2 are unrelated to the risk of bleeding.
Test-Taking Strategy: Use the process of elimination. Note that the WBC count is normal and that the platelet count is low. Recall that a low platelet count places the client at risk for bleeding. This will assist you with eliminating options 1, 2, and 4. Review normal WBC and platelet counts if you had difficulty with this question.
Level of Cognitive Ability: Analysis
Client Needs: Physiological Integrity
Integrated Process: Nursing Process/Planning
Content Area: Child Health
References: McKinney, E., James, S., Murray, S., & Ashwill, J. (2005). *Maternal-child nursing* (2nd ed., pp. 1324-1325). Philadelphia: Saunders.

403. 4
Rationale: The nurse needs to stress the importance of immunizations, dental hygiene, and routine well-child care. Options 1, 2, and 3 are appropriate statements. The parents are also provided instructions regarding measures to take in the event of blunt trauma (especially trauma that involves the joints), and they are instructed to apply prolonged pressure to superficial wounds until the bleeding has stopped.
Test-Taking Strategy: Use the process of elimination, and note the strategic words "need for further instructions." These words indicate a negative event query and ask you to select an option that is an incorrect statement. Recalling that bleeding is a concern among clients with this disorder will assist you with eliminating options 1, 2, and 3, because they include measures of protection and safety for the child. Review the home-care measures for the child with hemophilia if you had difficulty with this question.
Level of Cognitive Ability: Comprehension
Client Needs: Health Promotion and Maintenance
Integrated Process: Teaching and Learning
Content Area: Child Health
Reference: Price, D., & Gwin, J. (2008). *Pediatric nursing: An introductory text* (10th ed., p. 247). St. Louis: Saunders.

404. 2
Rationale: The risk of injury to the fragile mucous membranes is so great in the child with leukemia that only oral, axillary, or tympanic temperatures should be taken. Rectal abscesses can easily occur in damaged rectal tissue, so no rectal temperatures should be taken. In addition, oral temperatures should be avoided if the child has oral ulcers. Options 1, 3, and 4 are appropriate teaching measures.
Test-Taking Strategy: Use the process of elimination, and note the strategic words "need for further instructions." These words indicate a negative event query and ask you to select an option that is an incorrect statement. Options 1 and 3 can be easily eliminated first. From the remaining options, note the word "rectal" in option 2. Recalling that rectal temperatures should be avoided will direct you to this option. Review the home-care instructions for infection in the leukemic child if you had difficulty with this question.
Level of Cognitive Ability: Comprehension
Client Needs: Safe and Effective Care Environment
Integrated Process: Teaching and Learning
Content Area: Child Health
Reference: Wong, D., Perry, S., Hockenberry, M., Lowdermilk, D., & Wilson, D. (2006). *Maternal-child nursing care* (3rd ed., p. 1622). St. Louis: Mosby.

405. 4
Rationale: Clinical manifestations specifically associated with Hodgkin's disease include painless, firm, and movable adenopathy in the cervical and supraclavicular areas. Hepatosplenomegaly is also noted. Although anorexia, weight loss, fever, and malaise are associated with Hodgkin's disease, these manifestations are seen with many disorders.
Test-Taking Strategy: Note the strategic words "most characteristic." Eliminate options 1 and 2 first, because these symptoms are general and vague. Recalling that painless adenopathy is associated with Hodgkin's disease will direct you to option 4. Review the clinical manifestations of Hodgkin's disease if you had difficulty with this question.
Level of Cognitive Ability: Comprehension
Client Needs: Physiological Integrity
Integrated Process: Nursing Process/Data Collection
Content Area: Child Health
Reference: Price, D., & Gwin, J. (2008). *Pediatric nursing: An introductory text* (10th ed., p. 340). St. Louis: Elsevier.

406. 1
Rationale: Wilms' tumor is a tumor of the kidney. If Wilms' tumor is suspected, the mass should not be palpated. Excessive manipulation can cause seeding of the tumor and thus cause the spread of the cancerous cells. Fever, hematuria, and hypertension are clinical manifestations that are associated with Wilms' tumor.
Test-Taking Strategy: Use the process of elimination, and note the strategic words, "questions which intervention." These words indicate a negative event query and ask you to select an option that is an incorrect intervention. Knowledge that Wilms' tumor is located in the kidney will assist you with eliminating options 2, 3, and 4 because of the relationship of these options to renal function. Review the nursing interventions for the child with Wilms' tumor if you had difficulty with this question.
Level of Cognitive Ability: Analysis
Client Needs: Safe and Effective Care Environment
Integrated Process: Nursing Process/Implementation
Content Area: Child Health
Reference: Price, D., & Gwin, J. (2008). *Pediatric nursing: An introductory text* (10th ed., p. 214). St. Louis: Saunders.

407. 2
Rationale: A clinical manifestation of osteogenic sarcoma is progressive, insidious, intermittent pain at the tumor site. By the time these children receive medical attention, they may be in considerable pain from the tumor. Options 1, 3, and 4 are accurate regarding osteogenic sarcoma.
Test-Taking Strategy: Note the strategic words "need to further research." Recalling that osteogenic sarcoma is a malignant tumor of the bone will direct you to option 2. Review the clinical manifestations associated with osteogenic sarcoma if you had difficulty with this question.
Level of Cognitive Ability: Comprehension
Client Needs: Physiological Integrity
Integrated Process: Teaching and Learning
Content Area: Child Health
Reference: Leifer, G. (2007). *Introduction to maternity and pediatric nursing* (5th ed., p. 561). Philadelphia: Saunders.

408. 2
Rationale: Colorless drainage on the dressing would indicate the presence of cerebrospinal fluid and should be reported to the RN immediately; the RN would then contact the physician. Options 1, 3, and 4 delay required immediate interventions.
Test-Taking Strategy: Use the process of elimination. Note the strategic words "colorless drainage." This should quickly alert you to the possibility of the presence of cerebrospinal fluid.

Therefore, eliminate options 1, 3, and 4. Review the care of the child with a brain tumor if you had difficulty with this question.
Level of Cognitive Ability: Application
Client Needs: Physiological Integrity
Integrated Process: Nursing Process/Implementation
Content Area: Child Health
Reference: Hockenberry, M., & Wilson, D. (2007). *Nursing care of infants and children* (8th ed., p. 1594). St. Louis: Mosby.

ALTERNATE ITEM FORMAT: MULTIPLE RESPONSE

409. 1, 6

Rationale: Sickle cell anemia is one of a group of diseases called hemoglobinopathies in which hemoglobin A is partly or completely replaced by abnormal sickle hemoglobin S. It is caused by the inheritance of a gene for a structurally abnormal portion of the hemoglobin chain. Hemoglobin S is sensitive to changes in the oxygen content of the red blood cell, and insufficient oxygen causes the cells to assume a sickle shape; the cells become rigid and clumped together, thus obstructing capillary blood flow. Oral and intravenous fluids are important parts of treatment. Meperidine (Demerol) is not recommended for the child with sickle cell disease because of the risk for normeperidine-induced seizures. Normeperidine, which is a metabolite of meperidine, is a central nervous system stimulant that produces anxiety, tremors, myoclonus, and generalized seizures when it accumulates with repetitive dosing. Therefore, the nurse would question the orders for restricted fluids and meperidine for pain control. Positioning for comfort, avoiding strain in painful joints, oxygen, and a high-calorie, high-protein diet are also important parts of the treatment plan.
Test-Taking Strategy: Focus on the pathophysiology that occurs with sickle cell disease to assist you with identifying the orders that need to be questioned. Recalling that fluids are an important component of the treatment plan will help you to identify that a fluid-restriction order would need to be questioned. Recalling the effects of meperidine will assist you with identifying that this order needs to be questioned. Review the care of the child with sickle cell anemia who is experiencing a crisis if you had difficulty with this question.
Level of Cognitive Ability: Analysis
Client Needs: Physiological Integrity
Integrated Process: Nursing Process/Implementation
Content Area: Child Health
Reference: Hockenberry, M., & Wilson, D. (2007). *Nursing care of infants and children* (8th ed., pp.1523-1525.). St. Louis: Mosby.

REFERENCES

Leifer, G. (2007). *Introduction to maternity and pediatric nursing* (5th ed.). Philadelphia: Saunders.
McKinney, E., James, S., Murray, S., & Ashwill, J. (2005). *Maternal-child nursing* (2nd ed.). St. Louis: Saunders.
National Council of State Boards of Nursing (Eds.). (2008). *2008 Detailed Test Plan for the NCLEX-PN® Examination, National Council of State Boards of Nursing*. Chicago: Author.
National Council of State Boards of Nursing. *NCSBN home page.* www.ncsbn.org. Accessed July 27, 2008.
Price, D., & Gwin, J. (2008). *Pediatric nursing: An introductory text* (10th ed.). St. Louis: Saunders.
Wong, D., Perry, S., Hockenberry, M., Lowdermilk, D., & Wilson, D. (2006). *Maternal-child nursing care* (3rd ed.). St. Louis: Mosby.

CHAPTER 38

Communicable Diseases and Acquired Immunodeficiency Syndrome

I. RUBEOLA (MEASLES)
A. Description
1. Agent: Paramyxovirus virus
2. Incubation period: 10 to 20 days
3. Communicable period: From 4 days before to 5 days after the rash appears; mainly during the prodromal stage (this pertains to early symptoms that may mark the onset of disease)
4. Source: Respiratory tract secretions, blood, or urine of an infected person
5. Transmission: Airborne particles, direct contact with infectious droplets, or transplacental transmission
B. Data collection
1. Fever
2. Malaise
3. The "three Cs": Coryza, cough, and conjunctivitis
4. Rash appears as red, erythematous, discrete maculopapular eruption that starts on the face and spreads downward to the feet, that blanches easily with pressure, and that gradually turns a brownish color after 6 to 7 days; the rash begins behind the ears and spreads downward to the feet, and it may involve desquamation
5. Koplik spots: Small, red spots with a bluish-white center and a red base; they are located on the buccal mucosa and last for 3 days
C. Interventions
1. Use respiratory airborne droplet precautions if the child is hospitalized
2. Restrict the child to quiet activities and bedrest
3. Use a cool-mist vaporizer for cough and coryza
4. Dim the lights if photophobia is present
5. Administer antipyretics for fever, as prescribed

II. ROSEOLA (EXANTHEMA SUBITUM)
A. Description
1. Agent: Human herpesvirus type 6
2. Incubation period: 5 to 15 days
3. Communicable period: Unknown but thought to extend from the febrile stage to the time that the rash first appears

4. Source: Unknown
5. Transmission: Unknown
B. Data collection
1. Sudden high fever (greater than 102° F) of 3 to 5 days' duration in a child who appears well, followed by a rash (rose-pink maculas that blanch with pressure)
2. The rash appears several hours to 2 days after the fever subsides and lasts 1 to 2 days
C. Interventions: Supportive

III. RUBELLA (GERMAN MEASLES)
A. Description
1. Agent: Rubella virus
2. Incubation period: 14 to 21 days
3. Communicable period: 7 days before to about 5 days after the rash appears
4. Source: Nasopharyngeal secretions; the virus is also present in the blood, stool, and urine
5. Transmission
   a. Airborne or direct contact with infectious droplets
   b. Indirectly via articles that have been freshly contaminated with nasopharyngeal secretions, feces, or urine
   c. Transplacental
B. Data collection
1. Low-grade fever
2. Malaise
3. Pinkish-red maculopapular rash that begins on the face and spreads to the entire body within 1 to 3 days
4. Petechial red, pinpoint spots may occur on the soft palate
C. Interventions
1. Provide supportive treatment
2. Isolate the infected child from pregnant women

IV. MUMPS
A. Description
1. Agent: Paramyxovirus
2. Incubation period: 14 to 21 days
3. Communicable period: Immediately before and after parotid gland swelling begins

4. Source: The saliva and possibly the urine of an infected person
5. Transmission: Direct contact or droplet spread from an infected person

B. Data collection
1. Fever
2. Headache and malaise
3. Anorexia
4. Jaw or ear pain or ache aggravated by chewing and followed by parotid glandular swelling
5. Orchitis may occur

C. Interventions
1. Institute droplet respiratory precautions
2. Provide bedrest until the parotid gland swelling subsides
3. Avoid foods that require chewing
4. Apply hot or cold compresses to the neck, as prescribed
5. Apply warmth and local support with tight-fitting underpants to relieve orchitis

V. CHICKENPOX (VARICELLA)
A. Description
1. Agent: Varicella zoster virus (VZV)
2. Incubation period: 13 to 17 days
3. Communicable period: 1 to 2 days before the onset of the rash to 6 days after the first crop of vesicles, when crusts have formed
4. Source: Respiratory tract secretions of an infected person; skin lesions
5. Transmission: Direct contact, droplet (airborne) spread, and contaminated objects

B. Data collection
1. Slight fever, malaise, and anorexia are followed by a macular rash that first appears on the trunk and scalp and then moves to the extremities
2. Lesions become pustules, begin to dry, and develop a crust
3. Lesions may appear on the mucous membranes of the mouth, the genital area, and the rectal area

C. Interventions
1. In the hospital setting, ensure strict isolation (i.e., contact and droplet precautions)
2. In the home setting, isolate the infected child until the vesicles have dried; isolate high-risk children from the infected child
3. Supportive care

VI. PERTUSSIS (WHOOPING COUGH)
A. Description
1. Agent: Bordetella pertussis
2. Incubation period: 5 to 21 days (usually 10 days)
3. Communicable period: Greatest during the catarrhal stage (i.e., when discharge from respiratory secretions occurs)
4. Source: Discharge from the respiratory tract of the infected person
5. Transmission: Direct contact or droplet spread from the infected person; indirect contact with freshly contaminated articles

B. Data collection
1. Symptoms of respiratory infection followed by increased severity of cough with a loud whooping inspiration
2. May experience **cyanosis,** respiratory distress, and tongue protrusion
3. Listlessness, irritability, and anorexia

C. Interventions
1. Isolate the child during the catarrhal stage; if the child is hospitalized, institute droplet precautions
2. Administer antimicrobial therapy, as prescribed
3. Administer pertussis immune globulin, as prescribed
4. Reduce environmental factors that cause coughing spasms, such as dust, smoke, and sudden changes in temperature
5. Ensure adequate hydration and nutrition
6. Provide suction and humidified oxygen, if needed
7. Monitor the cardiopulmonary status via a monitor, as prescribed
8. Monitor the pulse oximetry
9. Infants do not receive maternal immunity to pertussis

VII. DIPHTHERIA
A. Description
1. Agent: *Corynebacterium diphtheriae*
2. Incubation period: 2 to 5 days
3. Communicable period: Variable; until virulent bacilli are no longer present (three negative cultures of discharge from the nose, nasopharynx, skin, and other lesions); usually 2 weeks but can be as long as 4 weeks
4. Source: Discharge from the mucous membrane of the nose, nasopharynx, skin, and other lesions of the infected person
5. Transmission: Direct contact with an infected person, carrier, or contaminated articles

B. Data collection
1. Low-grade fever, malaise, and sore throat
2. Foul-smelling and mucopurulent nasal discharge
3. Dense pseudomembrane formation of the throat that may interfere with eating, drinking, and breathing
4. Lymphadenitis, neck edema, and "bull neck"

C. Interventions
1. Ensure strict isolation for the hospitalized child
2. Administer diphtheria antitoxin, as prescribed, and after a skin or conjunctival test to rule out sensitivity to horse serum
3. Provide bedrest
4. Administer antibiotics, as prescribed
5. Provide suction and humidified oxygen, as needed
6. Provide tracheostomy care if a tracheostomy is necessary

VIII. POLIOMYELITIS
A. Description
1. Agent: Enteroviruses
2. Incubation period: 7 to 14 days
3. Communicable period: Not exactly known; the virus is present in the throat and feces shortly after infection and persists for about 1 week in the throat and 4 to 6 weeks in the feces
4. Source: The oropharyngeal secretions and feces of an infected person
5. Transmission: Direct contact with an infected person; fecal-oral and oropharyngeal routes
B. Data collection
1. Fever, malaise, anorexia, nausea, headache, and sore throat
2. Abdominal pain followed by soreness and stiffness of the trunk, neck, and limbs that may progress to central nervous system paralysis
C. Interventions
1. Enteric precautions
2. Supportive treatment
3. Bedrest
4. Monitoring for respiratory paralysis
5. Physical therapy

IX. SCARLET FEVER
A. Description
1. Agent: Group A β-hemolytic streptococci
2. Incubation period: 1 to 7 days
3. Communicable period: During the incubation period and clinical illness, which lasts about 10 days; during the first 2 weeks of the carrier stage, although this stage may persist for months
4. Source: Nasopharyngeal secretions of an infected person or carrier
5. Transmission: Direct contact with an infected person or droplet spread; indirectly by contact with contaminated articles or the ingestion of contaminated milk or other foods
B. Data collection
1. Abrupt high fever, flushed cheeks, vomiting, headache, enlarged lymph nodes in the neck, malaise, and abdominal pain
2. A red, fine, sandpaper-like papular rash develops in the axilla, groin, and neck and spreads to cover the entire body, except the face
3. The rash blanches with pressure (Schultz-Charlton reaction) except in areas of deep creases and folds of the joints (Pastia's sign).
4. Desquamation and sheet-like sloughing of the skin of the palms and soles by week 1 to week 3
5. The tongue is initially coated with a white, furry covering with red projecting papillae (white strawberry tongue); by the third to fifth day, the white coat sloughs off and leaves a red, swollen tongue (red strawberry tongue)
6. Tonsils are reddened, edematous, and covered with a gray-white exudate
7. Pharynx is edematous and beefy red
C. Interventions
1. Institute respiratory precautions until 24 hours after the initiation of antibiotic therapy
2. Provide supportive therapy
3. Provide bedrest
4. Encourage fluid intake

X. ERYTHEMA INFECTIOSUM (FIFTH DISEASE)
A. Description
1. Agent: Human parvovirus B19
2. Incubation period: 4 to 14 days; may be as long as 20 days
3. Communicable period: Uncertain, but before the onset of symptoms in most children
4. Source: Infected person
5. Transmission: Unknown; possibly respiratory secretions and blood
B. Data collection
1. Before rash, asymptomatic or mild fever, malaise, headache, and runny nose
2. Stages of the rash
a. Erythema of the face (slapped-cheek appearance) develops, chiefly on the cheeks, and disappears by 1 to 4 days
b. About 1 day after the rash appears on the face, maculopapular red spots appear and are symmetrically distributed on the extremities; the rash progresses from the proximal to distal surfaces and may last a week or more
c. The rash subsides but may reappear if the skin is irritated or traumatized by factors such as the sun, heat, cold, exercise, or friction
C. Interventions
1. Child is not usually hospitalized
2. Pregnant women should avoid the infected individual
3. Provide supportive care
4. Administer antipyretics, analgesics, and anti-inflammatory medications, as prescribed

XI. INFECTIOUS MONONUCLEOSIS
A. Description
1. Agent: Epstein-Barr virus
2. Incubation period: 4 to 6 weeks
3. Communicable period: Unknown; the virus is shed before the onset of the disease and until 6 months or longer after recovery
4. Source: Oral secretions
5. Transmission: Direct intimate contact, infected blood
B. Data collection
1. Fever, sore throat, malaise, headache, fatigue, nausea, abdominal pain, sore throat, and enlarged, red tonsils
2. Lymphadenopathy and hepatosplenomegaly
3. A discrete macular rash that is most prominent over the trunk may occur

C. Interventions

1. Provide supportive care
2. Monitor for signs of splenic rupture, which include abdominal pain, left upper quadrant pain, and left shoulder pain

XII. ROCKY MOUNTAIN SPOTTED FEVER

A. Description

1. Agent: *Rickettsia rickettsii*
2. Incubation period: 2 to 14 days
3. Source: Tick from a mammal source, most often from wild rodents and dogs
4. Transmission: The bite of an infected tick

B. Data collection

1. Fever, malaise, anorexia, vomiting, headache, and myalgia
2. A maculopapular or petechial rash primarily on the extremities (ankles and wrists) but that may spread to other areas; characteristically on the palms and soles

C. Interventions

1. Provide vigorous supportive care
2. Administer antibiotics, as prescribed
3. Teach the child and parents about protection from tick bites (Box 38-1)

XIII. ENTEROBIASIS (PINWORM)

A. Description

1. Agent: *Enterobius vermicularis*
2. Source: Common pinworm
   a. The nematode is universally present in temperate climatic zones
   b. The eggs are ingested or inhaled (transferred from the hands to the mouth); the worms infect the large intestine; the females then mate, deposit eggs in the perianal area, migrate out through the anus
3. Transmission
   a. Occurs most often in crowded conditions, such as classrooms and day-care centers
   b. Ingestion or inhalation of eggs
   c. Hands to mouth or fecal-oral route
   d. Contaminated items (pinworm eggs remain viable for several days)

B. Data collection: Intense perianal itching, irritability, restlessness, poor sleep, bed-wetting, distractibility, short attention span; in females, the worm may migrate to the vagina and urethra and cause infection

C. Interventions

1. Identify the worms
   a. Use a flashlight to inspect the anal area 2 to 3 hours after the child is asleep
   b. Tape test: Lightly press transparent sticky tape against the child's perianal skin; the tape is then examined for eggs microscopically; the specimen should be collected in the morning as soon as the child awakens and before a bowel movement or bath
2. Use enteric precautions
3. Administer antihelminthic medications (all household members are treated), as prescribed; the course of medication is repeated 2 weeks after the first course to prevent reinfection
4. Teach home-care measures to prevent reinfection

XIV. IMMUNIZATIONS

A. Guidelines

1. In the United States, the recommended age for beginning primary immunizations of infants is at birth
2. Children born prematurely should receive the full dose of each **vaccine** at the appropriate **chronological age**
3. Children who began primary immunizations at the recommended age but failed to receive all of the required doses do not need to begin the series again; rather, they need to receive only the missed doses
4. If there is a suspicion that the parent will not bring the child to the pediatrician or health care clinic for follow-up immunizations according to the optimal immunization schedule, any of the recommended **vaccines** can be administered simultaneously

B. General contraindications and precautions (Box 38-2)

C. Guidelines for administration (Box 38-3)

BOX 38-1 **Protection From Tick Bites**

Wear long-sleeved shirts, long pants tucked into long socks, and a hat when walking in tick-infested areas.
Wear light-colored clothing to make ticks more visible.
Avoid walking in tall grass and shrubs; follow paths.
Apply insect repellents that contain diethyltoluamide (DEET) and permethrin before possible exposure; should be used with caution for infants and small children.
Keep yards trimmed and free of brush.
Apply tick repellent to dogs.
Check children for the presence of ticks after they have been in high-risk or tick-infested areas.
Save the tick for later identification if it is removed from the body.

BOX 38-2 **General Contraindications and Precautions to Immunizations**

- Anaphylactic reaction to a previously administered vaccine or a component of the vaccine
- Live virus vaccines: A severely deficient immune system, a marked sensitivity to gelatin, or pregnancy

Precautions

- Moderate or severe acute illness with or without fever

Modified from Centers for Disease Control and Prevention. *Contraindications to vaccines chart.* www.cdc.gov/nip/recs/contraindications_vacc.htm. Accessed July 29, 2008.

▲ **XV. RECOMMENDED IMMUNIZATIONS: CHILDHOOD AND ADOLESCENT IMMUNIZATIONS** (Box 38-4)
A. Hepatitis B **vaccine** (HepB)
  1. The **vaccine** protects against HepB
  2. Administered by the intramuscular route
  3. The first dose of the HepB **vaccine** (monovalent) should be administered soon after birth and before hospital discharge; the birth dose can be delayed in rare circumstances if the infant's mother tests negative for HepB surface antigen (HBsAg)

  4. Monovalent HepB or a combination **vaccine** that contains HepB may be used to complete the series
  5. The second dose is administered at the age of 1 to 2 months
  6. The final dose should be given at 24 weeks (6 to 18 months)
  7. Contraindications: Severe allergic reaction to the previous dose or to one of the **vaccine** components, which include aluminum hydroxide and yeast protein
  8. Precautions: An infant who weighs less than 2000 g; moderate or severe acute illness with or without fever
  9. HBsAg-positive mothers
    a. Infant should receive the HepB **vaccine** and HepB immune globulin (HBIG) within 12 hours of birth

BOX 38-3 Guidelines for the Administration of Vaccines

Follow the manufacturer's recommendations for the route of administration, storage, and the reconstitution of the vaccine.
If refrigeration is necessary, store the vaccine on a center shelf and not on the door; frequent temperature increases from opening the refrigerator door can alter the potency of the vaccine.
For protection against light, wrap the vial in aluminum foil.
A vaccine information statement needs to be given to the parents or the individual, and informed consent for administration needs to be obtained.
Check the expiration date on the vaccine bottle.
Parenteral vaccines are given from separate syringes at different injection sites.
Vaccines that are administered intramuscularly are given in the vastus lateralis muscle (best site) or the ventrogluteal muscle; the deltoid can be used for older infants and children 36 months and older, and the dorsogluteal site (the buttocks) is avoided.
Vaccines that are administered subcutaneously are given into the fatty areas in the lateral upper arms and the anterior thighs.
Adequate needle length and gauge are as follows: intramuscular, 1 inch, 23 to 25 gauge; subcutaneous, ⅝ inch, 25 gauge.
Mild side effects may include fever, soreness, swelling, or redness at the injection site.
A topical anesthetic may be applied to the injection site before the injection.
For painful or red injection sites, advise the parent to apply cool compresses for the first 24 hours and to then use warm or cold compresses as long as needed.
An age-appropriate dose of acetaminophen (Tylenol) may be administered every 4 to 6 hours for vaccine-associated discomfort.
Maintain an immunization record: document the day, month, and year of administration; the manufacturer and lot number of vaccine; the name, address, and title of the person who administered the vaccine; and the site and route of administration.
A Vaccine Adverse Event Report needs to be filed and the health department needs to be notified if an adverse reaction to an immunization occurs.

BOX 38-4 Recommended Childhood and Adolescent Immunizations

Birth	Hepatitis B vaccine (HepB)
1 month	HepB
2 months	Inactivated poliovirus vaccine (IPV); diphtheria, tetanus, and acellular pertussis (DTaP) vaccine, *Haemophilus influenzae* type b (Hib) conjugate vaccine, and pneumococcal conjugate vaccine (PCV)
4 months	DTaP, Hib, IPV, and PCV
6 months	DTaP, HepB, Hib, IPV, and PCV
12 to 15 months	Hib; measles, mumps, and rubella (MMR) vaccine; PCV; first dose of hepatitis A vaccine (the second dose is given 6 months after the first dose)
12 to 18 months	Varicella vaccine
15 to 18 months	DTaP
18 to 21 months	Second dose of hepatitis A vaccine (given 6 months after the first dose)
4 to 6 years	DTaP, IPV, and MMR
11 to 12 years	MMR (if not administered at 4 to 6 years); Tdap (diphtheria, tetanus, and acellular pertussis adolescent preparation), and meningococcal vaccine (MCV4)
9 to 26 years	Gardasil (quadrivalent human papillomavirus types 6, 11, 16, and 18 recombinant vaccine) series may be recommended and administered as three injections over 6 months; the first dose is given, followed by the second dose 2 months after the first dose and the third dose 6 months after the first dose

b. Infant should be tested for HBsAg and anti-body to HBsAg after completion of the HepB series (between 9 to 18 months of age)

10. Mother whose HBsAg status is unknown

a. Infant should receive the first dose of the HepB **vaccine** series within 12 hours of birth

b. Maternal blood should be drawn as soon as possible to determine the mother's HBsAg status

c. If the mother's HBsAg test is positive, the infant should receive HBIG as soon as possible (no later than the age of 1 week)

B. Diphtheria, tetanus, acellular pertussis (DTaP), and tetanus toxoid; reduced diphtheria toxoid and acellular pertussis **vaccine** (Tdap adolescent preparation)

1. Protect against diphtheria, tetanus, and pertussis

2. Administered by the intramuscular route

3. The DTaP **vaccine** is administered at 2 months, 4 months, 6 months, between 15 and 18 months of age, and between 4 and 6 years of age

4. The fourth dose of DTaP can be given at 12 months of age if 6 months have elapsed since the third dose and if the child may not return for follow-up at 12 to 18 months of age

5. The fifth (final) dose is administered at the age of 4 years or older

6. The Tdap (adolescent preparation) is recommended to be given at 11 to 12 years of age to those who completed the recommended childhood DTaP series but who have not received a tetanus and diphtheria toxoid (Td) booster dose

7. Subsequent routine Td boosters are recommended every 10 years

8. Encephalopathy within 7 days of the administration of the previous dose of DTaP is a complication

9. Contraindication: Severe allergic reaction to a previous dose or to a **vaccine** component

C. *Haemophilus influenzae* type b (Hib) conjugate **vaccine**

1. The **vaccine** protects against a number of serious infections caused by Hib, such as bacterial meningitis, epiglottitis, bacterial pneumonia, septic arthritis, and sepsis

2. Administered by the intramuscular route

3. The Hib **vaccine** is administered at 2 months, 4 months, 6 months, and between 12 and 15 months of age

4. Depending on the brand of Hib **vaccine** used for the first and second doses, a dose at 6 months of age may not be needed

5. The DTaP-Hib combination products should not be used for primary immunization in infants aged 2, 4, or 6 months, but they can be used as boosters after any Hib **vaccine**

6. Contraindications: Severe allergic reaction to a previous dose or **vaccine** component

D. Influenza **vaccine**

1. Recommended annually for children from the age of 6 months with certain risk factors, such as asthma, cardiac disease, sickle cell disease, human immunodeficiency virus (HIV) infection, diabetes mellitus, and conditions that can compromise respiratory function; health care workers and others in close contact with those in high-risk groups should also be immunized

2. Healthy children between the ages of 6 and 23 months are encouraged to receive influenza **vaccine** because of their increased risk for influenza-related hospitalization

E. Inactivated poliovirus **vaccine** (IPV)

1. The IPV protects against polio

2. Administered by the subcutaneous route but may also be given by the intramuscular route

3. The IPV is administered at 2 months, 4 months, 6 to 18 months, and between 4 and 6 years of age

4. Contraindications: Severe allergic reaction to a previous dose or to **vaccine** components, which may include: formalin, neomycin, streptomycin, and polymyxin B

F. Measles, mumps, and rubella (MMR) **vaccine**

1. The MMR **vaccine** protects against measles, mumps, and rubella

2. Administered by the subcutaneous route

3. The first dose of the MMR **vaccine** is administered between 12 and 15 months of age; the second dose is recommended at 4 to 6 years of age, but it may be administered during any visit as long as at least 4 weeks have elapsed since the first dose

4. Those who have not received the second dose previously should complete the schedule at the 11- to 12-year-old pediatric or health care clinic visit

5. Contraindications: Severe allergic reaction to a previous dose or a **vaccine** component such as gelatin, neomycin, or sorbitol; pregnancy; known immunodeficiency

G. Varicella **vaccine**

1. Protects against chickenpox

2. Administered by the subcutaneous route

3. Administered between 12 and 18 months of age

4. Susceptible children 13 years old and older (i.e., those who have not had chickenpox or have not been previously vaccinated) need two doses given at least 4 weeks apart

5. **Vaccine** should be kept frozen and used within 30 minutes of reconstitution to ensure maximum potency

6. Contraindications: Severe allergic reaction to a previous dose or **vaccine** component, such as gelatin, bovine albumin, or neomycin; substantial suppression of cellular immunity; pregnancy

H. Pneumococcal conjugate **vaccine** (PCV)
   1. Prevents infection with *Streptococcus pneumoniae*, which may cause meningitis, pneumonia, septicemia, sinusitis, and otitis media
   2. Administered by the intramuscular route
   3. Can be given concurrently with other childhood **vaccines** at 2 months, 4 months, 6 months, and 12 to 15 months of age; the final dose in the series is to be given at the age of 12 months or older
   4. Pneumococcal polysaccharide **vaccine** (PPV) is recommended in addition to PCV for certain high-risk groups, such as children with chronic illnesses that are specifically associated with an increased risk of pneumococcal disease or its complications; anatomic or functional asplenia; hemoglobinopathies; nephrotic syndrome; cerebrospinal fluid leaks; and conditions associated with immunosuppression (PPV is given at least 8 weeks after the last dose of PCV)
   5. Contraindications: Severe allergic reaction to a previous dose or **vaccine** component

I. Hepatitis A **vaccine**
   1. Protects against hepatitis A
   2. Recommended for all children at the age of 1 year (12 to 23 months); the two doses should be administered at least 6 months apart
   3. Administered via the intramuscular route
   4. Contraindications: Severe allergic reaction to a previous dose or a **vaccine** component, such as aluminum hydroxide, bovine albumin or serum, or formalin

J. Meningococcal **vaccine**
   1. Protects against *Neisseria meningitidis*
   2. The meningococcal polysaccharide (MPSV4) vaccination is given subcutaneously; the meningococcal **vaccine** (MCV4) is given intramuscularly; (MPSV4 is used for children between the ages of 2 and 10 years, whereas MCV4 is used for older children)
   3. MCV4 should be administered to all children at the age of 11 to 12 years and to unvaccinated adolescents at high school entry (age of 15 years); all college freshman living in dormitories should be vaccinated
   4. Safety during pregnancy has not been established

K. Gardasil (quadrivalent human papillomavirus [HPV] types 6, 11, 16, and 18 recombinant **vaccine**)
   1. Guards against diseases that are caused by HPV types 6, 11, 16, and 18, such as cervical cancer, cervical abnormalities that can lead to cervical cancer, and genital warts

2. May be recommended for girls and women between the ages of 9 and 26 years
3. Administered as three injections over 6 months; the first dose is given, with the second dose given 2 months after the first dose and the third dose given 6 months after the first dose
4. Can cause pain, swelling, itching, and redness at the injection site; fever; nausea; and dizziness
5. Contraindicated in those with a reaction to a previous injection and in pregnant women

XVI. **REACTIONS TO A VACCINE**

A. Local reactions
   1. Tenderness, erythema, and swelling at the injection site
   2. Low-grade fever
   3. Behavioral changes, such as drowsiness, unusual crying, and eating less

B. Minimizing local reactions
   1. Select a needle of adequate length to deposit the **vaccine** deep into the muscle or subcutaneous mass
   2. Inject the **vaccine** into the appropriate, recommended site

C. Anaphylactic reactions
   1. The goals of treatment are to secure and protect the airway, restore adequate circulation, and prevent further exposure to the antigen
   2. For a mild reaction with no evidence of respiratory distress or cardiovascular compromise, a subcutaneous injection of an antihistamine such as diphenhydramine (Benadryl) or epinephrine (Adrenalin) may be administered
   3. For moderate or severe distress, establish an airway; provide cardiopulmonary resuscitation if the child is not breathing; elevate the head; administer epinephrine, fluids, and vasopressors, as prescribed; monitor the vital signs and the urine output

XVII. **CARE OF THE CHILD WITH HUMAN IMMUNODEFICIENCY VIRUS/ACQUIRED IMMUNODEFICIENCY SYNDROME**

A. Prophylaxis
   1. Provide prophylaxis, as prescribed, against pneumonia during the first year of life to the infant born to an HIV-infected woman; after 1 year of age, the need for prophylaxis is determined by the presence of severe immunosuppression or a history of *pneumocystis jiroveci* pneumonia
   2. Provide continued prophylaxis through 12 months of age for children who have been diagnosed with HIV
   3. For HIV-infected children who are more than 12 months old, continued prophylaxis is based on CD4 counts and whether pneumonia has previously occurred

B. Antiretroviral therapy: The goal is to suppress viral replication to preserve immune function and delay disease progression

C. Highly active antiretroviral therapy (HAART)
   1. HAART is a combination therapy that usually includes two nucleoside analogues, which target viral replication during the reverse transcription phase, and a protease inhibitor, which targets viral replication during a different phase
   2. Usually prescribed for an HIV-infected infant or child who exhibits clinical signs of infection or whose immune status is depressed or for an HIV-infected infant less than 1 year old when the diagnosis is confirmed

D. Parent instructions
   1. Encourage routine good hygiene and frequent handwashing
   2. Monitor for fever, malaise, fatigue, weight loss, vomiting, diarrhea, altered activity level, and oral lesions; notify the physician if these occur
   3. Monitor for signs and symptoms of opportunistic infections
   4. Administer antiretroviral medications, as prescribed; emphasize the importance of strict adherence to the treatment regimen
   5. The child should avoid exposure to other illnesses
   6. Keep immunizations up to date
   7. Keep the child home when he or she is sick
   8. Avoid direct unprotected contact with body fluids
   9. Monitor the weight
   10. Provide a high-calorie, high-protein diet
   11. Avoid fresh fruits, fresh vegetables, and raw fish (neutropenic diet if immunosuppressed)
   12. Avoid sharing objects that may become contaminated with blood, such as toothbrushes
   13. Avoid sharing eating utensils; wash eating utensils in the dishwasher
   14. Cover unused food and formula, and refrigerate them
   15. Discard unused refrigerated formula and food after 24 hours
   16. Wear gloves for care, especially when in contact with body fluids and changing diapers
   17. Change diapers frequently and away from food areas
   18. Fold soiled disposable diapers inward, close with tabs, and dispose in a tightly covered plastic-lined container
   19. Dispose of trash daily
   20. Clean up spills with bleach solution (10:1 ratio of water to bleach) or commercial disinfectants
   21. Encourage the use of barrier protection for a sexually active adolescent
   22. Provide family and individual support and counseling

E. Immunizations
   1. Immunizations against common childhood illnesses are recommended for all children exposed to or infected with HIV
   2. The varicella (chickenpox) **vaccine** is avoided
   3. Pneumococcal and influenza **vaccines** are administered
   4. The MMR **vaccine** is administered if the child is not severely immunocompromised; the child who is receiving intravenous gamma globulin prophylaxis may not respond to the MMR **vaccine**

PRACTICE QUESTIONS

More questions on the companion CD!

410. A child with rubeola (measles) is being admitted to the hospital. When preparing for the admission of the child, which precautions should be implemented?
   1. Enteric
   2. Contact
   3. Protective
   4. Respiratory

411. The nurse provides instructions regarding respiratory precautions to the mother of a child with mumps. The mother asks the nurse about the length of time required for the respiratory precautions. Which response by the nurse is accurate?
   1. Respiratory isolation is not necessary.
   2. Mumps is not transmitted by the respiratory system.
   3. Respiratory precautions are indicated during the period of communicability.
   4. Respiratory precautions are indicated for 18 days after the onset of parotid swelling.

412. A 6-month-old infant receives a diphtheria, tetanus, and acellular pertussis (DTap) immunization at the well-baby clinic. The mother returns home and calls the clinic to report that the infant has developed swelling and redness at the site of injection. Which instruction by the nurse is appropriate?
   1. Monitor the infant for a fever.
   2. Bring the infant back to the clinic.
   3. Apply an ice pack to the injection site.
   4. Leave the injection site alone, because this always occurs.

413. A child is diagnosed with scarlet fever. A nurse collects data regarding the child. Which of the following is a clinical manifestation of scarlet fever?
   1. Pastia's sign
   2. Abdominal pain and flaccid paralysis
   3. Gray membrane on the tonsils and pharynx
   4. Foul-smelling and mucopurulent nasal drainage

414. A child is diagnosed with infectious mononucleosis. The nurse provides home-care instructions to

the parents about the care of the child. Which information given by the nurse is accurate?
1. Maintain the child on bedrest for 2 weeks.
2. Maintain respiratory precautions for 1 week.
3. Notify the physician if the child develops a fever.
4. Notify the physician if the child develops abdominal or left shoulder pain.

415. A mother of a preschooler who attends day care reports that the child is constantly itching the perianal area and that the area is irritated. The nurse suspects the possibility of pinworm infection (enterobiasis). The nurse instructs the mother to obtain a rectal specimen with the use of the tape test. When is the best time to obtain the specimen?
1. After bathing
2. After toileting
3. When the child is put to bed
4. In the morning, when the child awakens

416. A nursing student is assigned to help administer immunizations to children in a clinic. The nursing instructor asks the student about the contraindications to receiving an immunization. Immunization is contraindicated in the presence of which condition?
1. A cold
2. Otitis media
3. Mild diarrhea
4. A severe febrile illness

417. A mother with human immunodeficiency virus (HIV) infection brings her 10-month-old infant to the clinic for a routine checkup. A physician has documented that the infant is asymptomatic for HIV infection. After the checkup, the mother tells the nurse that she is so pleased that the infant will not get HIV. Which response by the nurse is appropriate?
1. "I am also so pleased that everything has turned out fine."
2. "Since symptoms have not developed, it is unlikely that the infant will develop HIV infection."

3. "Everything looks great, but be sure that you return with your infant next month for the scheduled visit."
4. "Most children infected with HIV develop symptoms within the first 9 months of life, and some become symptomatic at some point before the age of 3 years."

418. A child is scheduled to receive a measles, mumps, and rubella (MMR) vaccine. The nurse who is preparing to administer the vaccine reviews the child's record. Which finding should make the nurse question the physician's order?
1. Recent recovery from a cold
2. A history of frequent respiratory infections
3. A history of an anaphylactoid reaction to neomycin
4. A local reaction at the site of a previous MMR vaccine injection

ALTERNATE ITEM FORMAT: MULTIPLE RESPONSE

419. Choose the home-care instructions that the nurse would provide to the mother of a child with acquired immunodeficiency syndrome (AIDS). Select all that apply.
☐ 1. Frequent handwashing is important.
☐ 2. The child should avoid exposure to other illnesses.
☐ 3. The child's immunization schedule will need revision.
☐ 4. Kissing the child on the mouth will never transmit the virus.
☐ 5. Clean up body fluid spills with bleach solution (10:1 ratio of water to bleach).
☐ 6. Fever, malaise, fatigue, weight loss, vomiting, and diarrhea are expected to occur and do not require special intervention.

ANSWERS

410. **4**
Rationale: Rubeola is transmitted via airborne particles or direct contact with infectious droplets. Respiratory precautions are required, and a mask is worn by those who come in contact with the child. Gowns and gloves are not indicated. Articles that are contaminated should be bagged and labeled. Options 1, 2, and 3 are not indicated for rubeola.
Test-Taking Strategy: Use the process of elimination. Recalling that rubeola is transmitted via the airborne route will direct you to option 4. Review the route of transmission and the therapeutic management of rubeola if you had difficulty with this question.

Level of Cognitive Ability: Application
Client Needs: Safe and Effective Care Environment
Integrated Process: Nursing Process/Planning
Content Area: Child Health
Reference: Hockenberry, M., & Wilson, D. (2007). *Nursing care of infants and children* (8th ed., pp. 670-671). St. Louis: Mosby.

411. **3**
Rationale: Mumps is transmitted via direct contact or droplets spread from an infected person and possibly by contact with urine. Respiratory precautions are indicated during the period of communicability. Options 1, 2, and 4 are incorrect.

Test-Taking Strategy: Use the process of elimination. Options 1 and 2 can be eliminated first, because they are comparable or alike. From the remaining options, select option 3, because it is the umbrella option, and it addresses communicability. In addition, the time frame indicated in option 4 seems rather lengthy. Review the infectious period of mumps if you had difficulty with this question.
Level of Cognitive Ability: Application
Client Needs: Safe and Effective Care Environment
Integrated Process: Teaching and Learning
Content Area: Child Health
Reference: Hockenberry, M., & Wilson, D. (2007). *Nursing care of infants and children* (8th ed., p. 673). St. Louis: Mosby.

412. **3**
Rationale: Occasionally tenderness, redness, or swelling may occur at the site of the injection. This can be relieved with ice packs for the first 24 hours and followed by warm compresses if the inflammation persists. It is not necessary to bring the infant back to the clinic. Option 1 may be an appropriate intervention, but it is not specific to the subject of the question.
Test-Taking Strategy: Use the process of elimination. Option 4 can be eliminated first because of the close-ended word "always." Eliminate option 1 next, because it does not relate specifically to the subject of the question. Next, eliminate option 2 as an unnecessary intervention. Review interventions after immunizations and injections if you had difficulty with this question.
Level of Cognitive Ability: Application
Client Needs: Health Promotion and Maintenance
Integrated Process: Nursing Process/Implementation
Content Area: Child Health
Reference: McKinney, E., James, S., Murray, S., & Ashwill, J. (2005). *Maternal-child nursing* (2nd ed., p. 71). Philadelphia: Saunders.

413. **1**
Rationale: Pastia's sign is a rash seen among children with scarlet fever that will blanch with pressure except in areas of deep creases and in the folds of joints. The tongue is initially coated with a white furry covering with red projecting papillae (white strawberry tongue). By the fourth to fifth day, the white strawberry tongue sloughs off and leaves a red, swollen tongue (strawberry tongue). The pharynx is edematous and beefy red in color. Option 2 is associated with poliomyelitis. Options 3 and 4 are characteristics of diphtheria.
Test-Taking Strategy: Focus on the subject—the clinical manifestations associated with scarlet fever. Remember that Pastia's sign describes the rash noted with scarlet fever. Review the clinical manifestations of scarlet fever if you had difficulty with this question.
Level of Cognitive Ability: Analysis
Client Needs: Physiological Integrity
Integrated Process: Nursing Process/Data Collection
Content Area: Child Health
References: Leifer, G. (2007). *Introduction to maternity and pediatric nursing* (5th ed., p. 715). Philadelphia: Saunders.
McKinney, E., James, S., Murray, S., & Ashwill, J. (2005). *Maternal-child nursing* (2nd ed., p. 1035). Philadelphia: Saunders.

414. **4**
Rationale: The parents need to be instructed to notify the physician if abdominal pain (especially in the left upper quadrant) or it left shoulder pain occurs, because this may indicate splenic rupture. Children with enlarged spleens are also instructed to avoid contact sports until the splenomegaly resolves. Bedrest is not necessary, and children usually self-limit their activity. Respiratory precautions are not required, although transmission can occur via direct intimate contact or contact with infected blood. Fever is treated with acetaminophen (Tylenol).
Test-Taking Strategy: Use the process of elimination and your knowledge regarding the organs that are affected in clients with mononucleosis. Options 1 and 2 can be eliminated first, because they are unnecessary interventions for this disease. From the remaining options, knowledge that splenic rupture is a concern will direct you to option 4. Review the complications associated with mononucleosis if you had difficulty with this question.
Level of Cognitive Ability: Application
Client Needs: Physiological Integrity
Integrated Process: Teaching and Learning
Content Area: Child Health
Reference: Hockenberry, M., & Wilson, D. (2007). *Nursing care of infants and children* (8th ed., p. 1324). St. Louis: Mosby.

415. **4**
Rationale: Diagnosis is confirmed by direct visualization of the worms. Parents can view the sleeping child's anus with a flashlight. The worm is white, thin, and about half an inch long, and it moves. The tape test, which is a simple technique, is used to capture worms and eggs. Transparent tape is lightly touched to the anus and then applied to a slide for examination. The best specimens are obtained as the child awakens, before toileting or bathing.
Test-Taking Strategy: Use the process of elimination. Thinking about the test and its purpose (to obtain a specimen that contains worms and eggs) will direct you to option 4. Review the procedure for the tape test if you had difficulty with this question.
Level of Cognitive Ability: Application
Client Needs: Physiological Integrity
Integrated Process: Nursing Process/Implementation
Content Area: Child Health
Reference: Price, D., & Gwin, J. (2008). *Pediatric nursing: An introductory text* (10th ed., pp. 201-202). St. Louis: Saunders.

416. **4**
Rationale: A severe febrile illness is a reason to delay immunization, but only until the child has recovered from the acute stage of the illness. Minor illnesses such as a cold, otitis media, or mild diarrhea are not contraindications to immunization.
Test-Taking Strategy: Use the process of elimination, and focus on the subject of a contraindication to receiving an immunization. Noting the word "severe" in option 4 will direct you to this option. If you had difficulty with this question, review the contraindications associated with immunizations.
Level of Cognitive Ability: Comprehension
Client Needs: Physiological Integrity

Integrated Process: Teaching and Learning
Content Area: Child Health
Reference: Price, D., & Gwin, J. (2008). *Pediatric nursing: An introductory text* (10th ed., p. 129). St. Louis: Saunders.

417. 4
Rationale: Most children who are infected with HIV develop symptoms within the first 9 months of life. The remainder of these infected children become symptomatic sometime before the age of 3 years. Children, with their immature immune systems, have a much shorter incubation period than adults. Options 1, 2, and 3 are incorrect.
Test-Taking Strategy: Use the process of elimination. Eliminate options 1, 2, and 3, because they are comparable or alike in content. Option 4 is the only option that provides specific and accurate data regarding HIV infection in the infant. Review the assessment findings associated with HIV infection if you had difficulty with this question.
Level of Cognitive Ability: Application
Client Needs: Psychosocial Integrity
Integrated Process: Nursing Process/Implementation
Content Area: Child Health
Reference: Price, D., & Gwin, J. (2008). *Pediatric nursing: An introductory text* (10th ed., p. 86). St. Louis: Saunders.

418. 3
Rationale: The MMR vaccine contains minute amounts of neomycin. A history of an anaphylactoid reaction to neomycin is considered a contraindication to the MMR vaccine. The general contraindication to all immunizations is a severe febrile illness. The presence of a minor illness such as the common cold is not a contraindication. In addition, a history of frequent respiratory infections is not a contraindication to receiving a vaccine. A local reaction to an immunization is treated with ice packs for the first 24 hours after injection, and this is followed by warm compresses if the inflammation persists.
Test-Taking Strategy: Use the process of elimination. Recalling that a general contraindication to all immunizations is a severe febrile illness will assist you with eliminating options 1 and 2. From the remaining options, note that option 4 identifies a local reaction. This will direct you to option 3, which is a systemic reaction and a potentially life-threatening condition. Review the contraindications to receiving immunizations if you had difficulty with this question.
Level of Cognitive Ability: Analysis
Client Needs: Physiological Integrity
Integrated Process: Nursing Process/Implementation
Content Area: Child Health

Reference: Price, D., & Gwin, J. (2008). *Pediatric nursing: An introductory text* (10th ed., p. 130). St. Louis: Saunders.

ALTERNATE ITEM FORMAT: MULTIPLE RESPONSE
419. 1, 2, 5
Rationale: AIDS is a disorder that is caused by the human immunodeficiency virus (HIV) and that is characterized by a generalized dysfunction of the immune system. Both cellular and humoral immunity are compromised. The horizontal transmission of HIV occurs through intimate sexual contact or parenteral exposure to blood or body fluids that contain visible blood. Vertical (perinatal) transmission occurs when an HIV-infected pregnant woman passes the infection to her infant. Home-care instructions include the following: frequent handwashing; monitoring for fever, malaise, fatigue, weight loss, vomiting, diarrhea, altered activity level, and oral lesions and notifying the physician if these occur; monitoring for signs and symptoms of opportunistic infections; administering antiretroviral medications, as prescribed; avoiding exposure to other illnesses; keeping immunizations up to date; avoiding kissing the child on the mouth; monitoring the weight and providing a high-calorie, high-protein diet; washing eating utensils in the dishwasher; and avoiding the sharing of eating utensils. Gloves are worn for care, especially when in contact with body fluids or changing diapers. Diapers are changed frequently and away from food areas, and soiled disposable diapers are folded inward, closed with their tabs, and disposed of in a tightly covered plastic-lined container. Any body fluid spills are cleaned with a bleach solution made up of a 10:1 ratio of water to bleach.
Test-Taking Strategy: Focus on the subject: the care of the child with AIDS. Recalling that this disorder is characterized by a generalized dysfunction of the immune system and the modes of transmission will assist you with selecting the home-care instructions. Review instructions regarding preventing the transmission of HIV/AIDS if you had difficulty with this question.
Level of Cognitive Ability: Application
Client Needs: Safe and Effective Care Environment
Integrated Process: Teaching and Learning
Content Area: Child Health
References: Hockenberry, M., & Wilson, D. (2007). *Nursing care of infants and children* (8th ed., pp. 1551-1552). St. Louis: Mosby.
Price, D., & Gwin, J. (2008). *Pediatric nursing: An introductory text* (10th ed., pp. 87-88). St. Louis: Saunders.

REFERENCES

Department of Health and Human Services, Centers for Disease Control and Prevention. *Immunization Schedules.* www.cdc.gov/vaccines/. Accessed October 26, 2008.

Hockenberry, M., & Wilson, D. (2007). *Nursing care of infants and children* (8th ed.). St. Louis: Mosby.

Ianelli, V., for About.com. *Combination vaccines.* pediatrics.about.com/cs/immunizations/a/combo_vaccines.htm. Accessed July 29, 2008.

Immunization Action Coalition. *Immunization Action Coalition home page.* www.immunize.org. Accessed July 29, 2008.

Leifer, G. (2007). *Introduction to maternity and pediatric nursing* (5th ed.). Philadelphia: Saunders.

McKinney, E., James, S., Murray, S., & Ashwill, J. (2005). *Maternal-child nursing* (2nd ed.). Philadelphia: Saunders.

National Council of State Boards of Nursing (Eds.). (2008). *2008 Detailed Test Plan for the NCLEX-PN® Examination, National Council of State Boards of Nursing.* Chicago: Author.

National Council of State Boards of Nursing. *NCSBN home page.* www.ncsbn.org. Accessed July 29, 2008.

Price, D., & Gwin, J. (2008). *Pediatric nursing: An introductory text* (10th ed.). St. Louis: Saunders.

Pediatric Medication Administration

I. MEDICATIONS AND THE PEDIATRIC CLIENT

A. Pediatric clients are smaller than adult clients, and their medications have to be adapted to their sizes and ages

B. Neonates and premature infants have immature body systems

C. The absorption, distribution, metabolism, and excretion of medications differ substantially, and the pediatric client will react more quickly to medication than an adult client will; also, their renal and hepatic function needs to be assessed before medications are administered (Figure 39-1)

D. Medication reactions are not as predictable in pediatric clients as they are in adult clients

II. ADMINISTERING ORAL MEDICATIONS

A. Most oral pediatric medications are in liquid or suspension form, because children usually cannot swallow a tablet

B. Solutions may be measured with the use of an oral syringe; if an oral syringe is not available, hypodermic syringes without needles can be used for dosage measurement

C. When volumes are extremely small, oral liquids are measured with the use of a calibrated medication dropper

D. Medications in suspension settle to the bottom of the bottle between uses, so thorough mixing is required before the pouring of the medication

E. Suspensions must be administered immediately after measurement to prevent settling and thus the administration of an incomplete dose

F. Administer oral medications with the child sitting in an upright position with the head elevated to prevent aspiration if the child cries or resists

G. Never pinch the infant or child's nostrils when administering medication

H. Do not place medication into a baby's bottle

I. Draw the required dose of an unpleasant medication into a small syringe, and place the syringe into the side and toward the back of the infant's mouth; administer the medication slowly, allowing the infant to swallow

J. Place the small child sideways on the adult's lap; the child's closest arm should be placed under the adult's arm and behind the adult's back; cradle the child's head, hold his or her hand, and administer the medication slowly with a plastic spoon or a small plastic cup

K. Mix liquid medications with less than 1 oz of fluid to disguise the taste, if necessary

L. If a tablet or capsule has been administered, check the child's mouth to ensure that it has been swallowed; if swallowing is a problem, some tablets can be crushed and given in small amounts of pureed food or flavored syrup; however, enteric-coated tablets, timed-release tablets, and capsules cannot be crushed

III. ADMINISTERING PARENTERAL MEDICATIONS

A. Subcutaneous and intramuscularly administered medications

1. Medications usually given via the subcutaneous route are insulin and some immunizations

2. Any site with sufficient subcutaneous tissue may be used for subcutaneous injections; common sites include the central third of the lateral aspect of the upper arm, the abdomen, and the center third of the anterior thigh

3. The safe use of all injection sites is based on normal muscle development and the size of the child; the preferred site for intramuscular injections in infants is the vastus lateralis (Figure 39-2)

4. Usually not more than 0.5 mL (infant) to 2.0 mL (child) is injected per intramuscular or subcutaneous site; the site of injection is rotated if frequent injections are necessary

5. For pediatric clients, the usual needle length is ½ to 1 inch, and the needle gauge is 22 to 25

6. Needle length can also be estimated by grasping the muscle for injection between the thumb and forefinger; half of the resulting distance between thumb and forefinger would be the needle length

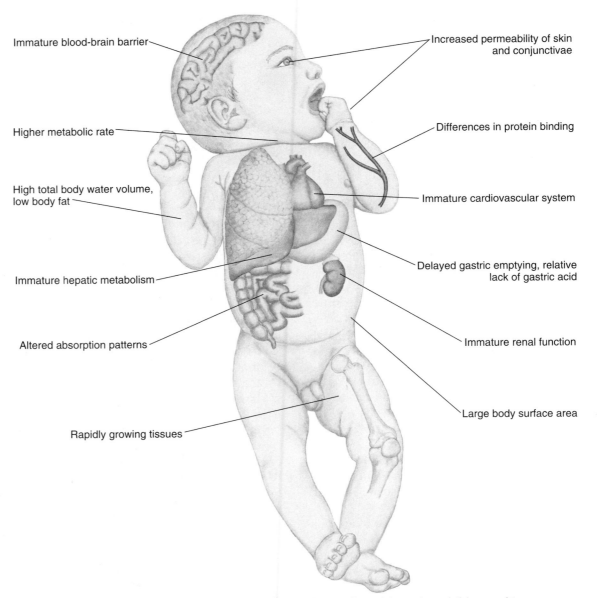

Immature blood-brain barrier

Increased permeability of skin and conjunctivae

Higher metabolic rate

Differences in protein binding

High total body water volume, low body fat

Immature cardiovascular system

Immature hepatic metabolism

Delayed gastric emptying, relative lack of gastric acid

Altered absorption patterns

Immature renal function

Rapidly growing tissues

Large body surface area

FIG. 39-1 Some factors that affect drug disposition in children. (From Price, D., & Gwin, J. [2005]. *Thompson's pediatric nursing* [9th ed.]. Philadelphia: Saunders.)

7. Pediatric dosages for subcutaneous and intramuscular administration are calculated to the nearest hundredth and measured with the use of a tuberculin syringe
8. For the toddler or preschooler, place an adhesive bandage or decorated Band-Aid over the puncture site

B. Monitoring intravenous (IV) medications
1. When an infant or a child is receiving an IV medication, the IV site needs to be assessed for signs of infiltration and inflammation immediately before, during, and after the completion of the administration of each medication (Box 39-1)
2. Signs of infiltration or inflammation need to be reported

IV. CALCULATION OF MEDICATION DOSAGE BY BODY WEIGHT
A. Conversion of body weight (Box 39-2)
B. Calculating daily dosages
1. Abbreviations (Box 39-3)
2. Dosages are expressed in terms of mg/kg/day, mg/lb/day, or mg/kg/dose
3. The total daily dosage is usually administered in divided doses (i.e., more than one) per day
4. Express the child's body weight in kilograms or pounds to correlate with the dosage specifications
5. Calculate the total daily dosage
6. Divide the total daily dosage by the number of doses to be administered over the course of 1 day

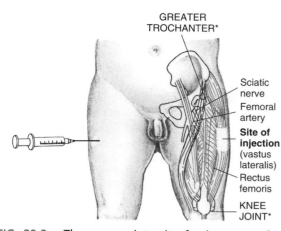

GREATER
TROCHANTER*

Sciatic
nerve

Femoral
artery

**Site of
injection**
(vastus
lateralis)

Rectus
femoris

KNEE
JOINT*

FIG. 39-2 The appropriate site for intramuscular injections in children: the vastus lateralis. (From Hockenberry, M. [2005]. *Wong's essentials of pediatric nursing* [7th ed.]. St. Louis: Saunders.)

| BOX 39-1 | Intravenous Site: Signs of Inflammation and Infiltration |

Inflammation: Redness, heat, swelling, and tenderness
Infiltration: Swelling, coolness, pain, and lack of blood return

| BOX 39-2 | Conversion of Body Weight |

Pounds to Kilograms
1 kg = 2.2 lbs
To convert pounds to kilograms, divide by 2.2.
Kilograms are expressed to the nearest tenth.
Kilograms to Pounds
1 kg = 2.2 lbs
To convert kilograms to pounds, multiply by 2.2.
Pounds are expressed to the nearest tenth.

V. CALCULATION OF BODY SURFACE AREA

A. The body surface area (BSA) is determined by comparing body weight and height with averages or norms on a graph called a nomogram
B. Not all children are the same size at the same age; therefore, the nomogram chart is used to determine the BSA of the child
C. Look at the nomogram chart (Figure 39-3); the height is on the left-hand side of the chart, and the weight is on the right-hand side
D. Place a ruler on the chart
E. Line up the left side of the ruler on the height and the right side of the ruler on the weight; read the BSA at the point where the straight edge of the ruler intersects the surface area (SA) column
F. The estimated SA is given in square meters (m^2)
G. See Box 39-4 for an example

| BOX 39-3 | Abbreviations |

gr = grain(s)
g = gram(s)
mcg = microgram(s)
mg = milligram(s)
kg = kilogram(s)
lb = pound(s)
mL = milliliter(s)
BSA = body surface area
SA = surface area
m^2 = square meters

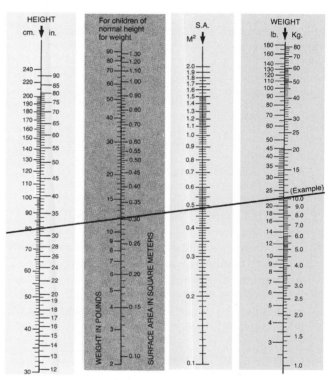

FIG. 39-3 Nomogram chart for estimating body surface area. (From Price, D., & Gwin, J. [2005]. *Thompson's pediatric nursing* [9th ed.]. Philadelphia: Saunders.)

| BOX 39-4 | How to Use the Nomogram |

Example: Use the nomogram to estimate the body surface area (BSA) of a child whose height is 58 inches and whose weight is 12 kg.

Look at the nomogram chart; note that the height is on the left-hand side of the chart and the weight is on the right-hand side of the chart.

Place a ruler on the chart, and line up the left side of the ruler on the height and the right side of the ruler on the weight. Read the BSA at the point where the straight edge of the ruler intersects the surface area (SA) column.

The estimated SA is given in square meters (m^2).

Answer: This child's BSA is 0.66 m^2

BOX 39-5   Calculating Medication Dosage

When dosage recommendations for children specify mg, mcg, or unit/m², calculating the dosage is simple multiplication.
Example: The dosage recommendation is 4 mg/m². The child has a body surface area of 1.1 m². What is the dosage to be administered?
Answer: 1.1 × 4 mg = 4.4 mg

BOX 39-6   Calculating a Child's Dosage From the Adult Dosage

When dosages are specified only for adults, a formula is used to calculate a child's dosage from the adult dosage.
Example: A physician has prescribed an antibiotic for a child. The average adult dose is 250 mg. The child has a body surface area (BSA) of 0.41 m². What is the dose for the child?
Formula:

$$\frac{\text{BSA of child (m}^2)}{1.73 \text{ m}^2} \times \text{Adult dose} = \text{Child's dose}$$

Thus,

$$\frac{0.41}{1.73} \times 250 \text{ mg} = 59.24 \text{ mg}$$

Answer: This child's dose is 59.24 mg.

VI. CALCULATIONS BASED ON BODY SURFACE AREA

A. When dosage recommendations for children specify mg, mcg, or unit per m², calculating the dosage is simple multiplication (Box 39-5)

B. When dosages are specified only for adults, a formula is used to calculate the child's dosage from the adult dosage (Box 39-6)

PRACTICE QUESTIONS

More questions on the companion CD!

420. Morphine sulfate, 2.5 mg, is prescribed for a child with cancer. The safe pediatric dose is 0.05 to 0.1 mg/kg/dose. The child weighs 50 kg. Which statement most accurately describes the prescribed dosage for this child?
   1. The dose is too low.
   2. The dose is too high.
   3. The dose is within the safe dosage range.
   4. There is not enough information to determine the safe dosage range.

421. A physician's order reads as follows: "Ampicillin (Omnipen), 125 mg intramuscular every 6 hours." The medication label reads "1 gram and reconstitute with 7.4 mL of bacteriostatic water." How many milliliters should the nurse draw up for one dose?
   1. 0.54 mL
   2. 0.92 mL
   3. 1.1 mL
   4. 7.4 mL

422. A physician has prescribed phenobarbital sodium (Luminal Sodium), 25 mg orally twice daily, for a child with febrile seizures. The medication label reads as follows: "Phenobarbital sodium, 20 mg/5 mL." The nurse has determined that the dose prescribed is a safe dose for the child. How many milliliters per dose should the nurse administer to the child?
   1. 2 mL
   2. 4.5 mL
   3. 6.25 mL
   4. 7 mL

423. Sulfisoxazole (Gantrisin), 1.0 g orally four times daily, is prescribed for an adolescent with a urinary tract infection. The medication label reads "500-mg tablets." The nurse has determined that the prescribed dose is safe. How many tablets per dose should the nurse administer to the adolescent?
   1. 0.5 tablet
   2. 1 tablet
   3. 2 tablets
   4. 3 tablets

424. Diphenhydramine hydrochloride (Benadryl), 25 mg orally every 6 hours, is prescribed for a child with an allergic reaction. The child weighs 25 kg. The safe pediatric dosage is 5 mg/kg/day. The nurse determines that:
   1. The dose is too low.
   2. The dose is too high.
   3. The dose is within the safe dosage range.
   4. There is not enough information to determine the safe dose.

425. Penicillin G procaine (Wycillin), 1,000,000 units given intramuscularly, is prescribed for an adolescent with an infection. The medication label reads as follows: "1,200,000 units/2 mL." The nurse has determined that the prescribed dose is safe. How many milliliters per dose should the nurse administer to the adolescent?
   1. 0.8 mL
   2. 1.2 mL
   3. 1.44 mL
   4. 1.66 mL

426. A pediatric client with a ventricular septal defect repair is placed on a maintenance dose of digoxin (Lanoxin) elixir. The safe dose is 0.03 mg/kg/day, and the client's weight is 7.2 kg. The physician orders the digoxin to be given twice daily. How much digoxin should the nurse administer to the client at each dose?
   1. 0.1 mg
   2. 0.37 mg
   3. 0.5 mg
   4. 2.5 mg

ALTERNATE ITEM FORMAT: FILL IN THE BLANK

427. Atropine sulfate, 0.2 mg given intramuscularly, is prescribed for a child preoperatively. The medication label reads as follows: "0.4 mg/mL." The nurse has determined that the prescribed dose is safe. How many milliliters should the nurse administer to the child?

Answer: __0.5__ mL

ANSWERS

420. 3
Rationale: Use the formula for calculating a safe dosage range. Dosage parameters:

$$0.05 \text{ mg/kg/dose} \times 50 \text{ kg} = 2.5 \text{ mg/dose}$$
$$0.1 \text{ mg/kg/dose} \times 50 \text{ kg} = 5 \text{ mg/dose}$$

The dose is within the safe dosage range.
Test-Taking Strategy: Identify the strategic components of the question and what the question is asking. In this case, the question asks for the safe dosage range of the medication. Calculate the dosage parameters with the use of the safe dosage range identified in the question and the child's weight in kilograms. Verify the answer with the use of a calculator. Review pediatric medication calculations if you had difficulty with this question.
Level of Cognitive Ability: Analysis
Client Needs: Physiological Integrity
Integrated Process: Nursing Process/Planning
Content Area: Child Health
Reference: Kee, J., & Marshall, S. (2009). *Clinical calculations: With applications to general and specialty areas* (6th ed., pp. 126, 170). Philadelphia: Saunders.

421. 2
Rationale: Convert grams to milligrams. With the metric system, to convert larger to smaller, multiply by 1000 or move the decimal three places to the right. Then, use the medication calculation formula:
1 g = 1000 mg
Formula:

$$\frac{\text{Desired}}{\text{Available}} \times \text{Volume} = \frac{125 \text{ mg}}{1000 \text{ mg}} \times 7.4 \text{ mL} = 0.925 \text{ mL/dose}$$

Test-Taking Strategy: Identify the strategic components of the question and what the question is asking. In this case, the question asks for milliliters per dose. First, convert grams to milligrams. Next, use the formula to determine the correct dosage, knowing that 1000 mg = 7.4 mL. Verify the answer with the use of a calculator. Review pediatric medication calculations if you had difficulty with this question.
Level of Cognitive Ability: Application
Client Needs: Physiological Integrity
Integrated Process: Nursing Process/Implementation
Content Area: Fundamental Skills
References: Asperheim, M. (2005). *Introduction to pharmacology* (10th ed., p. 15). Philadelphia: Saunders.
Kee, J., & Marshall, S. (2009). *Clinical calculations: With applications to general and specialty areas* (6th ed., pp. 126, 170). Philadelphia: Saunders.

422. 3
Rationale: Use the medication calculation formula.
Formula:

$$\frac{\text{Desired}}{\text{Available}} \times \text{Volume} = \frac{25 \text{ mg}}{20 \text{ mg}} \times 5 \text{ mL} = 6.25 \text{ mL/dose}$$

Test-Taking Strategy: Identify the strategic components of the question and what the question is asking. In this case, the question asks for milliliters per dose. Use the formula to determine the correct dosage, and use a calculator to verify the answer. Review pediatric medication calculations if you had difficulty with this question.
Level of Cognitive Ability: Application
Client Needs: Physiological Integrity
Integrated Process: Nursing Process/Implementation
Content Area: Child Health
Reference: Kee, J., & Marshall, S. (2009). *Clinical calculations: With applications to general and specialty areas* (6th ed., pp. 126, 170). Philadelphia: Saunders.

423. 3
Rationale: Change grams to milligrams, knowing that 1000 mg = 1 g. When converting from grams to milligrams (larger to smaller), move the decimal point three places to the right; thus, 1.0 g = 1000 mg. Then, use the medication calculation formula.
Formula:

$$\frac{\text{Desired}}{\text{Available}} \times \text{Tablet} = \frac{1000 \text{ mg}}{500 \text{ mg}} \times 1 \text{ tablet} = 2 \text{ tablets}$$

Test-Taking Strategy: Identify the strategic components of the question and what the question is asking. In this case, the question asks for tablets per dose. Change grams to milligrams first. Then, use the formula to determine the correct dosage. Remember to verify the answer with the use of a calculator. Review pediatric medication calculations if you had difficulty with this question.
Level of Cognitive Ability: Application
Client Needs: Physiological Integrity
Integrated Process: Nursing Process/Implementation
Content Area: Child Health
References: Asperheim, M. (2005). *Introduction to pharmacology* (10th ed., p. 15). Philadelphia: Saunders.
Kee, J., & Marshall, S. (2009). *Clinical calculations: With applications to general and specialty areas* (6th ed., pp. 126, 170). Philadelphia: Saunders.

424. 3
Rationale: Use the formula for calculating a safe dosage range.
Safe dose parameter:

$$5 \text{ mg/kg/day} \times 25 \text{ kg} = 125 \text{ mg/day}$$

Dosage frequency:

25 mg × 4 doses (every 6 hours) = 100 mg/day

The dose is within the safe dosage range.

Test-Taking Strategy: Identify the strategic components of the question and what the question is asking. In this case, the question asks for the safe dose of the medication. Calculate the dosage parameters using the safe dose identified in the question and the child's weight in kilograms. Use a calculator to verify the answer, and remember to determine the total daily dosage before selecting an option. Review pediatric medication calculations if you had difficulty with this question.

Level of Cognitive Ability: Analysis
Client Needs: Physiological Integrity
Integrated Process: Nursing Process/Planning
Content Area: Child Health
Reference: Kee, J., & Marshall, S. (2009). *Clinical calculations: With applications to general and specialty areas* (6th ed., pp. 126, 170). Philadelphia: Saunders.

425. 4
Rationale: Use the medication calculation formula.
Formula:

$$\frac{\text{Desired}}{\text{Available}} \times \text{Volume} = \frac{1,000,000}{1,200,000} \times 2 \text{ mL} = 1.66 \text{ mL/dose}$$

Test-Taking Strategy: Identify the strategic components of the question and what the question is asking. In this case, the question asks for milliliters per dose. Use the formula to determine the correct dose, and verify the answer with a calculator. Review pediatric medication calculations if you had difficulty with this question.

Level of Cognitive Ability: Application
Client Needs: Physiological Integrity
Integrated Process: Nursing Process/Implementation
Content Area: Child Health
Reference: Kee, J., & Marshall, S. (2009). *Clinical calculations: With applications to general and specialty areas* (6th ed., pp. 126, 170). Philadelphia: Saunders.

426. 1
Rationale: Calculate the dosage by weight first: therefore, 0.03 mg/day × 7.2 kg = 0.21 mg/day. Next, note that the physician orders digoxin to be given twice daily; thus, two doses in 24 hours will be administered, and 0.21 mg/day divided by 2 doses = 0.1 mg for each dose.

Test-Taking Strategy: Identify the strategic components of the question and what the question is asking. Read the question carefully, and note the strategic words "twice daily" and "each dose." Calculate the dosage by weight first, and then determine the milligrams per each dose. Verify the answer with the use of a calculator. Review pediatric medication calculations if you had difficulty with this question.

Level of Cognitive Ability: Application
Client Needs: Physiological Integrity
Integrated Process: Nursing Process/Implementation
Content Area: Child Health
Reference: Kee, J., & Marshall, S. (2009). *Clinical calculations: With applications to general and specialty areas* (6th ed., pp. 126, 170). Philadelphia: Saunders.

ALTERNATE ITEM FORMAT: FILL IN THE BLANK
427. 0.5
Rationale: Use the formula for calculating medication dosage.
Formula:

$$\frac{\text{Desired}}{\text{Available}} \times \text{Volume} = \frac{0.2 \text{ mg}}{0.4 \text{ mg}} \times 1 \text{ mL} = 0.5 \text{ mL}$$

Test-Taking Strategy: Identify what the question is asking. In this case, the question asks for the milliliters to be administered. Use the formula to determine the correct dose, and use a calculator to verify your answer. Review this formula if you had difficulty with this question.

Level of Cognitive Ability: Application
Client Needs: Physiological Integrity
Integrated Process: Nursing Process/Implementation
Content Area: Child Health
Reference: Kee, J., & Marshall, S. (2009). *Clinical calculations: With applications to general and specialty areas* (6th ed., pp. 126, 170). Philadelphia: Saunders.

REFERENCES

Asperheim, M. (2005). *Introduction to pharmacology* (10th ed.). Philadelphia: Saunders.

Hockenberry, M. (2005). *Wong's essentials of pediatric nursing* (7th ed.). St. Louis: Saunders.

Kee, J., & Marshall, S. (2009). *Clinical calculations: With applications to general and specialty areas* (6th ed.). Philadelphia: Saunders.

National Council of State Boards of Nursing (Eds.) (2008). *2008 Detailed Test Plan for the NCLEX-PN® Examination, National Council of State Boards of Nursing.* Chicago: Author.

National Council of State Boards of Nursing. *NCSBN home page.* www.ncsbn.org. Accessed July 27, 2008.

Price, D., & Gwin, J. (2005). *Thompson's pediatric nursing* (9th ed.). Philadelphia: Saunders.

The Adult Client With an Integumentary Disorder

PYRAMID TERMS

burns The cell destruction of the layers of the skin and the resultant depletion of fluid and electrolytes as a result of thermal or chemical injury.

carbon monoxide poisoning Carbon monoxide is a colorless, odorless, and tasteless gas that has an affinity for hemoglobin that is 200 times greater than that of oxygen. Oxygen molecules are displaced, and carbon monoxide reversibly binds to hemoglobin to form carboxyhemoglobin. Tissue hypoxia occurs.

chemical burn Tissue destruction caused by contact with strong acids, alkalis, or organic compounds. Systemic toxicity from cutaneous absorption can occur.

deep full-thickness burn A burn injury that involves damage of the muscle, bone, and tendons. The injured area appears black, and the eschar is hard and inelastic.

deep-partial thickness burn A burn injury that extends into the skin dermis. The wound is red and dry, with white areas in parts that are more deeply injured. Can convert to a full-thickness injury when tissue damage increases with infection, hypoxia, or ischemia.

electrical burn Tissue destruction caused by heat generated from electrical energy as it passes through the body and results in internal tissue damage.

full-thickness burn The injured area appears waxy white, deep red, yellow, brown, or black, and the injured surface appears dry. Edema is present under the eschar.

herpes zoster (shingles) An acute viral infection of the nerve structure caused by the varicella zoster virus. Herpes zoster is contagious to individuals who have not had chickenpox.

pressure ulcer A localized area of skin breakdown that occurs as a result of poor circulation to the area due to pressure betweeen a surface and a bony prominence.

skin cancer A malignant lesion of the skin that may or may not metastasize. Causes include chronic friction and irritation to a skin area and exposure to ultraviolet rays. Diagnosis is confirmed by a skin biopsy that is positive for cancer cells.

smoke inhalation injury Injury that results when the victim is trapped in an enclosed, smoke-filled space.

superficial-thickness burn A burn injury that involves damage of the upper third of the dermis. Mild to severe erythema is noted, and the skin blanches with pressure. The burn is painful.

superficial partial-thickness burn A mottled red base and a broken epidermis and a wet, shiny, and weeping surface are present. Large blisters cover an extensive area. The skin is edematous and painful.

thermal burn Tissue injury caused by exposure to flames, hot liquids, steam, or hot objects.

PYRAMID TO SUCCESS

The Pyramid to Success focuses on the concept that the integumentary system provides the first line of defense against infections. Focus on the protective measures that are necessary to prevent infection. The pyramid points address the risk factors related to the development of integumentary disorders and the preventive measures related to skin cancer. Focus on the emergency measures related to a client with a burn, fluid resuscitation, monitoring for complications, and skin grafting. Psychosocial issues relate to the body-image disturbances that can occur as a result of an integumentary disorder. The Integrated Processes addressed in this unit include Caring, the Clinical Problem-Solving Process (Nursing Process), Communication and Documentation, and Teaching and Learning.

CLIENT NEEDS

Safe and Effective Care Environment

Consulting with members of the health care team regarding treatments
Establishing priorities of care
Handling hazardous and infectious materials
Instituting standard and other precautions
Maintaining confidentiality related to a disorder
Making referrals to appropriate care providers
Obtaining informed consent for treatments and procedures
Practicing medical and surgical asepsis
Preventing infection

Health Promotion and Maintenance

Implementing disease prevention measures
Performing data collection regarding the integumentary system
Promoting health screening and health promotion programs to prevent skin disorders
Providing instructions to the client regarding care for an integumentary disorder

Psychosocial Integrity

Addressing end-of-life issues
Discussing unexpected body-image changes
Identifying coping mechanisms
Identifying situational role changes
Using support systems

Physiological Integrity

Assessing for alterations in body systems
Providing adequate nutrition for healing
Providing basic care and comfort
Providing emergency care
Monitoring for the expected effects of treatments
Monitoring for fluid and electrolyte imbalances and other complications
Monitoring laboratory values

REFERENCES

Chernecky, C., & Berger, B. (2008). *Laboratory tests and diagnostic procedures* (5th ed.). Philadelphia: Saunders.

Christensen, B., & Kockrow, E. (2006). *Adult health nursing* (5th ed.). St. Louis: Mosby.

Christensen, B., & Kockrow, E. (2006). *Foundations of nursing* (5th ed.). St. Louis: Mosby.

deWit, S. (2009). *Medical-surgical nursing: Concepts & practice.* Philadelphia: Saunders.

Hodgson, B., & Kizior, R. (2008). *Saunders nursing drug handbook 2008.* Philadelphia: Saunders.

Ignatavicius, D., & Workman, M. (2006). *Medical-surgical nursing: Critical thinking for collaborative care* (5th ed.). Philadelphia: Saunders.

Kee, J., Hayes, E., & McCuistion, L. (2006). *Pharmacology: A nursing process approach* (5th ed.). Philadelphia: Saunders.

Lehne, R. (2007). *Pharmacology for nursing care* (6th ed.). Philadelphia: Saunders.

Lewis, S., Heitkemper, M., Dirksen, S., & Bucher, L. (2007). *Medical-surgical nursing: Assessment and management of clinical problems* (7th ed.). St. Louis: Mosby.

Linton, A. (2007). *Introduction to medical-surgical nursing* (4th ed.). Philadelphia: Saunders.

McKenry, L., Tessier, E., & Hogan, M. (2006). *Mosby's pharmacology in nursing* (22nd ed.). St. Louis: Mosby.

Monahan, F., Sands, J., Marek, J., Neighbors, M., & Green, C. (2007). *Phipps' medical-surgical nursing: Health and illness perspectives* (8th ed.). St. Louis: Mosby.

National Council of State Boards of Nursing (Eds.). (2008). *2008 Detailed Test Plan for the NCLEX-PN® Examination, National Council of State Boards of Nursing.* Chicago: Author.

National Council of State Boards of Nursing. *NCSBN home page.* www.ncsbn.org. Accessed July 29, 2008.

Perry, A., & Potter, P. (2006). *Clinical nursing skills & techniques* (6th ed.). St. Louis: Mosby.

Skidmore-Roth, L. (2008). *2008 Mosby's nursing drug reference* (21st ed.). St. Louis: Mosby.

CHAPTER 40

Integumentary System

I. ANATOMY AND PHYSIOLOGY

A. The skin is the largest sensory organ of the body, with a surface area of 15 to 20 square feet and a weight of about 9 lbs

B. Functions
1. Provides the first line of defense against infection
2. Protects underlying tissues and organs from injury
3. Receives stimuli from the external environment; detects touch, pressure, pain, and temperature stimuli and relays that information to the nervous system
4. Maintains the normal body temperature
5. Excretes salts, water, and organic wastes
6. Protects the body from excessive water loss
7. Synthesizes vitamin D_3, which converts to calcitriol, for normal calcium metabolism
8. Stores nutrients

C. Layers
1. Epidermis
2. Dermis
3. Hypodermis (subcutaneous fat)

D. Epidermal appendages
1. Nails
2. Hair
3. Glands
   a. Sebaceous
   b. Sweat

E. Normal bacterial flora
1. Types of normal bacterial flora include the following:
   a. Gram-positive and gram-negative staphylococci
   b. Pseudomonas
   c. Streptococcus
2. Organisms are shed with normal exfoliation
3. A pH of 4.2 to 5.6 halts the growth of bacteria

II. RISK FACTORS FOR INTEGUMENTARY DISORDERS

A. Exposure to chemical and environmental pollutants
B. Exposure to radiation
C. Exposure to the sun
D. Lack of personal hygiene habits
E. Use of cosmetics and harsh soaps
F. Medications, such as long-term corticosteroid and anticoagulant therapy
G. Nutritional deficiencies
H. Moderate to severe emotional stress
I. Infection, with injured areas as the potential entry points for infection
J. Changes associated with developmental stages and aging

III. PSYCHOSOCIAL IMPACT

A. Changes in body image and decreased self-esteem
B. Social isolation and fear of rejection from embarrassment about changes in skin appearance
C. Restrictions in physical activity
D. Pain
E. Disruption or loss of employment
F. Cost of medications, hospitalizations, and follow-up care, including dressing supplies

IV. DIAGNOSTIC TESTS

A. Skin biopsy
1. Description
   a. Skin biopsy is the collection of a small piece of skin tissue for histopathologic study
   b. Methods include punch, excisional, incisional, and shave
2. Preprocedure interventions
   a. Obtain informed consent
   b. Cleanse site, as prescribed
3. Postprocedure interventions
   a. Place specimen, when obtained by physician, in the appropriate container and send to pathology laboratory for analysis
   b. Use surgically aseptic technique for biopsy site dressings
   c. Assess the biopsy site for bleeding and infection
   d. Instruct the client to keep the dressing dry and in place for at least 8 hours and to then clean the area daily and use antibiotic ointment, as prescribed

B. Skin cultures
1. Description
    a. Noninvasive procedure
    b. A small skin culture sample is obtained with the use of a sterile applicator and the appropriate type of culture tube (bacterial versus viral)
    c. Viral culture is immediately placed on ice
    d. Sample is sent to the laboratory to identify an existing organism
2. Preprocedure intervention: Obtain skin culture samples before instituting antibiotic therapy
3. Postprocedure intervention: Send the skin culture sample to the laboratory
C. Wood's light examination
1. Description: The skin is viewed under ultraviolet light through a special glass (Wood's glass) to identify superficial infections of the skin
2. Preprocedure intervention: Darken the room before the examination
3. Postprocedure intervention: Assist the client during adjusting to light after being in a darkened room

V. **SKIN DISORDERS**
A. Skin cancer
1. Description
    a. **Skin cancer** is a malignant lesion of the skin that may or may not metastasize
    b. **Skin cancer** causes include chronic friction and irritation to a skin area and exposure to ultraviolet rays
    c. Diagnosis is confirmed by a skin biopsy that is positive for cancer cells
2. Types
    a. Basal cell: The most common type; basal cell cancer arises from the basal cells contained in the epidermis
    b. Squamous cell: The second most common type of **skin cancer** among whites; squamous cell cancer is a tumor of the epidermal keratinocytes that can infiltrate surrounding structures, metastasize to lymph nodes, and subsequently be fatal
    c. Malignant melanoma: May occur anyplace on the body, especially where birthmarks or new moles are apparent; cancer of the melanocytes can metastasize to the brain, lungs, bone, liver, and skin and is ultimately fatal
3. Data collection (Box 40-1)
    a. Change in color, size, or shape of preexisting lesion
    b. Pruritus
    c. Local soreness
4. Interventions
    a. Instruct the client regarding preventive measures

> **BOX 40-1** Characteristics of Skin Cancer Lesions
>
> **Basal Cell Carcinoma**
> - Waxy border
> - Papule, with a red, central crater
> - Rarely metastasizes
>
> **Squamous Cell Carcinoma**
> - Oozing, bleeding, crusting lesion
> - Potentially metastatic
> - Larger tumors associated with higher risk for metastasis
>
> **Melanoma**
> - Irregular, circular, bordered lesion with hues of tan, black, or blue
> - Rapid infiltration into tissue
> - Rapid metastasis
> - Significant rates of morbidity and mortality

    b. Instruct the client to monitor for lesions that do not heal or that change characteristics
    c. Instruct the client to have moles or lesions that are subject to chronic irritation removed
    d. Instruct the client to avoid contact with chemical irritants
    e. Instruct the client to wear layered clothing and to use sunscreen with an appropriate skin protection factor when outdoors
    f. Instruct the client to avoid sun exposure between 10:00 AM and 3:00 PM
    g. Assist with the surgical excision of the lesion, as prescribed
B. Contact dermatitis
1. Description: An inflammatory response of the skin that produces skin changes after contact with a specific antigen
2. Data collection
    a. Pruritus and burning
    b. Edema
    c. Erythema at the point of contact
    d. Signs of infection
    e. Vesicles with drainage
3. Interventions
    a. Elevate the extremity to reduce edema
    b. Apply cool, wet dressings and tepid baths, as prescribed
    c. Maintain a cool environment
    d. Protect the affected area from trauma
    e. Prevent scratching and rubbing of the affected area
    f. Assist with skin testing, as prescribed, to determine allergen(s)
    g. Instruct the client to avoid contact with the allergen after it has been determined
    h. Instruct the client to avoid harsh soaps
    i. Instruct the client to avoid using heating pads or blankets

j. Administer antibiotics for infection, antipruritics or antihistamines for itching, and corticosteroids for inflammation, as prescribed

C. Poison ivy, poison oak, and poison sumac
   1. Description: A dermatitis that develops from contact with urushiol from poison ivy, oak, or sumac plants
   2. Data collection
      a. Papulovesicular lesions
      b. Severe itching
   3. Interventions
      a. Cleanse the skin of the plant oils immediately.
      b. Apply cool, wet dressings with Burow's solution, as prescribed, to relieve the itching
      c. Apply lotion or topical corticosteroids, as prescribed
      d. Administer oral corticosteroids, as prescribed, for a severe reaction

D. Erysipelas and cellulitis
   1. Description
      a. Erysipelas is an acute, superficial, rapidly spreading inflammation of the dermis and lymphatics caused by β-hemolytic streptococcus group A that enters the tissue via an abrasion, bite, trauma, or wound
      b. Cellulitis is a skin infection into the deeper dermis and subcutaneous fat; the causative organism is usually *Streptococcus pyogenes*
   2. Data collection
      a. Pain
      b. Itching
      c. Swelling
      d. Redness and warmth
   3. Interventions
      a. Promote rest
      b. Apply warm compresses, as prescribed (usually twice a day), to promote circulation and to decrease discomfort, erythema, and edema
      c. Administer antibiotics, as prescribed, for infection after a culture of the area
      d. Clean the skin daily with an antibacterial soap, as prescribed

E. Psoriasis
   1. Description
      a. Psoriasis is a chronic, noninfectious skin inflammation that involves keratin synthesis and that results in psoriatic patches
      b. Various forms exist, with psoriasis vulgaris being the most common
      c. Possible causes of the disorder include stress, trauma, infection, and changes in climate
      d. The disorder may also be exacerbated by the use of certain medications
      e. Koebner's phenomenon is the development of psoriatic lesions at a site of injury, such as a scratched or sunburned area
   2. Data collection
      a. Pruritus
      b. Shedding, silvery, white scales on a raised, reddened, round plaque that usually affects the scalp, the knees, the elbows, the extensor surfaces of the arms and legs, and the sacral regions
      c. A yellow discoloration, pitting, and thickening of the nails occurs if they are affected
      d. Joint inflammation with psoriatic arthritis
   3. Interventions
      a. Administer daily soaks and tepid, wet compresses to the affected areas to remove the scales; oils or coal-tar preparations may be added to the bath water
      b. Assist the client with removing the scales during the soak with the use of a soft washcloth and gentle, circular motions; emollient creams or salicylic acid may be applied to affected areas after the bath to continue to soften thick scales
   4. Topical pharmacological therapy
      a. Pharmacological therapy includes tar preparations, anthralin, salicylic acid, and corticosteroids; vitamin D preparation, calcipotriene (Dovonex), and the retinoid compound tazarotene (Tazorac) suppress epidermopoiesis and cause sloughing of the rapidly growing epidermal cells
      b. Occlusive dressings may be applied after the application of the corticosteroid to increase its effectiveness
      c. Use plastic wrap or bags as the occlusive dressing, and use rubber gloves on the client's hands, plastic bags on the feet, and a shower cap on the head, if these areas are affected; a plastic vinyl jogging suit may be used for the client who is being treated at home
   5. Intralesional therapy involves injections of triamcinolone acetonide (Aristocort, Kenalog-10) into highly visible or isolated patches of psoriasis that are resistant to other forms of therapy
   6. Systemic therapy
      a. Systemic medications may be prescribed to treat extensive psoriasis that does not respond to other forms of therapy
      b. Prescribed medications may include methotrexate, hydroxyurea (Hydrea), and cyclosporine
   7. Photochemotherapy
      a. A combination of psoralens and ultraviolet A light therapy decreases cellular proliferation

b. The client takes a photosensitizing medication (8-methoxypsoralen) and is subsequently exposed to long-wave ultraviolet light

8. Client education
   a. Instruct the client not to scratch the affected areas and to keep the skin lubricated to minimize itching
   b. Monitor for and instruct the client to recognize the signs and symptoms of infection
   c. Instruct the client to wear light cotton clothing over affected areas
   d. Instruct the client regarding prescribed treatments and medications and to avoid over-the-counter medications
   e. Assist the client with identifying ways to reduce stress

F. **Herpes zoster (shingles)**
   1. Description
      a. Among clients with a history of chickenpox, shingles is caused by the reactivation of the varicella zoster virus; shingles can occur during any immunocompromised state in these clients
      b. The dormant virus is located in the dorsal nerve root ganglion of the sensory cranial and spinal nerves
      c. The diagnosis is determined by visual examination, skin cultures, and skin stains that identify the organism and by an antinuclear antibody blood test that will produce a positive result
      d. Culture provides the definitive diagnosis
      e. **Herpes zoster** is contagious to individuals who have not had chickenpox
   2. Data collection
      a. Unilaterally clustered skin vesicles along the peripheral sensory nerves on the trunk, thorax, or face
      b. Fever
      c. Burning and neuralgia
      d. Pruritus
      e. Paresthesia
   3. Interventions
      a. Isolate the client, because exudate from the lesions contains the virus; maintain standard and other precautions, such as contact precautions
      b. Assess the neurovascular status and seventh cranial nerve function
      c. Assess for signs and symptoms of infection
      d. Keep blisters intact, if they have formed
      e. Assist the client with acetic acid compresses; cool, wet compresses; and tepid baths, as prescribed.
      f. Prepare to assist the physician with a nerve block using lidocaine (Xylocaine), if prescribed

g. Administer antiviral agents, analgesics, antianxiety agents, antipruritics, and corticosteroids, as prescribed.
   h. Use an air mattress and a bed cradle on the client's bed, and keep the environment cool; warmth and touch aggravate pain
   i. Prevent the client from scratching and rubbing the affected area
   j. Instruct the client to wear lightweight, loose cotton clothing and to avoid wool and synthetic clothing

G. Paronychia
   1. Description: An infection of the tissue around the nail plate that most commonly occurs among middle-aged women and clients with diabetes mellitus
   2. Data collection
      a. Redness and swelling around the nail bed
      b. Soreness of the nail bed
   3. Interventions
      a. Monitor the temperature
      b. Monitor for infection around the nails
      c. Monitor for cellulitis in the affected area
      d. Assist the client with warm soaks, as prescribed
      e. Prepare to assist with the incision and drainage of the infected area, if prescribed
      f. Administer antibiotic or fungicidal ointments, as prescribed.

H. Impetigo: See Chapter 35 for information about this disorder

I. Frostbite
   1. Description
      a. Damage to tissues and blood vessels as a result of prolonged exposure to cold
      b. The fingers, toes, nose, and ears are often affected
   2. Data collection
      a. Numbness
      b. Paresthesia
      c. Pallor
      d. Severe pain, swelling, erythema, and blistering that occur after the client is moved to a warm environment
      e. Necrosis and gangrene may develop in severe cases
   3. Interventions
      a. Handle the tissues gently
      b. Rewarm the affected part rapidly and continuously with a warm water bath (90° F to 107° F) for 15 to 20 minutes or until skin flushing occurs
      c. Avoid slow thawing, interrupted periods of warmth, or massage (these may result in further tissue damage)
      d. Do not débride blisters

e. Leave the area exposed initially for continued assessment, and then apply bulky dressings, as prescribed, to provide protection

J. Scabies

1. Description
   a. Scabies is a parasitic skin disorder caused by an infestation of *Sarcoptes scabiei* (itch mite)
   b. Scabies is endemic among schoolchildren and institutionalized populations as a result of close personal contact
   c. Risk factors include close personal contact with an infected person or a contaminated article
   d. Usually a 1-month delay occurs between the initial infestation and the onset of pruritus in the host

2. Data collection
   a. Erythematous papules and pustules
   b. Threadlike, brownish, linear burrows up to 1-cm long
   c. Burrows are most common between the fingers, on the palms, and on the inner aspect of the wrist
   d. Secondary lesions consist of vesicles, crusts, reddish-brown nodules, and excoriations
   e. Intense pruritus that worsens at night

3. Interventions
   a. Administer antihistamines or topical steroids to relieve itching, as prescribed.
   b. Apply topical anti-scabies creams or lotions such as lindane, crotamiton (Eurax), or permethrin (Elimite, Acticin), as prescribed.
   c. Lindane should not be used with children less than 2 years old because of the risk of neurotoxicity and seizures
   d. Instruct the client to apply the anti-scabies preparation thinly to the entire skin from the neck down (the face and scalp are not affected by scabies) and to leave it on for 12 to 24 hours, as prescribed
   e. Instruct the client to apply anti-scabies preparations to dry skin; moist skin increases absorption and thus the potential for central nervous system side effects such as seizures
   f. After treatment with anti-scabies preparations, instruct the client to remove the medication by thoroughly washing with soap and water
   g. Contact precautions need to be maintained, and all family members and close contacts should be treated simultaneously
   h. Instruct the client that all bedding and clothing should be washed in hot water and dried on the hot dryer cycle or dry-cleaned (mites can survive up to 36 hours on linen)

K. Acne vulgaris

1. Description
   a. Acne is a common, self-limiting, multifactorial disorder
   b. Acne requires active treatment for control until it spontaneously resolves
   c. The types of lesions include comedones (open and closed), pustules, papules, and nodules
   d. The exact cause is unknown but may include androgenic influence on the sebaceous glands, increased sebum production, and the proliferation of *Propionibacterium acnes* (the enzymes of which reduce lipids to irritating fatty acids)
   e. Exacerbations coincide with the menstrual cycle as a result of hormonal activity
   f. Heat, humidity, and excessive perspiration have roles in increased acne

2. Data collection
   a. Closed comedones are whiteheads and noninflamed lesions that develop in a follicle and enlarge with the retention of horny cells
   b. Open comedones are blackheads that result from the continuing accumulation of horny cells and sebum, which dilates the follicles
   c. Pustules and papules result as the inflammatory process progresses
   d. Nodules result from the total disintegration of a comedone and the subsequent collapse of the follicle
   e. Deep scarring can result from nodules

3. Interventions
   a. Instruct the client regarding the administration of topical or oral antibiotics, as prescribed; provide written instructions
   b. Instruct the client in the use of isotretinoin (Accutane) or other medications, if prescribed, to inhibit sebum production and reduce the size of the sebaceous glands
   c. Instruct the client about the adverse effects of isotretinoin, which include cheilitis (lip inflammation), skin dryness, elevated triglycerides, eye discomfort, and depression in some cases
   d. Instruct the client to stop taking vitamin A supplements during treatment with isotretinoin
   e. Inform the client that improvement may not be apparent for 4 to 6 weeks
   f. Instruct the client in appropriate skin-cleansing methods, with emphasis on not scrubbing the face and using only the prescribed topical agents
   g. Instruct the client not to squeeze, prick, or pick at lesions

h. Instruct the client to use products labeled noncomedogenic and cosmetics that are water-based and to avoid contact with excessively oil-based products

i. Instruct the client regarding the importance of follow-up treatment

L. **Pressure ulcer**
1. Description
   a. A **pressure ulcer** is an impairment of the skin integrity; occurs as a result of presure between the skin surface and a bony prominence
   b. The prevention of skin breakdown is a major role of the nurse, particularly when caring for the bedridden or immobile client
2. Risk factors
   a. Malnutrition
   b. Incontinence
   c. Immobility
   d. Skin shearing
   e. Decreased sensory perception
3. Data collection (Box 40-2)
4. Interventions
   a. Institute measures to prevent **pressure ulcers**
   b. Assess the nutritional status of the client
   c. Provide adequate nutritional intake to promote tissue integrity
   d. Monitor for alterations in skin integrity
   e. Relieve or remove pressure on the skin
   f. Turn and reposition the immobile client every 2 hours or more frequently, if necessary

---

BOX 40-2 **Stages of Pressure Ulcers**

Stage I
The skin is intact.
The area is red and does not blanch with external pressure.
Area may be painful, firm, soft, warm, or cool compared with adjacent tissue.

Stage II
The skin is not intact.
Partial-thickness skin loss of the epidermis or dermis occurs.
Presents as a shallow open ulcer with a red-pink wound bed or as an intact or open/ruptured serum-filled blister.

Stage III
Full-thickness skin loss is present and extends into the dermis and subcutaneous tissues and slough may be present.
The subcutaneous tissue may be visible.
Purulent drainage is common.
Undermining and tunneling may or may not be present.

Stage IV
Full-thickness skin loss is present and extends into the muscle, bone, or other supporting structures.
Slough or escar may be present.
Purulent, foul-smelling drainage is common.
Undermining and tunneling may develop.

---

g. Help the client to ambulate
h. Provide active and passive exercises every 8 hours
i. Keep the skin clean and dry and the sheets free of wrinkles
j. Apply a moisture barrier, as prescribed, to protect the skin
k. Use pressure reduction or relief devices to prevent pressure, such as a special mattress (i.e., an alternating air-pressure mattress), a mattress overlay, or wheelchair cushions
l. Apply medications or dressings to the wound, as prescribed

VI. **BURN INJURIES**
A. Description: Cell destruction of the layers of the skin and the resultant depletion of fluid and electrolytes
B. Burn size
   1. Small **burns**: The response of the body to injury is localized to the injured area
   2. Large or extensive **burns**
      a. Large **burns** consist of 25% or more of the total body surface area
      b. The response of the body to the injury is systemic.
      c. The **burn** affects all of the major systems of the body.
C. Estimating the extent of injury (Box 40-3 and Figure 40-1)
D. Burn depth
   1. **Superficial-thickness burn**
      a. Involves injury to the upper third of the dermis; the blood supply to the dermis is still intact
      b. Mild to severe erythema (pink to red) is present, but there are no blisters
      c. The skin blanches with pressure

BOX 40-3 **Methods to Estimate the Extent of Burn Injury**

Rule of Nines (Adult)
- Head: 9%
- Anterior trunk: 18%
- Posterior trunk: 18%
- Arms (9% each) 18%
- Legs (18% each): 36%
- Perineum: 1%

Lund-Browder and Berkow Classifications
- Modify percentages for body segments according to age
- Provide a more accurate estimate of the burn size
- Make use of a diagram of the body that is divided into sections, with the representative percentages of the total body surface area from birth throughout adulthood
- Burn size should be reevaluated after initial wound débridement.

d. The **burn** is painful, with a tingling sensation and pain that is eased with cooling

e. The discomfort lasts about 48 hours; healing occurs in about 3 to 5 days

f. There is no scarring, and skin grafts are not required

2. **Superficial partial-thickness burn**

a. Involves injury deeper into the dermis; the blood supply is reduced

b. Large blisters may cover an extensive area

c. Edema is present

d. The **burn** has a mottled pink to red base and a broken epidermis, with a wet, shiny, and weeping surface

e. The **burn** is painful and sensitive to cold air

f. Healing occurs in 10 to 21 days with no scarring, but some minor pigment changes may occur

g. Grafts may be used if the healing process is prolonged

3. **Deep partial-thickness burn**

a. Extends into the skin dermis

b. Blister formation usually does not occur, because the dead tissue layer is thick and sticks to the underlying viable dermis

c. The wound surface is red and dry, with white areas in deeper parts

d. The area may or may not blanch, and edema is moderate

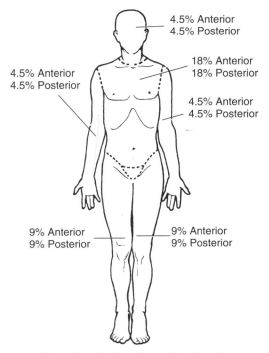

FIG. 40-1 The rule of nines for estimating burn percentage. (From Ignatavicius, D., & Workman, M. [2006]. *Medical surgical nursing: Critical thinking for collaborative care* [5th ed.]. Philadelphia: Saunders.)

4.5% Anterior
4.5% Posterior

4.5% Anterior
4.5% Posterior

18% Anterior
18% Posterior

4.5% Anterior
4.5% Posterior

9% Anterior
9% Posterior

9% Anterior
9% Posterior

e. Can convert to a **full-thickness burn** when tissue damage increases with infection, hypoxia, or ischemia

f. Generally heals in 3 to 6 weeks, but scar formation results, and skin grafting may be necessary

4. **Full-thickness burn**

a. Involves the injury and destruction of the epidermis and the dermis; the wound will not heal by re-epithelialization, and grafting may be required

b. Appears as a dry, hard, leathery eschar; this burn crust or dead tissue must slough off or be removed from the wound before healing can occur

c. Appears waxy white, deep red, yellow, brown, or black

d. Injured surface appears dry

e. Edema is present under the eschar

f. Sensation is reduced or absent as a result of the destruction of nerve endings

g. Healing may take weeks to months and depends on the establishment of an adequate blood supply

h. Treatment requires the removal of eschar and split- or **full-thickness** skin grafting

i. Scarring and wound contractures are likely to develop without preventive measures

5. **Deep full-thickness burn**

a. Extends beyond the skin into the underlying fascia and tissues; damage to the muscles, bones, and tendons occurs

b. The injured area appears black, and sensation is completely absent

c. The eschar is hard and inelastic

d. Healing takes months, and grafts are required

E. Age and general health

1. Mortality rates are higher for children less than 4 years old (particularly in the birth to 1-year-old age group) and for clients more than 65 years old

2. Debilitating disorders (i.e., cardiac, respiratory, endocrine, and renal disorders) negatively influence the client's response to injury and treatment

3. The mortality rate is higher when the client has a preexisting disorder at the time of the burn injury

F. **Burn** location

1. **Burns** of the head, neck, and chest are associated with pulmonary complications

2. **Burns** of the face are associated with corneal abrasion

3. **Burns** of the ear are associated with auricular chondritis

4. **Burns** of the hands and joints require intensive therapy to prevent disability

5. **Burns** of the perineal area are prone to auto-contamination by urine and feces
6. Circumferential **burns** of the extremities can produce a tourniquet-like effect and lead to vascular compromise (compartment syndrome)
7. Circumferential thorax **burns** lead to inadequate chest wall expansion and pulmonary insufficiency

VII. TYPES OF BURNS

A. **Thermal burns** are caused by exposure to flames, hot liquids, steam, and hot objects
B. **Chemical burns**
   1. **Burns** are caused by tissue contact with strong acids, alkalis, and organic compounds
   2. Systemic toxicity from cutaneous absorption can occur
C. **Electrical burns**
   1. **Burns** are caused by heat generated by electrical energy as it passes through the body
   2. **Electrical burns** result in internal tissue damage
   3. Cutaneous **burns** cause muscle and soft tissue damage that may be extensive, particularly with high-voltage electrical injuries
   4. The voltage, type of current, contact site, and duration of contact are important to identify
   5. Alternating current is more dangerous than direct current, because it is associated with cardiopulmonary arrest, ventricular fibrillation, tetanic muscle contractions, and long-bone or vertebral fractures
D. Radiation **burns** are caused by exposure to ultraviolet light, x-rays, and radioactive sources

VIII. INHALATION INJURIES

A. **Smoke inhalation injury**
   1. Description: Injury results when the victim is trapped in an enclosed, hot, smoke-filled space
   2. Data collection
      a. Facial burns
      b. Erythema
      c. Swelling of the oropharynx and nasopharynx
      d. Singed nasal hairs
      e. Flaring nostrils
      f. Stridor, wheezing, and dyspnea
      g. Hoarse voice
      h. Sooty (carbonaceous) sputum and cough
      i. Tachycardia
      j. Agitation and anxiety
B. **Carbon monoxide poisoning**
   1. Description
      a. Carbon monoxide is a colorless, odorless, and tasteless gas that has an affinity for hemoglobin 200 times greater than that of oxygen

      b. Oxygen molecules are displaced, and carbon monoxide reversibly binds to hemoglobin to form carboxyhemoglobin
      c. Tissue hypoxia occurs
   2. Data collection (Table 40-1)
C. Smoke poisoning
   1. Description
      a. Smoke poisoning is caused by the inhalation of the byproducts of combustion
      b. A localized inflammatory reaction occurs and causes a decrease in bronchial ciliary action and in surfactant
   2. Data collection
      a. Mucosal edema occurs in the airways
      b. Wheezing is evident on auscultation
      c. After several hours, sloughing of the tracheobronchial epithelium may occur, and hemorrhagic bronchitis may develop
      d. Adult respiratory distress syndrome can result
D. Direct thermal heat injury
   1. Description
      a. Thermal heat injury can occur to the lower airways as a result of the inhalation of steam or explosive gases or the aspiration of scalding liquids
      b. Injury can occur to the upper airways, which appear erythematous and edematous, with mucosal blisters and ulcerations
      c. Mucosal edema can lead to upper airway obstruction, especially during the first 24 to 48 hours
      d. All clients with head or neck burns should be monitored closely for the development of

TABLE 40-1	Carbon Monoxide Poisoning
Blood Level (%)	**Clinical Manifestations**
1-10	Normal level
11-20 (mild poisoning)	Headache
	Flushing
	Decreased visual acuity
	Decreased cerebral functioning
	Slight breathlessness
21-40 (moderate poisoning)	Headache
	Nausea and vomiting
	Drowsiness
	Tinnitus and vertigo
	Confusion and stupor
	Pale to reddish-purple skin
	Decreased blood pressure
	Increased and irregular heart rate
41-60 (severe poisoning)	Coma
	Seizures
61-80 (fatal poisoning)	Death

Modified from Ignatavicius, D., & Workman, M. (2006). *Medical surgical nursing: Critical thinking for collaborative care* (5th ed.). Philadelphia: Saunders.

airway obstruction; these clients are considered immediately for endotracheal intubation if obstruction occurs

2. Data collection
   a. Erythema and edema of the upper airways
   b. Mucosal blisters and ulcerations

IX. PATHOPHYSIOLOGY OF BURNS

A. After the burn, vasoactive substances are released from the injured tissue; these substances cause an increase in the capillary permeability, thus allowing plasma to seep into the surrounding tissues

B. The direct injury to the vessels increases capillary permeability; capillary permeability decreases 18 to 26 hours after the burn, but it does not normalize until 2 to 3 weeks after the injury

C. Extensive burns result in generalized body edema and a decrease in circulating intravascular blood volume

D. The fluid losses result in a decrease in organ perfusion

E. The heart rate increases, cardiac output decreases, and the blood pressure drops

F. Initially hyponatremia and hyperkalemia occur

G. The hematocrit level increases as a result of plasma loss; this initial increase falls to below normal on the third to fourth day after the burn as a result of red blood cell damage and loss at the time of injury

H. Initially the body shunts blood from the kidneys, thereby causing oliguria; the body then begins to reabsorb fluid, and diuresis of the excess fluid occurs over the next days to weeks

I. Blood flow to the gastrointestinal tract is diminished, which leads to intestinal ileus and gastrointestinal dysfunction

J. Immune system function is depressed, which results in immunosuppression and thus increases the risk of infection and sepsis

K. Pulmonary hypertension can develop, which results in decreases in the arterial oxygen tension level and lung compliance

L. Evaporative fluid losses through the burn wound are greater than normal, and the losses continue until complete wound closure occurs

M. If the intravascular space is not replenished with intravenous (IV) fluids, hypovolemic shock and ultimately death will occur

X. MANAGEMENT OF THE BURN INJURY

A. Emergent phase (Table 40-2)
   1. Description
      a. The emergent phase begins at the time of injury and ends with the restoration of capillary permeability (fluid resuscitation), usually at 48 to 72 hours after the injury; the phase includes prehospital and emergency department care
      b. The primary goals are to prevent hypovolemic shock and to preserve vital organ functioning
   2. Prehospital care
      a. Prehospital care begins at the scene of the accident and ends when emergency care is obtained

TABLE 40-2 Phases of Management of a Burn Injury

Phase	Goal
Emergent Phase • Begins at the time of injury • Ends with the restoration of capillary permeability • Duration is usually 48 to 72 hours • Includes prehospital care and emergency department care	The primary goals are to prevent hypovolemic shock and to preserve vital organ functioning.
Resuscitative Phase • Begins with the initiation of fluids • Ends when capillary integrity returns to near-normal levels and the large fluid shifts have decreased • Amount of fluid administered is based on the client's weight and the extent of injury (Note: Most fluid-replacement formulas are calculated from the time of injury rather than from the time of arrival at the hospital.)	The goal is to prevent shock by maintaining adequate circulating blood volume and vital organ perfusion.
Acute Phase • Begins when the client is hemodynamically stable, capillary permeability is restored, and diuresis has begun • Usually begins 48 to 72 hours after the time of injury • Focus is on infection control, wound care, wound closure, nutritional support, pain management, and physical therapy	The goal during this phase is restorative therapy, and the phase continues until wound closure is achieved.
Rehabilitative Phase • Overlaps the acute phase of care • Extends beyond hospitalization	The goals of this phase are designed so that the client can gain independence and achieve maximal function.

b. Remove the victim from the source of the burn

c. Remove the source of heat

d. Assess airway, breathing, and circulation

e. Assess for associated trauma

f. Conserve body heat

g. Cover **burns** with sterile or clean cloths

h. Remove constrictive jewelry and clothing

i. Assess the need for IV fluids

j. Transport the client

3. Emergency department care is a continuation of the care administered at the scene of the injury

4. Major **burns**

a. Evaluate the degree and extent of the **burn**, and treat life-threatening conditions

b. Ensure a patent airway, and administer 100% oxygen, as prescribed, if the **burn** occurred in an enclosed area

c. Monitor for respiratory distress, and assess the need for intubation

d. Assess the oropharynx for blisters and erythema

e. Monitor the arterial blood gases and the carboxyhemoglobin level

f. For an inhalation injury, administer 100% oxygen via a tight-fitting non-rebreather face mask, as prescribed, until the carboxyhemoglobin level falls below 15%

g. Initiate peripheral IV access to nonburned skin proximal to any extremity **burn**, or prepare for the insertion of a central venous line, as prescribed

h. Assess for hypovolemia, and prepare to administer IV fluids to maintain the fluid balance

i. Monitor the vital signs closely

j. Insert a Foley catheter, as prescribed, and maintain urine output at 30 to 50 mL per hour

k. Maintain nothing-by-mouth (NPO) status

l. Insert a nasogastric tube, as prescribed, to remove gastric secretions and to prevent aspiration

m. Administer tetanus prophylaxis, as prescribed

n. Administer pain medication, as prescribed, via the IV route

o. Prepare the client for an escharotomy or fasciotomy, as prescribed

5. Minor **burns**

a. Administer pain medication with small doses of morphine sulfate or meperidine (Demerol), as prescribed

b. Instruct the client regarding the use of oral analgesics, as prescribed

c. Administer tetanus prophylaxis, as prescribed

d. Administer wound care, as prescribed; this may include cleansing, débriding loose tissue, removing any damaging agents, and applying topical antimicrobial cream and a sterile dressing

e. Instruct the client regarding follow-up care, including active range-of-motion exercises and wound care treatments

B. Resuscitative phase (see Table 40-2)

1. Description

a. The resuscitative phase begins with the initiation of fluids and ends when capillary integrity returns to near-normal levels and the large fluid shifts have decreased

b. The amount of fluid administered is based on the client's weight and the extent of injury

c. Most fluid-replacement formulas are calculated from the time of injury rather than from the time of arrival at the hospital

d. The goal is to prevent shock by maintaining adequate circulating blood volume and vital organ perfusion

2. Fluid resuscitation (Table 40-3)

a. The amount of fluid administered depends on how much IV fluid is required to maintain a urinary output of 30 to 50 mL per hour

b. Successful fluid resuscitation is evaluated by stable vital signs, an adequate urine output, palpable peripheral pulses, and a clear sensorium

c. Urinary output is the most common and most sensitive noninvasive assessment parameter for cardiac output and tissue perfusion

d. IV fluid replacement may be titrated (adjusted) on the basis of urinary output plus serum electrolyte levels to meet the perfusion needs of the client with **burns**

e. If the hemoglobin and hematocrit levels decrease or if the urinary output exceeds 50 mL/hour, the rate of IV fluid administration may be decreased

3. Interventions

a. Monitor for tracheal or laryngeal edema, and administer respiratory treatments, as prescribed

b. Monitor the pulse oximetry, and prepare to obtain arterial blood gas and carboxyhemoglobin levels if inhalation injury is suspected

c. Elevate the head of the bed to 30 degrees or more for clients with **burns** of the face and head

d. Initiate electrocardiogram monitoring

e. Monitor the temperature, and assess for infection

TABLE 40-3	Common Fluid Resuscitation Formulas for the First 24 Hours After a Burn Injury		
	Formula	Solution	Rate of Administration
Modified Brooke	0.5 mL/kg/% TBSA burn 1.5 mL/kg/% TBSA burn	Protenate or 5% albumin in isotonic saline lactated Ringer's solution without dextrose	Half given during the first 8 hours; half given during the next 16 hours
Parkland (Baxter)	4 mL/kg/% TBSA burn per 24-hour period	Crystalloid only (lactated Ringer's solution)	Half given during the first 8 hours; half given during the next 16 hours
Monafo		Crystalloid (hypertonic saline: sodium = 250 mEq/L)	Adjust to maintain a urine output of 30 mL/hour
Modified Parkland	4 mL/kg/% TBSA burn + 15 mL/m² of TBSA	Crystalloid only (lactated Ringer's solution)	Half given during the first 8 hours; half given during the next 16 hours
Winski	2 mL/kg/% burn + maintenance fluid	Crystalloid only (lactated Ringer's solution)	Half given during the first 8 hours; half given during the next 16 hours

TBSA, Total body surface area.
Modified from Ignatavicius, D., & Workman, M. (2006). *Medical surgical nursing: Critical thinking for collaborative care* (5th ed.). Philadelphia: Saunders.

f. Initiate protective isolation techniques; maintain strict handwashing; use sterile sheets and linens when caring for the client; and wear gloves, cap, masks, shoe covers, scrub clothes, and plastic aprons

g. Shave or cut the body hair around wound margins

h. Monitor the client's daily weights; expect a weight gain of 15 to 20 lbs during the first 72 hours

i. Monitor the gastric output and pH levels and for gastric discomfort and bleeding, which indicate a stress ulcer

j. Administer antacids, H_2-receptor antagonists, and antiulcer medications such as sucralfate (Carafate), as prescribed

k. Auscultate the bowel sounds for ileus, and monitor for abdominal distention and gastrointestinal dysfunction

l. Monitor the stools for occult blood

m. Obtain a urine specimen for myoglobin and hemoglobin levels

n. Monitor IV fluids and hourly intake and output to determine the adequacy of fluid replacement therapy; notify the physician if urine output is less than 30 mL/hour or greater than 50 mL/hour

o. Elevate circumferential **burns** of the extremities on pillows above the level of the heart to reduce dependent edema if no obvious fractures are present; diuretics increase the risk of hypovolemia and are generally avoided as a means of decreasing edema

p. Monitor the pulses and capillary refill of the affected extremities, and assess the perfusion of the distal extremity with a circumferential **burn**

q. Prepare for chest and other radiographs to rule out fractures or associated trauma

r. Keep the room temperature warm

s. Place the client on an air-fluidized bed, and use a bed cradle to keep the sheets off of the client's skin

4. Pain management

a. Administer morphine sulfate or meperidine (Demerol), as prescribed, via the IV route

b. Avoid intramuscular or subcutaneous medication routes, because absorption through the soft tissue is unreliable when hypovolemia and large fluid shifts are occurring

c. Avoid administering medication by the oral route because of the possibility of gastrointestinal dysfunction

d. Medicate the client before painful procedures

5. Nutrition

a. Proper nutrition is essential to promote wound healing and prevent infection

b. The basal metabolic rate is 40 to 100 times higher than normal in a client with a **burn** injury

c. Maintain NPO status until bowel sounds are heard and then advance to clear liquids, as prescribed

d. Nutrition may be provided via enteral tube feedings or parenteral nutrition

e. Provide a diet that is high in protein, carbohydrates, fats, and vitamins

f. Monitor the calorie intake

6. Escharotomy

a. A lengthwise incision is made through the **burn** eschar to relieve constriction and pressure and to improve circulation

b. Escharotomy is performed for circulatory compromise caused by circumferential **burns**

c. Escharotomy is performed at the bedside without anesthesia, because nerve endings have been destroyed by the **burn** injury

d. Escharotomy can be performed on the thorax to improve ventilation

e. After the escharotomy, assess the pulses, color, movement, and sensation of the affected extremity, and control any bleeding with pressure

f. Pack the incision gently with fine-mesh gauze for 24 hours after escharotomy, as prescribed

g. Apply topical antimicrobial agents to the area, as prescribed, after the procedure

7. Fasciotomy

a. An incision is made that extends through the subcutaneous tissue and fascia

b. The procedure is performed if adequate tissue perfusion does not return after an escharotomy

c. Fasciotomy is performed in the operating department with the client under general anesthesia

d. After the procedure, assess the pulses, color, movement, and sensation of the affected extremity, and control any bleeding with pressure.

e. Apply topical antimicrobial agents and dressings to the area, as prescribed, after the procedure

C. Acute phase (see Table 40-2)

1. Description

a. The acute phase begins when the client is hemodynamically stable, capillary permeability is restored, and diuresis has begun

b. The acute phase usually begins 48 to 72 hours after the time of injury

c. Emphasis during this phase is placed on restorative therapy, and the phase continues until wound closure is achieved

d. The focus is on infection control, wound care, wound closure, nutritional support, pain management, and physical therapy

2. Interventions

a. Continue with protective isolation techniques

b. Provide wound care, as prescribed, and prepare for wound closure.

c. Provide pain management

d. Provide adequate nutrition, as prescribed

e. Prepare the client for rehabilitation

D. Wound care (Table 40-4)

1. Description: The cleansing, débridement, and dressing of the **burn** wounds

2. Hydrotherapy

a. Wounds are cleansed by immersion, showering, or spraying.

b. Hydrotherapy occurs for 30 minutes or less to prevent increased sodium loss through the **burn** wound, heat loss, pain, and stress

c. The client should be medicated before the procedure

d. Hydrotherapy is generally not used for clients who are hemodynamically unstable or for those with new skin grafts

e. Care is taken to minimize bleeding and to maintain body temperature during the procedure

f. If hydrotherapy is not used, wounds are washed and rinsed while the client is in bed before the application of antimicrobial agents.

TABLE 40-4 Open Versus Closed Method of Wound Care

Method	Advantages	Disadvantages
Open		
Antimicrobial cream is applied, and the wound is left open to the air without a dressing; antimicrobial cream may be prescribed every 12 hours	Visualization of the wound; easier mobility and joint range of motion; simplicity of wound care	Increased chance of hypothermia from exposure
Closed		
Gauze dressings are carefully wrapped from the distal to the proximal area of the extremity to ensure that circulation is not compromised; no two burn surfaces should be allowed to touch; touching can promote the webbing of digits, contractures, and a poor cosmetic outcome; dressings are usually changed every 8 to 12 hours	Decreases evaporative fluid and heat loss; aids in debridement	Mobility limitations; prevents effective range-of-motion exercises; wound assessment is limited

3. Débridement (Box 40-4)
   a. Débridement is the removal of eschar or necrotic tissue to prevent bacterial proliferation under the eschar and to promote wound healing
   b. Débridement may be mechanical, enzymatic, or surgical
   c. **Deep partial-** or **full-thickness burns:** The wound is cleansed and débrided, and topical antimicrobial agents are applied once or twice daily
E. Wound closure
   1. Description
      a. Wound closure prevents infection and the loss of fluid
      b. Closure promotes healing
      c. Closure prevents contractures
      d. Wound closure is performed on day 5 to 21 after the injury, depending on the extent of the **burn**
   2. Wound coverings (Box 40-5)
   3. Autografting (see Box 40-5)
      a. Autografting provides permanent wound coverage
      b. Autografting is the surgical removal of a thin layer of the client's own unburned skin, which is then applied to the excised burn wound
      c. Autografting is performed in the operating department with the client under anesthesia

BOX 40-4 Débridement

Mechanical
- Performed during hydrotherapy
- Involves the use of washcloths or sponges to débride eschar and the use of scissors and forceps to lift and trim away loose eschar
- Wet-to-dry or wet-to-wet dressing changes may be used
- Painful procedure that may cause bleeding

Enzymatic
- Application of topical enzyme agents directly to the wound that digest collagen in necrotic tissue

Surgical
- Excision of eschar or necrotic tissue via a surgical procedure in the operating department
- *Tangential technique:* Very thin layers of the necrotic burn surface are excised until bleeding occurs; bleeding indicates that a level of healthy dermis or subcutaneous fat has been reached
- *Fascial technique:* The burn wound is excised to the level of the superficial fascia; this technique is usually reserved for very deep and extensive burns

d. Monitor for bleeding after the graft, because bleeding beneath an autograft can prevent adherence
e. If prescribed, small amounts of blood or serum can be removed by gently rolling the fluid from the center of the graft to the periphery with a sterile gauze pad, where it can be absorbed
f. For large accumulations of blood, the physician will aspirate the blood with the use of a small-gauge needle and syringe
g. Autografts are immobilized after surgery for 3 to 7 days to allow time for the graft to adhere and attach to the wound bed
h. Position the client for the immobilization and elevation of the graft site to prevent the movement and shearing of the graft
4. Care of the graft site
   a. Elevate and immobilize the graft site
   b. Keep the site free from pressure
   c. Avoid weight bearing
   d. When the graft takes, roll a cotton-tipped applicator over the graft to remove exudate, because exudate can lead to infection and prevent graft adherence
   e. Monitor for foul-smelling drainage, increased temperature, increased white blood cell count, hematoma, and fluid accumulation
   f. Instruct the client to avoid using fabric softeners and harsh detergents in his or her laundry
   g. Instruct the client to lubricate the healing skin with prescribed agents
   h. Instruct the client to protect the affected area from sunlight
   i. Instruct the client to use splints and support garments, as prescribed
5. Care of the donor site
   a. The method of care varies, depending on the physician's preference
   b. A moist gauze dressing is applied at the time of surgery to maintain pressure and to stop any oozing
   c. The physician may prescribe site treatment with single-layer gauze impregnated with petrolatum or with a biosynthetic dressing (e.g., Biobrane)
   d. Keep the donor site clean, dry, and free from pressure
   e. Prevent the client from scratching the donor site
   f. Apply lubricating lotions to soften the area and to reduce the itching after the donor site is healed
   g. The donor site can be reused after healing has occurred; it should heal spontaneously within 7 to 14 days with proper care

BOX 40-5　Wound Coverings

Biological

Amnion

Amniotic membranes from human placentas are used to adhere to the wound.

This is effective as a dressing until epithelial cell regrowth occurs.

Frequent changes are required, because amnion does not develop a blood supply, and it disintegrates in about 48 hours.

Allograft or Homograft (Human Tissue)

Donated human cadaver skin is provided through a skin bank.

Monitor for wound exudate and signs of infection.

Rejection can occur within 24 hours.

The risk of transmitting a blood-borne infection exists with the use of this covering.

Xenograft or Heterograft (Animal Tissue)

Pigskin is harvested after slaughter and preserved for storage.

Monitor for infection and wound adherence.

Rejection can occur within 24 to 72 hours.

This tissue is placed over granulation tissue and replaced every 2 to 5 days until the wound heals naturally or until closure with an autograft is complete.

Cultured Skin

Cultured skin is grown in a laboratory from a small specimen of epidermal cells from an unburned portion of the client's body.

Cell sheets are grafted onto the client to generate a permanent skin surface.

Cell sheets are not durable; care must be taken when applying them to ensure adherence and prevent sloughing.

Artificial Skin

Artificial skin consists of two layers: a Silastic epidermis and a porous dermis made from bovine hide collagen and shark cartilage.

After application, fibroblasts move into the collagen part of the artificial skin and create a structure that is similar to that of normal dermis.

The artificial dermis then dissolves and is replaced with normal blood vessels and connective tissue called neodermis.

The neodermis supports a standard autograft that is placed over it when the Silastic layer is removed.

Biosynthetic

This type of covering is made of a combination of biosynthetic and synthetic materials.

It is placed in contact with the wound surface, and it forms an adherent bond until epithelialization has occurred.

Its porous substance allows exudate to pass through it.

Monitor for wound exudate and signs of infection.

Synthetic

Synthetic coverings are applied directly to the surface of a clean or surgically prepared wound, and they remain in place until they fall off or are removed.

The covering is transparent or translucent; therefore, the wound can be inspected without removing the dressing.

Pain at the wound site is reduced, because the covering prevents the contact of the wound with air.

Autograft

Skin is taken from a remote, unburned area of the client's own body and transplanted to cover the burn wound.

The graft is placed either on a clean granulated bed or over a surgically excised area of the burn.

Autograft provides for permanent skin coverage.

F. Physical therapy
1. An individualized program of splinting, positioning, exercises, ambulation, and activities of daily living is implemented early during the acute phase of recovery to maximize the functional and cosmetic outcomes
2. Perform range-of-motion exercises, as prescribed, to reduce edema and to maintain strength and joint function
3. Ambulate the client, as prescribed, to maintain the strength of the lower extremities
4. Apply splints, as prescribed, to maintain proper joint position and to prevent contractures
   a. Static splints immobilize the joint and are applied for periods of immobilization, during sleeping, and for clients who cannot maintain proper positioning
   b. Dynamic splints exercise the affected joint
   c. Avoid pressure to skin areas when applying splints, which could lead to further tissue and nerve damage
5. Scarring is controlled by elastic wraps and bandages that apply continuous pressure to the healing skin during the period of time when the skin is vulnerable to shearing
6. Anti–burn scar support garments are usually worn 23 hours a day until the **burn** scar tissue has matured, which takes 18 months to 2 years

G. Rehabilitative phase (see Table 40-2)
1. Description
   a. Rehabilitation is the final phase of **burn** care
   b. Rehabilitation overlaps with the acute care phase and goes well beyond hospitalization
   c. The goals of this phase are designed so that the client can gain independence and achieve maximal function
2. Goals
   a. Promote wound healing
   b. Minimize deformities
   c. Increase strength and function
   d. Provide emotional support

PRACTICE QUESTIONS

More questions on the companion CD!

428. A nurse is assigned to care for a client with herpes zoster. Which of the following characteristics would the nurse expect to note when assessing the lesions of this infection?
1. Clustered skin vesicles
2. A generalized body rash
3. Small blue-white spots with red bases
4. A fiery red edematous rash on the cheeks

429. A nurse who is employed in a long-term care facility is planning the clinical assignments for the day. The nurse avoids assigning which staff member to the client with a diagnosis of herpes zoster?
1. A staff member who has never had roseola
2. A staff member who has never had mumps
3. A nursing assistant who has never had German measles
4. An experienced nursing assistant who has never had chickenpox

430. A client returns to the clinic for follow-up treatment after a skin biopsy of a suspicious lesion that was performed 1 week ago. The biopsy report indicates that the lesion is a melanoma. The nurse understands that which of the following describes a characteristic of this type of a lesion?
1. Metastasis is rare.
2. It is encapsulated.
3. It is highly metastatic.
4. It is characterized by local invasion.

431. A nurse is reviewing the health care record of a client with a lesion that has been diagnosed as malignant melanoma. The nurse would expect which characteristic of this type of lesion to be documented in the client's record?
1. An irregularly shaped lesion
2. A small papule with a dry, rough scale
3. A firm nodular lesion topped with a crust
4. A pearly papule with a central crater and a waxy border

432. A nurse reinforces instructions to a group of clients regarding measures that will assist with the prevention of skin cancer. Which statement by a client indicates the need for further instruction?
1. "I need to wear sunscreen when participating in outdoor activities."
2. "I need to avoid sun exposure before 10:00 AM and after 3:00 PM."
3. "I need to wear a hat, opaque clothing, and sunglasses when in the sun."
4. "I need to examine my body monthly for any lesions that may be suspicious."

433. A client arrives at the emergency department and has experienced frostbite to the right hand. Which of the following would the nurse note when performing data collection regarding the client's hand?
1. A pink, edematous hand
2. Fiery red skin with edema in the nail beds
3. Black fingertips surrounded by an erythematous rash
4. A white color of the skin, which is insensitive to touch

434. An evening nurse reviews the nursing documentation in the client's chart and notes that the day nurse has documented that the client has a stage 2 pressure ulcer in the sacral area. Which of the following would the nurse expect to note when checking the client's sacral area?
1. Intact skin
2. The presence of tunneling
3. A deep, crater-like appearance
4. Partial-thickness skin loss of the epidermis

435. A nurse inspects the skin of a client who is suspected of having scabies. Which of the following findings would the nurse note if this disorder was present?
1. Patchy hair loss and round, red macules with scales
2. The presence of white patches scattered about the trunk
3. Multiple straight or wavy threadlike lines beneath the skin
4. The appearance of vesicles or pustules with a thick, honey-colored crust

436. A nurse is told that an assigned client is suspected of having scabies. Which of the following precautions will the nurse institute during the care of the client?
1. Wear gloves only.
2. Wear a mask and gloves.
3. Wear a gown and gloves.
4. Avoid touching the client's clothes.

437. The client arrives at the emergency department after a burn injury that occurred in the basement at home, and an inhalation injury is suspected. Which of the following would the nurse anticipate as being prescribed for the client?
1. Oxygen via nasal cannula at 10 L
2. Oxygen via nasal cannula at 15 L
3. 100% oxygen via an aerosol mask
4. 100% oxygen via a tight-fitting, nonrebreather face mask

438. A nurse is caring for a client who has just been admitted to the nursing unit after receiving flame burns to the face and chest. The nurse notes a hoarse cough and that the client is expectorating sputum with black flecks. The client's eyelashes and eyebrows are singed, and the eyelids are swollen. The client suddenly becomes restless, and his

color becomes dusky. The nurse interprets this data as indicating which of the following?
1. The client is hypotensive.
2. Pain is present from the burn injury.
3. The burn has probably caused laryngeal edema, which has occluded the airway.
4. The client is afraid and is having a panic attack as a result of the unfamiliar surroundings.

439. Which of the following would be the anticipated therapeutic outcome of an escharotomy procedure performed for a circumferential arm burn?
1. The return of distal pulses
2. Decreasing edema formation
3. Brisk bleeding from the injury site
4. The formation of granulation tissue

440. A nurse is caring for a client with circumferential burns of both legs. Which of the following leg positions is appropriate for this type of a burn?
1. A dependent position
2. Elevation of the knees
3. Flat, without elevation
4. Elevation above the level of the heart

441. A nurse is assisting with caring for a client who is receiving intravenous fluids and who has sustained full-thickness burn injuries of the back and legs. The nurse understands that which of the following would provide the most reliable indicator for determining the adequacy of the fluid resuscitation?
1. Vital signs
2. Urine output
3. Mental status
4. Peripheral pulses

442. A nurse is caring for a client after an autograft and grafting of a burn wound on the right knee. Which of the following would the nurse anticipate being prescribed for the client?
1. Placing the affected leg flat
2. Elevating and immobilizing the affected leg
3. Placing the affected leg in a dependent position
4. Immobilizing the client in a dependent position

443. A nurse reinforces discharge instructions regarding skin care to a client after the grafting of burn injuries of the left chest and left arm. Which statement by the client indicates the need for further instructions?
1. "I need to bathe using a mild soap and to rinse thoroughly."
2. "I need to avoid direct sunlight on the newly healed skin area."
3. "I should never wear warm clothing over the newly healed skin area."
4. "I need to avoid the use of lanolin products to the newly healed skin area."

444. Which of the following individuals would be at the greatest risk for development of an integumentary disorder?
1. An adolescent
2. An older female
3. A physical education teacher
4. An outdoor construction worker

445. A nurse has reinforced discharge instructions to a client who had a skin biopsy. Which statement by the client indicates the need for further instruction?
1. "I will use the antibiotic ointment, as prescribed."
2. "I will return in 7 days to have the sutures removed."
3. "I will call the physician if I see any drainage from the wound."
4. "I will remove the dressing when I get home and wash the site with tap water."

446. A nurse prepares to help a physician examine the client's skin with a Wood's light. Which of the following would be included in the plan for this procedure?
1. Prepare a local anesthetic.
2. Obtain an informed consent.
3. Darken the room for the examination.
4. Shave the skin and scrub it with a povidone-iodine (Betadine) solution.

447. A nurse reinforces instructions to a client who has complained of chronic dry skin and episodes of pruritus. Which of the following, if stated by the client, indicates the need for further instructions?
1. "I should drink 8 to 10 glasses of water a day."
2. "I need to avoid using astringents on my skin."
3. "I should use a dehumidifier, especially during the winter months."
4. "I should limit myself to one shower per day and apply an emollient to my skin after the shower."

448. A client calls the emergency department and tells the nurse that he has been cleaning a wooded area and that he came into direct contact with poison ivy shrubs. The client tells the nurse that he cannot see anything on the skin and asks the nurse what to do. The nurse makes which statement to the client?
1. "Come to the emergency department."
2. "Apply calamine lotion immediately to the exposed skin areas."
3. "Take a shower immediately, and lather and rinse several times."
4. "It is not necessary to do anything if you cannot see anything on your skin."

449. A client is being admitted to the hospital for the treatment of acute cellulitis of the lower left leg. The client asks the nurse to explain what

cellulitis means. The nurse bases the response on the understanding that the characteristics of cellulitis include:

1. An acute superficial infection
2. An inflammation of the lymphatics
3. A superficial infection caused by *Staphylococcus*
4. A skin infection into the deep dermis and subcutaneous fat

450. A nurse prepares to care for a client with acute cellulitis of the lower leg. Which of the following would the nurse anticipate being prescribed for the client?

1. Cold compresses to the affected area
2. Warm compresses to the affected area
3. Alternating hot and cold compresses continuously
4. Intermittent heat-lamp treatments four times per day

451. A nurse notes that the physician has documented a diagnosis of herpes zoster in the client's chart. On the basis of an understanding of the cause of this disorder, the nurse would determine that this diagnosis was made after the use of which diagnostic test?

1. Patch test
2. Skin biopsy
3. Culture of the lesion
4. Wood's light examination

ALTERNATE ITEM FORMAT: FILL IN THE BLANK

452. An adult client was burned as a result of an explosion. The burn initially affected the client's entire face (the anterior half of the head) and the upper half of the anterior torso, and there were circumferential burns to the lower half of both of the arms. The client's clothes caught on fire, and the client ran, which caused subsequent burn injuries of the posterior surface of the head and the upper half of the posterior torso. According to the rule of nines, what is the extent of this client's burn injury?

Answer: _____%

ANSWERS

428. **1**
Rationale: The primary lesion of herpes zoster is a vesicle. The classic presentation is grouped vesicles on a erythematous base along a dermatome. Because they follow nerve pathways, the lesions do not cross the body's midline. Options 2, 3, and 4 are incorrect descriptions.
Test-Taking Strategy: Use the process of elimination. Remembering that these lesions occur as grouped vesicles along a nerve pathway will assist you with answering the question. Review the characteristics of herpes zoster lesions if you had difficulty with this question.
Level of Cognitive Ability: Comprehension
Client Needs: Physiological Integrity
Integrated Process: Nursing Process/Data Collection
Content Area: Adult Health/Integumentary
Reference: Linton, A. (2007). *Introduction to medical-surgical nursing* (4th ed., p. 1140). Philadelphia: Saunders.

429. **4**
Rationale: Herpes zoster is caused by a reactivation of the varicella zoster virus, which is the causative virus of chickenpox. Individuals who have not been exposed to the varicella zoster virus are susceptible to chickenpox. Options 1, 2, and 3 are not associated with the herpes zoster virus.
Test-Taking Strategy: Use the process of elimination, and note the strategic word "avoids." Recalling that herpes zoster is caused by a reactivation of the varicella zoster virus will assist you with answering the question. Review the relationship between herpes zoster and chickenpox if you had difficulty with this question.
Level of Cognitive Ability: Application
Client Needs: Safe and Effective Care Environment
Integrated Process: Nursing Process/Planning
Content Area: Delegating/Prioritizing

Reference: Linton, A. (2007). *Introduction to medical-surgical nursing* (4th ed., p. 1140). Philadelphia: Saunders.

430. **3**
Rationale: Melanomas are pigmented malignant lesions that originate in the melanin-producing cells of the epidermis. This skin cancer is highly metastatic, and a person's survival depends on early diagnosis and treatment. Basal cell carcinomas arise in the basal cell layer of the epidermis. Early malignant basal cell lesions often go unnoticed, and, although metastasis is rare, underlying tissue destruction can progress to include vital structures. Squamous cell carcinomas are malignant neoplasms of the epidermis. They are characterized by local invasion and the potential for metastasis.
Test-Taking Strategy: Knowledge regarding the various types of skin cancers and recalling that melanomas are highly metastatic will direct you to the correct option. Review the characteristics of skin cancers if you had difficulty with this question.
Level of Cognitive Ability: Comprehension
Client Needs: Physiological Integrity
Integrated Process: Nursing Process/Data Collection
Content Area: Adult Health/Integumentary
Reference: Christensen, B., & Kockrow, E. (2006). *Adult health nursing* (5th ed., p. 100). St. Louis: Mosby.

431. **1**
Rationale: A melanoma is a irregularly shaped pigmented papule or plaque with a red, white, or blue color. Basal cell carcinoma appears as a pearly papule with a central crater and a rolled, waxy border. Squamous cell carcinoma is a firm nodular lesion that is topped with a crust or a central area of ulceration. Actinic keratosis, which is a premalignant lesion, appears as a small macule or papule with a dry, rough, adherent yellow or brown scale.

Test-Taking Strategy: Use the process of elimination. Remembering that irregularly shaped lesions are a cause for concern will assist you with answering the question. Review the characteristics of malignant skin lesions if you had difficulty with this question.
Level of Cognitive Ability: Comprehension
Client Needs: Physiological Integrity
Integrated Process: Nursing Process/Data Collection
Content Area: Adult Health/Integumentary
Reference: Christensen, B., & Kockrow, E. (2006). *Adult health nursing* (5th ed., p. 101). St. Louis: Mosby.

432. 2
Rationale: The client should be instructed to avoid sun exposure between the hours of approximately 10:00 AM and 3:00 PM. Sunscreen, a hat, opaque clothing, and sunglasses should be worn for outdoor activities. The client should be instructed to examine the body monthly for the appearance of any possible cancerous or precancerous lesions.
Test-Taking Strategy: Use the process of elimination. Note the strategic words "need for further instruction." These words indicate a negative event query and ask you to select an option that is an incorrect statement. A careful reading of the question will direct you to option 2. Review client teaching for the prevention of skin cancer if you had difficulty with this question.
Level of Cognitive Ability: Comprehension
Client Needs: Health Promotion and Maintenance
Integrated Process: Teaching and Learning
Content Area: Adult Health/Integumentary
Reference: Christensen, B., & Kockrow, E. (2006). *Adult health nursing* (5th ed., p. 101). St. Louis: Mosby.

433. 4
Rationale: The findings related to frostbite include a white or blue skin color and skin that is hard, cold, and insensitive to touch. As thawing occurs, so does flushing of the skin, the development of blisters or blebs, or tissue edema. Gangrene can develop in 9 to 15 days.
Test-Taking Strategy: Use the process of elimination, and focus on the diagnosis of frostbite. The words "insensitive to touch" should assist with directing you to option 4. Review the characteristics associated with frostbite if you had difficulty with this question.
Level of Cognitive Ability: Comprehension
Client Needs: Physiological Integrity
Integrated Process: Nursing Process/Data Collection
Content Area: Adult Health/Integumentary
Reference: Christensen, B., & Kochrow, E. (2006). *Foundations of nursing* (5th ed., p. 763). St. Louis: Mosby.

434. 4
Rationale: With a stage 2 pressure ulcer, the skin is not intact. There is partial-thickness skin loss of the epidermis or dermis. The ulcer is superficial, and it may look like an abrasion, blister, or shallow crater. The skin is intact with a stage 1 pressure ulcer. A deep, crater-like appearance occurs during stage 3, and tunneling develop during stage 4.
Test-Taking Strategy: Use the process of elimination and your knowledge of the characteristics associated with each stage of pressure ulcers. Remember, with a stage 2 pressure ulcer, the

skin is not intact. Review the characteristics associated with each stage of pressure ulcers if you had difficulty with this question.
Level of Cognitive Ability: Comprehension
Client Needs: Physiological Integrity
Integrated Process: Nursing Process/Data Collection
Content Area: Adult Health/Integumentary
Reference: Linton, A. (2007). *Introduction to medical-surgical nursing* (4th ed., pp. 316-317). Philadelphia: Saunders.

435. 3
Rationale: Scabies can be identified by the multiple straight or wavy threadlike lines noted beneath the skin. The skin lesions are caused by the female, which burrows beneath the skin and lays its eggs. The eggs hatch in a few days, and the baby mites find their way to the skin surface, where they mate and complete the life cycle. Options 1, 2, and 4 are not characteristics of scabies.
Test-Taking Strategy: Recalling that scabies mites burrow beneath the skin surface will assist you with the process of elimination and provide direction for selecting the correct option. Review the characteristics associated with scabies if you had difficulty with this question.
Level of Cognitive Ability: Comprehension
Client Needs: Physiological Integrity
Integrated Process: Nursing Process/Data Collection
Content Area: Adult Health/Integumentary
Reference: Linton, A. (2007). *Introduction to medical-surgical nursing* (4th ed., p. 1142). Philadelphia: Saunders.

436. 3
Rationale: The Centers for Disease Control and Prevention recommend the wearing of gowns and gloves when in close contact with a person who is infested with scabies. Masks are not necessary. Transmission via clothing and other inanimate objects is uncommon. Scabies is usually transmitted from person to person by direct skin contact. All contacts that the client has had should be treated at the same time.
Test-Taking Strategy: Consider the mode of transmission of scabies, and use the process of elimination. Because scabies is transmitted by direct skin contact, eliminate options 1, 2, and 4. Review standard precautions and the transmission mode of scabies if you had difficulty with question.
Level of Cognitive Ability: Application
Client Needs: Safe and Effective Care Environment
Integrated Process: Nursing Process/Implementation
Content Area: Adult Health/Integumentary
Reference: Christensen, B., & Kockrow, E. (2006). *Foundations of nursing* (5th ed., pp. 279-281). St. Louis: Mosby.

437. 4
Rationale: If an inhalation injury is suspected, the administration of 100% oxygen via a tight-fitting, nonrebreather face mask is prescribed until the carboxyhemoglobin level falls below 15%. With inhalation injuries, the oropharynx is inspected for evidence of erythema, blisters, or ulcerations. The need for endotracheal intubation is also assessed. Options 1, 2, and 3 are incorrect.
Test-Taking Strategy: Use the process of elimination. Recalling that 100% oxygen is required after an inhalation injury will assist you with eliminating options 1 and 2. From the

remaining options, recall that a tight-fitting nonrebreather mask is preferred so that the client will not rebreathe exhaled air. Review the care of the client after an inhalation injury if you had difficulty with this question.
Level of Cognitive Ability: Analysis
Client Needs: Physiological Integrity
Integrated Process: Nursing Process/Planning
Content Area: Adult Health/Integumentary
Reference: Monahan, F., Sands, J., Marek, J., Neighbors, M., & Green, C. (2007). *Phipps' medical-surgical nursing: Health and illness perspectives* (8th ed., pp. 1923-1924). St. Louis: Mosby.

438. **3**
Rationale: The client exhibits several warning signs of an inhalation injury: a history of a flame burn to the face, hoarseness, cough, carbonaceous sputum, singed facial hair, facial edema, and color change. Additionally, one of the cardinal signs of hypoxia is restlessness.
Test-Taking Strategy: Use the ABCs—airway, breathing, and circulation—to answer the question. The only option that addresses the airway is option 3. Review the clinical manifestations associated with burns of the face if you had difficulty with this question.
Level of Cognitive Ability: Analysis
Client Needs: Physiological Integrity
Integrated Process: Nursing Process/Data Collection
Content Area: Adult Health/Integumentary
Reference: Monahan, F., Sands, J., Marek, J., Neighbors, M., & Green, C. (2007). *Phipps' medical-surgical nursing: Health and illness perspectives* (8th ed., pp. 1911, 1923). St. Louis: Mosby.

439. **1**
Rationale: Escharotomies are performed to alleviate the compartment syndrome that can occur when edema forms under nondistensible eschar in a circumferential burn. Escharotomies are performed through avascular eschar to subcutaneous fat. Although bleeding may occur from the site, it is considered a complication rather than an anticipated therapeutic outcome. The formation of granulation tissue is not the intent of an escharotomy, and escharotomy will not affect the formation of edema.
Test-Taking Strategy: Note the subject of the question—a therapeutic outcome. Use the ABCs—airway, breathing, and circulation—to answer the question. The only option that addresses circulation is option 1. Review the purpose of an escharotomy if you had difficulty with this question.
Level of Cognitive Ability: Analysis
Client Needs: Physiological Integrity
Integrated Process: Nursing Process/Evaluation
Content Area: Adult Health/Integumentary
Reference: Christensen, B., & Kockrow, E. (2006). *Adult health nursing* (5th ed., p. 109). St. Louis: Mosby.

440. **4**
Rationale: Circumferential burns of the extremities may compromise circulation. Elevating injured extremities above the level of the heart and performing active exercise help to reduce dependent edema formation. Options 1, 2, and 3 are incorrect.
Test-Taking Strategy: Use the process of elimination. Remember that when an injury such as a burn occurs,

edema occurs. Option 4 addresses a position that will reduce edema. Review the care of the client with a circumferential burn injury if you had difficulty with this question.
Level of Cognitive Ability: Application
Client Needs: Physiological Integrity
Integrated Process: Nursing Process/Implementation
Content Area: Adult Health/Integumentary
Reference: Lewis, S., Heitkemper, M., Dirksen, S., & Bucher, L. (2007). *Medical-surgical nursing: Assessment and management of clinical problems* (7th ed., p. 498). St. Louis: Mosby.

441. **2**
Rationale: Successful or adequate fluid resuscitation in the adult is signaled by stable vital signs, adequate urine output, palpable peripheral pulses, and a clear sensorium. The most reliable indicator for determining the adequacy of fluid resuscitation is the urine output. For an adult, the hourly urine volume should be 30 mL to 50 mL.
Test-Taking Strategy: Use the process of elimination. Note the strategic word "reliable" and the subject of fluid resuscitation. Urine output is similar to the subject of administering fluids. Review the care of the burn client during fluid resuscitation if you had difficulty with this question.
Level of Cognitive Ability: Analysis
Client Needs: Physiological Integrity
Integrated Process: Nursing Process/Evaluation
Content Area: Adult Health/Integumentary
References: Lewis, S., Heitkemper, M., Dirksen, S., & Bucher, L. (2007). *Medical-surgical nursing: Assessment and management of clinical problems* (7th ed., p. 496). St. Louis: Mosby.
Linton, A. (2007). *Introduction to medical-surgical nursing* (4th ed., p. 1146). Philadelphia: Saunders.

442. **2**
Rationale: Autografts placed over joints or on the lower extremities are often elevated and immobilized after surgery for 3 to 7 days. This period of immobilization allows time for the autograft to adhere and attach to the wound bed.
Test-Taking Strategy: Use the process of elimination. Eliminate options 1 and 3 first, because they are comparable or alike. Note that the autograft was placed over a joint; this should direct you to the option that identifies elevation and immobilization. Review the care of an autograft placed over a joint if you had difficulty with this question.
Level of Cognitive Ability: Application
Client Needs: Physiological Integrity
Integrated Process: Nursing Process/Planning
Content Area: Adult Health/Integumentary
Reference: Linton, A. (2007). *Introduction to medical-surgical nursing* (4th ed., p. 1148). Philadelphia: Saunders.

443. **3**
Rationale: Newly healed skin is more sensitive to the cold, and the client should be instructed to wear warm clothing. The client should wash with a mild soap, rinse thoroughly, and pat the skin dry with a clean towel. Newly healed skin sunburns easily, and direct sunlight needs to be avoided. Products that contain perfume, alcohol, or lanolin should be avoided, because they tend to irritate newly healed skin.
Test-Taking Strategy: Use the process of elimination, and note the strategic words "need for further instructions."

These words indicate a negative event query and ask you to select an option that is an incorrect statement. Read each option carefully, and note that the correct option uses the close-ended word "never." Review the home-care instructions regarding the care of newly healed skin if you had difficulty with this question.
Level of Cognitive Ability: Application
Client Needs: Physiological Integrity
Integrated Process: Teaching and Learning
Content Area: Adult Health/Integumentary
Reference: Ignatavicius, D., & Workman, M. (2006). *Medical-surgical nursing: Critical thinking for collaborative care* (5th ed., pp. 1646-1648). Philadelphia: Saunders.

444. **4**
Rationale: Prolonged exposure to the sun, unusual cold, or other conditions can damage the skin. An older client may be at a higher risk than a younger individual, because immobility and lack of nutrition may increase the older person's risk. An adolescent may be prone to the development of acne, but this does not occur in all adolescents. The physical education teacher is at low or no risk of developing an integumentary problem.
Test-Taking Strategy: Use the process of elimination, and note the strategic words "greatest risk." Eliminate option 3 first. Eliminate options 1 and 2 next, because not all older persons or adolescents are at risk for the development of integumentary disorders. Review the risk factors associated with integumentary disorders if you had difficulty with this question.
Level of Cognitive Ability: Comprehension
Client Needs: Health Promotion and Maintenance
Integrated Process: Nursing Process/Data Collection
Content Area: Adult Health/Integumentary
References: deWit, S. (2009). *Medical-surgical nursing: Concepts & practice* (pp. 1012-1013). Philadelphia: Saunders.
Ignatavicius, D., & Workman, M. (2006). *Medical-surgical nursing: Critical thinking for collaborative care* (5th ed., p. 1652). Philadelphia: Saunders.
Monahan, F., Sands, J., Marek, J., Neighbors, M., & Green, C. (2007). *Phipps' medical-surgical nursing: Health and illness perspectives* (8th ed., p. 1861). St. Louis: Mosby.

445. **4**
Rationale: After a skin biopsy, the nurse instructs the client to keep the dressing dry and in place for a minimum of 8 hours. After the dressing is removed, the site is cleaned once a day with tap water or saline to remove any dry blood or crusts. The physician may prescribe an antibiotic ointment to minimize local bacterial colonization. The nurse instructs the client to report any redness or excessive drainage at the site. Sutures are usually removed 7 to 10 days after biopsy.
Test-Taking Strategy: Use the process of elimination, and note the strategic words "need for further instruction." These words indicate a negative event query and ask you to select an option that is an incorrect statement. Eliminate option 1 first, because the client verbalizes the physician's prescription. Eliminate options 2 and 3 next. The client needs to report signs of drainage and to return to the physician for follow-up and suture removal. Consider the alteration in skin integrity that occurs with a skin biopsy; this should direct you to

option 4. Review the client instructions after a skin biopsy if you had difficulty with this question.
Level of Cognitive Ability: Comprehension
Client Needs: Health Promotion and Maintenance
Integrated Process: Teaching and Learning
Content Area: Adult Health/Integumentary
References: Chernecky, C., & Berger, B. (2008). *Laboratory tests and diagnostic procedures* (5th ed., p. 668). Philadelphia: Saunders.
Ignatavicius, D., & Workman, M. (2006). *Medical-surgical nursing: Critical thinking for collaborative care* (5th ed., p. 1573). Philadelphia: Saunders.

446. **3**
Rationale: The examination of the skin under a Wood's light is always carried out in a darkened room. This is a noninvasive examination; therefore, informed consent is not required. A handheld long-wavelength ultraviolet light or Wood's light is used. The skin does not need to be shaved, and a local anesthetic is not necessary. Areas of blue-green or red fluorescence are associated with certain skin infections. The procedure is painless.
Test-Taking Strategy: Use the process of elimination. Recalling that this is a noninvasive procedure will assist you with eliminating options 1, 2, and 4. Review examination with a Wood's light if you had difficulty with this question.
Level of Cognitive Ability: Application
Client Needs: Physiological Integrity
Integrated Process: Nursing Process/Planning
Content Area: Adult Health/Integumentary
Reference: Linton, A. (2007). *Introduction to medical-surgical nursing* (4th ed., p. 1129). Philadelphia: Saunders.

447. **3**
Rationale: The client should avoid using a dehumidifier, because this will further dry the room air. Instead, the client should use a room humidifier during the winter months or whenever the furnace is in use. The client should be taught to maintain a daily fluid intake of 3000 mL, unless contraindicated, and to avoid alcohol and caffeine. The client should avoid applying rubbing alcohol, astringents, or other drying agents to the skin. One bath or shower per day for 15 to 20 minutes with warm water and a mild soap should be immediately followed by the application of an emollient to prevent the evaporation of water from the hydrated epidermis.
Test-Taking Strategy: Use the process of elimination, and note the strategic words "need for further instructions." These words indicate a negative event query and ask you to select an option that is an incorrect client statement. Recalling that a dehumidifier is going to dry the air in the environment will assist with directing you to option 3. Review the client teaching points related to dry skin and pruritus if you had difficulty with this question.
Level of Cognitive Ability: Comprehension
Client Needs: Health Promotion and Maintenance
Integrated Process: Teaching and Learning
Content Area: Adult Health/Integumentary
References: Ignatavicius, D., & Workman, M. (2006). *Medical-surgical nursing: Critical thinking for collaborative care* (5th ed., p. 1576). Philadelphia: Saunders.

Linton, A. (2007). *Introduction to medical-surgical nursing* (4th ed., p. 1132). Philadelphia: Saunders.

448. 3
Rationale: When an individual comes in contact with a poison ivy plant, the sap from the plant forms an invisible film on the skin. The client should be instructed to shower immediately, to lather the skin several times, and to rinse each time in running water. Calamine lotion is a treatment that is used if dermatitis develops. It is not necessary for the client to be seen in the emergency department at this time.
Test-Taking Strategy: Recall that dermatitis can develop from contact with an allergen. In addition, recalling that contact with poison ivy results in an invisible film will directing you to option 3. Review the immediate treatment for contact with poison ivy if you had difficulty with this question.
Level of Cognitive Ability: Application
Client Needs: Health Promotion and Maintenance
Integrated Process: Nursing Process/Implementation
Content Area: Adult Health/Integumentary
Reference: Monahan, F., Sands, J., Marek, J., Neighbors, M. & Green, C. (2007). *Phipps' medical-surgical nursing: Health and illness perspectives* (8th ed., p.1884). St. Louis: Mosby.

449. 4
Rationale: Cellulitis is a skin infection into the deeper dermis and the subcutaneous fat; usually caused by *Streptococcus pyogeries*; it results in deep red erythema without sharp borders, and it spreads widely through tissue spaces. The skin is erythematous, edematous, tender, and sometimes nodular. Erysipelas is an acute, superficial, rapidly spreading inflammation of the dermis and the lymphatics.
Test-Taking Strategy: Knowledge regarding the characteristics of cellulitis is required to answer the question. Remember that cellulitis is a skin infection into the deeper dermis and the subcutaneous fat. Review the characteristics of cellulitis and erysipelas if you had difficulty with this question.
Level of Cognitive Ability: Comprehension
Client Needs: Physiological Integrity
Integrated Process: Nursing Process/Implementation
Content Area: Adult Health/Integumentary
Reference: Christensen, B., & Kockrow, E. (2006). *Adult health nursing* (5th ed., p. 82). St. Louis: Mosby.

450. 2
Rationale: Warm compresses may be used to decrease discomfort, erythema, and edema. After tissue and blood cultures are obtained, antibiotics are initiated. Heat lamps can cause more disruption to tissue that is already inflamed. Continuous cold and hot compresses are not the best measures.
Test-Taking Strategy: Use the process of elimination, and note that option 2 is different from the other options. Option 2 addresses warm compresses, whereas options 1, 3, and 4 address either cold or hot measures. Review the treatment of cellulitis if you had difficulty with this question.
Level of Cognitive Ability: Application

Client Needs: Physiological Integrity
Integrated Process: Nursing Process/Planning
Content Area: Adult Health/Integumentary
Reference: Christensen, B., & Kockrow, E. (2006). *Adult health nursing* (5th ed., p. 83). St. Louis: Mosby.

451. 3
Rationale: Herpes zoster is caused by a reactivation of the varicella zoster virus, which is the cause of chickenpox. A viral culture of the lesion provides the definitive diagnosis. During a Wood's light examination, the skin is viewed under ultraviolet light to identify superficial infections of the skin. A patch test is a skin test that involves the administration of an allergen to the skin's surface to identify specific allergies. A biopsy will determine tissue type.
Test-Taking Strategy: Use the process of elimination, and focus on the diagnosis of herpes zoster. Recall that herpes zoster is caused by a virus; this will assist you with eliminating options 1 and 4. From the remaining options, remember that a biopsy will determine tissue type, whereas a culture will identify an organism. Review herpes zoster if you had difficulty with this question.
Level of Cognitive Ability: Comprehension
Client Needs: Physiological Integrity
Integrated Process: Nursing Process/Data Collection
Content Area: Adult Health/Integumentary
References: Christensen, B., & Kockrow, E. (2006). *Adult health nursing* (5th ed., pp. 79-80). St. Louis: Mosby.
Linton, A. (2007). *Introduction to medical-surgical nursing* (4th ed., p. 1140). Philadelphia: Saunders.

ALTERNATE ITEM FORMAT: FILL IN THE BLANK
452. 36
Rationale: According to the rule of nines, with the initial burn, the anterior half of the head equals 4.5%, the upper half of the anterior torso equals 9%, and the lower halves of both arms equals 9%. The subsequent burn included the posterior half of the head, which equals 4.5%, and the upper half of the posterior torso, which equals 9%. This totals 36%.
Test-Taking Strategy: Knowledge regarding the rule of nines is required to answer this question. According to the rule, the entire head equals 9%, each arm equals 9% (both arms, 18%), the anterior and posterior torso each equal 18% (entire torso, 36%), each leg equals 18% (both legs, 36%), and the perineum equals 1%. Remember the following: 9% (head) + 18% (arms) + 36% (torso) + 36% (legs) + 1% (perineum) = 100%. Review the rule of nines if you had difficulty with this question.
Level of Cognitive Ability: Analysis
Client Needs: Physiological Integrity
Integrated Process: Nursing Process/Data Collection
Content Area: Adult Health/Integumentary
Reference: Christensen, B., & Kockrow, E. (2006). *Adult health nursing* (5th ed., p. 109). St. Louis: Mosby.

REFERENCES

Chernecky, C., & Berger, B. (2008). *Laboratory tests and diagnostic procedures* (5th ed.). Philadelphia: Saunders.

Christensen, B., & Kockrow, E. (2006). *Adult health nursing* (5th ed.). St. Louis: Mosby.

Christensen, B., & Kochrow, E. (2006). *Foundations of nursing* (5th ed.). St. Louis: Mosby.

deWit, S. (2009). *Medical-surgical nursing: Concepts & practice* Philadelphia: Saunders.

Ignatavicius, D., & Workman, M. (2006). *Medical-surgical nursing: Critical thinking for collaborative care* (5th ed.). Philadelphia: Saunders..

Lehne, R. (2007). *Pharmacology for nursing care* (6th ed.). Philadelphia: Saunders.

Lewis, S., Heitkemper, M., Dirksen, S., & Bucher, L. (2007). *Medical-surgical nursing: Assessment and management of clinical problems* (7th ed.). St. Louis: Mosby.

Linton, A. (2007). *Introduction to medical-surgical nursing* (4th ed.). Philadelphia: Saunders.

Monahan, F., Sands, J., Marek, J., Neighbors, M., & Green, C. (2007). *Phipps' medical-surgical nursing: Health and illness perspectives* (8th ed.). St. Louis: Mosby.

Perry, A., & Potter, P. (2006). *Clinical nursing skills & techniques* (6th ed.). St. Louis: Mosby.

CHAPTER 41

Integumentary Medications

I. EMOLLIENTS AND LOTIONS
A. Emollients (Box 41-1)
   1. Oily or fatty substances that soften and soothe irritated skin by allowing the skin to retain water
   2. Available as creams or ointments
   3. Used for dry, scaly, and itchy inflammatory conditions
B. Solutions and lotions (Box 41-2)
   1. Liquid suspensions or dispersions
   2. Require shaking before application
   3. Although lotions are predominantly water, they have a drying effect on the skin when the water evaporates
   4. Used as a wash for the skin, as soaks, or as wet dressings on ulcers or **burns**
   5. Used for subacute inflammatory lesions after the severe exudate phase has ceased
   6. Medicated lotions are often used as anti-inflammatory agents, because they provide a drying, protective, and cooling effect
C. Therapeutic baths (Box 41-3)
   1. Relieve itching
   2. Soothe and lubricate
   3. Reduce skin bacteria
   4. Clean skin and add moisture
   5. Loosen scaled skin
   6. Support ultraviolet A or B light therapy

II. RUBS AND LINIMENTS (Box 41-4)
A. Used for the temporary relief of muscular aches, rheumatism, arthritis, sprains, and neuralgia
B. Over-the-counter products contain combinations of antiseptics, local anesthetics, analgesics, and counterirritants
C. Some products contain salicylates, and, if they are used over a large area of the skin, may cause salicylate side effects, such as tinnitus, nausea, and vomiting
D. A heating pad is not used with these products, because irritation or burning of the skin may occur

III. ANTI-INFECTIVE AGENTS
A. Description
   1. Include antiseptics and antibacterial, antifungal, antiviral, and antiparasitic medications

2. Topical antibiotics are safe and effective for certain conditions, but extensive use may encourage the emergence of resistant bacteria
B. Antiseptics: These substances pose a risk for caustic adverse effects; care should be taken to prevent irritation and injury
   1. Sodium hypochlorite (Dakin's solution)
      a. Dakin's solution is a diluted 0.5% sodium hypochlorite solution that loosens, dissolves, and deodorizes necrotic tissue and blood clots
      b. The solution kills most common bacteria, including spores, amoebas, fungi, protozoa, viruses, and yeast
      c. The solution is used for irrigating, cleaning, and deodorizing necrotic or purulent wounds
      d. The solution loses its potency during storage, so fresh solution is prepared frequently
      e. The solution should not be in contact with healing or normal tissue, because its mechanism of action results in clotting delays
      f. To keep tissue irritation to a minimum, the solution should be rinsed off immediately after irrigation
   2. Chlorhexidine gluconate (Hibiclens)
      a. Effective for cleaning wounds caused by most staphylococci and other gram-positive bacteria
      b. Used for irrigating and cleansing wounds but not for packing wounds, because it may cause contact dermatitis
      c. Its effectiveness is decreased in wounds in which soap, blood, or pus is present
   3. Acetic acid preparations
      a. Acetic acid is effective for irrigating, cleansing, and packing wounds infected by *Pseudomonas aeruginosa*
      b. Healthy skin surrounding the wound must be protected with a petroleum barrier, because acetic acid excoriates the skin
   4. Hydrogen peroxide
      a. As a 3% solution, hydrogen peroxide has effervescent action that releases gas and breaks up necrotic tissue

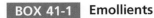

BOX 41-1 **Emollients**

- Cold cream
- Glycerin
- Lanolin
- Lubriderm
- Petrolatum
- Vitamin A & D ointment
- Zinc ointment

BOX 41-2 **Solutions and Lotions**

- Aluminum acetate solution (Burow's solution)
- Calamine lotion (Caladryl Lotion)

BOX 41-3 **Therapeutic Baths**

Antipruritics (to relieve itching)
- Aveeno colloidal oatmeal
- Aveeno oilated colloidal oatmeal
- Starch and baking soda

Antibacterial Baths (to reduce skin bacteria)
- Potassium permanganate

Emollient Baths (to clean the skin and add moisture)
- Bath emollient (Alpha Keri Therapeutic Bath Oil)
- Bath oils
- Mineral oil

Tar Baths (to loosen scaled skin and to support ultraviolet A or B light therapy)
- Coal tar (Balnetar, Zetar shampoo)
- Coal tar solution (Polytar soap and shampoo)
- Other coal tar preparations

BOX 41-4 **Rubs and Liniments**

- Menthyl salicylate, menthol (Ben-Gay, Icy Hot)
- Trolamine salicylate (Aspercreme, Myoflex)

BOX 41-5 **Antibacterials, Antifungals, and Antiparasitics**

Antibacterials
- Bacitracin preparations
- Chloramphenicol
- Chlortetracycline
- Erythromycin
- Gentamicin sulfate
- Mupirocin calcium (Bactroban)
- Neomycin preparations

Antifungals
- Amphotericin B (Fungizone) intravenous preparation
- Betamethasone dipropionate, clotrimazole (Lotrisone)
- Ciclopirox olamine (Loprox)
- Clotrimazole (Lotrimin AF, Desenex, Mycelex troches)
- Econazole nitrate (Spectazole)
- Haloprogin
- Ketoconazole (Ketoderm)
- Miconazole nitrate (Micatin)
- Nystatin (Mycostatin)
- Tolnaftate (Tinactin)
- Triacetin
- Undecylenic acid (Desenex)

Antivirals
- Acyclovir (Zovirax)

Antiparasitics
- Crotamiton (Eurax)
- Ivermectin
- Lindane
- Malathion (Ovide)
- Permethrin (Elimite, Nix, Acticin)

---

b. Used to irrigate and clean necrotic tissue and pus from open wounds

c. Not used to pack wounds, because it decomposes too rapidly

d. When epithelial tissue begins to form, the use of hydrogen peroxide is discontinued, because it inhibits tissue formation

5. Hexachlorophene (pHisoHex, Septisol)

a. A combination of hexachlorophene and alcohol

b. A bacteriostatic agent with activity against staphylococci and other gram-positive bacteria

c. Absorbs through broken skin and can cause neurotoxicity; it should not be used on wounds

d. The alcohol component dries and irritates tissue; it is not an effective germicide, and it forms a film that actually can promote infection

e. All hexachlorophene products should be rinsed well from the skin after their use to prevent systemic absorption

C. Antibacterials (Box 41-5)

1. Description: Used for superficial skin infections

2. Mupirocin calcium (Bactroban)

a. Topical antibacterial that is active against *Staphylococcus aureus*, β-hemolytic streptococci, and *Streptococcus pyogenes*

b. Usually applied 3 times daily; if improvement is not observed within 3 to 5 days, use is discontinued

D. Antifungal agents

1. May cause erythema, stinging, blistering, peeling, pruritus, urticaria, and general skin irritation

2. The client is reevaluated if no results are obtained after 4 weeks of treatment

E. Antiviral: Acyclovir (Zovirax)

1. Inhibits DNA replication in the virus

2. Used for herpes simplex types 1 and 2, varicella zoster virus, Epstein-Barr virus, and cytomegalovirus

BOX 41-6 **Antipruritics**

- Calamine lotion (Caladryl Lotion)
- Colloidal oatmeal (Aveeno)
- Starch and baking soda

3. Can cause mild pain and transient burning and stinging
4. Applied completely over the lesion, usually every 3 hours 6 times daily for 1 week
5. Rubber gloves are used to apply the ointment to prevent the spread of infection

F. Antiparasitics
  1. Used to treat scabies (mites) and pediculosis (lice)
  2. May be harmful during pregnancy and in young children
  3. May irritate the skin, eyes, and mucous membranes
  4. May cause allergic reactions
  5. Antiparasitic agents such as permethrin (Elimite, Nix, Acticin), which are used for the treatment of pediculosis capitis, are removed with a warm water rinse 10 minutes after application
  6. Antiparasitic agents such as malathion (Ovide), which are used for the treatment of pediculosis capitis, are washed off with shampoo 8 to 12 hours after application
  7. Antiparasitic agents such as lindane, which are used for the treatment of scabies, are washed off of the affected areas 8 to 12 hours after application

IV. **ANTIPRURITICS** (Box 41-6)
A. Used to allay itching
B. Applied as wet dressings, pastes, lotions, creams, or ointments or used in a bath
C. Persons with dry skin should be instructed to bathe less frequently

V. **KERATOLYTICS** (Box 41-7)
A. Description
  1. Preparations that dissolve keratin
  2. Soften scales and loosen the horny layer of the skin, thereby resulting in minimal peeling or extensive desquamation
  3. Used to treat superficial fungal infections, psoriasis, and localized dermatitis
B. Salicylic acid
  1. Used to treat seborrheic dermatitis, acne, and psoriasis and to thin and remove calluses
  2. Can be absorbed systemically and can cause salicylism, which is characterized by dizziness and tinnitus; it is not applied to large surface areas or open wounds
C. Podophyllum resin and imiquimod (Aldara)
  1. Used to treat various types of **skin cancer**
  2. Causes lesions to slough off, thereby leaving a superficial ulcer and moderate dermatitis

BOX 41-7 **Keratolytics**

- Cantharidin
- Imiquimod (Aldara)
- Masoprocol
- Podophyllum resin
- Podofilox (Condylox)
- Salicylic acid

BOX 41-8 **Stimulants and Irritants**

- Benzoin compound
- Coal tar

  3. After the therapy is discontinued, the lesions are treated with a mild antiseptic ointment; healing usually occurs within a few days
D. Cantharidin, podofilox (Condylox), and imiquimod (Aldara)
  1. Used to treat warts
  2. Have an exfoliation effect only on the epidermal cells
  3. May cause tingling, itching, and burning
  4. Site may be tender for 2 to 6 days
E. Masoprocol
  1. Has antiproliferative activity against keratinocytes
  2. Used to treat keratosis
  3. Occlusive dressings are not to be used with masoprocol
  4. Client may experience transient burning after administration

VI. **STIMULANTS AND IRRITANTS** (Box 41-8)
A. Description: Produce a mild irritation of the surface of the skin, thereby causing hyperemia and inflammation, which promote the healing process
B. Coal tar
  1. Used to treat psoriasis, seborrheic dermatitis, and atopic dermatitis
  2. Has an unpleasant odor and frequently stains the skin and hair
  3. Can cause phototoxicity
C. Benzoin compound
  1. Protects the skin when the client has sores, cracked nipples, or fissures of any orifice
  2. Causes a mild irritation that produces increased blood flow and healing

VII. **PROTECTIVES** (Box 41-9)
A. Description
  1. Preparations that provide a film on the skin to protect it from irritations such as light, moisture, air, and dust
  2. Promote natural healing without the usual formation of a dry crust over the wound
  3. Allow exudate to collect beneath the dressing, thus forming an artificial blister

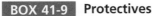

BOX 41-9 **Protectives**

Transparents
- Bio-occlusive membrane dressing
- OpSite
- Tegaderm

Hydrocolloids
- DuoDERM
- Tegasorb

Alginates
- Alginate
- Algosteril
- Comfeel

Biological
- AlloDerm
- Allograft
- Xenograft

BOX 41-10 **Enzymes to Débride and Remove Exudates**

- Collagenase (Santyl)
- Dextranomer (Debrisan)
- Fibrinolysin and desoxyribonuclease (Elase)
- Sutilains (Travase)

4. Transparent and hydrocolloidal protectives are designed to be left in place for up to 7 days or until leakage around the dressing occurs
5. Transparent protectives provide visualization of the wound; however, they can be difficult to apply and are nonabsorbent
6. Hydrocolloidal protectives provide wound protection for the wound bed and protection from bacterial contamination as well as wound débridement by autolysis; these protectives can soften and lose shape with heat, friction, and pressure, and wound visualization is not possible
7. Alginates absorb heavy drainage and provide protection for the wound bed; the advantages of alginates include high absorbency and easy application; however, wound visualization is not possible
8. Biological dressings provide protection for the wound bed and conform to uneven surfaces within the wound

B. Sunscreens
1. Act by absorbing ultraviolet rays
2. Most effective when applied about 30 minutes to 1 hour before exposure to the sun; should be reapplied every 2 to 3 hours after swimming or sweating
3. Can cause contact dermatitis and photosensitivity reactions

C. Nonadherent dressings
1. Woven or nonwoven dressings that may be impregnated with saline, petrolatum, or antimicrobials
2. Some nonadherent dressings include Telfa, Vaseline gauze, and Xeroform

VIII. ENZYMES
A. Description
1. Used to promote the healing of wounds and to débride necrotic tissue and skin ulcers
2. Reduce the inflammation that results from trauma and infection

3. Dissolve fibrin clots, which helps to reduce the size of surface hematomas
4. To be effective, enzymes must be in contact with the affected tissue in adequate concentrations for a sufficient length of time
5. Uninfected wounds with necrotic tissue may be débrided by enzymes over the course of 2 to 3 days to liquefy the necrotic tissue

B. Enzymes to débride and remove exudates (Box 41-10)
1. Description
   a. Enzymes digest or alter the thick, purulent drainage and turn it into a thin, liquid material that can be wiped away or irrigated easily off of the wound
   b. Enzyme contact with necrotic tissue within the wound is necessary
   c. Enzymes to débride wounds are discontinued when bleeding occurs or granulation tissue is apparent
2. Sutilains (Travase)
   a. Used to remove nonviable or necrotic tissue and purulent enzymes from **burns,** ulcers, traumatic injury, and peripheral vascular disease wounds
   b. Inactive on viable tissue
3. Collagenase (Santyl)
   a. Used as a topical débriding agent
   b. Provides effective débridement of the collagen tissue at the wound edges, where necrotic tissue is anchored
   c. Encourages the formation of granulation tissue at the wound edges and the quicker epithelization of wounds
   d. Apply with a tongue depressor directly into deep wounds
   e. Before application, cleanse the wound of debris by gently rubbing it with a gauze pad with sterile water or Dakin's solution, followed by sterile normal saline
   f. Remove all excess ointment each time the dressing is changed
   g. Apply only to the injured area; collagenase causes erythema in healthy tissues
   h. Protect healthy tissues by applying zinc oxide paste
   i. Use is discontinued when the necrotic tissue is gone

4. Fibrinolysin and desoxyribonuclease (Elase)
   a. Used to débride wounds, including **burns, pressure ulcers,** and inflamed or infected lesions
   b. Clean the wound with sterile normal saline to flush away necrotic debris, pat the area dry, and then apply a thin layer of fibrinolysin and desoxyribonuclease (Elase) and cover the area with petrolatum gauze
5. Dextranomer (Debrisan)
   a. Not a débriding agent; rather, it is a cleansing agent that actually absorbs peptides and proteins
   b. Effective in wet wounds only
   c. Not packed tightly into the wound, because the maceration of surrounding tissue may occur from contact with the agent
6. Papain (Accuzyme)
   a. Does not injure or affect healthy tissue or cells
   b. Must be in immediate contact with the purulent wound material
   c. Dressings are changed once a day

IX. **CORTICOSTEROIDS**
A. Topical corticosteroids have anti-inflammatory, antipruritic, and vasoconstrictive actions
B. Contraindications
   1. Clients demonstrating previous sensitivity to corticosteroids
   2. Clients with current systemic fungal, viral, or bacterial infections
   3. Clients with current complications related to corticosteroid therapy
C. Local adverse effects
   1. Hypopigmentation
   2. Acneiform eruptions
   3. Contact dermatitis
   4. Burning, dryness, irritation, and itching
   5. Overgrowth of bacteria, fungi, and viruses
   6. Skin atrophy
D. Systemic adverse effects
   1. Rare occurrence
   2. Adrenal suppression
   3. Cushing's syndrome
   4. Striae and skin atrophy
   5. Ocular effects such as glaucoma and cataracts
E. Interventions
   1. Monitor the plasma cortisol levels if prolonged therapy is necessary
   2. Wash the area just before application to increase the penetration of the medication
   3. Apply the medication sparingly in a thin film, rubbing gently
   4. May apply to the skin alone or with a dry occlusive dressing, as prescribed
   5. Instruct the client to report burning, irritation, or signs of infection to the physician

BOX 41-11 Acne Products

Cleansers
- Aluminum oxide (Brasivol)
- Salicylate acid and alcohol (Clearasil)

Drying Agents
- Sulfur, resorcinol, alcohol (Acnomel)
- Benzalkonium chloride (Ionax)

Miscellaneous
- Adapalene (Differin)
- Antibiotics
- Azelaic acid (Azelex)
- Benzoyl peroxide wash or gel
- Isotretinoin (Accutane)
- Resorcinol (as an ingredient in other preparations)
- Salicylic acid (as an ingredient in other preparations)
- Tazarotene
- Tretinoin (Retin-A)

X. **ACNE PRODUCTS** (Box 41-11)
A. Description
   1. Mild acne can be treated with bar soaps, soap-free cakes, liquid cleansers, lotions, gels, and creams
   2. For moderate acne, topical anti-inflammatory medications such as benzoyl peroxide, tretinoin (Retin-A), isotretinoin (Accutane), azelaic acid (Azelex), and adapalene (Differin) may be prescribed; antibiotics also may be prescribed
   3. Side effects can include excessive redness, extreme dryness of the skin leading to blistering and crusting, temporary pigmentation changes, and peeling of the skin
   4. All products are kept away from the eyes, the inside of the nose, the mucous membranes, and the hair
B. Benzoyl peroxide is a keratolytic agent that is bacteriostatic and that may decrease the production of irritant-free fatty acids in the follicle
C. Tretinoin and adapalene are acids of vitamin A that are used to treat acne vulgaris and that also may be used to treat **skin cancer** and the aging of the skin
D. Tretinoin (Retin-A)
   1. Decreases the cohesiveness of the epithelial cells, thereby increasing cell mitosis and turnover; tretinoin is potentially irritating, and mild redness and skin peeling are expected with topical use
   2. Within 48 hours of use, the skin generally becomes red and begins to peel
   3. Temporary hyperpigmentation and hypopigmentation can occur
   4. The client should avoid sun exposure, because photosensitivity may occur
   5. Applied liberally to the skin; the hands should be washed thoroughly immediately after application

6. Therapeutic results should be seen after 2 to 3 weeks but may not be optimal until after 6 weeks
7. The client may use cosmetics, but the skin needs to be cleaned thoroughly beforehand

E. Isotretinoin (Accutane)
1. A metabolite of vitamin A
2. Used to treat severe cystic acne; its use is reserved for persons who have not responded to other therapies, including systemic antibiotics
3. Can cause xerosis, facial and palmoplantar desquamation, pruritus, brittle nails, and hair loss
4. Administered with meals 2 times daily for a 15- to 20-week course; if another course of therapy is needed, an 8-week lapse of time should occur
5. Photosensitivity may occur, so the client needs to be instructed to decrease sun exposure
6. May cause depression in some cases
7. Alcohol consumption should be eliminated during therapy, because alcohol may potentiate serum triglyceride elevation

F. Local antibiotics
1. May be used to treat acne
2. Therapeutic response generally requires 6 to 12 weeks of therapy
3. Side effects include acute contact dermatitis, transient stinging or burning, staining of the skin, erythema, and skin tenderness

XI. POISON IVY TREATMENT (Box 41-12)
A. The treatment of lesions includes calamine lotion and other products that soothe the lesions, Burow's solution compresses, and/or Aveeno baths to relieve discomfort
B. Topical corticosteroids are effective to prevent or relieve inflammation, especially when they are used before blisters form
C. Oral corticosteroids may be prescribed for severe reactions, and a sedative such as diphenhydramine (Benadryl) may be prescribed

XII. BURN PRODUCTS (Box 41-13)
A. Nitrofurazone (Furacin)
1. Applied topically to the burn as a solution, ointment, or cream
2. Has a broad spectrum of antibacterial activity
3. Used in **burns** when bacterial resistance to other agents is a problem

4. Topical: Apply a 1/16-inch film directly to the burn
5. Side effects: Contact dermatitis and rash
6. Less common side effects: Pruritus and local edema

B. Mafenide acetate (Sulfamylon)
1. A water-soluble cream that is bacteriostatic for gram-negative and gram-positive organisms
2. Used to treat **burns** to reduce the bacteria present in avascular tissues
3. Diffuses through the devascularized areas of the skin; may precipitate metabolic acidosis (this is usually compensated for by hyperventilation)
4. Apply a 1/16-inch film directly to the **burn**
5. Side effects can include local pain and rash
6. Systemic effects include bone marrow depression, hemolytic anemia, and metabolic acidosis
7. Keep the **burn** covered with mafenide acetate at all times
8. Notify the physician if hyperventilation occurs; if acidosis develops, the mafenide acetate is washed off of the skin

C. Silver sulfadiazine (Silvadene)
1. Has a broad spectrum of activity against gram-negative bacteria, gram-positive bacteria, and yeast
2. Released slowly from the cream, which is selectively toxic to bacteria
3. Used primarily to prevent sepsis among clients with **burns**
4. Not a carbonic anhydrase inhibitor; therefore does not cause acidosis
5. Apply a 1/16-inch film, and keep the **burn** covered with silver sulfadiazine at all times
6. Side effects include rash and itching
7. Systemic effects include leukopenia and interstitial nephritis
8. Monitor the complete blood cell count, particularly the white blood cells, frequently; if leukopenia develops, the medication is discontinued

D. Silver nitrate
1. An antiseptic solution that is active against gram-negative bacteria
2. Dressings are applied to the **burn** and then kept moist with silver nitrate, which stains anything with which it comes in contact; however, this discoloration is not usually permanent

BOX 41-12 Poison Ivy Treatment Products

- Bentoquatam (for preventive use; Ivy Block)
- Calamine lotion (Caladryl Lotion)
- Hydrocortisone (Ivy Soothe; Ivy Stat)
- Isopropanol, cetyl alcohol (Ivy Cleanse)
- Zinc acetate, isopropanol (Ivy Dry)
- Zinc acetate, isopropanol, benzyl alcohol (Ivy Super Dry)

BOX 41-13 Burn Products

- Mafenide acetate (Sulfamylon)
- Nitrofurazone (Furacin)
- Silver nitrate
- Silver sulfadiazine (Silvadene)

3. May be prescribed for use on extensive **burns** that may precipitate fluid and electrolyte imbalances
4. Apply silver nitrate to the dressing; do not apply it directly to wounds, cuts, or broken skin

PRACTICE QUESTIONS

More questions on the companion CD!

453. Isotretinoin (Accutane) is prescribed for a client with severe acne. Before the administration of this medication, the nurse would expect that which laboratory test will be prescribed?
 1. Platelet count
 2. Triglyceride level
 3. Complete blood count
 4. White blood cell count
454. A client with severe acne is seen at the physician's office. The physician prescribes isotretinoin (Accutane). The nurse reviews the client's health record and would notify the physician if the client is presently taking which of the following medications?
 1. Vitamin A
 2. Digoxin (Lanoxin)
 3. Furosemide (Lasix)
 4. Phenytoin (Dilantin)
455. A nurse who is employed in a physician's office is collecting data from a client. The nurse notes that the client is taking azelaic acid (Azelex). Because of the medication prescription, the nurse suspects that the client is being treated for:
 1. Acne
 2. Eczema
 3. Hair loss
 4. Herpes simplex
456. A client is diagnosed with herpes simplex. The physician tells the nurse that a topical medication for treatment will be prescribed. The nurse expects that which of the following medications will be prescribed?
 1. Triple antibiotic
 2. Acyclovir (Zovirax)
 3. Masoprocol (Actinex)
 4. Mupirocin (Bactroban)
457. Salicylic acid is prescribed for a client with a diagnosis of psoriasis. The nurse suspects the presence of systemic toxicity from this medication if which of the following occurs in the client?
 1. Tinnitus
 2. Diarrhea
 3. Constipation
 4. Decreased respirations
458. A hospitalized client with severe seborrheic dermatitis is receiving treatments of topical glucocorticoid applications followed by the application of an occlusive dressing. The nurse monitors for

which systemic effect that can occur as a result of this treatment?
 1. Local infection
 2. Adrenal suppression
 3. Thinning of the skin
 4. Adrenal hyperactivity
459. A topical glucocorticoid is prescribed for a client with dermatitis. The nurse provides instructions to the client regarding the use of the medication. Which of the following, if stated by the client, would indicate the need for further instructions?
 1. "I need to apply the medication in a thin film."
 2. "I should gently rub the medication into the skin."
 3. "The medication will help to relieve the inflammation and itching."
 4. "I should place a bandage over the site after applying the medication."
460. Lindane is prescribed for the treatment of scabies. The nurse would question the order if the medication were prescribed for which of the following clients?
 1. An older client
 2. A 6-year-old child
 3. A 42-year-old female
 4. A 52-year-old male with hypertension
461. An outbreak of pediculosis capitis has occurred at a local school. A nurse is helping to provide instructions to the parents of the children attending the school regarding the application of permethrin 5% (Elimite). The nurse tells the parents to:
 1. Apply it before washing the hair.
 2. Apply it at bedtime, and rinse it off in the morning.
 3. Avoid saturating the hair and scalp when applying it.
 4. Allow it to remain on the hair for 10 minutes, and then rinse with water.
462. The physician has prescribed Myoflex topical cream for a client with a diagnosis of rheumatism who is complaining of muscular aches. Which of the following information does the nurse provide to the client regarding this medication?
 1. The medication will act as a local anesthetic.
 2. The medication acts by decreasing muscle spasms.
 3. The medication is prescribed to cause the skin to peel.
 4. Apply a heating pad to the area after applying the medication.
463. A camp nurse asks the children who are preparing to swim in the lake if they have applied sunscreen. The nurse tells the children that sunscreen is most effective when applied:
 1. Immediately after swimming
 2. One hour before exposure to the sun

3. Immediately before exposure to the sun
4. Fifteen minutes before exposure to the sun

464. Mafenide (Sulfamylon) is prescribed for the client with a burn injury. When applying the medication, the client complains of local discomfort and burning. The nurse would:
1. Discontinue the medication.
2. Inform the client that this is normal.
3. Notify the registered nurse immediately.
4. Apply a thinner film than prescribed to the burn site.

465. A burn client is receiving treatments of topical mafenide (Sulfamylon) to the site of injury. The nurse would suspect that a systemic effect has occurred if which of the following is noted in the client?
1. Hyperventilation
2. Elevated blood pressure
3. Localized rash at the burn site
4. Localized pain at the burn site

466. Tretinoin (Retin-A) is prescribed for a client with acne. The client calls the physician's office and

tells the nurse that the skin has become very red and is beginning to peel. The nurse responds by telling the client:
1. To notify the physician
2. To discontinue the medication
3. To come to the clinic immediately
4. That this is a normal occurrence with the use of this medication

ALTERNATE ITEM FORMAT: FILL IN THE BLANK

467. A nurse is caring for a client who has an ulcer on the medial aspect of the left ankle that is being treated with DuoDERM. The nurse removes the DuoDERM, cleanses the wound as prescribed, and reapplies the DuoDERM. The nurse documents that the DuoDERM needs to be changed in how many days?

Answer: _____ days

ANSWERS

453. **2**
Rationale: Isotretinoin can elevate triglyceride levels. Blood triglyceride levels should be measured before treatment and periodically thereafter until the effects of the medication on the triglycerides have been evaluated.
Test-Taking Strategy: Use the process of elimination. Eliminate options 3 and 4 first, because a complete blood count will also measure the white blood cell count. From the remaining options, it is necessary to know that the medication can affect triglyceride levels in the client. Review isotretinoin if you had difficulty with this question.
Level of Cognitive Ability: Analysis
Client Needs: Physiological Integrity
Integrated Process: Nursing Process/Planning
Content Area: Pharmacology
References: Kee, J., Hayes, E., & McCuistion, L. (2006). *Pharmacology: A nursing process approach* (5th ed., p. 742). Philadelphia: Saunders.
Lehne, R. (2007). *Pharmacology for nursing care* (6th ed., pp. 1205-1206). Philadelphia: Saunders.

454. **1**
Rationale: Vitamin A, from which isotretinoin is derived, can produce the generalized intensification of isotretinoin toxicity. Because of the potential for increased toxicity, vitamin A supplements should be discontinued before isotretinoin therapy. Options 2, 3, and 4 are not a concern.
Test-Taking Strategy: Use the process of elimination. Recalling that isotretinoin is a derivative of vitamin A will easily direct you to the correct option. Review the contraindications associated with the use of isotretinoin therapy if you had difficulty with this question.
Level of Cognitive Ability: Application
Client Needs: Safe and Effective Care Environment
Integrated Process: Nursing Process/Implementation

Content Area: Pharmacology
Reference: Lehne, R. (2007). *Pharmacology for nursing care* (6th ed., p.1206). Philadelphia: Saunders.

455. **1**
Rationale: Azelaic acid is a topical medication that is used to treat mild to moderate acne. It appears to work by suppressing the growth of *Propionibacterium acnes* and by decreasing the proliferation of keratinocytes.
Test-Taking Strategy: Knowledge regarding the use of azelaic acid is required to answer this question. Remember that azelaic acid is a topical medication that is used to treat mild to moderate acne. Review azelaic acid if you had difficulty with this question.
Level of Cognitive Ability: Analysis
Client Needs: Physiological Integrity
Integrated Process: Nursing Process/Data Collection
Content Area: Pharmacology
Reference: Lehne, R. (2007). *Pharmacology for nursing care* (6th ed., pp. 1204-1205). Philadelphia: Saunders.

456. **2**
Rationale: Acyclovir is a topical antiviral agent that inhibits DNA replication in the virus. It has activity against herpes simplex virus types 1 and 2, varicella zoster virus, Epstein-Barr virus, and cytomegalovirus. Triple antibiotic would not be effective for the treatment of herpes virus. Mupirocin is a topical antibacterial that is active against impetigo caused by *Staphylococcus* or *Streptococcus*. Masoprocol is a keratolytic.
Test-Taking Strategy: Use the process of elimination. Recalling that herpes simplex is a virus will direct you to the option that identifies an antiviral medication. Review acyclovir if you had difficulty with this question.
Level of Cognitive Ability: Analysis
Client Needs: Physiological Integrity

Integrated Process: Nursing Process/Planning
Content Area: Pharmacology
References: Hodgson, B., & Kizior, R. (2008). *Saunders nursing drug handbook 2008* (p. 19). Philadelphia: Saunders. Skidmore-Roth, L. (2008). *2008 Mosby's nursing drug reference* (21st ed., p. 1109). St. Louis: Mosby.

457. 1
Rationale: Salicylic acid is readily absorbed through the skin, and systemic toxicity (salicylism) can result. Symptoms include tinnitus, hyperpnea, dizziness, and psychological disturbances. Constipation and diarrhea are not associated with salicylism.
Test-Taking Strategy: Use the process of elimination. Noting the name of the medication will assist with directing you to the correct option if you can recall the toxic effects that occur with acetylsalicylic acid (aspirin). Review the toxic effects of salicylic acid if you had difficulty with this question.
Level of Cognitive Ability: Analysis
Client Needs: Physiological Integrity
Integrated Process: Nursing Process/Data Collection
Content Area: Pharmacology
Reference: Lehne, R. (2007). *Pharmacology for nursing care* (6th ed., p. 1202). Philadelphia: Saunders.

458. 2
Rationale: Topical glucocorticoids can be absorbed in sufficient amounts to produce systemic toxicity. The principal concerns are growth retardation in children and adrenal suppression in all age groups. Options 1 and 3 identify local rather than systemic reactions.
Test-Taking Strategy: Use the process of elimination. Options 1 and 3 can be eliminated first, because they are local reactions. From the remaining options, the ability to recall the concerns related to systemic toxicity is required to answer the question. Review these systemic effects if you had difficulty with this question.
Level of Cognitive Ability: Analysis
Client Needs: Physiological Integrity
Integrated Process: Nursing Process/Data Collection
Content Area: Pharmacology
Reference: Lehne, R. (2007). *Pharmacology for nursing care* (6th ed., pp. 1201-1202). Philadelphia: Saunders.

459. 4
Rationale: Clients should be advised to not use occlusive dressings (i.e., bandages or plastic wraps) to cover the affected site after the application of a topical glucocorticoid, unless the physician specifically prescribes wound coverage. Options 1, 2, and 3 are accurate statements related to the use of this medication.
Test-Taking Strategy: Use the process of elimination, and note the strategic words "need for further instructions." Eliminate option 3, knowing that this is the action for glucocorticoids. The words "thin" in option 1 and "gently" in option 2 should assist you with eliminating these options. Review the use of topical glucocorticoids if you had difficulty with this question.
Level of Cognitive Ability: Analysis
Client Needs: Physiological Integrity
Integrated Process: Teaching and Learning
Content Area: Pharmacology

Reference: Lehne, R. (2007). *Pharmacology for nursing care* (6th ed., p. 1202). Philadelphia: Saunders.

460. 2
Rationale: Lindane can penetrate the intact skin and cause convulsions if it is absorbed in sufficient quantities. The clients who are at highest risk for convulsions are premature infants, children, and clients with preexisting seizure disorders. Lindane should not be used on pediatric clients unless safer medications have failed to control the infection.
Test-Taking Strategy: Knowledge regarding the contraindications associated with the use of lindane is required to answer this question. Remember that lindane should not be used on pediatric clients unless safer medications have failed to control the infection. Review the contraindications for the use of lindane if you had difficulty with this question.
Level of Cognitive Ability: Analysis
Client Needs: Safe and Effective Care Environment
Integrated Process: Nursing Process/Implementation
Content Area: Pharmacology
Reference: Lehne, R. (2007). *Pharmacology for nursing care* (6th ed., p. 1141). Philadelphia: Saunders.

461. 4
Rationale: The instructions for the use of permethrin include washing, rinsing, and towel drying the hair; applying a sufficient volume to saturate the hair and scalp; allowing the medication to remain on the hair for 10 minutes; and then rinsing with water. Options 1, 2, and 3 are incorrect instructions.
Test-Taking Strategy: Note that both options 2 and 4 address a time frame for allowing the permethrin to remain on the hair; recognizing this may provide you with the clue that one of these options is correct. From this point, it is necessary to know the procedure for permethrin treatment. Review treatment with permethrin if you had difficulty with this question.
Level of Cognitive Ability: Application
Client Needs: Physiological Integrity
Integrated Process: Nursing Process/Implementation
Content Area: Pharmacology
Reference: Lehne, R. (2007). *Pharmacology for nursing care* (6th ed., p. 1140). Philadelphia: Saunders.

462. 1
Rationale: Myoflex is one of the many products that are used for the temporary relief of muscular aches, rheumatism, arthritis, sprains, and neuralgia. These types of products contain combinations of antiseptics, local anesthetics, analgesics, and counterirritants. A heating pad should not be applied, because irritation or burning of the skin may occur. These medications do not act in a systemic manner (option 2). They are not prescribed to cause the skin to peel; if this sort of reaction occurs, the physician should be notified.
Test-Taking Strategy: Use the process of elimination. Noting the strategic words "topical cream" may assist you with eliminating option 2. Eliminate option 3 knowing that this is not an expected therapeutic effect. Recalling the principles related to the application of heat will assist you with eliminating option 4. Review Myoflex if you had difficulty with this question.
Level of Cognitive Ability: Application
Client Needs: Physiological Integrity

Integrated Process: Teaching and Learning
Content Area: Pharmacology
Reference: Lewis, S., Heitkemper, M., Dirksen, S., & Bucher, L. (2007). *Medical-surgical nursing: Assessment and management of clinical problems* (7th ed., p. 141). St. Louis: Mosby.

463. 2
Rationale: Sunscreens are most effective when they are applied about 30 to 60 minutes before exposure to the sun so that they can penetrate the skin. All sunscreens should be reapplied after swimming or sweating.
Test-Taking Strategy: Use the process of elimination. Recalling that sunscreens need to penetrate the skin will assist you with eliminating options 3 and 4. From the remaining options, noting the strategic words "most effective" will direct you to option 2. Review protective skin measures if you had difficulty with this question.
Level of Cognitive Ability: Application
Client Needs: Health Promotion and Maintenance
Integrated Process: Nursing Process/Implementation
Content Area: Pharmacology
Reference: Lehne, R. (2007). *Pharmacology for nursing care* (6th ed., p. 1208). Philadelphia: Saunders.

464. 2
Rationale: Mafenide acetate is bacteriostatic for both gram-negative and gram-positive organisms. It is used to treat burn injuries and to reduce bacteria that are present in avascular tissues. The client should be informed that the medication will cause local discomfort and burning.
Test-Taking Strategy: Use the process of elimination. Eliminate options 1 and 4, because it is not within the scope of nursing practice to alter or discontinue a medication. From the remaining options, recalling that local discomfort and burning are normal and expected occurrences will direct you to option 2. Review mafenide acetate if you had difficulty with this question.
Level of Cognitive Ability: Application
Client Needs: Physiological Integrity
Integrated Process: Nursing Process/Implementation
Content Area: Pharmacology
Reference: McKenry, L., Tessier, E., & Hogan, M. (2006). *Mosby's pharmacology in nursing* (22nd ed., p. 1188). St. Louis: Mosby.

465. 1
Rationale: Mafenide acetate can suppress the renal excretion of acid and cause acidosis, which is evidenced by hyperventilation. The acid-base status of clients who are receiving this treatment should be monitored. If the acidosis becomes severe, the medication is discontinued for 1 to 2 days. Options 3 and 4 describe local rather than systemic effects.

An elevated blood pressure may be expected in the client with pain.
Test-Taking Strategy: Use the process of elimination, and note the strategic words "systemic effect." Options 3 and 4 can be eliminated, because these are local rather than systemic effects. From the remaining options, recall that the client in pain is likely to have an elevated blood pressure; this should direct you to option 1. Review the systemic effects of mafenide acetate if you had difficulty with this question.
Level of Cognitive Ability: Analysis
Client Needs: Physiological Integrity
Integrated Process: Nursing Process/Data Collection
Content Area: Pharmacology
Reference: Lehne, R. (2007). *Pharmacology for nursing care* (6th ed., pp. 1004-1005). Philadelphia: Saunders.

466. 4
Rationale: Tretinoin decreases the cohesiveness of the epithelial cells, thereby increasing cell mitosis and turnover. It is potentially irritating, particularly when it is used correctly. Within 48 hours of use, the skin generally becomes red and begins to peel.
Test-Taking Strategy: Use the process of elimination. Options 1 and 3 can be eliminated first, because they are comparable or alike. Eliminate option 2 next, because it is not within the scope of nursing practice to advise a client to discontinue a medication. Review the effects of tretinoin if you had difficulty with this question.
Level of Cognitive Ability: Application
Client Needs: Physiological Integrity
Integrated Process: Nursing Process/Implementation
Content Area: Pharmacology
Reference: Lehne, R. (2007). *Pharmacology for nursing care* (6th ed., pp. 1024-1025). Philadelphia: Saunders.

ALTERNATE ITEM FORMAT: FILL IN THE BLANK
467. 7
Rationale: Protective dressings such as DuoDERM are designed to be left in place for 7 days unless leakage occurs around the dressing.
Test-Taking Strategy: Note the strategic word "DuoDERM." Recalling that these dressings are designed to be left in place for 7 days will assist you with answering this question. Review the purpose and procedure for using protective dressings if you had difficulty with this question.
Level of Cognitive Ability: Application
Client Needs: Physiological Integrity
Integrated Process: Nursing Process/Planning
Content Area: Pharmacology
Reference: McKenry, L., Tessier, E., & Hogan, M. (2006). *Mosby's pharmacology in nursing* (22nd ed., p. 1204). St. Louis: Mosby.

REFERENCES

deWit, S. (2009). *Medical-surgical nursing: Concepts & practice*. St. Louis: Saunders.

Hodgson, B., & Kizior, R. (2008). *Saunders nursing drug handbook 2008*. Philadelphia: Saunders.

Ignatavicius, D., & Workman, M. (2006). *Medical-surgical nursing: Critical thinking for collaborative care* (5th ed.). Philadelphia: Saunders.

Kee, J., Hayes, E., & McCuistion, L. (2006). *Pharmacology: A nursing process approach* (5th ed.). Philadelphia: Saunders.

Lehne, R. (2007). *Pharmacology for nursing care* (6th ed.). Philadelphia: Saunders.

Linton, A. (2007). *Introduction to medical-surgical nursing* (4th ed.). Philadelphia: Saunders.

Lewis, S., Heitkemper, M., Dirksen, S., & Bucher, L. (2007). *Medical-surgical nursing: Assessment and management of clinical problems* (7th ed.). St. Louis: Mosby.

McKenry, L., Tessier, E., & Hogan, M. (2006). *Mosby's pharmacology in nursing* (22nd ed.). St. Louis: Mosby.

Skidmore-Roth, L. (2008). *2008 Mosby's nursing drug reference* (21st ed.). St. Louis: Mosby.

The Adult Client With an Oncological Disorder

PYRAMID TERMS

adenocarcinoma Cancer that arises from glandular tissues.

benign Usually refers to growths that are encapsulated, that remain localized, and that are slow-growing.

cancer A neoplastic disorder that can involve all body organs. Cells lose their normal growth-controlling mechanism, and the growth of cells is uncontrolled.

carcinogen A physical, chemical, or biological stressor that causes neoplastic changes in normal cells.

carcinoma A new growth or malignant tumor that originates from the epithelial cells, the skin, the gastrointestinal tract, the lungs, the uterus, the breast, or other organs.

carcinoma in situ A lesion with all of the histological characteristics of a malignancy except invasion.

dysplasia An alteration in the size, shape, and organization of differentiated cells. Cells lose their regularity and show variability in size and shape.

hospice A concept of care for terminally ill clients that includes the idea of intensive caring rather than intensive care. The family and the client are the focus of nursing care, and the goals are to relieve pain and to facilitate an optimal quality of life.

hyperplasia An increase in the number of normal cells in a body part that results from an increased rate of cellular division.

leukemias and myelomas Neoplasms that originate from blood-forming organs.

lymphomas Neoplasms that originate from lymphoid tissue.

malignant Refers to growths that are not encapsulated but that metastasize and grow. These growths are cancerous lesions that have the characteristics of disorderly, uncontrolled, and chaotic proliferations of cells.

metastasis The transfer of disease from one organ or part to another organ or part that is not directly connected with it. Secondary malignant lesions, which originate from the primary tumor, are located in anatomically distant places.

nadir The period of time during which an antineoplastic medication has its most profound effects on the bone marrow.

neoplasm A new growth that may be benign or malignant.

sarcomas Neoplasms that originate from muscle, bone, fat, the lymph system, or connective tissues.

staging A method of classifying malignancies on the basis of the presence and extent of the tumor within the body.

tumor marker A specific body substance that seems to indicate tumor progression or regression.

undifferentiated cell A cell that has lost the capacity for specialized function.

PYRAMID TO SUCCESS

The pyramid points focus on the treatment modalities related to an oncological disorder (e.g., pain management, internal and external radiation, chemotherapy) and on oncological disorders such as skin cancer, leukemia, breast cancer, and lung cancer. The specific foci relate to the nursing care related to these treatment modalities and disorders, to client adaptation, and to the impact of the treatment or the disorder. Specifically, the emphasis is on the complications related to chemotherapy, the nursing measures required to monitor for these complications, and the prevention of life-threatening conditions such as infection and bleeding. Specific laboratory values include the white blood cell (WBC) count and the platelet count. The Integrated Processes addressed in this unit include Caring, the Clinical Problem-Solving Process (Nursing Process), Communication and Documentation, and Teaching and Learning.

CLIENT NEEDS

Safe and Effective Care Environment

Discussing oncology-related consultations and referrals

Ensuring that advance directives are in the client's medical record

Ensuring advocacy related to the client's decisions

Establishing priorities

Ensuring ethical practices

Handling hazardous and infectious materials related to radiation and chemotherapy safely

Implementing protective, standard, and other precautions

Maintaining medical and surgical asepsis

Preventing disease related to infection

Providing confidentiality regarding the client's diagnosis

Providing informed consent for treatments and procedures

Upholding client's rights

Health Promotion and Maintenance

Discussing expected body-image changes related to chemotherapy and treatments

Providing client and family instructions regarding home care

Providing instructions regarding monthly breast or testicular self-examinations

Respecting client lifestyle choices

Teaching about health promotion programs regarding risks for cancer

Teaching about health screening measures for cancer

Psychosocial Integrity

Assessing the client's ability to cope, adapt, and/or problem solve during illness or stressful events

Assisting the client and family with coping with alterations in body image

Discussing end-of-life and grief and loss issues related to death and the dying process

Mobilizing the appropriate support and resource systems

Promoting a positive environment to maintain an optimal quality of life

Respecting religious and cultural preferences

Physiological Integrity

Administering blood and blood products

Caring for central venous access devices

Caring for the client who is receiving chemotherapy

Caring for the client who is receiving radiation therapy

Managing pain

Monitoring diagnostic tests and laboratory values, such as white blood cell and platelet counts

Monitoring for expected and unexpected responses to radiation and chemotherapy

Protecting the client from the life-threatening adverse effects of treatments

Providing basic care and comfort

Providing nutrition

REFERENCES

Black, J., & Hawks, J. (2005). *Medical-surgical nursing: Clinical management for positive outcomes* (7th ed.). Philadelphia: Saunders.

Chernecky, C., & Berger, B. (2008). *Laboratory tests and diagnostic procedures* (5th ed.). Philadelphia: Saunders.

Christensen, B., & Kockrow, E. (2006). *Adult health nursing* (5th ed.). St. Louis: Mosby.

Christensen, B., & Kockrow, E. (2006). *Foundations of nursing* (5th ed.). St. Louis: Mosby.

deWit, S. (2009). *Medical-surgical nursing: Concepts & practice.* Philadelphia: Saunders.

Hodgson, B., & Kizior, R. (2008). *Saunders nursing drug handbook 2008.* Philadelphia: Saunders.

Ignatavicius, D., & Workman, M. (2006). *Medical-surgical nursing: Critical thinking for collaborative care* (5th ed.). Philadelphia: Saunders.

Kee, J., Hayes, E., & McCuistion, L. (2006). *Pharmacology: A nursing process approach* (5th ed.). Philadelphia: Saunders.

Lehne, R. (2007). *Pharmacology for nursing care* (6th ed.). Philadelphia: Saunders.

Lewis, S., Heitkemper, M., Dirksen, S., & Bucher, L. (2007). *Medical-surgical nursing: Assessment and management of clinical problems* (7th ed.). St. Louis: Mosby.

Linton, A. (2007). *Introduction to medical-surgical nursing* (4th ed.). Philadelphia: Saunders.

McKenry, L., Tessier, E., & Hogan, M. (2006). *Mosby's pharmacology in nursing* (22nd ed.). St. Louis: Mosby.

Monahan, F., Sands, J., Marek, J., Neighbors, M., & Green, C. (2007). *Phipps' medical-surgical nursing: Health and illness perspectives* (8th ed.). St. Louis: Mosby.

National Council of State Boards of Nursing (Eds.). (2008). *2008 Detailed Test Plan for the NCLEX-PN® Examination,* National Council of State Boards of Nursing. Chicago: Author.

National Council of State Boards of Nursing. *NCSBN home page.* www.ncsbn.org. Accessed August 1, 2008.

Perry, A., & Potter, P. (2006). *Clinical nursing skills & techniques* (6th ed.). St. Louis: Mosby.

Skidmore-Roth, L. (2008). *2008 Mosby's nursing drug reference* (21st ed.). St. Louis: Mosby.

Oncological Disorders

CHAPTER

42

I. CANCER

A. Description
1. A neoplastic disorder that can involve any body organ
2. Cells lose their normal growth-controlling mechanism, and the growth of cells is uncontrolled
3. **Cancer** produces serious health problems such as impaired immune and hematopoietic (blood-producing) function; altered gastrointestinal (GI) tract structure and function; motor and sensory deficits; and decreased respiratory function

B. **Metastasis** (Box 42-1)
1. **Cancer** cells move from their original location to other sites
2. Routes of **metastasis**
   a. Local seeding: Distribution of shed **cancer** cells occurs in the local area of the primary tumor
   b. Blood-borne **metastasis**: Tumor cells enter the blood; this is the most common cause of **cancer** spread
   c. Lymphatic spread: Primary sites rich in lymphatics are more susceptible to early metastatic spread

C. **Cancer** classification
1. Solid tumors: Associated with the organs from which they develop, such as breast **cancer** or lung **cancer**
2. Hematologic **cancers**: Originate from blood cell–forming tissues, such as the **leukemias** and the **lymphomas**

D. Grading and **staging** (Box 42-2)
1. A method used to describe the tumor
2. Includes the extent of the tumor, the extent to which malignancy has increased in size, the involvement of regional nodes, and metastatic development
3. Grading classifies the cellular aspects of the **cancer**
4. **Staging** classifies the clinical aspects of the **cancer**

E. Factors that influence **cancer** development
1. Environmental factors
   a. Chemical **carcinogens**: Industrial chemicals, drugs, and tobacco
   b. Physical **carcinogens**: Ionizing radiation (diagnostic and therapeutic x-rays) and ultraviolet radiation (sun, tanning beds, and germicidal lights); chronic irritation and tissue trauma
   c. Viral **carcinogens**: Viruses capable of causing **cancer** are known as oncoviruses (e.g., Epstein-Barr virus, hepatitis B virus, human papillomavirus)
2. Dietary factors: High-fat and low-fiber diets; high animal-fat intake; preservatives, contaminants, additives, and nitrates
3. Genetic predisposition: Inherited predisposition to specific **cancers,** inherited conditions associated with **cancer,** familial clustering, and chromosomal aberrations
4. Age: Advancing age is a significant risk factor for the development of **cancer**
5. Immune function: Incidences of **cancer** are higher among immunosuppressed individuals, organ transplant recipients who are taking immunosuppressive medication, and individuals with acquired immunodeficiency syndrome

F. Prevention
1. Avoidance of known or potential **carcinogens** and avoidance or modification of the factors associated with the development of **cancer** cells
2. Minimize the intake of red meat and eat more cruciferous vegetables, such as broccoli, cauliflower, brussels sprouts, and cabbage
3. Eat foods high in vitamin A (e.g., apricots, carrots, cauliflower, leafy green vegetables) and vitamin C (e.g., fresh fruits and vegetables, especially citrus fruits)

G. Early detection (Box 42-3)
1. Mammography
2. Papanicolaou (Pap) test
3. Stools for occult blood
4. Sigmoidoscopy

BOX 42-1 Common Sites of Metastasis

Breast Cancer
- Bone
- Lung

Lung Cancer
- Brain

Colorectal Cancer
- Liver

Prostate Cancer
- Bone
- Spine and legs

Brain Tumors
- Central nervous system

BOX 42-2 Grading and Staging

Grading
- *Grade I:* Cells differ slightly from normal cells and are well differentiated (mild dysplasia)
- *Grade II:* Cells are more abnormal and are moderately differentiated (moderate dysplasia)
- *Grade III:* Cells are very abnormal and are poorly differentiated (severe dysplasia)
- *Grade IV:* Cells are immature (anaplasia) and undifferentiated; the cell of origin is difficult to determine

Staging
- *Stage 0:* Cancer in situ
- *Stage I:* Tumor limited to the tissue of origin; localized tumor growth
- *Stage II:* Limited local spread
- *Stage III:* Extensive local and regional spread
- *Stage IV:* Metastasis

BOX 42-3 Seven Warning Signs of Cancer: "CAUTION"

Change in bowel or bladder habits
Any sore that does not heal
Unusual bleeding or discharge
Thickening or lump in the breast or elsewhere
Indigestion
Obvious change in wart or mole
Nagging cough or hoarseness

5. Breast self-examination
6. Testicular self-examination
7. Skin inspection

II. **BREAST SELF-EXAMINATION**
A. Performing breast self-examination (BSE)
   1. Perform 7 to 10 days after menses
   2. Postmenopausal clients or clients who have had a hysterectomy should select a specific day of the month and perform a BSE monthly on that day
B. Procedure (Figure 42-1)

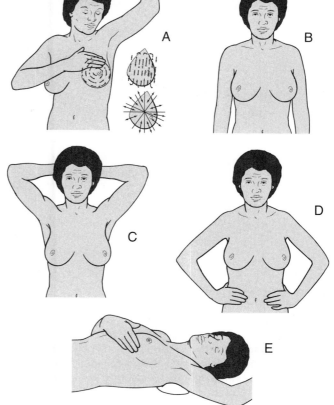

FIG. 42-1 Breast self-examination (BSE). **A,** While in the shower or bath, when the skin is slippery with soap and water, examine your breasts. Use the pads of your second, third, and fourth fingers to firmly press every part of the breast. Use your right hand to examine your left breast and your left hand to examine your right breast. Using the pads of the fingers on your left hand, examine the entire breast with the use of small circular motions in a spiral or in an up-and-down motion so that the entire breast area is examined. Repeat the procedure using your right hand to examine your left breast. Repeat the pattern of palpation under the arm. Check for any lump, hard knot, or thickening of the tissue. **B,** Look at your breasts in a mirror. Stand with your arms at your side. **C,** Raise your arms overhead and check for any changes in the shape of your breasts, any dimpling of the skin, or any changes in the nipple. **D,** Place your hands on your hips and press down firmly, tightening the pectoral muscles. Observe for asymmetry or changes, keeping in mind that your breasts probably do not match exactly. **E,** While lying down, feel your breasts as described in part A. When examining your right breast, place a folded towel under your right shoulder, and put your right hand behind your head. Repeat the procedure when examining your left breast. Mark on your calendar that you have completed your BSE; note any changes or unique characteristics that you want to discuss with your health care provider. (From Lewis, S., Heitkemper, M., Dirksen, S., & Bucher, L. [2007]. *Medical-surgical nursing: Assessment and management of clinical problems* [7th ed.]. St. Louis: Mosby.)

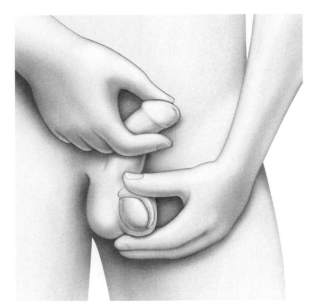

FIG. 42-2 Testicular self-examination. (1) The best time to perform this examination is right after a shower when your scrotal skin is moist and relaxed, thus making the testicles easy to feel. (2) Gently lift each testicle. Each one should feel like an egg; it should be firm but not hard and smooth with no lumps. (3) Using both hands, place your middle fingers on the underside of each testicle and your thumbs on top. (4) Gently roll each testicle between the thumb and fingers to feel for any lumps, swellings, or masses. (5) If you notice any changes from one month to the next, notify your health care provider. (From Harkreader, H., & Hogan, M. A. [2007]. *Fundamentals of nursing: Caring and clinical judgment* [3rd ed.]. Philadelphia: Saunders.)

▲ **III. TESTICULAR SELF-EXAMINATION**

A. Performing testicular self-examination (TSE): Select a day of the month and perform the examination on the same day each month

B. Procedure (Figure 42-2)

IV. DIAGNOSTIC TESTS

A. Diagnostic tests to be performed depend on the suspected primary or metastatic sites of the **cancer** (Box 42-4)

▲ B. Biopsy

1. Description
   a. Definitive means of diagnosing **cancer**; provides histologic proof of malignancy
   b. Involves the surgical incision of a small piece of tissue for microscopic examination
2. Types
   a. Needle: Aspiration of cells
   b. Incisional: Wedge of suspected tissue is removed from a larger mass
   c. Excisional: Complete removal of the entire lesion
   d. **Staging**: Multiple needle or incisional biopsies in tissues in which **metastasis** is suspected or likely (see Boxes 42-1 and 42-2)

BOX 42-4 **Diagnostic Tests**

- Biopsy
- Bone marrow examination (if a hematolymphoid malignancy is suspected)
- Chest x-ray
- Complete blood count
- Computed tomography scan
- Cytology studies (Papanicolaou smear)
- Liver function studies
- Magnetic resonance imaging
- Presence of oncofetal antigens such as carcinoembryonic antigen and alpha-fetoprotein
- Proctoscopic examination (including guaiac for occult blood)
- Radiographic studies (mammography)
- Radioisotope scans (e.g., liver, brain, bone, lung)

---

3. Tissue examination
   a. After excision, a frozen section or a permanent paraffin section is obtained to examine the specimen
   b. The advantage of the frozen section is the speed with which the section can be prepared and the diagnosis made; only minutes are required for this test
   c. A permanent paraffin section takes about 24 hours; however, it provides clearer details than the frozen section
4. Interventions
   a. The procedure is usually performed in an outpatient surgical setting
   b. Prepare the client for the diagnostic procedure in accordance with the physician's instructions
   c. Obtain informed consent

V. PAIN CONTROL ▲

A. Causes of pain
   1. Bone destruction
   2. Obstruction of an organ
   3. Compression of peripheral nerves
   4. Infiltration and distention of tissue
   5. Inflammation and necrosis
   6. Psychological causes (e.g., fear, anxiety)

B. Interventions ▲
   1. Assess the client's pain; pain is what the client describes or says that it is; medicate on the basis of the client's pain assessment
   2. Collaborate with other members of the health care team to develop a pain-management program
   3. Administer oral preparations, if possible and if they provide adequate relief of pain
   4. Mild or moderate pain may be treated with salicylates, acetaminophen (Tylenol), and nonsteroidal anti-inflammatory drugs

5. Severe pain is treated with opioids such as codeine sulfate, meperidine (Demerol), morphine sulfate, and hydromorphone hydrochloride (Dilaudid)
6. Subcutaneous injections and continuous intravenous (IV) infusions of opioids provide the best pain control
7. Monitor the vital signs for side effects of medications
8. Monitor for the effectiveness of medications
9. Provide nonpharmacological techniques of pain control, such as relaxation, guided imagery, biofeedback, and diversion
10. Do not undermedicate the client with **cancer** who is in pain

VI. SURGERY

A. Description: Used to diagnose, stage, and treat **cancer**
B. Prophylactic surgery
   1. Performed in clients with an existing premalignant condition or a known family history that strongly predisposes the person to the development of **cancer**
   2. An attempt is made to remove the tissue or organ at risk and thus prevent the development of **cancer**
C. Curative surgery: All gross and microscopic tumor is either removed or destroyed
D. Control (cytoreductive) surgery
   1. A debulking procedure that consists of removing part of the tumor
   2. It decreases the number of **cancer** cells and increases the chance that other therapies will be successful
E. Palliative surgery
   1. Performed to improve the quality of life during the survival time
   2. Performed to reduce pain, relieve airway obstruction, relieve obstructions in the GI and urinary tracts, relieve pressure on the brain or spinal cord, prevent hemorrhage, remove infected or ulcerated tumors, or drain abscesses
F. Reconstructive or rehabilitative surgery: Performed to improve the quality of life by restoring maximal function and appearance (e.g., breast reconstruction after mastectomy)
G. Side effects of surgery
   1. Loss of a specific body part
   2. Reduced function as a result of organ loss
   3. Scarring or disfigurement
   4. Grieving about an altered body image or an imposed change in lifestyle

▲ VII. CHEMOTHERAPY

A. Description
   1. Kills or inhibits the reproduction of neoplastic cells; also attacks and kills normal cells
   2. Effects are systemic; affects both healthy cells and cancerous cells
   3. Normal cells most profoundly affected include those of the skin, the hair, the lining of the GI tract, the spermatocytes, and the hematopoietic cells
   4. Cell cycle phase–specific medications affect cells only during a certain phase of the reproductive cycle, and cell cycle phase–nonspecific medications affect cells during any phase of the reproductive cycle
   5. Usually several medications are used in combination (combination therapy) to increase the therapeutic response
   6. Combination chemotherapy is planned to avoid prescribing medications with **nadirs** (the times during which bone marrow activity and white blood cell counts are at their lowest) at or near the same time to minimize immunosuppression
   7. Antineoplastic therapy may be combined with other treatments, such as surgery and radiation
   8. The preferred route of administration is the IV route
   9. Side effects include alopecia, nausea, vomiting, mucositis, skin changes, immunosuppression, anemia, and thrombocytopenia
   10. See Chapter 43 for information about the care of the client who is receiving chemotherapy

VIII. RADIATION THERAPY

A. Description
   1. Radiation therapy destroys **cancer** cells with minimal exposure of normal cells to the damaging effects of radiation; the cells that are damaged die or become unable to divide
   2. Radiation therapy is effective on tissues directly within the path of the radiation beam
   3. Side effects include local skin changes and irritation, alopecia (hair loss), fatigue (most common side effect of radiation), duplicate and altered taste sensation; the effects vary according to the site of treatment
   4. External-beam radiation (also called teletherapy) and brachytherapy are the types of radiation therapy that are most commonly used to treat **cancer**
B. External-beam radiation (the actual radiation source is external to the client)
   1. Instruct the client regarding skin care (Box 42-5)
   2. The client does not emit radiation and does not pose a hazard to anyone else
C. Brachytherapy
   1. The radiation source comes into direct, continuous contact with tumor tissues for a specific time

2. The radiation source is within the client; for a period of time, the client emits radiation and can pose a hazard to others

3. Brachytherapy includes a sealed or unsealed source of radiation

4. Unsealed radiation source
   a. Administration is via the oral or IV route or by instillation into the body cavities
   b. The source is not confined completely to one body area; it enters body fluids and eventually is eliminated via various excreta, which are radioactive and harmful to others; most of the source is eliminated from the body within 48 hours, at which time neither the client nor the excreta are radioactive or harmful

5. Sealed radiation source (Boxes 42-6 and 42-7)
   a. A sealed temporary or permanent radiation source (solid implant) is implanted within the tumor target tissues
   b. The client emits radiation while the implant is in place, but the excreta are not radioactive

6. Removal of sealed radiation sources
   a. The client is no longer radioactive
   b. Inform the client that sexual partners cannot "catch" **cancer**
   c. Inform the female client that she may resume sexual intercourse after 7 to 10 days if the implant was cervical or vaginal
   d. Provide a povidone-iodine douche, if prescribed, if the implant was placed in the cervix
   e. Administer a Fleet enema, as prescribed

f. Advise the client who had a cervical or vaginal implant to notify the physician if nausea, vomiting, diarrhea, frequent urination, vaginal or rectal bleeding, hematuria, foul-smelling vaginal discharge, abdominal pain or distention, or a fever occurs

IX. **BONE MARROW TRANSPLANTATION**
A. Description
   1. Used for the treatment of **leukemia** for clients who have closely matched donors and who are experiencing temporary remission with chemotherapy
   2. The goal of treatment is to rid the client of **malignant** cells through treatment with high doses of chemotherapy
   3. Because these treatments are lethal to the bone marrow, without the replacement of bone marrow function through transplantation, the client would die of infection or hemorrhage

BOX 42-8 **Classification of Leukemia**

Acute Lymphocytic Leukemia
- Mostly lymphoblasts present in the bone marrow
- Age of onset is usually younger than 15 years

Acute Myelogenous Leukemia
- Mostly myeloblasts present in the bone marrow
- Age of onset is usually between 15 and 39 years

Chronic Myelogenous Leukemia
- Mostly granulocytes present in the bone marrow
- Age of onset is usually older than 50 years

Chronic Lymphocytic Leukemia
- Mostly lymphocytes present in the bone marrow
- Age of onset is usually older than 50 years

B. Transplantation: Bone marrow is administered through the client's central line in a manner similar to that of a blood transfusion

C. Post-transplantation period
   1. The client remains without any natural immunity until the donor marrow begins to proliferate and engraftment occurs
   2. Infection and severe thrombocytopenia are major concerns until engraftment occurs

D. Complications: Major complications include failure to engraft and graft-versus-host disease

X. SKIN CANCER (see Chapter 40)

XI. LEUKEMIA (Box 42-8)
   A. Description
      1. **Malignant** exacerbation in the number of leukocytes, usually at an immature stage, in the bone marrow
      2. May be acute, with a sudden onset and short duration, or chronic, with a slow onset and persistent symptoms over a period of years
      3. Affects the bone marrow, thereby causing anemia, leukopenia, the production of immature cells, thrombocytopenia, and a decline in immunity
      4. The cause is unknown but appears to involve gene damage of the cells, thus leading to the transformation of cells from a normal state to a **malignant** state
      5. Risk factors include genetic, viral, immunological, and environmental factors as well as exposure to radiation, chemicals, and medications
   B. Data collection
      1. Anorexia, fatigue, weakness, dyspnea on exertion, and weight loss
      2. Bleeding: Nosebleeds, gum bleeding, rectal bleeding, hematuria, and increased menstrual flow
      3. Petechiae
      4. Prolonged bleeding after minor abrasions or lacerations
      5. Elevated temperature and fever
      6. Lymphadenopathy and splenomegaly
      7. Normal, elevated, or reduced white blood cell (WBC) count
      8. Decreased hemoglobin and hematocrit levels
      9. Decreased platelet count
      10. Positive bone marrow biopsy identifying leukemic blast-phase cells

   C. Infection
      1. A major cause of death in the immunosuppressed client
      2. Can occur through autocontamination or cross-contamination
      3. Common sites of infection are the skin, the respiratory tract, and the GI tract
      4. Initiate protective isolation procedures
      5. Ensure frequent and thorough handwashing
      6. Ensure that anyone entering the client's room is wearing a mask
      7. Use strict aseptic technique for all procedures
      8. Keep supplies for the client separate from supplies for other clients; keep frequently used equipment in the room for the client's use only
      9. Limit the number of caregivers that enter the client's room
      10. Maintain the client in a private room
      11. Place the client in a room with high-efficiency particulate air filtration system or a laminar airflow system, if possible
      12. Reduce exposure to environmental organisms by eliminating raw fruits and vegetables (low-bacteria diet) from the diet and fresh flowers from the client's room and by not leaving standing water in the client's room
      13. Be sure that the client's room is cleaned daily
      14. Assist the client with daily bathing with the use of an antimicrobial soap
      15. Assist the client with performing oral hygiene frequently
      16. Initiate a bowel program to prevent constipation and rectal trauma
      17. Avoid invasive procedures (e.g., injections, rectal temperatures, urinary catheterization)
      18. Change wound dressings daily, and inspect the wounds for redness, swelling, or drainage
      19. Monitor the urine for color and cloudiness
      20. Monitor the skin and oral mucous membranes for signs of infection (Box 42-9)
      21. Encourage the client to cough and deep breathe
      22. Monitor the vital signs
      23. Monitor the white blood cell, neutrophil, and absolute granulocyte counts as well as the differential results
      24. The physician is notified if signs of infection are present; prepare to obtain specimens for the culture of open lesions, urine, and sputum

BOX 42-9　**Mouth Care for the Client With Mucositis**

Inspect the mouth daily.
Offer complete mouth care before and after every meal and at bedtime.
Brush the teeth and tongue with a soft-bristled toothbrush or sponges.
Provide mouth rinses every 12 hours (saline or sodium bicarbonate and water, as prescribed).
Administer topical anesthetic agents to mouth sores, as prescribed.
Avoid the use of alcohol- or glycerin-based mouthwashes or swabs.
Avoid foods that are hard or spicy.

25. Antibiotic, antifungal, and antiviral medication may be prescribed
26. Instruct the client to avoid crowds and those with infections
27. Instruct the client regarding a low-bacteria diet and to avoid drinking water that has been standing for longer than 15 minutes
28. Instruct the client to avoid activities that expose him or her to infection, such as changing a pet's litter box or working with houseplants or in the garden
29. Instruct clients that neither they nor their household contacts should receive immunization with a live virus, including influenza; measles, mumps, rubella; varicella zoster, Bacille-Calmette-Guerin; typhoid; vaccinia (smallpox); and yellow fever vaccines

D. Bleeding
   1. During the period of greatest bone marrow suppression (the **nadir**), the platelet count may be extremely low
   2. The client is at risk for bleeding when the platelet count falls below 50,000/mm^3; spontaneous bleeding frequently occurs when the platelet count is less than 20,000/mm^3
   3. Clients with platelet counts less than 20,000/mm^3 may need a platelet transfusion
   4. For clients with anemia and fatigue, packed red blood cells may be prescribed
   5. Monitor the laboratory values (e.g., partial thromboplastin time, international normalized ratio, fibrinogen, fibrin degradation/split products, and platelet counts, as appropriate)
   6. Examine the client for signs and symptoms of bleeding; examine all body fluids and excrement for the presence of blood
   7. Handle the client gently; use caution when obtaining blood pressure measurements to prevent skin injury
   8. Measure the abdominal girth, which can provide an indication of internal hemorrhage

9. Provide soft foods at moderate temperatures; avoid foods that are at extreme temperatures
10. Avoid injections, if possible, to prevent trauma to the skin and bleeding; apply firm and gentle pressure to a needle-stick site for at least 10 minutes
11. Pad the side rails and sharp corners of the bed and furniture
12. Avoid rectal suppositories, enemas, and thermometers
13. If the female client is menstruating, count the number of pads or tampons used
14. Blood products may be prescribed
15. Instruct the client to use a soft toothbrush and to avoid dental floss
16. Instruct the client to use only an electric razor for shaving
17. Instruct the client to avoid blowing the nose
18. Instruct the client to avoid constrictive or tight clothing or shoes
19. Discourage the client from engaging in activities that involve the use of sharp objects
20. Instruct the client to avoid using nonsteroidal anti-inflammatory drugs and products that contain aspirin

E. Fatigue and nutrition
   1. Assist the client with selecting a well-balanced diet
   2. Provide small, frequent, high-calorie, high-protein, high-carbohydrate meals that require little chewing
   3. Assist the client with self-care and mobility activities
   4. Allow for adequate rest periods during care
   5. Do not perform activities unless they are essential
   6. Administer blood products for anemia, as prescribed

F. Additional interventions
   1. Chemotherapy
   2. Prepare the client for transplantation, as prescribed
   3. Administer colony-stimulating factors, as prescribed
   4. Provide psychosocial support and support services for home care

XII. LYMPHOMA: HODGKIN'S DISEASE
A. Description
   1. A malignancy of the lymph nodes that originates in a single lymph node or a single chain of nodes
   2. **Metastasis** occurs to other, adjacent lymph structures and eventually invades nonlymphoid tissue
   3. Usually involves the lymph nodes, tonsils, spleen, and bone marrow; it is characterized

by the presence of Reed-Sternberg cells in the nodes

4. Possible causes include viral infections and previous exposure to alkylating chemical agents
5. Prognosis is dependent on the stage of the disease (Box 42-10)

B. Data collection
1. Fever
2. Malaise, fatigue, and weakness
3. Night sweats
4. Loss of appetite and significant weight loss
5. Anemia and thrombocytopenia
6. Enlarged lymph nodes, spleen, and liver
7. Positive biopsy of lymph nodes, with cervical nodes most often affected first
8. Presence of Reed-Sternberg cells in nodes
9. Positive computed tomography scan of the liver and spleen

C. Interventions
1. For stages 1 and 2 without mediastinal node involvement, the treatment of choice is extensive external radiation of the involved lymph node regions
2. With more extensive disease, radiation along with multiagent chemotherapy is used
3. Monitor for side effects related to chemotherapy (drug-induced pancytopenia) or radiation
4. Monitor for signs of infection and bleeding
5. Maintain infection and bleeding precautions
6. Discuss the possibility of sterility with the client who is receiving radiation; inform the male client of options related to sperm banks

XIII. MULTIPLE MYELOMA
A. Description
1. A **malignant** proliferation of plasma cells and tumors within the bone
2. An excessive number of abnormal plasma cells invade the bone marrow, develop into tumors, and ultimately destroy the bone; the invasion of the lymph nodes, spleen, and liver occurs

3. The abnormal plasma cells produce an abnormal antibody (**myeloma** protein or the Bence Jones protein) that is found in the blood and urine
4. Causes the decreased production of immunoglobulin and antibodies and increased levels of uric acid and calcium, which can lead to renal failure
5. Multiple **myeloma** cells also produce excess cytokines that increase the **cancer** cell growth rates and destroy bone
6. The cause is unknown

B. Data collection
1. Bone (skeletal) pain, especially in the pelvis, spine, and ribs
2. Weakness and fatigue
3. Recurrent infections
4. Anemia
5. Bence Jones proteinuria and elevated total serum protein level
6. Osteoporosis (bone loss and the development of pathological fractures)
7. Thrombocytopenia and granulocytopenia
8. Elevated calcium and uric acid levels
9. Renal failure
10. Spinal cord compression and paraplegia

C. Interventions
1. Administer chemotherapy, as prescribed; autologous bone marrow transplantation may also be an option
2. Provide supportive care to control symptoms and prevent complications, especially bone fractures, renal failure, and infections
3. Maintain neutropenic and bleeding precautions, as necessary
4. Monitor for signs of bleeding, infection, and skeletal fractures
5. Encourage at least 2L of fluid per day to offset potential problems associated with hypercalcemia, hyperuricemia, and proteinuria
6. Monitor for signs of renal failure
7. Encourage ambulation to prevent renal problems and to slow down bone resorption
8. Provide skeletal support during moving, turning, and ambulating to prevent pathological fractures; provide a hazard-free environment
9. IV fluids and diuretics may be prescribed to increase the renal excretion of calcium
10. Blood transfusions may be prescribed for anemia
11. Administer analgesics, as prescribed, to control pain
12. Administer antibiotics, as prescribed, for infection
13. Prepare the client for local radiation therapy, if prescribed

14. Instruct the client regarding home-care measures and the signs and symptoms of infection

XIV. TESTICULAR CANCER

A. Description
1. Arises from the germinal epithelium of the sperm-producing germ cells or from the nongerminal epithelium of other structures in the testicles (Box 42-11)
2. Incidence is higher among males who have an undescended testis (cryptorchidism)
3. Most often occurs between the ages of 15 and 40 years
4. **Metastasis** to the lung, liver, bone, and adrenal glands occurs

B. Prevention: Routine TSE

C. Data collection
1. Painless testicular swelling
2. Dragging sensation in the scrotum as well as discomfort such as heaviness in the lower abdomen
3. Palpable lymphadenopathy, abdominal masses, and gynecomastia may indicate **metastasis**
4. Late signs include back or bone pain and respiratory symptoms
5. Common **tumor markers** for testicular **cancer** are alpha-fetoprotein (the β subunit of human chorionic gonadotropin)

D. Interventions
1. Chemotherapy will be prescribed
2. Prepare the client for radiation therapy, as prescribed
3. Prepare the client for unilateral orchiectomy, if prescribed, for diagnosis and primary surgical management
4. Prepare the client for radical retroperitoneal lymph node dissection, if prescribed, to stage the disease and reduce the tumor volume so that chemotherapy and radiation therapy are more effective
5. Discuss reproduction, sexuality, and fertility information and options with the client
6. Identify reproductive options such as sperm storage, donor insemination, and adoption

E. Postoperative interventions
1. Monitor for signs of bleeding and wound infection
2. Monitor the intake and output (I&O)

3. The physician is notified if chills, fever, increasing pain or tenderness at the incision site, or drainage of the incision occurs
4. Instruct the client that he may resume normal activities within 1 week, except for lifting objects heavier than 20 pounds and climbing stairs
5. Instruct the client to perform a monthly TSE on the remaining testicle
6. Inform the client that sutures will be removed, usually 7 to 10 days after surgery

XV. CERVICAL CANCER

A. Description
1. Preinvasive **cancer** is limited to the cervix and often asymptomatic (Box 42-12)
2. Invasive **cancer** is in the cervix and other pelvic structures
3. **Metastasis** is usually confined to the pelvis, but distant **metastasis** occurs through lymphatic spread
4. Premalignant changes are described on a continuum from **dysplasia,** which is the earliest premalignancy change, to **carcinoma** in situ, which is the most advanced premalignant change

B. Risk factors
1. Human papillomavirus (HPV) infection (vaccination against HPV-16 and HPV-18 is effective to avoid HPV infection and thus cervical **cancer**).
2. Cigarette smoking, both active and passive
3. Reproductive behavior, including early first intercourse (before age 17), multiple sex partners, or male partners with multiple sex partners
4. Screening via regular gynecologic examinations and Pap tests with the treatment of precancerous abnormalities decreases the incidence and mortality of cervical **cancer**

C. Data collection
1. Painless vaginal bleeding, postmenstrually and postcoitally
2. Watery, blood-tinged vaginal discharge that becomes dark and foul-smelling or serosanguineous vaginal discharge
3. Pelvic, lower back, leg, or groin pain
4. Anorexia and weight loss
5. Leakage of urine and feces from the vagina
6. Dysuria

BOX 42-11 **Types of Testicular Cancer**

Germinal Tumors
- Seminomas
- Nonseminomas

Nongerminal Tumors
- Interstitial cell tumors
- Androblastoma

BOX 42-12 **Preinvasive Cancers: Cervical Intraepithelial Neoplasia**

- CIN I: Mild dysplasia
- CIN II: Moderate dysplasia
- CIN III: Severe dysplasia to cancer in situ

7. Hematuria
8. Cytological changes on Pap test
9. Indication of recurrence or **metastasis** includes unexplained weight loss, dysuria (painful urination), hematuria, rectal bleeding, chest pain, and cough

D. Interventions (Box 42-13)

E. Laser therapy
1. Used when all boundaries of the lesion are visible during colposcopic examination
2. Energy from the beam is absorbed by fluid in the tissues, which causes them to vaporize
3. Minimal bleeding is associated with the procedure
4. Slight vaginal discharge is expected after the procedure; healing occurs in 6 to 12 weeks

F. Cryosurgery
1. Freezing of the tissues by a probe with subsequent necrosis
2. No anesthesia is required, although cramping may occur during the procedure
3. A heavy, watery discharge will occur for several weeks after the procedure
4. Instruct the client to avoid intercourse and the use of tampons while the discharge is present
5. Explain to the client that she should expect a heavy watery discharge for several weeks after the procedure

G. Conization
1. A cone-shaped area of the cervix is removed
2. Performed for women who want to preserve their fertility
3. Long-term follow-up care is needed, because new lesions can develop
4. The risks of the procedure include hemorrhage, uterine perforation, incompetent cervix, cervical stenosis, and preterm labor in future pregnancies

H. Hysterectomy
1. Description
   a. For microinvasive **cancer** if childbearing is not desired
   b. A vaginal approach is most commonly performed
   c. A radical hysterectomy and bilateral lymph node dissection may be performed for **cancer** that has spread beyond the cervix but not to the pelvic wall
2. Postoperative interventions
   a. Monitor the vital signs
   b. Assist with coughing and deep-breathing exercises and the use of an incentive spirometer
   c. Assist with range-of-motion (ROM) exercises and provide early ambulation
   d. Apply antiembolism stockings, as prescribed
   e. Monitor the I&O, Foley catheter drainage, and hydration status
   f. Monitor the bowel sounds
   g. Monitor vaginal bleeding; more than one saturated pad per hour may indicate excessive bleeding
   h. Monitor the incision site for signs of infection
   i. Administer pain medication, as prescribed
   j. Instruct the client to avoid tub baths, sitting for long periods, and stair climbing for 1 month
   k. Avoid strenuous activity or lifting anything that weighs more than 10 to 20 pounds
   l. Instruct the client to consume foods that aid in healing
   m. Instruct the client to avoid sexual intercourse for 3 to 6 weeks, as prescribed
   n. Instruct the client regarding the signs that are associated with complications

I. Pelvic exenteration (Box 42-14)
1. Description
   a. A radical surgical procedure that involves removal of all pelvic contents and is performed for recurrent **cancer** if there is no evidence of tumor outside of the pelvis and no lymph node involvement
   b. When the bladder is removed, an ileal conduit will be created and located on the right side of the abdomen to divert urine
   c. A colostomy may need to be created and will be located of the left side of the abdomen for the passage of feces

BOX 42-13 Treatment for Cervical Cancer

Nonsurgical
- Chemotherapy
- Cryosurgery
- External radiation
- Internal radiation implants (intracavitary)
- Laser therapy

Surgical
- Conization
- Hysterectomy
- Pelvic exenteration

BOX 42-14 Types of Pelvic Exenteration

Anterior
Removal of the uterus, ovaries, fallopian tubes, vagina, bladder, urethra, and pelvic lymph nodes

Posterior
Removal of the uterus, ovaries, fallopian tubes, descending colon, rectum, and anal canal

Total
Combination of anterior and posterior

2. Postoperative interventions
   a. Nursing care measures are similar to postoperative care after hysterectomy
   b. Monitor the incision site for infection
   c. Administer perineal irrigations with half-normal saline and hydrogen peroxide, as prescribed
   d. Provide sitz baths, as prescribed
   e. Instruct the client that the perineal opening, if present, may drain for several months
   f. Instruct the client regarding the care of the ileal conduit and colostomy, if created
   g. Provide sexual counseling; vaginal intercourse is not possible after anterior and total pelvic exenteration

XVI. OVARIAN CANCER

A. Description
   1. Grows rapidly, spreads fast, and is often bilateral
   2. **Metastasis** occurs by direct spread to the organs in the pelvis, by distal spread through the lymphatic drainage, or by peritoneal seeding
   3. Prognosis is usually poor, because the tumor is usually detected late
   4. An exploratory laparotomy is performed to diagnose and stage the tumor

B. Data collection
   1. Abdominal discomfort or swelling
   2. GI disturbances with dyspepsia, indigestion, flatus, and distention
   3. Dysfunctional vaginal bleeding
   4. Abdominal mass
   5. **Tumor marker** CA-125 may be elevated if ovarian **cancer** is present

C. Interventions
   1. External radiation is used if the tumor has invaded other organs
   2. Chemotherapy is used postoperatively for all stages of ovarian **cancer**
   3. Intraperitoneal chemotherapy, which involves the instillation of chemotherapy into the abdominal cavity, may be prescribed
   4. Immunotherapy, which alters the immunological response of the ovary and promotes tumor resistance, may be prescribed
   5. Total abdominal hysterectomy and bilateral salpingo-oophorectomy may be necessary

XVII. ENDOMETRIAL CANCER

A. Description
   1. A slow-growing tumor that is associated with the menopausal years
   2. **Metastasis** occurs through the lymphatic system to the ovaries and pelvis and via the blood to the lungs, liver, and bone, or intra-abdominally to the peritoneal cavity

B. Risk factors
   1. Use of estrogen replacement therapy
   2. Nulliparity
   3. Polycystic ovary disease
   4. Increased age
   5. Late menopause
   6. Family history of uterine **cancer** or hereditary nonpolyposis colorectal **cancer**
   7. Obesity
   8. Hypertension
   9. Diabetes mellitus

C. Data collection
   1. Postmenopausal bleeding
   2. Watery, serosanguineous discharge
   3. Low back, pelvic, or abdominal pain
   4. Enlarged uterus in advanced stages
   5. **Tumor marker** CA-125 is used to rule out the ovarian involvement

D. Nonsurgical interventions
   1. External radiation or internal radiation (intracavitary radiation) used alone or in combination with surgery, depending on the stage of **cancer**
   2. Chemotherapy to treat advanced or recurrent disease
   3. Progestational therapy with medication such as medroxyprogesterone (Depo-Provera) or megestrol acetate (Megace) for estrogen-dependent tumors
   4. Tamoxifen (Nolvadex), an antiestrogen, may also be prescribed

E. Surgical interventions: Total abdominal hysterectomy and bilateral salpingo-oophorectomy

XVIII. BREAST CANCER

A. Description
   1. Classified as invasive when it penetrates the tissue that surrounds the mammary duct and grows in an irregular pattern
   2. **Metastasis** occurs via lymph nodes
   3. Common sites of **metastasis** are the bones, and lungs
   4. Diagnosis is made by breast biopsy through a needle aspiration or by the surgical removal of the tumor with a microscopic examination for **malignant** cells

B. Risk factors
   1. Age
   2. Family history of breast **cancer**
   3. Early menarche and late menopause
   4. Previous **cancer** of the breast, uterus, or ovaries
   5. Nulliparity or late first birth
   6. Obesity
   7. High-dose radiation exposure of the chest

C. Data collection
   1. Mass felt during BSE
   2. Mass usually felt in the upper outer quadrant or beneath the nipple
   3. A fixed, irregular, nonencapsulated mass
   4. A painless mass, except during the very late stages
   5. Nipple retraction or elevation

6. Asymmetry, with the affected breast being higher
7. Bloody or clear nipple discharge
8. Skin dimpling, retraction, or ulceration
9. Skin edema or peau d'orange skin, which may indicate lymphatic involvement (blocked skin drainage causes skin edema and an "orange peel" appearance)
10. Axillary lymphadenopathy
11. Lymphedema of the affected arm
12. Symptoms of bone or lung **metastasis**
13. Presence of the lesion on mammography

D. Prevention: Monthly BSE
E. Nonsurgical interventions
   1. Chemotherapy
   2. Radiation therapy
   3. Hormonal manipulation via the use of medication in postmenopausal women or other medications (e.g., tamoxifen [Nolvadex]) for estrogen receptor–positive tumors
F. Surgical interventions: Surgical breast procedures with possible breast reconstruction (Box 42-15)
G. Postoperative interventions
   1. Monitor the vital signs
   2. Position the client in a semi-Fowler's position; turn her from the back to the unaffected side, with the affected arm elevated above the level of the heart to promote drainage and prevent lymphedema
   3. Encourage coughing and deep breathing
   4. If a drain (usually a Jackson-Pratt) is in place, maintain suction, and record the amount of drainage and the drainage characteristics
   5. Monitor the operative site for infection, swelling, or the presence of fluid collection under the skin flaps
   6. Monitor the incision site for constriction from the dressings, impaired sensation, or color changes of the skin
   7. If breast reconstruction was performed, the client will return from surgery with a surgical brassiere and the temporary prosthesis in place
   8. Place a sign above the bed that states the following: "No IVs, no injections, no blood pressure readings, and no venipunctures in the affected arm"; the affected arm is protected for life, and any intervention that could traumatize the affected arm should be avoided
   9. Provide the use of a pressure sleeve, as prescribed, if edema is severe
   10. Administer diuretics and provide a low-salt diet, as prescribed, for severe lymphedema
   11. Consult with the physician and the physical therapist regarding the appropriate exercise program
   12. Assist with exercise, as prescribed, to decrease lymphedema and muscle weakness
   13. Instruct the client regarding home-care measures (Box 42-16)

XIX. GASTRIC CANCER
A. Description
   1. A **malignant** growth in the stomach
   2. Risk factors include *Helicobacter pylori* infection; a diet of smoked, highly salted, processed, or spiced foods; smoking; alcohol and nitrate ingestion; and a history of gastric ulcers.
   3. Complications include hemorrhage, obstruction, **metastasis,** and dumping syndrome
   4. The goals of treatment are to remove the tumor and to provide a nutritional program
B. Data collection
   1. Fatigue
   2. Anorexia and weight loss
   3. Nausea and vomiting

BOX 42-16 Client Instructions After Mastectomy

Avoid overuse of the arm during the first few months.
To prevent lymphedema, keep the affected arm elevated.
Provide incision care with lanolin to soften and prevent wound contracture.
Encourage the use of Reach for Recovery volunteers.
Encourage the client to perform a monthly breast self-examination on the remaining breast.
Protect the affected hand and arm.
Avoid exposure of the affected arm to strong sunlight.
Do not let the affected arm hang dependent.
Do not carry a handbag or anything heavy over the affected arm.
Avoid trauma, cuts, bruises, or burns to the affected side.
Avoid wearing constricting clothing or jewelry on the affected side.
Wear gloves when gardening.
Use thick oven mitts when cooking.
Use a thimble when sewing.
Apply lanolin hand cream several times daily.
Use cream cuticle remover.
Call the physician if signs of inflammation occur in the affected arm.
Wear a Medic-Alert bracelet that identifies the arm with lymphedema.

BOX 42-15 Surgical Breast Procedures

Lumpectomy
The tumor is excised and removed.
Lymph node dissection may also be performed.
Simple Mastectomy
Breast tissue and the nipple are removed.
The lymph nodes are left intact.
Modified Radical Mastectomy
Breast tissue, the nipple, and the lymph nodes are removed.
The muscles are left intact.

4. Indigestion and epigastric discomfort
5. A sensation of pressure in the stomach
6. Dysphagia
7. Anemia
8. Ascites
9. Palpable mass

C. Interventions
1. Monitor the vital signs
2. Monitor the hemoglobin and hematocrit levels; blood transfusions may be prescribed
3. Monitor the weight daily
4. Monitor the nutritional status; encourage small, bland, easily digestible meals with vitamin and mineral supplements
5. Administer pain medication, as prescribed
6. Prepare the client for chemotherapy or radiation therapy, as prescribed
7. Prepare the client for surgical resection of the tumor, as prescribed (Box 42-17)

D. Postoperative interventions (see Chapter 46 for information regarding postoperative care)

XX. PANCREATIC CANCER

A. Description
1. Most pancreatic tumors are highly **malignant**, rapidly growing **adenocarcinomas** that originate from the epithelium of the ductal system
2. Pancreatic **cancer** is associated with increased age, a history of diabetes mellitus, alcohol use, a history of previous pancreatitis, smoking, the ingestion of a high-fat diet, and exposure to environmental chemicals
3. Symptoms usually do not occur until the tumor is large; therefore, the prognosis is poor

B. Data collection
1. Nausea and vomiting
2. Jaundice
3. Unexplained weight loss
4. Clay-colored stools
5. Glucose intolerance

6. Abdominal pain
7. Endoscopic retrograde cholangiopancreatography for visualization of the pancreatic duct and biliary system and for the collection of tissue and secretions

C. Interventions
1. Radiation
2. Chemotherapy
3. Whipple procedure, which involves a pancreaticoduodenectomy with the removal of the distal third of the stomach, a pancreaticojejunostomy, a gastrojejunostomy, and a choledochojejunostomy (Figure 42-3)
4. Postoperative care measures are similar to those for the care of a client with pancreatitis and for a client after gastric surgery; monitor the blood glucose levels for transient hyperglycemia or hypoglycemia that results from the surgical manipulation of the pancreas

XXI. INTESTINAL TUMORS

A. Description
1. **Malignant** lesions that develop in the cells lining the bowel wall or that develop as polyps in the colon or rectum
2. Complications include bowel perforation with peritonitis, abscess and/or fistula formation, hemorrhage, and complete intestinal obstruction
3. **Metastasis** occurs via the circulatory or lymphatic system or by direct extension to other areas in the colon or other organs

B. Data collection
1. Blood in the stool
2. Anorexia, vomiting, and weight loss
3. Malaise
4. Anemia

BOX 42-17	**Surgical Interventions for Gastric Cancer**

Subtotal Gastrectomy
Billroth I
- Also called gastroduodenostomy
- Partial gastrectomy; the remaining segment is anastomosed to the duodenum

Billroth II
- Also called gastrojejunostomy
- Partial gastrectomy; the remaining segment is anastomosed to the jejunum

Total Gastrectomy
- Also called esophagojejunostomy
- Removal of the stomach, with the attachment of the esophagus to the jejunum or the duodenum

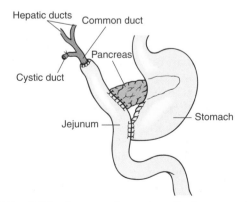

FIG. 42-3 Whipple procedure or radical pancreaticoduodenectomy. (From Lewis, S., Heitkemper, M., Dirksen, S., & Bucher, L. [2007]. *Medical-surgical nursing: Assessment and management of clinical problems* [7th ed.]. St. Louis: Mosby.)

5. Abnormal stools
   a. Ascending colon tumor: Diarrhea
   b. Descending colon tumor: Constipation, some diarrhea, or flat, ribbon-like stool as a result of a partial obstruction
   c. Rectal tumor: Alternating constipation and diarrhea
6. Guarding or abdominal distention
7. Abdominal mass (late sign)
8. Cachexia (late sign)

C. Interventions
   1. Monitor for signs of complications, which include bowel perforation with peritonitis, abscess and/or fistula formation, hemorrhage, and complete intestinal obstruction
   2. Monitor for signs of intestinal perforation, which include low blood pressure, rapid and weak pulse, distended abdomen, and elevated temperature
   3. Monitor for signs of intestinal obstruction, which include vomiting (may be fecal contents), pain, constipation, and abdominal distention
   4. Note that an early sign of intestinal obstruction is increased peristaltic activity, which produces an increase in bowel sounds; as the obstruction progresses, hypoactive sounds are heard
   5. Prepare for radiation preoperatively to facilitate surgical resection and postoperatively to decrease the risk of recurrence or to reduce pain, hemorrhage, bowel obstruction, or **metastasis**
   6. Chemotherapy is used postoperatively to assist with the control of symptoms and the spread of the disease

D. Surgical interventions: Bowel resection and the creation of a colostomy or an ileostomy

E. Colostomy or ileostomy
   1. Preoperative interventions
      a. Consult with the enterostomal therapist to assist with identifying the optimal placement of ostomy
      b. Instruct the client to eat a low-residue diet for a day or two before surgery, as prescribed
      c. Administer intestinal antiseptics and antibiotics, as prescribed, to decrease the bacterial content of the colon and to reduce the risk of infection from the surgical procedure
      d. Administer laxatives and enemas, as prescribed
   2. Postoperative: Colostomy
      a. Place a petroleum jelly gauze over the stoma to keep it moist, and keep it covered by a dry sterile dressing if a pouch system is not in place
      b. Place a pouch system on the stoma as soon as possible

   c. Monitor the stoma for size, unusual bleeding, and necrotic tissue
   d. Monitor for color changes in the stoma
   e. Note that the normal stoma color is red or pink, which indicates high vascularity
   f. Note that a pale pink stoma indicates low hemoglobin and hematocrit levels and that a purple-black stoma indicates compromised circulation that requires physician notification
   g. Monitor the pouch system for proper fit and signs of leakage
   h. Assess the functioning of the colostomy
   i. Expect that stool will be liquid postoperatively but that it will become more solid, depending on the area of the colostomy
   j. Ascending colon colostomy: Expect liquid stool
   k. Transverse colon colostomy: Expect loose to semiformed stool
   l. Descending colon colostomy: Expect close-to-normal stool
   m. Fecal matter should not be allowed to remain on the skin
   n. Empty the pouch when it is one-third full
   o. Administer analgesics and antibiotics, as prescribed
   p. Irrigate the perineal wound, if present and if prescribed, and monitor for signs of infection
   q. Instruct the client to avoid foods that cause excessive gas formation and odor
   r. Instruct the client regarding stoma care and irrigations, as prescribed (Box 42-18)
   s. Instruct the client that normal activities may be resumed when approved by the physician

---

BOX 42-18   Colostomy Irrigation

Purpose
An enema is given through the stoma to stimulate bowel emptying.

Description
Lukewarm tap water (500 to 1000 mL) is infused through the stoma; the water and stool are allowed to drain into a collection bag.

Procedure
If the client is ambulatory, position him or her sitting on a toilet.
If the client is on bedrest, position him or her on his or her side.
Hang the irrigation bag so that the bottom of the bag is at the level of the client's shoulder or slightly higher.
Insert the irrigation tube carefully, without force.
Begin the flow of irrigation.
Clamp the tubing if cramping occurs; release the tubing as cramping subsides.
Perform irrigation around the same time each day.
It is preferable to perform irrigation 1 hour after a meal.

3. Postoperative: Ileostomy
   a. A healthy stoma is red; a color change to dark blue or black should be reported to the physician
   b. Postoperative drainage will be dark green and progress to yellow as the client begins to eat
   c. Stool is liquid
   d. The risk for dehydration and electrolyte imbalance exists
   e. Do not give suppositories through the ileostomy

XXII. LUNG CANCER
A. Description
   1. A **malignant** tumor of the lung that may be primary or metastatic
   2. The lungs are a common target for **metastasis** from other organs
   3. Bronchogenic **carcinoma** spreads through direct extension and lymphatic dissemination
   4. The four major types of lung **cancer** are small cell (oat cell), epidermal (squamous cell), **adenocarcinoma**, and large cell anaplastic **carcinoma**
   5. Diagnosis is made by a chest x-ray, which will show a lesion or mass, and bronchoscopy and sputum studies, which will demonstrate a positive cytology for **cancer** cells

B. Causes
   1. Cigarette smoking
   2. Exposure to environmental pollutants
   3. Exposure to occupational pollutants

C. Data collection
   1. Cough
   2. Dyspnea
   3. Hoarseness
   4. Hemoptysis
   5. Chest pain
   6. Anorexia and weight loss
   7. Weakness

D. Interventions
   1. Monitor the vital signs
   2. Monitor the breathing patterns and breath sounds and for signs of respiratory impairment
   3. Monitor for tracheal deviation
   4. Administer analgesics, as prescribed, for pain management
   5. Place the client in Fowler's position for ease of breathing
   6. Administer oxygen, as prescribed, and humidification to moisten and loosen secretions
   7. Monitor the pulse oximetry
   8. Provide respiratory treatments, as prescribed
   9. Administer bronchodilators and corticosteroids, as prescribed, to decrease bronchospasm, inflammation, and edema

10. Provide a high-calorie, high-protein, high-vitamin diet
11. Provide activity (as tolerated), rest periods, and active and passive range-of-motion (ROM) exercises
12. Monitor for bleeding, infection, and electrolyte imbalances

E. Nonsurgical interventions
   1. Radiation therapy for localized intrathoracic lung **cancers** and for the palliation of hemoptysis, obstructions, dysphagia, and pain
   2. Chemotherapy may be prescribed for the treatment of nonresectable tumors or as adjuvant therapy

F. Surgical interventions
   1. Laser therapy: To relieve endobronchial obstruction
   2. Thoracentesis and pleurodesis: To remove pleural fluid and relieve hypoxia
   3. Thoracotomy (opening into the thoracic cavity) with pneumonectomy: Surgical removal of a lung
   4. Thoracotomy with lobectomy: Surgical removal of one lobe of the lung for tumors that are confined to a single lobe
   5. Thoracotomy with segmental resection: Surgical removal of a lobe segment

G. Preoperative interventions
   1. Explain the potential postoperative need for chest tubes
   2. Note that closed-chest drainage is not usually used for a pneumonectomy and that the serum fluid that accumulates in the empty thoracic cavity eventually consolidates, thus preventing shifts of the mediastinum, heart, and remaining lung

H. Postoperative interventions
   1. Monitor the vital signs
   2. Monitor the cardiac and respiratory statuses; monitor for the absence or presence of lung sounds
   3. Monitor the chest tube drainage system, which will drain air and/or blood that accumulates in the pleural space
   4. Monitor the chest tube insertion site for crepitus (subcutaneous air) and drainage
   5. Administer oxygen, as prescribed
   6. Check the physician's orders regarding client positioning; complete lateral turning must be avoided
   7. Monitor the pulse oximetry
   8. Provide activity, as tolerated
   9. Encourage active ROM exercises of the operative shoulder, as prescribed
   10. See Chapter 19 for the care of the client with a chest tube

XXIII. LARYNGEAL CANCER

A. Description
   1. A **malignant** tumor of the larynx
   2. Laryngeal **cancer** presents as **malignant** ulcerations with underlying infiltration
   3. **Metastasis** to the lung is common
   4. Diagnosis is made by laryngoscopy and biopsy showing a positive cytology for **cancer** cells

B. Risk factors
   1. Cigarette smoking
   2. Exposure to environmental pollutants
   3. Exposure to radiation
   4. Voice strain

C. Data collection
   1. Persistent hoarseness and sore throat
   2. Painless neck mass
   3. The feeling of a lump in the throat
   4. Burning sensation in the throat
   5. Dysphagia
   6. Change in voice quality
   7. Dyspnea
   8. Weakness and weight loss
   9. Hemoptysis
   10. Foul breath odor

D. Interventions
   1. Place the client in Fowler's position to promote optimal air exchange
   2. Monitor the respiratory status
   3. Monitor for signs of food and fluid aspiration
   4. Administer oxygen, as prescribed
   5. Provide respiratory treatments, as prescribed
   6. Provide activity, as tolerated
   7. Provide a high-calorie, high-protein, high-vitamin diet
   8. Prepare to provide nutritional support via parenteral nutrition or nasogastric, gastrostomy, or jejunostomy tube, as prescribed
   9. Administer analgesics for pain, as prescribed

E. Nonsurgical interventions
   1. Radiation therapy if the **cancer** is limited to a small area in one vocal cord
   2. Chemotherapy, which may be performed in combination with radiation and surgery

F. Surgical interventions
   1. Depend on the tumor size and the amount of tissue to be resected
   2. Types of resection include cordal stripping, cordectomy, partial laryngectomy, and total laryngectomy
   3. A tracheostomy is performed with a total laryngectomy; this airway opening is always permanent and is referred to as a laryngectomy stoma

G. Preoperative interventions
   1. Establish communication methods for the client
   2. Encourage the client to express feelings about changes in body image and the loss of the voice
   3. Describe the rehabilitation program and provide information about the tracheostomy and suctioning

H. Postoperative interventions
   1. Monitor the vital signs
   2. Monitor the respiratory status and airway patency, and provide frequent suctioning to remove bloody secretions
   3. Place the client in high Fowler's position
   4. Maintain mechanical ventilator support or a tracheostomy collar with humidification, as prescribed
   5. Monitor the pulse oximetry
   6. Maintain surgical drains in the neck area, if present
   7. Observe for hemorrhage and edema in the neck
   8. Monitor IV fluids or parenteral nutrition, if prescribed, until nutrition is administered via nasogastric, gastrostomy, or jejunostomy tube
   9. Provide oral hygiene
   10. Monitor the gag and cough reflexes and the ability to swallow
   11. Increase activity, as tolerated
   12. Monitor the color, amount, and consistency of the sputum
   13. Provide stoma and laryngectomy care (Box 42-19)
   14. Provide consultation with a speech and language pathologist, as prescribed
   15. Reinforce the method of communication that is established preoperatively
   16. Prepare the client for rehabilitation and speech therapy (Box 42-20)

BOX 42-19 **Stoma Care After Laryngectomy**

Teach the client clean suctioning technique.
Instruct the client regarding cleaning the incision and providing stoma care.
Protect the neck from injury.
Instruct the client to wear a stoma guard to shield the stoma.
Avoid swimming, showering, and using aerosol sprays.
Demonstrate ways to prevent debris from entering the stoma.
Advise the client to wear loose-fitting, high-collar clothing to hide the stoma.
Advise the client to increase the humidity in the home.
Instruct the client in range-of-motion exercises for the arms, shoulders, and neck, as prescribed.
Avoid exposure to people with infections.
Alternate rest periods with activity.
Increase the fluid intake to 3000 mL/day, as prescribed.
Advise the client to obtain a Medic-Alert bracelet.

| BOX 42-20 | **Speech Rehabilitation After Laryngectomy** |

Esophageal Speech
- Client produces esophageal speech by "burping" the air that is swallowed
- Voice produced is monotone; it cannot be raised or lowered, and it carries no pitch
- Client must have adequate hearing, because he or she uses the mouth to shape words as they are heard

Mechanical Devices
- Known as electrolarynges
- Placed against the side of the neck; air inside the neck and pharynx is vibrated, and the client articulates
- Cooper-Rand device: Consists of a plastic tube that is placed inside the client's mouth and that vibrates on articulation

Tracheoesophageal Fistula
- Surgical creation of a fistula between the trachea and the esophagus, with the eventual placement of a prosthesis that is used to produce speech
- Prosthesis provides the client with a means to divert the air from the lungs through the trachea, into the esophagus, and out of the mouth
- Speech is produced by lip and tongue movement

XXIV. CANCER OF THE PROSTATE
A. Description
1. A slow-growing **cancer** of the prostate gland, which is usually an androgen-dependent type of **adenocarcinoma**
2. The risk increases in men with each decade, usually after the age of 50 years
3. Prostate **cancer** can spread via the direct invasion of surrounding tissues or by **metastasis** through the bloodstream and lymphatics to the bony pelvis and spine
4. Bone **metastasis** is a concern
B. Data collection
1. Asymptomatic during the early stages
2. Hard, pea-sized nodule palpated on rectal examination
3. Hematuria (painless)
4. Late symptoms include weight loss, urinary obstruction, and pain radiating from the lumbosacral area down the leg
5. Prostate-specific antigen level is elevated in various noncancerous conditions and therefore should not be used as a screening test without a digital rectal exam; it is routinely used to monitor response to therapy
6. Diagnosis is made through biopsy of the prostate
C. Nonsurgical interventions
1. Prepare the client for hormone manipulation therapy, as prescribed

2. Administer luteinizing hormone (e.g., leuprolide acetate [Lupron]), flutamide (Eulexin), or estrogens (e.g., diethylstilbestrol), as prescribed, to slow the rate of growth of the tumor
3. Pain medication, radiation therapy, corticosteroids, and bisphosphonates may be prescribed for palliation in clients with advanced prostate **cancer**
4. Prepare the client for external-beam radiation or brachytherapy , which may be prescribed alone or along with surgery and which may be prescribed preoperatively or postoperatively to reduce the lesion and limit **metastasis**
5. Prepare the client for the administration of chemotherapy in cases of hormone-resistant tumors
D. Surgical interventions
1. Prepare the client for orchiectomy (palliative), if prescribed, which will limit the production of testosterone
2. Prepare the client for prostatectomy, if prescribed
3. The radical prostatectomy can be performed via a retropubic, perineal, or suprapubic approach
4. Cryosurgical ablation is a minimally invasive procedure that may be an alternative to radical prostatectomy; liquid nitrogen freezes the gland, and the dead cells are absorbed by the body
E. Transurethral resection of the prostate (TURP)
1. Insertion of a scope into the urethra to excise prostatic tissue
2. Bleeding is common after TURP, and monitoring for hemorrhage is an important nursing intervention
3. Continuous bladder irrigation (CBI) will be prescribed postoperatively to maintain the urine at a pink color (Box 42-21)
4. Bladder spasms are common after surgery, and antispasmodics may be prescribed
5. Dribbling or incontinence may occur postoperatively, and it is important for the nurse to instruct the client to monitor for these occurrences
6. Sterility may or may not occur after the surgical procedure
F. Suprapubic prostatectomy
1. The removal of the prostate by an abdominal incision with a bladder incision
2. The client will have an abdominal dressing that may drain copious amounts of urine; this dressing will need to be frequently changed
3. Severe hemorrhage is possible, and monitoring for blood loss is an important nursing intervention

BOX 42-21 Postoperative Care After Transurethral Resection of the Prostate

Continuous Bladder Irrigation
Three-way (lumen) irrigation to decrease bleeding and to keep the bladder free from clots:
- One lumen for inflating the balloon (30 mL)
- One lumen for instillation (inflow)
- One lumen for outflow

Interventions
Maintain traction on the catheter, if applied to prevent bleeding, by pulling the catheter taut and taping it to the abdomen or thigh.

Instruct the client to keep the leg straight if traction is applied to the catheter and it is taped to the thigh.

Catheter traction is not released without a physician's order; it is usually released after any bright-red drainage has diminished.

Use only normal saline or a prescribed solution to prevent water intoxication.

Run the solution at the prescribed rate to keep the urine pink.

Run the solution rapidly if bright-red drainage or clots are present.

Run the solution at about 40 gtt/minute when the bright-red drainage clears.

If the urinary catheter becomes obstructed, turn off the continuous bladder irrigation and irrigate the catheter with 30 to 50 mL of normal saline, if prescribed; notify the physician if the obstruction does not resolve.

Monitor for transurethral resection syndrome or severe hyponatremia (water intoxication) caused by the excessive absorption of bladder irrigation (i.e., altered mental status, bradycardia, increased blood pressure, and confusion).

Discontinue continuous bladder irrigation and Foley catheterization as prescribed, usually 24 to 48 hours after surgery.

Monitor for continence and urinary retention when the catheter is removed.

Inform the client that some burning, frequency, and dribbling may occur after catheter removal.

Inform the client that he should be voiding 150 to 200 mL of clear yellow urine every 3 to 4 hours by 3 days after surgery.

Inform the client that he may pass small clots and tissue debris for several days.

Teach the client to avoid heavy lifting, stressful exercise, driving, Valsalva's maneuver, and sexual intercourse for 2 to 6 weeks to prevent strain.

Instruct the client to call the physician if bleeding occurs or if there is a decrease in the urinary stream.

Instruct the client to drink 2400 to 3000 mL of fluid each day, preferably before 8:00 PM.

Instruct the client to avoid alcohol, caffeinated beverages, and spicy foods to prevent the overstimulation of the bladder.

Instruct the client that, if the urine becomes bloody, he should rest and increase the fluid intake; if the bleeding does not subside, he should notify the physician.

---

4. Bladder spasms are common, and antispasmodics may be prescribed
5. CBI will be prescribed and administered to keep the urine pink
6. A longer healing process is involved as compared with TURP
7. Sterility occurs with this procedure

G. Retropubic prostatectomy
1. Removal of the prostate gland by a low abdominal incision without opening the bladder
2. Less bleeding occurs with this procedure as compared with suprapubic prostatectomy, and the client experiences fewer bladder spasms
3. There is minimal abdominal drainage
4. CBI may be used
5. Sterility occurs with this procedure

H. Perineal prostatectomy
1. The prostate gland is removed through an incision made between the scrotum and the anus
2. Minimal bleeding occurs with this procedure
3. The client needs to be monitored closely for infection, because the risk of infection is increased with this type of prostatectomy
4. Urinary incontinence is common
5. The procedure causes sterility

6. Teach the client how to perform perineal exercises
7. Avoid inserting rectal tubes, taking the temperature rectally, or administering enemas

I. Postoperative interventions
1. Monitor the vital signs
2. Monitor the urinary output
3. Monitor the urine for hemorrhage and clots
4. Increase fluids to 2400 to 3000 mL/day, unless contraindicated
5. Monitor for arterial bleeding as evidenced by bright red urine with numerous clots; if it occurs, increase the CBI and notify the physician immediately
6. Monitor for venous bleeding as evidenced by burgundy-colored urine output; if it occurs, notify the physician, who may apply traction on the catheter
7. Monitor the hemoglobin and hematocrit levels daily or per the physician's orders
8. Expect red to light-pink urine for 24 hours; it should turn amber in 3 days
9. Ambulate the client as early as possible and as soon as the client's urine begins to clear in color

10. Inform the client that the continuous feeling of an urge to void is normal
11. Instruct the client to avoid attempts to void around the catheter, because this will cause bladder spasms
12. Administer antibiotics, analgesics, stool softeners, and antispasmodics, as prescribed
13. Monitor the three-way Foley catheter, which will have a 30- to 45-mL retention balloon
14. Maintain CBI with a sterile bladder irrigation solution, as prescribed, to keep the catheter free of obstruction and to maintain the urine at a pink color

J. Postoperative: Suprapubic prostatectomy
1. Monitor the suprapubic and Foley catheter drainage
2. Monitor the CBI, if prescribed
3. Note that the Foley catheter will be removed 2 to 4 days postoperatively if the client has a suprapubic catheter
4. If prescribed, clamp the suprapubic catheter after the Foley catheter is removed, and instruct client to attempt to void; after the client has voided, check the amount of residual urine in the bladder by unclamping the suprapubic catheter and measuring the output
5. Prepare for the removal of the suprapubic catheter when the client consistently empties the bladder and the residual urine is 75 mL or less
6. Monitor the suprapubic incision dressing, which may become saturated with urine, until the incision heals

K. Postoperative: Retropubic prostatectomy
1. Note that because the bladder is not entered, there is no urinary drainage on the abdominal dressing
2. Check for urinary or purulent drainage on the dressing; if this occurs, notify the physician
3. Monitor for fever and increased pain, which may indicate infection

L. Postoperative: Perineal prostatectomy
1. Note that the client will have an incision, which may or may not have a drain
2. Avoid rectal thermometers, rectal tubes, and enemas, because they may cause trauma and bleeding

XXV. BLADDER CANCER
A. Description
1. Papillomatous growths in the bladder urothelium that undergo **malignant** changes and that may infiltrate the bladder wall
2. Predisposing factors include cigarette smoking, exposure to industrial chemicals, and exposure to radiation
3. Common sites of **metastasis** include the liver, bones, and lungs
4. As the tumor progresses, it can extend into the rectum, vagina, other pelvic soft tissues, and retroperitoneal structures

B. Data collection
1. Gross, painless hematuria
2. Frequency, urgency, and dysuria
3. Clot-induced obstruction
4. Bladder biopsy confirms the diagnosis

C. Radiation
1. Most bladder **cancers** are poorly radiosensitive and require high doses of radiation
2. Radiation therapy is more acceptable for advanced disease that cannot be eradicated by surgery
3. Palliative radiation may be used to relieve pain and bowel obstruction and to control potential hemorrhage and leg edema secondary to venous or lymphatic obstruction
4. Intracavitary radiation may be prescribed, which protects adjacent tissue
5. External radiation combined with chemotherapy or surgery may be prescribed, because the external radiation alone may not be effective
6. Complications of radiation
   a. Abacterial cystitis
   b. Proctitis
   c. Fistula formation
   d. Ileitis or colitis
   e. Bladder ulceration and hemorrhage

D. Chemotherapy
1. Intravesical instillation
   a. An alkylating chemotherapeutic agent is instilled into the bladder
   b. This method provides a concentrated topical treatment with little systemic absorption
   c. The medication is injected into a urethral catheter and retained for 2 hours
   d. After instillation, the client's position is rotated every 15 to 30 minutes, starting in the supine position, to avoid lying on a full bladder
   e. After 2 hours, the client voids in a sitting position and is instructed to increase fluids to flush the bladder
   f. Treat the urine as a biohazard, and send it to the radioisotope laboratory for monitoring
   g. For 6 hours after intravesical chemotherapy, disinfect the toilet with household bleach after the client has voided
2. Systemic chemotherapy: Used to treat inoperable or late tumors
3. Complications of chemotherapy
   a. Bladder irritation
   b. Hemorrhagic cystitis

E. Surgical interventions
1. Transurethral resection of the bladder tumor

a. Local resection and fulguration (destruction of tissue by electrical current through electrodes placed in direct contact with the tissue)

b. Performed for very early tumors for cure or for inoperable tumors for palliation

2. Partial cystectomy
   a. The removal of up to half of the bladder
   b. Performed for early tumors and for clients who cannot tolerate a radical cystectomy
   c. During the initial postoperative period, the bladder capacity is markedly reduced to about 60 mL; however, as the bladder tissue expands, the capacity increases to 200 to 400 mL
   d. Maintenance of a continuous output of urine after surgery is critical to prevent bladder distention and stress on the suture line
   e. A urethral catheter and a suprapubic catheter may be in place, and the suprapubic catheter may be left in place for 2 weeks until healing occurs

3. Cystectomy and urinary diversion (Figure 42-4)
   a. Various surgical procedures performed to create alternate pathways for urine collection and excretion
   b. Urinary diversion may be performed with or without cystectomy (bladder removal)
   c. The surgery may be performed in two stages if the tumor is extensive, with the creation of the urinary diversion first and the cystectomy several weeks later
   d. If a radical cystectomy is performed, lower-extremity lymphedema may occur as a result of lymph node dissection, and male impotence may occur

4. Ileal conduit
   a. Also called ureteroileostomy or Bricker's procedure
   b. Ureters are implanted into a segment of the ileum, with the formation of an abdominal stoma
   c. The urine flows into the conduit and is continually propelled out through the stoma by peristalsis
   d. The client is required to wear an appliance over the stoma to collect the urine (Box 42-22)
   e. Complications include obstruction, pyelonephritis, leakage at the anastomosis site, stenosis, hydronephrosis, calculi, skin irritation and ulceration, and stomal defects

5. Kock pouch
   a. A continent internal ileal reservoir created from a segment of the ileum and the ascending colon

b. The ureters are implanted into the side of the reservoir, and a special nipple valve is constructed to attach the reservoir to the skin

c. Postoperatively, the client will have a size 24 to 26 Foley catheter in place to drain urine continuously until the pouch has healed

d. The catheter is irrigated gently with normal saline to prevent obstruction caused by mucus or clots

e. After the removal of the catheter, the client is instructed in how to self-catheterize and to drain the reservoir at 4- to 6-hour intervals (Box 42-23)

6. Indiana pouch
   a. A continent reservoir is created from the ascending colon and the terminal ileum, thus making a pouch larger than the Kock pouch (additional continent reservoirs include the Mainz and Florida pouch systems)
   b. Postoperatively, the client will have a size 24 to 26 Foley catheter in place to drain urine continuously until the pouch has healed
   c. The Foley catheter is irrigated gently with normal saline to prevent obstruction caused by mucus or clots
   d. After the removal of the Foley catheter, the client is instructed in how to self-catheterize and to drain the reservoir at 4- to 6-hour intervals (see Box 42-23)

7. Creation of a neobladder
   a. Similar to the creation of an internal reservoir but different because, instead of emptying through an abdominal stoma, it empties through a pelvic outlet into the urethra
   b. The client empties the neobladder by relaxing the external sphincter and creating abdominal pressure or by intermittent self-catheterization

8. Percutaneous nephrostomy or pyelostomy
   a. Used when the **cancer** is inoperable, to prevent obstruction
   b. Involves a percutaneous or surgical insertion of a nephrostomy tube into the kidney for drainage
   c. Nursing interventions involve stabilizing the tube to prevent dislodgment and monitoring output

9. Ureterostomy
   a. May be performed as a palliative procedure if the ureters are obstructed by the tumor
   b. The ureters are attached to the surface of the abdomen, where the urine flows directly into a drainage appliance without a conduit
   c. Potential problems include infection, skin irritation, and the obstruction of urinary flow as a result of strictures at the opening

Ureterostomies divert urine directly to the skin surface through a ureteral skin opening (stoma). After ureterostomy, the client must wear a pouch.

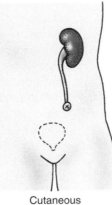

Cutaneous ureterostomy

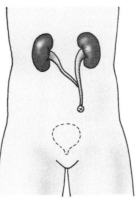

Cutaneous ureteroureterostomy

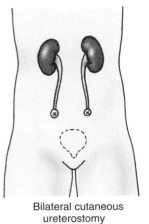

Bilateral cutaneous ureterostomy

Conduits collect urine in a portion of the intestine, which is then opened onto the skin surface as a stoma. After the creation of a conduit, the client must wear a pouch.

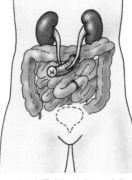

Ileal (Bricker's) conduit

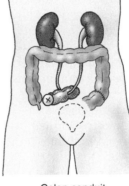

Colon conduit

Ileal reservoirs divert urine into a surgically created pouch, or pocket, that functions as a bladder. The stoma is continent, and the client removes urine by regular self-catheterization.

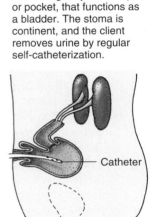

Catheter

Continent internal ileal reservoir (Kock's pouch)

Sigmoidostomies divert urine to the large intestine, so no stoma is required. The client excretes urine with bowel movements, and bowel incontinence may result.

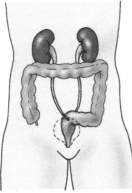

Ureterosigmoidostomy

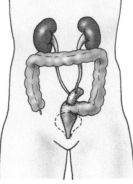

Ureteroileosigmoidostomy

FIG. 42-4 Urinary diversion procedures used for the treatment of bladder cancer. (From Ignatavicius, D., & Workman, M. [2006]. *Medical-surgical nursing: Critical thinking for collaborative care* [5th ed.]. Philadelphia: Saunders.)

10. Vesicostomy
    a. The bladder is sutured to the abdomen, and a stoma is created in the bladder wall
    b. The bladder empties through the stoma
F. Preoperative interventions
    1. Administer bowel preparation, as prescribed, which may include a clear liquid diet 12 to 24 hours before the surgical procedure, laxatives and enemas, and antibiotics to lower the bacterial count in the bowel
    2. Assist the surgeon and the enterostomal nurse with selecting an appropriate skin site for the creation of the abdominal stoma
    3. Encourage the client to talk about his or her feelings related to the stoma creation

G. Postoperative interventions
1. Monitor the vital signs
2. Monitor the incision site
3. Assess the stoma (it should be red and moist) every hour for the first 24 hours
4. Monitor for edema in the stoma, which may be present during the immediate postoperative period

---

BOX 42-22 **Urinary Stoma Care**

Instruct the client to change the appliance in the morning, when urinary production is slowest.

Collect the equipment, remove the collection bag, and use water or a commercial solvent to loosen the adhesive.

Hold a rolled gauze pad against the stoma to collect and absorb urine during the procedure.

Cleanse the skin around the stoma and under the drainage bag with a mild, nonresidue soap and water.

Inspect the skin for excoriation, and instruct the client to prevent urine from coming into contact with the skin.

After the skin is dry, apply skin adhesive around the appliance.

Instruct the client to cut the stoma opening of the skin barrier just large enough to fit over the stoma (i.e., no more that 3 mm larger than the stoma).

Instruct the client that the stoma will begin to shrink, thus requiring a smaller stoma opening on the skin barrier.

Apply the skin barrier before attaching the pouch or faceplate.

Place the appliance over the stoma, and secure it in place.

Encourage self-care; teach the client to use a mirror.

Instruct the client that the pouch may be drained by a bedside bag or a leg bag, especially at night.

Instruct the client to empty the urinary collection bag when it is one-third to one-half full to prevent pulling of the appliance and leakage.

Instruct the client to check the appliance seal if perspiring occurs.

Instruct the client to leave the urinary pouch in place as long as it is not leaking and to change it every 5 to 7 days.

During appliance changes, leave the skin open to air as long as possible.

Use a non–karaya gum product, because urine erodes karaya gum.

To control odor, instruct the client to drink adequate fluids, to wash the appliance thoroughly with soap and lukewarm water, and to soak the collection pouch in dilute white vinegar for 20 to 30 minutes or to place a special deodorant tablet into the pouch while it is being worn.

Instruct the client who takes baths to keep the level of the water below the stoma and to avoid oily soaps.

If the client plans to shower, instruct him or her to direct the flow of water away from the stoma.

---

5. If the stoma appears dark and dusky, notify the physician immediately, because this indicates necrosis
6. Monitor for the prolapse or retraction of the stoma
7. Monitor for the return of bowel function; monitor for peristalsis, which will return in 3 to 4 days
8. Maintain nothing-by-mouth status, as prescribed, until bowel sounds return
9. Monitor the urine flow, which is continuous (30 to 60 mL/hour) after surgery
10. The physician is notified if the urine output is less than 30 mL/hour or if there is no urine output for more than 15 minutes
11. Ureteral stents or catheters may be in place for 2 to 3 weeks or until healing occurs; maintain stability of catheters to prevent dislodgment
12. Monitor the urinary output closely and irrigate the catheter gently to prevent obstruction, as prescribed
13. Monitor for hematuria
14. Monitor for signs of peritonitis

BOX 42-23 **Self-Irrigation and Catheterization of a Stoma**

Irrigation

Instruct the client to wash the hands and to use clean technique

Instruct the client to use a catheter and syringe and to instill 60 mL of normal saline or water into the reservoir and to gently aspirate it or allow it to drain.

Instruct the client to irrigate until the drainage remains free of mucus but to be cautious to not overirrigate.

Catheterization

Instruct the client to wash the hands and to use clean technique.

Initially the client is taught to insert a catheter every 2 to 3 hours to drain the reservoir; during each week thereafter, the interval is increased by 1 hour until the catheterization is performed every 4 to 6 hours.

Lubricate the catheter well with water-soluble lubricant, and instruct the client never to force the catheter into the reservoir.

If resistance is met, instruct the client to pause, rotate the catheter, and apply gentle pressure to complete the insertion.

Instruct the client to notify the physician if he or she is unable to insert the catheter.

When the urine has stopped, instruct the client to take several deep breaths and to move the catheter in and out 2 to 3 inches to ensure that the pouch is empty.

Instruct the client to withdraw the catheter slowly and to pinch the catheter when it is withdrawn so that it does not leak urine.

Instruct the client to carry catheterization supplies with him or her.

15. Monitor for bladder distention after a partial cystectomy
16. Monitor for shock, hemorrhage, thrombophlebitis, and lower-extremity lymphedema after a radical cystectomy
17. Monitor the urinary drainage pouch for leaks, and check the skin integrity
18. Monitor the pH of the urine (do not place the dipstick into the stoma), because strong alkaline urine can cause skin irritation and facilitate crystal formation
19. Instruct the client regarding the potential for urinary tract infection or the development of calculi
20. Instruct the client to check the skin for irritation and to monitor the urinary drainage pouch for any leakage
21. Encourage the client to express feelings about changes in body image and sexual function as well as embarrassment

XXVI. ONCOLOGICAL EMERGENCIES

A. Sepsis and disseminated intravascular coagulation (DIC)
   1. Description: The client with an oncological disorder is at increased risk for infection; DIC is caused by sepsis
   2. Interventions
      a. Maintain strict aseptic technique with the immunocompromised client, and monitor closely for infection
      b. IV antibiotics may be prescribed
      c. Anticoagulants may be prescribed during the early phase of DIC
      d. Cryoprecipitated clotting factors may be prescribed when DIC progresses and hemorrhage is the primary problem

B. Syndrome of inappropriate antidiuretic hormone
   1. Description
      a. Tumors can produce, secrete, or stimulate the brain to synthesize antidiuretic hormone
      b. Mild symptoms include weakness, muscle cramps, loss of appetite, and fatigue; serum sodium levels range from 115 to 120 mEq/L
      c. More serious signs and symptoms relate to water intoxication and include weight gain, personality changes, confusion, and extreme muscle weakness
      d. As the serum sodium level approaches 110 mEq/L, seizures, coma, and eventually death will occur unless the condition is rapidly treated
   2. Interventions
      a. Initiate fluid restriction and increased sodium intake, as prescribed
      b. Demeclocycline (Declomycin) may be prescribed; this is an antagonist to antidiuretic hormone
      c. Monitor the serum sodium levels

C. Spinal cord compression
   1. Description
      a. Occurs when a tumor directly enters the spinal cord or when the vertebral column collapses as a result of tumor entry
      b. Causes back pain, usually before neurological deficits occur
      c. Neurological deficits relate to the spinal level of compression and include numbness and tingling; the loss of urethral, vaginal, and rectal sensation; and muscle weakness
   2. Interventions
      a. Monitor for back pain and neurological deficits
      b. Prepare the client for radiation and/or chemotherapy to reduce the size of the tumor and relieve compression
      c. Surgery may need to be performed to remove the tumor and relieve the pressure on the spinal cord
      d. Instruct the client regarding the use of neck or back braces, if prescribed
      e. High doses of corticosteroids may be given to reduce the edema around the spinal cord

D. Hypercalcemia
   1. Description
      a. A late manifestation of extensive malignancy that occurs most often in clients with bone **metastasis**
      b. Decreased physical mobility contributes to or worsens hypercalcemia
      c. Early signs include fatigue, anorexia, nausea, vomiting, constipation, confusion, and polyuria
      d. More serious signs and symptoms include severe muscle weakness, diminished deep tendon reflexes, paralytic ileus, dehydration, and electrocardiography changes
   2. Interventions
      a. Monitor the serum calcium level
      b. Oral or parenteral (normal saline) fluids may be prescribed
      c. Medications to lower the calcium level may be prescribed
      d. Prepare the client for dialysis if the condition becomes life threatening or is accompanied by renal impairment

E. Superior vena cava (SVC) syndrome
   1. Description
      a. Occurs when the SVC is compressed or obstructed by tumor growth
      b. Signs and symptoms result from the blockage of blood flow in the venous system of the head, neck, and upper trunk
      c. Early signs and symptoms generally occur in the morning and include edema of the face

(especially around the eyes) and tightness of the shirt or blouse collar (Stokes' sign)

  d. As the condition worsens, edema in the arms and hands, dyspnea, erythema of the upper body, and epistaxis (nosebleed) occur

  e. Life-threatening signs and symptoms include hemorrhage, cyanosis, mental status changes, decreased cardiac output, and hypotension

  2. Interventions

  a. Monitor for signs and symptoms of SVC syndrome

  b. Prepare the client for radiation therapy to the mediastinal area

F. Tumor lysis syndrome (TLS)

  1. Description

  a. Occurs when large quantities of tumor cells are destroyed rapidly and released into the bloodstream faster than the body's homeostatic mechanisms can handle them

  b. TLS is a positive sign that **cancer** treatment is effective; however, if left untreated, it can cause severe tissue damage and death

  c. Hyperkalemia and hyperuricemia occur; hyperuricemia can lead to acute renal failure

  2. Interventions

  a. Encourage oral hydration (at least 3 L for 3 days after treatment); IV hydration may be prescribed for the client who is experiencing nausea

  b. Instruct the client regarding the importance of fluid intake during chemotherapy

  c. Diuretics may be prescribed to increase the urine flow through the kidneys

  d. Medications that increase the excretion of purines (e.g., allopurinol [Zyloprim]), may be prescribed

  e. The IV infusion of glucose and insulin may be prescribed to treat hyperkalemia

  f. Prepare the client for dialysis if hyperkalemia and hyperuricemia persist despite treatment

  g. Provide antiemetics, as prescribed, to prevent dehydration as a result of nausea and vomiting

PRACTICE QUESTIONS

More questions on the companion CD!

468. A nurse is assisting with developing a plan of care for the client with multiple myeloma. Which of the following is a priority nursing intervention for this client?
  1. Encouraging fluids
  2. Providing frequent oral care
  3. Coughing and deep breathing
  4. Monitoring the red blood cell count

469. A nurse is assisting with conducting a health-promotion program to community members regarding testicular cancer. The nurse determines that further teaching is needed if a community member states that which of the following is a sign of testicular cancer?
  1. Alopecia
  2. Back pain
  3. Painless testicular swelling
  4. A heavy sensation in the scrotum

470. A nurse is reviewing the laboratory results of a client with leukemia who has received a regimen of chemotherapy. Which laboratory value would the nurse specifically note as a result of the massive cell destruction that occurs with the chemotherapy?
  1. Anemia
  2. Decreased platelets
  3. Increased uric acid level
  4. Decreased leukocyte count

471. A client is receiving external radiation to the neck for cancer of the larynx. The nurse plans the client's care knowing that the most likely side effect to be expected is:
  1. Dyspnea
  2. Diarrhea
  3. Sore throat
  4. Constipation

472. A nurse is providing instructions to a client receiving external radiation therapy. The nurse determines that the client needs further instructions if the client states an intention to:
  1. Eat a high-protein diet.
  2. Avoid exposure to sunlight.
  3. Wash the skin with a mild soap and pat it dry.
  4. Apply pressure on the radiated area to prevent bleeding.

473. A nurse is caring for a client with an internal radiation implant. When caring for the client, the nurse should observe which principle?
  1. Pregnant women are not allowed into the client's room.
  2. Limit the time with the client to 1 hour per 8-hour shift.
  3. Remove the dosimeter badge when entering the client's room.
  4. Individuals less than 16 years old may be allowed to go in the room as long as they are 6 feet away from the client.

474. A nurse teaches skin care to the client who is receiving external radiation therapy. Which of the following statements, if made by the client, would indicate the need for further instruction?
  1. "I will handle the area gently."
  2. "I will wear loose-fitting clothing."
  3. "I will avoid the use of deodorants."
  4. "I will limit sun exposure to 1 hour daily."

475. A client is hospitalized for the insertion of an internal cervical radiation implant. While giving care, the nurse finds the radiation implant in the bed. The nurse would immediately:
    1. Call the physician.
    2. Reinsert the implant into the vagina immediately.
    3. Pick up the implant with gloved hands and flush it down the toilet.
    4. Pick up the implant with long-handled forceps and place into a lead container.

476. A nurse is assisting with developing a plan of care for a client who is experiencing hematological toxicity as a result of chemotherapy. The nurse suggests including which of the following in the plan of care?
    1. Restricting all visitors
    2. Restricting fluid intake
    3. Restricting fresh fruits and vegetables in the diet
    4. Inserting an indwelling urinary catheter to prevent skin breakdown

477. A nurse is reviewing the laboratory results of a client who is receiving chemotherapy and notes that the platelet count is 10,000/mm^3. On the basis of this laboratory value, the priority action is to monitor which of the following?
    1. Skin turgor
    2. Temperature
    3. Bowel sounds
    4. Level of consciousness

478. A client is admitted to the hospital with a diagnosis of suspected Hodgkin's disease. Which of the following findings would the nurse most likely expect to find documented in the client's record?
    1. Fatigue
    2. Weakness
    3. Weight gain
    4. Enlarged lymph nodes

479. When reviewing the health care record of a client with ovarian cancer, the nurse recognizes which symptom as being typical of the disease?
    1. Diarrhea
    2. Hypermenorrhea
    3. Abnormal bleeding
    4. Abdominal distention

480. A nurse is caring for a client after a modified radical mastectomy. Which of the following findings would indicate that the client is experiencing a complication related to the surgery?
    1. Mild pain at the incisional site
    2. Arm edema on the operative side
    3. Sanguineous drainage in the drainage tube
    4. Complaints of decreased sensation near the operative site

481. A nurse is caring for a client with cancer of the prostate after a prostatectomy. The nurse provides discharge instructions and plans to include which of the following?
    1. Avoid driving the car for 1 week.
    2. Restrict fluid intake to prevent incontinence.
    3. Avoid lifting objects heavier than 20 pounds for at least 6 weeks.
    4. Notify the physician if small blood clots are noticed during urination.

482. A nurse is assisting with providing a teaching session to a community group regarding the risks and causes of bladder cancer. The nurse determines that additional teaching is needed if a member of the community group states which of the following regarding this type of cancer?
    1. It most often occurs in women.
    2. It is generally seen in clients who are older than 40 years old.
    3. Environmental health hazards have been found to be a cause of this disease.
    4. Using cigarettes, artificial sweeteners, and coffee drinking can increase the risk for this cancer.

483. A nurse is reviewing the history of a client with bladder cancer. The nurse would expect to note which most common symptom of this type of cancer as being documented in the client's record?
    1. Dysuria
    2. Hematuria
    3. Urgency of urination
    4. Frequency of urination

484. A nurse is inspecting the stoma of a client after a ureterostomy. Which of the following would the nurse expect to note?
    1. A dry stoma
    2. A pale stoma
    3. A dark-colored stoma
    4. A red and moist stoma

485. A nurse is caring for a client after a radical mastectomy. Which nursing intervention would assist with preventing lymphedema of the affected arm?
    1. Placing cool compresses on the affected arm
    2. Elevating the affected arm on a pillow above heart level
    3. Avoiding arm exercises during the immediate postoperative period
    4. Maintaining an intravenous (IV) insertion site below the antecubital area on the affected side

486. A nurse is instructing a client to perform a testicular self-examination (TSE). Which instruction would the nurse provide to the client?
    1. Examine the testicles while lying down.
    2. The best time for the examination is after a shower.
    3. Gently touch the testicle with one finger to feel for a growth.

4. Testicular examinations should be done at least every 6 months.

487. A nurse is assisting with conducting a health-promotion program at a local school. The nurse determines that additional teaching is needed if a student identifies which of the following as a risk factor associated with cancer?
  1. Stress
  2. Viral factors
  3. Exposure to radiation
  4. Low-fat and high-fiber diets

488. A client with cancer is receiving chemotherapy and develops thrombocytopenia. Which intervention is a priority in the nursing plan of care?
  1. Monitor the client for bleeding.
  2. Monitor the client's temperature.
  3. Ambulate the client three times daily.
  4. Monitor the client for pathological fractures.

489. A nurse is instructing a group of female clients about breast self-examination (BSE). The nurse would instruct the clients to perform the examination:
  1. At the onset of menstruation
  2. Every month during ovulation
  3. Weekly at the same time of day
  4. One week after menstruation begins

490. A client who has been diagnosed with multiple myeloma asks the nurse about the diagnosis. The nurse bases the response on which characteristic of the disorder?
  1. Altered red blood cell production
  2. Altered production of lymph nodes
  3. Malignant exacerbation in the number of leukocytes
  4. Malignant proliferation of plasma cells and tumors within the bone

491. A nurse is reviewing the laboratory results of a client who has been diagnosed with multiple myeloma. Which of the following would the nurse expect to specifically note with this diagnosis?
  1. Increased calcium level
  2. Increased white blood cells
  3. Decreased blood urea nitrogen (BUN) level
  4. Decreased number of plasma cells in the bone marrow

ALTERNATE ITEM FORMAT: MULTIPLE RESPONSE

492. A client with carcinoma of the lung develops the syndrome of inappropriate antidiuretic hormone (SIADH) as a complication of the cancer. The nurse anticipates that which of the following may be prescribed?
  ☐ **1.** Radiation
  ☐ **2.** Chemotherapy
  ☐ **3.** Increased fluid intake
  ☐ **4.** Serum sodium blood levels
  ☐ **5.** Decreased oral sodium intake
  ☐ **6.** Medication that is antagonistic to antidiuretic hormone (ADH)

ANSWERS

468. **1**
Rationale: Hypercalcemia secondary to bone destruction is a priority concern in the client with multiple myeloma. The nurse should encourage fluids in adequate amounts to maintain an output of 1.5 to 2 L/day. Clients require about 3 L of fluid per day. The fluid is needed not only to dilute the calcium but also to prevent protein from precipitating in the renal tubules. Options 2, 3, and 4 may be components of the plan of care, but they are not the priorities for this client.
Test-Taking Strategy: Knowledge regarding the clinical manifestations that occur in clients with multiple myeloma is required to answer the question. Recalling that encouraging fluids is specific to the care of a client with this disorder will direct you to option 1. Review the specific manifestations of this disorder if you had difficulty with this question.
Level of Cognitive Ability: Application
Client Needs: Physiological Integrity
Integrated Process: Nursing Process/Planning
Content Area: Adult Health/Oncology
References: Christensen, B., & Kockrow, E. (2006). *Adult health nursing* (5th ed., p. 317). St. Louis: Mosby.
Lewis, S., Heitkemper, M., Dirksen, S., & Bucher, L. (2007). *Medical-surgical nursing: Assessment and management of clinical problems* (7th ed., p. 728). St. Louis: Mosby.

469. **1**
Rationale: Alopecia is not a finding in clients with testicular cancer. However, it may occur as a result of radiation or chemotherapy. Options 2, 3, and 4 are findings in clients with testicular cancer. Back pain may indicate metastasis to the retroperitoneal lymph nodes.
Test-Taking Strategy: Note the strategic words "further teaching is needed." These words indicate a negative event query and ask you to select an option that is an incorrect sign. Use the process of elimination, and remember that alopecia occurs as a result of chemotherapy rather than of the disease. Review the manifestations associated with testicular cancer if you had difficulty with this question.
Level of Cognitive Ability: Comprehension
Client Needs: Health Promotion and Maintenance
Integrated Process: Teaching and Learning
Content Area: Adult Health/Oncology
Reference: Christensen, B., & Kockrow, E. (2006). *Adult health nursing* (5th ed., p. 618). St. Louis: Mosby.

470. **3**
Rationale: Hyperuricemia is especially common after treatment for leukemias and lymphomas, because the therapy results in massive cell destruction. Although options 1, 2, and 4 may also be noted, an increased uric acid level is specifically related to cell destruction.

Test-Taking Strategy: Note the strategic words "specifically note" and "massive cell destruction." Recalling the cell response to destruction will assist with directing you to option 3. Review this concept if you had difficulty with this question.

Level of Cognitive Ability: Comprehension
Client Needs: Physiological Integrity
Integrated Process: Nursing Process/Data Collection
Content Area: Adult Health/Oncology
Reference: Christensen, B., & Kockrow, E. (2006). *Adult health nursing* (5th ed., p. 839). St. Louis: Mosby.

471. **3**
Rationale: In general, only the area in the treatment field is affected by the radiation. Skin reactions, fatigue, nausea, and anorexia may occur with radiation to any site, whereas other side effects occur only when specific areas are involved in treatment. A client who is receiving radiation to the larynx is most likely to experience a sore throat. Options 2 and 4 may occur with radiation to the gastrointestinal (GI) tract. Dyspnea may occur with lung involvement.
Test-Taking Strategy: Use the process of elimination, and note the strategic words "most likely." Eliminate options 2 and 4 first, because they are comparable or alike, and both are GI related. Consider the anatomical location of the radiation therapy to direct you to option 3. Review the effects of radiation therapy if you had difficulty with this question.
Level of Cognitive Ability: Application
Client Needs: Physiological Integrity
Integrated Process: Nursing Process/Planning
Content Area: Adult Health/Oncology
Reference: Christensen, B., & Kockrow, E. (2006). *Adult health nursing* (5th ed., p. 417). St. Louis: Mosby.

472. **4**
Rationale: The client should avoid pressure on the radiated area and should wear loose-fitting clothing. Options 1, 2, and 3 are accurate instructions regarding radiation therapy.
Test-Taking Strategy: Use the process of elimination and note the strategic words "needs further instructions." These words indicate a negative event query and ask you to select an option that is an incorrect statement. The word "pressure" in option 4 should be an indication that this is an inappropriate measure. Review the client teaching points related to skin care and radiation therapy if you had difficulty with this question.
Level of Cognitive Ability: Comprehension
Client Needs: Physiological Integrity
Integrated Process: Teaching and Learning
Content Area: Adult Health/Oncology
Reference: Monahan, F., Sands, J., Marek, J., Neighbors, M., & Green, C. (2007). *Phipps' medical-surgical nursing: Health and illness perspectives* (8th ed., p. 541). St. Louis: Mosby.

473. **1**
Rationale: The time that the nurse spends in the room of a client with an internal radiation implant is 30 minutes per 8-hour shift. The dosimeter badge must be worn when in the client's room. Children less than 16 years old and pregnant women are not allowed in the client's room.
Test-Taking Strategy: Use the process of elimination. Option 3 can be eliminated first. Knowledge of the time frame related

to exposure to the client will assist you with eliminating option 2. From the remaining options, select option 1 because of the possible risks associated with exposure to the mother and fetus. Review the principles of radiation exposure if you had difficulty with this question.
Level of Cognitive Ability: Application
Client Needs: Safe and Effective Care Environment
Integrated Process: Nursing Process/Implementation
Content Area: Adult Health/Oncology
References: Christensen, B., & Kockrow, E. (2006). *Adult health nursing* (5th ed., p. 829). St. Louis: Mosby.
Ignatavicius, D., & Workman, M. (2006). *Medical-surgical nursing: Critical thinking for collaborative care* (5th ed., p. 490). Philadelphia: Saunders.
Linton, A. (2007). *Introduction to medical-surgical nursing* (4th ed., p. 377). Philadelphia: Saunders.

474. **4**
Rationale: The client needs to be instructed to avoid exposure to the sun. Options 1, 2, and 3 are accurate measures for the care of a client who is receiving external radiation therapy.
Test-Taking Strategy: Note the strategic words "need for further instruction." These words indicate a negative event query and ask you to select an option that is an incorrect statement. Eliminate option 1 because of the word "gently" and option 2 because of the word "loose." From the remaining options, recalling that sun exposure is to be avoided will assist you with answering the question. Review skin care measures for the client who is receiving external radiation if you had difficulty with this question.
Level of Cognitive Ability: Comprehension
Client Needs: Physiological Integrity
Integrated Process: Teaching and Learning
Content Area: Adult Health/Oncology
Reference: Christensen, B., & Kockrow, E. (2006). *Adult health nursing* (5th ed., p. 828). St. Louis: Mosby.

475. **4**
Rationale: A lead container and long-handled forceps should be kept in the client's room at all times during internal radiation therapy. If the implant becomes dislodged, the nurse should pick up the implant with long-handled forceps and place it into the lead container. Options 1, 2, and 3 are inaccurate interventions.
Test-Taking Strategy: Use the process of elimination. Note the strategic word "immediately." Option 2 is not an appropriate action. Eliminate option 3 next, because the implant would not be discarded. Although the physician would be notified, the immediate action is option 4. Review the measures related to a dislodged implant if you had difficulty with this question.
Level of Cognitive Ability: Application
Client Needs: Safe and Effective Care Environment
Integrated Process: Nursing Process/Implementation
Content Area: Adult Health/Oncology
References: Christensen, B., & Kockrow, E. (2006). *Adult health nursing* (5th ed., p. 829). St. Louis: Mosby.
Ignatavicius, D., & Workman, M. (2006). *Medical-surgical nursing: Critical thinking for collaborative care* (5th ed., p. 490). Philadelphia: Saunders.

476. 3

Rationale: In a client who is experiencing hematological toxicity, a low-bacteria diet is implemented. This includes avoiding fresh fruits and vegetables and performing a thorough cooking of all foods. Not all visitors are restricted, but the client is protected from people with known infections. Fluids should be encouraged. Invasive measures such as an indwelling urinary catheter should be avoided to prevent infections.

Test-Taking Strategy: Use the process of elimination. Eliminate option 1 because of the word "all." Next, eliminate option 2; it is not reasonable to restrict fluids for a client who is receiving chemotherapy, because he or she is already at risk for fluid and electrolyte imbalances. Eliminate option 4 because of the risk of infection that exists with this measure. Review the interventions for the client with hematological toxicity if you had difficulty with this question.

Level of Cognitive Ability: Application
Client Needs: Safe and Effective Care Environment
Integrated Process: Nursing Process/Planning
Content Area: Adult Health/Oncology
Reference: Christensen, B., & Kockrow, E. (2006). *Adult health nursing* (5th ed., p. 833). St. Louis: Mosby.

477. 4

Rationale: A high risk of hemorrhage exists when the platelet count is less than 20,000/mm³. Fatal central nervous system hemorrhage or massive gastrointestinal hemorrhage can occur when the platelet count is less than 10,000/mm³. The client should be monitored for changes in the level of consciousness, which may be an early indication of an intracranial hemorrhage. Option 2 is a priority when the white blood cell count is low and the client is at risk for an infection. Although options 1 and 3 are important, they are not the priority in this situation.

Test-Taking Strategy: Use the process of elimination, and note the strategic word "priority." Recalling the normal platelet count and determining that a low count places the client at risk for bleeding will assist you with eliminating options 1, 2, and 3. Review the normal platelet count and the nursing interventions for a client with a low count if you had difficulty with this question.

Level of Cognitive Ability: Analysis
Client Needs: Physiological Integrity
Integrated Process: Nursing Process/Implementation
Content Area: Adult Health/Oncology
References: Christensen, B., & Kockrow, E. (2006). *Adult health nursing* (5th ed., p. 833). St. Louis: Mosby.
Ignatavicius, D., & Workman, M. (2006). *Medical-surgical nursing: Critical thinking for collaborative care* (5th ed., p. 496). Philadelphia: Saunders.
Lewis, S., Heitkemper, M., Dirksen, S., & Bucher, L., (2007). *Medical-surgical nursing: Assessment and management of clinical problems* (7th ed., pp. 296-297). St. Louis: Mosby.

478. 4

Rationale: Hodgkin's disease is a chronic progressive neoplastic disorder of the lymphoid tissue that is characterized by the painless enlargement of the lymph nodes with progression to extralymphatic sites, such as the spleen and liver. Weight loss is most likely to be noted. Fatigue and weakness may occur, but they are not significantly related to the disease.

Test-Taking Strategy: Use the process of elimination, and note the strategic words "most likely." Option 3 can be eliminated first, because, in clients with such a disorder, weight loss is most likely to occur. Options 1 and 2 are comparable or alike and rather vague symptoms that can occur with many disorders. In addition, recalling that Hodgkin's disease affects the lymph nodes will direct you to option 4. Review the manifestations associated with Hodgkin's disease if you had difficulty with this question.

Level of Cognitive Ability: Comprehension
Client Needs: Physiological Integrity
Integrated Process: Nursing Process/Data Collection
Content Area: Adult Health/Oncology
Reference: Christensen, B., & Kockrow, E. (2006). *Adult health nursing* (5th ed., pp. 318-319). St. Louis: Mosby.

479. 4

Rationale: Clinical manifestations of ovarian cancer include abdominal distention, urinary frequency and urgency, pain from pressure caused by the growing tumor and the effects of urinary or bowel obstruction, and constipation. Abnormal bleeding is associated with uterine cancer and often results in hypermenorrhea.

Test-Taking Strategy: Use the process of elimination. Eliminate options 2 and 3 first, because they are comparable or alike. From the remaining options, consider the anatomical location of the diagnosis. This will assist with directing you to option 4. Review the manifestations associated with ovarian cancer if you had difficulty with this question.

Level of Cognitive Ability: Comprehension
Client Needs: Physiological Integrity
Integrated Process: Nursing Process/Data Collection
Content Area: Adult Health/Oncology
References: Christensen, B., & Kockrow, E. (2006). *Adult health nursing* (5th ed., pp. 600-601). St. Louis: Mosby.
Linton, A. (2007). *Introduction to medical-surgical nursing* (4th ed., p. 1068). Philadelphia: Saunders.

480. 2

Rationale: Arm edema on the operative side (lymphedema) is a complication after mastectomy that can occur immediately, months, or even years after surgery. Options 1, 3, and 4 are expected occurrences after mastectomy and are not indicative of a complication.

Test-Taking Strategy: Use the process of elimination, and consider the normal and expected occurrences after a mastectomy. This will direct you to the correct option. Review the complications after mastectomy if you had difficulty with this question.

Level of Cognitive Ability: Comprehension
Client Needs: Physiological Integrity
Integrated Process: Nursing Process/Data Collection
Content Area: Adult Health/Oncology
Reference: Linton, A. (2007). *Introduction to medical-surgical nursing* (4th ed., p. 1066). Philadelphia: Saunders.

481. 3

Rationale: Small pieces of tissue or blood clots can be passed during urination for up to 2 weeks after surgery. Driving a car and sitting for long periods of time are restricted for at least 3 weeks. A daily fluid intake of 2 to 2.5 L/day should be maintained to limit clot formation and prevent infection. Option 3 is an accurate discharge instruction after prostatectomy.

Test-Taking Strategy: Use the process of elimination. Option 2 can easily be eliminated first. Eliminate option 1 next, because 1 week is a rather short time period. Recalling that blood clots are expected after this type of surgery will direct you to option 3. Review the client teaching points after prostatectomy if you had difficulty with this question.

Level of Cognitive Ability: Application
Client Needs: Physiological Integrity
Integrated Process: Teaching and Learning
Content Area: Adult Health/Oncology
Reference: Monahan, F., Sand, J., Neighbors, M., Marek, J., & Green, C. (2007). *Phipps' medical-surgical nursing: Health and illness perspectives* (8th ed., p. 1741). St. Louis: Mosby.

482. 1
Rationale: The incidence of bladder cancer is three times greater among men than among women, and it affects the white population twice as often as the black population. Options 2, 3, and 4 are associated with the incidence of bladder cancer.

Test-Taking Strategy: Use the process of elimination, and note the strategic words "additional teaching is needed." Basic information regarding the risks associated with cancer will assist you with eliminating options 3 and 4. From the remaining options, knowledge regarding the risk factors associated with bladder cancer will direct you to option 1. Review these risks if you had difficulty with this question.

Level of Cognitive Ability: Comprehension
Client Needs: Health Promotion and Maintenance
Integrated Process: Teaching and Learning
Content Area: Adult Health/Oncology
Reference: Monahan, F., Sand, J., Neighbors, M., Marek, J., & Green, C. (2007). *Phipps' medical-surgical nursing: Health and illness perspectives* (8th ed., p. 984). St. Louis: Mosby.

483. 2
Rationale: The most common symptom among clients with cancer of the bladder is hematuria. The client may also experience irritative voiding symptoms such as frequency, urgency, and dysuria; these symptoms are often associated with cancer in situ.

Test-Taking Strategy: Use the process of elimination, and note the strategic words "most common." Options 1, 3, and 4 are symptoms that are associated with bladder infection. Review the clinical manifestations associated with bladder cancer if you had difficulty with this question.

Level of Cognitive Ability: Comprehension
Client Needs: Physiological Integrity
Integrated Process: Nursing Process/Data Collection
Content Area: Adult Health/Oncology
Reference: Monahan, F., Sand, J., Neighbors, M., Marek, J., & Green, C. (2007). *Phipps' medical-surgical nursing: Health and illness perspectives* (8th ed., p. 985). St. Louis: Mosby.

484. 4
Rationale: After ureterostomy, the stoma should be red and moist. A pale stoma may indicate an inadequate amount of vascular supply, and a dry stoma may indicate body fluid

deficit. Any sign of darkness or duskiness in the stoma may mean a loss of vascular supply and must be corrected immediately, or necrosis can occur.

Test-Taking Strategy: Use the process of elimination. You should easily be able to eliminate options 2 and 3. From the remaining options, note the strategic word "moist" in option 4. This should indicate that this is an expected and positive finding. Review expected and unexpected findings after ureterostomy if you had difficulty with this question.

Level of Cognitive Ability: Comprehension
Client Needs: Physiological Integrity
Integrated Process: Nursing Process/Data Collection
Content Area: Adult Health/Oncology
Reference: Linton, A. (2007). *Introduction to medical-surgical nursing* (4th ed., pp. 409, 413). Philadelphia: Saunders.

485. 2
Rationale: After mastectomy, the arm should be elevated above the level of the heart, and simple arm exercises should be encouraged. No blood pressure readings, injections, IV line insertions, or blood draws should be performed on the affected arm. Cool compresses are not a suggested measure to prevent lymphedema from occurring.

Test-Taking Strategy: Note the strategic words "assist with preventing." Use the process of elimination, and note the relationship between the words "lymphedema" in the question and "elevating" in the correct option. Review treatment measures after mastectomy if you had difficulty with this question.

Level of Cognitive Ability: Application
Client Needs: Physiological Integrity
Integrated Process: Nursing Process/Implementation
Content Area: Adult Health/Oncology
Reference: Linton, A. (2007). *Introduction to medical-surgical nursing* (4th ed., p. 1066). Philadelphia: Saunders.

486. 2
Rationale: The TSE is recommended monthly after a warm bath or shower, when the scrotal skin is relaxed. The client should stand to examine the testicles. Using both hands, with the fingers under the scrotum and the thumbs on top, the client should gently roll the testicles, feeling for any lumps. The TSE should be performed monthly.

Test-Taking Strategy: Use the process of elimination. Eliminate option 4 first because of the words "6 months." Next, eliminate option 3 because of the word "one." From the remaining options, eliminate option 1 by trying to visualize the process of the TSE. Review the TSE if you had difficulty with this question.

Level of Cognitive Ability: Application
Client Needs: Health Promotion and Maintenance
Integrated Process: Teaching and Learning
Content Area: Adult Health/Oncology
References: Christensen, B., & Kockrow, E. (2006). *Adult health nursing* (5th ed. pp. 618-619). St. Louis: Mosby.
Potter, P., & Perry, A. (2005). *Fundamentals of nursing* (6th ed., p. 752). St. Louis: Mosby.

487. 4
Rationale: Viruses may be one of multiple agents that act to initiate carcinogenesis and that have been associated with several types of cancer. Increased stress has been associated with

causing the growth and proliferation of cancer cells. Two forms of radiation, ultraviolet and ionizing, can lead to cancer. High-fiber diets may reduce the risk of colon cancer. A diet that is high in fat may increase the risk of the development of certain cancers.

Test-Taking Strategy: Note the strategic words "additional teaching is needed." These words indicate a negative event query and ask you to select an option that is an incorrect statement. Read each option carefully, and use the process of elimination. Recalling the risk factors related to cancer will direct you to option 4. Review these risk factors if you had difficulty with this question.

Level of Cognitive Ability: Comprehension
Client Needs: Health Promotion and Maintenance
Integrated Process: Teaching and Learning
Content Area: Adult Health/Oncology
References: Ignatavicius, D., & Workman, M. (2006). *Medical-surgical nursing: Critical thinking for collaborative care* (5th ed., pp. 478-479). Philadelphia: Saunders.
Linton, A. (2007). *Introduction to medical-surgical nursing* (4th ed., p. 372). Philadelphia: Saunders.
Phipps, W., Monahan, F., Sands, J., Neighbors, M., Marek, J., & Green, C. (2007). *Phipps' medical-surgical nursing: Health and illness perspectives* (8th ed., p. 513). St. Louis: Mosby.

488. 1
Rationale: Thrombocytopenia indicates a decrease in the number of platelets in the circulating blood. A major concern is monitoring for and preventing bleeding. Option 2 relates to monitoring for infection, particularly if leukopenia is present. Options 3 and 4, although important to the plan of care, are not directly related to thrombocytopenia.

Test-Taking Strategy: Use the process of elimination, and note the strategic word "thrombocytopenia." Recalling that this condition places the client at risk for bleeding will assist you with eliminating options 2, 3, and 4. Review the nursing interventions related to thrombocytopenia if you had difficulty with this question.

Level of Cognitive Ability: Application
Client Needs: Physiological Integrity
Integrated Process: Nursing Process/Planning
Content Area: Adult Health/Oncology
Reference: Linton, A. (2007). *Introduction to medical-surgical nursing* (4th ed., p. 587). Philadelphia: Saunders.

489. 4
Rationale: The BSE should be performed monthly about 7 days after the menstrual period begins. It is not recommended to perform the examination weekly; at the onset of menstruation and during ovulation, hormonal changes occur that may alter breast tissue.

Test-Taking Strategy: Use the process of elimination. Option 3 can be eliminated first because of the word "weekly." Eliminate options 1 and 2 next because of the similarity that exists with regard to the hormonal changes that occur during these times. Review the procedure for performing the BSE if you had difficulty with this question.

Level of Cognitive Ability: Application
Client Needs: Health Promotion and Maintenance
Integrated Process: Teaching and Learning
Content Area: Adult Health/Oncology

References: Linton, A. (2007). *Introduction to medical-surgical nursing* (4th ed., p. 1038). Philadelphia: Saunders.
Potter, P., & Perry, A. (2005). *Fundamentals of nursing* (6th ed., p. 736). St. Louis: Mosby.

490. 4
Rationale: Multiple myeloma is a neoplastic condition that is characterized by the abnormal malignant proliferation of plasma cells and the accumulation of mature plasma cells in the bone marrow. Options 1 and 2 are not characteristics of multiple myeloma, and option 3 describes the leukemic process.

Test-Taking Strategy: Use the process of elimination and your knowledge regarding the pathophysiology associated with multiple myeloma to answer the question. Focusing on the name of the diagnosis will direct you to option 4. Review the pathophysiology of multiple myeloma if you had difficulty with this question.

Level of Cognitive Ability: Comprehension
Client Needs: Physiological Integrity
Integrated Process: Nursing Process/Planning
Content Area: Adult Health/Oncology
Reference: Christensen, B., & Kockrow, E. (2006). *Adult health nursing* (5th ed., pp. 316-317). St. Louis: Mosby.

491. 1
Rationale: Findings that are indicative of multiple myeloma are an increased number of plasma cells in the bone marrow, anemia, hypercalcemia as a result of the release of calcium from the deteriorating bone tissue, and an elevated BUN level. An increased white blood cell count may or may not be present, but this is not specifically related to multiple myeloma.

Test-Taking Strategy: Knowledge regarding the pathophysiology associated with multiple myeloma and its effects on the body is required to answer the question. Remember, hypercalcemia occurs as a result of the release of calcium from the deteriorating bone tissue. Review the pathophysiology of multiple myeloma if you had difficulty with this question.

Level of Cognitive Ability: Comprehension
Client Needs: Physiological Integrity
Integrated Process: Nursing Process/Data Collection
Content Area: Adult Health/Oncology
Reference: Lewis, S., Heitkemper, M., Dirksen, S., & Bucher, L. (2007). *Medical-surgical nursing: Assessment and management of clinical problems* (7th ed., p. 728). St. Louis: Mosby.

ALTERNATE ITEM FORMAT: MULTIPLE RESPONSE

492. 1, 2, 4, 6
Rationale: Cancer is a common cause of SIADH. In clients with SIADH, excessive amounts of water are reabsorbed by the kidney and put into the systemic circulation. The increased water causes hyponatremia (decreased serum sodium levels) and some degree of fluid retention. SIADH is managed by treating the condition and its cause, and treatment usually includes fluid restriction, increased sodium intake, and a medication with a mechanism of action that is antagonistic to ADH. Sodium levels are monitored closely, because hypernatremia can suddenly develop as a

result of treatment. The immediate institution of appropriate cancer therapy (usually either radiation or chemotherapy) can cause such tumor regression that ADH synthesis and release processes return to normal.

Test-Taking Strategy: Focus on the client's diagnosis, and recall that in clients with SIADH, excessive amounts of water are reabsorbed by the kidney and put into the systemic circulation. Review the treatment for SIADH if you had difficulty with this question.

Level of Cognitive Ability: Analysis

Client Needs: Physiological Integrity
Integrated Process: Nursing Process/Planning
Content Area: Adult Health/Oncology
References: Ignatavicius, D., & Workman, M. (2006). *Medical-surgical nursing: Critical thinking for collaborative care* (5th ed., pp. 1469-1470). Philadelphia: Saunders.
Linton, A. (2007). *Introduction to medical-surgical nursing* (4th ed., p. 393). Philadelphia: Saunders.

REFERENCES

Black, J., & Hawks, J. (2005). *Medical-surgical nursing: Clinical management for positive outcomes* (7th ed.). Philadelphia: Saunders.

Christensen, B., & Kockrow, E. (2006). *Adult health nursing* (5th ed.). St. Louis: Mosby.

Christensen, B., & Kockrow, E. (2006). *Foundations of nursing* (5th ed.). St. Louis: Mosby.

Ignatavicius, D., & Workman, M. (2006). *Medical-surgical nursing: Critical thinking for collaborative care* (5th ed.). Philadelphia: Saunders.

Lewis, S., Heitkemper, M., Dirksen, S., & Bucher, L. (2007). *Medical-surgical nursing: Assessment and management of clinical problems* (7th ed.). St. Louis: Mosby.

Lilley, L., Harrington, S., & Snyder, J. (2007). *Pharmacology and the nursing process* (5th ed.). St. Louis: Mosby.

Linton, A. (2007). *Introduction to medical-surgical nursing* (4th ed.). Philadelphia: Saunders.

Monahan, F., Sands, J., Neighbors, M., Marek, J., & Green, C. (2007). *Phipps' medical-surgical nursing: Health and illness perspectives* (8th ed.). Louis: Mosby.

Pagana, K., & Pagana, T. (2005). *Mosby's diagnostic and laboratory test reference* (7th ed.). St. Louis: Mosby.

CHAPTER

43

Antineoplastic Medications

I. ANTINEOPLASTIC MEDICATIONS

A. Description
   1. Antineoplastic medications kill or inhibit the reproduction of neoplastic cells
   2. Antineoplastic medications are used to cure, increase survival time, and decrease life-threatening complications
   3. The effect of antineoplastic medications may not be limited to neoplastic cells; normal cells are also affected by the medication
   4. Cell cycle phase–specific medications affect cells only during a certain phase of the reproductive cycle (Figure 43-1)
   5. Cell cycle phase–nonspecific medications affect cells during any phase of the reproductive cycle (see Figure 43-1)
   6. Usually several medications are used in combination to increase the therapeutic response
   7. Antineoplastic medications may be combined with other treatments, such as surgery and radiation
   8. Although the intravenous (IV) route is the most common for administration, antineoplastic medications may be given by the oral, intra-arterial, isolated limb perfusion, and intracavitary routes; dosing is typically based on the client's body surface area (BSA) and the type of **cancer**
   9. Chemotherapy dosing is usually based on total BSA; calculating this measurement requires a current and accurate height and weight before each medication administration to ensure that the client receives the optimal doses of the chemotherapy medications
   10. Side effects result from the effects of the antineoplastic medication on normal cells

B. Side effects
   1. Mucositis
   2. Alopecia
   3. Anorexia, nausea, and vomiting
   4. Diarrhea
   5. Anemia
   6. Low white blood cell count (neutropenia)
   7. Thrombocytopenia
   8. Infertility and sexual alterations

C. Interventions
   1. Physiological Integrity
      a. Monitor the complete blood count (CBC), the white blood cell count, the platelet count, and the electrolyte levels
      b. Initiate bleeding precautions if thrombocytopenia occurs
      c. When the platelet count is less than 50,000 cells/mm^3, minor trauma can lead to episodes of prolonged bleeding; when it is less than 20,000 cells/mm^3, spontaneous and uncontrollable bleeding can occur
      d. Monitor for petechiae, ecchymosis, bleeding of the gums, and nosebleeds, because the decreased platelet count can precipitate bleeding tendencies
      e. Avoid intramuscular injections and venipunctures as much as possible to prevent bleeding
      f. Initiate neutropenic precautions if the white blood cell count decreases
      g. Monitor for fever, sore throat, unusual bleeding, and signs and symptoms of infection
      h. Inform the client that loss of appetite may also be the result of taste changes or a bitter taste in the mouth from the medications
      i. Monitor for nausea and vomiting, and provide a high-calorie diet with protein supplements
      j. Administer antiemetics several hours before chemotherapy and for 12 to 48 hours after, as prescribed, because antineoplastic medications stimulate the vomiting center in the brain; delayed nausea and vomiting can continue for as long as 7 days
      k. Encourage hydration; IV fluids will be administered before and during therapy
      l. Promote a fluid intake of at least 2000 mL per day to maintain adequate renal function

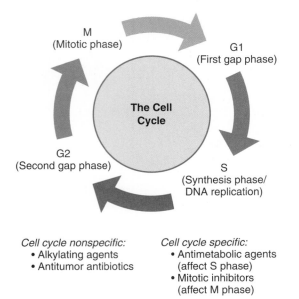

FIG. 43-1 The cell cycle. *G1*, the cell is preparing for division. *S* (synthesis phase/DNA replication), the cell doubles its DNA content through DNA synthesis. *G2*, the cell produces proteins to be used in cell division and in normal physiologic function after cell division is complete. *M* (mitotic phase), the single cell splits apart into two cells. (Created by Ellen Matthews. Legend by Linda Silvestri)

m. Administer allopurinol (Zyloprim), as prescribed, to lower the serum uric acid that occurs as a result of the rapid destruction of cells by the antineoplastic medications

2. Safe and Effective Care Environment

a. Prepare IV chemotherapy in an air-vented space (e.g., biohazard cabinet area)

b. Wear gloves, a gown, eye protectors, and a mask when handling IV medications

c. Nurses who are pregnant should consider avoiding chemotherapy preparation or the administration of IV chemotherapy

d. Discard IV equipment in designated (biohazard) containers

e. Administer the antineoplastic medication precisely as prescribed to maximize the antineoplastic effects while allowing normal cells to recover

f. Monitor for phlebitis with IV administration, because these medications may irritate the veins

g. Monitor for extravasation (the leakage of medication into the surrounding skin and subcutaneous tissue), which causes tissue necrosis; notify the registered nurse or physician if this occurs; heat or ice is applied, depending on the medication, and an antidote may be injected into the site

3. Psychosocial Integrity

a. Instruct the client regarding the potential for hair loss; inform him or her that varying degrees of hair loss may occur after the first or second treatment

b. Discuss the purchase of a wig before treatment starts

c. Inform the client that new hair growth will occur several months after the final treatment

d. Instruct the client about the need for contraception, because these medications have teratogenic effects

e. Discuss the potential effects of infertility, which may be irreversible

f. Encourage pretreatment counseling

4. Health Promotion and Maintenance

a. Instruct the client that if diarrhea is a problem, avoid hot foods and high-fiber foods, which increase peristalsis

b. Instruct the client to frequently inspect the oral mucosa for erythema and ulcers, to rinse the mouth after meals, and to perform good oral hygiene

c. Instruct the client to use saline or sodium bicarbonate mouth rinses for mouth sores, if necessary

d. Instruct the client in the use of antifungal medications for mouth sores, if they are prescribed, for the development of a fungal superinfection

e. Instruct the client to avoid crowds and persons with infections and to report signs of infection such as a low-grade fever, chills, or sore throat

f. Instruct individuals with colds or infections to wear a mask when visiting or to avoid visiting the client

g. Instruct the client to use a soft toothbrush and an electric razor to minimize the risk of bleeding

h. Instruct the client to avoid aspirin-containing products to minimize the risk of bleeding

i. Instruct the client to avoid alcohol to minimize the risk of toxicity

j. Instruct the client to consult the physician before receiving vaccinations; live vaccines should not be administered

D. Anaphylactic reactions

1. Precautions

a. Obtain an allergy history

b. Administer a test dose, when prescribed by the physician

c. Stay with the client during the administration of the medication

d. Monitor the vital signs

e. Have emergency equipment and medications readily available

f. Ensure that an IV line is available for the administration of emergency medications, if needed

2. Signs of anaphylactic reaction
   a. Dyspnea
   b. Chest tightness or pain
   c. Pruritus or urticaria
   d. Tachycardia
   e. Dizziness
   f. Anxiety or agitation
   g. Flushed appearance
   h. Hypotension
   i. Decreased sensorium
   j. Cyanosis
3. Interventions for an anaphylactic reaction
   a. Stop the medication
   b. Maintain the airway
   c. Notify the physician
   d. Maintain the IV access with 0.9% normal saline
   e. Place the client in a supine position with the legs elevated, if not contraindicated
   f. Monitor the vital signs
   g. Administer prescribed emergency medications.

II. ALKYLATING MEDICATIONS (Box 43-1)

A. Description
   1. These medications break the DNA helix, thereby interfering with DNA replication
   2. They are cell cycle phase–nonspecific medications
B. Side effects
   1. Anorexia, nausea, and vomiting may occur
   2. Stomatitis may occur
   3. Rash may occur
   4. Client may feel IV site pain during IV administration
   5. Busulfan (Myleran, Busulfex) may cause hyperuricemia
   6. Chlorambucil (Leukeran) and mechlorethamine (Mustargen) may cause gonadal suppression and hyperuricemia
   7. Cisplatin (Platinol) may cause ototoxicity, tinnitus, hypokalemia, hypocalcemia, hypomagnesemia, and nephrotoxicity
   8. Cyclophosphamide (Cytoxan, Neosar) may cause alopecia, gonadal suppression, hemorrhagic cystitis, and hematuria
C. Interventions
   1. Assess the vital signs and the temperature for signs of infection
   2. Monitor the CBC, the white blood cell count, the platelet count, and the uric acid and electrolyte levels
   3. Withhold the medication if the platelet count is less than 75,000 cells/L or the neutrophil count is less than 2000 cells/L; notify the registered nurse and the physician (this may vary, depending on the alkylating agent and agency policy)
   4. Assess the results of pulmonary function tests

BOX 43-1 **Alkylating Medications**

Nitrogen Mustards
- Chlorambucil (Leukeran)
- Cyclophosphamide (Cytoxan, Neosar)
- Ifosfamide (Ifex)
- Mechlorethamine (Mustargen)
- Melphalan (Alkeran)

Nitrosoureas
- Carmustine (BiCNU, Gliadel)
- Lomustine (CeeNU)
- Streptozocin (Zanosar)

Alkylating-Like Medications
- Altretamine (Hexalen)
- Busulfan (Myleran, Busulfex)
- Carboplatin (Paraplatin)
- Cisplatin (Platinol)
- Dacarbazine (DTIC-Dome)
- Oxaliplatin (Eloxatin)
- Temozolomide (Temodar)
- Thiotepa (Thioplex)

---

5. Assess the results of chest radiographs and renal and liver function studies
6. Hydrate the client with IV and oral fluids before administering the antineoplastic medication, as prescribed
7. Administer an antiemetic 30 to 60 minutes before the antineoplastic medication, as prescribed
8. Reduce IV site pain by altering IV rates, diluting the medication, or warming the injection site to distend the vein and increase blood flow, as prescribed
9. Monitor the IV site for irritation and phlebitis, and change the site, as needed.
10. When administering cisplatin (Platinol), assess the client for dizziness, tinnitus, hearing loss, incoordination, and numbness or tingling of the extremities
11. Monitor for signs of hemorrhagic cystitis, such as hematuria or dysuria, during cyclophosphamide (Cytoxan, Neosar) or ifosfamide (Ifex) therapy; encourage the client to drink increased fluids (2 to 3 L per day)
12. Mesna (Mesnex) may be administered with ifosfamide (Ifex) to reduce the potential of ifosfamide-induced cystitis
13. Instruct the client that cyclophosphamide (Cytoxan, Neosar), when prescribed orally, is administered without food
14. Instruct the client to follow a diet low in purine to alkalize urine and lower uric acid blood levels
15. Instruct the client regarding how to avoid infection
16. Instruct the client to report signs of infection or bleeding
17. Instruct the client about good oral hygiene and the use of a soft toothbrush

III. ANTITUMOR ANTIBIOTIC MEDICATIONS
   (Box 43-2)
   A. Description
      1. Interfere with DNA and RNA synthesis
      2. Cell cycle phase–nonspecific medications
   B. Side effects
      1. Nausea and vomiting
      2. Fever
      3. Bone marrow depression
      4. Rash
      5. Alopecia
      6. Stomatitis
      7. Gonadal suppression
      8. Hyperuricemia
      9. Vesication (blistering of tissue at the IV site)
     10. Plicamycin (Mithracin) affects bleeding time
     11. Daunorubicin (DaunoXome) may cause congestive heart failure and dysrhythmias
     12. Doxorubicin (Adriamycin, Doxil) and idarubicin (Idamycin) may cause cardiotoxicity, cardiomyopathy, and electrocardiographic changes; Dexrazoxane (Zinecard) may be administered with doxorubicin to reduce cardiomyopathy
     13. Pulmonary toxicity can occur with bleomycin (Blenoxane)
   C. Interventions
      1. Assess the vital signs and temperature for signs of infection
      2. Monitor the CBC, the white blood cell count, the platelet count, the uric acid level, the bleeding time, and electrolyte levels
      3. Withhold the medication if the platelet count is less than 75,000 cells/L or the neutrophil count is less than 2000 cells/L; notify the registered nurse and physician (this may vary, depending on the alkylating agent and agency policy)
      4. Assess the results of pulmonary function tests
      5. Monitor for electrocardiographic changes
      6. Assess the lung sounds for crackles
      7. Assess for signs of congestive heart failure, including dyspnea, crackles, peripheral edema, and weight gain
      8. Assess the results of chest radiographs and renal and liver function studies
      9. Hydrate the client with IV and/or oral fluids before the antineoplastic medication

     10. Administer an antiemetic 30 to 60 minutes before the antineoplastic medication
     11. Reduce IV site pain by altering IV rates, diluting the medication, or warming the injection site to distend the vein and increase blood flow, as prescribed
     12. Monitor the IV site for irritation, phlebitis, and vesication, and change the site, as needed
     13. Assess for myocardial toxicity, dyspnea, dysrhythmias, hypotension, and weight gain when administering doxorubicin (Adriamycin, Doxil) or idarubicin (Idamycin)
     14. Monitor the pulmonary status when administering bleomycin (Blenoxane)
     15. Avoid the use of aspirin, anticoagulants, and thrombolytic agents with plicamycin (Mithracin)

IV. ANTIMETABOLITE MEDICATIONS (Box 43-3)
   A. Description
      1. Antimetabolite medications halt the synthesis of cell protein; as "counterfeit" metabolites, their presence impairs cell division
      2. Antimetabolite medications replace the normal proteins required for DNA synthesis
      3. Antimetabolite medications are cell cycle phase–specific; they affect the S phase
   B. Side effects
      1. Anorexia, nausea, and vomiting
      2. Diarrhea
      3. Alopecia
      4. Stomatitis
      5. Depression of the bone marrow
      6. Cytarabine (Cytosar-U, DepoCyt, Tarabine PFS) may cause alopecia, stomatitis, hyperuricemia, and hepatotoxicity
      7. Fluorouracil (Adrucil) may cause alopecia, stomatitis, diarrhea, phototoxicity reactions, and cerebellar dysfunction
      8. Mercaptopurine (Purinethol) may cause hyperuricemia and hepatotoxicity
      9. Methotrexate may cause alopecia, stomatitis, hyperuricemia, photosensitivity, hepatotoxicity, and hematological, gastrointestinal, and skin toxicity

---

BOX 43-2 **Antitumor Antibiotic Medications**

- Bleomycin sulfate (Blenoxane)
- Dactinomycin (Cosmegen)
- Daunorubicin (DaunoXome)
- Doxorubicin (Adriamycin, Doxil)
- Epirubicin (Ellence)
- Idarubicin (Idamycin)
- Mitomycin (Mutamycin)
- Mitoxantrone (Novantrone)
- Plicamycin (Mithracin)

BOX 43-3 **Antimetabolite Medications**

- Capecitabine (Xeloda)
- Cladribine (Leustatin)
- Cytarabine (Cytosar-U, DepoCyt, Tarabine PFS)
- Floxuridine (FUDR)
- Fludarabine (Fludara)
- Fluorouracil (Adrucil)
- Gemcitabine (Gemzar)
- Hydroxyurea (Hydrea, Mylocel)
- Mercaptopurine (Purinethol)
- Methotrexate (Rheumatrex, Trexall)
- Pentostatin (Nipent)
- Thioguanine (Tabloid)

C. Interventions
1. Monitor the vital signs and temperature for signs of infection
2. Assess the CBC, the white blood cell count, the uric acid level, and the platelet count
3. Hold the medication if the neutrophil count is less than 2000 cells/L or the platelet count is less than 75,000 cells/L; notify the registered nurse and physician (this may vary depending on the alkylating agent and agency policy)
4. Monitor the renal function studies
5. Monitor for cerebellar dysfunction
6. Assess for photosensitivity
7. Administer antiemetics 30 to 60 minutes before the antineoplastic medication, as prescribed
8. Monitor the IV site for extravasation
9. Encourage a fluid intake of 2 to 3 L per day
10. Encourage good oral hygiene
11. Instruct the client regarding how to avoid infections and bleeding
12. When administering fluorouracil (Adrucil), assess for signs of cerebellar dysfunction, such as dizziness, weakness, and ataxia; assess for stomatitis and diarrhea, which may necessitate medication discontinuation
13. When administering methotrexate in large doses, prepare to administer leucovorin (folinic acid or citrovorum factor), as prescribed, to prevent toxicity (also called leucovorin rescue).
14. When administering fluorouracil (Adrucil) or methotrexate, instruct the client to use sunscreen and to wear protective clothing to prevent photosensitivity reactions

V. ANTIMITOTIC MEDICATIONS (VINCA ALKALOIDS) (Box 43-4)
A. Description
1. Mitotic inhibitors prevent mitosis (cell division), thus causing cell death
2. Mitotic inhibitors are cell cycle phase–specific and act during the M phase
B. Side effects
1. Leukopenia
2. Neurotoxicity with vincristine (Oncovin, Vincasar), which is manifested as numbness and tingling in the fingers and toes, constipation, and paralytic ileus

3. Ptosis
4. Hoarseness
5. Motor instability
6. Anorexia, nausea, and vomiting
7. Constipation
8. Peripheral neuropathy
9. Alopecia
10. Stomatitis
11. Hyperuricemia
12. Phlebitis at the IV site
C. Interventions
1. Monitor the vital signs
2. Monitor the white blood cell count, the CBC, the uric acid level, and the platelet count
3. Monitor for hoarseness.
4. Assess the eyes for ptosis
5. Assess the client's motor stability and initiate safety precautions, as necessary
6. Monitor for neurotoxicity with vincristine sulfate (Oncovin, Vincasar), which is manifested as numbness and tingling in the fingers and toes
7. Monitor for constipation and paralytic ileus

VI. TOPOISOMERASE INHIBITORS (Box 43-5)
A. Description
1. These drugs block the enzyme needed for DNA synthesis and cell division
2. They are cell cycle phase–specific and act during the G2 and S phases
B. Side effects
1. Leukopenia, thrombocytopenia, and anemia
2. Anorexia, nausea, and vomiting
3. Diarrhea
4. Alopecia
5. Orthostatic hypotension
6. Hypersensitivity reaction
C. Interventions
1. Monitor the vital signs
2. Monitor the white blood cell count, the CBC, and the platelet count

VII. HORMONAL MEDICATIONS AND ENZYMES (Box 43-6)
A. Description
1. Suppress the immune system and block the normal hormones in the hormone-sensitive tumors
2. Change the hormonal balance and slow the growth rates of certain tumors

---

BOX 43-4 **Mitotic Inhibitors**

Vinca Alkaloids
- Vinblastine sulfate (Velban)
- Vincristine sulfate (Oncovin, Vincasar)
- Vinorelbine (Navelbine)

Taxanes
- Docetaxel (Taxotere)
- Paclitaxel (Abraxane, Taxol, Onxol)

BOX 43-5 **Topoisomerase Inhibitors**

- Etoposide (VePesid, Toposar, Etopophos)
- Irinotecan (Camptosar)
- Teniposide (Vumon)
- Topotecan (Hycamtin)

BOX 43-6 **Hormonal Medications and Enzymes**

Estrogens
- Diethylstilbestrol
- Estramustine (Emcyt)
- Ethinyl estradiol (Estinyl)

Antiestrogens
- Anastrozole (Arimidex)
- Exemestane (Aromasin)
- Fulvestrant (Faslodex)
- Letrozole (Femara)
- Raloxifene (Evista)
- Tamoxifen citrate (Nolvadex)
- Testolactone (Teslac)
- Toremifene (Fareston)

Androgens
- Fluoxymesterone (Halotestin)
- Testosterone

Antiandrogens
- Bicalutamide (Casodex)
- Flutamide (Eulexin)
- Goserelin acetate (Zoladex)
- Nilutamide (Nilandron)
- Triptorelin (Trelstar)

Progestins
- Medroxyprogesterone (Depo-Provera)
- Megestrol acetate (Megace)

Other Hormonal Antagonists and Enzymes
- Aminoglutethimide (Cytadren)
- Asparaginase (Elspar)
- Leuprolide acetate (Lupron)
- Mitotane (Lysodren)

BOX 43-7 **Immunomodulator Agents**

- Aldesleukin (Proleukin, interleukin-2)
- Interferon alfa-2a
- Interferon alfa-2b
- Interferon alfa-n3 (Alferon N)
- Levamisole (Ergamisole)
- Recombinant interferon-α-2b (Intron A)
- Recombinant interferon-α-2a (Roferon-A)

Common Monoclonal Antibodies
- Alemtuzumab (Campath)
- Gemtuzumab ozogamicin (Mylotarg)
- Ibritumomab (Zevalin)
- Rituximab (Rituxan)
- Trastuzumab (Herceptin)

B. Side effects
1. Anorexia, nausea, and vomiting
2. Leukopenia
3. Impaired pancreatic function with asparaginase (Elspar)
4. Sex-characteristic alterations
   a. Masculinizing effects in women: chest and facial hair develop, and menses stops (androgens and antiestrogen receptor drugs)
   b. Feminine manifestations in men: gynecomastia (estrogens, progestins, or antiestrogen receptors)
5. Breast swelling
6. Hot flashes
7. Weight gain
8. Hemorrhagic cystitis, hypouricemia, and hypercholesterolemia, with mitotane (Lysodren)
9. Hypertension
10. Thromboembolytic disorders
11. Edema
12. Electrolyte imbalances
13. Tamoxifen citrate (Nolvadex) may cause edema, hypercalcemia, and elevated cholesterol and triglyceride levels
14. Tamoxifen citrate decreases the effects of estrogen
15. Diethylstilbestrol may cause impotence and gynecomastia in men
16. Diethylstilbestrol may alter the effects of insulin, orally administered anticoagulants, and orally administered hypoglycemic agents

C. Interventions
1. Monitor the vital signs
2. Assess the medications that the client is currently taking
3. Monitor the serum calcium levels with androgens
4. Monitor for signs of alterations in sexual characteristics
5. Monitor pancreatic function with asparaginase (Elspar)
6. Encourage an oral intake of 2 to 3 L of fluid per day
7. Monitor the uric acid and cholesterol levels
8. Monitor for signs of hemorrhagic cystitis

VIII. **IMMUNOMODULATOR AGENTS: BIOLOGICAL RESPONSE MODIFIERS** (Box 43-7)

A. Description
1. Immunomodulators stimulate the immune system to recognize **cancer** cells and to take action to eliminate or destroy them
2. Interleukins help different immune system cells to recognize and destroy abnormal body cells
3. Interferons slow down tumor cell division, stimulate proliferation, and cause **cancer** cells to differentiate into nonproliferative forms

B. Colony-stimulating factors induce more rapid bone-marrow recovery after suppression by chemotherapy (Box 43-8)

IX. **GENE THERAPY**

A. Description
1. Gene therapy is experimental, but early response rates indicate a potential for this therapy
2. Gene therapy is used to render tumor cells more susceptible to damage by other treatments and to make the client's immune system better able to recognize **cancer** cells as nonself

Colony-Stimulating Factors

Granulocyte-Macrophage Colony-Stimulating Factor
- Sargramostim (Leukine, Prokine)

Granulocyte Colony-Stimulating Factor
- Filgrastim (Neupogen)

Erythropoietin
- Epoetin alfa (Epogen)
- Darbepoetin (Aranesp)

BOX 43-9 **Other Antineoplastic Medications**
- Asparaginase (Elspar)
- Arsenic trioxide (Trisenox)
- Bexarotene (Targretin)
- Bortezomib (Velcade)
- Imatinib (Gleevec)
- Procarbazine (Natulan)
- Temozolomide (Temodar)

X. TARGETED THERAPY
A. Description
  1. Medications used as targeted therapies are either monoclonal antibodies that "target" a cellular element of the **cancer** cell or "antisense" medications that work at the gene level
  2. Some examples of monoclonal antibodies are rituximab (Rituxan), tositumomab (Bexxar), trastuzumab (Herceptin), alemtuzumab (Campath), and cetuximab (Erbitux)
B. Side effects: Allergic reactions (monoclonal antibodies)

XI. OTHER ANTINEOPLASTIC MEDICATIONS
(Box 43-9)
A. Altretamine (Hexalen): A cytotoxic agent used to treat ovarian **cancer**
B. Denileukin diftitox (Ontak): A recombinant DNA–derived medication used to treat cutaneous T-cell **lymphoma**
C. Gemcitabine (Gemzar): FDA approved to treat non–small cell lung **cancer,** adenocarcinoma of the pancreas, metastatic breast **cancer,** and lung **cancer** (in combination with paclitaxel [Abraxane, Taxol, Onxol])
D. Irinotecan (Camptosar): Used to treat colorectal or rectal **cancer**
E. Paclitaxel (Abraxane, Taxol, Onxol): Used to treat ovarian or metastatic breast **cancer**
F. Pegaspargase (Oncaspar): Used in combination chemotherapies for acute lymphoblastic leukemia for clients who are unable to take asparaginase (Elspar)
G. Topotecan (Hycamtin): Indicated for the treatment of relapsed or refractory metastatic ovarian **cancer** after other therapies have failed
H. Trastuzumab (Herceptin): Used in combination chemotherapy to treat breast **cancer**
I. Tretinoin (Vesanoid): Used to treat acute promyelocytic leukemia
J. Bexarotene (Targretin): Use to treat advanced-stage cutaneous T-cell **lymphoma**

PRACTICE QUESTIONS
More questions on the companion CD!

493. A nurse is instructed to initiate bleeding precautions for a client who is receiving an antineoplastic medication intravenously. The nurse reviews the laboratory results and would expect to note which of the following?
    1. A clotting time of 10 minutes
    2. An ammonia level of 20 mcg/dL
    3. A platelet count of 70,000 cells/μL
    4. A white blood cell (WBC) of 5000 cells/μL

494. A nurse is caring for a client who is receiving an intravenous (IV) infusion of an antineoplastic medication. During the infusion, the client complains of pain at the insertion site. During an inspection of the site, the nurse notes redness and swelling and that the rate of infusion of the medication has slowed. The nurse takes which appropriate action?
    1. Notify the registered nurse.
    2. Administer pain medication to reduce the discomfort.
    3. Apply ice and maintain the infusion rate, as prescribed.
    4. Elevate the extremity of the IV site, and slow the infusion.

495. A client with leukemia is receiving busulfan (Myleran). Allopurinol (Zyloprim) is prescribed for the client. The nurse administers the allopurinol, knowing that its purpose is to prevent:
    1. Diarrhea
    2. Stomatitis
    3. Gouty arthritis
    4. Hyperuricemia

496. A nurse is providing medication instructions to a client with breast cancer who will be taking cyclophosphamide (Cytoxan). Which of the following would the nurse include in the instructions?
    1. Take the medication with food.
    2. Increase the fluid intake to 2000 to 3000 mL/day.
    3. Decrease the sodium intake while taking the medication.
    4. Increase the potassium intake while taking the medication.

497. A nurse is assigned to care for a client with non-Hodgkin's lymphoma who is receiving

daunorubicin (Cerubidine). Which of the following signs would indicate to the nurse that the client is experiencing a toxic effect related to the medication?
1. Fever
2. Dyspnea
3. Diarrhea
4. Nausea and vomiting

498. A nurse who has been assigned to care for a client with testicular cancer who is receiving plicamycin (Mithracin) is preparing to administer the prescribed daily medications to the client. The nurse would question which of the following medications if it was noted on the client's medication record?
1. Warfarin (Coumadin)
2. Ondansetron (Zofran)
3. Allopurinol (Zyloprim)
4. Acetaminophen (Tylenol)

499. A client with squamous cell carcinoma of the larynx is receiving bleomycin sulfate (Blenoxane) intravenously. The nurse anticipates that which diagnostic study will be prescribed for this client?
1. Echocardiography
2. Electrocardiography
3. Cervical x-ray studies
4. Pulmonary function studies

500. Cytarabine hydrochloride is prescribed for the client with acute lymphocytic leukemia. The nurse plans care, knowing that this is a:
1. Hormone medication
2. Cell cycle phase–specific medication
3. Cell cycle phase–nonspecific medication
4. A medication that affects cells during any phase of the reproductive cycle

501. The nurse is assisting in the preparation of a teaching plan for a client who is receiving an antineoplastic medication. The nurse suggests including which of the following in the plan of care?
1. Be sure to receive the influenza and pneumonia vaccines.
2. Drink beverages that contain alcohol in moderate amounts.
3. Consult with the physician before receiving immunizations.
4. Take aspirin (acetylsalicylic acid), as needed, for headaches.

502. A client with ovarian cancer is being treated with vincristine sulfate (Oncovin). The nurse who is caring for the client monitors for which side effect that is specific to this medication?
1. Diarrhea
2. Hair loss
3. Chest pain
4. Numbness and tingling in the fingers and toes

503. Asparaginase (Elspar), which is an antineoplastic agent, is prescribed for a client. The nurse who has been assigned to care for the client collects data from the client. The nurse would report which of the following conditions, with which the administration of asparaginase is contraindicated?
1. Pancreatitis
2. Diabetes mellitus
3. Myocardial infarction
4. Chronic obstructive pulmonary disease

504. The client with metastatic breast cancer is receiving tamoxifen (Nolvadex). The nurse who is assigned to care for the client monitors for signs of which of the following during therapy with this medication?
1. Weight loss
2. Leukocytosis
3. Hypotension
4. Hypercalcemia

505. Megestrol acetate (Megace), which is an antineoplastic medication, is prescribed for a client with metastatic endometrial carcinoma. The nurse who has been assigned to the client collects data regarding the client's medical history. The nurse would report which of the following conditions, which requires caution with the administration of megestrol acetate?
1. Gout
2. Asthma
3. Thrombophlebitis
4. Myocardial infarction

506. A client with acute myelocytic leukemia is being treated with busulfan (Myleran). The nurse monitors for signs of which of the following, which specifically occurs as a result of the administration of this medication?
1. Renal failure
2. Hyperkalemia
3. Hyperglycemia
4. Congestive heart failure

ALTERNATE ITEM FORMAT: MULTIPLE RESPONSE

507. A nurse is assisting with caring for a client with cancer who is receiving cisplatin (Platinol). Select the toxic effects that the nurse monitors for and that are associated with this medication. Select all that apply.
☑ 1. Tinnitus
☐ 2. Ototoxicity
☐ 3. Hyperkalemia
☐ 4. Hypercalcemia
☑ 5. Nephrotoxicity
☑ 6. Hypomagnesemia

ANSWERS

493. 3

Rationale: Bleeding precautions need to be initiated when the platelet count drops. Bleeding precautions include avoiding all trauma (e.g., rectal temperatures, injections). The normal platelet count is 150,000 to 450,000 cells/mm^3, and the normal WBC count is 5000 to 10,000/mm^3. When the WBC count drops, neutropenic precautions need to be implemented. The normal clotting time is 8 to 15 minutes, and the normal ammonia value is 15 to 45 mcg/dL.

Test-Taking Strategy: Use the process of elimination and your knowledge regarding normal laboratory values. Options 1, 2, and 4 identify normal laboratory values. Remember, correlate a low platelet count with the need for bleeding precautions and a low WBC count with the need for neutropenic precautions. Review these normal laboratory values if you had difficulty with this question.

Level of Cognitive Ability: Analysis
Client Needs: Safe and Effective Care Environment
Integrated Process: Nursing Process/Data Collection
Content Area: Pharmacology
Reference: Lilley, L., Harrington, S., & Snyder, J. (2007). *Pharmacology and the nursing process* (5th ed., pp. 758, 761). St. Louis: Mosby.

494. 1

Rationale: When antineoplastic medications are administered via IV, great care must be taken to prevent the medication from escaping into the tissues surrounding the injection site, because pain, tissue damage, and necrosis can result. The nurse monitors for signs of extravasation, such as redness or swelling at the insertion site and a decreased infusion rate. If extravasation occurs, the registered nurse needs to be notified; he or she will then contact the physician.

Test-Taking Strategy: Use the process of elimination, and focus on the data in the question. Eliminate options 3 and 4 first. The nurse would not slow the IV rate, and the nurse would not be able to maintain the prescribed rate in this situation. Administering pain medication to reduce discomfort at an IV site is not an appropriate action. Further investigation of the cause of the discomfort is required. This leaves option 1 as the correct nursing action. Review the care of the client who is receiving IV chemotherapy if you had difficulty with this question.

Level of Cognitive Ability: Application
Client Needs: Physiological Integrity
Integrated Process: Nursing Process/Implementation
Content Area: Pharmacology
Reference: Lilley, L., Harrington, S., & Snyder, J. (2007). *Pharmacology and the nursing process* (5th ed., pp. 743-745, 753). St. Louis: Mosby.

495. 4

Rationale: Busulfan is as alkylating medication that is used for the treatment of acute myelocytic leukemia and for the palliative treatment of chronic myelogenous leukemia. Hyperuricemia can result from the use of this medication, and may produce uric acid nephropathy, renal stones, and acute renal failure. Allopurinol, which is an antigout medication, is used with chemotherapy to prevent or treat hyperuricemia. It may be prescribed for use in mouthwash after fluorouracil (Adrucil) therapy to prevent stomatitis. Allopurinol is not used to prevent diarrhea.

Test-Taking Strategy: Knowledge regarding the side effects associated with busulfan and the purpose of administering allopurinol during the administration of an antineoplastic medication is needed to answer this question. Recalling that allopurinol is an antigout medication and that it is used to prevent increased uric acid levels will direct you to the correct option. Review busulfan and allopurinol if you had difficulty with this question.

Level of Cognitive Ability: Application
Client Needs: Physiological Integrity
Integrated Process: Nursing Process/Implementation
Content Area: Pharmacology
Reference: Mosby. (2008). *2008 Mosby's nursing drug reference* (21st ed., pp. 99-100, 204-206). St. Louis: Mosby.

496. 2

Rationale: Hemorrhagic cystitis is a toxic effect that can occur with the use of cyclophosphamide. The client needs to be instructed to drink copious amounts of fluid during the administration of this medication. Clients should also monitor the urine output for hematuria. The medication should be taken on an empty stomach, unless gastrointestinal upset occurs. Hyperkalemia can result from the use of the medication; therefore, the client would not be encouraged to increase the potassium intake. The client would not be instructed to alter his or her sodium intake.

Test-Taking Strategy: Use the process of elimination. Correlate cyclophosphamide with hemorrhagic cystitis; this will direct you to option 2. Review the toxic effects associated with cyclophosphamide if you had difficulty with this question.

Level of Cognitive Ability: Application
Client Needs: Physiological Integrity
Integrated Process: Teaching and Learning
Content Area: Pharmacology
Reference: Kee, J., Hayes, E., & McCuistion, L. (2006). *Pharmacology: A nursing process approach* (5th ed., p. 537). Philadelphia: Saunders.

497. 2

Rationale: Cardiotoxicity and/or cardiomyopathy manifested as congestive heart failure (CHF) is a toxic effect of daunorubicin. Bone marrow depression is also a toxic effect. Nausea and vomiting are frequent side effects associated with the medication that begin a few hours after administration and that last for 24 to 48 hours. Fever is a frequent side effect, and diarrhea can also occasionally occur.

Test-Taking Strategy: Use the process of elimination, and keep in mind that the question is asking for a toxic effect; this concept should direct you to the option of addressing a sign of CHF. Additionally, the correct option presents the most serious concern. Review the toxic effects associated with daunorubicin if you had difficulty with this question.

Level of Cognitive Ability: Analysis
Client Needs: Physiological Integrity
Integrated Process: Nursing Process/Data Collection
Content Area: Pharmacology
Reference: Kee, J., Hayes, E., & McCuistion, L. (2006). *Pharmacology: A nursing process approach* (5th ed., pp. 544, 546). Philadelphia: Saunders.

498. 1
Rationale: Plicamycin is an antitumor and antibiotic agent. Because plicamycin affects the bleeding time, the use of aspirin, anticoagulants, and thrombolytic agents should be avoided. Warfarin is an anticoagulant, and the risk of hemorrhage is increased if it is administered during plicamycin therapy. Allopurinol, which is an antigout medication, may be used with chemotherapy to prevent or treat hyperuricemia secondary to blood dyscrasias caused by cancer chemotherapy. Acetaminophen may be used to treat mild discomfort. Ondansetron is an antiemetic that is used to prevent or treat nausea and vomiting during chemotherapy.
Test-Taking Strategy: Focus on the subject, the medication that the nurse would question. Remember that plicamycin affects the bleeding time. Review plicamycin and the other medications identified in the options if you had difficulty with this question.
Level of Cognitive Ability: Analysis
Client Needs: Physiological Integrity
Integrated Process: Nursing Process/Implementation
Content Area: Pharmacology
Reference: Kee, J., Hayes, E., & McCuistion, L. (2006). *Pharmacology: A nursing process approach* (5th ed., p. 542). Philadelphia: Saunders.

499. 4
Rationale: Bleomycin sulfate is an antineoplastic medication that can cause interstitial pneumonitis, which can progress to pulmonary fibrosis. Pulmonary function studies—along with hematologic, hepatic, and renal function tests—need to be monitored. The nurse needs to monitor for dyspnea, which may indicate pulmonary toxicity. The medication will be discontinued immediately if pulmonary toxicity occurs.
Test-Taking Strategy: Use the process of elimination. Eliminate options 1 and 2 first, because they are comparable or alike and are both cardiac-related. From the remaining options, select option 4, because it relates to the airway. Review the toxic effects of bleomycin sulfate if you had difficulty with this question.
Level of Cognitive Ability: Analysis
Client Needs: Physiological Integrity
Integrated Process: Nursing Process/Planning
Content Area: Pharmacology
Reference: Gahart, B., & Nazareno, A. (2006) *Intravenous medications* (22nd ed., pp. 185-186). St. Louis: Mosby.

500. 2
Rationale: Cytarabine is an antimetabolite, and antimetabolites are classified as cell cycle phase–specific. Alkylating medications affect all phases of the cell reproductive cycle. Hormone medications suppress the immune system and block the normal hormones in hormone-sensitive tumors.
Test-Taking Strategy: Use the process of elimination. Eliminate options 3 and 4 first, because they are comparable or alike. From the remaining options, recalling that this medication is an antimetabolite will direct you to the correct option. Review the action of cytarabine if you had difficulty with this question.
Level of Cognitive Ability: Application
Client Needs: Physiological Integrity
Integrated Process: Nursing Process/Planning

Content Area: Pharmacology
Reference: Mosby. (2008). *2008 Mosby's nursing drug reference* (21st ed., p. 320). St. Louis: Mosby.

501. 3
Rationale: Because antineoplastic medications lower the body's resistance, clients must be informed not to receive immunizations or vaccines without a physician's approval. Aspirin and aspirin-containing products need to be avoided to minimize the risk of bleeding. Alcohol needs to be avoided to minimize the risk of toxicity.
Test-Taking Strategy: Use the general guidelines related to medication administration. Also, remembering that antineoplastic medications lower the body's resistance will direct you to option 3. Review client teaching points regarding antineoplastic medications if you had difficulty with this question.
Level of Cognitive Ability: Application
Client Needs: Health Promotion and Maintenance
Integrated Process: Nursing Process/Planning
Content Area: Pharmacology
References: Kee, J., Hayes, E., & McCuistion, L. (2006). *Pharmacology: A nursing process approach* (5th ed., p. 537). Philadelphia: Saunders.
Lilley, L., Harrington, S., & Snyder, J. (2007). *Pharmacology and the nursing process* (5th ed., p. 731). St. Louis: Mosby.

502. 4
Rationale: A side effect that is specific to vincristine sulfate is peripheral neuropathy, which occurs in nearly every client. This can be manifested as numbness and tingling in the fingers and toes. Constipation rather than diarrhea is more likely to occur with this medication, although diarrhea may occur occasionally. Hair loss occurs with nearly all of the antineoplastic medications. Chest pain is unrelated to this medication.
Test-Taking Strategy: Use the process of elimination. Eliminate options 1 and 2 first, because these side effects are associated with many of the antineoplastic agents. Next, note that the question asks for the side effect that is "specific" to vincristine. Correlate peripheral neuropathy with this medication. Review the side effects of vincristine if you had difficulty with this question.
Level of Cognitive Ability: Analysis
Client Needs: Physiological Integrity
Integrated Process: Nursing Process/Data Collection
Content Area: Pharmacology
Reference: Lehne, R. (2007). *Pharmacology for nursing care* (6th ed., p. 1168). Philadelphia: Saunders.

503. 1
Rationale: Asparaginase is contraindicated if hypersensitivity exists, among clients with pancreatitis, or if the client has a history of pancreatitis. The medication impairs pancreatic function, and pancreatic function tests should be performed before therapy begins and when a week or more has elapsed between the administration of the doses. The client needs to be monitored for signs of pancreatitis, which include nausea, vomiting, and abdominal pain.
Test-Taking Strategy: Focus on the name of the medication and remember that asparaginase is contraindicated in pancreatitis or if the client has a history of pancreatitis. Review asparaginase if you had difficulty with this question.

Level of Cognitive Ability: Analysis
Client Needs: Physiological Integrity
Integrated Process: Nursing Process/Implementation
Content Area: Pharmacology
Reference: Lehne, R. (2007). *Pharmacology for nursing care* (6th ed., p. 1170). Philadelphia: Saunders.

504. **4**
Rationale: Tamoxifen may increase calcium, cholesterol, and triglyceride levels. The nurse should monitor for hypercalcemia while the client is taking this medication. Signs of hypercalcemia include increased urine volume, excessive thirst, nausea, vomiting, constipation, hypotonicity of the muscles, and deep bone or flank pain. Leukopenia, weight gain, and hypertension are most likely to occur.
Test-Taking Strategy: Focus on the name of the medication and remember that tamoxifen can increase the calcium level. Review tamoxifen if you had difficulty with this question.
Level of Cognitive Ability: Analysis
Client Needs: Physiological Integrity
Integrated Process: Nursing Process/Data Collection
Content Area: Pharmacology
Reference: Stidmore-Roth, L. (2008). *2008 Mosby's nursing drug reference* (21st ed., p. 963). St. Louis: Mosby.

505. **3**
Rationale: Megestrol acetate suppresses the release of luteinizing hormone from the anterior pituitary by inhibiting pituitary function and regressing tumor size. It is used with caution if the client has a history of thrombophlebitis. Options 1, 2 and 4 are not a concern.
Test-Taking Strategy: Focus on the name of the medication and recall that megastrol acetate is used with caution in a clinet with thrombophlebitis. Review megestrol acetate if you had difficulty with this question.
Level of Cognitive Ability: Application
Client Needs: Physiological Integrity
Integrated Process: Nursing Process/Implementation
Content Area: Pharmacology
Reference: Skidmore-Roth, L. (2008). *2008 Mosby's nursing drug reference* (21st ed., p. 645). St. Louis: Mosby.

506. **1**
Rationale: Busulfan can cause an increase in the uric acid level. Hyperuricemia can produce uric acid nephropathy, renal stones, and acute renal failure. Options 2, 3, and 4 are unrelated to the administration of this medication.
Test-Taking Strategy: Focus on the name of the medication. Recalling that busulfan causes hyperuricemia will direct you to option 1. Review the effects of busulfan if you had difficulty with this question.
Level of Cognitive Ability: Analysis
Client Needs: Physiological Integrity
Integrated Process: Nursing Process/Data Collection
Content Area: Pharmacology
Reference: Skidmore-Roth, L. (2008). *2008 Mosby's nursing drug reference* (21st ed., p. 205). St. Louis: Mosby.

ALTERNATE ITEM FORMAT: MULTIPLE RESPONSE

507. **1, 2, 5, 6**
Rationale: Cisplatin is an alkylating medication. Alkylating medications are cell cycle phase–nonspecific medications that affect the synthesis of DNA by causing the cross-linking of DNA to inhibit cell reproduction. Cisplatin may cause ototoxicity, tinnitus, hypokalemia, hypocalcemia, hypomagnesemia, and nephrotoxicity. Amifostine (Ethyol) may be administered before cisplatin to reduce the potential for renal toxicity.
Test-Taking Strategy: Note that cisplatin is an antineoplastic medication. Recall that most antineoplastic medications affect the bone marrow and the hematological system. This concept will assist you with determining that "hypo-" rather than "hyper-" conditions would occur. In addition, recall that this medication affects the ears (ototoxicity and tinnitus) and the kidneys (nephrotoxicity). Review the toxic effects of cisplatin if you had difficulty with this question.
Level of Cognitive Ability: Analysis
Client Needs: Physiological Integrity
Integrated Process: Nursing Process/Data Collection
Content Area: Pharmacology
Reference: Mosby. (2008). *2008 Mosby's nursing drug reference* (21st ed., pp. 277-278). St. Louis: Mosby.

REFERENCES

Gahart, B., & Nazareno, A. (2006). *Intravenous medications* (22nd ed.). St. Louis: Mosby.

Kee, J., Hayes, E., & McCuistion, L. (2006). *Pharmacology: A nursing process approach* (5th ed.). Philadelphia: Saunders.

Lehne, R. (2007). *Pharmacology for nursing care* (6th ed.). Philadelphia: Saunders.

Lilley, L., Harrington, S., & Snyder, J. (2007). *Pharmacology and the nursing process* (5th ed.). St. Louis: Mosby.

Skidmore-Roth, L. (2008). *2008 Mosby's nursing drug reference* (21st ed.). St. Louis: Mosby.

The Adult Client With an Endocrine Disorder

PYRAMID TERMS

addisonian crisis A life-threatening disorder caused by adrenal hormone insufficiency. It is precipitated by infection, trauma, stress, or surgery. Death can occur from shock, vascular collapse, or hyperkalemia.

Addison's disease The hyposecretion of adrenal cortex hormones (glucocorticoids and mineralocorticoids) from the adrenal gland that results in a deficiency of the steroid hormones. The condition is fatal if left untreated.

adrenalectomy The surgical removal of an adrenal gland. The lifelong replacement of glucocorticoids and mineralocorticoids is necessary with a bilateral adrenalectomy. Temporary replacement may be necessary for up to 2 years for a unilateral adrenalectomy.

Chvostek's sign A spasm of the facial muscles elicited by tapping the facial nerve just anterior to the ear. It is noted in clients with hypocalcemia.

Cushing's syndrome A condition that results from the hypersecretion of glucocorticoids from the adrenal cortex.

dawn phenomenon A condition that results from a nocturnal release of growth hormone, which may cause blood glucose level elevations before breakfast. Treatment includes administering an evening dose of intermediate-acting insulin at 10:00 PM.

diabetes insipidus The hyposecretion of antidiuretic hormone from the posterior pituitary gland, which results in the failure of the tubular reabsorption of water in the kidneys.

diabetes mellitus A chronic disorder of glucose intolerance and impaired carbohydrate, protein, and lipid metabolism caused by a deficiency of insulin or resistance to the action of insulin. A deficiency of effective insulin results in hyperglycemia.

diabetic ketoacidosis A life-threatening complication of diabetes mellitus that develops when a severe insulin deficiency occurs. Hyperglycemia progresses to ketoacidosis over a period of several hours to several days. It occurs in clients with type 1 diabetes mellitus, individuals with undiagnosed diabetes, and persons who stop taking the prescribed treatment for diabetes.

hyperglycemia An elevated blood glucose level.

hyperglycemic hyperosmolar nonketotic syndrome Extreme hyperglycemia without acidosis. It is a complication of type 2 diabetes mellitus, which may result in dehydration or vascular collapse. The onset is usually slow, taking from hours to days.

hyperthyroidism A condition that occurs as a result of excessive thyroid hormone secretion.

hypoglycemia A low blood glucose level (<60 mg/dL) that results from too much insulin, not enough food, or excess activity.

hypophysectomy The removal of the pituitary gland.

myxedema (hypothyroidism) A hypothyroid state that results from the hyposecretion of thyroid hormone. The condition occurs during adulthood.

myxedema coma A rare but serious disorder that results from the persistently low production of thyroid hormones. It can be precipitated by acute illness, the rapid withdrawal of thyroid medication, anesthesia, surgery, hypothermia, and the use of sedatives and opioids.

Somogyi phenomenon A rebound phenomenon that occurs in clients with type 1 diabetes mellitus. Normal or elevated blood glucose levels are present at bedtime, and hypoglycemia occurs at about 2:00 AM to 3:00 AM. Counterregulatory hormones, which are produced to prevent further hypoglycemia, result in hyperglycemia; this is evident in the prebreakfast blood glucose level. Treatment includes decreasing the evening (predinner or bedtime) dose of intermediate-acting insulin or increasing the bedtime snack.

thyroid storm An acute, potentially fatal exacerbation of hyperthyroidism. It may result from the manipulation of the thyroid gland during surgery, severe infection, or stress.

thyroidectomy The surgical removal of the thyroid gland to treat persistent hyperthyroidism or thyroid tumors.

Trousseau's sign A sign of hypocalcemia. Carpal spasm can be elicited by compressing the brachial artery with a blood pressure cuff for 3 minutes.

PYRAMID TO SUCCESS

The endocrine system is made up of organs or glands that secrete hormones and release them directly into the circulation. The endocrine system can be easily understood if you remember that basically one of two situations can occur: either the hypersecretion or the hyposecretion of hormones from the organ or gland. When an excess of the hormone occurs, treatment is aimed at blocking the hormone release through medication or surgery. When a deficit of the hormone exists, treatment is aimed at replacement therapy. The pyramid points focus on diabetes mellitus, including the prevention and treatment of complications, insulin therapy, hypoglycemic and hyperglycemic reactions, and diabetic ketoacidosis; Addison's disease and addisonian crisis; Cushing's syndrome; thyroid disorders and thyroid storm; and care of the client after thyroidectomy or adrenalectomy. The Integrated Processes addressed in this unit include Caring, the Clinical Problem-Solving Process (Nursing Process), Communication and Documentation, and Teaching and Learning.

▲ CLIENT NEEDS

Safe and Effective Care Environment

Acting as a client advocate
Collaborating with a multidisciplinary team regarding treatment
Consulting with appropriate care providers
Delegating care activities to others
Establishing priorities of care
Handling hazardous and infectious materials
Obtaining informed consent for treatments and procedures
Maintaining confidentiality related to the disorder
Preventing accidents and client injury
Using medical and surgical asepsis to prevent infection

Health Promotion and Maintenance

Discussing expected body-image changes
Identifying lifestyle choices related to treatment
Performing data collection techniques related to the endocrine system
Preventing disease
Providing health screening
Teaching about self-care measures

Psychosocial Integrity

Discussing grief and loss issues related to complications of the disorder
Discussing situational role changes related to the disorder
Discussing unexpected body-image changes
Identifying coping mechanisms
Monitoring for sensory/perceptual alterations as a result of the disorder
Making use of support systems

Physiological Integrity

Administering medications safely
Monitoring for alterations in body systems as a result of the disorder

Monitoring for expected outcomes/effects of pharmacological therapy
Monitoring for fluid and electrolyte imbalances that can occur
Monitoring the laboratory values
Monitoring for potential complications of diagnostic tests, treatments, and procedures
Monitoring for potential complications from surgical procedures and health alterations
Monitoring for problems with elimination as a result of the disorder
Monitoring for unexpected responses to therapies
Performing dosage calculations related to medication administration
Preparing the client for diagnostic tests
Providing nonpharmacological comfort interventions
Providing nutrition and oral hydration measures
Providing emergency care to the client

REFERENCES

American Diabetic Association. (2006). *Standards of medical care in diabetes—2006*. care.diabetesjournals.org/cgi/content/full/29/suppl_1/s4. Accessed August 6, 2008.

Black, J., & Hawks, J. (2005). *Medical-surgical nursing: Clinical management for positive outcomes* (7th ed.). Philadelphia: Saunders.

Chernecky, C., & Berger, B. (2008). *Laboratory tests and diagnostic procedures* (5th ed.). Philadelphia: Saunders.

Christensen, B., & Kockrow, E. (2006). *Adult health nursing* (5th ed.). St. Louis: Mosby.

Christensen, B., & Kockrow, E. (2006). *Foundations of nursing* (5th ed.). St. Louis: Mosby.

deWit, S. (2009). *Medical-surgical nursing: Concepts & practice*. Philadelphia: Saunders.

Hodgson, B., & Kizior, R. (2008). *Saunders nursing drug handbook 2008*. Philadelphia: Saunders.

Ignatavicius, D., & Workman, M. (2006). *Medical-surgical nursing: Critical thinking for collaborative care* (5th ed.). Philadelphia: Saunders.

Kee, J., Hayes, E., & McCuistion, L. (2006). *Pharmacology: A nursing process approach* (5th ed.). Philadelphia: Saunders.

Lehne, R. (2007). *Pharmacology for nursing care* (6th ed.). Philadelphia: Saunders.

Lewis, S., Heitkemper, M., Dirksen, S., & Bucher, L. (2007). *Medical-surgical nursing: Assessment and management of clinical problems* (7th ed.). St. Louis: Mosby.

Linton, A. (2007). *Introduction to medical-surgical nursing* (4th ed.). Philadelphia: Saunders.

McKenry, L., Tessier, E., & Hogan, M. (2006). *Mosby's pharmacology in nursing* (22nd ed.). St. Louis: Mosby.

Monahan, F., Sands, J., Marek, J., Neighbors, M., & Green, C. (2007). *Phipps' medical-surgical nursing: Health and illness perspectives* (8th ed.). St. Louis: Mosby.

National Council of State Boards of Nursing (Eds.). (2008). *2008 Detailed Test Plan for the NCLEX-PN® Examination, National Council of State Boards of Nursing*. Chicago: Author.

National Council of State Boards of Nursing. *NCSBN home page*. www.ncsbn.org. Accessed August 6, 2008.

Perry, A., & Potter, P. (2006). *Clinical nursing skills & techniques* (6th ed.). St. Louis: Mosby.

Skidmore-Roth, L. (2008). *2008 Mosby's nursing drug reference* (21st ed.). St. Louis: Mosby.

CHAPTER 44

Endocrine System

I. ANATOMY AND PHYSIOLOGY OF THE ENDOCRINE GLANDS (Box 44-1)
- A. Functions (Box 44-2)
  1. Maintenance and regulation of vital functions
  2. Response to stress and injury
  3. Growth and development
  4. Energy metabolism
  5. Reproduction
  6. Fluid, electrolyte, and acid-base balance
- B. Hypothalamus (Box 44-3)
  1. A portion of the diencephalon of the brain that forms the floor and part of the lateral wall of the third ventricle
  2. Activates, controls, and integrates the peripheral autonomic nervous system, the endocrine processes, and many somatic functions, such as body temperature, sleep, and appetite
- C. Pituitary gland (Box 44-4 and Figure 44-1)
  1. The master gland; located at the base of the brain
  2. Influenced by the hypothalamus; directly affects the function of the other endocrine glands
  3. Promotes the growth of body tissue, influences water absorption by the kidney, and controls sexual development and function
- D. Adrenal gland
  1. One adrenal gland is on top of each kidney
  2. Regulates sodium and electrolyte balance; affects carbohydrate, fat, and protein metabolism; influences the development of sexual characteristics; and sustains the "fight-or-flight" response
  3. Adrenal cortex
     a. The outer shell of the adrenal gland
     b. Synthesizes glucocorticoids and mineralocorticoids; secretes small amounts of sex hormones (i.e., androgens and estrogens; Box 44-5)
  4. Adrenal medulla
     a. The inner core of the adrenal gland
     b. Works as part of the sympathetic nervous system; produces epinephrine and norepinephrine
- E. Thyroid gland
  1. Located in the anterior part of the neck
  2. Controls the rate of body metabolism and growth; produces thyroxine (T_4), triiodothyronine (T_3), and thyrocalcitonin
- F. Parathyroid glands
  1. Located on the thyroid gland
  2. Control calcium and phosphorus metabolism; produce parathyroid hormone
- G. Pancreas
  1. Located posterior to the stomach
  2. Influences carbohydrate metabolism; indirectly influences fat and protein metabolism; and produces insulin and glucagon
- H. Ovaries and testes
  1. The ovaries are located in the pelvic cavity and produce estrogen and progesterone
  2. The testes are located in the scrotum; they control the development of the secondary sex characteristics and produce testosterone
- I. Negative feedback loop
  1. Regulates hormone secretion by the hypothalamus and the pituitary gland
  2. Increased amounts of target gland hormones in the bloodstream decrease the secretion of the same hormones and other hormones that stimulate their release

II. DIAGNOSTIC TESTS
- A. Stimulation and suppression tests
  1. Stimulation testing
     a. For the client with suspected underactivity of an endocrine gland, a stimulus may be provided to determine whether the gland is capable of normal hormone production.
     b. Measured amounts of selected hormones or substances are administered to stimulate the target gland to produce its hormone
     c. Hormone levels produced by the target gland are measured
     d. The failure of the hormone level to increase with stimulation indicates hypofunction

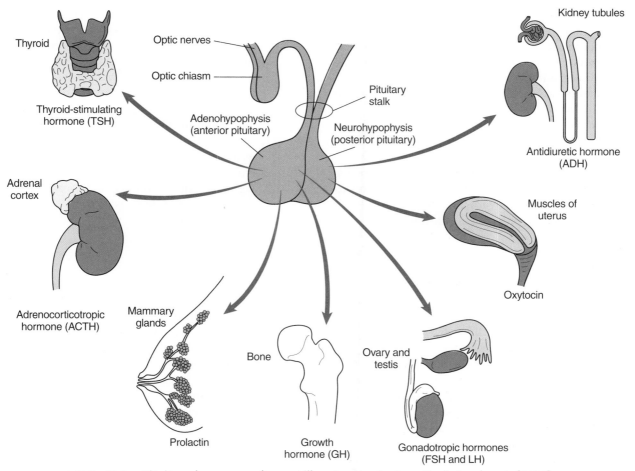

FIG. 44-1 Pituitary hormones. (From Lilley, L., Harrington, S., & Snyder, J. [2005]. *Pharmacology and the nursing process* [4th ed.]. St. Louis: Mosby.)

BOX 44-5 **Adrenal Cortex**

Glucocorticoids: Cortisol, Cortisone, and Corticosterone
Responsible for glucose metabolism, protein metabolism, fluid and electrolyte balance, the suppression of the inflammatory response to injury, the protective immune response to invasion by infectious agents, and resistance to stress
Mineralocorticoids: Aldosterone
Regulate electrolyte balance by promoting sodium retention and potassium excretion

2. Suppression tests
   a. Suppression tests are used when hormone levels are high or in the upper range of normal
   b. Agents that normally induce a suppressed response are administered to determine whether normal negative feedback is intact
   c. The failure of hormone production to be suppressed during standardized testing indicates hyperfunction
B. Radioactive iodine uptake
   1. This thyroid function test measures the absorption of the iodine isotope to determine how the thyroid gland is functioning
   2. A small dose of radioactive iodine is given by mouth or by the intravenous (IV) route; the amount of radioactivity is measured in 2 to 4 hours and again at 24 hours
   3. Normal values are 3% to 10% at 2 to 4 hours and 5% to 30% at 24 hours
   4. Elevated values indicate **hyperthyroidism,** decreased iodine intake, or increased iodine excretion
   5. Decreased values indicate a low T_4 level, the use of antithyroid medications, thyroiditis, **myxedema,** or **hypothyroidism**
   6. The test is contraindicated during pregnancy
C. T_3 and T_4 resin uptake test
   1. Blood tests are used to diagnose thyroid disorders
   2. T_3 and T_4 regulate thyroid-stimulating hormone
   3. Normal values (normal findings vary between laboratory settings)
      a. T_3: 80 to 230 ng/dL
      b. T_4: 5 to 12 mcg/dL
      c. Thyroxine, free (FT_4): 0.8 to 2.4 ng/dL
   4. The T_3 is elevated in **hyperthyroidism**; it decreases with the aging process and may be decreased in **hypothyroidism.**
   5. The T_4 is elevated in **hyperthyroidism** and decreased in **hypothyroidism**
D. Thyroid-stimulating hormone
   1. Blood test is used to differentiate the diagnosis of primary **hypothyroidism**

2. Normal value is 0.2 to 5.4 microunits/mL normal findings vary among laboratory settings
3. Elevated values indicate primary **hypothyroidism**
4. Decreased values indicate **hyperthyroidism** or secondary **hypothyroidism**
E. Thyroid scan
   1. A thyroid scan is performed to identify nodules or growths in the thyroid gland
   2. A radioisotope of iodine or technetium is administered before the scanning of the thyroid gland
   3. Reassure the client that the level of radioactive medication is not dangerous to the self or others
   4. Determine whether the client has received radiographic contrast agents within the past 3 months, because these may invalidate the scan
   5. Check with the physician regarding discontinuing medications that contain iodine for 14 days before the test and regarding the need to discontinue thyroid medication before the test
   6. Instruct the client to maintain nothing-by-mouth status after midnight on the day before the test; if iodine is used, the client will fast for an additional 45 minutes after the ingestion of the oral isotope, and the scan will be performed in 24 hours
   7. If technetium is used, it is administered by the IV route 30 minutes before the scan
   8. The test is contraindicated during pregnancy
F. Needle aspiration of thyroid tissue
   1. Aspiration of thyroid tissue is done for cytological examination
   2. No client preparation is necessary
   3. Light pressure is applied to the aspiration site after the procedure
G. Glucose tolerance test
   1. The glucose tolerance test aids in the diagnosis of **diabetes mellitus**
   2. A 2-hour post-load glucose level (2 hours after the injection or ingestion of glucose) greater than 200 mg/dL confirms the diagnosis of **diabetes mellitus**
   3. Client preparation (Box 44-6)
   4. Many factors can alter the results; therefore, this is not always a reliable test
H. Glycosylated hemoglobin
   1. Description
      a. Glycosylated hemoglobin is blood glucose that is bound to hemoglobin
      b. Glycosylated hemoglobin A (HbA_{1c}) is a reflection of how well the blood glucose levels have been controlled for the prior 3 to 4 months

BOX 44-6 Client Preparation: Glucose Tolerance Test

Eat a diet that includes at least 150 g of carbohydrates for 3 days before the test.
Avoid alcohol, coffee, and smoking for 36 hours before testing.
Fast for 10 to 12 hours before the test.
Avoid strenuous exercise for 8 hours before and after the test.
If you have diabetes mellitus, withhold the morning insulin or oral hypoglycemic medication.
A fasting blood glucose is drawn, and you will be given a high-glucose drink
Blood samples will be drawn at 30-minute intervals for a minimum of 2 hours

BOX 44-7 Disorders of the Pituitary Gland

Anterior Pituitary
• Hyperpituitarism
• Hypopituitarism

Posterior Pituitary
These disorders can be caused by damage to the posterior pituitary gland or the hypothalamus:
• Diabetes insipidus
• Syndrome of inappropriate antidiuretic hormone

---

c. **Hyperglycemia** in a client with **diabetes mellitus** is usually the cause of an increase in HbA$_{1c}$

2. Values
   a. Values are expressed as a percentage of the total hemoglobin
   b. The goal for clients with **diabetes mellitus** is 7% or less
   c. For clients without **diabetes mellitus,** the normal range is 4% to 6%

3. Nursing consideration: Fasting is not required

I. Glycosylated serum albumin (fructosamine)
   1. Reflects average serum glucose levels over a period of 2 to 3 weeks
   2. More sensitive to recent changes than the HbA$_{1c}$
   3. Normal ranges vary according to the method of testing used; for a nondiabetic client, the normal range is 1.5 to 2.7 mmol/L, and, for a diabetic client, it is 2.0 to 5.0 mmol/L

III. DISORDERS OF THE PITUITARY GLAND
   (Box 44-7)
A. Hypopituitarism
   1. Description: The hyposecretion of one or more of the pituitary hormones caused by tumors, trauma, encephalitis, autoimmunity, or stroke
   2. The hormones that are most often affected are growth hormone (GH) and the gonadotropins (luteinizing hormone and follicle-stimulating hormone), but thyroid-stimulating hormone (TSH), adrenocorticotropic hormone (ACTH), and antidiuretic hormone (ADH) may be involved
   3. Data collection
      a. Mild to moderate obesity (GH, TSH)
      b. Reduced cardiac output (GH, ADH)
      c. Infertility and sexual dysfunction (gonadotropins, ACTH)
      d. Fatigue and low blood pressure (TSH, ADH, ACTH, GH)

e. Tumors of the pituitary may also cause headaches and visual defects (the pituitary is located near the optic nerve)

4. Interventions
   a. Provide emotional support to the client and family
   b. Encourage the client and family to express feelings related to disturbed body image or sexual dysfunction
   c. Client may need hormone replacement for specific deficient hormones
   d. Client may require education regarding the signs and symptoms of both hypo- and hyperfunction related to insufficient or excess hormone replacement

B. Hyperpituitarism
   1. Description
      a. The hypersecretion of growth hormone by the anterior pituitary gland in an adult and is caused primarily by pituitary tumors
      b. Leads to conditions such as acromegaly and **Cushing's disease**
   2. Data collection
      a. Large hands and feet
      b. Thickening and protrusion of the jaw
      c. Arthritic changes
      d. Visual disturbances
      e. Diaphoresis
      f. Oily, rough skin
      g. Organomegaly
      h. Hypertension
      i. Dysphagia
      j. Deepening of the voice
   3. Interventions
      a. Provide emotional support to the client and family, and encourage the client and family to express feelings related to disturbed body image
      b. Provide frequent skin care
      c. Provide pharmacological and nonpharmacological interventions for joint pain
      d. Prepare the client for radiation of the pituitary gland, if prescribed
      e. Prepare the client for **hypophysectomy**, if planned

C. **Hypophysectomy** (pituitary adenectomy, transsphenoidal pituitary surgery)
   1. Description
      a. The removal of the pituitary tumor via craniotomy or via transsphenoidal (endoscopic transnasal) approach; the latter approach is preferred, because it is associated with fewer complications
      b. Complications of craniotomy include increased intracranial pressure, bleeding, meningitis, and hypopituitarism
      c. Complications of the transsphenoidal surgery include cerebrospinal fluid leak, infection, and hypopituitarism
   2. Postoperative interventions
      a. Initiate postoperative care similar to craniotomy care
      b. Monitor the vital signs, neurological status, and level of consciousness
      c. Elevate the head of the bed
      d. Monitor for increased intracranial pressure
      e. Monitor for bleeding
      f. Monitor for any postnasal drip or nasal drainage, which may indicate the leakage of cerebrospinal fluid after the transsphenoidal approach; check the nasal drainage for glucose
      g. Instruct the client to avoid sneezing, coughing, and blowing the nose
      h. Monitor electrolyte values for temporary **diabetes insipidus** or syndrome of inappropriate ADH as a result of ADH disturbances
      i. Monitor the intake and output (I&O), and avoid water intoxication
      j. Administer glucocorticoids and other hormone replacements, as prescribed
      k. Administer antibiotics, analgesics, and antipyretics, as prescribed
      l. Instruct the client regarding the administration of prescribed medications, which may include vasopressin (synthetic ADH), levothyroxine (Synthroid), gonadotropic hormones, growth hormone (somatotropin), and glucocorticoids if the entire gland was removed

D. **Diabetes insipidus**
   1. Description
      a. The hyposecretion of ADH caused by strokes, trauma, or idiopathic causes
      b. The kidney tubules fail to reabsorb water
   2. Data collection
      a. Polyuria of 4 to 24 L per day
      b. Polydipsia
      c. Dehydration (e.g., decreased skin turgor, dry mucous membranes)
      d. Inability to concentrate urine
      e. A low urinary specific gravity (1.006 or less)
      f. Fatigue
      g. Muscle pain and weakness
      h. Headache
      i. Postural hypotension that may progress to vascular collapse without rehydration
      j. Tachycardia
   3. Interventions
      a. Monitor the vital signs and the neurological and cardiovascular statuses
      b. Provide a safe environment, particularly for the client with postural hypotension
      c. Monitor the electrolyte values and for signs of dehydration
      d. Maintain the intake of adequate fluids
      e. Monitor the I&O, weight, serum osmolality, and specific gravity of urine
      f. Instruct the client to avoid foods or liquids that produce diuresis
      g. Chlorpropamide (Diabinese) may be prescribed for mild **diabetes insipidus**
      h. Vasopressin tannate (Pitressin) or desmopressin acetate (DDAVP, Stimate) may be prescribed; these are used when the ADH deficiency is severe or chronic
      i. Instruct the client regarding the administration of medications, as prescribed; DDAVP may be administered by injection, intranasally, or orally
      j. Instruct the client to wear a Medic-Alert bracelet

E. Syndrome of inappropriate antidiuretic hormone
   1. Description
      a. Excess ADH is released, but not in response to a bodily need for it
      b. Causes include trauma, stroke, malignancies (often in the lungs or pancreas), medications, and stress
      c. The syndrome results in water intoxication and hyponatremia
   2. Data collection
      a. Signs of fluid volume overload
      b. Changes in the level of consciousness and mental status changes
      c. Weight gain
      d. Hypertension
      e. Tachycardia
      f. Anorexia, nausea, and vomiting
      g. Hyponatremia
   3. Interventions
      a. Monitor the vital signs and the cardiac and neurological statuses
      b. Provide a safe environment, particularly for the client with changes in the level of consciousness or mental status
      c. Monitor the I&O and obtain a daily weight
      d. Monitor the fluid and electrolyte balance
      e. Monitor the serum and urine osmolality

f. Restrict fluid intake, as prescribed

g. Administer diuretics and IV fluids (normal saline or hypertonic saline), as prescribed; monitor IV fluids carefully because of the risk for fluid volume overload (IV solutions containing water are contraindicated because of the risk of water intoxication)

h. Demeclocycline (Declomycin) may be prescribed; it inhibits ADH-induced water reabsorption and produces water diuresis

IV. DISORDERS OF THE ADRENAL GLANDS (Box 44-8)

A. Addison's disease
1. Description
   a. Hyposecretion of adrenal cortex hormones (glucocorticoids and mineralocorticoids)
   b. Can be primary or secondary
   c. The condition is fatal if left untreated
2. Data collection (Table 44-1)
3. Interventions
   a. Monitor the vital signs, particularly blood pressure, weight, and I&O
   b. Monitor the blood glucose and potassium levels
   c. Administer glucocorticoid or mineralocorticoid medications, as prescribed
   d. Observe for addisonian crisis caused by stress, infection, trauma, or surgery
4. Client education
   a. Avoid individuals with infections
   b. Diet: High protein and carbohydrate intake; normal sodium intake
   c. Avoid strenuous exercise and stressful situations
   d. Need for lifelong glucocorticoid therapy
   e. Avoid over-the-counter medications
   f. Wear a Medic-Alert bracelet
   g. Signs and symptoms related to the under- and over-replacement of hormones

B. Addisonian crisis
1. Description (Box 44-9)
2. Data collection
   a. Severe headache
   b. Severe abdominal, leg, and lower back pain

c. Generalized weakness
d. Irritability and confusion
e. Severe hypotension
f. Shock
3. Interventions
   a. Prepare to administer IV glucocorticoids, as prescribed; hydrocortisone sodium succinate (Solu-Cortef) is usually prescribed initially
   b. After the resolution of the crisis, administer glucocorticoids and mineralocorticoids orally, as prescribed
   c. Monitor the vital signs, particularly blood pressure
   d. Monitor the neurological status, noting irritability and confusion
   e. Monitor the I&O

TABLE 44-1	Data Collection: Addison's Disease and Cushing's Disease (Cushing's Syndrome)
Addison's Disease	**Cushing's Disease and Syndrome**
Lethargy, fatigue, and muscle weakness	Generalized muscle wasting and weakness
Gastrointestinal disturbances	Moonface and buffalo hump
Weight loss	Truncal obesity with thin extremities, supraclavicular fat pads, and weight gain
Menstrual changes in women; impotence in men	Hirsutism (masculine characteristics in females)
Hypoglycemia and hyponatremia	Hyperglycemia and hypernatremia
Hyperkalemia and hypercalcemia	Hypokalemia and hypocalcemia
Postural hypotension	Hypertension
Hyperpigmentation of the skin (bronzed) with primary disease	Fragile skin that easily bruises
	Reddish-purple striae on the abdomen and upper thighs

BOX 44-8 Disorders of the Adrenal Glands

Adrenal Cortex
- Addison's disease
- Primary hyperaldosteronism (Conn's syndrome)
- Cushing's disease
- Cushing's syndrome

Adrenal Medulla
- Pheochromocytoma

BOX 44-9 Addisonian Crisis

- A life-threatening disorder caused by acute adrenal insufficiency
- Precipitated by stress, infection, trauma, surgery, or the abrupt withdrawal of exogenous corticosteroid use
- Can cause hyponatremia, hyperkalemia, hypoglycemia, and shock

f. Monitor the laboratory values, particularly sodium, potassium, and blood glucose

g. Administer IV fluids, as prescribed, to restore electrolyte balance

h. Protect the client from infection

i. Maintain the client on bedrest and provide a quiet environment

C. Cushing's disease and Cushing's syndrome (hypercortisolism)

1. Description

a. Characterized by a hypersecretion of glucocorticoids from the adrenal cortex

b. Cushing's disease is a metabolic disorder characterized by the abnormally increased secretion (endogenous) of adrenocortical steroids, particularly cortisol, caused by increased amounts of ACTH secreted by the pituitary gland

c. Cushing's syndrome is a metabolic disorder that results from the chronic and excessive production of cortisol by the adrenal cortex or from the administration of glucocorticoids in large doses for several weeks or longer (exogenous or iatrogenic)

2. Data collection (see Table 44-1)

3. Interventions

a. Monitor the vital signs, particularly blood pressure

b. Monitor the I&O and weight

c. Monitory the laboratory values, particularly the serum glucose level, the white blood cell count, and the sodium, potassium, and calcium levels

d. Provide good skin care

e. Allow the client to discuss feelings related to body appearance

f. Administer chemotherapeutic agents, as prescribed, for inoperable adrenal tumors

g. Prepare the client for radiation, as prescribed, if the condition results from a pituitary adenoma

h. Prepare the client for the removal of pituitary tumor (hypophysectomy, transsphenoidal adenectomy) if the condition results from the increased pituitary secretion of ACTH

i. Prepare the client for adrenalectomy if the condition results from an adrenal adenoma; glucocorticoid replacement may be required after adrenalectomy

D. Primary hyperaldosteronism (Conn's syndrome)

1. Description

a. A hypersecretion of mineralocorticoids (aldosterone) from the adrenal cortex of the adrenal gland

b. Most commonly caused by an adenoma

2. Data collection

a. Symptoms related to hypokalemia, hypernatremia, and hypertension

b. Headache, fatigue, muscle weakness, and nocturia

c. Polydipsia and polyuria

d. Paresthesias

e. Visual changes

f. Low urine specific gravity and increased urinary aldosterone

g. Elevated serum aldosterone levels

h. Metabolic alkalosis

3. Interventions

a. Monitor the vital signs, particularly blood pressure

b. Monitor for signs of hypokalemia and hypernatremia

c. Monitor the I&O and the urine for specific gravity

d. Spironolactone (Aldactone) may be prescribed to promote fluid balance and to control hypertension; the medication is a potassium-sparing diuretic and an aldosterone antagonist, and the client needs to be monitored for hyperkalemia, particularly in the presence of impaired renal function or excessive potassium intake

e. Administer potassium supplements, as prescribed

f. Prepare the client for adrenalectomy

g. Maintain sodium restriction preoperatively, if prescribed

h. Administer glucocorticoids preoperatively, as prescribed, to prevent adrenal hypofunction

i. Monitor the client for adrenal insufficiency postoperatively

j. Instruct the client regarding the need for glucocorticoid therapy after adrenalectomy

k. Instruct the client about the need to wear a Medic-Alert bracelet

E. Pheochromocytoma

1. Description

a. A catecholamine-producing tumor that is usually found in the adrenal medulla; extra-adrenal locations include the chest, bladder, abdomen, and brain; it is typically a benign tumor, but it can be malignant.

b. Excessive amounts of epinephrine and norepinephrine are secreted

c. Diagnostic tests include a 24-hour urine collection for vanillylmandelic acid (a product of catecholamine metabolism), metanephrine, and catecholamines, all of which are elevated in the presence of pheochromocytoma; the normal range of urinary catecholamines is up to 14 mcg/100 mL of urine, with higher levels occurring in clients with pheochromocytoma

    d. The surgical removal of the adrenal gland is the primary treatment

    e. Symptomatic treatment is initiated if surgical removal is not possible

    f. The complications associated with pheochromocytoma include hypertensive crisis including hypertensive retinopathy and nephropathy; cardiac enlargement and dysrhythmias; congestive heart failure; myocardial infarction; increased platelet aggregation; and brain attack (stroke)

    g. Death can occur from shock, cerebrovascular stroke, renal failure, dysrhythmias, or dissecting aortic aneurysm

  2. Data collection

    a. Paroxysmal or sustained hypertension

    b. Severe headaches

    c. Palpitations

    d. Flushing and profuse diaphoresis

    e. Pain in the chest or abdomen with nausea and vomiting

    f. Heat intolerance

    g. Weight loss

    h. Tremors

    i. Hyperglycemia

  3. Interventions

    a. Monitor the vital signs, particularly the blood pressure and heart rate

    b. Monitor for hypertensive crisis and for complications that can occur with hypertensive crisis, such as stroke, cardiac dysrhythmias, and myocardial infarction

    c. Be alert to stimuli that can precipitate a hypertensive crisis, such as increased abdominal pressure, urination, and vigorous abdominal palpation; avoid these stimuli

    d. Instruct the client not to smoke, drink caffeine-containing beverages, or change position suddenly

    e. Prepare to administer an α-adrenergic blocking agent (e.g., phenoxybenzamine [Dibenzyline]), as prescribed, to control hypertension

    f. Monitor the serum glucose level

    g. Promote rest and a nonstressful environment

    h. Provide a diet high in calories, vitamins, and minerals

    i. Prepare the client for adrenalectomy

F. Adrenalectomy

  1. Description (Box 44-10)

  2. Preoperative interventions

    a. Monitor the electrolytes and correct electrolyte imbalances

    b. Assess for dysrhythmias

BOX 44-10   **Adrenalectomy**

This procedure involves the surgical removal of an adrenal gland.

Lifelong glucocorticoid and mineralocorticoid replacement are necessary with a bilateral adrenalectomy.

Temporary glucocorticoid replacement for up to 2 years is necessary for a unilateral adrenalectomy.

Catecholamine levels drop as a result of surgery, which can result in cardiovascular collapse, hypotension, and shock; the client needs to be monitored closely.

Hemorrhage also can occur as a result of the high vascularity of the adrenal glands.

---

    c. Monitor for hyperglycemia

    d. Protect the client from infections

    e. Administer glucocorticoids, as prescribed

  3. Postoperative interventions

    a. Monitor the vital signs

    b. Monitor the I&O; if the urinary output is less that 30 mL/hour, notify the physician, because this may indicate renal failure and impending shock

    c. Monitor the weight daily

    d. Monitor the electrolyte and serum glucose levels

    e. Monitor for signs of shock and hemorrhage, particularly during the first 24 to 48 hours

    f. Monitor for manifestations of adrenal insufficiency

    g. Assess the dressing for drainage

    h. Monitor for paralytic ileus, which is manifested by abdominal distention and pain, nausea, vomiting, and diminished or absent bowel sounds; this condition can develop from internal bleeding, anesthesia effects, and bowel manipulation

    i. Administer IV fluids, as prescribed, to maintain blood volume

    j. Administer glucocorticoids and mineralocorticoids, as prescribed

    k. Administer pain medication, as prescribed

    l. Provide pulmonary interventions to prevent atelectasis (e.g., coughing, deep breathing, incentive spirometry, splinting of the incision)

    m. Instruct the client regarding the importance of hormone replacement therapy after surgery

    n. Instruct the client regarding the signs and symptoms of the under- and over-replacement of hormones

    o. Instruct the client regarding the need to wear a Medic-Alert bracelet

V. DISORDERS OF THE THYROID GLAND
(Box 44-11)

A. Hypothyroidism
1. Description
   a. A hypothyroid state that results from the hyposecretion of the thyroid hormones T_4 and T_3
   b. Characterized by a decreased rate of body metabolism
2. Data collection
   a. Lethargy and fatigue
   b. Weakness, muscle aches, and paresthesias
   c. Intolerance to cold
   d. Weight gain
   e. Dry skin and hair and loss of body hair
   f. Bradycardia
   g. Constipation
   h. Generalized puffiness and edema around the eyes and face (myxedema)
   i. Forgetfulness and loss of memory
   j. Menstrual disturbances
   k. Cardiac enlargement and the tendency to develop congestive heart failure
   l. Goiter may or may not be present
3. Interventions
   a. Monitor the vital signs, including heart rate and rhythm
   b. Administer thyroid replacement; levothyroxine sodium (Synthroid) is most commonly prescribed
   c. Instruct the client about thyroid replacement therapy and about the clinical manifestations of both hypo- and hyperthyroidism related to the under- or over-replacement of the hormone
   d. Instruct the client in a low-calorie, low-cholesterol, and low–saturated-fat diet
   e. Assess the client for constipation; provide roughage and fluids to prevent constipation
   f. Provide a warm environment for the client
   g. Avoid sedatives and opioid analgesics because of the client's increased sensitivity to these medications
   h. Monitor for the overdose of thyroid medications, which is characterized by tachycardia, chest pain, restlessness, nervousness, and insomnia
   i. Instruct the client to report episodes of chest pain or other signs of overdose immediately

---

BOX 44-11   **Disorders of the Thyroid Gland**

- Hyperthyroidism
- Hypothyroidism

B. Myxedema coma
1. Description (Box 44-12)
2. Data collection
   a. Hypotension
   b. Bradycardia
   c. Hypothermia
   d. Hyponatremia
   e. Hypoglycemia
   f. Generalized edema
   g. Respiratory failure
   h. Coma
3. Interventions
   a. Maintain a patent airway
   b. Administer IV fluids (normal or hypertonic saline), as prescribed
   c. Administer IV levothyroxine sodium (Synthroid), as prescribed
   d. Administer IV glucose, as prescribed
   e. Administer corticosteroids, as prescribed
   f. Assess the client's temperature hourly
   g. Monitor the blood pressure frequently
   h. Keep the client warm
   i. Monitor for changes in mental status
   j. Monitor the electrolyte and glucose levels
   k. Institute aspiration precautions

C. Hyperthyroidism
1. Description
   a. A hyperthyroid state that results from the hypersecretion of the thyroid hormones T_3 and T_4
   b. Characterized by an increased rate of body metabolism
   c. A common cause is Graves' disease, which is also known as toxic diffuse goiter
   d. Clinical manifestations are referred to as thyrotoxicosis
2. Data collection for hyperthyroidism caused by Graves' disease
   a. Enlarged thyroid gland (goiter)
   b. Palpitations and cardiac dysrhythmias, such as tachycardia or atrial fibrillation
   c. Protruding eyeballs (exophthalmos) are possibly present
   d. Hypertension
   e. Heat intolerance
   f. Diaphoresis
   g. Weight loss

BOX 44-12   **Myxedema Coma**

This is a rare but serious disorder that results from persistently low thyroid production.
Coma can be precipitated by acute illness, the rapid withdrawal of thyroid medication, anesthesia, surgery, hypothermia, or the use of sedatives and opioid analgesics.

h. Diarrhea
i. Smooth, soft skin and hair
j. Nervousness and fine tremors of the hands
k. Personality changes, such as irritability, agitation, and mood swings
3. Interventions
a. Provide adequate rest
b. Administer sedatives, as prescribed
c. Provide a cool and quiet environment
d. Obtain the weight daily
e. Provide a high-calorie diet
f. Avoid the administration of stimulants
g. Administer antithyroid medications (e.g., propylthiouracil) that block thyroid synthesis, as prescribed
h. Administer iodine preparations that inhibit the release of thyroid hormone, as prescribed
i. Administer propranolol (Inderal) for tachycardia, as prescribed
j. Prepare the client for radioactive iodine therapy, as prescribed, to destroy thyroid cells
k. Prepare the client for thyroidectomy, if prescribed
D. Thyroid storm
1. Description (Box 44-13)
2. Data collection
a. Elevated temperature (fever)
b. Tachycardia
c. Systolic hypertension
d. Nausea, vomiting, and diarrhea
e. Agitation, tremors, and anxiety
f. Irritability, agitation, restlessness, confusion, and seizures as the condition progresses
g. Delirium and coma
3. Interventions
a. Maintain a patent airway and adequate ventilation
b. Administer antithyroid medications, sodium iodide solution, propranolol (Inderal), and glucocorticoids, as prescribed
c. Monitor the vital signs
d. Monitor continually for cardiac dysrhythmias

e. Administer nonsalicylate antipyretics, as prescribed; (salicylates increase free thyroid hormone levels)
f. Use a cooling blanket to decrease the client's temperature, as prescribed
E. Thyroidectomy
1. Description
a. Removal of the thyroid gland
b. Performed when persistent hyperthyroidism exists
2. Preoperative interventions
a. Obtain the vital signs and weight
b. Assess the electrolyte levels
c. Assess for hyperglycemia
d. Instruct the client regarding how to perform coughing and deep-breathing exercises and how to support the neck during the postoperative period when coughing and moving
e. Administer antithyroid medications, sodium iodide solution, propranolol (Inderal), and glucocorticoids, as prescribed, to prevent the occurrence of thyroid storm
3. Postoperative interventions
a. Monitor for respiratory distress
b. Have a tracheotomy set, oxygen, and suction at the bedside
c. Maintain the client in a semi-Fowler's position
d. Monitor the surgical site for edema and signs of bleeding; check the dressing anteriorly and at the back of the neck
e. Limit client talking, and assess the level of hoarseness
f. Monitor for laryngeal nerve damage as evidenced by respiratory obstruction, dysphonia, high-pitched voice, stridor, dysphagia, and restlessness
g. Monitor for signs of hypocalcemia and tetany, which can be the result of trauma to the parathyroid gland (Box 44-14)
h. Prepare to administer calcium gluconate, as prescribed, for tetany
i. Monitor for thyroid storm

BOX 44-13 Thyroid Storm

Thyroid storm is an acute and life-threatening condition that occurs in a client with uncontrollable hyperthyroidism.
It can occur as a result of the manipulation of the thyroid gland during surgery and the release of thyroid hormone into the bloodstream; it also can occur as a result of severe infection and stress.
Antithyroid medications, β-blockers, glucocorticoids, and iodides are administered to the client before thyroid surgery to prevent its occurrence.

BOX 44-14 Signs of Tetany

- Cardiac dysrhythmias
- Carpopedal spasm
- Dysphagia
- Muscle and abdominal cramps
- Numbness and tingling of the face and extremities
- Positive Chvostek's sign
- Positive Trousseau's sign
- Visual disturbances (photophobia)
- Wheezing and dyspnea (bronchospasm, laryngospasm)
- Seizures

BOX 44-15   Disorders of the Parathyroid Gland

- Hyperparathyroidism
- Hypoparathyroidism

VI. DISORDERS OF THE PARATHYROID GLAND
    (Box 44-15)
  A. Hypoparathyroidism
    1. Description
      a. A condition caused by the hyposecretion of parathyroid hormone by the parathyroid gland
      b. Can occur after **thyroidectomy** because of the removal of parathyroid tissue
    2. Data collection
      a. Hypocalcemia and hyperphosphatemia
      b. Numbness and tingling in the face
      c. Muscle cramps and cramps in the abdomen or in the extremities
      d. Positive **Trousseau's sign** or **Chvostek's sign**
      e. Signs of overt tetany, such as bronchospasm, laryngospasm, carpopedal spasm, dysphagia, photophobia, cardiac dysrhythmias, and seizures
      f. Hypotension
      g. Anxiety, irritability, and depression
    3. Interventions
      a. Monitor the vital signs
      b. Monitor for signs of hypocalcemia and tetany
      c. Initiate seizure precautions
      d. Place a tracheotomy set, oxygen, and suctioning equipment at the bedside
      e. Prepare to administer IV calcium gluconate for hypocalcemia
      f. Provide a high-calcium, low-phosphorus diet
      g. Instruct the client regarding the administration of calcium supplements, as prescribed
      h. Instruct the client regarding the administration of vitamin D supplements, as prescribed; vitamin D enhances the absorption of calcium from the gastrointestinal tract
      i. Instruct the client regarding the administration of phosphate binders, as prescribed, to promote the excretion of phosphate through the gastrointestinal tract
      j. Instruct the client to wear a Medic-Alert bracelet
  B. Hyperparathyroidism
    1. Description: A condition caused by the hypersecretion of parathyroid hormone by the parathyroid gland
    2. Data collection
      a. Hypercalcemia and hypophosphatemia
      b. Fatigue and muscle weakness

      c. Skeletal pain and tenderness
      d. Bone deformities that result in pathological fractures
      e. Anorexia, nausea, vomiting, and epigastric pain
      f. Weight loss
      g. Constipation
      h. Hypertension
      i. Cardiac dysrhythmias
      j. Renal stones
    3. Interventions
      a. Monitor the vital signs, particularly the blood pressure
      b. Monitor for cardiac dysrhythmias
      c. Monitor the I&O and for signs of renal stones
      d. Monitor for skeletal pain; move the client slowly and carefully
      e. Encourage fluid intake
      f. Administer furosemide (Lasix), as prescribed, to lower calcium levels
      g. Administer IV normal saline, as prescribed, to maintain hydration
      h. Administer phosphates, as prescribed; they interfere with calcium resorption
      i. Administer calcitonin (Calcimar), as prescribed, to decrease skeletal calcium release and increase the renal clearance of calcium
      j. Monitor the calcium and phosphorus levels
      k. Notify the physician immediately if a precipitous drop in the calcium level occurs; assess for tingling and numbness in the face and extremities and for other signs of hypocalcemia
      l. Prepare the client for parathyroidectomy, as prescribed
  C. Parathyroidectomy
    1. Description: The removal of one or more of the parathyroid glands
    2. Preoperative interventions
      a. Monitor the electrolyte, calcium, phosphate, and magnesium levels
      b. Ensure that calcium levels are decreased to near normal
      c. Inform the client that talking may be painful for the first day or two after surgery
    3. Postoperative interventions
      a. Monitor for respiratory distress
      b. Place a tracheotomy set, oxygen, and suctioning equipment at the bedside
      c. Monitor the vital signs
      d. Position the client in a semi-Fowler's position
      e. Assess the neck dressing for bleeding
      f. Monitor for hypocalcemic crisis as evidenced by tingling and twitching in the extremities and face

g. Assess for positive **Trousseau's sign** or **Chvostek's sign**; these signal the potential for tetany

h. Monitor for changes in voice pattern and hoarseness

i. Monitor for laryngeal nerve damage

j. Instruct the client regarding the administration of calcium and vitamin D supplements, as prescribed

VII. DISORDERS OF THE PANCREAS

A. **Diabetes mellitus** (Box 44-16)

1. Description
   a. A chronic disorder of impaired carbohydrate, protein, and lipid metabolism that is caused by a deficiency of insulin
   b. An absolute or relative deficiency of insulin results in **hyperglycemia**
   c. Type 1 **diabetes mellitus** is a nearly absolute deficiency of insulin; if insulin is not given, fats are metabolized for energy, which results in ketonemia (acidosis)
   d. Type 2 **diabetes mellitus** is a relative lack of insulin or resistance to the action of insulin; insulin is usually sufficient to stabilize fat and protein metabolism but not to deal with carbohydrate metabolism; obesity is a major risk factor for type 2 **diabetes mellitus**
   e. Macrovascular complications include coronary artery disease, cardiomyopathy, hypertension, cerebrovascular disease, peripheral vascular disease, and infection
   f. Microvascular complications include retinopathy, nephropathy, and neuropathy

2. Data collection
   a. Polyuria, polydipsia, and polyphagia (more common with type 1 **diabetes mellitus**)
   b. **Hyperglycemia**
   c. Weight loss (common with type 1 **diabetes mellitus,** rare with type 2 **diabetes mellitus**)
   d. Blurred vision
   e. Slow wound healing
   f. Vaginal infections
   g. Weakness and paresthesias
   h. Signs of inadequate circulation to the feet
   i. Signs of accelerated atherosclerosis (renal, cerebral, cardiac, and peripheral)

3. Diet
   a. The total number of calories is individualized on the basis of the client's current or desired weight and the presence of other existing health problems
   b. Day-to-day consistency in timing and amount of food intake helps control the blood glucose level
   c. As prescribed by the physician, the client may be advised to follow the food exchange

---

BOX 44-16 **Major Types of Diabetes Mellitus**

Type 1: Primary β-cell destruction that leads to absolute insulin deficiency
Type 2: Ranges from insulin resistance with an insulin deficiency to secretory deficit with insulin resistance

---

from the American Diabetic Association diet or the dietary guidelines for Americans (MyPyramid) issued by the U.S. Departments of Agriculture and Health and Human Services

d. Carbohydrate counting may be a more simpler approach: it focuses on the total grams of carbohydrates eaten per meal; the client may be more compliant with carbohydrate counting, which results in better glycemic control and which is usually necessary for clients making use of intense insulin therapy

e. Incorporate the diet into individual client needs, lifestyle, and cultural and socioeconomic patterns

4. Exercise
   a. Exercise lowers the blood glucose level, encourages weight loss, reduces cardiovascular risks, improves circulation and muscle tone, decreases total cholesterol and triglyceride levels, and decreases insulin resistance and glucose intolerance
   b. Instruct the client regarding dietary adjustments when exercising; dietary adjustments are individualized
   c. Instruct the client to monitor the blood glucose level before exercising; if the client plans to participate in extended periods of exercise, blood glucose levels should be checked before, during, and after the exercise period
   d. If the client requires extra food during exercise to prevent **hypoglycemia,** it need not be deducted from the regular meal plan
   e. If the blood glucose level is greater than 250 mg/dL and urinary ketones are present in a client with type 1 **diabetes mellitus,** then the client is instructed not to exercise until the blood glucose is closer to normal and urinary ketones are absent

5. Oral hypoglycemic medications
   a. Oral medications are prescribed for clients with type 2 **diabetes mellitus** when diet and weight control therapy have failed to maintain satisfactory blood glucose levels
   b. Assess the client's knowledge of **diabetes mellitus** and the use of oral hypoglycemic agents

c. Assess the vital signs and blood glucose levels

d. Assess the medications that the client is currently taking

e. Aspirin, alcohol, sulfonamides, oral contraceptives, and monoamine oxidase inhibitors increase the hypoglycemic effect, thereby causing a decrease in blood glucose levels

f. Glucocorticoids, thiazide diuretics, and estrogen increase blood glucose levels

g. Teach the client to recognize symptoms of **hypoglycemia** and **hyperglycemia**

h. Teach the client to avoid over-the-counter medications, unless prescribed by the physician

i. Teach the client to avoid alcohol if taking sulfonylureas

j. Inform the client with type 2 **diabetes mellitus** that insulin may be needed during stress, surgery, or infection

k. Teach the client about the importance of compliance with the prescribed medication

l. Advise the client to wear a Medic-Alert bracelet

6. Insulin

a. Insulin is used to treat both type 1 and 2 **diabetes mellitus** when diet, weight-control therapy, and oral hypoglycemic agents have failed to maintain satisfactory blood glucose levels

b. Regular insulin is the only insulin that can be administered by IV for the emergency treatment of **diabetic ketoacidosis**

c. Aspirin, alcohol, oral anticoagulants, oral hypoglycemic medications, β-blockers, tricyclic antidepressants, tetracycline, and monoamine oxidase inhibitors increase the hypoglycemic effect of insulin, thus causing a further decrease in blood glucose levels

d. Glucocorticoids, thiazide diuretics, thyroid agents, oral contraceptives, and estrogen increase blood glucose levels

e. Illness, infection, and stress increase blood glucose levels and the need for insulin; insulin should not be withheld during illness, infection, or stress, because **hyperglycemia** and ketoacidosis can result

f. Instruct the client to recognize symptoms of **hypoglycemia** and **hyperglycemia**

g. The peak action time of insulin is important because of the possibility of hypoglycemic reactions occurring during that time

B. Complications of insulin therapy

1. Local allergic reactions

a. Redness, swelling, tenderness, and an induration or wheal at the site of injection may occur 1 to 2 hours after administration

b. Reactions usually occur during the early stages of insulin therapy

c. Instruct the client to cleanse the skin with alcohol before injection

2. Insulin lipodystrophy

a. Lipoatrophy is a loss of subcutaneous fat, and it appears as a slight dimpling or a more serious pitting of the subcutaneous fat; the use of human insulin helps to prevent this complication

b. Lipohypertrophy is the development of fibrous fatty masses at the injection site; it is caused by the repeated use of an injection site

c. Instruct the client to avoid injecting insulin into affected sites

d. Instruct the client about the importance of rotating insulin injections within one anatomic site

3. Insulin resistance

a. The client who is receiving insulin develops immune antibodies that bind the insulin, thereby decreasing the insulin available for use in the body

b. Treatment consists of administering a purer insulin preparation

c. Insulin resistance is also the term used for the lack of tissue sensitivity to the insulin from the body, which results in **hyperglycemia**

4. **Dawn phenomenon**

a. **Dawn phenomenon** results from reduced tissue sensitivity to insulin that develops between 5:00 AM and 8:00 AM (prebreakfast **hyperglycemia** occurs) and that may be caused by the nocturnal release of growth hormone

b. Treatment includes administering an evening dose (or increasing the amount of a current dose) of intermediate-acting insulin at 10:00 PM

5. **Somogyi phenomenon**

a. Normal or elevated blood glucose levels are present at bedtime; **hypoglycemia** occurs at 2:00 AM to 3:00 AM, which causes an increase in the production of counterregulatory hormones

b. By 7:00 AM, in response to the counterregulatory hormones, the blood glucose rebounds significantly to the hyperglycemic range

c. Treatment includes decreasing the evening (predinner or bedtime) dose of intermediate-acting insulin or increasing the bedtime snack

C. Insulin administration

1. See Chapter 45 for information about subcutaneous injections and mixing insulin

2. Insulin pens
   a. An insulin pen is a device that uses a small, prefilled insulin cartridge that is loaded into a pen-like holder; a disposable needle is attached to the device for injection, and the dosage is selected by dialing in the desired amount
   b. The client inserts the needle for injection, and the insulin is delivered by pushing a button
3. Jet injectors
   a. A jet injector is a device that delivers insulin through the skin under pressure in an extremely fine stream
   b. Insulin administered by this device is usually absorbed faster
   c. The injector can cause bruising at the site of insulin delivery
4. Insulin pumps
   a. Continuous subcutaneous insulin infusion is administered by an externally worn device that contains a syringe attached to a long, thin, narrow-lumen tube with a needle or Teflon catheter attached to the end
   b. The client inserts the needle or Teflon catheter into the subcutaneous tissue (usually on the abdomen) and secures it with tape or a transparent dressing; the pump is worn on a belt or in a pocket; the needle or Teflon catheter is changed at least every 3 days
   c. A continuous basal rate of insulin infuses; in addition, on the basis of the blood glucose level, the anticipated food intake, and the activity level, the client delivers a bolus of insulin before each meal
   d. Both rapid-acting and regular insulin (buffered to prevent the precipitation of insulin crystals within the catheter) are appropriate for use in these pumps
5. Implantable insulin delivery
   a. An insulin pump is implanted in the peritoneal cavity, where insulin can be absorbed in a more physiological manner
   b. Implants are not widely used because of mechanical problems associated with the pump, the catheter, and the insulin delivery
6. Newer methods of insulin administration
   a. Inhaled insulin: Insulin contained in a pellet is vaporized in an inhaler or delivered as a dry powder that is inhaled through a mouthpiece; insulin particles quickly dissolve in the alveoli and pass into the circulation
   b. Transdermal insulin: The administration of insulin via the skin through a patch (this is currently being tested)

7. Pancreas transplants
   a. The goal of pancreatic transplantation is to halt or reverse the complications of **diabetes mellitus**
   b. Transplants are performed on a limited number of clients, particularly clients who are receiving kidney transplantations simultaneously
   c. Immunosuppressive therapy is prescribed to prevent and treat rejection
D. Self-monitoring of blood glucose
   1. Self-monitoring provides the client with the current blood glucose level and with information to maintain good glycemic control
   2. Monitoring requires a finger prick to obtain a drop of blood for testing
   3. Alternative site testing (i.e., obtaining blood from the forearm, upper arm, abdomen, thigh, or calf) is now available with specific meters; these sites are not as reliable as the fingertip site when blood glucose levels are changing rapidly
   4. Tests must be used with caution among clients with diabetic neuropathy
   5. Client instructions (Box 44-17)
E. Urine testing
   1. Urine testing for glucose is not a reliable indicator of blood glucose and is therefore no longer used for monitoring purposes
   2. Instruct the client regarding the procedure for testing urine ketones
   3. The presence of ketones may indicate impending ketoacidosis
   4. Urine ketone testing should be performed during illness and whenever the client with type 1 **diabetes mellitus** has persistently elevated blood glucose levels (greater than 240 mg/dL for two consecutive testing periods)

BOX 44-17 | **Client Instructions: Monitoring of Blood Glucose**

Use the proper procedure for obtaining the blood glucose level.
Perform the procedure precisely to obtain accurate results.
Follow the manufacturer's instructions for the glucometer.
Wash your hands before and after performing the procedure to prevent infection.
Calibrate the monitor as instructed by the manufacturer.
Check the expiration date on the test strips.
If the blood glucose results do not seem reasonable, reread the instructions, reassess your technique, check the expiration date of the test strips, and perform the procedure again to verify your results.
Use only the fingertip collection site when glucose levels are changing rapidly, because alternative testing sites may not be accurate.

VIII. ACUTE COMPLICATIONS OF DIABETES MELLITUS

A. Hypoglycemia
  1. Description
     a. Hypoglycemia occurs when the blood glucose level falls to less than 60 mg/dL or when the blood glucose drops rapidly from an elevated level
     b. Hypoglycemia is caused by too much insulin or oral hypoglycemic agents, too little food, or excessive activity
     c. The client needs to be instructed to always carry some form of fast-acting simple carbohydrate with them
     d. If the client has a hypoglycemic reaction and does not have any of the recommended emergency foods available, any available food should be eaten; high-fat foods slow the absorption of glucose, and the hypoglycemic symptoms may not resolve quickly
  2. Data collection (Box 44-18)
     a. Mild hypoglycemia: Client remains fully awake but displays adrenergic symptoms (e.g., diaphoresis, irritability, weakness, headache, and shakiness); the blood glucose level is usually less than 60 mg/dL
     b. Moderate hypoglycemia: Client displays symptoms of worsening hypoglycemia (e.g., cold and clammy skin, pale and rapid pulse, rapid and shallow respirations, marked change in mood, and drowsiness); the blood glucose level is usually less than 40 mg/dL
     c. Severe hypoglycemia: Client displays severe neuroglycopenic symptoms (e.g., inability to swallow, unconsciousness, and seizures); the blood glucose level is usually less than 20 mg/dL
  3. Interventions: Mild hypoglycemia
     a. Give 10 to 15 g of a fast-acting simple carbohydrate (Box 44-19)
     b. Retest the blood glucose level in 15 minutes, and repeat the treatment if symptoms do not resolve
     c. After symptoms resolve, a snack that contains protein and carbohydrates (e.g., milk or cheese and crackers) is recommended unless the client plans to eat a regular meal within 60 minutes
  4. Interventions: Moderate hypoglycemia
     a. Administer 15 to 30 g of a fast-acting simple carbohydrate
     b. Administer additional food (e.g., low-fat milk or cheese) after 10 to 15 minutes
  5. Interventions for severe hypoglycemia
     a. If the client is unconscious and cannot swallow, an injection of glucagon is administered subcutaneously or intramuscularly
     b. Administer a second dose in 10 minutes if the client remains unconscious
     c. A small meal is given to the client when he or she awakens as long as he or she is not nauseated
     d. The physician is notified if a severe hypoglycemic reaction occurs
     e. In the hospital or emergency department, the client may be treated with an IV injection of 25 to 50 mL of 50% dextrose in water
     f. Family members need to be instructed regarding the administration of glucagon
B. Diabetic ketoacidosis (DKA)
  1. Description (Figure 44-2)
     a. DKA is a life-threatening complication of type 1 **diabetes mellitus** that develops when a severe insulin deficiency occurs
     b. The main clinical manifestations include hyperglycemia, dehydration, electrolyte imbalance, and acidosis
  2. Data collection (Table 44-2)
  3. Interventions
     a. Restore circulating blood volume and protect against cerebral, coronary, and renal hypoperfusion

BOX 44-18 Data Collection: Hypoglycemia

Mild
- Hunger
- Nervousness
- Palpitations
- Sweating
- Tachycardia
- Tremor

Moderate
- Confusion
- Double vision
- Drowsiness
- Emotional changes
- Headache
- Impaired coordination
- Inability to concentrate
- Irrational or combative behavior
- Lightheadedness
- Numbness of the lips and tongue
- Slurred speech

Severe
- Difficulty arousing
- Disoriented behavior
- Loss of consciousness
- Seizures

BOX 44-19 Simple Carbohydrates to Treat Hypoglycemia

- Commercially prepared glucose tablets
- 6 to 10 Life Savers or hard candies
- 4 tsp of sugar
- 4 sugar cubes
- 1 Tbsp of honey or syrup
- ½ cup of fruit juice or regular (nondiet) soft drink
- 8 oz low-fat milk
- 6 saltine crackers
- 3 graham crackers

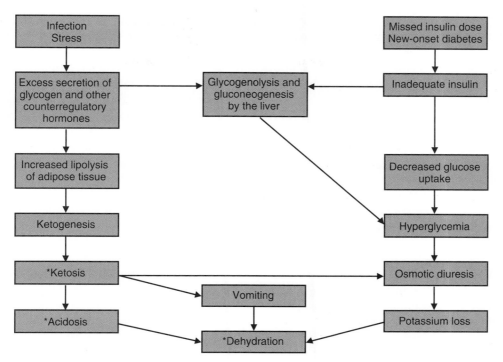

*Hallmarks of DKA

FIG. 44-2 The pathophysiology of diabetic ketoacidosis. (From Black, J., & Hawks, J. [2005]. *Medical-surgical nursing: Clinical management for positive outcomes* [7th ed.]. Philadelphia: Saunders.)

TABLE 44-2	Differences Between Diabetic Ketoacidosis and Hyperglycemic-Hyperosmolar Nonketotic Syndrome	
	Diabetic Ketoacidosis	**Hyperglycemic-Hyperosmolar Nonketotic Syndrome**
Onset	Sudden	Gradual
Precipitating factors	Infection	Infection
	Other stressors	Other stressors
	Inadequate insulin dose	Poor fluid intake
Manifestations	*Ketosis:* Kussmaul's respirations, fruity odor of the breath, nausea, and abdominal pain	Altered central nervous system function with neurologic symptoms
	Dehydration or electrolyte loss: polyuria, polydipsia, weight loss, dry skin, sunken eyes, soft eyeballs, lethargy, and coma	Dehydration or electrolyte loss; same as for DKA
Laboratory Findings		
Serum glucose	>300 mg/dL (16.7 mmol/L)	>800 mg/dL (44.5 mmol/L)
Osmolarity	Variable	>350 mOsm/L
Serum ketones	Positive at 1:2 dilutions	Negative
Serum pH	<7.35	>7.4
Serum HCO_3	<15 mEq/L	>20 mEq/L
Serum Na	Low, normal, or high	Normal or low
Serum K	Normal; elevated with acidosis, low after dehydration	Normal or low
BUN	>20 mg/dL; elevated because of dehydration	Elevated
Creatinine	>1.5 mg/dL; elevated because of dehydration	Elevated
Urine ketones	Positive	Negative

BUN, Blood urea nitrogen; *DKA,* diabetic ketoacidosis; *HCO_3,* bicarbonate; *K,* potassium; *Na,* sodium.
Modified from Ignatavicius, D., & Workman, M. (2006). *Medical-surgical nursing: Critical thinking for collaborative care* (5th ed.). Philadelphia: Saunders.

b. Treat dehydration with rapid IV infusions of 0.9% or 0.45% normal saline, as prescribed; dextrose is added to IV fluids (D_5NS or 5% dextrose in 0.45% saline) when the blood glucose level reaches 250 to 300 mg/dL

c. Treat hyperglycemia with regular insulin administered by IV, as prescribed

d. Correct electrolyte imbalances (the potassium level may be elevated as a result of dehydration and acidosis)

e. Monitor the potassium level closely, because, when the client receives treatment for the dehydration and acidosis, the serum potassium will decrease, and potassium replacement may be required

4. Insulin IV administration

a. Use regular insulin only

b. A dose of 5 to 10 units of regular insulin by IV bolus may be prescribed before a continuous infusion is begun

c. Mix the prescribed IV dose of regular insulin for continuous infusion in 0.9% or 0.45% normal saline, as prescribed

d. Flush the insulin solution through the entire IV infusion set, and discard the first 50 to 100 mL of solution before connecting and administering it to the client; insulin molecules adhere to the plastic of IV infusion sets

e. Always place the insulin infusion on an IV infusion controller

f. Insulin is infused continuously until subcutaneous administration resumes

g. Monitor the vital signs

h. Monitor the urinary output and for signs of fluid overload

i. Monitor the potassium and glucose levels and for signs of increased intracranial pressure

j. If the blood glucose level falls too far or too fast before the brain has time to equilibrate, water is pulled from the blood to the cerebrospinal fluid and the brain, thereby causing cerebral edema and increased intracranial pressure

k. The potassium level will fall rapidly within the first hour of treatment as the dehydration and the acidosis are treated

l. Potassium is administered by IV in a diluted solution, as prescribed, when the potassium reaches a normal level in order to prevent hypokalemia; ensure adequate renal function before administering potassium

5. Client education (Box 44-20)

C. Hyperglycemic hyperosmolar nonketotic syndrome (HHNS)

1. Description

a. Extreme hyperglycemia occurs without ketosis and acidosis

b. The syndrome occurs most often among individuals with type 2 **diabetes mellitus**

c. The major difference between HHNS and DKA is that ketosis and acidosis do not occur with HHNS; enough insulin is present with HHNS to prevent the breakdown of fats for energy, thus preventing ketosis

2. Data collection (see Table 44-2)

3. Interventions

a. Treatment is similar to that for DKA

b. Treatment includes fluid replacement, the correction of electrolyte imbalances, and insulin administration

c. Fluid replacement in the older client must be done very carefully secondary to the potential for heart failure

d. Insulin plays a less critical role in the treatment of HHNS than it does for the treatment of DKA, because ketosis and acidosis do not occur; rehydration alone may decrease glucose levels

IX. CHRONIC COMPLICATIONS OF DIABETES MELLITUS

A. Diabetic retinopathy

1. Description

a. A chronic and progressive impairment of the retinal circulation that eventually causes hemorrhage

b. Permanent vision changes and blindness can occur

c. The client has difficulty with carrying out the daily tasks of blood glucose testing and insulin injections

BOX 44-20 **Client Education: Guidelines During Illness**

Take insulin or oral antidiabetic medications, as prescribed.

Test the blood glucose level and the urine for ketones every 3 to 4 hours.

If the usual meal plan cannot be followed, substitute soft foods 6 to 8 times a day.

If vomiting, diarrhea, or fever occurs, consume liquids every 30 minutes to 1 hour to prevent dehydration and to provide calories.

Notify the physician if vomiting, diarrhea, or fever persists; if blood glucose levels are greater than 250 to 300 mg/dL; when ketonuria is present for more than 24 hours; when you are unable to take food or fluids for a period of 4 hours; or when illness persists for more than 2 days.

2. Data collection
   a. A change in vision is caused by the rupture of small microaneurysms in the retinal blood vessels
   b. Blurred vision results from macular edema
   c. A sudden loss of vision results from retinal detachment
   d. Cataracts result from lens opacity
3. Interventions
   a. Maintain safety
   b. Early prevention via the control of hypertension and blood glucose levels
   c. Photocoagulation (laser therapy) removes hemorrhagic tissue to decrease scarring and prevent the progression of the disease process
   d. Vitrectomy removes vitreous hemorrhages and decreases tension on the retina, thus preventing detachment
   e. Cataract removal with a lens implant improves vision

B. Diabetic nephropathy
   1. Description: A progressive decrease in kidney function
   2. Data collection
      a. Microalbuminuria
      b. Thirst
      c. Fatigue
      d. Anemia
      e. Weight loss
      f. Signs of malnutrition
      g. Frequent urinary tract infections
      h. Signs of a neurogenic bladder
   3. Interventions
      a. Early prevention measures include the control of hypertension and blood glucose levels
      b. Assess the vital signs
      c. Monitor the I&O
      d. Monitor the serum blood urea nitrogen, creatinine, and urine albumin levels
      e. Restrict dietary protein, sodium, and potassium intake, as prescribed
      f. Avoid nephrotoxic medications
      g. Prepare the client for dialysis procedures, as prescribed
      h. Prepare the client for kidney transplant, as prescribed
      i. Prepare the client for pancreas transplant, as prescribed

C. Diabetic neuropathy
   1. Description
      a. A general deterioration of the nervous system throughout the body
      b. Complications include the development of nonhealing ulcers of the feet, gastric paresis, and erectile dysfunction
   2. Classifications
      a. Focal or mononeuropathy: Involves a single nerve or a group of nerves, most frequently cranial nerves III (oculomotor) and VI (abducens), and results in diplopia; it usually resolves spontaneously
      b. Sensory or peripheral neuropathy: Affects the distal portion of the nerves, most frequently in the lower extremities
      c. Autonomic neuropathy: Symptoms vary according to the organ system involved
      d. Cardiovascular: Cardiac denervation syndrome (i.e., the heart rate does not respond to changes in oxygenation needs) and orthostatic hypotension occur
      e. Pupillary: Pupil does not dilate in response to decreased light
      f. Gastric: Decreased gastric emptying (gastroparesis)
      g. Urinary: Neurogenic bladder
      h. Sudomotor: Decreased sweating
      i. Adrenal: Hypoglycemic unawareness
      j. Reproductive: Impotence (male) and painful intercourse (female)
   3. Data collection
      a. Paresthesias
      b. Decreased or absent reflexes
      c. Decreased sensation to vibration or light touch
      d. Pain, aching, and burning in the lower extremities
      e. Poor peripheral pulses
      f. Skin breakdown and signs of infection
      g. Weakness or loss of sensation in cranial nerves III (oculomotor), IV (trochlear), V (trigeminal), or VI (abducens)
      h. Dizziness and postural hypotension
      i. Nausea and vomiting
      j. Diarrhea or constipation
      k. Incontinence
      l. Dyspareunia
      m. Impotence
      n. Hypoglycemic unawareness
   4. Interventions
      a. Early prevention measures include the control of hypertension and blood glucose levels
      b. Careful foot care is required to prevent trauma (Box 44-21)
      c. Administer medications for pain relief, as prescribed
      d. Initiate bladder-training programs
      e. Instruct the client regarding the use of estrogen-containing lubricants for women with dyspareunia
      f. Prepare the male client with impotence for penile injections or implantable devices, as prescribed

BOX 44-21 Preventive Foot Care Instructions

Provide meticulous skin care and proper foot care.

Inspect the feet daily and monitor them for redness, swelling, or breaks in skin integrity.

Notify the physician if redness or a break in the skin occurs.

Avoid thermal injuries from hot water, heating pads, and baths.

Wash the feet with warm (not hot) water, and dry them thoroughly.

Avoid foot soaks

Consult a podiatrist for treating corns, blisters, or ingrown toenails.

Do not cross the legs or wear tight garments that may constrict blood flow.

Apply moisturizing lotion to the feet, but not between the toes.

Prevent moisture from accumulating between the toes.

Wear loose socks and well-fitting (not tight) shoes.

Do not go barefoot.

Wear clean cotton socks to keep the feet warm, and change the socks daily.

Do not wear the same pair of shoes 2 days in a row.

Do not wear open-toed shoes or shoes with a strap that goes between the toes.

Check the shoes for cracks or tears in the lining and for foreign objects before putting them on.

Break in new shoes gradually.

Cut the toenails straight across, and smooth the nails with an emery board.

Do not smoke.

g. Prepare for surgical decompression of compression lesions related to the cranial nerves, as prescribed

X. CARE OF THE DIABETIC CLIENT UNDERGOING SURGERY

A. Preoperative care
1. Check with the physician regarding withholding oral hypoglycemic medications or insulin
2. Some long-acting oral antidiabetic medications are discontinued 24 to 48 hours before surgery
3. Metformin (Glucophage) may need to be discontinued 48 hours before surgery, and it may not be restarted until renal function is normal postoperatively
4. All other oral antidiabetic medications are stopped the day of surgery
5. The insulin dose may be adjusted or withheld if IV insulin administration during surgery is planned
6. Monitor the blood glucose level
7. Administer IV fluids, as prescribed

B. Intraoperative care
1. Monitor the blood glucose levels frequently
2. Administer IV short- or rapid-acting insulin, as prescribed, to maintain blood glucose levels less than 200 mg/dL

C. Postoperative care
1. Administer IV glucose and regular insulin infusions, as prescribed, until the client can tolerate oral feedings
2. Administer supplemental short-acting insulin, as prescribed, on the basis of blood glucose results
3. Monitor blood glucose levels frequently if the client is receiving parenteral nutrition
4. When the client is tolerating food, ensure that he or she receives an adequate amount of carbohydrates daily to prevent **hypoglycemia** and ketosis
5. The client is at higher risk for cardiovascular and renal complications postoperatively
6. The client is also at risk for impaired wound healing

PRACTICE QUESTIONS

More questions on the companion CD!

508. A nurse is caring for a client after thyroidectomy and notes that calcium gluconate is prescribed for the client. The nurse determines that this medication has been prescribed to:
 1. Treat thyroid storm.
 2. Prevent cardiac irritability.
 3. Treat hypocalcemic tetany.
 4. Stimulate the release of parathyroid hormone.

509. A nurse is collecting data regarding a client after a thyroidectomy and notes that the client has developed hoarseness and a weak voice. Which nursing action is appropriate?
 1. Check for signs of bleeding.
 2. Administer calcium gluconate.
 3. Notify the registered nurse immediately.
 4. Reassure the client that this is usually a temporary condition.

510. A client is admitted to the emergency department, and a diagnosis of myxedema coma is made. Which nursing action would the nurse prepare to carry out initially?
 1. Warm the client.
 2. Maintain a patent airway.
 3. Infuse intravenous fluids.
 4. Administer thyroid hormone.

511. A nurse is assisting with preparing a teaching plan for the client with diabetes mellitus regarding proper foot care. Which instruction should be included in the plan of care?
 1. Soak the feet in hot water.
 2. Avoid using soap to wash the feet.
 3. Apply a moisturizing lotion to dry feet, but not between the toes.

4. Always have a podiatrist cut your toenails; never cut them yourself.

512. A nurse provides dietary instructions to a client with diabetes mellitus regarding the prescribed diabetic diet. Which statement, if made by the client, indicates the need for further teaching?
1. "I'll eat a balanced meal plan."
2. "I need to drink diet soft drinks."
3. "I need to buy special dietetic foods."
4. "I will snack on fruit instead of cake."

513. A client who has been newly diagnosed with diabetes mellitus has been stabilized with daily insulin injections. Which information should the nurse teach when carrying out plans for discharge?
1. Keep insulin vials refrigerated at all times.
2. Rotate the insulin injection sites systematically.
3. Increase the amount of insulin before unusual exercise.
4. Monitor the urine acetone level to determine the insulin dosage.

514. A nurse reinforces teaching with a client with diabetes mellitus regarding differentiating between hypoglycemia and ketoacidosis. The client demonstrates an understanding of the teaching by stating that glucose will be taken if which symptom develops?
1. Polyuria
2. Shakiness
3. Blurred vision
4. Fruity breath odor

515. When the nurse is teaching a client who has been newly diagnosed with type 1 diabetes mellitus, which statement by the client would indicate that teaching has been effective?
1. "I will stop taking my insulin if I'm too sick to eat."
2. "I will decrease my insulin dose during times of illness."
3. "I will adjust my insulin dose according to the level of glucose in my urine."
4. "I will notify my physician if my blood glucose level is greater than 250 mg/dL."

516. A nurse is monitoring a client who has been newly diagnosed with diabetes mellitus for sign of complications. Which of the following, if exhibited by the client, would indicate hyperglycemia and thus warrant physician notification?
1. Polyuria
2. Bradycardia
3. Diaphoresis
4. Hypertension

517. A nurse is reinforcing instructions with a client with diabetes mellitus who is recovering from diabetic ketoacidosis (DKA) regarding measures to prevent a recurrence. Which instruction is important for the nurse to emphasize?
1. Eat six small meals daily.
2. Test the urine ketone levels.
3. Monitor blood glucose levels frequently.
4. Receive appropriate follow-up health care.

518. A nurse is reviewing discharge teaching with a client who has Cushing's syndrome. Which statement by the client indicates that the instructions related to dietary management were understood?
1. "I can eat foods that contain potassium."
2. "I will need to limit the amount of protein in my diet."
3. "I am fortunate that I can eat all the salty foods I enjoy."
4. "I am fortunate that I do not need to follow any special diet."

519. A client with type 1 diabetes mellitus calls the nurse to report recurrent episodes of hypoglycemia. Which statement by the client indicates a correct understanding of NPH insulin and exercise?
1. "I should not exercise after lunch."
2. "I should not exercise after breakfast."
3. "I should not exercise in the late evening."
4. "I should not exercise in the late afternoon."

520. A nurse is caring for a postoperative parathyroidectomy client. Which of the following would require the nurse's immediate attention?
1. Incisional pain
2. Laryngeal stridor
3. Difficulty voiding
4. Abdominal cramps

521. When a nurse notes that a client with type 1 diabetes mellitus has lipodystrophy on both upper thighs, what information should the nurse obtain from the client?
1. Plan of injection rotation
2. Consistency of aspiration
3. Preparation of the injection site
4. Angle at which the medication is administered

522. Which client complaint would alert the nurse to a possible hypoglycemic reaction?
1. Tremors
2. Anorexia
3. Hot, dry skin
4. Muscle cramps

523. Which nursing action would be appropriate to implement when a client has a diagnosis of pheochromocytoma?
1. Weigh the client.
2. Test the client's urine for glucose.
3. Monitor the client's blood pressure.
4. Palpate the client's skin to determine warmth.

524. A nurse is caring for a client with pheochromocytoma. The client is scheduled for an adrenalectomy. During the preoperative period, the priority nursing action would be to monitor:
    1. The vital signs
    2. The intake and output
    3. The blood urea nitrogen level
    4. The urine for glucose and acetone

525. A nurse is caring for a client with pheochromocytoma. The client asks for a snack and something warm to drink. The appropriate choice for this client to meet nutritional needs would be which of the following?
    1. Crackers with cheese and tea
    2. Graham crackers and warm milk
    3. Toast with peanut butter and cocoa
    4. Vanilla wafers and coffee with cream and sugar

526. A nurse is caring for a client with pheochromocytoma. Which data would indicate a potential complication associated with this disorder?
    1. A urinary output of 50 mL/hour
    2. A coagulation time of 5 minutes
    3. Congestion heard on auscultation of the lungs
    4. A blood urea nitrogen (BUN) level of 20 mg/dL

527. A nurse is caring for a client after thyroidectomy and monitoring for signs of thyroid storm. The nurse understands that which of the following is a manifestation associated with this disorder?
    1. Bradycardia
    2. Hypotension
    3. Constipation
    4. Hypothermia

528. When caring for a client who is having clear drainage from his nares after transsphenoidal hypophysectomy, which action by the nurse is appropriate?
    1. Lower the head of the bed.
    2. Test the drainage for glucose.
    3. Obtain a culture of the drainage.

    4. Continue to observe the drainage.

529. After several diagnostic tests, a client is diagnosed with diabetes insipidus. The nurse understands that which symptom is indicative of this disorder?
    1. Diarrhea
    2. Polydipsia
    3. Weight gain
    4. Blurred vision

530. Which clinical manifestation should the nurse expect to note when assessing a client with Addison's disease?
    1. Edema
    2. Obesity
    3. Hirsutism
    4. Hypotension

531. What would the nurse anticipate being included in the plan of care for a client who has been diagnosed with Graves' disease?
    1. Provide a high-fiber diet.
    2. Provide a restful environment.
    3. Provide three small meals per day.
    4. Provide the client with extra blankets.

ALTERNATE ITEM FORMAT: PRIORITIZING (ORDERED RESPONSE)

532. A hospitalized client with type 1 diabetes mellitus received NPH and regular insulin 2 hours ago at 7:30 AM. The client calls the nurse and reports that he is feeling hungry, shaky, and weak. The client ate breakfast at 8:00 and is due to eat lunch at noon. List, in order of priority, the actions that the nurse would take. (Number 1 is the first action.)
    ___ Take the client's vital signs.
    ___ Retest the client's blood glucose level.
    ___ Check the client's blood glucose level.
    ___ Give the client half a cup of fruit juice to drink.
    ___ Give the client a small snack of carbohydrate and protein.
    ___ Document the client's complaints, the actions taken, and the outcome.

ANSWERS

508. **3**
Rationale: Hypocalcemia can develop after thyroidectomy if the parathyroid glands are accidentally removed or injured during surgery. Manifestations develop 1 to 7 days after surgery. If the client develops numbness and tingling around the mouth, fingertips, or toes or muscle spasms or twitching, the physician is notified immediately. Calcium gluconate should be kept at the bedside.

Test-Taking Strategy: Noting the name of the medication (calcium gluconate) should easily direct you to option 3. Calcium is given if hypocalcemic tetany occurs. Review calcium gluconate if you had difficulty with this question.
Level of Cognitive Ability: Analysis
Client Needs: Physiological Integrity
Integrated Process: Nursing Process/Planning
Content Area: Pharmacology
Reference: Linton, A. (2007). *Introduction to medical-surgical nursing* (4th ed., p. 987). Philadelphia: Saunders.

509. 4

Rationale: Weakness and hoarseness of the voice can occur as a result of trauma of the laryngeal nerve. If this develops, the client should be reassured that the problem will subside in a few days. Unnecessary talking should be discouraged. It is not necessary to notify the registered nurse immediately. These signs do not indicate bleeding or the need to administer calcium gluconate.

Test-Taking Strategy: Use the process of elimination. Options 1 and 2 can easily be eliminated, because they are unrelated to the signs presented in the question. From the remaining options, recall that these signs indicate a temporary condition. Review the expected findings after thyroidectomy if you had difficulty with this question.

Level of Cognitive Ability: Application
Client Needs: Physiological Integrity
Integrated Process: Nursing Process/Implementation
Content Area: Adult Health/Endocrine
References: Linton, A. (2007). *Introduction to medical-surgical nursing* (4th ed., p. 987). Philadelphia: Saunders.
Monahan, F., Sands, J., Marek, J., Neighbors, M., & Green, C. (2007). *Phipps' medical-surgical nursing: Health and illness perspectives* (8th ed., p. 1087). St. Louis: Mosby.

510. 2

Rationale: The initial nursing action would be to maintain a patent airway. Oxygen would be administered, followed by fluid replacement. The nurse would also keep the client warm, monitor the vital signs, and administer thyroid hormones.

Test-Taking Strategy: Note the strategic words "carry out initially." All of the options are appropriate interventions, but the use of the ABCs—airway, breathing, and circulation—will direct you to option 2. Review the care of the client with myxedema coma if you had difficulty with this question.

Level of Cognitive Ability: Application
Client Needs: Physiological Integrity
Integrated Process: Nursing Process/Implementation
Content Area: Delegating/Prioritizing
Reference: Fultz, J., & Sturt, P. (2005). *Emergency nursing reference* (3rd ed., p. 328). St. Louis: Mosby.

511. 3

Rationale: The client should use a moisturizing lotion on his or her feet but should avoid applying the lotion between the toes. The client should also be instructed to not soak the feet and to avoid hot water to prevent burns. The client may cut the toenails straight and even with the toe itself, but he or she should consult a podiatrist if the toenails are thick or hard to cut or if his or her vision is poor. The client should be instructed to wash the feet daily with a mild soap.

Test-Taking Strategy: Use the process of elimination. Eliminate option 4 first because of the word "always," and eliminate option 1 because of the word "hot." From the remaining options, recalling the concern related to skin infection will assist you with eliminating option 2. Review diabetic foot care instructions if you had difficulty with this question.

Level of Cognitive Ability: Application

Client Needs: Health Promotion and Maintenance
Integrated Process: Nursing Process/Planning
Content Area: Adult Health/Endocrine
References: Christensen, B., & Kockrow, E. (2006). *Adult health nursing* (5th ed., p. 555). St. Louis: Mosby.
Monahan, F., Sands, J., Marek, J., Neighbors, M., & Green, C. (2007). *Phipps' medical-surgical nursing: Health and illness perspectives* (8th ed., p. 1154). St. Louis: Mosby.

512. 3

Rationale: It is important to emphasize to the client and family that they are not eating a diabetic diet but rather following a balanced meal plan. Adherence to nutrition principles is an important component of diabetic management, and an individualized meal plan should be developed for the client. It is not necessary for the client to purchase special dietetic foods.

Test-Taking Strategy: Note the strategic words "indicates the need for further teaching." These words indicate a negative event query and ask you to select an option that is an incorrect statement. Basic principles related to the diabetic diet will direct you to option 3. Review these principles if you had difficulty with this question.

Level of Cognitive Ability: Comprehension
Client Needs: Physiological Integrity
Integrated Process: Teaching and Learning
Content Area: Adult Health/Endocrine
Reference: Christensen, B., & Kockrow, E. (2006). *Adult health nursing* (5th ed., p. 561). St. Louis: Mosby.

513. 2

Rationale: Insulin dosages should not be adjusted or increased before unusual exercise. If acetone is found in the urine, it may possibly indicate the need for additional insulin. To minimize the discomfort associated with insulin injections, the insulin should be administered at room temperature. Injection sites should be systematically rotated from one area to another. The client should be instructed to give injections in one area, about 1 inch apart, until the whole area has been used and to then change to another site. This prevents dramatic changes in daily insulin absorption.

Test-Taking Strategy: Use the process of elimination. Eliminate option 1 first because of the words "at all times." Knowledge regarding insulin administration and the significance of acetone in the urine will assist you with eliminating options 3 and 4. Review insulin management if you had difficulty with this question.

Level of Cognitive Ability: Application
Client Needs: Physiological Integrity
Integrated Process: Nursing Process/Planning
Content Area: Pharmacology
Reference: Linton, A. (2007). *Introduction to medical-surgical nursing* (4th ed., p. 1012-1014). Philadelphia: Saunders.

514. 2

Rationale: Shakiness is a sign of hypoglycemia, and it would indicate the need for food or glucose. Fruity breath odor, blurred vision, and polyuria are signs of hyperglycemia.

Test-Taking Strategy: Knowledge regarding the signs and symptoms of hypoglycemia and hyperglycemia is required to answer this question. Remember that shakiness is a sign of

hypoglycemia. Review the signs and symptoms of hypoglycemia and hyperglycemia if you had difficulty with this question.
Level of Cognitive Ability: Comprehension
Client Needs: Physiological Integrity
Integrated Process: Nursing Process/Evaluation
Content Area: Adult Health/Endocrine
Reference: deWit, S. (2009). *Medical-surgical nursing: Concepts & practice* (p. 926). Philadelphia: Saunders.

515. 4
Rationale: During illness, the client should monitor the blood glucose level, and he or she should notify the physician if the level is greater than 250 mg/dL. Insulin should never be stopped. In fact, insulin may need to be increased during times of illness. Doses should not be adjusted without the physician's advice.
Test-Taking Strategy: Use the process of elimination. Note that options 1, 2, and 3 all relate to the adjustment of insulin doses; therefore, eliminate these options. Review diabetic management during illness if you had difficulty with this question.
Level of Cognitive Ability: Comprehension
Client Needs: Physiological Integrity
Integrated Process: Nursing Process/Evaluation
Content Area: Adult Health/Endocrine
Reference: Linton, A. (2007). *Introduction to medical-surgical nursing* (4th ed., p. 1017). Philadelphia: Saunders.

516. 1
Rationale: The classic symptoms of hyperglycemia include polydipsia, polyuria, and polyphagia. Options 2, 3, and 4 are not signs of hyperglycemia.
Test-Taking Strategy: Focus on the subject of hyperglycemia. Remember the 3 Ps—polyuria, polydipsia, polyphagia. Review the signs of hyperglycemia if you had difficulty with this question.
Level of Cognitive Ability: Comprehension
Client Needs: Physiological Integrity
Integrated Process: Nursing Process/Data Collection
Content Area: Adult Health/Endocrine
Reference: Linton, A. (2007). *Introduction to medical-surgical nursing* (4th ed., p. 1009). Philadelphia: Saunders.

517. 3
Rationale: Client education after DKA should emphasize the need for home glucose monitoring four to five times per day. It is also important to instruct the client to notify the health care provider when illness occurs. The presence of urinary ketones indicates that DKA has already occurred. The client should eat well-balanced meals with snacks, as prescribed.
Test-Taking Strategy: Focus on the subject of preventing DKA. Recall that the treatment of DKA focuses on the maintenance of an appropriate blood glucose level. Option 1 is not an accurate component of diabetic care. Option 4 will not prevent DKA. Option 2 does not prevent DKA but rather confirms the diagnosis. Review DKA if you had difficulty with this question.
Level of Cognitive Ability: Application
Client Needs: Health Promotion and Maintenance
Integrated Process: Teaching and Learning

Content Area: Adult Health/Endocrine
Reference: deWit, S. (2009). *Medical-surgical Nursing: Concepts & practice* (p. 925). Philadelphia: Saunders.

518. 1
Rationale: A diet that is low in calories, carbohydrates, and sodium but ample in protein and potassium content is encouraged for a client with Cushing's syndrome. Such a diet promotes weight loss, the reduction of edema and hypertension, the control of hypokalemia, and the rebuilding of wasted tissue.
Test-Taking Strategy: Note the strategic words "instructions related to dietary management were understood." Eliminate option 4, because it indicates that no dietary change is necessary. Eliminate option 2 next, because protein is usually only limited with renal disorders. Excess sodium is not healthy in general, so eliminate option 3. Review the dietary management of Cushing's syndrome if you had difficulty with this question.
Level of Cognitive Ability: Comprehension
Client Needs: Physiological Integrity
Integrated Process: Nursing Process/Evaluation
Content Area: Adult Health/Endocrine
Reference: Christensen, B., & Kockrow, E. (2006). *Adult health nursing* (5th ed., pp. 538-539). St. Louis: Mosby.

519. 4
Rationale: A hypoglycemic reaction may occur in response to increased exercise. Clients should avoid exercise during the peak time of insulin. NPH insulin peaks at 6 to 14 hours; therefore, late afternoon exercise would occur during the peak of the medication.
Test-Taking Strategy: Use the process of elimination, and note the strategic words "a correct understanding." Recalling the peak time of insulin will direct you to option 4. Review the measures to prevent hypoglycemia if you had difficulty with this question.
Level of Cognitive Ability: Comprehension
Client Needs: Physiological Integrity
Integrated Process: Nursing Process/Evaluation
Content Area: Adult Health/Endocrine
Reference: Linton, A. (2007). *Introduction to medical-surgical nursing* (4th ed., pp. 1006, 1027). Philadelphia: Saunders.

520. 2
Rationale: During the postoperative period, the nurse carefully observes the client for signs of hemorrhage, which cause swelling and the compression of adjacent tissue. Laryngeal stridor is a harsh, high-pitched sound heard on inspiration and expiration that is caused by the compression of the trachea and that leads to respiratory distress. It is an acute emergency situation that requires immediate attention to avoid the complete obstruction of the airway.
Test-Taking Strategy: Consider the anatomical location of the surgical procedure, and use the ABCs—airway, breathing, and circulation—to select the correct option. Options 1, 3, and 4 are usual postoperative problems that are not life threatening. Option 2 addresses the airway. Review the care of the client after parathyroidectomy if you had difficulty with this question.
Level of Cognitive Ability: Analysis

Client Needs: Physiological Integrity
Integrated Process: Nursing Process/Data Collection
Content Area: Adult Health/Endocrine
Reference: Linton, A. (2007). *Introduction to medical-surgical nursing* (4th ed., pp. 996, 998). Philadelphia: Saunders.

521. **1**
Rationale: Lipodystrophy (i.e., the hypertrophy of subcutaneous tissue at the injection site) occurs in some diabetic clients when the same injection sites are used for prolonged periods of time. Thus, clients are instructed to adhere to a rotating injection site plan to avoid tissue changes. Preparation of the site, aspiration, and the angle of insulin administration do not produce tissue damage.
Test-Taking Strategy: Recalling the definition of lipodystrophy will direct you to the correct option. Remember that lipodystrophy is the hypertrophy of subcutaneous tissue at the injection site. Review this potential complication of insulin therapy if you had difficulty with this question.
Level of Cognitive Ability: Application
Client Needs: Physiological Integrity
Integrated Process: Nursing Process/Data Collection
Content Area: Adult Health/Endocrine
Reference: Christensen, B., & Kockrow, E. (2006). *Adult health nursing* (5th ed., p. 551). St. Louis: Mosby.

522. **1**
Rationale: Decreased blood glucose levels produce automatic nervous system symptoms, which are classically manifested as nervousness, irritability, and tremors. Option 3 is more likely to occur with hyperglycemia. Options 2 and 4 are unrelated to the signs of hypoglycemia.
Test-Taking Strategy: Focus on the subject of a hypoglycemic reaction. Recalling the signs associated with this reaction will direct you to option 1. Review hypoglycemia if you had difficulty with this question.
Level of Cognitive Ability: Comprehension
Client Needs: Physiological Integrity
Integrated Process: Nursing Process/Data Collection
Content Area: Adult Health/Endocrine
Reference: Linton, A. (2007). *Introduction to medical-surgical nursing* (4th ed., p. 1005). Philadelphia: Saunders.

523. **3**
Rationale: Hypertension is the major symptom that is associated with pheochromocytoma. The blood pressure status is monitored by taking the client's blood pressure. Glycosuria, weight loss, and diaphoresis are also clinical manifestations of pheochromocytoma, but hypertension is the major symptom.
Test-Taking Strategy: Use the principles associated with prioritizing and the ABCs—airway, breathing, and circulation. A method of assessing circulation is to take the blood pressure. Review the manifestations of pheochromocytoma if you had difficulty with this question.
Level of Cognitive Ability: Application
Client Needs: Physiological Integrity
Integrated Process: Nursing Process/Implementation
Content Area: Adult Health/Endocrine
Reference: Christensen, B., & Kockrow, E. (2006). *Adult health nursing* (5th ed., p. 541). St. Louis: Mosby.

524. **1**
Rationale: Hypertension is the hallmark of pheochromocytoma. Severe hypertension can precipitate a brain attack (stroke) accident or sudden blindness. Although all of the options are accurate nursing interventions for the client with pheochromocytoma, the priority nursing action is to monitor the vital signs, particularly the blood pressure.
Test-Taking Strategy: Note the strategic words "priority nursing action." Monitoring the vital signs is the nursing action that would assess the ABCs—airway, breathing, and circulation. In addition, note that options 2, 3, and 4 all refer to the assessment of the renal system. Review the care of the client with pheochromocytoma if you had difficulty with this question.
Level of Cognitive Ability: Application
Client Needs: Physiological Integrity
Integrated Process: Nursing Process/Implementation
Content Area: Delegating/Prioritizing
Reference: Christensen, B., & Kockrow, E. (2006). *Adult health nursing* (5th ed., p. 541). St. Louis: Mosby.

525. **2**
Rationale: The client with pheochromocytoma needs to be provided with a diet that is high in vitamins, minerals, and calories. Of particular importance is that food or beverages that contain caffeine (e.g., chocolate, coffee, tea, cola) are prohibited.
Test-Taking Strategy: Use the process of elimination. Eliminate options 1, 3, and 4, because they are comparable or alike and include food items that contain caffeine. Review dietary measures for the client with pheochromocytoma if you had difficulty with this question.
Level of Cognitive Ability: Application
Client Needs: Physiological Integrity
Integrated Process: Nursing Process/Implementation
Content Area: Adult Health/Endocrine
Reference: Linton, A. (2007). *Introduction to medical-surgical nursing* (4th ed., p. 976). Philadelphia: Saunders.

526. **3**
Rationale: The complications associated with pheochromocytoma include hypertensive retinopathy and nephropathy, myocarditis, congestive heart failure (CHF), increased platelet aggregation, and stroke. Death can occur from shock, stroke, renal failure, dysrhythmias, or dissecting aortic aneurysm. Congestion heard on auscultation of the lungs is indicative of CHF. A urinary output of 50 mL/hour is an appropriate output; the nurse would become concerned if the output was less than 30 mL/hour. A BUN level of 20 mg/dL is a normal finding. A coagulation time of 5 minutes is normal.
Test-Taking Strategy: Use the ABCs—airway, breathing, and circulation. Congestion heard on auscultation of the lungs is associated with the airway. In addition, if you know the normal hourly urinary output, the normal laboratory values for coagulation time, and the BUN level, you can determine that option 3 is correct by the process of elimination. Review the complications associated with pheochromocytoma if you had difficulty with this question.

Level of Cognitive Ability: Analysis
Client Needs: Physiological Integrity
Integrated Process: Nursing Process/Data Collection
Content Area: Adult Health/Endocrine
Reference: Christensen, B., & Kockrow, E. (2006). *Adult health nursing* (5th ed., p. 541). St. Louis: Mosby.

527. 2
Rationale: Clinical manifestations associated with thyroid storm include a fever as high as 106° F (41.1° C), severe tachycardia, profuse diarrhea, extreme vasodilation, hypotension, atrial fibrillation, hyperreflexia, abdominal pain, diarrhea, and dehydration. With this disorder, the client's condition can rapidly progress to coma and cardiovascular collapse.
Test-Taking Strategy: Knowledge regarding the manifestations associated with thyroid storm is required to answer the question. Remember that this condition is a rare but potentially fatal hypermetabolic state. Review thyroid storm if you had difficulty with this question.
Level of Cognitive Ability: Comprehension
Client Needs: Physiological Integrity
Integrated Process: Nursing Process/Data Collection
Content Area: Adult Health/Endocrine
Reference: Linton, A. (2007). *Introduction to medical-surgical nursing* (4th ed., p. 988). Philadelphia: Saunders.

528. 2
Rationale: After hypophysectomy, the client should be monitored for rhinorrhea, which could indicate a cerebrospinal fluid (CSF) leak. If this occurs, the drainage should be collected and tested for glucose, indicating the presence of CSF. The head of the bed should not be lowered to prevent increased intracranial pressure. Clear nasal drainage would not indicate the need for a culture. Continuing to observe the drainage without taking action could result in a serious complication.
Test-Taking Strategy: Use the process of elimination. Option 1 can be eliminated first. Option 3 can be eliminated, because the drainage is clear. Because an action is required, eliminate option 4. Review the complications after hypophysectomy if you had difficulty with this question.
Level of Cognitive Ability: Application
Client Needs: Physiological Integrity
Integrated Process: Nursing Process/Implementation
Content Area: Adult Health/Endocrine
References: Ignatavicius, D., & Workman, M. (2006). *Medical-surgical nursing: Critical thinking for collaborative care* (5th ed., p. 1464). Philadelphia: Saunders.
Linton, A. (2007). *Introduction to medical-surgical nursing* (4th ed., p. 430). Philadelphia: Saunders.

529. 2
Rationale: Polydipsia and polyuria are classic symptoms of diabetes insipidus. The urine is pale in color, and its specific gravity is low. Anorexia and weight loss occur.
Test-Taking Strategy: Use the process of elimination and your knowledge of the manifestations of diabetes insipidus. Remember that polydipsia and polyuria are classic symptoms. Review the clinical manifestations associated with diabetes insipidus if you had difficulty with this question.

Level of Cognitive Ability: Comprehension
Client Needs: Physiological Integrity
Integrated Process: Nursing Process/Data Collection
Content Area: Adult Health/Endocrine
References: Christensen, B., & Kockrow, E. (2006). *Adult health nursing* (5th ed., p. 524). St. Louis: Mosby.
Linton, A. (2007). *Introduction to medical-surgical nursing* (4th ed., p. 961). Philadelphia: Saunders.
Monahan, F., Sands, J., Marek, J., Neighbors, M., & Green, C. (2007). *Phipps' medical-surgical nursing: Health and illness perspectives* (8th ed., p. 1072). St. Louis: Mosby.

530. 4
Rationale: Common manifestations of Addison's disease include postural hypotension from fluid loss, syncope, muscle weakness, anorexia, nausea, vomiting, abdominal cramps, weight loss, depression, and irritability.
Test-Taking Strategy: Knowledge regarding the clinical manifestations associated with Addison's disease is required to answer this question. Remember that hypotension occurs with Addison's disease. Review Addison's disease if you had difficulty with this question.
Level of Cognitive Ability: Comprehension
Client Needs: Physiological Integrity
Integrated Process: Nursing Process/Data Collection
Content Area: Adult Health/Endocrine
Reference: Linton, A. (2007). *Introduction to medical-surgical nursing* (4th ed., p. 971). Philadelphia: Saunders.

531. 2
Rationale: Because of the hypermetabolic state, the client with Graves' disease needs to be provided with an environment that is restful both physically and mentally. Six full meals a day that are well balanced and high in calories are required because of the accelerated metabolic rate. Foods that increase peristalsis (e.g., high-fiber foods) need to be avoided. These clients suffer from heat intolerance and require a cool environment.
Test-Taking Strategy: The strategic concept to bear in mind when answering this question is that clients with Graves' disease experience an accelerated metabolic rate. This concept should assist you with eliminating options 1, 3, and 4. Review the care of the client with Graves' disease if you had difficulty with this question.
Level of Cognitive Ability: Application
Client Needs: Physiological Integrity
Integrated Process: Nursing Process/Planning
Content Area: Adult Health/Endocrine
Reference: Linton, A. (2007). *Introduction to medical-surgical nursing* (4th ed., p. 985). Philadelphia: Saunders.

ALTERNATE ITEM FORMAT:
PRIORITIZING (ORDERED RESPONSE)
532. 3, 4, 1, 2, 5, 6
Rationale: The client is experiencing symptoms of mild hypoglycemia. If symptoms such as hunger, irritability, shakiness, or weakness occur, the nurse first would check the client's blood glucose level to verify that the client is experiencing hypoglycemia. After this is verified, the nurse would give the client 10 to 15 g of carbohydrates and then retest the blood

glucose level in 15 minutes. In the meantime, the nurse would check the client's vital signs. The nurse would give the client another food item containing 10 to 15 g of carbohydrate if the client's symptoms do not resolve. Otherwise, the nurse would provide a small snack of carbohydrates and protein if the client's next scheduled meal is more than an hour away from the time of the occurrence. After treatment and the resolution of the hypoglycemic event, the nurse would document the occurrence, the actions taken, and the outcome. *Test-Taking Strategy:* Focus on the client's symptoms. Noting that the client is hospitalized will assist you with determining that the first action would be to check the client's blood glucose level. After this has been done, treating the hypoglycemia is necessary. Recalling that an outcome cannot be determined until treatment has been instituted will assist you with

selecting the documentation action as the last action. From the remaining three actions, select taking the vital signs as the third action. The nurse would not give the client a carbohydrate and protein item immediately after giving the client a 10- to 15-g carbohydrate item or before retesting the blood glucose level. Review the management of hypoglycemia if you had difficulty with this question.
Level of Cognitive Ability: Application
Client Needs: Physiological Integrity
Integrated Process: Nursing Process/Implementation
Content Area: Delegating/Prioritizing
Reference: Ignatavicius, D., & Workman, M. (2006). *Medical-surgical nursing: Critical thinking for collaborative care* (5th ed., p. 1540-1541). Philadelphia: Saunders.

REFERENCES

Chernecky, C., & Berger, B. (2008). *Laboratory tests and diagnostic procedures* (5th ed.). Philadelphia: Saunders.

Christensen, B., & Kockrow, E. (2006). *Adult health nursing* (5th ed.). St. Louis: Mosby.

Christensen, B., & Kockrow, E. (2006). *Foundations of nursing* (5th ed.). St. Louis: Mosby.

deWit, S. (2009). *Medical-surgical nursing: Concepts & practice.* Philadelphia: Saunders.

Fultz, J., & Sturt, P. (2005). *Emergency nursing reference* (3rd ed.). St. Louis: Mosby.

Ignatavicius, D., & Workman, M. (2006). *Medical-surgical nursing: Critical thinking for collaborative care* (5th ed.). Philadelphia: Saunders.

Lehne, R. (2007). *Pharmacology for nursing care* (6th ed.). Philadelphia: Saunders.

Linton, A. (2007). *Introduction to medical-surgical nursing* (4th ed.). Philadelphia: Saunders.

Monahan, F., Sands, J., Marek, J., Neighbors, M., & Green, C. (2007). *Phipps' medical-surgical nursing: Health and illness perspectives* (8th ed.). St. Louis: Mosby.

Skidmore-Roth, L. (2008). *2008 Mosby's nursing drug reference* (21st ed.). St. Louis: Mosby.

Endocrine Medications

I. PITUITARY MEDICATIONS

A. Description

1. The anterior pituitary gland secretes growth hormone (GH), thyroid-stimulating hormone (TSH), adrenocorticotropic hormone (ACTH), prolactin, melanocyte-stimulating hormone (MSH), and gonadotropins (follicle-stimulating hormone [FSH] and luteinizing hormone [LH])
2. The posterior pituitary gland secretes antidiuretic hormone (vasopressin) and oxytocin

B. Growth hormones and related medications

1. Uses and side effects (Table 45-1)
2. Interventions
   a. Assess child's physical growth and compare growth with standards
   b. Recommend annual bone age determinations for children receiving growth hormones
   c. Monitor blood glucose levels and thyroid function tests
   d. Teach the client and family about the clinical manifestations of **hyperglycemia** and the importance of follow-up regarding periodic blood tests

II. ANTIDIURETIC HORMONES (Box 45-1)

A. Description

1. Antidiuretic hormones enhance reabsorption of water in the kidneys, promoting an antidiuretic effect and regulating fluid balance
2. Antidiuretic hormones are used in **diabetes insipidus**

B. Side effects

1. Flushing
2. Headache
3. Nausea and abdominal cramps
4. Water intoxication
5. Hypertension with water intoxication
6. Nasal congestion with nasal administration

C. Interventions

1. Monitor weight
2. Monitor intake and output and urine osmolality
3. Monitor electrolytes
4. Monitor for signs of dehydration, indicating need to increase dosage

5. Monitor for signs of water intoxication (drowsiness, listlessness, shortness of breath, and headache), indicating need to decrease dosage
6. Monitor blood pressure
7. Instruct the client on how to use the intranasal medication
8. Instruct the client to weigh himself or herself daily to identify weight gain
9. Instruct the client to report signs of water intoxication or symptoms of headache or shortness of breath

III. THYROID HORMONES (Box 45-2)

A. Description

1. Thyroid hormones control the metabolic rate of tissues and accelerate heat production and oxygen consumption
2. Thyroid hormones are used to replace the thyroid hormone deficit in conditions such as **hypothyroidism** or **myxedema**
3. Thyroid hormones enhance the action of oral anticoagulants, sympathomimetics, and antidepressants, and they decrease the action of insulin, oral hypoglycemics, and digitalis preparations; the action of thyroid hormones is decreased by phenytoin (Dilantin) and carbamazepine (Tegretol)
4. Thyroid hormones should be given at least 4 hours apart from multivitamins, aluminum hydroxide and magnesium hydroxide, simethicone, calcium carbonate, bile acid sequestrants, iron, and sucralfate (Carafate) because these medications decrease the absorption of thyroid replacements

B. Side effects

1. Nausea and decreased appetite
2. Abdominal cramps and diarrhea
3. Weight loss
4. Nervousness and tremors
5. Insomnia
6. Sweating and heat intolerance
7. Tachycardia, dysrhythmias, palpitations, and chest pain
8. Hypertension

TABLE 45-1	Growth Hormones and Related Medications		
Medication(s)	**Use**	**Side Effects**	
Somatrem (Protropin)	Growth failure (children)	Development of antibodies to growth hormone	
Somatropin (Humatrope)	Growth failure (children and adults)	Headache, muscle pain, weakness, mild hyperglycemia, hypertension, allergic reaction (rash, swelling), pain at injection site	
Bromocriptine mesylate (Parlodel)	Acromegaly	Nausea, headache, dizziness	
Octreotide acetate (Sandostatin)	Acromegaly	Diarrhea, nausea, abdominal discomfort, increased or decreased glucose	
Cabergoline (Dostinex)	Acromegaly	Abdominal pain, vertigo	
Pegvisomant (Somavert)	Acromegaly	AST and ALT elevations, injection site reactions, flu syndrome, weight gain, infection, dizziness, peripheral edema, sinusitis, nausea, diarrhea, pain	

ALT, Alanine aminotranferase; *AST*, aspartate aminotranferase.

9. Headache
10. Toxicity: **hyperthyroidism**
C. Interventions
  1. Assess client for history of medications currently being taken
  2. Monitor vital signs
  3. Monitor weight
  4. Monitor triiodothyronine, thyroxine, and TSH levels
  5. Instruct the client to take the medication at the same time each day, preferably in the morning without food
  6. Instruct the client on how to monitor pulse rate
  7. Advise the client to report symptoms of **hyperthyroidism,** such as tachycardia, chest pain, palpitations, and excessive sweating
  8. Instruct the client to avoid foods that can inhibit thyroid secretion, such as strawberries, peaches, pears, cabbage, turnips, spinach, kale, brussels sprouts, cauliflower, radishes, and peas
  9. Advise the client to avoid over-the-counter medications
  10. Instruct the client to wear a Medic-Alert bracelet
IV. ANTITHYROID MEDICATIONS (Box 45-3)
A. Description
  1. Antithyroid medications inhibit the synthesis of thyroid hormone
  2. Antithyroid medications are used for **hyperthyroidism,** or Graves' disease
B. Side effects
  1. Nausea and vomiting
  2. Diarrhea
  3. Drowsiness, headache, and fever
  4. Hypersensitivity with rash
  5. Agranulocytosis with leukopenia and thrombocytopenia
  6. Alopecia and hyperpigmentation
  7. Toxicity: **hypothyroidism**
  8. Iodism: characterized by vomiting, abdominal pain, metallic or brassy taste in the mouth, rash, and sore gums and salivary glands

BOX 45-1	Antidiuretic Hormones

Desmopressin acetate (DDAVP)
Lypressin
Vasopressin (Pitressin)

BOX 45-2	Thyroid Hormones

Levothyroxine sodium (Synthroid, Levothroid, Levoxyl)
Liothyronine sodium (Cytomel)
Liotrix (Thyrolar)

BOX 45-3	Antithyroid Medications

Methimazole (Tapazole)
Propylthiouracil (PTU)
Potassium iodide (Lugol's solution)
Radioactive iodine (sodium iodide ^{131}I)

C. Interventions
  1. Monitor vital signs
  2. Monitor triiodothyronine, thyroxine, and TSH levels
  3. Monitor weight
  4. Instruct the client to take medication with meals to avoid gastrointestinal upset
  5. Instruct the client on how to monitor the pulse rate
  6. Inform the client of side effects and when to notify the physician
  7. Advise the client to contact the physician if a fever or sore throat develops
  8. Instruct the client on the signs of **hypothyroidism**
  9. Instruct the client regarding the importance of medication compliance and that abruptly stopping the medication could cause **thyroid storm**
  10. Instruct the client to monitor for signs and symptoms of **thyroid storm** (fever, flushed

skin, confusion and behavioral changes, tachycardia, dysrhythmias, and signs of heart failure)
11. Instruct the client to monitor for signs of iodism
12. Advise the client to consult a physician before eating iodized salt and iodine-rich foods
13. Instruct the client to avoid acetylsalicylic acid (aspirin) and medications containing iodine

V. PARATHYROID MEDICATIONS (Box 45-4)

A. Description
1. Parathyroid hormone regulates serum calcium levels
2. Low serum levels of calcium stimulate parathyroid hormone release
3. Hyperparathyroidism results in a high serum calcium level and bone demineralization, and medication is used to lower the serum calcium level
4. Hypoparathyroidism results in a low serum calcium level, which increases neuromuscular excitability; the treatment includes calcium and vitamin D supplements
5. Administration of calcium salts with digoxin (Lanoxin) increases the risk of digoxin toxicity
6. Oral calcium salts reduce the absorption of tetracycline hydrochloride

B. Interventions
1. Monitor electrolyte and calcium levels
2. Assess for signs and symptoms of hypocalcemia and hypercalcemia

---

BOX 45-4 **Medications to Treat Calcium Disorders**

Calcium Supplements
Calcium carbonate (Caltrate 600, Rolaids, Tums)
Calcium carbonate (OsCal, Oysco, Oyst-Cal)
Calcium citrate (Citracal)
Calcium glubionate (Calcionate)
Calcium gluconate
Calcium lactate
Dibasic calcium phosphate
Tribasic calcium phosphate (Posture)
Vitamin D Supplements
Calcitriol (Calcijex, Rocaltrol)
Ergocalciferol (Calciferol, Drisdol)
Calcium Regulators
Alendronate sodium (Fosamax)
Calcitonin human (Cibacalcin)
Calcitonin salmon (Calcimar, Miacalcin)
Etidronate disodium (Didronel)
Pamidronate disodium (Aredia)
Risedronate sodium (Actonel)
Tiludronate disodium (Skelid)
Antihypercalcemics
Cinacalcet hydrochloride (Sensipar)
Doxercalciferol (Hectorol)
Gallium nitrate (Ganite)
Paricalcitol (Zemplar)

---

3. Assess for symptoms of tetany in the client with hypocalcemia
4. Assess for renal calculi in the client with hypercalcemia
5. Instruct the client in the signs and symptoms of hypercalcemia and hypocalcemia
6. Instruct the client to check over-the-counter medication labels for the possibility of calcium content
7. Instruct the client receiving oral calcium supplements to maintain an adequate intake of vitamin D because vitamin D enhances absorption of calcium
8. Instruct the client receiving calcium regulators such as alendronate sodium (Fosamax) to swallow the tablet whole with water at least 30 minutes before breakfast and not to lie down for at least 30 minutes
9. Instruct the client using nasal spray of Miacalcin (calcitonin) to alternate nares during administration
10. Instruct the client using antihypercalcemic agents to avoid foods rich in calcium, such as green, leafy vegetables, dairy products, shellfish, and soy
11. Instruct the client not to take other medications within 1 hour of calcium salts
12. Instruct the client to increase fluid and fiber in diet to prevent constipation associated with calcium supplements

VI. CORTICOSTEROIDS (MINERALOCORTICOIDS) (Box 45-5)

A. Description
1. Mineralocorticoids are steroid hormones that enhance the reabsorption of sodium and chloride and promote the excretion of potassium and hydrogen from the renal tubules, thereby helping to maintain fluid and electrolyte balance
2. Mineralocorticoids are used for replacement therapy in primary and secondary adrenal insufficiency in **Addison's disease**

B. Side effects
1. Sodium and water retention (hypernatremia and edema), as well as hypertension
2. Hypokalemia
3. Hypocalcemia
4. Osteoporosis and compression fractures
5. Weight gain
6. Heart failure

C. Interventions
1. Monitor vital signs
2. Monitor intake and output and weight, and monitor for edema

---

BOX 45-5 **Corticosteroid: Mineralocorticoid**

Fludrocortisone acetate (Florinef Acetate)

3. Monitor electrolytes and calcium level
4. Instruct the client to take medication with food or milk
5. Instruct the client to consume a high-potassium diet
6. Instruct the client not to stop the medication abruptly
7. Instruct the client to report illness, such as severe diarrhea, vomiting, and fever
8. Instruct the client to notify the physician if low blood pressure, weakness, cramping, or palpitations occur, as well as changes in mental status
9. Instruct the client to wear a Medic-Alert bracelet

VII. CORTICOSTEROIDS (GLUCOCORTICOIDS) (Box 45-6)
A. Description
 1. Glucocorticoids affect glucose, protein, and bone metabolism; alter the normal immune response and suppress inflammation; and produce anti-inflammatory, anti-allergic, and antistress effects
 2. Glucocorticoids may be used as a replacement in adrenocortical insufficiency
B. Side effects
 1. **Hyperglycemia**
 2. Hypokalemia
 3. Hypocalcemia and osteoporosis
 4. Sodium and fluid retention
 5. Weight gain
 6. Mood swings
 7. Moon face, buffalo hump, and truncal obesity
 8. Increased susceptibility to infection and masking of the signs and symptoms of infection
 9. Cataracts
 10. Hirsutism, acne, fragile skin, and bruising
 11. Growth retardation in children
 12. Gastrointestinal (GI) irritation, peptic ulcer, and pancreatitis
 13. Seizures and psychosis
C. Contraindications and cautions
 1. Contraindicated in clients with hypersensitivity, psychosis, and fungal infections
 2. Should be used with caution in clients with **diabetes mellitus**
 3. Use with extreme caution in clients with infections because they mask the signs and symptoms of an infection

BOX 45-6 **Corticosteroids: Glucocorticoids**

Dexamethasone (Decadron)
Hydrocortisone (Cortef)
Methylprednisolone (Medrol dose pack, Depo-Medrol, Solu-Medrol)
Prednisolone (Delta-Cortef, Prelone, Orapred, Pediapred)
Prednisone (Orasone, Deltasone, Meticorten)
Triamcinolone (Aristocort)

4. Increase the potency of medications taken concurrently, such as aspirin, and nonsteroidal anti-inflammatory drugs, thus increasing the risk of GI bleeding and ulceration
5. Use of potassium-wasting diuretics increases potassium loss, resulting in hypokalemia
6. Dexamethasone (Decadron) decreases the effects of orally administered anticoagulants and antidiabetic agents
7. Barbiturates, phenytoin (Dilantin), and rifampin (Rifadin) decrease the effect of prednisone

D. Interventions
 1. Monitor vital signs
 2. Monitor serum electrolytes and blood glucose level
 3. Monitor for hypokalemia and **hyperglycemia**
 4. Monitor intake and output and weight, and monitor for edema
 5. Monitor for hypertension
 6. Assess medical history for glaucoma, cataracts, peptic ulcer, mental health disorders, or **diabetes mellitus**
 7. Monitor the older client for signs and symptoms of increased osteoporosis
 8. Assess for changes in muscle strength
 9. Prepare a schedule for the client on short-term, tapered doses
 10. Instruct the client to take medications at mealtime or with food
 11. Advise the client to eat foods high in potassium
 12. Instruct the client to avoid individuals with respiratory infections
 13. Advise the client to inform all health care providers of the medication regimen
 14. Instruct the client to report signs and symptoms of a medication overdose or **Cushing's syndrome,** including a moon face, puffy eyelids, edema in the feet, increased bruising, dizziness, bleeding, and menstrual irregularities
 15. Note that the client may need additional doses during periods of stress, such as surgery
 16. Instruct the client not to stop the medication abruptly because abrupt withdrawal can result in severe adrenal insufficiency
 17. Advise the client to consult with the physician before receiving vaccinations
 18. Advise the client to wear a Medic-Alert bracelet

VIII. ANDROGENS (Box 45-7)
A. Description
 1. Used to replace deficient hormones or to treat hormone-sensitive disorders
 2. Can cause bleeding if the client is taking oral anticoagulants (increase the effect of anticoagulants)
 3. Can cause decreased serum glucose concentration, thereby reducing insulin requirements in the client with **diabetes mellitus**

BOX 45-7 **Androgens**

Fluoxymesterone
Methytestasterone (Testred, Virilon)
Testosterone preparations
  Testosterone, pellets (Testopel)
  Testosterone, transdermal (Androderm)
  Testosterone cypionate (Depo-Testosterone)
  Testosterone enanthate (Delatestryl)

BOX 45-8 **Estrogens**

Diethylstibestrol (DES)
Estradiol (Estrace, Climara, Estraderm, Vivelle)
Estradiol cypionate (Depo-Estradiol)
Estradiol hemihydrate (Estrasorb)
Estradiol valerate (Delestrogen)
Estrogens, conjugated (Premarin)
Estropipate (Ogen Ogestrel 0.5/50)
Ethinyl estradiol

BOX 45-9 **Progestins**

Hydroxyprogesterone
Levonorgestrel
Medroxyprogesterone acetate (Depo-Provera, Provera)
Medroxyprogesterone and conjugated estrogens
  (Premphase, Prempro)
Megestrol acetate (Megace)
Norethindrone acetate (Aygestin)
Progesterone (Crinone, Progestasert, Prometrium)

4. Hepatotoxic medications are avoided with the use of androgens because of the risk of additive damage to the liver
5. Androgens usually are avoided in men with known prostatic or breast carcinoma because androgens often stimulate growth of these tumors

B. Side effects
  1. Masculine secondary sexual characteristics (body hair growth, lowered voice, muscle growth)
  2. Bladder irritation and urinary tract infections
  3. Breast tenderness
  4. Gynecomastia
  5. Priapism
  6. Menstrual irregularities
  7. Virilism
  8. Sodium and water retention with edema
  9. Nausea, vomiting, or diarrhea
  10. Acne
  11. Changes in libido
  12. Hepatotoxicity and jaundice
  13. Hypercalcemia

C. Interventions
  1. Monitor vital signs
  2. Monitor for edema, weight gain, and skin changes
  3. Assess mental status and neurological function
  4. Assess for signs of liver dysfunction, including right upper quadrant abdominal pain, malaise, fever, jaundice, and pruritus
  5. Assess for the development of secondary sexual characteristics
  6. Instruct the client to take with meals or a snack
  7. Instruct the client to notify the physician if priapism develops
  8. Instruct the client to notify the physician if fluid retention occurs
  9. Instruct women to use a nonhormonal contraceptive while on therapy
  10. For women, monitor for menstrual irregularities and decreased breast size

IX. **ESTROGENS AND PROGESTINS**
 A. Description
  1. Estrogens are steroids that stimulate female reproductive tissue

2. Progestins are steroids that specifically stimulate the uterine lining
3. Estrogen and progestin preparations may be used to stimulate the endogenous hormones to restore hormonal balance or to treat hormone-sensitive tumors (suppress tumor growth) or for contraception (Boxes 45-8 and 45-9)

B. Contraindications and cautions
  1. Estrogens
    a. Estrogens are contraindicated in clients with breast cancer, endometrial hyperplasia, endometrial cancer, history of thromboembolism, or known or suspected pregnancy, or in clients who are lactating
    b. Use estrogens with caution in clients with hypertension, gallbladder disease, or liver or kidney dysfunction
    c. Estrogens increase the risk of toxicity when used with hepatotoxic medications
    d. Barbiturates, phenytoin (Dilantin), and rifampin (Rifadin) decrease the effectiveness of estrogen
  2. Progestins are contraindicated in clients with thromboembolitic disorders and should be avoided in clients with breast tumors or hepatic disease

C. Side effects
  1. Breast tenderness and menstrual changes
  2. Nausea, vomiting, and diarrhea
  3. Malaise, depression, and excessive irritability
  4. Weight gain
  5. Edema and fluid retention
  6. Atherosclerosis
  7. Hypertension, stroke, and myocardial infarction

8. Thromboembolism (estrogen)
9. Migraine headaches and vomiting (estrogen)

D. Interventions
1. Monitor vital signs
2. Monitor for hypertension
3. Assess for edema and weight gain
4. Advise the client not to smoke
5. Advise the client to undergo routine breast and pelvic examinations

X. CONTRACEPTIVES

A. Description
1. These medications contain a combination of estrogen and a progestin or a progestin alone
2. Estrogen-progestin combinations suppress ovulation and change the cervical mucus, making it difficult for sperm to enter
3. Medications that contain only progestins are less effective than the combined medications
4. Contraceptives are usually taken for 21 consecutive days and stopped for 7 days; then the administration cycle is repeated
5. Contraceptives provide reversible prevention of pregnancy
6. Contraceptives are useful in controlling irregular or excessive menstrual cycles
7. Risk factors associated with the development of complications related to the use of contraceptives include smoking, obesity, and hypertension
8. Contraceptives are contraindicated in women with hypertension, thromboembolitic disease, cerebrovascular or coronary artery disease, estrogen-dependent cancers, and pregnancy
9. Contraceptives should be avoided with the use of hepatotoxic medications
10. Contraceptives interfere with the activity of bromocriptine mesylate (Parlodel) and anticoagulants and increase the toxicity of tricyclic antidepressants
11. Contraceptives may alter blood glucose levels
12. Antibiotics may decrease the absorption and effectiveness of oral contraceptives

B. Side effects
1. Breakthrough bleeding
2. Excessive cervical mucus formation
3. Breast tenderness
4. Hypertension
5. Nausea or vomiting

C. Interventions
1. Monitor vital signs and weight
2. Instruct the client in the administration of the medication (it may take up to 1 week for full contraceptive effect to occur when the medication is begun)
3. Instruct the client with **diabetes mellitus** to monitor blood glucose levels carefully

4. Instruct the client to report signs of thromboembolitic complications
5. Instruct the client to notify the physician if vaginal bleeding or menstrual irregularities occur or if pregnancy is suspected
6. Advise the client to use an alternative method of birth control when taking antibiotics because antibiotics may decrease absorption of the oral contraceptive
7. Instruct the client to perform breast self-examination monthly and about the importance of yearly physical examinations
8. If the client decides to discontinue the contraceptive to become pregnant, recommend that the client use an alternative form of birth control for 2 months after discontinuation to ensure more complete excretion of hormonal agents before conception
9. Contraceptive patches
   a. Designed to be worn for 3 weeks and removed for a 1-week period
   b. Applied on clean, dry, intact skin on the buttocks, abdomen, upper outer arm, or upper torso
   c. Instruct the client to peel away one half of backing on patch, apply the sticky surface to the skin, remove the other half of the backing, and then press down on the patch with the palm for 10 seconds
   d. Instruct the client to change the patch weekly, using a new location for each patch
   e. If the patch falls off and remains off for less than 24 hours (such as when the client is sleeping or is unaware that it has fallen off), it can be reapplied if still sticky, or it can be replaced with a new patch
   f. If the patch is off for more than 24 hours, a new 4-week cycle must be started immediately
10. Vaginal ring
    a. Inserted into the vagina by the client, left in place for 3 weeks, and removed for 1 week
    b. The medication is absorbed through the mucous membranes of the vagina
    c. Removed rings should be wrapped in a foil pouch and discarded, not flushed down the toilet
11. Implants and depot injections provide long-acting forms of birth control, from 3 months to 5 years

XI. FERTILITY MEDICATIONS (Box 45-10)

A. Description
1. Fertility medications act to stimulate follicle development and ovulation in functioning ovaries and are combined with human chorionic gonadotropin to maintain the follicles once ovulation has occurred

BOX 45-10 **Fertility Medications**

Bromocriptine mesylate (Parlodel)
Chorionic gonadotropin (Profasi)
Clomiphene citrate (Clomid)
Follitropin alfa (Gonal-F)
Follitropin beta (Follistim)
Menotropins (Pergonal)

2. Fertility medications are contraindicated in the presence of primary ovarian dysfunction, thyroid or adrenal dysfunction, ovarian cysts, pregnancy, or idiopathic uterine bleeding
3. Fertility medications should be used with caution in clients with thromboembolitic or respiratory diseases
B. Side effects
1. Risk of multiple births and birth defects
2. Ovarian overstimulation (abdominal pain, distention, ascites, pleural effusion)
3. Headache or irritability
4. Fluid retention and bloating
5. Nausea or vomiting
6. Uterine bleeding
7. Ovarian enlargement
8. Gynecomastia
9. Rash
10. Orthostatic hypotension
11. Febrile reactions
C. Interventions
1. Instruct the client regarding administration of the medication
2. Provide a calendar of treatment days and instructions on when intercourse should occur to increase therapeutic effectiveness of the medication
3. Provide information about the risks and hazards of multiple births
4. Instruct the client to notify the physician if signs of ovarian overstimulation occur
5. Inform the client about the need for regular follow-up for evaluation

XII. MEDICATIONS FOR PENILE ERECTION DYSFUNCTION
A. Description
1. Alprostadil (Caverject, Muse) is a prostaglandin that relaxes smooth muscle and promotes blood flow into the corpus cavernosum
2. Sildenafil (Viagra), tadalafil (Cialis), and vardenafil (Levitra) cause smooth muscle relaxation and allow blood flow into the corpus cavernosum
3. Erectile dysfunction medications are contraindicated in the presence of any anatomical obstruction or condition that might predispose to priapism and in clients with penile implants

4. Caution should be used in clients with bleeding disorders
5. Sildenafil, tadalafil, and vardenafil are used cautiously in clients with coronary artery disease, active peptic ulcer disease, bleeding disorders, or retinitis pigmentosa
6. Sildenafil, tadalafil, and vardenafil cannot be administered to clients taking nitrates, nitroprusside, or β-blockers
B. Side effects
1. Alprostadil: Pain at the injection site, infection, priapism, fibrosis, rash, hypertension
2. Sildenafil, tadalafil, and vardenafil: Headache, flushing, dyspepsia, urinary tract infection, diarrhea, hypotension, dizziness, rash, neuralgia, insomnia
3. Blurred vision and changes in color vision
C. Interventions
1. Perform a thorough assessment of health and medication history
2. Instruct the client regarding administration of the medication; alprostadil is injected intracavernously or inserted urogenitally as a suppository; sildenafil, tadalafil, and vardenafil are taken orally
3. Inform the client of the side effects necessitating the need to notify the physician.

XIII. MEDICATIONS FOR DIABETES MELLITUS
A. Insulin and oral hypoglycemic medications
1. Description
a. Insulin increases glucose transport into cells and promotes conversion of glucose to glycogen, decreasing serum glucose levels
b. Oral hypoglycemic agents stimulate the pancreas to produce more insulin, increase the sensitivity of peripheral receptors to insulin, decrease hepatic glucose output, or delay intestinal absorption of glucose, thus decreasing serum glucose levels
2. Contraindications and concerns
a. Insulin is contraindicated in clients with hypersensitivity
b. Oral hypoglycemic agents are contraindicated in type 1 **diabetes mellitus**
c. β-Adrenergic blocking agents may mask signs and symptoms of **hypoglycemia** associated with hypoglycemic medications
d. Anticoagulants, chloramphenicol (Chloromycetin), salicylates, propranolol (Inderal), monoamine oxidase inhibitors, pentamidine (Pentam 300), and sulfonamides may cause **hypoglycemia**
e. Corticosteroids, sympathomimetics, thiazide diuretics, phenytoin (Dilantin), thyroid preparations, oral contraceptives, and estrogen compounds may cause **hyperglycemia**

f. Side effects of the sulfonylureas include gastrointestinal symptoms and dermatological reactions; **hypoglycemia** can occur when an excessive dose is administered or when meals are omitted or delayed, food intake is decreased, or activity is increased

g. Sulfonylureas, such as chlorpropamide (Diabinese), can cause a disulfiram (Antabuse) type of reaction when alcohol is ingested

B. Oral hypoglycemic medications
1. Prescribed for clients with type 2 **diabetes mellitus**
2. Sulfonylureas (Box 45-11)
   a. Sulfonylureas may be classified as first- or second-generation sulfonylureas
   b. Sulfonylureas stimulate the beta cells to produce more insulin
3. Biguanides (see Box 45-11)
   a. May be used alone or in combination with a sulfonylurea
   b. Suppress hepatic production of glucose and increases insulin sensitivity
   c. Side effects: diarrhea (most common) and lactic acidosis (most serious)
4. α-Glucosidase inhibitors (see Box 45-11)
   a. Delay absorption of ingested carbohydrates (sucrose and complex carbohydrates), resulting in smaller rise in blood glucose after meals
   b. Do not increase insulin production
   c. Can be given alone or in combination with sulfonylureas
   d. Will not cause **hypoglycemia** when given alone
   e. Given with first bite of meal
5. Thiazolidinediones (see Box 45-11)
   a. Insulin-sensitizing agents that lower blood glucose by decreasing hepatic glucose production and improving target cell response to insulin
   b. May cause liver toxicity
6. Meglitinides (see Box 45-11)
   a. Stimulate pancreatic insulin secretion
   b. Quicker and shorter duration of action, therefore less chance of **hypoglycemia** because blood glucose lowering effect wears off quickly
   c. Very fast onset of action allows clients to take the medication with meals and skip a dose when they skip a meal
7. Interventions
   a. Assess the client's knowledge of **diabetes mellitus** and the use of oral antidiabetic agents
   b. Obtain a medication history regarding the medications that the client is taking currently

---

BOX 45-11 **Oral Hypoglycemic Agents**

Sulfonylureas
Acetohexamide (Dymelor)
Chlorpropamide (Diabinese)
Glimepiride (Amaryl)
Glipizide (Glucotrol)
Glyburide (DiaBeta, Micronase)
Tolazamide (Tolinase)
Tolbutamide (Orinase)
Biguanides
Metformin (Glucophage)
α-Glucosidase Inhibitors
Acarbose (Precose)
Miglitol (Glyset)
Thiazolidinediones
Pioglitazone (Actos)
Rosiglitazone (Avandia)
Meglitinides
Nateglinide (Starlix)
Repaglinide (Prandin)
Dipeptidyl peptidase-4 Inhibitor (Dpp-4 Inhibitor)
Silagliptin (Januvia)

---

   c. Assess vital signs and blood glucose levels
   d. Instruct the client to recognize the signs and symptoms of **hypoglycemia** and **hyperglycemia**
   e. Instruct the client to avoid over-the-counter medications unless prescribed by the health care provider
   f. Instruct the client not to ingest alcohol with sulfonylureas
   g. Inform the client that insulin may be needed during stress, surgery, or infection
   h. Instruct the client in the necessity of compliance with prescribed medication
   i. Instruct the client on how to take each specific medication, such as with the first bite of the meal for meglitinides and α-glucosidase inhibitors
   j. Advise the client to wear a Medic-Alert bracelet

C. Insulin
1. Insulin primarily acts in the liver, muscle, and adipose tissue by attaching to receptors on cellular membranes and facilitating the passage of glucose, potassium, and magnesium
2. Insulin is prescribed for clients with type 1 and type 2 **diabetes mellitus** whose blood glucose is not controlled with oral hypoglycemic agents
3. The onset, peak, and duration of action depends on the insulin type (Table 45-2)
4. Storing of insulin (Box 45-12)

TABLE 45-2 Time Activity of Subcutaneous Human Insulin

Preparation	Brand	Onset (hr)	Peak (hr)	Duration (hr)
Rapid Acting				
Insulin aspart injection	NovoLog	0.25	1-3	3-5
Insulin lispro injection	Humalog	0.25	0.5-1.5	3-4
Insulin glulisine injection	Apidra	0.3	0.5-1.5	5
Short Acting				
Regular human insulin injection	Humulin R	0.5	2-4	6-8
	Novolin R	0.5	2.5-5	8
Buffered regular human insulin injection	Velosulin BR	0.5	1-3	8
Intermediate Acting				
Human insulin isophane suspension	NPH	1.5	4-12	24
Human insulin zinc suspension	Lente	2.5	7-15	22
Long Acting				
Human insulin extended zinc suspension	Ultralente	4-6	8-20	28
Insulin glargine injection	Lantus	2-4	None	24
Combination Insulin				
70% Insulin aspart protamine suspension/30% insulin aspart injection	NovoLog Mix 70/30	0.25	1-4	24
70% Insulin lispro protamine suspension/25% insulin lispro injection	Humalog Mix 75/25	0.25	1-2	24
70% Human insulin isophane suspension (NPH)/30% human insulin injection (regular)	Humulin 70/30	0.5	2-12	24
	Novolin 70/30	0.5	2-12	24
50% Human insulin isophane suspension (NPH)/50% human insulin injection (regular)	Humulin 50/50	0.5	3-5	24

From Ignatavicius, D., & Workman, M. (2006). *Medical-surgical nursing: Critical thinking for collaborative care* (5th ed). Philadelphia: Saunders.

BOX 45-12 Storing Insulin

Avoid exposing insulin to extremes in temperature.
Insulin should not be frozen or kept in direct sunlight or a hot car.
Before injection, insulin should be kept at room temperature.
If a vial of insulin will be used up in a month, it may be kept at room temperature; otherwise, the vial should be refrigerated.

5. Insulin injection sites
   a. The main areas for injections are the abdomen, arms (posterior surface), thighs (anterior surface), and hips (Figure 45-1)
   b. Insulin injected into the abdomen may absorb more evenly and rapidly than at other sites
   c. Systematic rotation within one anatomical area is recommended to prevent lipodystrophy; the client should be instructed not to use the same site more than once in a 2- to 3-week period
   d. Injections should be 1.5 inches apart within the anatomical area
   e. Heat, massage, and exercise of the injected area can increase absorption rates and may result in **hypoglycemia**
   f. Injection into scar tissue may delay absorption of insulin

6. Administering insulin
   a. To prevent dosage errors, be certain that there is a match between the insulin concentration noted on the vial and the calibration of units on the insulin syringe; the usual concentration of insulin is U 100 (100 units/mL)
   b. Most insulin syringes have a 27- to 29-gauge needle that is about ½-inch long
   c. Before use, swirl insulin vial gently or rotate between palms to ensure that the insulin and ingredients are mixed well; otherwise, an inaccurate dose will be drawn; vigorously shaking the bottle will cause bubbles to form
   d. Premixed insulins (NPH and regular insulin) are available as 70/30 (most commonly used) and 50/50; premixed insulin lispro protamine and insulin lispro 75/25 are also available
   e. Inject air into the insulin bottle (a vacuum makes it difficult to draw up the insulin)
   f. When mixing insulins, draw up the regular (shorter-acting) insulin first (Figure 45-2)
   g. Regular insulin may be mixed with NPH or lente insulin
   h. Lispro insulin may be mixed with Humulin N or Humulin U (ultralente)

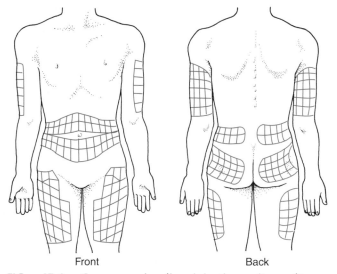

FIG. 45-1 Common insulin injection sites. (From Ignatavicius, D. & Workman, M. [2006]. *Medical-surgical nursing: Critical thinking for collaborative care* [5th ed.]. Philadelphia: Saunders.)

1. Wash hands.
2. Gently rotate NPH insulin bottle.
3. Wipe off tops of insulin vials with alcohol sponge.
4. Draw back amount of air into the syringe that equals total dose.

5. Inject air equal to NPH dose into NPH vial. Remove syringe from vial.

6. Inject air equal to regular dose into regular vial.

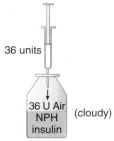

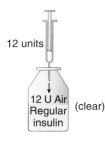

7. Invert regular insulin bottle and withdraw regular insulin dose.

8. Without adding more air to NPH vial, carefully withdraw NPH dose.

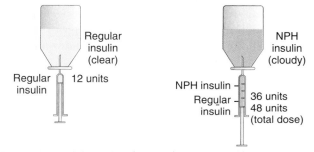

FIG. 45-2 Mixing insulins. This step-order process avoids the problem of contaminating regular insulin with intermediate-acting insulin. (From Lewis, S., Heitkemper, M., & Dirksen, S. [2007]. *Medical-surgical nursing: Assessment and management of clinical problems* [7th ed.]. St Louis: Mosby.)

  i. Insulin aspart may be mixed with NPH insulin only
  j. Insulin zinc suspensions may be mixed only with each other and regular insulin, not with other types of insulin
  k. Glargine insulin CANNOT be mixed with any other types of insulin
  l. Administer a mixed dose of insulin within 5 to 15 minutes of preparation; after this time the regular insulin binds with the NPH insulin and its action is reduced
  m. Aspiration generally is not recommended with self-injection of insulin
  n. Administer insulin at a 45- to 90-degree angle; administer at a 45- to 60-degree angle in clients with minimal subcutaneous mass
  o. Remember: Regular insulin is the only type of insulin that can be administered intravenously
 D. Exubera (insulin human [rDNA origin]) Inhalation Powder
  1. A short-acting inhaled insulin indicated for treatment of type 1 and type 2 **diabetes mellitus**
  2. Consists of a fine dry-powder insulin that enters the bloodstream more rapidly than by subcutaneous injection
  3. Inhaled 10 minutes before meals
  4. Causes a decrease in pulmonary function, and pulmonary function studies are performed before treatment starts and periodically during treatment

  5. Contraindicated in the client who smokes, starts smoking, or quits smoking less than 6 months prior to initiation of treatment; unstable or poorly controlled lung disease such as asthma, emphysema, or chronic obstructive pulmonary disease; in the pregnant client; and in individuals younger than 18 years of age
  6. Side effects include cough, dry mouth, chest discomfort, and **hypoglycemia**
  7. Teach the client about the side effects of the medication, how and when to use the inhaler, and how to care for the inhaler
 E. Exenatide (Byetta)
  1. A synthetic hormone classified as an incretin mimetic that is administered subcutaneously.
  2. Used for clients with type 2 **diabetes mellitus** (not recommended for clients taking insulin, nor should clients be taken off of insulin and given exenatide)
  3. Restores first-phase insulin response (first 10 minutes after food ingestion), lowers the

production of glucagon after meals, slows gastric emptying (which limits the rise in the blood glucose after a meal), reduces fasting and postprandal blood glucose, and reduces caloric intake, resulting in a weight loss.

    4. Packaged in premeasured doses (pen) that require refrigeration (cannot be frozen)

    5. Administered as a subcutaneous injection in the thigh, abdomen, or upper arm within 60 minutes before morning and evening meals; not taken after meals, and if a dose is missed, the treatment regimen is resumed as prescribed with the next scheduled dose

    6. Can cause mild to moderate nausea that abates with use

F. Pramlintide (Symlin)

    1. A synthetic form of amylin, a naturally occurring hormone that is secreted by the pancreas

    2. Used for clients with type 1 and type 2 **diabetes mellitus** who use insulin and is given before meals to lower blood glucose after meals, leading to less fluctuation during the day and better long-term glucose control

    3. Associated with an increased risk of insulin-induced severe **hypoglycemia,** particularly in clients with type 1 **diabetes mellitus**

    4. GI side effects including nausea can occur

    5. Unopened vials are refrigerated; opened vials can be refrigerated or kept at room temperature for up to 28 days

G. Glucagon

    1. A hormone secreted by the alpha cells of the islets of Langerhans in the pancreas

    2. Increases blood glucose by stimulating glycogenolysis in the liver

    3. Can be administered subcutaneously, intramuscularly, or intravenously

    4. Used to treat insulin-induced **hypoglycemia** when the client is semiconscious or unconscious and is unable to ingest liquids

    5. The blood glucose level begins to increase within 5 to 20 minutes after administration

    6. Instruct the family in the procedure for administration

    7. Refer to Chapter 44 for additional information regarding interventions for severe **hypoglycemia**

H. Diazoxide (Proglycem)

    1. Increases blood glucose by inhibiting insulin release from the beta cells and stimulating the release of epinephrine from the adrenal medulla

    2. Used to treat chronic **hypoglycemia** caused by hyperinsulinism resulting from islet cell cancer or hyperplasia

    3. Not used for hypoglycemic reactions from insulin

PRACTICE QUESTIONS

533. A nurse provides instructions to the client taking fludrocortisone (Florinef). The nurse tells the client to notify the physician if which of the following occurs?
    1. Nausea
    2. Fatigue
    3. Weight loss
    4. Swelling of the feet

534. Calcitriol (Rocaltrol) is prescribed for the client with hypocalcemia, and the nurse provides dietary instructions to the client. Which food item would the nurse instruct the client to avoid while taking this medication?
    1. Milk
    2. Oysters
    3. Sardines
    4. Whole-grain cereals

535. A daily dose of prednisone (Deltasone) is prescribed for a client. A nurse provides instructions to the client regarding administration of the medication and tells the client that the best time to take this medication is:
    1. At noon
    2. At bedtime
    3. Early morning
    4. Any time, at the same time, each day

536. Sildenafil citrate (Viagra) is prescribed to treat a client with erectile dysfunction. A nurse reviews the client's medical record and would question the prescription if which of the following is noted in the client's history?
    1. Insomnia
    2. Neuralgia
    3. Use of nitroglycerin
    4. Use of multivitamins

537. A nurse is teaching the client how to mix regular insulin and NPH insulin in the same syringe. Which of the following actions, if performed by the client, would indicate the need for further teaching?
    1. Withdraws the NPH insulin first
    2. Withdraws the regular insulin first
    3. Injects air into the NPH insulin vial first
    4. Injects the amount of air equal to the desired dose of insulin into the vial

538. A nurse is reinforcing home care instructions to a client recently diagnosed with diabetes mellitus. The client is taking NPH insulin daily and asks the nurse how to store the unopened vials of insulin. The nurse tells the client to:
    1. Freeze the insulin
    2. Refrigerate the insulin
    3. Keep the insulin in a dark, dry place
    4. Keep the insulin at room temperature

539. A client with diabetes mellitus is self-administering NPH insulin from a vial that is kept at

room temperature. The client asks the nurse about the length of time an unrefrigerated vial of insulin will maintain its potency. The appropriate response is which of the following?

1. Two weeks
2. Six months
3. One month
4. Two months

540. Lispro insulin (Humalog), a rapid-acting form of insulin, is prescribed for a client. The nurse instructs the client to administer the insulin:

1. 30 minutes before eating
2. 45 minutes before eating
3. 60 minutes before eating
4. Immediately before eating

541. Tolbutamide (Orinase) is prescribed for the client with diabetes mellitus. The nurse instructs the client to avoid which of the following while taking this medication?

1. Alcohol
2. Organ meats
3. Whole-grain cereals
4. Carbonated beverages

542. A nurse is monitoring a client receiving desmopressin (DDAVP). Which of the following, if noted in the client, would indicate an adverse effect of the medication?

1. Insomnia
2. Drowsiness
3. Weight loss
4. Increased urination

543. A nurse provides instructions to a client taking levothyroxine (Synthroid). The nurse determines that the teaching was effective if the client states that he or she will take the medication:

1. At bedtime
2. At lunch time
3. Two hours after a meal
4. One hour before breakfast

544. A nurse reinforces medication instructions to a client taking levothyroxine (Synthroid). The nurse

should instruct the client to notify the doctor if which problem occurs?

1. Fatigue
2. Tremors
3. Cold intolerance
4. Excessively dry skin

545. A nurse reviews the health record of a client seen in the physician's office and noted that the client is taking propylthiouracil (PTU) daily. The nurse suspects that the client is taking the medication for which condition?

1. Myxedema
2. Acromegaly
3. Graves' disease
4. Addison's disease

546. Propylthiouracil (PTU) is prescribed for a client with hyperthyroidism, and the nurse provides instructions to the client regarding the medication. The nurse informs the client to notify the physician if which of the following signs occur?

1. Polyuria
2. Dry mouth
3. Sore throat
4. Drowsiness

ALTERNATE FORMAT ITEM: FILL IN THE BLANK

547. A client with diabetes mellitus is preparing for discharge from the hospital and tells the nurse that syringes prefilled with NPH and regular insulin will be prepared by a home care nurse who will be visiting the client. The client asks the nurse how often the home care nurse will need to visit to fill syringes. Considering the stability of insulin, the nurse tells the client that how many prefilled syringes can be prepared by the home care nurse?

Answer: _____

ANSWERS

533. 4

Rationale: Excessive doses of fludrocortisone cause retention of sodium and water and excessive excretion of potassium, resulting in expansion of blood volume, hypertension, cardiac enlargement, edema, and hypokalemia. The client needs to be informed about the signs of sodium and water retention, such as unusual weight gain or swelling of the feet or lower legs. If these signs occur, the physician needs to be notified.

Test-Taking Strategy: Use the process of elimination. Recalling that fludrocortisone can cause water retention will direct you to option 4. If you are unfamiliar with the adverse effects associated with this medication, review this content.

Level of Cognitive Ability: Application

Client Needs: Physiological Integrity
Integrated Process: Teaching and Learning
Content Area: Pharmacology
Reference: Skidmore-Roth, L. (2008). *2008 Mosby's nursing drug reference* (21st ed., p. 470). St. Louis: Mosby.

534. 4

Rationale: The client taking an antihypocalcemic medication should be instructed to avoid eating foods that can suppress calcium absorption. These foods include Swiss chard, beets, bran, and whole-grain cereals.

Test-Taking Strategy: Use the process of elimination. Note that the client's diagnosis is "hypocalcemia" and note the strategic word "avoid." Eliminate options 2 and 3 first because they are comparable or alike. From the remaining options, recalling the food items that can suppress calcium absorption will

direct you to option 4. Review these foods if you had difficulty with this question.
Level of Cognitive Ability: Application
Client Needs: Physiological Integrity
Integrated Process: Teaching and Learning
Content Area: Pharmacology
Reference: Lehne, R. (2007). *Pharmacology for nursing care* (6th ed., p. 863). Philadelphia: Saunders.

535. **3**
Rationale: Glucocorticoids should be administered before 9:00 AM, and the client should be instructed to do so. Administration at this time helps minimize adrenal insufficiency and mimics the burst of glucocorticoids released naturally by the adrenals each morning.
Test-Taking Strategy: Knowledge regarding the administration of glucocorticoids is required to answer this question. Remember, glucocorticoids should be administered before 9:00 AM. If you had difficulty with this question, review the guidelines associated with administering glucocorticoids.
Level of Cognitive Ability: Application
Client Needs: Physiological Integrity
Integrated Process: Nursing Process/Implementation
Content Area: Pharmacology
Reference: Kee, J., Hayes, E., & McCuistion, L. (2006). *Pharmacology: A nursing process approach.* (5th ed., p. 765). Philadelphia: Saunders.

536. **3**
Rationale: Sildenafil citrate (Viagra) enhances the vasodilation effect of nitric oxide in the corpus cavernosus of the penis, thus sustaining an erection. Because of the effect of the medication, it is contraindicated with concurrent use of organic nitrates and nitroglycerin. It is not contraindicated with the use of vitamins. Neuralgia and insomnia are side effects of the medication.
Test-Taking Strategy: Use the process of elimination and note the strategic words "would question the prescription." Recalling the action of the medication will direct you to option 3. If you had difficulty with this question, review the contraindications associated with the use of this medication.
Level of Cognitive Ability: Analysis
Client Needs: Physiological Integrity
Integrated Process: Nursing Process/Implementation
Content Area: Pharmacology
Reference: Skidmore-Roth, L. (2008). *Mosby's nursing drug reference* (21st ed., p. 927). St. Louis: Mosby.

537. **1**
Rationale: When preparing a mixture of regular insulin with another insulin preparation, the regular insulin should be drawn into the syringe first. This sequence will avoid contaminating the vial of regular insulin with insulin of another type. Options 2, 3, and 4 are correct.
Test-Taking Strategy: Use the process of elimination and note the strategic words "need for further teaching." These words indicate a negative event query and the need to select the incorrect client statement. Recalling the appropriate method of preparing insulin for injection will direct you to option 1. Review this procedure if you had difficulty with this question.
Level of Cognitive Ability: Analysis

Client Needs: Physiological Integrity
Integrated Process: Teaching and Learning
Content Area: Pharmacology
References: Lehne, R. (2007). *Pharmacology for nursing care* (6th ed., p. 655). Philadelphia: Saunders.
Lewis, S., Heitkemper, M., Dirksen, S., & Bucher, L. (2007). *Medical-surgical nursing: Assessment and management of clinical problems* (7th ed., p. 1262). St. Louis: Mosby.

538. **2**
Rationale: Unopened vials of insulin should be stored under refrigeration until needed. Vials should not be frozen. Open vials in use may be kept at room temperature and should be kept away from heat and direct light.
Test-Taking Strategy: Use the process of elimination and note the strategic word "store" in the question. Remembering that insulin should not be frozen will assist in eliminating option 1. Eliminate options 3 and 4 next because they are comparable or alike. Review client teaching points related to insulin if you had difficulty with this question.
Level of Cognitive Ability: Application
Client Needs: Physiological Integrity
Integrated Process: Teaching and Learning
Content Area: Pharmacology
Reference: deWit, S. (2009). *Medical-surgical nursing: Concepts & practice* (1st ed., 917). Philadelphia: Saunders.

539. **3**
Rationale: An unrefrigerated insulin vial will maintain its potency for up to 1 month. Direct sunlight and heat must be avoided.
Test-Taking Strategy: Note the strategic word "unrefrigerated" to assist in directing you to the correct option. Review the concepts related to insulin stability if you had difficulty with this question.
Level of Cognitive Ability: Application
Client Needs: Physiological Integrity
Integrated Process: Nursing Process/Implementation
Content Area: Pharmacology
Reference: Lehne, R. (2007). *Pharmacology for nursing care* (6th ed., p. 657). Philadelphia: Saunders.

540. **4**
Rationale: The effect of lispro insulin begins within 5 minutes of subcutaneous injection and persists for 2 to 4 hours. Lispro insulin acts more rapidly than regular insulin but has a shorter duration of action. Because of its rapid onset, it can be administered immediately before eating. In contrast, regular insulin is generally administered 30 minutes before meals.
Test-Taking Strategy: Use the process of elimination. Noting the strategic words "rapid-acting" will assist in eliminating options 2 and 3. From the remaining options, remember that the question is asking about lispro, not regular, insulin. Review this type of insulin if you had difficulty with this question.
Level of Cognitive Ability: Application
Client Needs: Physiological Integrity
Integrated Process: Teaching and Learning
Content Area: Pharmacology

References: Black, J., & Hawks, J. (2005). *Medical-surgical nursing: Clinical management for positive outcomes* (7th ed., pp. 1254-1255). Philadelphia: W.B. Saunders.
Lehne, R. (2007). *Pharmacology for nursing care* (6th ed., p. 653). Philadelphia: Saunders.

541. **1**

Rationale: When alcohol is combined with tolbutamide, a disulfiram-like reaction may occur. This syndrome includes flushing, palpitations, and nausea. Also, alcohol can potentiate the hypoglycemic effects of tolbutamide. Clients must be warned about alcohol consumption while taking this medication.

Test-Taking Strategy: Use the process of elimination. Eliminate options 2, 3, and 4 because these food items are allowed in a diabetic diet. From the remaining options, remembering that alcohol can affect the action of many medications will assist in directing you to option 1. Review this medication if you had difficulty with this question.

Level of Cognitive Ability: Application
Client Needs: Physiological Integrity
Integrated Process: Teaching and Learning
Content Area: Pharmacology
Reference: Lehne, R. (2007). *Pharmacology for nursing care* (6th ed., p. 662). Philadelphia: Saunders.

542. **2**

Rationale: Water intoxication or hyponatremia is an adverse reaction to DDAVP. Early signs include drowsiness, listlessness, and headache. Decreased urination, rapid weight gain, confusion, seizures, and coma may also occur in overhydration.

Test-Taking Strategy: Use the process of elimination. Knowledge that this medication is used in the treatment of diabetes insipidus will assist in eliminating options 3 and 4. Recalling the action of the medication will assist you in determining that water intoxication is an adverse reaction. This thought process will assist in directing you to option 2. Review the adverse effects related to this medication if you had difficulty with this question.

Level of Cognitive Ability: Analysis
Client Needs: Physiological Integrity
Integrated Process: Nursing Process/Data Collection
Content Area: Pharmacology
Reference: Lilley, L., Harrington, S., & Snyder J. (2007). *Pharmacology and the nursing process* (5th ed., p. 460). St. Louis: Mosby.

543. **4**

Rationale: Oral doses of levothyroxine should be taken on an empty stomach to enhance absorption. The medication should be taken in the morning before breakfast.

Test-Taking Strategy: Use the process of elimination. Eliminate options 2 and 3 first because they are comparable or alike. From the remaining options, recalling the purpose of the medication and that it is administered in the morning will direct you to option 4. Review this medication if you had difficulty with this question.

Level of Cognitive Ability: Analysis
Client Needs: Physiological Integrity
Integrated Process: Nursing Process/Evaluation
Content Area: Pharmacology

References: Lilley, L., Harrington, S., & Snyder J. (2007). *Pharmacology and the nursing process* (5th ed., p. 471). St. Louis: Mosby.
Skidmore-Roth, L. *2008 Mosby's nursing drug reference* (21st ed., p. 611). St. Louis: Mosby.

544. **2**

Rationale: Excessive doses of levothyroxine can produce signs and symptoms of hyperthyroidism (thyrotoxicosis). These include tachycardia, angina, tremors, nervousness, insomnia, hyperthermia, heat intolerance, and sweating. The client should be instructed to notify the physician if these occur. Options 1, 3, and 4 are signs of hypothyroidism.

Test-Taking Strategy: Use the process of elimination, recalling the symptoms associated with hypothyroidism, the purpose of administering levothyroxine, and the effects of the medication. Options 1, 3, and 4 are symptoms related to hypothyroidism. Review the adverse effects of the medication if you are unfamiliar with it.

Level of Cognitive Ability: Application
Client Needs: Physiological Integrity
Integrated Process: Teaching and Learning
Content Area: Pharmacology
References: Kee, J., Hayes, E., & McCuistion, L. (2006). *Pharmacology: A nursing process approach* (5th ed., p. 765). Philadelphia: Saunders.
Lehne, R. (2007). *Pharmacology for nursing care* (6th ed., p. 679). Philadelphia: Saunders.

545. **3**

Rationale: PTU inhibits thyroid hormone synthesis and is used to treat hyperthyroidism or Graves' disease. Myxedema indicates hypothyroidism. Cushing's syndrome and Addison's disease are disorders related to adrenal function.

Test-Taking Strategy: Knowledge regarding the action of the medication and the treatment measures for Graves' disease is required to answer the question. Remember that PTU inhibits thyroid hormone synthesis and is used to treat hyperthyroidism or Graves' disease. Review this medication if you had difficulty with this question.

Level of Cognitive Ability: Analysis
Client Needs: Physiological Integrity
Integrated Process: Nursing Process/Data Collection
Content Area: Pharmacology
References: Lehne, R. (2007). *Pharmacology for nursing care* (6th ed., p. 680). Philadelphia: Saunders.
Lilley, L., Harrington, S., & Snyder J. (2007). *Pharmacology and the nursing process* (5th ed., p. 469). St. Louis: Mosby.

546. **3**

Rationale: An adverse effect of PTU is agranulocytosis. The client needs to be informed of the early signs of this adverse effect, which include fever or sore throat. Drowsiness is an occasional side effect of the medication. Polyuria and dry mouth are unrelated to this medication.

Test-Taking Strategy: Use the process of elimination. Recalling that agranulocytosis is an adverse effect of PTU will direct you to option 3. Review this medication if you had difficulty with this question.

Level of Cognitive Ability: Application
Client Needs: Physiological Integrity

Integrated Process: Nursing Process/Implementation
Content Area: Pharmacology
References: Lehne, R. (2007). *Pharmacology for nursing care* (6th ed., pp. 680-681). Philadelphia: Saunders.
Lilley, L., Harrington, S., & Snyder J. (2007). *Pharmacology and the nursing process* (5th ed., p. 471). St. Louis: Mosby.

ALTERNATE ITEM FORMAT: FILL IN THE BLANK

547. **7**
Rationale: Mixtures of insulin in prefilled syringes should be stored in a refrigerator, where they will be stable for 1 week. The syringe should be stored vertically, with the needle pointing up, to avoid clogging the needle. Prior to administration, the syringe should be agitated gently to resuspend the insulin.
Test-Taking Strategy: It is necessary to know the concepts related to insulin stability and storage to answer this question. Remember that mixtures of insulin in prefilled syringes are stable for 1 week. Review these concepts if you are unfamiliar with the principles related to prefilling insulin syringes.
Level of Cognitive Ability: Application
Client Needs: Physiological Integrity
Integrated Process: Nursing Process/Implementation
Content Area: Pharmacology
Reference: Lehne, R. (2007). *Pharmacology for nursing care* (6th ed., p. 670). Philadelphia: Saunders.

REFERENCES

Black, J., & Hawks, J. (2005). *Medical-surgical nursing: Clinical management for positive outcomes* (7th ed.). Philadelphia: Saunders.

deWit, S. (2009). *Medical-surgical nursing: Concepts & practice* (1st ed.). Philadelphia: Saunders.

Kee, J., Hayes, E., & McCuistion, L. (2006). *Pharmacology: A nursing process approach* (5th ed.). Philadelphia: Saunders.

Lehne, R. (2007). *Pharmacology for nursing care* (6th ed.). Philadelphia: Saunders.

Lewis, S., Heitkemper, M., Dirksen, S., & Bucher, L. (2007). *Medical-surgical nursing: Assessment and management of clinical problems* (7th ed.). St. Louis: Mosby.

Lilley, L., Harrington, S., & Snyder, J. (2007). *Pharmacology and the nursing process* (5th ed.). St. Louis: Mosby.

Linton, A., & Maebius, N. (2007). *Introduction to medical-surgical nursing* (4th ed.). Philadelphia: Saunders.

Skidmore-Roth, L. (2008). *2008 Mosby's nursing drug reference* (21st ed.). St. Louis: Mosby.

The Adult Client With a Gastrointestinal Disorder

PYRAMID TERMS

ascites The accumulation of fluid within the peritoneal cavity

asterixis A coarse tremor characterized by rapid, nonrhythmic extensions and flexions in the wrist and fingers; also termed liver flap

Billroth I Also called gastroduodenostomy; partial gastrectomy and remaining segment are anastomosed to the duodenum

Billroth II Also called gastrojejunostomy; partial gastrectomy and remaining segment are anastomosed to the jejunum

cholecystectomy Removal of the gallbladder

cholecystitis An inflammation of the gallbladder that may occur as an acute or chronic process. Acute inflammation is associated with gallstones (cholelithiasis). Chronic cholecystitis results when inefficient bile emptying and gallbladder muscle wall disease result in a fibrotic and contracted gallbladder

choledocholithotomy Incision into the common bile duct to remove a gallstone

cirrhosis A chronic, progressive disease of the liver in which liver cells are replaced by scar tissue

Crohn's disease An inflammatory disease that can occur anywhere in the gastrointestinal (GI) tract, but most often affects the terminal ileum and leads to thickening and scarring, a narrowed lumen, fistulas, ulcerations, and abscesses. It is characterized by remissions and exacerbations

Cullen's sign Bluish discoloration of the abdomen and periumbilical area seen in acute hemorrhagic pancreatitis

diverticulitis Inflammation of one or more diverticuli in the lining of the intestinal wall, caused by intestinal contents becoming lodged in diverticula

diverticulosis Outpouchings or herniations of the intestinal mucosa; this condition can occur in any part of the intestine but is most common in the sigmoid colon

dumping syndrome Rapid emptying of the gastric contents into the small intestine; occurs following gastric resection

esophageal varices Dilated veins in the submucosa of the esophagus; they are caused by portal hypertension, are often associated with liver cirrhosis, and are at high risk for rupture if portal circulation pressure rises

fetor hepaticus The fruity, musty breath odor associated with severe chronic liver disease

gastrectomy Also called esophagojejunostomy; involves removal of the stomach, with attachment of the esophagus to the jejunum or duodenum

gastric resection Also called antrectomy; involves removal of the lower half of the stomach and usually includes a vagotomy

hepatitis Inflammation of the liver that causes cell damage, often caused by a virus; viral types of hepatitis are classified as A, B, C, D, E, and G

hiatal hernia Also known as esophageal or diaphragmatic hernia; a portion of the stomach herniates through the diaphragm and into the thorax; hiatal hernia results from weakening of the muscles of the diaphragm and is aggravated by factors that increase abdominal pressure, such as pregnancy, ascites, obesity, tumors, and heavy lifting

Kock ileostomy (continent ileostomy) An intra-abdominal pouch is constructed from the terminal ileum; the pouch is connected to the stoma with a nipple-like valve constructed from a portion of the ileum; the stoma is flush with the skin

Murphy's sign A sign of gallbladder disease consisting of pain on taking a deep breath when the examiner's fingers are on the approximate location of the gallbladder

pancreatitis An acute or chronic inflammation of the pancreas, with associated escape of pancreatic enzymes into surrounding tissue; acute pancreatitis occurs suddenly as one attack or can be recurrent but resolves; chronic pancreatitis is a continual inflammation and destruction of the pancreas, with scar tissue replacing pancreatic tissue

peristalsis Wave-like rhythmic contractions that propel material through the GI tract

portal hypertension A persistent increase in pressure within the portal vein that develops as a result of obstruction to flow

pyloroplasty Enlarging the pylorus to prevent or decrease pyloric obstruction, thereby enhancing gastric emptying

Turner's sign A gray-blue discoloration of the flanks seen in acute hemorrhagic pancreatitis

ulcerative colitis Ulcerative and inflammatory disease of the bowel that results in poor absorption of nutrients; acute ulcerative colitis results in vascular congestion, hemorrhage, edema, and ulceration of the bowel mucosa; chronic ulcerative colitis causes muscular hypertrophy, fat deposits, and fibrous tissue with bowel thickening, shortening, and narrowing

vagotomy Surgical division of the vagus nerve to eliminate the vagal impulses that stimulate hydrochloric acid secretion in the stomach

▲ PYRAMID TO SUCCESS

Pyramid points focus on diagnostic tests, nursing care related to the various gastric or intestinal tubes, gastric surgery, cirrhosis, hepatitis, pancreatitis, and colostomy care. Focus on preprocedure and postprocedure care of the client undergoing a gastrointestinal diagnostic test. Remember that an informed consent is required for any invasive procedure. Focus on diet restrictions before and after the diagnostic test, and remember that the gag reflex or bowel sounds must return before allowing a client to consume food or fluids. Pyramid points include instructions to the client and family regarding the prevention of gastrointestinal disorders and the complications associated with the disorder. Focus on teaching the client and family about diet and nutrition specific to the disorder, tube and wound care, preventing the transmission of infection, and care of a colostomy or ileostomy. The Integrated Processes addressed in this unit include Caring, Clinical Problem-Solving Process (Nursing Process), Communication and Documentation, and Teaching and Learning.

▲ CLIENT NEEDS

Safe and Effective Care Environment

Consulting with other health care professionals regarding the client's nutritional status
Ensuring that confidentiality issues related to the gastrointestinal disorder are maintained
Establishing priorities of care
Handling infectious drainage and secretions safely
Maintaining standard precautions and other precautions as appropriate
Obtaining informed consent for treatments and surgical procedures
Obtaining referrals for home care and community services
Preventing disease transmission

Health Promotion and Maintenance

Performing data collection techniques of the gastrointestinal system
Preventing disease related to the gastrointestinal system
Providing health screening and health promotion programs related to gastrointestinal disorders
Teaching related to colostomy or ileostomy care
Teaching related to preventing the transmission of disease

Teaching related to prescribed dietary and other treatment measures

Psychosocial Integrity

Assessing coping mechanisms
Considering end-of-life and grief and loss issues
Identifying available support systems
Monitoring for expected body-image changes related to colostomy or ileostomy

Physiological Integrity

Administering medications as prescribed specific to the gastrointestinal disorder
Assessing for signs and symptoms of infectious diseases of the gastrointestinal tract
Assisting with personal hygiene
Monitoring elimination patterns
Monitoring for complications related to tests, procedures, and surgical interventions
Monitoring for fluid and electrolyte imbalances
Monitoring laboratory values related to gastrointestinal disorders
Monitoring parenterally administered fluids, including parenteral nutrition
Providing adequate nutrition and oral hydration
Providing care for gastrointestinal tubes
Providing nonpharmacological and pharmacological comfort measures
Providing preprocedure and postprocedure care for diagnostic tests related to the gastrointestinal system

REFERENCES

Black, J., & Hawks, J. (2005). *Medical-surgical nursing: Clinical management for positive outcomes* (7th ed.). Philadelphia: Saunders.
Chernecky, C., & Berger, B. (2008). *Laboratory tests and diagnostic procedures* (5th ed.). Philadelphia: Saunders.
Christensen, B., & Kockrow, E. (2006). *Adult health nursing* (5th ed.). St. Louis: Mosby.
Christensen, B., & Kockrow, E. (2006). *Foundations of nursing* (5th ed.). St. Louis: Mosby.
deWit, S. (2009). *Medical-surgical nursing: Concepts & practice.* (1st ed.). Philadelphia: Saunders.
Hodgson, B., & Kizior, R. (2008). *Saunders nursing drug handbook 2008.* Philadelphia: Saunders.
Ignatavicius, D., & Workman, M. (2006). *Medical-surgical nursing: Critical thinking for collaborative care* (5th ed.). Philadelphia: Saunders.
Kee, J., Hayes, E., & McCuistion, L. (2006). *Pharmacology: A nursing process approach* (5th ed.). Philadelphia: Saunders.
Lehne, R. (2007). *Pharmacology for nursing care* (6th ed.). Philadelphia: Saunders.
Lewis, S., Heitkemper, M., Dirksen, S., & Bucher, L. (2007). *Medical-surgical nursing: Assessment and management of clinical problems* (7th ed.). St. Louis: Mosby.
Linton, A., & Maebius, N. (2007). *Introduction to medical-surgical nursing* (4th ed.). Philadelphia: Saunders.
McKenry, L., Tessier, E., & Hogan, M. (2006). *Mosby's pharmacology in nursing* (22nd ed.). St. Louis: Mosby.

Monahan, F., Sands, J., Marek, J., et al. (2007). *Phipps' medical-surgical nursing: Health and illness perspectives* (8th ed.). St. Louis: Mosby.

National Council of State Boards of Nursing (eds.). *2008 Detailed Test Plan for the NCLEX-PN® Examination, National Council of State Boards of Nursing.* (2008). Chicago: Author.

National Council of State Boards of Nursing, Inc. Web site: http://www.ncsbn.org.

Perry, A., & Potter, P. (2006). *Clinical nursing skills & techniques* (6th ed.). St. Louis: Mosby.

Skidmore-Roth, L. (2008). *2008 Mosby's nursing drug reference* (21st ed.). St. Louis: Mosby.

Gastrointestinal System

I. ANATOMY AND PHYSIOLOGY

A. Functions of the gastrointestinal system
1. Process food substances
2. Absorb the products of digestion into the blood
3. Excrete unabsorbed materials
4. Provide an environment for microorganisms to synthesize nutrients, such as vitamin K
5. For risk factors associated with the gastrointestinal system, see Box 46-1

B. Mouth
1. Contains the lips, cheeks, palate, tongue, teeth, salivary glands, muscles, and maxillary bones
2. Saliva contains the amylase enzyme (ptyalin) that aids in digestion

C. Esophagus
1. A collapsible muscular tube about 10 inches long
2. Carries food from the pharynx to the stomach

D. The stomach
1. Contains the cardia, fundus, body, and pylorus
2. Mucous glands are located in the mucosa and prevent autodigestion by providing an alkaline protective covering
3. The lower esophageal (cardiac) sphincter prevents reflux of gastric contents into the esophagus
4. The pyloric sphincter regulates the rate of stomach emptying into the small intestine
5. Hydrochloric acid kills microorganisms, breaks food into small particles, and provides a chemical environment that facilitates gastric enzyme activation
6. Pepsin is the chief coenzyme of gastric juice, which converts proteins into proteases and peptones
7. Intrinsic factor is necessary for the absorption of vitamin B_{12}
8. Gastrin controls gastric acidity

E. Small intestine
1. The duodenum contains the openings of the bile and pancreatic ducts
2. The jejunum is about 8 feet long
3. The ileum is about 12 feet long
4. The small intestine terminates into the cecum

F. Pancreatic intestinal juice enzymes
1. Amylase digests starch to maltose
2. Maltase reduces maltose to monosaccharide glucose
3. Lactase splits lactose into galactose and glucose
4. Sucrase reduces sucrose to fructose and glucose
5. Nucleoses split nucleic acids to nucleotides
6. Enterokinase activates trypsinogen to trypsin

G. Large intestine
1. Is about 5 feet long
2. Absorbs water and eliminates wastes
3. Intestinal bacteria play a vital role in the synthesis of some B vitamins and vitamin K
4. Colon: includes the ascending, transverse, descending, sigmoid, and rectum
5. The ileocecal valve prevents contents of the large intestine from entering the ileum
6. The anal sphincters control/guard the anal canal

H. Peritoneum: lines the abdominal cavity and forms the mesentery that supports the intestines and blood supply

I. Liver
1. The largest gland in the body, weighing 3 to 4 lb
2. Contains Kupffer's cells, which remove bacteria in the portal venous blood
3. Removes excess glucose and amino acids from the portal blood
4. Synthesizes glucose, amino acids, and fats
5. Aids in the digestion of fats, carbohydrates, and proteins
6. Stores and filters blood (200 to 400 mL of blood stored)
7. Stores vitamins A, D, and B, as well as iron
8. Secretes bile to emulsify fats (500 to 1000 mL of bile a day)
9. Hepatic ducts
   a. Deliver bile to the gallbladder via the cystic duct and to the duodenum via the common bile duct

Risk Factors Associated with the Gastrointestinal (GI) System

Allergic reactions to food or medications
Cardiac, respiratory, and endocrine disorders that may lead to constipation
Chronic alcohol use
Chronic high stress levels
Chronic laxative use
Chronic use of aspirin or nonsteroidal anti-inflammatory drugs
Diabetes mellitus, which may predispose to oral candidal infections or other GI disorders
Family history of GI disorders
Long-term GI conditions, such as ulcerative colitis, that may predispose to colorectal cancer
Neurological disorders that can impair movement, particularly with chewing and swallowing
Previous abdominal surgery or trauma, which may lead to adhesions
Tobacco use

BOX 46-2 Gastrointestinal System Diagnostic Studies

Anoscopy, proctoscopy, and sigmoidoscopy
Cholecystography
Defecography
Endoscopic retrograde cholangiopancreatography (ERCP)
Fiberoptic colonoscopy
Gastric analysis
Gastrointestinal motility studies
Hydrogen and urea breath test
Laparoscopy (peritoneoscopy)
Liver and pancreas laboratory studies
Liver biopsy
Lower gastrointestinal tract study (barium enema)
Paracentesis
Percutaneous transhepatic cholangiography
Stool specimens
Upper gastrointestinal endoscopy or esophagogastroduodenoscopy (EGD)
Upper gastrointestinal tract study (barium swallow)

Note: Informed consent is obtained for a diagnostic study that is invasive.

b. The common bile duct opens into the duodenum with the pancreatic duct at the ampulla of Vater
c. The sphincter prevents the reflux of intestinal contents into the common bile duct and pancreatic duct

J. Gallbladder
1. Stores and concentrates bile and contracts to force bile into the duodenum during the digestion of fats
2. The cystic duct joins the hepatic duct to form the common bile duct
3. The sphincter of Oddi is located at the entrance into the duodenum
4. The presence of fatty materials in the duodenum stimulates the liberation of cholecystokinin, which causes contraction of the gallbladder and relaxation of the sphincter of Oddi

K. Pancreas
1. Exocrine gland
   a. Secretes sodium bicarbonate to neutralize the acidity of the stomach contents that enter the duodenum
   b. Pancreatic juices contain enzymes for digesting carbohydrates, fats, and proteins
2. Endocrine gland
   a. Secretes glucagon to raise blood glucose levels and secretes somatostatin to exert a hypoglycemic effect
   b. The islets of Langerhans secrete insulin
   c. Insulin is secreted into the bloodstream and is important for carbohydrate metabolism

II. DIAGNOSTIC PROCEDURES (Box 46-2)
A. Upper gastrointestinal tract study (barium swallow)
1. Description: An examination of the upper gastrointestinal tract under fluoroscopy after the client drinks barium sulfate
2. Preprocedure: NPO after midnight before the day of the test
3. Postprocedure
   a. A laxative may be prescribed
   b. Instruct the client to increase oral fluid intake to help pass the barium
   c. Monitor stools for the passage of barium (stools will appear chalky white) because barium can cause a bowel obstruction
B. Lower gastrointestinal tract study (barium enema)
1. Description
   a. A fluoroscopic and radiographic examination of the large intestine is performed after rectal instillation of barium sulfate
   b. The study may be done with or without air
2. Preprocedure
   a. A low-residue diet for 1 to 2 days before the test
   b. A clear liquid diet and a laxative the evening before the test
   c. NPO after midnight before the day of the test
   d. Cleansing enemas on the morning of the test
3. Postprocedure
   a. Instruct the client to increase oral fluid intake to help pass the barium
   b. Administer a mild laxative as prescribed to facilitate emptying of the barium

c. Monitor stools for the passage of barium

d. Notify the physician if a bowel movement does not occur within 2 days

C. Gastric analysis

1. Description

a. Gastric analysis requires the passage of a nasogastric tube into the stomach to aspirate gastric contents for the analysis of acidity (pH), appearance, and volume; the entire gastric contents are aspirated, and then specimens are collected every 15 minutes for 1 hour

b. Histamine or pentagastrin may be administered subcutaneously to stimulate gastric secretions; these medications may produce a flushed feeling

c. Esophageal reflux of gastric acid may be performed by ambulatory pH monitoring; a probe is placed just above the lower esophageal sphincter, is connected to an external recording device, and provides a computer analysis and graphic display of results

2. Preprocedure

a. Fasting for 8 to 12 hours is required before the test

b. Tobacco and chewing gum is avoided for 6 hours before the test

c. Medications that stimulate gastric secretions are withheld for 24 to 48 hours

3. Postprocedure

a. Client may resume normal activities

b. Refrigerate gastric samples if not tested within 4 hours

D. Upper gastrointestinal endoscopy

1. Description

a. Is also known as esophagogastroduodenoscopy

b. Following sedation, an endoscope is passed down the esophagus to view the gastric wall, sphincters, and duodenum; tissue specimens can be obtained

2. Preprocedure

a. The client must be NPO for 6 to 12 hours before the test

b. A local anesthetic (spray or gargle) is administered along with medication that provides conscious sedation and relieves anxiety, such as midazolam (Versed), intravenously, just before the scope is inserted

c. Atropine sulfate may be administered to reduce secretions, and glucagon may be administered to relax smooth muscle

d. Client is positioned on the left side to facilitate saliva drainage and to provide easy access of the endoscope

e. Airway patency is monitored during the test, and pulse oximetry is used to monitor oxygen saturation; emergency equipment should be readily available

3. Postprocedure

a. Client must be NPO until the gag reflex returns (1 to 2 hours)

b. Monitor for signs of perforation (pain, bleeding, unusual difficulty swallowing, elevated temperature)

c. Maintain bedrest for the sedated client until alert

d. Lozenges, saline gargles, or oral analgesics can relieve a minor sore throat (not given to the client until the gag reflex returns)

E. Anoscopy, proctoscopy, and sigmoidoscopy

1. Description

a. Anoscopy requires the use of a rigid scope to examine the anal canal; the client is placed in the knee-chest position with the back inclined at a 45-degree angle

b. Proctoscopy and sigmoidoscopy require the use of a flexible scope to examine the rectum and sigmoid colon; the client is placed on the left side with the right leg bent and placed anteriorly

c. Biopsies and polypectomies can be performed

2. Preprocedure: Enemas are given until the returns are clear

3. Postprocedure: Monitor for rectal bleeding and signs of perforation and peritonitis (Box 46-3)

F. Fiberoptic colonoscopy

1. Description

a. Colonoscopy is a fiberoptic endoscopy study in which the lining of the large intestine is visually examined; biopsies and polypectomies can be performed

b. Cardiac and respiratory functions are monitored continuously during the test

c. Colonoscopy is performed with the client lying on the left side with the knees drawn up to the chest; position may be changed during the test to facilitate passing of the scope

2. Preprocedure

a. Adequate cleansing of the colon is necessary, as prescribed by the physician

| BOX 46-3 | Signs of Bowel Perforation and Peritonitis |

Guarding of the abdomen
Increased fever and chills
Pallor
Progressive abdominal distention and abdominal pain
Restlessness
Tachycardia and tachypnea

b. A clear liquid diet is started on the day before the test

c. Consult with the physician regarding medications that must be withheld before the test

d. Client is NPO after midnight on the day before the test

e. Midazolam (Versed) is administered intravenously to provide sedation

f. Glucagon may be administered to relax smooth muscle

3. Postprocedure

a. Provide bedrest until alert

b. Monitor for signs of bowel perforation and peritonitis (see Box 46-3)

c. Instruct the client to report any bleeding to the physician

G. Laparoscopy (peritoneoscopy) is performed with a fiberoptic laparoscope that allows direct visualization of organs and structures within the abdomen; biopsies may be obtained

H. Cholecystography

1. Description: Performed to detect gallstones and to assess the ability of the gallbladder to fill, concentrate its contents, contract, and empty

2. Preprocedure

a. Assess for allergies to iodine or seafood

b. Contrast agents such as iopanoic acid (Telepaque), iodipamide meglumine (Cholografin), or sodium ipodate (Oragrafin) may be administered 10 to 12 hours (evening before) before the test

c. Client is NPO after the contrast agent is administered

d. Instruct the client to report to the emergency room if a rash, itching, hives, or difficulty in breathing occurs after taking the contrast agent.

3. Postprocedure

a. Inform the client that dysuria is common because the contrast agent is excreted in the urine

b. A normal diet may be resumed (a fatty meal may enhance excretion of the contrast agent)

I. Endoscopic retrograde cholangiopancreatography (ERCP)

1. Description

a. Examination of the hepatobiliary system is performed via a flexible endoscope inserted into the esophagus to the descending duodenum; multiple positions are required during the procedure to pass the endoscope

b. If medication is administered before the procedure, the client is monitored closely for signs of respiratory and central nervous system depression, hypotension, oversedation, and vomiting

2. Preprocedure

a. Client is NPO for several hours before the procedure

b. Sedation is administered before the procedure

3. Postprocedure

a. Monitor vital signs

b. Monitor for the return of the gag reflex

c. Monitor for signs of perforation (see Box 46-3) or peritonitis

J. Percutaneous transhepatic cholangiography

1. Description

a. The examination involves the injection of dye directly into the biliary tree

b. The hepatic ducts within the liver, the entire length of the common bile duct, the cystic duct, and the gallbladder are outlined clearly

2. Preprocedure

a. Client is NPO

b. Sedating medication is administered

3. Postprocedure

a. Monitor vital signs

b. Monitor for signs of bleeding, peritonitis (see Box 46-3), and septicemia; report the presence of pain immediately

c. Administer antibiotics as prescribed to reduce the risk of sepsis

K. Paracentesis

1. Description: transabdominal removal of fluid from the peritoneal cavity for analysis

2. Preprocedure

a. Have client void before the start of procedure to empty the bladder and to move the bladder out of the way of the paracentesis needle

b. Measure abdominal girth, weight, and baseline vital signs

c. Note that the client is positioned upright on the edge of the bed with the back supported and the feet resting on a stool (Fowler's position is used for the client confined to bed)

3. Postprocedure

a. Monitor vital signs

b. Measure fluid collected, describe, and record

c. Label fluid samples and send to the laboratory for analysis

d. Apply a dry sterile dressing to the insertion site; monitor site for bleeding

e. Measure abdominal girth and weight

f. Monitor for hypovolemia, electrolyte loss, mental status changes, or encephalopathy

g. Monitor for hematuria caused by bladder trauma

h. Instruct the client to notify the physician if the urine becomes bloody, pink, or red

L. Liver biopsy
1. Description: A needle is inserted through the abdominal wall to the liver to obtain a tissue sample for biopsy and microscopic examination
2. Preprocedure
   a. Assess results of coagulation tests (prothrombin time, partial thromboplastin time, platelet count)
   b. Administer a sedative as prescribed
   c. Note that the client is placed in the supine or left lateral position during the procedure to expose the right side of the upper abdomen
3. Postprocedure
   a. Assess vital signs
   b. Assess biopsy site for bleeding
   c. Monitor for peritonitis (see Box 46-3)
   d. Maintain bedrest for several hours
   e. Place the client on the right side with a pillow under the costal margin to decrease the risk of hemorrhage, and instruct the client to avoid coughing and straining
   f. Instruct the client to avoid heavy lifting and strenuous exercise for 1 week
M. Stool specimens
1. Testing of stool specimens includes inspecting the specimen for consistency and color and testing for occult blood
2. Tests for fecal urobilinogen, fat, nitrogen, parasites, pathogens, food substances, and other substances may be performed; these tests require that the specimen be sent to the laboratory
3. Random specimens are sent promptly to the laboratory
4. Quantitative 24- to 72-hour collections must be kept refrigerated until they are taken to the laboratory
5. Some specimens require that a certain diet be followed or that certain medications be withheld; check agency guidelines regarding specific procedures
N. Urea breath test
1. The urea breath test detects the presence of *Helicobacter pylori*, the bacteria that causes peptic ulcer disease
2. The client consumes a capsule of carbon-labeled urea and provides a breath sample 10 to 20 minutes later
3. Certain medications may need to be avoided before testing and these may include the following: antibiotics or bismuth subsalicylate (Pepto-Bismol) for 1 month before the test; sucralfate (Carafate) and omeprazole (Prilosec) for 1 week before the test; and cimetidine (Tagamet), famotidine (Pepcid), ranitidine (Zantac), or nizatidine (Axid) for 24 hours before breath testing

4. *H. pylori* can also be detected by assessing serum antibody levels
O. Liver and pancreas laboratory studies (refer to Chapter 11)
1. Alkaline phosphatase is released during liver damage or biliary obstruction
2. Prothrombin time is prolonged with liver damage
3. Serum ammonia assesses the ability of the liver to deaminate protein by-products
4. Liver enzymes (transaminase studies) are elevated with liver damage
5. An increase in cholesterol indicates **pancreatitis** or biliary obstruction
6. An increase in bilirubin indicates liver damage or biliary obstruction
7. Increased values for amylase and lipase indicate **pancreatitis**

III. **DATA COLLECTION**
A. Abdominal assessment (Box 46-4)
1. Inspect the skin for color, abnormalities, contour, and tautness, and the abdomen for distention
2. Auscultate for bowel sounds
3. Percuss for air or solids
4. Palpate for tenderness
B. Bowel sounds
1. Auscultate bowel sounds before percussion and palpation
2. Normal bowel sounds occur 5 to 30 times a minute or every 5 to 15 seconds
3. Auscultate in all abdominal quadrants
4. Listen at least 5 minutes in each quadrant before assuming sounds are absent
IV. **GASTROINTESTINAL TUBES** (Refer to Chapter 19 for information regarding care of the client with these tubes.)
V. **GASTROESOPHAGEAL REFLUX DISEASE**
A. Description
1. Gastroesophageal reflux is the backflow of gastric and duodenal contents into the esophagus
2. The reflux is caused by an incompetent lower esophageal sphincter, pyloric stenosis, or a motility disorder
B. Data collection
1. Pyrosis
2. Dyspepsia
3. Regurgitation

BOX 46-4 | **Order for Performing the Abdominal Assessment**

1. Inspect
2. Auscultate
3. Percuss
4. Palpate

4. Pain and difficulty with swallowing
5. Hypersalivation
C. Interventions
   1. Instruct the client to avoid factors that decrease lower esophageal sphincter pressure or cause esophageal irritation
   2. Instruct the client to eat a low-fat, high-fiber diet; avoid caffeine, tobacco, and carbonated beverages; avoid eating and drinking 2 hours before bedtime; avoid wearing tight clothes; and elevate the head of the bed on 6- to 8-inch blocks
   3. Avoid the use of anticholinergics, which delay stomach emptying
   4. Instruct the client regarding prescribed medications, such as antacids, histamine 2 (H_2)-receptor antagonists, or proton pump inhibitors
   5. Instruct the client regarding the administration of prokinetic medications, if prescribed, which accelerate gastric emptying
   6. If medical management is unsuccessful, surgery may be required and involves a fundoplication (wrapping a portion of the gastric fundus around the sphincter area of the esophagus); surgery may be performed by laparoscopy

VI. HIATAL HERNIA

A. Description
   1. A **hiatal hernia** is also known as esophageal or diaphragmatic hernia
   2. A portion of the stomach herniates through the diaphragm and into the thorax
   3. Herniation results from weakening of the muscles of the diaphragm and is aggravated by factors that increase abdominal pressure such as pregnancy, **ascites,** obesity, tumors, and heavy lifting
   4. Complications include ulceration, hemorrhage, regurgitation and aspiration of stomach contents, strangulation, and incarceration of the stomach in the chest with possible necrosis, peritonitis, and mediastinitis
B. Data collection
   1. Heartburn
   2. Regurgitation or vomiting
   3. Dysphagia
   4. Feeling of fullness
C. Interventions
   1. Medical and surgical management is similar to that for gastroesophageal reflux disease
   2. Provide small frequent meals and limit the amount of liquids taken with meals
   3. Advise the client not to recline for 1 hour after eating
   4. Avoid anticholinergics, which delay stomach emptying

VII. GASTRITIS

A. Description
   1. Inflammation of the stomach or gastric mucosa
   2. Acute gastritis is caused by the ingestion of food contaminated with disease-causing microorganisms or food that is irritating or too highly seasoned, the overuse of aspirin or other non-steroidal anti-inflammatory drugs (NSAIDs), excessive alcohol intake, bile reflux, or radiation therapy
   3. Chronic gastritis is caused by benign or malignant ulcers or by the bacteria *H. pylori*, and it may be caused by autoimmune diseases, dietary factors, medications, alcohol, smoking, or reflux
B. Data collection (Box 46-5)
C. Interventions
   1. Acute gastritis: Food and fluids may be withheld until symptoms subside; afterward, ice chips, followed by clear liquids, and then solid food is introduced
   2. Monitor for signs of hemorrhagic gastritis such as hematemesis, tachycardia, and hypotension; notify the physician if these signs occur
   3. Instruct the client to avoid irritating foods, fluids, and other substances such as spicy and highly seasoned foods, caffeine, alcohol, and nicotine
   4. Instruct the client on the use of prescribed medications, such as antibiotics and bismuth salts (Pepto-Bismol)
   5. Provide the client with information about the importance of vitamin B_{12} injections, if a deficiency is present

VIII. PEPTIC ULCER DISEASE

A. Description
   1. A peptic ulcer is an ulceration in the mucosal wall of the stomach, pylorus, duodenum, or esophagus in portions that are accessible to gastric secretions; erosion may extend through the muscle

---

BOX 46-5	Data Collection: Acute and Chronic Gastritis

Acute Gastritis
Abdominal discomfort
Anorexia, nausea, and vomiting
Headache
Hiccuping
Chronic Gastritis
Anorexia, nausea, and vomiting
Belching
Heartburn after eating
Sour taste in the mouth
Vitamin B_{12} deficiency

2. The ulcer may be referred to as gastric, duodenal, or esophageal depending on its location
3. The most common peptic ulcers are gastric ulcers and duodenal ulcers

B. Gastric ulcers
1. Description
   a. A gastric ulcer involves ulceration of the mucosal lining that extends to the submucosal layer of the stomach
   b. Predisposing factors include stress, smoking, the use of corticosteroids, NSAIDs, alcohol, a history of gastritis, a family history of gastric ulcers, or infection with *H. pylori*
   c. Complications include hemorrhage, perforation, and pyloric obstruction
2. Data collection (Box 46-6)
3. Interventions
   a. Monitor vital signs and signs of bleeding
   b. Administer small, frequent bland feedings during the active phase
   c. Administer H_2-receptor antagonists as prescribed to decrease the secretion of gastric acid
   d. Administer antacids as prescribed to neutralize gastric secretions
   e. Administer anticholinergics as prescribed to reduce gastric motility
   f. Administer mucosal barrier protectants as prescribed 1 hour before each meal
   g. Administer prostaglandins as prescribed for their protective and antisecretory actions
4. Client education
   a. Avoid consuming alcohol and substances that contain caffeine or chocolate
   b. Avoid smoking
   c. Avoid aspirin or NSAIDs
   d. Obtain adequate rest and reduce stress
5. Interventions during active bleeding
   a. Monitor vital signs closely
   b. Assess for signs of dehydration, hypovolemic shock, sepsis, and respiratory insufficiency

c. Maintain NPO status and administer intravenous (IV) fluid replacement as prescribed; monitor intake and output (I&O)
d. Monitor hemoglobin and hematocrit
e. Administer blood transfusions as prescribed
f. Assist with the insertion of a nasogastric tube for decompression and for lavage access
g. Assist with normal saline or tap water lavage at room temperature to reduce active bleeding
h. Prepare to assist with administering vasopressin (Pitressin) intravenously as prescribed to induce vasoconstriction and reduce bleeding

6. Surgical interventions
   a. Total **gastrectomy**: removal of the stomach with attachment of the esophagus to the jejunum or duodenum; also called esophagojejunostomy or esophagoduodenostomy
   b. **Vagotomy**: surgical division of the vagus nerve to eliminate the vagal impulses that stimulate hydrochloric acid secretion in the stomach
   c. **Gastric resection**: removal of the lower half of the stomach and usually includes a **vagotomy**; also called antrectomy
   d. **Billroth I**: partial **gastrectomy**, with the remaining segment anastomosed to the duodenum; also called gastroduodenostomy
   e. **Billroth II**: partial **gastrectomy**, with the remaining segment anastomosed to the jejunum; also called gastrojejunostomy
   f. **Pyloroplasty**: enlargement of the pylorus to prevent or decrease pyloric obstruction, thereby enhancing gastric emptying

7. Postoperative interventions
   a. Monitor vital signs
   b. Position in Fowler's for comfort and to promote drainage
   c. Administer fluids and electrolyte replacements intravenously as prescribed; monitor I&O
   d. Assess bowel sounds
   e. Monitor nasogastric suction as prescribed
   f. Do not irrigate or remove the nasogastric tube; assist the physician with nasogastric tube irrigation or removal
   g. Maintain NPO status as prescribed for 1 to 3 days until **peristalsis** returns
   h. Progress the diet from NPO to sips of clear water to six small, bland meals a day as prescribed when bowel sounds return
   i. Monitor for postoperative complications of hemorrhage, **dumping syndrome**, diarrhea, hypoglycemia, and vitamin B_{12} deficiency

---

| **BOX 46-6** | **Data Collection: Gastric and Duodenal Ulcers** |

Gastric Ulcers
Gnawing, sharp pain in or left of the midepigastric region occurs 30 to 60 minutes after a meal (food ingestion accentuates the pain)
Hematemesis is more common than melena
Duodenal Ulcers
Burning pain in the midepigastric area 1.5 to 3 hours after a meal and during the night (often awakens the client)
Melena is more common than hematemesis
Pain is often relieved by the ingestion of food

C. Duodenal ulcers
1. Description
   a. A duodenal ulcer is a break in the mucosa of the duodenum
   b. Risk factors and causes include alcohol intake; smoking; stress; caffeine; the use of aspirin, corticosteroids, and NSAIDs; and infection with *H. pylori*
   c. Complications include bleeding, perforation, gastric outlet obstruction, and intractable disease
2. Data collection (see Box 46-6)
3. Interventions
   a. Monitor vital signs
   b. Instruct the client in a bland diet with small frequent meals
   c. Provide for adequate rest
   d. Encourage the cessation of smoking
   e. Instruct the client to avoid alcohol intake, caffeine, and the use of aspirin, corticosteroids, and NSAIDs
   f. Administer antacids as prescribed to neutralize acid secretions
   g. Administer H_2-receptor antagonists as prescribed to block the secretion of acid
4. Surgical interventions: Surgery is performed only if the ulcer is unresponsive to medications or if hemorrhage, obstruction, or perforation occurs

D. **Dumping syndrome**
1. Description: the rapid emptying of the gastric contents into the small intestine that occurs following **gastric resection**
2. Data collection
   a. Symptoms occurring 30 minutes after eating
   b. Nausea and vomiting
   c. Feelings of abdominal fullness and abdominal cramping
   d. Diarrhea
   e. Palpitations and tachycardia
   f. Perspiration
   g. Weakness and dizziness
   h. Borborygmi (loud gurgles indicating hyperperistalsis, or stomach growling)
3. Client education (Box 46-7)

IX. VITAMIN B_{12} DEFICIENCY
A. Description
1. Vitamin B_{12} deficiency results from an inadequate intake of vitamin B_{12} or a lack of absorption of ingested vitamin B_{12} from the intestinal tract
2. Pernicious anemia results from a deficiency of intrinsic factor, which is necessary for intestinal absorption of vitamin B_{12}; gastric disease or surgery can result in a lack of intrinsic factor
3. Vitamin B_{12} deficiency can also result from disease or surgery of the ileum because vitamin B_{12} is absorbed from the ileum in the presence of intrinsic factor

B. Data collection
1. Severe pallor
2. Fatigue
3. Weight loss
4. Smooth, beefy red tongue
5. Slight jaundice
6. Paresthesias of the hands and feet
7. Disturbances with gait and balance

C. Interventions
1. Increase dietary intake of foods rich in vitamin B_{12} if the anemia is the result of a dietary deficiency (Box 46-8)
2. Initially administer vitamin B_{12} injections as prescribed weekly and then monthly for maintenance (lifelong) if the anemia is the result of a deficiency of the intrinsic factor or disease or surgery of the ileum

X. BARIATRIC SURGERY
A. Description
1. Surgical reduction of gastric capacity that may be performed on a client with morbid obesity to produce permanent weight loss
2. Surgery may be performed by laparoscope, and the decision is based on the client's weight, body build, history of abdominal surgery, and current medical disorders
3. Obese clients are at increased postoperative risk for pulmonary and thromboembolitic complications and death
4. Surgery can prevent the complications of obesity such as diabetes mellitus, hypertension and other cardiovascular disorders, depression, or sleep apnea

---

BOX 46-7 **Client Education: Preventing Dumping Syndrome**

Avoid sugar, salt, and milk.
Eat a high-protein, high-fat, low-carbohydrate diet.
Eat small meals and avoid consuming fluids with meals.
Lie down after meals.
Take antispasmodic medications as prescribed to delay gastric emptying.

BOX 46-8 **Foods Rich in Vitamin B_{12}**

Brewer's yeast
Citrus fruits
Dried beans
Green, leafy vegetables
Liver
Nuts
Organ meats

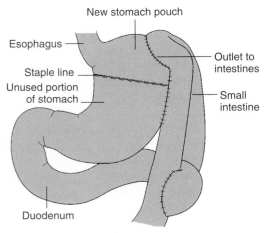

Gastric Bypass

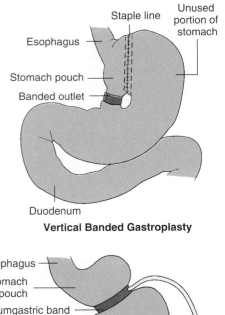

Vertical Banded Gastroplasty

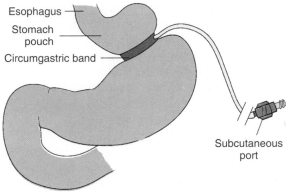

Circumgastric Banding

FIG. 46-1 Bariatric surgical procedures. (From Ignatavicius, D., & Workman, M. [2006]. *Medical-surgical nursing: Critical thinking for collaborative care* [5th ed.]. St. Louis: Saunders.)

5. The client needs to agree to modify his or her lifestyle, to lose weight and keep the weight off, and to obtain support from available community resources (Box 46-9)

B. Types (Figure 46-1)
   1. Gastric restrictive surgery
      a. Allows for normal digestion without the risk of nutritional deficiency
      b. A vertical banded gastroplasty may be performed in which the surgeon places a vertical line of staples to create a small stomach pouch to which the band is connected to provide an outlet to the small intestine
      c. A circumgastric banding may be performed in which an inflatable band is placed around the stomach to limit stomach size; the band can be inflated or deflated through a subcutaneous port to change the size of the stomach as the client loses weight
   2. Gastric restriction combined with malabsorption surgery
      a. Known as a gastric bypass or Roux-en-Y gastric bypass
      b. In addition to stapling, the stomach, duodenum, and part of the ileum is bypassed so that fewer calories can be absorbed
C. Postoperative interventions
   1. Care is similar as for the client undergoing abdominal surgery
   2. Clear liquids are introduced slowly once bowel sounds have returned and the client passes flatus (1-ounce cups are used for each serving)
   3. Clear fluids are followed by pureed foods, juices, thin soups, and milk 24 to 48 hours after clear fluids are tolerated (the diet is limited to liquids or pureed foods for 6 weeks); then the diet is progressed to nutrient-dense regular food
D. Client teaching points about diet are provided (Box 46-10)
XI. GASTRIC CANCER (Refer to Chapter 42)
XII. ESOPHAGEAL VARICES
A. Description

BOX 46-10 **Dietary Measures for the Client Following Bariatric Surgery**

Avoid alcohol, high-protein foods, and foods high in sugar and fat.
Eat slowly and chew food well.
Progress food types and amounts as prescribed.
Take nutritional supplements as prescribed, which may include calcium, iron, multivitamins, and vitamin B_{12}.
Monitor and report signs and symptoms of complications such as dehydration.

1. Dilated and tortuous veins in the submucosa of the esophagus
2. Caused by **portal hypertension,** are often associated with liver **cirrhosis,** and are at high risk for rupture if portal circulation pressure rises
3. Bleeding varices are an emergency
4. The goal of treatment is to control bleeding, prevent complications, and prevent the reoccurrence of bleeding

B. Data collection
1. Hematemesis
2. Melena
3. Tarry stools
4. **Ascites**
5. Jaundice
6. Hepatomegaly and splenomegaly
7. Dilated abdominal veins
8. Signs of shock

C. Interventions
1. Monitor vital signs
2. Elevate the head of the bed
3. Monitor for orthostatic hypotension
4. Monitor lung sounds and for the presence of respiratory distress
5. Administer oxygen as prescribed to prevent tissue hypoxia
6. Monitor level of consciousness
7. Maintain NPO status
8. Administer fluids intravenously as prescribed to restore fluid volume and electrolyte imbalances; monitor I&O
9. Monitor hemoglobin, hematocrit, and coagulation factors
10. Administer blood transfusions or clotting factors as prescribed
11. Assist in inserting a nasogastric tube or a balloon tamponade as prescribed
12. Assist with the administration of iced saline irrigations to achieve vasoconstriction of the varices
13. Prepare to assist with administering vasopressin (Pitressin) by IV or intra-arterial infusion as prescribed to induce vasoconstriction and reduce bleeding
14. Prepare to assist with administering nitroglycerin with the vasopressin (Pitressin) if prescribed to prevent vasoconstriction of the coronary arteries
15. Instruct the client to avoid activities that will initiate vasovagal responses
16. Prepare the client for endoscopic procedures or surgical procedures as prescribed

D. Endoscopic injection (sclerotherapy)
1. The procedure involves the injection of a sclerosing agent into and around bleeding varices

2. Complications include chest pain, pleural effusion, aspiration pneumonia, esophageal stricture, and perforation of the esophagus

E. Endoscopic variceal ligation
1. The procedure involves ligation of the varices with an elastic rubber band
2. Sloughing, followed by superficial ulceration, occurs in the area of ligation within 3 to 7 days

F. Surgical shunting procedures
1. Description: shunt blood away from the **esophageal varices**
2. Distal splenorenal shunt
   a. The shunt involves splenectomy, with anastomosis of the splenic vein to the left renal vein
   b. The splenic vein conducts blood from the high-pressure varices to the low-pressure renal vein
3. Portacaval shunting involves anastomosis of the portal vein to the inferior vena cava, diverting blood from the portal system to the systemic circulation
4. Mesocaval shunting involves a side anastomosis of the superior mesenteric vein to the proximal end of the inferior vena cava
5. Transjugular intrahepatic portal/systemic shunt (TIPS)
   a. The nonsurgical procedure uses the normal vascular anatomy of the liver to create a shunt with the use of a metallic stent
   b. The shunt is between the portal and systemic venous system within the liver and is aimed at relieving **portal hypertension**

XIII. ULCERATIVE COLITIS
A. Description
1. An ulcerative and inflammatory disease of the bowel that results in poor absorption of nutrients
2. Commonly begins in the rectum and spreads upward toward the cecum
3. The colon becomes edematous and may develop bleeding lesions and ulcers; the ulcers may lead to perforation
4. Scar tissue develops and causes loss of elasticity and loss of the ability to absorb nutrients
5. Colitis is characterized by various periods of remissions and exacerbations
6. Acute **ulcerative colitis** results in vascular congestion, hemorrhage, edema, and ulceration of the bowel mucosa
7. Chronic **ulcerative colitis** causes muscular hypertrophy, fat deposits, and fibrous tissue with bowel thickening, shortening, and narrowing
8. Surgical intervention involves creation of an ostomy; the ostomy can be created within

the ileum or at various sites within the large bowel

9. An ileostomy is the surgical creation of an opening into the ileum or small intestine that allows for drainage of fecal matter from the ileum to the outside of the body

10. A colostomy is the surgical creation of an opening into the colon that allows for drainage of fecal matter from the colon to the outside of the body

B. Data collection
1. Anorexia
2. Weight loss
3. Malaise
4. Abdominal tenderness and cramping
5. Severe diarrhea that may contain blood and mucus
6. Dehydration and electrolyte imbalances
7. Anemia
8. Vitamin K deficiency

C. Interventions
1. Acute phase: Maintain NPO status and administer fluids and electrolytes intravenously or parenteral nutrition as prescribed.
2. Restrict the client's activity to reduce intestinal activity.
3. Monitor bowel sounds and for abdominal tenderness and cramping.
4. Monitor stools, noting color, consistency, and the presence or absence of blood.
5. Monitor for bowel perforation, peritonitis (see Box 46-3), and hemorrhage.

6. Following the acute phase, the diet progresses from clear liquids to low residue as tolerated.
7. Instruct the client to consume a low-residue, high-protein diet; vitamins and iron supplements may be prescribed
8. Instruct the client to avoid gas-forming foods and milk products, and foods such as whole grains, nuts, raw fruits and vegetables, pepper, alcohol, and caffeine-containing products
9. Instruct the client to avoid smoking
10. Administer medications as prescribed, which may include a combination of medications such as salicylate compounds, corticosteroids, immunosuppressants, and antidiarrheals

D. Surgical interventions
1. Total proctocolectomy with permanent ileostomy
   a. The procedure is curative and involves the removal of the entire colon (colon, rectum, and anus with anal closure)
   b. The end of the terminal ileum forms the stoma, which is located in the right lower quadrant
2. **Kock ileostomy (continent ileostomy)** (Figure 46-2)
   a. The **Kock ileostomy** is an intra-abdominal pouch that stores the feces and is constructed from the terminal ileum
   b. The pouch is connected to the stoma with a nipple-like valve constructed from a portion of the ileum; the stoma is flush with the skin

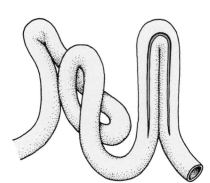

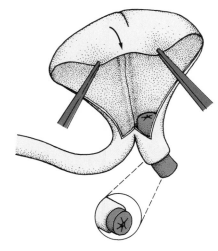

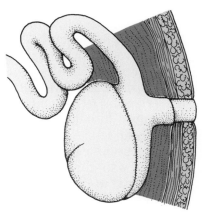

1. A reservoir, in which the client will retain stool until draining it, is constructed from a loop of ileum folded and sutured together, then cut.

2. A portion of the ileum is intussuscepted to form a nipple valve, and the upper part of the stitched and cut ileum is pulled down and sutured to form a pouch.

3. The nipple valve, which shuts tight against pressure from a filled pouch, is pulled through the stoma and sutured flush with the abdomen.

FIG. 46-2 The creation of a Kock's (continent) ileostomy. (From Ignatavicius, D., & Workman, M. [2006]. *Medical-surgical nursing: Critical thinking for collaborative care* [5th ed.]. St. Louis: Saunders.)

c. A catheter is used to empty the pouch, and a small dressing or adhesive bandage is worn over the stoma between emptyings

3. Ileoanal reservoir (Figure 46-3)
   a. Creation of an ileoanal reservoir is a two-stage procedure that involves the excision of the rectal mucosa, an abdominal colectomy, construction of a reservoir to the anal canal, and a temporary loop ileostomy
   b. The ileostomy is closed 3 to 4 months after the capacity of the reservoir is increased and has had time to heal

4. Ileoanal anastomosis (ileorectostomy)
   a. Ileorectostomy does not require an ileostomy
   b. A 12- to 15-cm rectal stump is left after the colon is removed, and the small intestine is inserted into this rectal sleeve and anastomosed
   c. Ileorectostomy requires a large, compliant rectum

5. Preoperative colostomy/ileostomy interventions
   a. Consult with enterostomal therapist to assist in identifying optimal placement of the ostomy
   b. Instruct the client to eat a low-residue diet for 1 to 2 days before surgery as prescribed
   c. Administer intestinal antiseptics and antibiotics as prescribed to cleanse the bowel and to decrease the bacterial content of the colon
   d. Administer laxatives and enemas as prescribed

6. Postoperative colostomy interventions
   a. Place a petrolatum gauze over the stoma as prescribed to keep it moist, followed by a dry sterile dressing if a pouch (external) system is not in place
   b. Place a pouch system on the stoma as soon as possible
   c. Monitor the stoma for size, unusual bleeding, or necrotic tissue
   d. Monitor for color changes in the stoma
   e. Note that the normal stoma color is pink to bright red and shiny, indicating high vascularity
   f. Note that a pale pink stoma indicates low hemoglobin and hematocrit levels, and a purple-black stoma indicates compromised circulation, requiring physician notification
   g. Assess the functioning of the colostomy
   h. Expect that stool is liquid in the immediate postoperative period but becomes more solid depending on the area of the colostomy: ascending colon—liquid; transverse

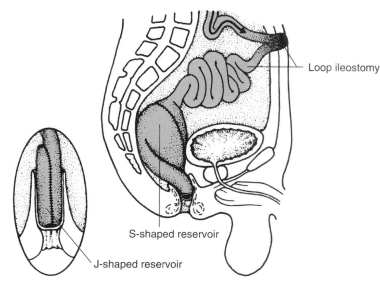

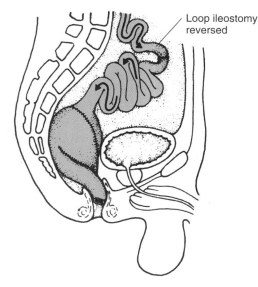

Stage 1
After removal of the colon, a temporary loop ileostomy is created and an ileoanal reservoir is formed. The reservoir is created in an S-shaped reservoir (using three loops of ileum) or a J-shaped reservoir (suturing a portion of ileum to the rectal cuff, with an upward loop).

Stage 2
After the reservoir has had time to heal—usually several months—the temporary loop ileostomy is reversed, and stool is allowed to drain into the reservoir.

FIG. 46-3 The creation of an ileoanal reservoir. (From Ignatavicius, D., & Workman, M. [2006]. *Medical-surgical nursing: Critical thinking for collaborative care* [5th ed.]. St. Louis: Saunders.)

colon—loose to semiformed; and descending colon—close to normal

    i. Monitor the pouch system for proper fit and signs of leakage

    j. Empty the pouch when it is one-third full

    k. Fecal matter should not be allowed to remain on the skin

    l. Administer analgesics and antibiotics as prescribed

    m. Irrigate the perineal wound (if present) as prescribed and monitor for signs of infection

    n. Instruct the client to avoid foods that cause excess gas formation and odor

    o. Instruct the client about stoma care and irrigations as prescribed (refer to Chapter 42 for information on colostomy irrigation)

    p. Instruct the client that normal activities may be resumed when approved by the physician

  7. Postoperative ileostomy interventions

    a. Note that normal stool is liquid

    b. Monitor for dehydration and electrolyte imbalance

    c. Do not give suppositories through an ileostomy

XIV. CROHN'S DISEASE

A. Description

  1. An inflammatory disease that can occur anywhere in the gastrointestinal tract but most often affects the terminal ileum and leads to thickening and scarring, a narrowed lumen, fistulas, ulcerations, and abscesses

  2. Characterized by remissions and exacerbations

B. Data collection

  1. Fever

  2. Cramp-like and colicky pain after meals

  3. Diarrhea (semisolid), which may contain mucus and pus

  4. Abdominal distention

  5. Anorexia, nausea, and vomiting

  6. Weight loss

  7. Anemia

  8. Dehydration

  9. Electrolyte imbalances

C. Interventions: Care is similar to the client with **ulcerative colitis**; however, surgery is avoided as much as possible because recurrence of the disease process in the same region is likely to occur

XV. PANCREATIC TUMORS, INTESTINAL TUMORS, AND BOWEL OBSTRUCTIONS (Refer to Chapter 42)

XVI. DIVERTICULOSIS AND DIVERTICULITIS

A. Description

  1. **Diverticulosis**

    a. **Diverticulosis** is an outpouching or herniation of the intestinal mucosa

    b. The disorder can occur in any part of the intestine but is most common in the sigmoid colon

  2. **Diverticulitis**

    a. **Diverticulitis** is the inflammation of one or more diverticula that occurs from penetration of fecal matter through the thin-walled diverticula and can result in local abscess formation and perforation

    b. A perforated diverticulum can progress to intra-abdominal perforation with generalized peritonitis

B. Data collection

  1. Left lower quadrant abdominal pain that increases with coughing, straining, or lifting

  2. Elevated temperature

  3. Nausea and vomiting

  4. Flatulence

  5. Cramp-like pain

  6. Abdominal distention and tenderness

  7. Palpable, tender rectal mass

  8. Blood in the stools

C. Interventions

  1. Provide bedrest during the acute phase

  2. Maintain NPO status or provide clear liquids during the acute phase as prescribed

  3. Introduce a fiber-containing diet gradually, when the inflammation has resolved

  4. Administer antibiotics, analgesics, and anticholinergics to reduce bowel spasms as prescribed

  5. Instruct the client to refrain from lifting, straining, coughing, or bending to avoid increased intra-abdominal pressure

  6. Monitor for perforation (see Box 46-3), hemorrhage, fistulas, and abscesses

  7. Instruct the client to increase fluid intake to 2500 to 3000 mL daily, unless contraindicated

  8. Instruct the client to eat soft, high-fiber foods such as whole grains

  9. Instruct the client to avoid gas-forming foods or foods containing indigestible roughage, seeds, or nuts because these food substances become trapped in diverticula and cause inflammation

  10. Instruct the client to consume a small amount of bran daily and to take bulk-forming laxatives as prescribed to increase stool mass

  11. Instruct the client to avoid high-fiber foods when inflammation occurs because these foods will further irritate the mucosa

D. Surgical interventions

  1. Colon resection with primary anastomosis may be an option

  2. Temporary or permanent colostomy may be required for increased bowel inflammation

XVII. HEMORRHOIDS

A. Description
1. Dilated varicose veins of the anal canal
2. May be internal, external, or prolapsed
3. Internal hemorrhoids lie above the anal sphincter and cannot be seen on inspection of the perianal area
4. External hemorrhoids lie below the anal sphincter and can be seen on inspection
5. Prolapsed hemorrhoids can become thrombosed or inflamed
6. Hemorrhoids are caused by **portal hypertension,** straining, irritation, or increased venous or abdominal pressure

B. Data collection
1. Bright red bleeding with defecation
2. Rectal pain
3. Rectal itching

C. Interventions
1. Apply cold packs to the anal/rectal area followed by sitz baths as prescribed
2. Apply witch hazel soaks and topical anesthetics as prescribed
3. Encourage a high-fiber diet and fluids to promote bowel movements without straining
4. Administer stool softeners as prescribed

D. Surgical interventions: May include ultrasound, sclerotherapy, circular stapling, or simple resection of the hemorrhoids (hemorrhoidectomy)

E. Postoperative interventions following hemorrhoidectomy
1. Assist the client to a prone or side-lying position to prevent bleeding
2. Maintain ice packs over the dressing as prescribed until the packing is removed by the physician
3. Monitor for urinary retention
4. Administer stool softeners as prescribed
5. Instruct the client to increase fluids and high-fiber foods
6. Instruct the client to limit sitting to short periods
7. Instruct the client in the use of sitz baths three to four times a day as prescribed

XVIII. APPENDICITIS

A. Description
1. Inflammation of the appendix
2. When the appendix becomes inflamed or infected, rupture may occur within a matter of hours, leading to peritonitis and sepsis

B. Data collection
1. Pain in the periumbilical area that descends to the right lower quadrant
2. Abdominal pain that is most intense at McBurney's point
3. Rebound tenderness and abdominal rigidity
4. Low-grade fever

5. Elevated white blood cell count
6. Anorexia, nausea, and vomiting
7. Client in side-lying position, with abdominal guarding and legs flexed
8. Constipation or diarrhea

C. Peritonitis: inflammation of the peritoneum (see Box 46-3)

D. Appendectomy: surgical removal of the appendix
1. Preoperative interventions
   a. Maintain NPO status
   b. Administer fluids intravenously to prevent dehydration
   c. Monitor for changes in level of pain
   d. Monitor for signs of ruptured appendix and peritonitis (see Box 46-3)
   e. Position right side–lying or low to semi-Fowler's position to promote comfort
   f. Monitor bowel sounds
   g. Avoid the application of heat to the abdomen
   h. Apply ice packs to the abdomen for 20 to 30 minutes every hour as prescribed
   i. Administer antibiotics as prescribed
   j. Avoid laxatives or enemas
2. Postoperative interventions
   a. Monitor temperature for signs of infection
   b. Assess incision for signs of infection such as redness, swelling, and pain
   c. Maintain NPO status until bowel function has returned
   d. Advance diet gradually as tolerated and as prescribed, when bowel sounds return
   e. If rupture of the appendix occurred, expect insertion of a Penrose drain, or the incision may be left open to heal from the inside out
   f. Expect that drainage from the Penrose drain may be profuse for the first 12 hours
   g. Position the client in a right side–lying or low to semi-Fowler's position, with legs flexed, to facilitate drainage
   h. Change the dressing as prescribed and record the type and amount of drainage
   i. Perform wound irrigations if prescribed
   j. Maintain nasogastric suction and patency of the nasogastric tube if present
   k. Administer antibiotics and analgesics as prescribed

XIX. CIRRHOSIS (Box 46-11)

A. Description
1. A chronic, progressive disease of the liver characterized by diffuse degeneration and destruction of hepatocytes
2. Repeated destruction of hepatic cells causes the formation of scar tissue

BOX 46-11 **Types of Cirrhosis**

Laënnec's Cirrhosis
Cirrhosis is alcohol induced, nutritional, or portal.
Cellular necrosis causes eventual widespread scar tissue, with fibrotic infiltration of the liver.

Postnecrotic Cirrhosis
Cirrhosis occurs after massive liver necrosis.
Cirrhosis results as a complication of acute viral hepatitis or exposure to hepatotoxins.
Scar tissue causes destruction of liver lobules and entire lobes.

Biliary Cirrhosis
Cirrhosis develops from chronic biliary obstruction, bile stasis, and inflammation resulting in severe obstructive jaundice.

Cardiac Cirrhosis
Cirrhosis is associated with severe, right-sided congestive heart failure and results in an enlarged, edematous, congested liver.
The liver becomes anoxic, resulting in liver cell necrosis and fibrosis.

B. Complications
  1. **Portal hypertension**: A persistent increase in pressure within the portal vein that develops as a result of obstruction to flow
  2. **Ascites**
     a. The accumulation of fluid within the peritoneal cavity that results from venous congestion of the hepatic capillaries
     b. Capillary congestion leads to plasma leaking directly from the liver surface and portal vein
  3. Bleeding **esophageal varices**: fragile, thin-walled, distended esophageal veins that become irritated and rupture
  4. Coagulation defects
     a. Decreased synthesis of bile fats in the liver prevents the absorption of fat-soluble vitamins
     b. Without vitamin K and clotting factors II, VII, IX, and X, the client is prone to bleeding
  5. Jaundice: Occurs because the liver is unable to metabolize bilirubin and because the edema, fibrosis, and scarring of the hepatic bile ducts interfere with normal bile and bilirubin secretion
  6. Portal systemic encephalopathy: End-stage hepatic failure and **cirrhosis** characterized by altered level of consciousness, neurological symptoms, impaired thinking, and neuromuscular disturbances
  7. Hepatorenal syndrome
     a. Progressive renal failure associated with hepatic failure
     b. Characterized by a sudden decrease in urinary output, elevated blood urea

nitrogen and creatinine, decreased urine sodium excretion, and increased urine osmolarity
C. Data collection (Figure 46-4)
D. Interventions
  1. Elevate the head of the bed to minimize shortness of breath
  2. If **ascites** and edema are absent and the client does not exhibit signs of impending coma, a high-protein diet supplemented with vitamins is prescribed
  3. Provide supplemental vitamins (B complex; vitamins A, C, and K; folic acid; and thiamine) as prescribed
  4. Restrict sodium intake and fluid intake as prescribed
  5. Initiate enteral feedings or parenteral nutrition as prescribed
  6. Administer diuretics as prescribed to treat **ascites**
  7. Monitor I&O and electrolyte balance
  8. Weigh client and measure abdominal girth daily
  9. Monitor level of consciousness; assess for pre-coma state (tremors, delirium)
  10. Monitor for **asterixis,** a course tremor characterized by rapid, nonrhythmic extension and flexions in the wrist and fingers
  11. Monitor for **fetor hepaticus**—the fruity, musty breath odor of severe chronic liver disease
  12. Maintain gastric intubation to assess bleeding or esophagogastric balloon tamponade to control bleeding varices if prescribed
  13. Administer blood products as prescribed
  14. Monitor coagulation laboratory results; administer vitamin K if prescribed
  15. Administer low-sodium antacids as prescribed
  16. Administer lactulose (Chronulac) as prescribed, which decreases the pH of the bowel, decreases production of ammonia by bacteria in the bowel, and facilitates the excretion of ammonia
  17. Administer neomycin (Mycifradin) or metronidazole (Flagyl) as prescribed to inhibit protein synthesis in bacteria and decrease the production of ammonia
  18. Avoid medications such as opioids, sedatives, and barbiturates and any hepatotoxic medications or substances
  19. Instruct the client about the restriction of alcohol intake
  20. Prepare the client for paracentesis to remove abdominal fluid
  21. Prepare the client for surgical shunting procedures if prescribed to divert fluid from **ascites** into the venous system

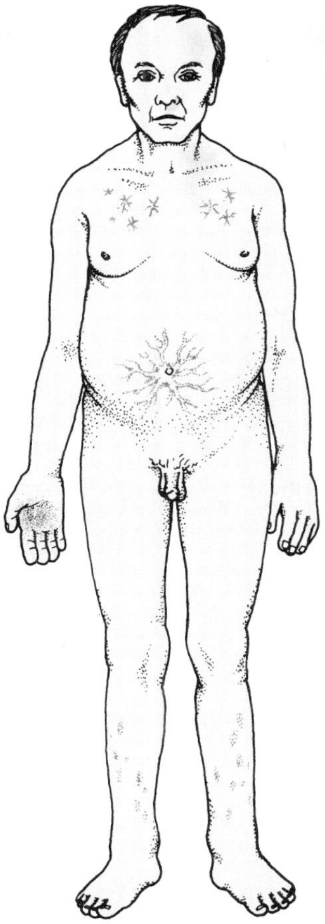

NEUROLOGICAL FINDINGS
Asterixis
Paresthesias of feet
Peripheral nerve degeneration
Portal-systemic encephalopathy
Reversal of sleep-wake pattern
Sensory disturbances

GASTROINTESTINAL (GI)
FINDINGS
Abdominal pain
Anorexia
Ascites
Clay-colored stools
Diarrhea
Esophageal varices
Fetor hepaticus
Gallstones
Gastritis
Gastrointestinal bleeding
Hemorrhoidal varices
Hepatomegaly
Hiatal hernia
Hypersplenism
Malnutrition
Nausea
Small nodular liver
Vomiting

RENAL FINDINGS
Hepatorenal syndrome
Increased urine bilirubin

ENDOCRINE FINDINGS
Increased aldosterone
Increased antidiuretic hormone
Increased circulating estrogens
Increased glucocorticoids
Gynecomastia

IMMUNE SYSTEM DISTURBANCES
Increased susceptibility to infection
Leukopenia

CARDIOVASCULAR FINDINGS
Cardiac dysrhythmias
Development of collateral circulation
Fatigue
Hyperkinetic circulation
Peripheral edema
Portal hypertension
Spider angiomas

PULMONARY FINDINGS
Dyspnea
Hydrothorax
Hyperventilation
Hypoxemia

HEMATOLOGICAL FINDINGS
Anemia
Disseminated intravascular
   coagulation
Impaired coagulation
Splenomegaly
Thrombocytopenia

DERMATOLOGICAL FINDINGS
Axillary and pubic hair changes
Caput medusae
Ecchymosis
Increased skin pigmentation
Jaundice
Palmar erythema
Pruritus
Spider angiomas

FLUID AND ELECTROLYTE
DISTURBANCES
Ascites
Decreased effective blood volume
Dilutional hyponatremia or
   hypernatremia
Hypocalcemia
Hypokalemia
Peripheral edema
Water retention

FIG. 46-4   The clinical picture of a client with liver dysfunction. Manifestations vary according to the progression of the disease. (From Ignatavicius, D., & Workman, M. [2006]. *Medical-surgical nursing: Critical thinking for collaborative care* [5th ed]. St. Louis: Saunders.)

XX. CHOLECYSTITIS

A. Description
1. An inflammation of the gallbladder that may occur as an acute or chronic process
2. Acute inflammation is associated with gallstones (cholelithiasis)
3. Chronic **cholecystitis** results when inefficient bile emptying and gallbladder muscle wall disease cause a fibrotic and contracted gallbladder
4. Acalculous **cholecystitis** occurs in the absence of gallstones and is due to bacterial invasion via the lymphatic or vascular systems

B. Data collection
1. Nausea and vomiting
2. Indigestion
3. Belching
4. Flatulence
5. Epigastric pain that radiates to the scapula 2 to 4 hours after eating fatty foods and may persist for 4 to 6 hours
6. Pain localized in right upper quadrant
7. Guarding, rigidity, and rebound tenderness
8. Mass palpated in the right upper quadrant
9. **Murphy's sign** (cannot take a deep breath when the examiner's fingers are passed below the hepatic margin because of pain)
10. Elevated temperature
11. Tachycardia
12. Signs of dehydration

C. Biliary obstruction
1. Jaundice
2. Dark orange and foamy urine
3. Steatorrhea and clay-colored feces
4. Pruritus

D. Interventions
1. Maintain NPO status during nausea and vomiting episodes
2. Maintain nasogastric decompression as prescribed for severe vomiting
3. Administer antiemetics as prescribed for nausea and vomiting
4. Administer analgesics as prescribed to relieve pain and reduce spasm (Note: Although morphine sulfate or codeine sulfate may be prescribed, they are generally avoided because they can cause spasm of the sphincter of Oddi and increase pain)
5. Administer antispasmodics (anticholinergics) as prescribed to relax smooth muscle
6. Instruct the client with chronic **cholecystitis** to eat small, low-fat meals
7. Instruct the client to avoid gas-forming foods
8. Prepare the client for nonsurgical and surgical procedures as prescribed

E. Surgical interventions
1. **Cholecystectomy** is the removal of the gallbladder
2. **Choledocholithotomy** requires incision into the common bile duct to remove the stone
3. Surgical procedures may be performed by laparoscopy

F. Postoperative interventions
1. Monitor for respiratory complications caused by pain at the incisional site
2. Encourage coughing and deep breathing
3. Encourage early ambulation
4. Instruct the client about splinting the abdomen to prevent discomfort during coughing
5. Administer antiemetics as prescribed for nausea and vomiting
6. Administer analgesics as prescribed for pain relief
7. Maintain NPO status and nasogastric tube suction as prescribed
8. Advance diet from clear liquids to solids when prescribed and as tolerated by the client
9. Maintain and monitor drainage from the T-tube, if present (Box 46-12)

XXI. PANCREATITIS
A. Description
1. An acute or chronic inflammation of the pancreas with associated escape of pancreatic enzymes into surrounding tissue
2. Acute **pancreatitis** occurs suddenly as one attack or can be recurrent with resolutions
3. Chronic **pancreatitis** is a continual inflammation and destruction of the pancreas, with scar tissue replacing pancreatic tissue
4. Precipitating factors include trauma, the use of alcohol, biliary tract disease, viral or bacterial disease, hyperlipidemia, cholelithiasis,

hyperparathyroidism, ischemic vascular disease, and peptic ulcer disease

B. Acute **pancreatitis**
1. Data collection
a. Abdominal pain, including a sudden onset at the midepigastric or left upper quadrant location with radiation to the back
b. Pain that is aggravated by a fatty meal or alcohol or by lying in a recumbent position
c. Abdominal tenderness and guarding
d. Nausea and vomiting
e. Weight loss
f. **Cullen's sign** (discoloration of the abdomen and periumbilical area)
g. **Turner's sign** (bluish discoloration of the flanks)
h. Absent or decreased bowel sounds
i. Elevated white blood cell count, glucose, bilirubin, alkaline phosphatase, or urinary amylase
j. Elevated serum lipase and amylase
2. Interventions
a. Maintain NPO status and maintain hydration with IV fluids as prescribed
b. Administer parenteral nutrition for severe nutritional depletion
c. Administer supplemental preparations and vitamins and minerals to increase caloric intake if prescribed

---

BOX 46-12 **Care of a T-Tube**

Purpose and Description

A T-tube is placed after surgical exploration of the common bile duct. The tube preserves the patency of the duct and ensures drainage of bile until edema resolves and bile is effectively draining into the duodenum. A gravity drainage bag is attached to the T-tube to collect the drainage.

Interventions

Position the client in a semi-Fowler's position to facilitate drainage.

Monitor the amount, color, consistency, and odor of the drainage.

Report sudden increases in bile output to the physician.

Monitor for inflammation and protect the skin from irritation.

Keep the drainage system below the level of the gallbladder.

Monitor for foul odor and purulent drainage and report its presence to the physician.

Avoid irrigation, aspiration, or clamping of the T-tube without a physician's order.

As prescribed, clamp the tube before a meal, and observe for abdominal discomfort and distention, nausea, chills, or fever; unclamp the tube if nausea or vomiting occurs.

d. Maintain nasogastric tube to decrease gastric distention and suppress pancreatic secretion

e. Administer meperidine hydrochloride (Demerol) as prescribed for pain because it causes less incidence of smooth muscle spasm of the pancreatic ducts and sphincter of Oddi (Note: Although morphine sulfate or codeine sulfate may be prescribed, they are generally avoided because they can cause spasm of the sphincter of Oddi and increase pain)

f. Administer antacids as prescribed to neutralize gastric secretions

g. Administer H_2-receptor antagonists as prescribed to decrease hydrochloric acid production and prevent activation of pancreatic enzymes

h. Administer anticholinergics as prescribed to decrease vagal stimulation, decrease gastrointestinal motility, and inhibit pancreatic enzyme secretion

i. Instruct the client on the importance of avoiding alcohol

j. Instruct the client on the importance of follow-up visits with the physician

k. Instruct the client to notify the physician if acute abdominal pain, jaundice, clay-colored stools, or dark urine develops

C. Chronic **pancreatitis**

1. Data collection
   a. Abdominal pain and tenderness
   b. Left upper quadrant mass
   c. Steatorrhea and foul-smelling stools that may increase in volume as pancreatic insufficiency increases
   d. Weight loss
   e. Muscle wasting
   f. Jaundice
   g. Signs and symptoms of diabetes mellitus

2. Interventions
   a. Instruct the client on the prescribed dietary measures (fat and protein intake may be limited)
   b. Instruct the client to avoid heavy meals
   c. Instruct the client about the importance of avoiding alcohol
   d. Provide supplemental preparations and vitamins and minerals to increase caloric intake
   e. Administer pancreatic enzymes as prescribed to aid in the digestion and absorption of fat and protein
   f. Administer insulin or oral hypoglycemic medications as prescribed to control diabetes mellitus, if present
   g. Instruct the client on the use of pancreatic enzyme medications

h. Instruct the client on the treatment plan for glucose management

i. Instruct the client to notify the physician if increased steatorrhea occurs or if abdominal distention or cramping and skin breakdown develops

j. Instruct the client in the importance of follow-up visits

XXII. HEPATITIS

A. Description

1. An inflammation of the liver caused by a virus, bacteria, or exposure to medications or hepatotoxins

2. The goals of treatment include resting the inflamed liver to reduce metabolic demands and increasing the blood supply, thus promoting cellular regeneration and preventing complications

B. Types of viral **hepatitis**

1. **Hepatitis** A virus (HAV): infectious **hepatitis**
2. **Hepatitis** B virus (HBV): serum **hepatitis**
3. **Hepatitis** C virus (HCV): non-A, non-B **hepatitis** or post-transfusion **hepatitis**
4. **Hepatitis** D virus (HDV): delta agent **hepatitis**
5. **Hepatitis** E virus (HEV): enterically transmitted or epidemic non-A, non-B **hepatitis**
6. **Hepatitis** G virus: non-A, non-B, non-C **hepatitis**

C. Stages of viral **hepatitis** (Box 46-13)

D. Data collection

1. Preicteric stage
   a. Flu-like symptoms: malaise, fatigue
   b. Anorexia, nausea, vomiting, or diarrhea
   c. Pain: headache, muscle aches, or polyarthritis
   d. Elevated serum bilirubin and enzyme levels

2. Icteric stage
   a. Jaundice
   b. Pruritus
   c. Brown urine
   d. Lighter-colored stools
   e. Decrease in preicteric-phase symptoms

BOX 46-13 **Stages of Viral Hepatitis**

Preicteric Stage
The first stage of hepatitis preceding the appearance of jaundice; includes flu-like symptoms
Icteric Stage
The second stage of hepatitis, which includes the appearance of jaundice and associated symptoms such as elevated bilirubin levels, dark or tea-colored urine, and clay-colored stools
Posticteric Stage
The convalescent stage in which the jaundice decreases and the color of the urine and stool returns to normal

3. Posticteric stage
   a. Increased energy levels
   b. Subsiding of pain
   c. Minimal to absent gastrointestinal symptoms
   d. Serum bilirubin and enzyme levels return to normal
E. Laboratory assessment
   1. Alanine aminotransferase: elevated into the thousands (normal is 4 to 36 international units/L)
   2. Aspartate aminotransferase: elevated into the thousands (normal is 8 to 33 units/L)
   3. Alkaline phosphatase levels: may be normal or mildly elevated (normal is 4.5 to 13 King-Armstrong units/dL)
   4. Total bilirubin levels: elevated in the serum and urine (normal is less than 1.5 mg/dL)

XXIII. HEPATITIS A

A. Description
   1. Formerly known as infectious **hepatitis**
   2. Commonly seen during the fall and early winter
B. Individuals at increased risk
   1. Commonly seen in young children
   2. Individuals in institutionalized settings
   3. Health care personnel
C. Transmission
   1. Fecal-oral route
   2. Person-to-person contact
   3. Parenteral
   4. Contaminated fruits, vegetables, or uncooked shellfish
   5. Contaminated water or milk
   6. Poorly washed utensils
D. Incubation and infectious period
   1. Incubation period: 2 to 6 weeks
   2. Infectious period: 2 to 3 weeks before and 1 week after development of jaundice
E. Testing
   1. Infection is established by the presence of HAV antibodies (anti-HAV) in the blood
   2. Immunoglobulin M (IgM) and G (IgG) are normally present in the blood, and increased levels indicate infection and inflammation
   3. Ongoing inflammation of the liver is evidenced by the presence of elevated IgM antibodies, which persist in the blood for 4 to 6 weeks
   4. Previous infection is indicated by the presence of elevated IgG antibodies
F. Complication: fulminant (severe acute and often fatal) **hepatitis**
G. Prevention
   1. Strict hand washing
   2. Stool and needle precautions
   3. Treatment of municipal water supplies

4. Serological screening of food handlers
5. **Hepatitis** A vaccine (Havrix)
6. Immune globulin: For individuals exposed to HAV who have never received the **hepatitis** A vaccine, administer immune globulin during the period of incubation and within 2 weeks of exposure
7. Immune globulin and **hepatitis** A vaccine are recommended for household members and sexual contacts of individuals with **hepatitis** A
8. Pre-exposure prophylaxis with immunoglobulin is recommended to individuals traveling to countries with poor or uncertain sanitation conditions

XXIV. HEPATITIS B

A. Description
   1. **Hepatitis** B is nonseasonal
   2. All age groups are affected
B. Individuals at increased risk
   1. Drug addicts
   2. Clients undergoing long-term hemodialysis
   3. Health care personnel
C. Transmission
   1. Blood or body fluid contact
   2. Infected blood products
   3. Infected saliva or semen
   4. Contaminated needles
   5. Sexual contact
   6. Parenteral
   7. Perinatal period
   8. Blood or body fluids contact at birth
D. Incubation period: 6 to 24 weeks
E. Testing
   1. Infection is established by the presence of **hepatitis** B antigen-antibody systems in the blood
   2. Presence of **hepatitis** B surface antigen (HBsAg) is the serological marker to establish the diagnosis of **hepatitis** B
   3. The client is considered infectious if these antigens are present in the blood
   4. If the serological marker (HBsAg) is present after 6 months, it indicates a carrier state or chronic **hepatitis**
   5. Normally the serological marker (HBsAg) level declines and disappears after the acute **hepatitis** B episode
   6. The presence of antibodies to HBsAg (anti-HBs) indicates recovery and immunity to **hepatitis** B
   7. **Hepatitis** B early antigen (HBeAg) is detected in the blood about 1 week after the appearance of HBsAg, and its presence determines the infective state of the client
F. Complications
   1. Fulminant **hepatitis**
   2. Chronic liver disease

3. **Cirrhosis**
4. Primary hepatocellular carcinoma
G. Prevention
1. Strict hand washing
2. Screening blood donors
3. Testing of all pregnant women
4. Needle precautions
5. Avoiding intimate sexual contact if test for HBsAg is positive in a person
6. **Hepatitis** B vaccine: Engerix-B, Recombivax HB
7. **Hepatitis** B immune globulin: for individuals exposed to HBV through sexual contact or through the percutaneous or transmucosal routes, who have never had **hepatitis** B, and who have never received **hepatitis** B vaccine

XXV. HEPATITIS C
A. Description
1. **Hepatitis** C virus infection occurs year-round
2. Infection can occur in any age group
3. Infection with HCV is common among drug abusers and is the major cause of post-transfusion **hepatitis**
4. Risk factors are similar to those for HBV because **hepatitis** C is also transmitted parenterally
B. Individuals at increased risk
1. Parenteral drug users
2. Clients receiving frequent transfusions
3. Health care personnel
C. Transmission: Same as for HBV; primarily through blood
D. Incubation period: 5 to 10 weeks
E. Testing: Anti-HCV is the antibody to HCV and is most accurate in detecting chronic states of **hepatitis** C
F. Complications
1. Chronic liver disease
3. **Cirrhosis**
3. Primary hepatocellular carcinoma
G. Prevention
1. Strict hand washing
2. Needle precautions
3. Screening of blood donors

XXVI. HEPATITIS D
A. Description
1. **Hepatitis** D is common in the Mediterranean and Middle Eastern areas
2. **Hepatitis** D occurs with **hepatitis** B and may cause infection only in the presence of active HBV infection
3. Coinfection with the delta-agent (HDV) intensifies the acute symptoms of **hepatitis** B
4. Transmission and risk of infection are the same as for HBV, via contact with blood and blood products
5. Prevention of HBV infection with vaccine also prevents HDV infection because HDV depends on HBV for replication

B. High-risk individuals
1. Drug users
2. Clients receiving hemodialysis
3. Clients receiving frequent blood transfusions
C. Transmission: Same as for HBV
D. Incubation period: 7 to 8 weeks
E. Testing: Serological HDV determination is made by detection of the **hepatitis** D antigen (HDAg) early in the course of the infection and by detection of anti-HDV antibody in the later disease stages
F. Complications
1. Chronic liver disease
2. Fulminant **hepatitis**
G. Prevention: Because **hepatitis** D must co-exist with **hepatitis** B, the precautions that help prevent **hepatitis** B are also useful in preventing delta **hepatitis**

XXVII. HEPATITIS E
A. Description
1. **Hepatitis** E is a waterborne virus
2. **Hepatitis** E is prevalent in areas where sewage disposal is inadequate or where communal bathing in contaminated rivers is practiced
3. Risk of infection is the same as for HAV
4. Infection with HEV presents as a mild disease except in infected women in the third trimester of pregnancy, with whom the mortality rate is high
B. Individuals with increased risk
1. Travelers to countries that have a high incidence of **hepatitis** E such as India, Burma (Myanmar), Afghanistan, Algeria, and Mexico
2. Eating or drinking of food or water contaminated with the virus
C. Transmission: Same as for HAV
D. Incubation period: 2 to 9 weeks
E. Testing: Specific serological tests for HEV include detection of IgM and IgG antibodies to **hepatitis** E (anti-HEV)
F. Complications
1. High mortality rate in pregnant women
2. Fetal demise
G. Prevention
1. Strict hand washing
2. Treatment of water supplies and sanitation measures

XXVIII. HEPATITIS G
A. **Hepatitis** G is non-A, non-B, non-C **hepatitis**
B. Risk factors are similar to those for **hepatitis** C
C. **Hepatitis** G virus has been found in some blood donors, IV drug users, hemodialysis clients, and clients with hemophilia; however, **hepatitis** G virus does not appear to cause significant liver disease

XXIX. CLIENT AND FAMILY HOME CARE INSTRUCTIONS FOR HEPATITIS (Box 46-14)

BOX 46-14   Home Care Instructions About Hepatitis

Hand washing must be strict and frequent.

Bathrooms should not be shared unless the client strictly adheres to personal hygiene measures.

Individual washcloths, towels, drinking and eating utensils, toothbrushes, and razors must be labeled and identified.

The client must not prepare food for other family members.

The client should avoid alcohol and over-the-counter medications, particularly acetaminophen (Tylenol) and sedatives because these medications are hepatotoxic.

The client should increase activity gradually to prevent fatigue.

The client should consume small, frequent, high-carbohydrate, low-fat foods.

The client is not to donate blood.

The client may maintain normal contact with persons as long as proper personal hygiene is maintained.

Close personal contact such as kissing should be discouraged until hepatitis B surface antigen test results are negative.

The client is to avoid sexual activity until hepatitis B surface antigen results are negative.

The client needs to carry a Medic-Alert card noting the date of hepatitis onset.

The client needs to inform other health professionals, such as medical or dental personnel, of the onset of hepatitis.

The client needs to keep follow-up appointments with the health care provider.

PRACTICE QUESTIONS

More questions on the companion CD!

548. A nurse is teaching the client about an upcoming colonoscopy procedure. The nurse would include in the instructions that the client will be placed in which of the following positions for the procedure?
   1. Left Sims' position
   2. Lithotomy position
   3. Knee-chest position
   4. Right Sims' position

549. A nurse is preparing to perform an abdominal examination. The initial step would be which of the following?
   1. Palpation
   2. Inspection
   3. Percussion
   4. Auscultation

550. A nurse provides instructions to a client following a liver biopsy. The nurse tells the client to:
   1. Avoid alcohol for 8 hours
   2. Remain NPO for 24 hours

   3. Lie on the right side for 2 hours
   4. Save all stools to be checked for blood

551. A nurse is caring for a client with a diagnosis of chronic gastritis. The nurse anticipates that this client is at risk for which vitamin deficiency?
   1. Vitamin A
   2. Vitamin C
   3. Vitamin E
   4. Vitamin B_{12}

552. A nurse is caring for a client following a Billroth II procedure. On review of the postoperative orders, which of the following, if prescribed, would the nurse question and verify?
   1. Leg exercises
   2. Early ambulation
   3. Irrigating the nasogastric (NG) tube
   4. Coughing and deep breathing exercises

553. The nurse is providing discharge instructions to a client following gastrectomy. Which measure will the nurse instruct the client to follow to help prevent dumping syndrome?
   1. Ambulate following a meal
   2. Eat high-carbohydrate foods
   3. Limit the fluids taken with meals
   4. Sit in a high Fowler's position during meals

554. A nurse is monitoring a client for the early signs and symptoms of dumping syndrome. Which of the following symptoms will indicate this occurrence?
   1. Sweating and pallor
   2. Dry skin and stomach pain
   3. Bradycardia and indigestion
   4. Double vision and chest pain

555. A nurse is reviewing the record of a client with Crohn's disease. Which of the following stool characteristics would the nurse expect to see documented in the record?
   1. Diarrhea
   2. Constipation
   3. Bloody stools
   4. Stool constantly oozing from the rectum

556. A client with ascites is scheduled for a paracentesis. The nurse is assisting the physician in performing the procedure. Which of the following positions will the nurse assist the client to assume for this procedure?
   1. Flat
   2. Upright
   3. Left side–lying
   4. Right side–lying

557. An ultrasound of the gallbladder is scheduled for the client with a suspected diagnosis of cholecystitis. The nurse explains to the client that this test:
   1. Is uncomfortable
   2. Requires that the client be NPO
   3. Requires the client to lie still for short intervals
   4. Is preceded by the administration of oral tablets

558. It has been determined that a client with hepatitis has contracted the infection from contaminated food. What type of hepatitis is this client most likely experiencing?
    1. Hepatitis A
    2. Hepatitis B
    3. Hepatitis C
    4. Hepatitis D

559. A nurse is reviewing the physician's orders written for a client admitted with acute pancreatitis. Which physician order would the nurse verify if noted on the client's chart?
    1. NPO status
    2. Morphine sulfate for pain
    3. An anticholinergic medication
    4. Prepare to insert a nasogastric tube

560. A client with hiatal hernia chronically experiences heartburn following meals. The nurse would teach the client to avoid which of the following, which is contraindicated with hiatal hernia?
    1. Lying recumbent following meals
    2. Eating small, frequent, bland meals
    3. Raising the head of the bed on 6-inch blocks
    4. Taking histamine receptor antagonist medication, as prescribed

561. A nurse is monitoring for stoma prolapse in a client with a colostomy. The nurse would observe which of the following appearances in the stoma if prolapse occurred?
    1. Dark and bluish
    2. Sunken and hidden
    3. Narrowed and flattened
    4. Protruding and swollen

562. A client with acute pancreatitis is experiencing severe pain from the disorder. The nurse tells the client to avoid which position that could aggravate the pain?
    1. Sitting up
    2. Lying flat
    3. Leaning forward
    4. Flexing the left leg

563. A nurse is evaluating the effect of dietary counseling on the client with cholecystitis. The nurse determines that the client understands the instructions given if the client states that which food item is acceptable to include in the diet?
    1. Beef chili
    2. Grilled steak
    3. Mashed potatoes
    4. Turkey and lettuce sandwich

564. A client is admitted to the hospital with acute viral hepatitis. Which of the following signs or symptoms would the nurse expect to note based upon this diagnosis?
    1. Fatigue
    2. Pale urine

3. Weight gain
4. Spider angiomas

565. Of the following infection control methods, which would be the priority to include in the plan of care to prevent hepatitis B in a client considered to be at high risk for exposure?
    1. Hepatitis B vaccine
    2. Proper personal hygiene
    3. Use of immune globulin
    4. Correct hand-washing technique

566. A client is admitted to the hospital with viral hepatitis and is complaining of a loss of appetite. In order to provide adequate nutrition, the nurse encourages the client to:
    1. Select foods high in fat
    2. Increase intake of fluids
    3. Eat less often, preferably only three large meals daily
    4. Eat a large supper when anorexia is most likely not as severe

567. A client presents to the emergency department with upper gastrointestinal (GI) bleeding and is in moderate distress. Which nursing action would be the priority for this client?
    1. Determination of vital signs
    2. Complete abdominal physical examination
    3. Thorough investigation of the precipitating events
    4. Insertion of a nasogastric tube and Hematest of the emesis

568. A nurse is caring for a client with acute pancreatitis and a history of alcoholism and is monitoring the client for complications. Which of the following data would be a sign of paralytic ileus?
    1. Inability to pass flatus
    2. Loss of anal sphincter control
    3. Severe, constant pain with rapid onset
    4. Firm, nontender mass palpable at the lower right costal margin

569. A client with viral hepatitis has no appetite, and food makes the client nauseated. Which nursing intervention would be appropriate?
    1. Offer small, frequent meals.
    2. Encourage foods low in calories
    3. Explain that high-fat diets are usually better tolerated
    4. Explain that the majority of calories need to be consumed in the evening hours

570. A nurse is participating in a health screening clinic and is preparing teaching materials about colorectal cancer. The nurse would plan to include which risk factor for colorectal cancer in the material?
    1. Age of 20 years
    2. High-fiber, low-fat diet
    3. Distant relative with colorectal cancer
    4. Personal history of ulcerative colitis or gastrointestinal polyps

571. A client has undergone esophagogastroduodenoscopy (EGD). The nurse places highest priority on which of the following items as part of the client's care plan?
    1. Monitoring the temperature
    2. Checking for return of a gag reflex
    3. Giving warm gargles for a sore throat
    4. Monitoring for complaints of heartburn

ALTERNATE ITEM FORMAT: MULTIPLE RESPONSE

572. A nurse is reviewing the orders of a client admitted to the hospital with a diagnosis of acute pancreatitis. Choose the interventions that the nurse would expect to be prescribed for the client. Select all that apply.
    ☐ **1.** Administer antacids, as prescribed
    ☐ **2.** Small, frequent high calorie feedings
    ☐ **3.** Encourage coughing and deep breathing
    ☐ **4.** Administer anticholinergics, as prescribed
    ☐ **5.** Meperidine (Demerol) as prescribed for pain
    ☐ **6.** Maintain the client in a supine and flat position

ANSWERS

548. **1**
Rationale: The client is placed in the left Sims' position for the procedure. This position takes the best advantage of the client's anatomy for ease in introducing the colonoscope. The other options are incorrect.
Test-Taking Strategy: Use concepts related to gastrointestinal anatomy to answer this question. The position would be the same as that used for giving the client an enema while lying down. When answering factual questions such as these, remember the guiding principles and attempt to visualize the procedure to help you select the correct option. Review this procedure if you had difficulty with this question.
Level of Cognitive Ability: Application
Client Needs: Physiological Integrity
Integrated Process: Nursing Process/Implementation
Content Area: Adult Health/Gastrointestinal
Reference: Chernecky, C., & Berger, B. (2008). *Laboratory tests and diagnostic procedures* (5th ed., pp. 358-359). Philadelphia: Saunders.

549. **2**
Rationale: The appropriate technique for abdominal examination is inspection, auscultation, percussion, and palpation. Auscultation is performed after inspection and before percussion and palpation to ensure that the motility of the bowel and bowel sounds are not altered. The sequence of maneuvers is inspect, auscultate, percuss, and palpate.
Test-Taking Strategy: Use the process of elimination and think about the procedure. Remember that the sequence for abdominal examination is different than the usual systematic approach. Review this technique if you had difficulty with this question.
Level of Cognitive Ability: Application
Client Needs: Health Promotion and Maintenance
Integrated Process: Nursing Process/Data Collection
Content Area: Adult Health/Gastrointestinal
Reference: Christensen, B., & Kochrow, E. (2006). *Foundations of nursing* (5th ed., pp. 73-74). St. Louis: Mosby.

550. **3**
Rationale: In order to splint the puncture site, the client is kept on his or her right side for a minimum of 2 hours. It is not necessary to remain NPO for 24 hours. Permission regarding the consumption of alcohol should be obtained from the physician. It is not necessary to save all stools.
Test-Taking Strategy: Use the process of elimination and focus on the subject: a liver biopsy. Recalling the anatomical location of this procedure will direct you to option 3. Review postprocedure instructions following a liver biopsy if you had difficulty with this question.
Level of Cognitive Ability: Application
Client Needs: Physiological Integrity
Integrated Process: Nursing Process/Implementation
Content Area: Adult Health/Gastrointestinal
Reference: Pagana, K., & Pagana, T. (2005). *Mosby's diagnostic and laboratory test reference* (7th ed., p. 597). St. Louis: Mosby.

551. **4**
Rationale: Deterioration and atrophy of the lining of the stomach lead to the loss of function of the parietal cells. When the acid secretion decreases, the source of the intrinsic factor is lost, which results in the inability to absorb vitamin B_{12}. This leads to the development of pernicious anemia. Options 1, 2, and 3 are incorrect.
Test-Taking Strategy: Use the process of elimination. Knowledge regarding the pathophysiology related to the lining of the stomach is required to answer this question. If you are unfamiliar with vitamin B_{12} deficiency and its relationship to gastric disorders, review this content.
Level of Cognitive Ability: Comprehension
Client Needs: Physiological Integrity
Integrated Process: Nursing Process/Data Collection
Content Area: Adult Health/Gastrointestinal
Reference: Linton, A., & Maebius, N. (2007). *Introduction to medical-surgical nursing* (4th ed., p. 764). Philadelphia: Saunders.

552. **3**
Rationale: In a Billroth II resection, the proximal remnant of the stomach is anastomosed to the proximal jejunum. Patency of the NG tube is critical for preventing the retention of gastric secretions. The nurse, however, should never irrigate or reposition the gastric tube after gastric surgery unless specifically ordered by the physician. In this situation, the nurse should clarify the order. Options 1, 2, and 4 are appropriate postoperative interventions.
Test-Taking Strategy: Use the process of elimination. Eliminate options 1, 2, and 4 because they are general

postoperative measures. Also, consider the anatomical location of the surgical procedure to assist in directing you to option 3. Review these postoperative measures if you had difficulty with this question.
Level of Cognitive Ability: Application
Client Needs: Safe and Effective Care Environment
Integrated Process: Nursing Process/Implementation
Content Area: Adult Health/Gastrointestinal
Reference: Christensen, B., & Kockrow, E. (2006). *Adult health nursing* (5th ed., pp. 218-219). St. Louis: Mosby.

553. **3**
Rationale: The client should be instructed to decrease the amount of fluid taken at meals. The client should also be instructed to avoid high-carbohydrate foods including fluids, such as fruit nectars; to assume a low Fowler's position during meals; to lie down for 30 minutes after eating to delay gastric emptying; and to take antispasmodics as prescribed.
Test-Taking Strategy: Use the process of elimination. Eliminate options 1 and 4 first because these measures will promote gastric emptying. From the remaining options, select option 3 because this measure will delay gastric emptying. If you are unfamiliar with this syndrome, review these client-teaching points.
Level of Cognitive Ability: Application
Client Needs: Physiological Integrity
Integrated Process: Teaching and Learning
Content Area: Adult Health/Gastrointestinal
Reference: Linton, A., & Maebius, N. (2007). *Introduction to medical-surgical nursing* (4th ed., p. 772). Philadelphia: Saunders.

554. **1**
Rationale: Early manifestations occur 5 to 30 minutes after eating. Symptoms include vertigo, tachycardia, syncope, sweating, pallor, palpitations, and the desire to lie down.
Test-Taking Strategy: Knowledge regarding the early manifestations associated with dumping syndrome is required to answer this question. Remember, sweating and pallor occur and are early signs of dumping syndrome. If you are unfamiliar with these manifestations, review this content.
Level of Cognitive Ability: Comprehension
Client Needs: Physiological Integrity
Integrated Process: Nursing Process/Data Collection
Content Area: Adult Health/Gastrointestinal
Reference: Linton, A., & Maebius, N. (2007). *Introduction to medical-surgical nursing* (4th ed., p. 742). Philadelphia: Saunders.

555. **1**
Rationale: Crohn's disease is characterized by non-bloody diarrhea of usually not more than four or five stools daily. Over time, the diarrhea episodes increase in frequency, duration, and severity. Options 2 and 4 are not characteristics of Crohn's disease.
Test-Taking Strategy: Use the process of elimination. Recalling the pathophysiology related to Crohn's disease will direct you to option 1. If you are unfamiliar with this disorder, review this content.
Level of Cognitive Ability: Comprehension

Client Needs: Physiological Integrity
Integrated Process: Nursing Process/Data Collection
Content Area: Adult Health/Gastrointestinal
Reference: Christensen, B., & Kockrow, E. (2006). *Adult health nursing* (5th ed., p. 231). St. Louis: Mosby.

556. **2**
Rationale: An upright position allows the intestine to float posteriorly and helps prevent intestinal laceration during catheter insertion. Options 1, 3, and 4 are incorrect positions.
Test-Taking Strategy: Use the process of elimination and visualize this procedure in selecting the correct option. Knowing that fluid will be aspirated from the abdominal cavity will assist in directing you to option 2. If you had difficulty with this question, review this procedure.
Level of Cognitive Ability: Application
Client Needs: Physiological Integrity
Integrated Process: Nursing Process/Implementation
Content Area: Adult Health/Gastrointestinal
References: Chernecky, C., & Berger, B. (2008). *Laboratory tests and diagnostic procedures* (5th ed., pp. 844-845). Philadelphia: Saunders.
Linton, A., & Maebius, N. (2007). *Introduction to medical-surgical nursing* (4th ed., p. 810). Philadelphia: Saunders.

557. **3**
Rationale: Ultrasound of the gallbladder is a noninvasive procedure and is frequently used for emergency diagnosis of acute cholecystitis. The client does not need to be NPO but may be instructed to avoid carbonated beverages for 48 hours before the test to help decrease intestinal gas. It is a painless test and does not require the administration of oral tablets as preparation.
Test-Taking Strategy: Focus on the subject—an ultrasound. Visualizing this procedure will direct you to option 3. Review this procedure if you had difficulty with this question.
Level of Cognitive Ability: Application
Client Needs: Physiological Integrity
Integrated Process: Nursing Process/Implementation
Content Area: Adult Health/Gastrointestinal
Reference: Chernecky, C., & Berger, B. (2008). *Laboratory tests and diagnostic procedures* (5th ed., pp. 548-549). Philadelphia: Saunders.

558. **1**
Rationale: Hepatitis A is transmitted by the fecal-oral route via contaminated food or infected food handlers. Hepatitis B, C, and D are most commonly transmitted via infected blood or body fluids.
Test-Taking Strategy: Knowledge regarding the modes of transmission of the various types of hepatitis is required to answer this question. Remember, hepatitis A is transmitted by the fecal-oral route via contaminated food or infected food handlers. If you are unfamiliar with the modes of transmission of hepatitis, review this content.
Level of Cognitive Ability: Comprehension
Client Needs: Physiological Integrity
Integrated Process: Nursing Process/Data Collection
Content Area: Adult Health/Gastrointestinal
Reference: Christensen, B., & Kockrow, E. (2006). *Foundations of nursing* (5th ed., p. 265). St. Louis: Mosby.

559. 2

Rationale: Meperidine (Demerol) rather than morphine sulfate is the medication of choice, because morphine sulfate can cause spasms in the sphincter of Oddi. Therefore, the nurse would verify this order. Options 1, 3, and 4 are appropriate interventions for the client with acute pancreatitis.

Test-Taking Strategy: Use the process of elimination and note the strategic word "acute" in the question. Recalling the treatment measures for acute pancreatitis and the contraindications in the care of the client will direct you to option 2. Review these measures if you had difficulty with this question.

Level of Cognitive Ability: Analysis
Client Needs: Safe and Effective Care Environment
Integrated Process: Nursing Process/Implementation
Content Area: Adult Health/Gastrointestinal
Reference: Christensen, B., & Kockrow, E. (2006). *Adult health nursing* (5th ed., p. 278). St. Louis: Mosby.

560. 1

Rationale: Hiatal hernia is due to a protrusion of a portion of the stomach above the diaphragm, where the esophagus usually is positioned. The client generally experiences pain caused by reflux resulting from ingestion of irritating foods, lying flat following meals or at night, and consuming large or fatty meals. Relief is obtained by eating small, frequent, and bland meals; by histamine antagonists and antacids; and by elevation of the thorax following meals and during sleep.

Test-Taking Strategy: Use the process of elimination. Note the strategic word "contraindicated." This tells you that the correct answer will be the option that represents an aggravating factor for hiatal hernia discomfort. Visualize each option and think about the anatomical location of a hiatal hernia to direct you to option 1. Review these teaching points if you had difficulty with this question.

Level of Cognitive Ability: Application
Client Needs: Physiological Integrity
Integrated Process: Teaching and Learning
Content Area: Adult Health/Gastrointestinal
Reference: Linton, A., & Maebius, N. (2007). *Introduction to medical-surgical nursing* (4th ed., p. 762). Philadelphia: Saunders.

561. 4

Rationale: A prolapsed stoma is one in which bowel protrudes through the stoma, with an elongated and swollen appearance. A stoma retraction is characterized by sinking of the stoma. Ischemia of the stoma would be associated with dusky or bluish color. A stoma with a narrowed opening, either at the level of the skin or fascia, is said to be stenosed.

Test-Taking Strategy: Use the process of elimination. Focusing on the strategic word "prolapse" will direct you to option 4. Review the different complications that can occur with ostomy formation if you had difficulty with this question.

Level of Cognitive Ability: Analysis
Client Needs: Physiological Integrity
Integrated Process: Nursing Process/Data Collection
Content Area: Adult Health/Gastrointestinal
Reference: Linton, A., & Maebius, N. (2007). *Introduction to medical-surgical nursing* (4th ed., pp. 405-406). Philadelphia: Saunders.

562. 2

Rationale: Positions such as sitting up, leaning forward, and flexing the legs (especially the left leg) may alleviate some of the pain associated with pancreatitis. The pain is aggravated by lying supine or walking. This is because the pancreas is located retroperitoneally, and the edema and inflammation intensify the irritation of the posterior peritoneal wall with these positions.

Test-Taking Strategy: Use the process of elimination. Eliminate options 1 and 3 first because they are comparable or alike. From the remaining options, visualize the pancreas and the potential effects of stretching associated with the various positions listed. This will direct you to option 2. Review care of the client with pancreatitis if you had difficulty with this question.

Level of Cognitive Ability: Application
Client Needs: Physiological Integrity
Integrated Process: Nursing Process/Implementation
Content Area: Adult Health/Gastrointestinal
Reference: Christensen, B., & Kockrow, E. (2006). *Adult health nursing* (5th ed., p. 278). St. Louis: Mosby.

563. 4

Rationale: The client with cholecystitis should decrease overall intake of dietary fat. Red meats (hamburger and steak) contain fat. Mashed potatoes are usually made with milk and butter. The correct food item that is low in fat is the turkey and lettuce sandwich.

Test-Taking Strategy: Use the process of elimination and recall that clients with cholecystitis should decrease fat intake. Also note that options 1, 2, and 3 are comparable or alike and are high in fat. Review dietary instructions for the client with cholecystitis if you had difficulty with this question.

Level of Cognitive Ability: Comprehension
Client Needs: Physiological Integrity
Integrated Process: Nursing Process/Evaluation
Content Area: Adult Health/Gastrointestinal
References: Christensen, B., & Kockrow, E. (2006). *Adult health nursing* (5th ed., p. 277). St. Louis: Mosby.
Grodner, M., Long, S. & Walkinshaw, B. (2007). *Foundations and clinical applications of nutrition: A nursing approach.* (4th ed., p. 414). St. Louis: Mosby.
Nix, S. (2005). *Williams' basic nutrition and diet therapy* (11th ed., p. 343). St. Louis: Mosby.

564. 1

Rationale: Common signs of acute viral hepatitis include weight loss, dark urine, and fatigue. The client is anorexic and finds food distasteful. The urine darkens because of excess bilirubin being excreted by the kidneys. Fatigue occurs during all phases of hepatitis. Spider angiomas—small, dilated blood vessels—are commonly seen in cirrhosis of the liver.

Test-Taking Strategy: Use the process of elimination. Recalling the function of the liver will direct you to option 1. Remember, lethargy is a classic symptom associated with hepatitis. If you had difficulty with this question, review the manifestations associated with hepatitis.

Level of Cognitive Ability: Analysis
Client Needs: Physiological Integrity
Integrated Process: Nursing Process/Data Collection

Content Area: Adult Health/Gastrointestinal
Reference: Linton, A., & Maebius, N. (2007). *Introduction to medical-surgical nursing* (4th ed., p. 806). Philadelphia: Saunders.

565. 1
Rationale: Immunization is the most effective method of preventing hepatitis B infection. Other general measures include hand washing. Immune globulin is used to prevent hepatitis A and is used for prophylaxis if the client is traveling to endemic areas. Personal hygiene, such as hand washing after a bowel movement and before eating, also helps prevent the transmission of hepatitis A.
Test-Taking Strategy: Use the process of elimination and note the strategic word "priority." Although more than one of the options is correct for preventing transmission of hepatitis B, the priority is immunization with hepatitis B vaccine. If you had difficulty with this question, review the content associated with hepatitis.
Level of Cognitive Ability: Application
Client Needs: Safe and Effective Care Environment
Integrated Process: Nursing Process/Planning
Content Area: Adult Health/Gastrointestinal
Reference: Linton, A., & Maebius, N. (2007). *Introduction to medical-surgical nursing* (4th ed., p. 804). Philadelphia: Saunders.

566. 2
Rationale: Although no special diet is required in the treatment of viral hepatitis, it is generally recommended that clients have a diet with low-fat content, since fat may be poorly tolerated because of decreased bile production. Small, frequent meals are preferable and may even prevent nausea. Frequently, the appetite is better in the morning, so it is easier to eat a healthy breakfast. An adequate fluid intake of 2500 to 3000 mL/day that includes nutritional fluids is also important.
Test-Taking Strategy: Use the process of elimination and focus on the subject: a lack of appetite. Eliminate option 1 because of the words "high in fat." Eliminate options 3 and 4 next because of the word "large." Review dietary measures for the client with hepatitis if you had difficulty with this question.
Level of Cognitive Ability: Application
Client Needs: Physiological Integrity
Integrated Process: Nursing Process/Implementation
Content Area: Adult Health/Gastrointestinal
References: Christensen, B., & Kockrow, E. (2006). *Adult health nursing* (5th ed., p. 262). St. Louis: Mosby.
Linton, A., & Maebius, N. (2007). *Introduction to medical-surgical nursing* (4th ed., p. 807). Philadelphia: Saunders.

567. 1
Rationale: The determination of vital signs indicates whether the client is in shock from blood loss and provides a baseline blood pressure and pulse by which to monitor the progress of treatment. Signs and symptoms of shock include low blood pressure; rapid, weak pulse; increased thirst; cold, clammy skin; and restlessness. Vital signs should be monitored at least every 15 to 30 minutes, and the physician should be informed of any significant changes. The client may not be able to provide subjective data until the immediate physical

needs are met. Although options 2 and 4 may be a component of care, they are not the priority.
Test-Taking Strategy: Note the word "priority" and use the ABCs—airway, breathing, and circulation. A client with an acute upper GI bleed is at risk for shock. Monitoring vital signs is the nursing action that will assess circulation, provide information about the client's circulating volume status, and alert the nurse to early stages of shock. Review care of the client with a GI bleed if you had difficulty with this question.
Level of Cognitive Ability: Application
Client Needs: Physiological Integrity
Integrated Process: Nursing Process/Implementation
Content Area: Adult Health/Gastrointestinal
References: Christensen, B., & Kockrow, E. (2006). *Adult health nursing* (5th ed., pp. 217-218). St. Louis: Mosby.
Linton, A., & Maebius, N. (2007). *Introduction to medical-surgical nursing* (4th ed., p. 293). Philadelphia: Saunders.

568. 1
Rationale: An inflammatory reaction such as acute pancreatitis can cause paralytic ileus, the most common form of nonmechanical obstruction. Inability to pass flatus is a clinical manifestation of paralytic ileus. Option 4 is the description of the physical finding of liver enlargement. The liver is usually enlarged in cases of cirrhosis or hepatitis. Although this client may have an enlarged liver, it is not a sign of paralytic ileus or intestinal obstruction. Pain is associated with paralytic ileus, but the pain usually presents as a more constant generalized discomfort. Pain that is severe, constant, and rapid in onset is more likely caused by strangulation of the bowel. Loss of sphincter control is not a sign of paralytic ileus.
Test-Taking Strategy: Use the process of elimination. Note the relationship between the words "paralytic ileus" and "inability to pass flatus" in option 1. Review these clinical manifestations if you had difficulty with this question.
Level of Cognitive Ability: Comprehension
Client Needs: Physiological Integrity
Integrated Process: Nursing Process/Data Collection
Content Area: Adult Health/Gastrointestinal
References: Christensen, B., & Kockrow, E. (2006). *Adult health nursing* (5th ed., p. 240). St. Louis: Mosby.
Linton, A., & Maebius, N. (2007). *Introduction to medical-surgical nursing* (4th ed., p. 263). Philadelphia: Saunders.

569. 1
Rationale: If nausea persists, the client will need to be assessed for fluid and electrolyte imbalances. It is important to explain to the client that the majority of calories should be eaten in the morning hours, because nausea most often occurs in the afternoon and evening. Clients should select a diet high in calories, because energy is required for healing. Changes in bilirubin interfere with fat absorption, so low-fat diets are better tolerated.
Test-Taking Strategy: Use the process of elimination. Recalling the nutritional aspects of care for clients with viral hepatitis will direct you to option 1. Review care of the client with viral hepatitis if you had difficulty answering this question.
Level of Cognitive Ability: Application
Client Needs: Physiological Integrity
Integrated Process: Nursing Process/Implementation
Content Area: Adult Health/Gastrointestinal

Reference: Christensen, B., & Kockrow, E. (2006). *Adult health nursing* (5th ed., p. 268). St. Louis: Mosby.

570. 4

Rationale: Common risk factors for colorectal cancer include age over 40 years; first-degree relative with colorectal cancer; high-fat, low-fiber diet; and history of bowel problems such as ulcerative colitis or familial polyposis.

Test-Taking Strategy: Use the process of elimination. Noting the strategic words "personal history" in option 4 will direct you to this option. Review these risk factors if you had difficulty with this question.

Level of Cognitive Ability: Application

Client Needs: Health Promotion and Maintenance

Integrated Process: Nursing Process/Planning

Content Area: Adult Health/Gastrointestinal

Reference: Linton, A., & Maebius, N. (2007). *Introduction to medical-surgical nursing* (4th ed., pp. 373, 791-792). Philadelphia: Saunders.

571. 2

Rationale: The nurse places highest priority on managing the client's airway. This includes assessing for return of the gag reflex. The client's vital signs are also monitored and a sudden sharp increase in temperature could indicate perforation of the gastrointestinal tract. This would be accompanied by other signs as well, such as pain. Monitoring for sore throat and heartburn are also important; the client's airway still takes priority, however.

Test-Taking Strategy: Use the process of elimination. Note that the question contains the strategic words "highest priority." Use the ABCs—airway, breathing, and circulation. This will direct you to option 2. Review postprocedure care following EGD if you had difficulty with this question.

Level of Cognitive Ability: Application

Client Needs: Physiological Integrity

Integrated Process: Nursing Process/Data Collection

Content Area: Delegating/Prioritizing

Reference: Chernecky, C., & Berger, B. (2008). *Laboratory tests and diagnostic procedures* (5th ed., p. 484). Philadelphia: Saunders.

ALTERNATE ITEM FORMAT: MULTIPLE RESPONSE

572. 1, 3, 4, 5

Rationale: The client with acute pancreatitis is normally placed on an NPO status to rest the pancreas and suppress GI secretions. Because abdominal pain is a prominent symptom of pancreatitis, pain medication such as meperidine will be prescribed. Some clients experience lessened pain by assuming positions that flex the trunk and draw the knees up to the chest. A side-lying position with the head elevated 45 degrees decreases tension on the abdomen and may also help ease the pain. The client is susceptible to respiratory infections because the retroperitoneal fluid raises the diaphragm, which causes the client to take shallow, guarded abdominal breaths. Therefore, measures such as turning, coughing, and deep breathing are instituted. Antacids and anticholinergics may be prescribed to suppress GI secretions.

Test-Taking Strategy: Focus on the pathophysiology associated with pancreatitis and note the word "acute" in the question. This will assist in selecting the correct interventions. Review treatment measures for acute pancreatitis if you had difficulty with this question.

Level of Cognitive Ability: Analysis

Client Needs: Physiological Integrity

Integrated Process: Nursing Process/Planning

Content Area: Adult Health/Gastrointestinal

Reference: Christensen, B., & Kockrow, E. (2006). *Adult health nursing* (5th ed., pp. 278-279). St. Louis: Mosby.

REFERENCES

Black, J., & Hawks, J. (2005). *Medical-surgical nursing: Clinical management for positive outcomes* (7th ed.). Philadelphia: Saunders.

Chernecky, C., & Berger, B. (2008). *Laboratory tests and diagnostic procedures* (5th ed.). Philadelphia: Saunders.

Christensen, B., & Kockrow, E. (2006). *Adult health nursing* (5th ed.). St. Louis: Mosby.

Christensen, B., & Kochrow, E. (2006). *Foundations of nursing* (5th ed.). St. Louis: Mosby.

Grodner, M., Long, S., & Walkinshaw, B. (2007). *Foundations and clinical applications of nutrition: A nursing approach* (4th ed.). St. Louis: Mosby.

Ignatavicius, D., & Workman, M. (2006). *Medical-surgical nursing: Critical thinking for collaborative care* (5th ed.). Philadelphia: Saunders.

Lewis, S., Heitkemper, M., Dirksen, S., & Bucher, L. (2007). *Medical-surgical nursing: Assessment and management of clinical problems* (7th ed.). St. Louis: Mosby.

Linton, A., & Maebius, N. (2007). *Introduction to medical-surgical nursing* (4th ed.). Philadelphia: Saunders.

Nix, S. (2005). *Williams' basic nutrition and diet therapy* (12th ed.). St. Louis: Mosby.

Pagana, K., & Pagana, T. (2005). *Mosby's diagnostic and laboratory test reference* (7th ed.). St. Louis: Mosby.

Schlenker, E., & Long, S. (2007). *Williams' essentials of nutrition & diet therapy* (9th ed.). St. Louis: Mosby.

Skidmore-Roth, L. (2008). *2008 Mosby's nursing drug reference* (21st ed.). St. Louis: Mosby.

CHAPTER 47

Gastrointestinal Medications

I. **ANTACIDS** (Figure 47-1 and Box 47-1)
A. Description
   1. React with gastric acid to produce neutral salts or salts of low acidity
   2. Inactivate pepsin and enhance mucosal protection but do not coat the ulcer crater to protect it from the acid and pepsin
   3. Used for peptic ulcer disease and gastroesophageal reflux disease
   4. Should be taken on a regular schedule; some are prescribed to be taken 1 and 3 hours after each meal and at bedtime
   5. To provide maximum benefit, treatment should elevate the gastric pH above 5
   6. Antacid tablets should be chewed thoroughly and followed with a glass of water or milk
   7. Liquid preparations should be shaken before dispensing
   8. To prevent interactions with other medications and interference with the action of other medications, allow 1 hour between antacid administration and the administration of other medications
B. Aluminum hydroxide preparations
   1. Are slow-acting
   2. Contain significant amounts of sodium and should be used with caution in clients with hypertension and heart failure
   3. The most common side effect is constipation
   4. Aluminum hydroxide can reduce the effects of tetracyclines, warfarin sodium (Coumadin), and digoxin (Lanoxin) and can reduce phosphate absorption and thereby cause hypophosphatemia
C. Calcium carbonate preparations
   1. Are rapid-acting and release carbon dioxide in the stomach, causing belching and flatulence
   2. A common side effect is constipation, and milk-alkali syndrome (headache, urinary frequency, anorexia, nausea/vomiting, fatigue) can occur
D. Magnesium hydroxide preparations
   1. Are rapid-acting
   2. Magnesium hydroxide is also a saline laxative, and the most prominent side effect is diarrhea;

it is usually administered in combination with aluminum hydroxide, an antacid that assists in preventing diarrhea
   3. Is contraindicated in clients with intestinal obstruction, appendicitis, or undiagnosed abdominal pain
   4. In clients with renal impairment, magnesium can accumulate to high levels, causing signs of toxicity
E. Sodium bicarbonate
   1. Has a rapid onset and liberates carbon dioxide, increases intra-abdominal pressure, and promotes flatulence
   2. Should be used with caution in clients with hypertension and heart failure
   3. Can cause systemic alkalosis in clients with renal impairment
   4. Is useful for treating acidosis and elevating urinary pH to promote excretion of acidic medications following overdose

II. **GASTRIC PROTECTANTS** (Box 47-2)
A. Misoprostol (Cytotec)
   1. Suppresses secretion of gastric acid
   2. Promotes secretion of bicarbonate and cytoprotective mucus
   3. Maintains submucosal blood flow by promoting vasodilation
   4. Is used to prevent gastric ulcers caused by long-term therapy with nonsteroidal anti-inflammatory drugs
   5. Is administered with meals
   6. Causes diarrhea and abdominal pain
   7. Is contraindicated for use in pregnancy
B. Sucralfate (Carafate)
   1. Creates a protective barrier against acid and pepsin
   2. Is administered orally and should be taken on an empty stomach
   3. May cause constipation
   4. May impede absorption of warfarin sodium (Coumadin), phenytoin (Dilantin), theophylline, digoxin (Lanoxin), and some antibiotics and should be administered at least 2 hours apart from these medications

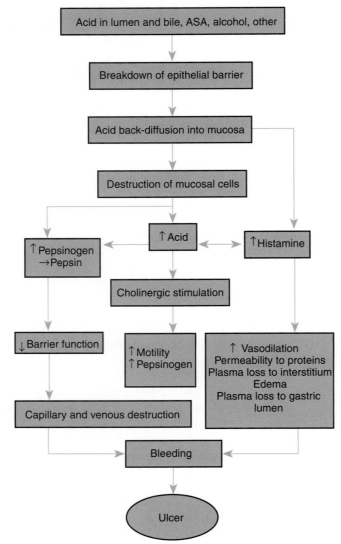

FIG. 47-1   Pathophysiological consequences of back diffusion of acid through the damaged mucosal barrier. (From Price, S. & Wilson, L. [2003]. *Pathophysiology: Clinical concepts of disease processes* [6th ed.]. St. Louis: Mosby.)

BOX 47-1   Antacids

Aluminum hydroxide gel (Alu-Cap, Alu-Tab, Amphojel, ALternaGEL, Dialume)
Aluminum hydroxide; magnesium hydroxide (Maalox oral suspension)
Calcium carbonate (Mylanta, Tums)
Magnesium hydroxide (Milk of Magnesia)
Sodium bicarbonate preparations

BOX 47-2   Gastric Protectants

Misoprostol (Cytotec)
Sucralfate (Carafate)

BOX 47-3   Histamine 2 (H$_2$)-Receptor Antagonists

Cimetidine (Tagamet)
Famotidine (Pepcid)
Nizatidine (Axid)
Ranitidine (Zantac)

2. Food reduces the rate of absorption; if taken with meals, absorption will be slowed.
3. By the IV piggyback route, a 300-mg dose can be diluted in 100 mL and infused over 15 to 20 minutes (always follow agency guidelines for its administration)
4. Antacids can decrease the absorption of oral cimetidine
5. Cimetidine and antacids should be administered at least 1 hour apart from each other
6. Cimetidine passes the blood-brain barrier, and central nervous system side effects can occur; may cause mental confusion, agitation, psychosis, depression, anxiety, and disorientation
7. Dosage should be reduced in clients with renal impairment
8. IV administration can cause hypotension and dysrhythmias
9. If cimetidine is administered with warfarin sodium (Coumadin), phenytoin (Dilantin), theophylline, or lidocaine, the dosages of these medications should be reduced
C. Ranitidine (Zantac)
1. Can be administered orally, intramuscularly, or intravenously
2. Side effects are uncommon and does not penetrate the blood-brain barrier as cimetidine does
3. Ranitidine is not affected by food
4. By the IV piggyback route, ranitidine should be diluted in 100 mL and administered over 15 to 20 minutes (always follow agency guidelines for its administration)

III. HISTAMINE 2 (H$_2$)-RECEPTOR ANTAGONISTS (Box 47-3)

A. Description
   1. Suppress secretion of gastric acid
   2. Alleviate symptoms of heartburn and assist in preventing complications of peptic ulcer disease
   3. Prevent stress ulcers and reduce the recurrence of all ulcers
   4. Promote healing in gastroesophageal reflux disease
   5. Are contraindicated in hypersensitive clients
   6. Should be used with caution in clients with impaired renal or hepatic function
B. Cimetidine (Tagamet)
   1. Can be administered orally, intramuscularly, or intravenously

D. Famotidine (Pepcid) and nizatidine (Axid)
1. Famotidine and nizatidine are similar to ranitidine and cimetidine
2. These medications do not need to be administered with food

IV. PROTON PUMP INHIBITORS (Box 47-4)
A. Suppress gastric acid secretion
B. Are used to treat active ulcer disease, erosive esophagitis, and pathological hypersecretory conditions
C. Are contraindicated in hypersensitivity
D. Common side effects include headache, diarrhea, abdominal pain, and nausea

V. MEDICATION REGIMENS TO TREAT *HELICOBACTER PYLORI* INFECTIONS (Box 47-5)
A. An antibacterial agent alone is not effective for eradicating *Helicobacter pylori* because the bacterium readily becomes resistant to the agent
B. Dual, triple, and quadruple therapy with a variety of medication combinations is used
C. The combinations can include antibacterial agents, proton pump inhibitors, histamine 2 (H_2)–receptor antagonists, and antacids
D. A common treatment protocol is triple therapy with two antibacterial agents and a proton pump inhibitor
E. If triple therapy fails, quadruple therapy is recommended with two antibacterial agents, a proton pump inhibitor, and a bismuth or H_2-receptor antagonist

---

BOX 47-4 **Proton Pump Inhibitors**

Esomeprazole (Nexium)
Lansoprazole (Prevacid)
Omeprazole (Prilosec)
Pantoprazole (Protonix)
Rabeprazole (Aciphex)

BOX 47-5 **Medication Regimens for Treating *Helicobacter Pylori* Infections**

Dual Therapy
Ranitidine bismuth citrate and clarithromycin (Biaxin)
Omeprazole (Prilosec) and clarithromycin (Biaxin)
Triple Therapy
Metronidazole (Flagyl), omeprazole (Prilosec), and clarithromycin (Biaxin)
Amoxicillin (Amoxil), lansoprazole (Prevacid), and clarithromycin (Biaxin)
Quadruple Therapy
Colloidal bismuth subcitrate, tetracycline (Achromycin), metronidazole (Flagyl), and omeprazole (Prilosec)

Note: Other combinations may be prescribed for each level of therapy.

VI. GASTROINTESTINAL STIMULANTS (Box 47-6)
A. Stimulate motility of the upper gastrointestinal tract and increase the rate of gastric emptying without stimulating gastric, biliary, or pancreatic secretions
B. Are used to treat gastroesophageal reflux and paralytic ileus
C. May cause restlessness, drowsiness, extrapyramidal reactions, dizziness, insomnia, and headache
D. Are usually administered 30 minutes before meals and at bedtime
E. Are contraindicated in clients with sensitivity and in clients with mechanical obstruction, perforation, or gastrointestinal hemorrhage
F. Can precipitate hypertensive crisis in clients with pheochromocytoma
G. Safety in pregnancy is not established
H. Metoclopramide (Reglan) can cause Parkinson-like reactions; if this occurs, the medication will be discontinued by the physician
I. Anticholinergics and opioid analgesics antagonize the effects of metoclopramide
J. Alcohol, sedatives, cyclosporine (Sandimmune), and tranquilizers produce an additive effect

VII. BILE ACID SEQUESTRANTS (Box 47-7)
A. Act by absorbing and combining with intestinal bile salts, which are then secreted in the feces, preventing intestinal reabsorption
B. Are used to treat hypercholesterolemia in adults, biliary obstruction, and pruritus associated with biliary disease
C. Taste and palatability are often reasons for noncompliance and can be improved by the use of flavored products or by mixing the medication with various juices
D. Should be used cautiously in clients with bowel obstruction or severe constipation because of the adverse gastrointestinal effects
E. Side effects include nausea, bloating, and constipation; fecal impaction and intestinal obstruction can result
F. Stool softeners and other sources of fiber can be used to abate the gastrointestinal side effects

---

BOX 47-6 **Gastrointestinal Stimulants**

Bethanechol chloride (Urecholine, Duvoid)
Dexpanthenol (Ilopan, Ilopan-Choline)
Metoclopramide (Reglan)
Neostigmine methylsulfate (Prostigmin)

BOX 47-7 **Bile Acid Sequestrants**

Cholestyramine (Questran, Prevalite)
Colestipol (Colestid)

BOX 47-8	Medications to Treat Hepatic Encephalopathy

Lactulose (Cholac, Chronulac, Duphalac)
Neomycin (Mycifradin)

BOX 47-9	Pancreatic Enzyme Replacements

Pancreatin
Pancrelipase (Pancrease, Viokase)

VIII. MEDICATIONS TO TREAT HEPATIC ENCEPHALOPATHY (Box 47-8)

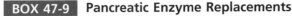

A. Lactulose (Cholac, Chronulac, Duphalac)
1. Reduces ammonia levels; lowers the colonic pH from 7 to 5, and this acidification pulls ammonia into the bowel to be excreted in the feces, thus lowering the ammonia level
2. Improves protein tolerance in clients with advanced hepatic cirrhosis
3. Is administered orally in the form of a syrup or rectally
B. Neomycin (Mycifradin)
1. Reduces the number of colonic bacteria that normally convert urea and amino acids into ammonia
2. Is administered orally or via nasogastric tube
3. Is used with caution in clients with kidney impairment

IX. PANCREATIC ENZYME REPLACEMENTS (Box 47-9)

A. These medications are used to supplement or replace pancreatic enzymes
B. They should be taken with meals or a snack (food helps to buffer the stomach acid)
C. A high-fiber diet may increase the efficacy of the medication
D. Side effects include abdominal cramps or pain, nausea, and diarrhea
E. Products that contain calcium carbonate or magnesium hydroxide interfere with the action of the medication

X. TREATMENT OF INFLAMMATORY BOWEL DISEASE (Box 47-10)

A. Antimicrobials: Prevent or treat secondary infection
B. 5-Aminosalicylates (5-ASA): Decrease gastrointestinal inflammation
C. Corticosteroids: Decrease gastrointestinal inflammation
D. Immunosuppressants: Suppress the immune system
E. Immunomodulators
1. Inhibit cytokine tumor necrosis factor-alpha, which reduces the degree of inflammation (infliximab [Remicade])
2. Interrupt the movement of leukocytes, which reduces the inflammatory process (natalizumab [Tysabri])

BOX 47-10	Medications to Treat Inflammatory Bowel Disease

Antimicrobials
Metronidazole (Flagyl)
5-Aminosalicylates
Sulfasalazine (Azulfidine)
Mesalamine (Rowasa, Asacol, Pentasa, Canasa)
Olsalazine (Dipentum)
Corticosteroids
Cortisone
Prednisone (Deltasone)
Budesonide (Entocort)
Hydrocortisone
Immunosuppressants
Azathioprine (Imuran)
Cyclosporine (Neoral)
Mercaptopurine (6 MP)
Immunomodulators
Infliximab (Remicade)
Natalizumab (Tysabri)

BOX 47-11	Commonly Administered Antiemetics

Diphenidol
Dolasetron (Anzemet)
Dronabinol (Marinol)
Granisetron (Kytril)
Hydroxyzine pamoate (Vistaril)
Meclizine hydrochloride (Antivert)
Metoclopramide (Reglan)
Ondansetron (Zofran)
Prochlorperazine (Compazine)
Promethazine hydrochloride (Phenergan)
Scopolamine transdermal (Transderm-Scop)
Thiethylperazine maleate (Torecan)
Trimethobenzamide hydrochloride (Tigan)

XI. ANTIEMETICS (Box 47-11)

A. Medications used to control vomiting and motion sickness
B. The choice of the antiemetic is determined by the cause of the nausea and vomiting
C. Monitor for drowsiness and protect the client from injury
D. Monitor vital signs and intake and output
E. Limit odors in the client's room when the client is nauseated or vomiting
F. Limit oral intake to clear liquids when the client is nauseated or vomiting

XII. LAXATIVES (Box 47-12)

A. Bulk-forming laxatives
1. Description
a. Absorb water into the feces and increase bulk to produce large and soft stools
b. Contraindicated in bowel obstruction
c. Dependency can occur with chronic use

BOX 47-12 Laxatives

Bulk-Forming Laxatives
Calcium polycarbophil (FiberCon)
Methylcellulose (Citrucel)
Psyllium hydrophilic mucilloid (Metamucil, Fiberall, Konsyl, Serutan)
Stimulant Cathartics
Bisacodyl (Modane)
Cascara sagrada
Castor oil (Neoloid)
Docusate sodium, sennosides (Ex-Lax)
Sennosides (Senexon, Senna-Gen, Senokot)
Saline (Osmotic) Cathartics
Lactulose (Constilac)
Magnesium citrate (Citrate of Magnesia)
Magnesium hydroxide (Milk of Magnesia)
Polyethylene glycol and electrolytes (GoLYTELY)
Sodium phosphates (Fleet Enema, Fleet Phospho-Soda)
Stool Softeners
Docusate calcium (Surfak)
Docusate sodium (Colace, Peri-Colace)
Lubricant
Mineral oil (Kondremul)

BOX 47-13 Medications to Control Diarrhea

Opioids And Related Medications
Codeine phosphate; codeine sulfate
Difenoxin with atropine sulfate (Motofen)
Diphenoxylate hydrochloride with atropine sulfate (Lomotil)
Loperamide hydrochloride (Imodium)
Tincture of opium
Adsorbent Antidiarrheals
Bismuth subsalicylate (Pepto-Bismol, Kaopectate)
Kaolin and pectin (Kapectolin)

BOX 47-14 Antispasmodic

Dicyclomine hydrochloride (Antispas, Bentyl)

2. Side effects include gastrointestinal disturbances, dehydration, and electrolyte imbalances
B. Stimulant cathartics: Stimulate motility of large intestine
C. Saline (osmotic) cathartics: Attract water into the large intestine to produce bulk and stimulate peristalsis.
D. Stool softeners
   1. Inhibit absorption of water so fecal mass remains large and soft
   2. Are used to avoid straining
E. Lubricants
   1. Act to soften the feces, ease the strain of passing stool, and lessen irritation to hemorrhoids
   2. Mineral oil: Interferes with absorption of fat-soluble vitamins A, D, E, and K and can cause lipid pneumonia if accidentally aspirated
XIII. MEDICATIONS TO CONTROL DIARRHEA (Box 47-13)
A. Opioids
   1. Opioids decrease intestinal motility and peristalsis
   2. When poisons, infections, or bacterial toxins are the cause of the diarrhea, opioids worsen the condition by delaying the elimination of toxins
   3. Tincture of opium has an unpleasant taste and can be diluted with 15 to 30 mL of water for administration
B. Other antidiarrheals: Refer to Box 47-13
XIV. ANTISPASMODICS (Box 47-14)
A. Description: Relax the smooth muscle of the gastrointestinal tract
B. Side effects include nausea, constipation or diarrhea, headache, drowsiness, weakness, dizziness, rash, and euphoria

PRACTICE QUESTIONS

More questions on the companion CD!

573. A client with a history of duodenal ulcer is taking calcium carbonate chewable tablets. The nurse determines that the client is experiencing optimal effects of the medication if:
   1. Heartburn is relieved
   2. Muscle twitching stops
   3. Serum calcium levels rise
   4. Serum phosphorus levels decrease

574. A hospitalized client asks the nurse for sodium bicarbonate to relieve heartburn following a meal. The nurse reviews the client's medical record, knowing that the medication is contraindicated in which of the following conditions?
   1. Urinary calculi
   2. Chronic bronchitis
   3. Metabolic alkalosis
   4. Respiratory acidosis

575. An 80-year-old client has recently been started on cimetidine (Tagamet). The nurse monitors the client for which most frequent central nervous system (CNS) side effect of this medication?
   1. Tremors
   2. Dizziness
   3. Confusion
   4. Hallucinations

576. A client with a gastric ulcer has an order for sucralfate (Carafate), 1 g orally four times a day. The nurse schedules the medication for which of the following times?
   1. With meals and at bedtime
   2. Every 6 hours around the clock
   3. One hour after meals and at bedtime
   4. One hour before meals and at bedtime

577. A physician has written an order for ranitidine (Zantac), once daily. The nurse schedules the medication for which of the following times?

1. At bedtime
2. After lunch
3. With supper
4. Before breakfast

578. A client has been taking omeprazole (Prilosec) for 4 weeks. The nurse determines that the client is receiving the optimal intended effect of the medication if the client reports absence of which of the following symptoms?
1. Diarrhea
2. Heartburn
3. Flatulence
4. Constipation

579. A physician prescribes bisacodyl (Dulcolax) for a client in preparation for a diagnostic test and wants the client to achieve a rapid effect from the medication. The nurse then tells the client to take the medication:
1. With a large meal
2. On an empty stomach
3. At bedtime with a snack
4. With two glasses of juice

580. A client has a PRN order for loperamide (Imodium). The nurse should plan to administer this medication if the client has:
1. Constipation
2. Abdominal pain
3. An episode of diarrhea
4. Hematest-positive nasogastric tube drainage

581. A client is taking docusate sodium (Colace). The nurse monitors which of the following to determine whether the client is having a therapeutic effect from this medication?
1. Abdominal pain
2. Reduction in steatorrhea
3. Hematest-negative stools
4. Regular bowel movements

582. A nurse teaches a client taking metoclopramide (Reglan) to discontinue the medication immediately and call the physician if which side effect occurs with long-term use?
1. Excessive excitability
2. Anxiety or irritability
3. Uncontrolled rhythmic movements of the face or limbs
4. Dry mouth not helped by the use of sugar-free hard candy

583. A client has just taken a dose of trimethobenzamide (Tigan). The nurse plans to monitor this client for relief of:
1. Heartburn
2. Constipation
3. Abdominal pain
4. Nausea and vomiting

584. A client has a PRN order for ondansetron (Zofran). The nurse would administer this medication to the postoperative client for relief of:
1. Paralytic ileus
2. Incisional pain
3. Urinary retention
4. Nausea and vomiting

585. A client has an order to take magnesium citrate to prevent constipation following a barium study of the upper gastrointestinal (GI) tract. The nurse plans to administer this medication:
1. Chilled
2. With fruit juice only
3. At room temperature
4. With a full glass of water

586. A client has begun medication therapy with pancrelipase (Pancrease). The nurse determines that the medication is having the optimal intended benefit if which effect is observed?
1. Weight loss
2. Relief of heartburn
3. Reduction of steatorrhea
4. Absence of abdominal pain

ALTERNATE ITEM FORMAT: MULTIPLE RESPONSE

587. A histamine (H_2)-receptor antagonist will be prescribed for a client. The nurse understands that which medications are H_2-receptor antagonists, one of which could be prescribed. Select all that apply.
☐ 1. Nizatidine (Axid)
☐ 2. Ranitidine (Zantac)
☐ 3. Famotidine (Pepcid)
☐ 4. Cimetidine (Tagamet)
☐ 5. Esomeprazole (Nexium)
☐ 6. Lansoprazole (Prevacid)

ANSWERS

573. **1**

Rationale: Calcium carbonate is used as an antacid for the relief of heartburn and indigestion in a client with a duodenal ulcer. It can also be used as a calcium supplement (option 3) or to bind phosphorus in the gastrointestinal tract with renal failure (option 4). Option 2 is incorrect, although proper calcium levels are needed for proper neurological function.

Test-Taking Strategy: Focus on the client's diagnosis. The strategic words in the question are "duodenal ulcer" and "optimal effects." Knowledge of the concepts related to duodenal ulcer will direct you to option 1. Review the actions and use of this medication if you had difficulty with this question.

Level of Cognitive Ability: Analysis
Client Needs: Physiological Integrity
Integrated Process: Nursing Process/Evaluation
Content Area: Pharmacology
Reference: Skidmore-Roth, L. (2008). *2008 Mosby's nursing drug reference* (21st ed., pp. 212-213). St. Louis: Mosby.

574. **3**
Rationale: Sodium bicarbonate is an electrolyte modifier and antacid. It would further aggravate metabolic alkalosis. The conditions identified in the other options are not contraindications for the use of sodium bicarbonate.
Test-Taking Strategy: Note the strategic word "contraindicated," and use knowledge of acid-base concepts to answer this question. Focus on the name of the medication to assist in eliminating options 1, 2, and 4. Review the contraindications associated with the use of this medication if you had difficulty with this question.
Level of Cognitive Ability: Analysis
Client Needs: Physiological Integrity
Integrated Process: Nursing Process/Data Collection
Content Area: Pharmacology
Reference: Skidmore-Roth, L. (2008). *2008 Mosby's nursing drug reference* (21st ed., p. 932). St. Louis: Mosby.

575. **3**
Rationale: Older clients are especially susceptible to the CNS side effects of cimetidine. The most frequent side effect is confusion. Less common CNS side effects include headache, dizziness, drowsiness, and hallucinations.
Test-Taking Strategy: Use the process of elimination. Note the strategic words "most frequent." Use knowledge of the concepts related to the older client and medication administration, as well as knowledge of this medication, to answer the question. Review this medication if you had difficulty with this question.
Level of Cognitive Ability: Application
Client Needs: Physiological Integrity
Integrated Process: Nursing Process/Implementation
Content Area: Pharmacology
Reference: Skidmore-Roth, L. (2008). *2008 Mosby's nursing drug reference* (21st ed., p. 273). St. Louis: Mosby.

576. **4**
Rationale: The medication should be scheduled for administration 1 hour before meals and at bedtime. The medication is timed to allow it to form a protective coating over the ulcer before food intake stimulates gastric acid production and mechanical irritation. The other options are incorrect.
Test-Taking Strategy: Use the process of elimination. Focusing on the client's diagnosis and recalling the action of the medication will direct you to option 4. Review this medication if you had difficulty with this question.
Level of Cognitive Ability: Application
Client Needs: Physiological Integrity
Integrated Process: Nursing Process/Implementation
Content Area: Pharmacology
Reference: Lehne, R. (2007). *Pharmacology for nursing care* (6th ed., p. 899). Philadelphia: Saunders.

577. **1**
Rationale: A single daily dose of ranitidine is scheduled to be given at bedtime. This allows for a prolonged effect, and the greatest protection of the gastric mucosa. The other options are incorrect.
Test-Taking Strategy: Specific knowledge of the timing of this medication is needed to answer this question. Also, recalling that ranitidine suppresses secretions of gastric acids will direct you to option 1. If you had difficulty with this question, review this medication.
Level of Cognitive Ability: Application
Client Needs: Physiological Integrity
Integrated Process: Nursing Process/Implementation
Content Area: Pharmacology
Reference: Lehne, R. (2007). *Pharmacology for nursing care* (6th ed., p. 897). Philadelphia: Saunders.

578. **2**
Rationale: Omeprazole is a proton pump inhibitor and is classified as an anti-ulcer agent. The intended effect of the medication is relief of pain from gastric irritation, often referred to as heartburn by clients. Options 1, 3, and 4 are incorrect.
Test-Taking Strategy: Use the process of elimination. Recalling the action and use of omeprazole will direct you to option 2. Review this medication if you had difficulty with this question.
Level of Cognitive Ability: Analysis
Client Needs: Physiological Integrity
Integrated Process: Nursing Process/Evaluation
Content Area: Pharmacology
Reference: Lilley, L., Harrington, S., & Snyder J. (2007). *Pharmacology and the nursing process* (5th ed., pp. 797-798). St. Louis: Mosby.

579. **2**
Rationale: Most rapid results from bisacodyl occur when it is taken on an empty stomach. It will not have a rapid effect if taken with a large meal. If it is taken at bedtime, the client will have a bowel movement in the morning. Taking the medication with two glasses of juice will not add to its effect.
Test-Taking Strategy: Use the process of elimination. Focus on the strategic words "rapid effect." Recalling that food generally slows the absorption of medication will assist in directing you to option 2. Review the administration of laxatives if you had difficulty with this question.
Level of Cognitive Ability: Application
Client Needs: Physiological Integrity
Integrated Process: Nursing Process/Implementation
Content Area: Pharmacology
Reference: Skidmore-Roth, L. (2005). *Mosby's drug guide for nurses* (6th ed., p. 103). St. Louis: Mosby.

580. **3**
Rationale: Loperamide is an antidiarrheal agent. It is commonly administered after loose stools. It is used in the management of acute diarrhea, as well as in chronic diarrhea, such as with inflammatory bowel disease. It can also be used to reduce the volume of drainage from an ileostomy. The other options are incorrect.

Test-Taking Strategy: Use the process of elimination. Knowledge that this medication is an antidiarrheal will direct you to the correct option. Review the action of this medication if you had difficulty with this question.
Level of Cognitive Ability: Application
Client Needs: Physiological Integrity
Integrated Process: Nursing Process/Planning
Content Area: Pharmacology
Reference: Skidmore-Roth, L. (2008). *2008 Mosby's nursing drug reference* (21st ed., p. 624). St. Louis: Mosby.

581. 4
Rationale: Docusate sodium is a stool softener that promotes the absorption of water into the stool, producing a softer consistency of stool. The intended effect is relief or prevention of constipation. The medication does not relieve abdominal pain, stop gastrointestinal bleeding, or decrease the amount of fat in the stools.
Test-Taking Strategy: Use the process of elimination. Recalling that docusate is a stool softener will direct you to option 4. Review the action of this medication if you had difficulty with this question.
Level of Cognitive Ability: Application
Client Needs: Physiological Integrity
Integrated Process: Nursing Process/Implementation
Content Area: Pharmacology
Reference: Skidmore-Roth, L. (2008). *2008 Mosby's nursing drug reference* (21st ed., pp. 381-382). St. Louis: Mosby.

582. 3
Rationale: If the client experiences tardive dyskinesia (rhythmic movements of the face or limbs), the client should stop the medication and call the physician. These side effects may be irreversible. Excitability is not a side effect of this medication. Anxiety, irritability, and dry mouth are side effects that are not as harmful to the client.
Test-Taking Strategy: Use the process of elimination and focus on the subject—to call the physician. Recalling that the medication can cause tardive dyskinesia will direct you to option 3. Review the side effects of this medication if you had difficulty with this question.
Level of Cognitive Ability: Application
Client Needs: Physiological Integrity
Integrated Process: Teaching and Learning
Content Area: Pharmacology
Reference: Skidmore-Roth, L. (2008). *2008 Mosby's nursing drug reference* (21st ed., p. 674). St. Louis: Mosby.

583. 4
Rationale: Trimethobenzamide is an antiemetic agent used in the treatment of nausea and vomiting. The other options are incorrect.
Test-Taking Strategy: Use the process of elimination. Recalling that trimethobenzamide is an antiemetic will direct you to option 4. Review the action and use of this medication if you had difficulty with this question.
Level of Cognitive Ability: Application
Client Needs: Physiological Integrity
Integrated Process: Nursing Process/Planning
Content Area: Pharmacology

Reference: Skidmore-Roth, L. (2008). *2008 Mosby's nursing drug reference* (21st ed., p. 1034). St. Louis: Mosby.

584. 4
Rationale: Ondansetron is an antiemetic used in the treatment of postoperative nausea and vomiting, as well as nausea and vomiting associated with chemotherapy. The other options are incorrect.
Test-Taking Strategy: Use the process of elimination. Recalling that ondansetron is an antiemetic will direct you to option 4. Review the action and use of this medication if you had difficulty with this question.
Level of Cognitive Ability: Application
Client Needs: Physiological Integrity
Integrated Process: Nursing Process/Implementation
Content Area: Pharmacology
Reference: Kee, J., Hayes, E., & McCuistion, L. (2006). *Pharmacology: A nursing process approach* (5th ed., p. 689). Philadelphia: Saunders.

585. 1
Rationale: Magnesium citrate is available as an oral solution. It is used commonly as a laxative before certain GI surgeries or following certain studies of the GI tract. It should be served chilled and should not be allowed to stand for prolonged periods. This would reduce the carbonation and make the solution even less palatable. Options 2, 3, and 4 are incorrect.
Test-Taking Strategy: Use the process of elimination. Eliminate options 2 and 4 first, knowing that magnesium citrate is itself a liquid. From the remaining options, it is necessary to know it should be given cold to enhance palatability. Review this medication if you had difficulty with this question.
Level of Cognitive Ability: Application
Client Needs: Physiological Integrity
Integrated Process: Nursing Process/Planning
Content Area: Pharmacology
Reference: Skidmore-Roth, L. (2008). *2008 Mosby's nursing drug reference* (21st ed., p. 636). St. Louis: Mosby.

586. 3
Rationale: Pancrelipase is a pancreatic enzyme used in clients with pancreatitis as a digestive aid. The medication should reduce the amount of fatty stools (steatorrhea). Another intended effect could be improved nutritional status. It is not used to treat abdominal pain or heartburn. It could result in weight gain but should not result in weight loss if it is aiding in digestion.
Test-Taking Strategy: Use the process of elimination. The name of the medication gives an indication of the possible uses of this medication. Use knowledge of the physiology of the pancreas to assist in directing you to the correct option. Review this medication if you had difficulty with this question.
Level of Cognitive Ability: Analysis
Client Needs: Physiological Integrity
Integrated Process: Nursing Process/Evaluation
Content Area: Pharmacology
Reference: Skidmore-Roth, L. (2008). *2008 Mosby's nursing drug reference* (21st ed., p. 783). St. Louis: Mosby.

ALTERNATE ITEM FORMAT: MULTIPLE RESPONSE

587. **1, 2, 3, 4**

Rationale: H_2-receptor antagonists suppress secretion of gastric acid, alleviate symptoms of heartburn, and assist in preventing complications of peptic ulcer disease. These medications also suppress gastric acid secretions and are used in active ulcer disease, erosive esophagitis, and pathological hypersecretory conditions. The other medications listed are proton pump inhibitors.

Test-Taking Strategy: Focus on the subject—H_2-receptor antagonists. Recalling that these medication names end with the letters "dine" will assist in answering this question. Also recall that proton pump inhibitor medication names end with the letters "zole." Review the H_2-receptor antagonists if you had difficulty with this question.

Level of Cognitive Ability: Analysis
Client Needs: Physiological Integrity
Integrated Process: Nursing Process/Analysis
Content Area: Pharmacology
Reference: Skidmore-Roth, L. (2008). *2008 Mosby's nursing drug reference* (21st ed., p. 666). St. Louis: Mosby.

REFERENCES

Kee, J., Hayes, E., & McCuistion, L. (2006). *Pharmacology: A nursing process approach* (5th ed.). Philadelphia: Saunders.

Lehne, R. (2007). *Pharmacology for nursing care* (6th ed.). Philadelphia: Saunders.

Lilley, L., Harrington, S., & Snyder, J. (2007). *Pharmacology and the nursing process* (5th ed.). St. Louis: Mosby.

Skidmore-Roth, L. (2008). *2008 Mosby's nursing drug reference* (21st ed.). St. Louis: Mosby.

Skidmore-Roth, L. (2005). *Mosby's drug guide for nurses* (6th ed.). St. Louis: Mosby.

The Adult Client With a Respiratory Disorder

PYRAMID TERMS

Bacille Calmette-Guérin vaccine A vaccine containing attenuated tubercle bacilli that may be given to persons in foreign countries or to those traveling to foreign countries to produce increased resistance to tuberculosis

chronic airflow limitation, chronic obstructive lung disease, chronic obstructive pulmonary disease A disease state characterized by pulmonary airflow obstruction that is usually progressive, not fully reversible, and sometimes accompanied by airway hyperreactivity; airflow obstruction may be caused by chronic bronchitis and/or emphysema; in chronic hypercapnia the stimulus to breathe is a low Po_2 instead of an increased Pco_2

emphysema A chronic pulmonary disease marked by a narrowing of the small airways and the trapping of air, with destructive changes in their walls; also known as chronic obstructive pulmonary disease; also described as an abnormal permanent enlargement of airspaces distal to the terminal bronchioles with destruction of alveolar walls, without obvious fibrosis

Mantoux test A skin rest that determines infection with tuberculosis; a small amount (0.1 mL) of intermediate-strength purified protein derivative containing 5 tuberculin units is given intradermally in the forearm; an area of induration measuring 10 mm or more in diameter, 48 to 72 hours after injection, indicates that the individual has been exposed to tuberculosis

mechanical ventilation The use of a ventilator to move room air or oxygen-enriched air into and out of the lungs mechanically if a client is unable to ventilate enough on his or her own to maintain proper levels of oxygen and carbon dioxide in the blood.

multidrug-resistant strain A multidrug-resistant strain of tuberculosis (MDR-TB) can occur as a result of improper or noncompliant use of prescribed treatment programs and the development of mutations in the tubercle bacilli

Mycobacterium tuberculosis The causative organism (bacillus) of tuberculosis; an aerobic bacterium that is a nonmotile, nonsporulating, acid-fast rod that secretes niacin

pneumothorax The accumulation of atmospheric air in the pleural space caused by a rupture in the visceral or parietal pleura, which results in a rise in intrathoracic pressure and reduced vital capacity; the loss of negative intrapleural pressure results in collapse of the lung; diagnosis of pneumothorax is made by chest radiography

suctioning A sterile procedure that involves the removal of respiratory secretions that accumulate in the tracheobronchial airway when the client is unable to expectorate secretions; performed to maintain a patent airway

tuberculosis A highly communicable disease caused by *Mycobacterium tuberculosis*; tuberculosis is transmitted by the airborne route via droplet infection

PYRAMID TO SUCCESS

The Pyramid to Success focuses on maintaining a patent airway. Pyramid points focus on infectious diseases, particularly tuberculosis, and on the client with pneumonia, respiratory failure, chronic obstructive pulmonary disease, or pneumothorax. The Pyramid to Success includes the care of the client with tuberculosis, especially with regard to the importance of the medication regimen, providing adequate nutrition and adequate rest to promote the healing process, and preventing disease progression. Focus on assisting the client to cope with the social isolation issues that exist during the period of illness and on teaching the client and family the critical measures of screening and of preventing respiratory disease and the transmission of disease. The Integrated Processes addressed in this unit include Caring, the Clinical Problem-Solving Process (Nursing Process), Communication and Documentation, and Teaching and Learning.

CLIENT NEEDS

Safe and Effective Care Environment

Collaborating with multidisciplinary team in the management of the respiratory disorder

Discussing consultations and referrals related to the respiratory disorder

Establishing priorities

Safely handling infectious materials such as sputum or body fluids

Maintaining asepsis when caring for wounds or tracheostomy sites and during suctioning

Maintaining confidentiality related to the respiratory disorder

Maintaining respiratory precautions, standard precautions, and other precautions

Obtaining informed consent related to diagnostic and surgical procedures

Upholding client rights

Health Promotion and Maintenance

Educating the client about adequate fluid and nutritional intake

Educating the client about breathing exercises and respiratory therapy and care

Educating the client about medication administration

Educating the client about the need for follow-up care

Educating the client about the prevention of transmission of infection

Informing the client about health promotion programs

Performing data collection techniques

Preventing respiratory disorders and infectious diseases

Providing health screening related to risks for respiratory disorders

Psychosocial Integrity

Considering religious, cultural, and spiritual influences when providing care

Discussing body image changes related to tracheostomy if performed

Discussing end-of-life and grief and loss issues

Discussing situational role changes

Identifying coping mechanisms

Identifying support systems

Informing the client about community resources

Physiological Integrity

Administering medications

Caring for the client on mechanical ventilation

Caring for the client receiving respiratory care and oxygen

Managing illnesses

Monitoring for acid-base imbalances

Monitoring for alterations in body systems

Monitoring for infectious diseases

Providing comfort

Providing nutrition and oral hygiene

Providing personal hygiene and promoting rest and sleep

REFERENCES

Black, J., & Hawks, J. (2005). *Medical-surgical nursing: Clinical management for positive outcomes* (7th ed.). Philadelphia: Saunders.

Chernecky, C., & Berger, B. (2008). *Laboratory tests and diagnostic procedures* (5th ed.). Philadelphia: Saunders.

Christensen, B., & Kockrow, E. (2006). *Adult health nursing* (5th ed.). St. Louis: Mosby.

Christensen, B., & Kockrow, E. (2006). *Foundations of nursing* (5th ed.). St. Louis: Mosby.

deWit, S. (2009). *Medical-surgical nursing: Concepts & practice* (1st ed.). Philadelphia: Saunders.

Hodgson, B., & Kizior, R. (2008). *Saunders nursing drug handbook 2008*. Philadelphia: Saunders.

Ignatavicius, D., & Workman, M. (2006). *Medical-surgical nursing: Critical thinking for collaborative care* (5th ed.). Philadelphia: Saunders.

Kee, J., Hayes, E., & McCuistion, L. (2006). *Pharmacology: A nursing process approach* (5th ed.). Philadelphia: Saunders.

Lehne, R. (2007). *Pharmacology for nursing care* (6th ed.). Philadelphia: Saunders.

Lewis, S., Heitkemper, M., Dirksen, S., & Bucher, L. (2007). *Medical-surgical nursing: Assessment and management of clinical problems* (7th ed.). St. Louis: Mosby.

Linton, A., & Maebius, N. (2007). *Introduction to medical-surgical nursing* (4th ed.). Philadelphia: Saunders.

McKenry, L., Tessier, E., & Hogan, M. (2006). *Mosby's pharmacology in nursing* (22nd ed.). St. Louis: Mosby.

Monahan, F., Sands, J., Marek, J., et al. (2007). *Phipps' medical-surgical nursing: Health and illness perspectives* (8th ed.). St. Louis: Mosby.

National Council of State Boards of Nursing (eds.) (2008). *2008 Detailed Test Plan for the NCLEX-PN® Examination, National Council of State Boards of Nursing*. Chicago: Author.

National Council of State Boards of Nursing, Inc. Web site: http://www.ncsbn.org.

Perry, A., & Potter, P. (2006). *Clinical nursing skills & techniques* (6th ed.). St. Louis: Mosby.

Skidmore-Roth, L. (2008). *2008 Mosby's nursing drug reference* (21st ed.). St. Louis: Mosby.

CHAPTER 48

Respiratory System

I. ANATOMY AND PHYSIOLOGY

A. Primary functions of the respiratory system
1. Provides oxygen for metabolism in the tissues
2. Removes carbon dioxide, the waste product of metabolism

B. Secondary functions of the respiratory system
1. Facilitates sense of smell
2. Produces speech
3. Maintains acid-base balance
4. Maintains body water levels
5. Maintains heat balance

C. Upper respiratory tract
1. Nose: humidifies, warms, and filters inspired air
2. Sinuses: air-filled cavities within the hollow bones that surround the nasal passages and provide resonance during speech
3. Pharynx
   a. A passageway for the respiratory and digestive tracts that is located behind the oral and nasal cavities
   b. Is divided into the nasopharynx, oropharynx, and laryngopharynx
4. Larynx
   a. Located above the trachea, just below the pharynx at the root of the tongue and commonly called the voice box
   b. Contains two pairs of vocal cords: the false and true cords
   c. The opening between the true vocal cords is the glottis
   d. The glottis plays an important role in coughing, which is the most fundamental defense mechanism of the lungs
5. Epiglottis
   a. A leaf-shaped elastic structure that is attached along one end to the top of the larynx
   b. Prevents food from entering the tracheobronchial tree by closing over the glottis during swallowing

D. Lower respiratory tract
1. Trachea: located in front of the esophagus, branching into the right and left mainstem bronchi at the carina

2. Mainstem bronchi
   a. Begin at the carina
   b. The right bronchus is slightly wider, shorter, and more vertical than the left bronchus
   c. The mainstem bronchi divide into secondary or lobar bronchi that enter each of the five lobes of the lung
   d. The bronchi are lined with cilia, which propel mucus up and away from the lower airway to the trachea, where it can be expectorated or swallowed
3. Bronchioles
   a. Branch from the secondary bronchi and subdivide into the small terminal and respiratory bronchioles
   b. The bronchioles contain no cartilage and depend on the elastic recoil of the lung for patency
   c. The terminal bronchioles contain no cilia and do not participate in gas exchange
4. Alveolar ducts and alveoli
   a. Acinus (plural acini) is a term used to indicate all structures distal to the terminal bronchiole
   b. Alveolar ducts branch from the respiratory bronchioles
   c. Alveolar sacs, which arise from the ducts, contain clusters of alveoli, which are the basic units of gas exchange
   d. Type II alveolar cells in the walls of the alveoli secrete surfactant, a phospholipid protein that reduces the surface tension in the alveoli; without surfactant, the alveoli would collapse
5. Lungs
   a. Located in the pleural cavity in the thorax
   b. Extend from just above the clavicles to the diaphragm, the major muscle of inspiration
   c. The right lung, which is larger than the left, is divided into three lobes: upper, middle, and lower
   d. The left lung, which is narrower than the right lung to accommodate the heart, is divided into two lobes

e. Innervation of the respiratory structures is accomplished by the phrenic nerve, the vagus nerve, and the thoracic nerves

f. The parietal pleura line the inside of the thoracic cavity, including the upper surface of the diaphragm

g. The visceral pleura cover the pulmonary surfaces

h. A thin fluid layer, which is produced by the cells lining the pleura, lubricates the visceral pleura and the parietal pleura, allowing them to glide smoothly and painlessly during respiration

i. Blood flow through the lungs occurs via the pulmonary system and the bronchial system

6. Accessory muscles of respiration include the scalene muscles, which elevate the first two ribs; the sternocleidomastoid muscles, which raise the sternum; and the trapezius and pectoralis muscles, which fix the shoulders

7. The respiratory process

a. The diaphragm descends into the abdominal cavity during inspiration, causing negative pressure in the lungs

b. The negative pressure draws air from the area of greater pressure, the atmosphere, into the area of lesser pressure, the lungs

c. In the lungs, air passes through the terminal bronchioles into the alveoli to oxygenate the body tissues

d. At the end of inspiration, the diaphragm and intercostal muscles relax and the lungs recoil

e. As the lungs recoil, pressure within the lungs becomes greater than atmospheric pressure, causing the air, which now contains the cellular waste products of carbon dioxide and water, to move from the alveoli in the lungs to the atmosphere

f. Effective gas exchange depends on distribution of gas (ventilation) and blood (perfusion) in all portions of the lungs

II. DIAGNOSTIC TESTS

A. Risk factors for respiratory disorders (Box 48-1)

B. Chest x-ray film (radiograph)

1. Description: provides information regarding the anatomical location and appearance of the lungs

2. Preprocedure

a. Remove all jewelry and other metal objects from the chest area

b. Assess the client's ability to inhale and hold breath

c. Question females regarding pregnancy or the possibility of pregnancy

3. Postprocedure: Assist the client to dress

C. Sputum specimen

1. Description: a specimen obtained by expectoration or tracheal **suctioning** to assist in the identification of organisms or abnormal cells (Box 48-2)

2. Preprocedure

a. Determine specific purpose of collection and check with institutional policy for appropriate collection of specimen

b. Obtain an early morning sterile specimen from **suctioning** or expectoration after a respiratory treatment, if a treatment is prescribed

c. Instruct the client to rinse the mouth with water before collection

d. Obtain 15 mL of sputum

e. Instruct the client to take several deep breaths and then cough deeply to obtain sputum

f. Always collect the specimen before the client begins antibiotic therapy

3. Postprocedure

a. If a culture of sputum is prescribed, transport the specimen to the laboratory immediately

b. Assist the client with mouth care

D. Bronchoscopy

1. Description: direct visual examination of the larynx, trachea, and bronchi with a fiberoptic bronchoscope

---

BOX 48-1 **Risk Factors for Respiratory Disorders**

Allergies
Chest injury
Crowded living conditions
Exposure to chemicals and environmental pollutants
Family history of infectious disease
Frequent respiratory illnesses
Geographic residence and travel to foreign countries
Smoking
Surgery
Use of chewing tobacco

BOX 48-2 **Suctioning Procedure**

Use aseptic technique.
Hyperoxygenate the client by a resuscitation bag, increasing the oxygen flow rate, or by asking the client to take deep breaths.
Lubricate the catheter with sterile water.
Tracheal suctioning: Insert the catheter 4 inches.
Nasotracheal suctioning: Insert the catheter to induce cough reflex.
Do not apply suction while inserting the catheter.
Apply suction intermittently for 10 seconds; rotate the catheter and withdraw.
Hyperoxygenate the client and encourage deep breaths.

2. Preprocedure
   a. Obtain informed consent
   b. Maintain NPO status for the client from midnight before the procedure
   c. Obtain vital signs
   d. Assess the results of coagulation studies
   e. Remove dentures or eyeglasses
   f. Prepare suction equipment
   g. Establish an intravenous (IV) access as necessary and administer medication for sedation as prescribed
   h. Have emergency resuscitation equipment readily available
3. Postprocedure
   a. Monitor vital signs
   b. Maintain the client in the semi-Fowler's position
   c. Assess for the return of the gag reflex
   d. Maintain NPO status until the gag reflex returns
   e. Have an emesis basin readily available for the client to expectorate sputum
   f. Monitor for bloody sputum
   g. Monitor respiratory status, particularly if sedation was administered
   h. Monitor for complications, such as bronchospasm, bronchial perforation indicated by facial or neck crepitus, dysrhythmias, fever, bacteremia, hemorrhage, hypoxemia, and **pneumothorax**
   i. Notify the physician if fever, difficulty in breathing, or other signs of complications occur following the procedure

E. Pulmonary angiography
1. Description
   a. An invasive fluoroscopic procedure in which a catheter is inserted through the antecubital or femoral vein into the pulmonary artery or one of its branches
   b. Involves an injection of iodine or radiopaque or contrast material
2. Preprocedure
   a. Obtain informed consent
   b. Assess for allergies to iodine, seafood, or other radiopaque dyes
   c. Maintain NPO status of the client for 8 hours before the procedure
   d. Monitor vital signs
   e. Assess results of coagulation studies
   f. Establish an IV access
   g. Administer sedation as prescribed
   h. Instruct the client to lie still during the procedure
   i. Instruct the client that he or she may feel an urge to cough, flushing, or nausea or experience a salty taste following injection of the dye

   j. Have emergency resuscitation equipment available
3. Postprocedure
   a. Monitor vital signs
   b. Avoid taking blood pressures for 24 hours in the extremity used for the injection
   c. Monitor peripheral neurovascular status of the affected extremity
   d. Assess insertion site for bleeding
   e. Monitor for delayed reaction to the dye

F. Thoracentesis
1. Description: removal of fluid or air from the pleural space via a transthoracic aspiration
2. Preprocedure
   a. Obtain informed consent
   b. Obtain vital signs
   c. Prepare the client for ultrasound or chest radiograph, if prescribed, before the procedure
   d. Assess results of coagulation studies
   e. Note that the client is positioned sitting upright, with the arms and shoulders supported by a table at the bedside during the procedure
   f. If the client cannot sit up, he or she is placed lying in bed toward the unaffected side with the head of the bed elevated.
   g. Instruct the client not to cough, breathe deeply, or move during the procedure
3. Postprocedure
   a. Monitor vital signs
   b. Monitor respiratory status
   c. Apply a pressure dressing, and assess the puncture site for bleeding and crepitus
   d. Monitor for signs of **pneumothorax**, air embolism, and pulmonary edema

G. Pulmonary function test
1. Description: a number of different tests used to evaluate lung mechanics, gas exchange, and acid-base disturbance through spirometric measurements, lung volumes, and arterial blood gases.
2. Preprocedure
   a. Determine whether an analgesic that may depress the respiratory function is being administered
   b. Consult with the physician regarding holding bronchodilators before testing
   c. Instruct the client to void before the procedure and to wear loose clothing
   d. Remove dentures
   e. Instruct the client to refrain from smoking; also, the client should avoid or eating a heavy meal for 4 to 6 hours before the test
3. Postprocedure: Client may resume a normal diet and any bronchodilators and respiratory treatments that were held before the procedure

H. Lung biopsy
   1. Description
      a. A percutaneous lung biopsy is performed to obtain tissue for analysis by culture or cytological examination
      b. A needle biopsy is done to identify pulmonary lesions, changes in lung tissue, and the cause of pleural effusion
   2. Preprocedure
      a. Obtain informed consent
      b. Maintain NPO status of the client before the procedure
      c. Inform the client that a local anesthetic will be used but that a sensation of pressure during needle insertion and aspiration may be felt
      d. Administer analgesics and sedatives as prescribed
   3. Postprocedure
      a. Monitor vital signs
      b. Apply a dressing to the biopsy site and monitor for drainage or bleeding
      c. Monitor for signs of respiratory distress, and notify the physician if they occur
      d. Monitor for signs of **pneumothorax** and air emboli, and notify the physician if they occur
      e. Prepare the client for chest radiography if prescribed
I. Ventilation-perfusion lung scan
   1. Description
      a. The perfusion scan evaluates blood flow to the lungs
      b. The ventilation scan determines the patency of the pulmonary airways and detects abnormalities in ventilation
      c. A radionuclide may be injected for the procedure
   2. Preprocedure
      a. Obtain informed consent
      b. Assess the client for allergies to dye, iodine, or seafood
      c. Remove jewelry around the chest area
      d. Review breathing methods that may be required during testing
      e. Establish an IV access
      f. Administer sedation if prescribed
      g. Have emergency resuscitation equipment available
   3. Postprocedure
      a. Monitor the client for reaction to the radionuclide
      b. Instruct the client that the radionuclide clears from the body in about 8 hours
J. Skin tests: A skin test is an intradermal injection used to assist in diagnosing various infectious diseases (Box 48-3)

BOX 48-3 Skin Test Procedure

Determine hypersensitivity or previous reactions to skin tests.

Use a skin site that is free of excessive body hair, dermatitis, and blemishes.

Apply the injection at the upper one third of the inner surface of the left arm.

Circle and mark the injection test site.

Document the date, time, and test site.

Advise the client not to scratch the test site in order to prevent infection and possible abscess formation.

Instruct the client to avoid washing the test site.

Interpret the reaction at the injection site 24 to 72 hours after administration of the test antigen.

Assess the test site for the amount of induration (hard swelling) in millimeters and for the presence of erythema and vesiculation (small blister-like elevations).

K. Arterial blood gases (ABGs)
   1. Description: measurement of the dissolved oxygen and carbon dioxide in the arterial blood to reveal the acid-base state and how well the oxygen is being carried to the body
   2. Preprocedure and postprocedure care (see Chapter 10)
L. Pulse oximetry
   1. Description
      a. Pulse oximetry is a noninvasive test that registers the oxygen saturation (SaO_2) of the client's hemoglobin
      b. The capillary SaO_2 is recorded as a percentage
      c. The normal value is 96% to 100%
      d. After a hypoxic client uses up the readily available oxygen (measured as the arterial oxygen pressure [PaO_2] on ABG testing), the reserve oxygen—that oxygen attached to the hemoglobin (SaO_2)—is drawn on to provide oxygen to the tissues
      e. A pulse oximeter reading can alert the nurse to hypoxemia before clinical signs occur
   2. Procedure
      a. A sensor is placed on the client's finger, toe, nose, ear lobe, or forehead to measure SaO_2, which is then displayed on a monitor
      b. Maintain the transducer at heart level
      c. Do not select an extremity with an impediment to blood flow
      d. Results lower than 91% necessitate immediate treatment
      e. If the SaO_2 is less than 85%, oxygenation to body tissues is compromised; an SaO_2 of less than 70% is life threatening

BOX 48-4 **Client Education: Breathing Retraining and Huff Coughing**

Breathing Retraining
Includes exercises to decrease the use of accessory muscles of breathing to decrease fatigue.
The main types of exercises include pursed-lip breathing and diaphragmatic breathing.
The client should inhale slowly through the nose.
The client should place the hand over the abdomen while inhaling; the abdomen should expand with inhalation and contract during exhalation.
The client should exhale three times longer than inhalation by blowing through pursed lips.

Huff Coughing
An effective coughing technique that conserves energy, reduces fatigue, and facilitates mobilization of secretions.
The client should perform three to four deep breaths using pursed lip and diaphragmatic breathing. Leaning slightly forward, the client should cough three to four times during exhalation.
The client may need to splint the thorax or abdomen to achieve a maximum cough.

BOX 48-5 **Chest Physiotherapy (CPT) Procedure**

Perform CPT in the morning on rising, 1 hour before meals, or 2-3 hours after meals.
Stop CPT if pain occurs.
If the client is receiving a tube feeding, stop the feeding and aspirate the residual before beginning CPT.
Administer the bronchodilator (if prescribed) 15 minutes before the procedure.
Place a layer of material (gown or pajamas) between the hands or percussion device and the client's skin.
Position the client for postural drainage based on assessment.
Percuss the area for 1-2 minutes.
Vibrate the same area while the client exhales four to five deep breaths.
Monitor for respiratory tolerance to the procedure.
Stop the procedure if cyanosis or exhaustion occurs.
Maintain the position for 5-20 minutes after the procedure.
Repeat in all necessary positions until the client no longer expectorates mucus.
Dispose of sputum properly.
Provide mouth care after the procedure.

III. RESPIRATORY TREATMENTS
A. Breathing retraining (Box 48-4)
B. Chest physiotherapy (CPT)
  1. Description: percussion, vibration, and postural drainage techniques performed over the thorax to loosen secretions in the affected area of the lungs and move them into more central airways
  2. Interventions (Box 48-5)
  3. Contraindications
    a. Unstable vital signs
    b. Increased intracranial pressure
    c. Increase in bronchospasm from CPT
    d. History of pathological fractures
    e. Rib fractures
    f. Chest incisions
C. Incentive spirometry (Box 48-6)
IV. OXYGEN
A. Interventions
  1. Assess color and vital signs before and during treatment
  2. Place an "OXYGEN IN USE" sign at the client's bedside
  3. Assess for chronic lung problems
  4. Humidify the oxygen if prescribed.
B. Nasal cannula (nasal prongs) (Box 48-7)
  1. Description
    a. A nasal cannula is used at flow rates of 1 to 6 L/min, providing approximate oxygen concentrations of 24% (at 1 L/min) to 44% (at 6 L/min)
    b. Flow rates higher than 6 L/min do not significantly increase oxygenation because the anatomical reserve or dead space (oral and nasal cavities) is full

BOX 48-6 **Client Instructions for Incentive Spirometry**

Instruct the client to assume a sitting or upright position.
Instruct the client to place the mouth tightly around the mouthpiece of the device.
Instruct the client to inhale slowly to raise and maintain the flow rate indicator between the 600 and 900 marks.
Instruct the client to hold the breath for 5 seconds and then to exhale through pursed lips.
Instruct the client to repeat this process 10 times every hour.

    c. A nasal cannula is used for the client with chronic airflow limitation and for long-term oxygen use
    d. A client who is hypoxemic and has chronic hypercapnia requires low levels of oxygen delivery at 1 to 2 L/min; a low arterial oxygen level is the client's primary drive for breathing
    e. Effective oxygen concentration can be delivered to nose breathers and mouth breathers with the use of a nasal cannula
  2. Interventions
    a. Place the nasal prongs in the nostrils, with the openings facing the client
    b. Add humidification if prescribed when a flow rate higher than 2 L/min is prescribed
    c. Check the water level and change the humidifier as needed.
    d. Assess the client for changes in respiratory rate or depth

BOX 48-7 — Fraction of Inspired Oxygen Delivered via Nasal Cannula

24% at 1 L/min	36% at 4 L/min
28% at 2 L/min	40% at 5 L/min
32% at 3 L/min	44% at 6 L/min

BOX 48-8 — Fraction of Inspired Oxygen Delivered via Simple Face Mask

40% at 5 L/min
45%-50% at 6 L/min
55%-60% at 8 L/min
Pyramid Point
Flow rate must be set to at least 5 L/min to flush the mask of carbon dioxide.

e. Assess the nasal mucosa because high flow rates have a drying effect and increase mucosal irritation
f. Assess skin integrity because the oxygen tubing can irritate the skin

C. Simple face mask (Box 48-8 and Figure 48-1)
1. Description
a. A face mask is used to deliver oxygen concentrations of 40% to 60% for short-term oxygen therapy or to deliver oxygen in an emergency
b. A minimal flow rate of 5 L/min is needed to prevent the rebreathing of exhaled air
2. Interventions
a. Be sure the mask fits securely over the nose and mouth because a poorly fitting mask reduces the fraction of inspired oxygen (FIO$_2$) delivered
b. Assess the skin and provide skin care to the area covered by the mask because pressure and moisture under the mask may cause skin breakdown (remove mucus and saliva from the mask)
c. Monitor the client closely for the risk of aspiration because the mask limits the client's ability to clear the mouth, especially if vomiting occurs
d. Provide emotional support to decrease anxiety in the client who feels claustrophobic
e. Consult with the physician regarding switching the client from a mask to a nasal cannula during eating

D. Partial rebreather mask (Figure 48-2 and Box 48-9)
1. Description
a. A partial rebreather mask consists of a mask with a reservoir bag that provides an oxygen concentration of 70% to 90% with flow rates of 6 to 15 L/min
b. The client rebreathes one third of the exhaled tidal volume, which is high in oxygen, thus providing a high FIO$_2$

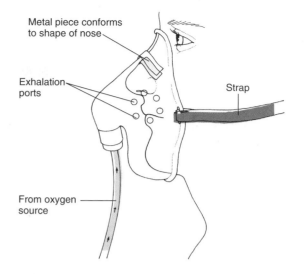

FIG. 48-1 Simple face mask used to deliver oxygen. (From Ignatavicius, D. & Workman, M. [2006]. *Medical-surgical nursing: Critical thinking for collaborative care* [5th ed.]. Philadelphia: Saunders.)

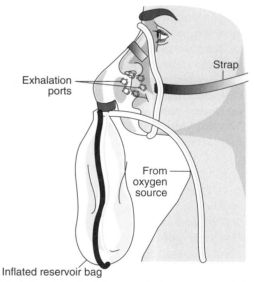

FIG. 48-2 Partial rebreather mask. (From Ignatavicius, D. & Workman, M. [2006]. *Medical-surgical nursing: Critical thinking for collaborative care* [5th ed.]. Philadelphia: Saunders.)

BOX 48-9 — Fraction of Inspired Oxygen Delivered via Partial Rebreather Mask

70%-90% FIO$_2$ delivered at 6 to 15 L/min
Pyramid Point
A flow rate high enough to maintain the bag two-thirds full during inspiration is needed.

2. Interventions
a. Make sure that the reservoir does not twist, kink, or become deflated.
b. Adjust the flow rate to keep the reservoir bag inflated two-thirds full during inspiration because deflation results in decreased

oxygen delivered and rebreathing of exhaled air

E. Non-rebreather mask (Figure 48-3)
1. Description
   a. A non-rebreather mask provides the highest concentration of the low-flow systems and can deliver an FIO_2 greater than 90%, depending on the client's ventilatory pattern
   b. A non-rebreather mask is used most frequently in the client with a deteriorating respiratory status who might require intubation
   c. The non-rebreather mask has a one-way valve between the mask and the reservoir and two flaps over the exhalation ports
   d. The valve allows the client to draw the entire quantity of oxygen from the reservoir bag
   e. The flaps prevent room air from entering through the exhalation ports
   f. During exhalation, air leaves through these exhalation ports while the one-way valve prevents exhaled air from reentering the reservoir bag
2. FIO_2 delivered: 60% to 100% FIO_2 at a liter flow that maintains the bag two-thirds full
3. Interventions
   a. Remove mucus or saliva from the mask
   b. Assess the client closely
   c. Ensure that the valve and flaps are intact and functional during each breath
   d. Valves should open during expiration and close during inhalation

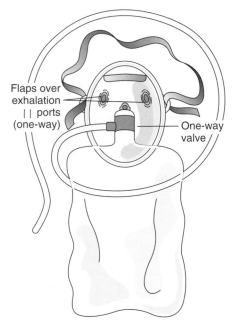

Flaps over exhalation || ports (one-way)

One-way valve

FIG. 48-3 Non-rebreather mask. (From Ignatavicius, D. & Workman, M. [2006]. *Medical-surgical nursing: Critical thinking for collaborative care* [5th ed.]. Philadelphia: Saunders.)

e. Suffocation can occur if the reservoir bag kinks or if the oxygen source disconnects

F. Face tent
1. A face tent fits over the client's chin, with the top extending halfway across the face
2. The oxygen concentration varies, but the face tent is useful instead of a tight-fitting mask for the client who has facial trauma or burns

G. Aerosol mask: used for the client who requires high humidity after extubation or upper airway surgery or for the client who has thick secretions

H. Tracheostomy collar and T piece
1. The tracheostomy collar can be used to deliver high humidity and the desired oxygen to the client with a tracheostomy
2. A special adapter, called the T piece, can be used to deliver any desired FIO_2 to the client with a tracheostomy, laryngectomy, or endotracheal tube
3. Refer to Chapter 19 for information on endotracheal and tracheostomy tubes

I. Interventions for face tent, aerosol mask, tracheostomy collar, and T piece
1. Change the delivery system to a nasal cannula during mealtimes if prescribed for the client with a face mask or aerosol mask
2. Ensure that the aerosol mist escapes from the vents of the delivery system during inspiration and expiration
3. Empty condensation from the tubing to prevent the client from being lavaged with water and to promote an adequate flow rate; remove and clean the tubing at least every 4 hours
4. Ensure that sufficient water is in the aerosol water container, and change the container as needed
5. Keep the exhalation port on the T piece open and uncovered (if the port is occluded, the client can suffocate)
6. Position the T piece so that it does not pull on the tracheostomy or endotracheal tube and cause erosion of the skin at the tracheostomy insertion site
7. Make sure the humidifier creates enough mist; a mist should be seen during inspiration and expiration

J. Venturi mask (Figure 48-4)
1. Description
   a. Provides a high-flow oxygen delivery system
   b. Operation of the Venturi mask is based on a mechanism that pulls in a specific proportional amount of room air for each liter flow of oxygen
   c. An adapter is located between the bottom of the mask and the oxygen source; the adapter contains holes of different sizes that allow only specific amounts of air to mix with the oxygen
   d. The adapter allows selection of the amount of oxygen desired

2. FIO_2 delivered: 24% to 55% FIO_2 with flow rates of 4 to 10 L/min
3. Interventions
   a. Monitor the client closely to ensure an accurate flow rate for specific FIO_2
   b. Keep the air entrapment port for the Venturi adapter open and uncovered to ensure adequate oxygen delivery
   c. Ensure that the mask fits snugly and that the tubing is free of kinks because the FIO_2 is altered if kinking occurs or if the mask fits poorly
   d. Assess the client for dry mucous membranes; humidity or aerosol can be added to the system

V. MECHANICAL VENTILATION

A. Description: used to overcome the client's inability to ventilate or oxygenate adequately
B. Interventions
   1. Assess the client first and the ventilator second
   2. Assess vital signs, lung sounds, respiratory status, and breathing patterns; the client will never breathe at a rate less than the rate set on the ventilator
   3. Monitor skin color, particularly in the lips and nailbeds
   4. Monitor chest for bilateral expansion
   5. Obtain pulse oximetry readings
   6. Monitor ABG results
   7. Assess the need for **suctioning** and observe the type, color, and amount of secretions

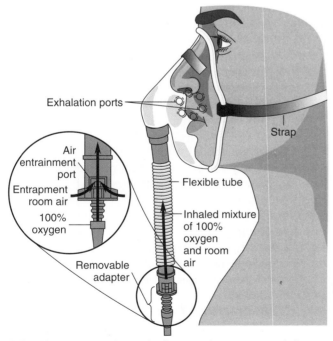

FIG. 48-4 Venturi mask for precise oxygen delivery. (From Ignatavicius, D. & Workman, M. [2006]. *Medical-surgical nursing: Critical thinking for collaborative care* [5th ed.]. Philadelphia: Saunders.)

8. Assess ventilator settings
9. Assess the level of water in the humidifier and the temperature of the humidification system because extremes in temperature can cause damage to the mucosa in the airway
10. Ensure that the alarms are set (never shut alarms off)
11. If a cause for an alarm cannot be determined, ventilate the client manually with a resuscitation bag until the problem is corrected
12. Empty the ventilator tubing when moisture collects
13. Turn the client at least every 2 hours or get the client out of bed, as prescribed, to prevent complications of immobility
14. Have resuscitation equipment available at the bedside

C. Causes of alarms (Box 48-10)
D. Complications
   1. Hypotension caused by the application of positive pressure, which increases intrathoracic pressure and inhibits blood returning to the heart
   2. Respiratory complications such as **pneumothorax** or subcutaneous **emphysema** as a result of positive pressure can occur
   3. Gastrointestinal alterations such as stress ulcers
   4. Malnutrition, if nutrition is not maintained
   5. Infections
   6. Muscular deconditioning
   7. Ventilator dependence or inability to wean
E. Weaning: the process of going from ventilator dependence to spontaneous breathing

VI. CHEST INJURIES

A. Rib fracture
   1. Description
      a. Results from direct blunt chest trauma and causes a potential for intrathoracic injury, such as **pneumothorax** or pulmonary contusion

BOX 48-10 Causes of Ventilator Alarms

High-Pressure Alarm
Increased secretions are in the airway.
Wheezing or bronchospasm causes decreased airway size.
The endotracheal tube is displaced.
The endotracheal tube is obstructed as a result of water or a kink in the tubing.
The client coughs, gags, or bites on the oral endotracheal tube.
The client is anxious or fights the ventilator.
Low-Pressure Alarm
Disconnection or leak in the ventilator or in the client's airway cuff occurs.
The client stops spontaneous breathing.

b. Pain with movement and chest splinting result in impaired ventilation and inadequate clearance of secretions

2. Data collection
   a. Pain at the injury site that increases with inspiration
   b. Tenderness at the site
   c. Shallow respirations
   d. Client splints chest
   e. Fractures noted on chest x-ray film
3. Interventions
   a. Note that the ribs usually unite spontaneously
   b. Place the client in the high Fowler's position
   c. Administer pain medication as prescribed to maintain adequate ventilatory status
   d. Monitor for increased respiratory distress
   e. Instruct the client to self-splint with hands and arms
   f. Prepare the client for an intercostal nerve block as prescribed if the pain is severe

B. Flail chest
1. Description
   a. Occurs from blunt chest trauma associated with accidents, which may result in hemothorax and rib fractures
   b. The loose segment of the chest wall becomes paradoxical to the expansion and contraction of the rest of the chest wall
2. Data collection
   a. Paradoxical respirations (inward movement of a segment of the thorax during inspiration with outward movement during expiration)
   b. Severe pain in the chest
   c. Dyspnea
   d. Cyanosis
   e. Tachycardia
   f. Hypotension
   g. Tachypnea; shallow respirations
   h. Diminished breath sounds
3. Interventions
   a. Place the client in the high Fowler's position
   b. Administer humidified oxygen as prescribed
   c. Monitor for increased respiratory distress
   d. Encourage coughing and deep breathing
   e. Administer pain medication as prescribed
   f. Maintain bedrest and limit activity to reduce oxygen demands
   g. Prepare for intubation with **mechanical ventilation** (positive end expiratory pressure [PEEP] is used for flail chest associated with respiratory failure and shock)

C. Pulmonary contusion
1. Description
   a. Is characterized by interstitial hemorrhage associated with intraalveolar hemorrhage, resulting in decreased pulmonary compliance

b. The major complication is acute respiratory distress syndrome

2. Data collection
   a. Dyspnea
   b. Hypoxemia
   c. Increased bronchial secretions
   d. Hemoptysis
   e. Restlessness
   f. Decreased breath sounds
   g. Crackles and wheezes
3. Interventions
   a. Maintain a patent airway and adequate ventilation
   b. Place the client in the high Fowler's position
   c. Administer oxygen as prescribed
   d. Monitor for increased respiratory distress
   e. Maintain bedrest and limit activity to reduce oxygen demands
   f. Prepare for **mechanical ventilation** with PEEP if required

D. Pneumothorax (Figure 48-5)
1. Description
   a. The accumulation of atmospheric air in the pleural space, which results in a rise in intrathoracic pressure and in a reduction in vital capacity
   b. The loss of negative intrapleural pressure results in collapse of the lung
   c. A spontaneous **pneumothorax** occurs with the rupture of a pulmonary bleb
   d. An open **pneumothorax** occurs when an opening through the chest wall allows the entrance of positive atmospheric air pressure into the pleural space
   e. A tension **pneumothorax** occurs from a blunt chest injury or from **mechanical ventilation** with PEEP when a buildup of positive pressure occurs in the pleural space
   f. Diagnosis of **pneumothorax** is made by chest x-ray film
2. Data collection (Box 48-11)
3. Interventions
   a. Apply a dressing over an open chest wound
   b. Administer oxygen as prescribed
   c. Place the client in the high Fowler's position
   d. Prepare for chest tube placement until the lung has expanded fully
   e. Monitor the chest tube drainage system
   f. Monitor for subcutaneous **emphysema**
   g. Refer to Chapter 19 for information on chest tubes

VII. **ACUTE RESPIRATORY FAILURE**
A. Description
1. Occurs when insufficient oxygen is transported to the blood or inadequate carbon dioxide is removed from the lungs and the client's compensatory mechanisms fail

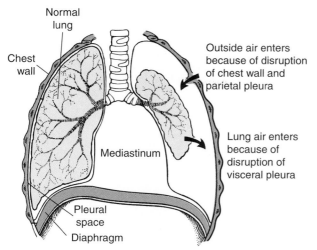

Normal lung

Chest wall

Outside air enters because of disruption of chest wall and parietal pleura

Lung air enters because of disruption of visceral pleura

Mediastinum

Pleural space

Diaphragm

FIG. 48-5   Pneumothorax. Air in the pleural space causes the lung to collapse around the hilus and may push mediastinal contents (heart and great vessels) toward the other lung. (From McCance, K. & Huether, S. [2006]. *Pathophysiology: The biologic basis for disease in adults and children* [5th ed.]. St.Louis: Mosby.)

BOX 48-11   Data Collection Findings: Pneumothorax

Absent breath sounds on affected side
Cyanosis
Decreased chest expansion unilaterally
Dyspnea
Hypotension
Sharp chest pain
Subcutaneous emphysema as evidenced by crepitus on palpation
Sucking sound with open chest wound
Tachycardia
Tachypnea
Tracheal deviation to the unaffected side with tension pneumothorax

---

2. Causes include a mechanical abnormality of the lungs or chest wall, a defect in the respiratory control center in the brain, or an impairment in the function of the respiratory muscles
3. In oxygenation failure, or hypoxemic respiratory failure, oxygen may reach the alveoli but cannot be absorbed or used properly, resulting in a Pao_2 less than 60 mm Hg, arterial Sao_2 lower than 90%, or partial pressure of arterial carbon dioxide ($Paco_2$) greater than 50 mm Hg occurring with acidemia
4. Many clients experience both hypoxemic and hypercapnic respiratory failure and retained carbon dioxide in the alveoli displaces oxygen contributing to the hypoxemia
5. Manifestations of respiratory failure are related to the extent and rapidity of change in Pao_2 and $Paco_2$

B. Data collection
   1. Dyspnea
   2. Headache
   3. Restlessness
   4. Confusion
   5. Tachycardia
   6. Hypertension
   7. Dysrhythmias
   8. Decreased level of consciousness
   9. Alterations in respirations and breath sounds
C. Interventions
   1. Identify and treat the cause of the respiratory failure
   2. Administer oxygen to maintain the Pao_2 level greater than 60 to 70 mm Hg
   3. Place the client in the high Fowler's position
   4. Encourage deep breathing
   5. Administer bronchodilators as prescribed
   6. Prepare the client for **mechanical ventilation** if supplemental oxygen cannot maintain acceptable Pao_2 and $Paco_2$ levels

VIII. ACUTE RESPIRATORY DISTRESS SYNDROME
A. Description
   1. A form of acute respiratory failure that occurs as a complication of some other condition; it is caused by a diffuse lung injury and leads to extravascular lung fluid
   2. The major site of injury is the alveolar capillary membrane
   3. The interstitial edema causes compression and obliteration of the terminal airways and leads to reduced lung volume and compliance
   4. The ABGs identify respiratory acidosis and hypoxemia that does not respond to an increased percentage of oxygen
   5. The chest x-ray film shows bilateral interstitial and alveolar infiltrates; interstitial edema may not show until there is a 30% increase in fluid content
   6. Some of the causes include sepsis, fluid overload, shock, trauma, neurological injuries, burns, disseminated intravascular coagulation, drug ingestion, aspiration, and the inhalation of toxic substances
B. Data collection
   1. Tachypnea
   2. Dyspnea
   3. Decreased breath sounds
   4. Deteriorating arterial blood gas levels
   5. Hypoxemia despite high concentrations of delivered oxygen
   6. Decreased pulmonary compliance
   7. Pulmonary infiltrates
C. Interventions
   1. Identify and treat the cause of the acute respiratory distress syndrome

2. Administer oxygen as prescribed
3. Place the client in the high Fowler's position
4. Restrict fluid intake as prescribed
5. Provide respiratory treatments as prescribed
6. Administer diuretics, anticoagulants, or corticosteroids as prescribed
7. Prepare the client for intubation and **mechanical ventilation** using PEEP

IX. ASTHMA (Refer to Chapter 31 for information on asthma)

X. CHRONIC OBSTRUCTIVE PULMONARY DISEASE

A. Description
1. Is also known as chronic obstructive lung disease and chronic airflow limitation
2. **Chronic obstructive pulmonary disease** is a disease state characterized by airflow obstruction caused by **emphysema,** or chronic bronchitis
3. Progressive airflow limitations occurs, associated with abnormal inflammatory response of the lungs that is not completely reversible
4. **Chronic obstructive pulmonary disease** leads to pulmonary insufficiency, pulmonary hypertension, and cor pulmonale

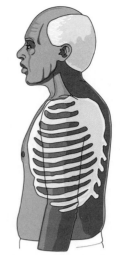

FIG. 48-6   Typical barrel chest in the client with chronic obstructive pulmonary disease. (From Ignatavicius, D. & Workman, M. [2006]. *Medical-surgical nursing: Critical thinking for collaborative care* [5th ed.]. Philadelphia: Saunders.)

B. Data collection
1. Cough
2. Exertional dyspnea
3. Wheezing and crackles
4. Sputum production
5. Weight loss
6. Barrel chest (**emphysema**) (Figure 48-6)
7. Use of accessory muscles for breathing
8. Prolonged expiration
9. Orthopnea
10. Cardiac dysrhythmias
11. Congestion and hyperinflation on chest x-ray film (Figure 48-7)
12. ABGs that indicate respiratory acidosis and hypoxemia
13. Pulmonary function tests that demonstrate decreased vital capacity

C. Interventions
1. Monitor vital signs
2. Administer a low concentration of oxygen (1-2 L/min) as prescribed; the stimulus to breathe is a low arterial Po_2 instead of an increased Pco_2
3. Monitor pulse oximetry
4. Provide respiratory treatments and CPT
5. Instruct the client in diaphragmatic or abdominal breathing techniques and pursed lip breathing techniques
6. Record the color, amount, and consistency of sputum
7. Suction fluids from the client's lungs, if necessary, to clear the airway and prevent infection
8. Monitor weight
9. Encourage small, frequent meals to maintain nutrition and prevent dyspnea
10. Provide a high-calorie, high-protein diet with supplements
11. Encourage fluid intake up to 3000 mL/day to keep secretions thin, unless contraindicated
12. Place the client in the high Fowler's position and leaning forward to aid in breathing
13. Allow activity as tolerated
14. Administer bronchodilators as prescribed, and instruct the client in the use of oral and inhalant medications
15. Short term use of oral corticosteroids or inhaled corticosteroids may be prescribed to treat exacerbation
16. Administer mucolytics to thin secretions as prescribed
17. Administer antibiotics for infection if prescribed

D. Client education (Box 48-12)

XI. SEVERE ACUTE RESPIRATORY SYNDROME (SARS)

A. A respiratory illness caused by the coronavirus, called SARS-associated coronavirus
B. The syndrome begins with a fever, an overall feeling of discomfort, body aches, and mild respiratory symptoms
C. After 2 to 7 days, the client may develop a dry cough and dyspnea
D. Infection is spread by close person-to-person contact by direct contact with infectious material (respiratory secretions or by contact with persons or objects infected with infectious droplets)
E. Prevention includes avoiding contact with those suspected of having SARS, avoiding travel to countries with an outbreak of SARS, avoiding close contact with crowds in areas where SARS exists, and frequent handwashing if in an area where SARS exists.

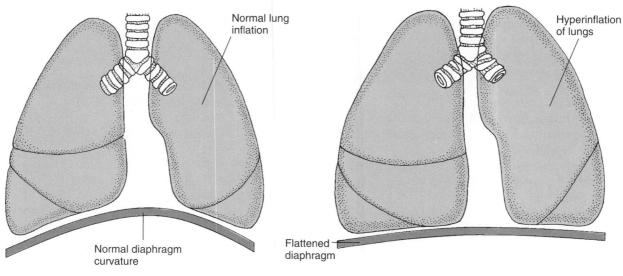

NORMAL

CHRONIC OBSTRUCTIVE PULMONARY DISEASE

FIG. 48-7 Diaphragm shape and lung inflation in the normal client and in the client with chronic obstructive pulmonary disease. (From Ignatavicius, D. & Workman, M. [2006]. *Medical-surgical nursing: Critical thinking for collaborative care* [5th ed.]. Philadelphia: Saunders.)

BOX 48-12	**Client Education: Chronic Obstructive Pulmonary Disease**

Adhere to activity limitations, alternating rest periods with activity.

Avoid gas-producing foods, spicy foods, and extremely hot or cold foods.

Avoid exposure to individuals with infections, and avoid crowds.

Avoid extremes in temperature.

Avoid fireplaces, pets, feather pillows, and other environmental allergens.

Avoid powerful odors.

Meet nutritional requirements.

Receive immunizations as recommended.

Recognize the signs and symptoms of respiratory infection and hypoxia.

Stop smoking.

Use medications and inhalers as prescribed.

Use oxygen therapy as prescribed.

Use pursed lip and diaphragmatic or abdominal breathing.

When dusting, use a wet cloth.

XII. PNEUMONIA

A. Description
   1. An infection of the pulmonary tissue, including the interstitial spaces, the alveoli, and the bronchioles
   2. The edema associated with inflammation stiffens the lung, decreases lung compliance and vital capacity, and causes hypoxemia
   3. Pneumonia can be community acquired or hospital acquired

4. The chest x-ray film shows lobar or segmental consolidation, pulmonary infiltrates, or pleural effusions
   5. A sputum culture identifies the organism
   6. The white blood cell count and the erythrocyte sedimentation rate are elevated
B. Data collection
   1. Chills
   2. Elevated temperature
   3. Pleuritic pain
   4. Tachypnea
   5. Rhonchi and wheezes
   6. Use of accessory muscles for breathing
   7. Mental status changes
   8. Sputum production
C. Interventions
   1. Administer oxygen as prescribed
   2. Monitor respiratory status
   3. Monitor for labored respirations, cyanosis, and cold and clammy skin
   4. Encourage coughing and deep breathing and use of the incentive spirometer
   5. Place the client in the semi-Fowler position to facilitate breathing and lung expansion
   6. Change the client's position frequently and ambulate as tolerated to mobilize secretions
   7. Provide CPT
   8. Perform nasotracheal **suctioning** if the client is unable to clear secretions
   9. Monitor pulse oximetry
   10. Monitor and record color, consistency, and amount of sputum

11. Provide a high-calorie, high-protein diet with small frequent meals
12. Encourage fluids up to 3 L a day to thin secretions unless contraindicated
13. Provide a balance of rest and activity, gradually increasing activity
14. Administer antibiotics as prescribed
15. Administer antipyretics, bronchodilators, cough suppressants, mucolytic agents, and expectorants as prescribed
16. Prevent the spread of infection by handwashing and the proper disposal of secretions

D. Client education
1. Instruct the client about the importance of rest, proper nutrition, and adequate fluid intake
2. Avoid chilling and exposure to individuals with respiratory infections or viruses
3. Instruct the client regarding medications and the use of inhalants as prescribed
4. Instruct the client to notify the physician if chills, fever, dyspnea, hemoptysis, or increased fatigue occurs
5. Instruct the client on the importance of receiving immunizations as recommended

XIII. INFLUENZA

A. Description
1. Is a highly contagious acute viral respiratory infection; also known as the flu
2. May be caused by several viruses usually known as A, B, and C
3. Yearly vaccination is recommended to prevent the disease, especially for those who are older than 50 years of age, individuals with chronic illness or immune compromise, those living in institutions, and health care individuals providing direct care to clients (the vaccination is contraindicated in the individual with egg allergies)
4. Additional prevention measures include avoiding those who developed influenza, frequent and proper handwashing, and cleaning and disinfecting surfaces that have become contaiminated with secretions
5. Avian influenza (bird flu)
   a. Affects birds; however, it can be transmitted to humans if the virus mutates and therefore a vaccine is not available since a human strain does not exist
   b. Reported symptoms are similar to those that are associated with influenza A, B, and C
   c. Prevention measures include thoroughly cooking poultry products, avoiding contact with wild animals, frequent and proper handwashing, and cleaning and disinfecting surfaces that have become contaminated with secretions

B. Data collection
1. Acute onset of fever and muscle aches
2. Headache
3. Fatigue, weakness, and anorexia
4. Sore throat, cough, and rhinorrhea

C. Interventions
1. Encourage rest
2. Encourage fluids to prevent pulmonary complications (unless contraindicated)
3. Monitor lung sounds
4. Provide supportive therapy such as antipyretics or antitussives as indicated
5. Administer antiviral medications as prescribed for current strain of influenza (refer to Chapter 49)

XIV. LEGIONNAIRE'S DISEASE

A. Description
1. An acute bacterial infection caused by *Legionella pneumophila*
2. Sources of the organism include contaminated air conditioner cooling towers and warm stagnant water supplies, including water vaporizers, water sonicators, whirlpool spas, and showers
3. Person-to-person contact does not occur and the risk for infection is increased by the presence of other conditions

B. Data collection: Influenza-like symptoms with a high fever, chills, muscle aches, and headache that may progress to dry cough, pleurisy, and sometimes diarrhea

C. Interventions: Treatment is supportive and antibiotics may be prescribed

XV. PLEURAL EFFUSION

A. Description
1. Pleural effusion is the collection of fluid in the pleural space
2. Any condition that interferes with secretion or drainage of fluid in the pleural space will lead to pleural effusion

B. Data collection
1. Pleuritic pain that is sharp and increases with inspiration
2. Progressive dyspnea with decreased movement of the chest wall on the affected side
3. Dry, nonproductive cough caused by bronchial irritation or mediastinal shift
4. Tachycardia
5. Elevated temperature
6. Decreased breath sounds over affected area
7. Chest x-ray film that shows pleural effusion and a mediastinal shift away from the fluid if the effusion is greater than 250 mL

C. Interventions
1. Identify and treat the underlying cause
2. Monitor breath sounds
3. Place the client in the high Fowler's position
4. Encourage coughing and deep breathing
5. Prepare the client for thoracentesis
6. If pleural effusion is recurrent, prepare the client for pleurectomy or pleurodesis as prescribed

D. Pleurectomy
1. Consists of surgically stripping the parietal pleura away from the visceral pleura
2. This produces an intense inflammatory reaction that promotes adhesion formation between the two layers during healing

E. Pleurodesis
1. Involves the instillation of a sclerosing substance into the pleural space via a thoracotomy tube
2. The substance creates an inflammatory response that scleroses tissues together

XVI. EMPYEMA
A. Description
1. The collection of pus within the pleural cavity
2. The fluid is thick, opaque, and foul smelling
3. The most common cause is pulmonary infection and lung abscess caused by thoracic surgery or chest trauma, in which bacteria are introduced directly into the pleural space
4. Treatment focuses on treating the infection, emptying the empyema cavity, re-expanding the lung, and controlling the infection

B. Data collection
1. Recent febrile illness or trauma
2. Chest pain
3. Cough
4. Dyspnea
5. Anorexia and weight loss
6. Malaise
7. Elevated temperature and chills
8. Night sweats
9. Pleural exudate on chest x-ray film

C. Interventions
1. Monitor breath sounds
2. Place the client in the semi-Fowler's or high Fowler's position
3. Encourage coughing and deep breathing
4. Administer antibiotics as prescribed
5. Instruct the client to splint the chest as necessary
6. Assist with thoracentesis or chest tube insertion to promote drainage and lung expansion
7. If marked pleural thickening occurs, prepare the client for decortication, if prescribed; this is a surgical procedure that involves removal of the restrictive mass of fibrin and inflammatory cells

XVII. PLEURISY
A. Description
1. The inflammation of the visceral and parietal membranes that may be caused by pulmonary infarction or pneumonia
2. The visceral and parietal membranes rub together during respiration and cause pain
3. Pleurisy usually occurs on one side of the chest, usually in the lower lateral portions in the chest wall

B. Data collection
1. Knife-like pain that is aggravated on deep breathing and coughing
2. Dyspnea
3. Pleural friction rub heard on auscultation
4. Apprehension

C. Interventions
1. Identify and treat the cause
2. Monitor lung sounds
3. Administer analgesics as prescribed
4. Apply hot or cold applications as prescribed
5. Encourage coughing and deep breathing
6. Instruct the client to lie on the affected side to splint the chest

XVIII. PULMONARY EMBOLISM
A. Description
1. Occurs when a thrombus forms (most commonly in a deep vein), detaches, and travels to the right side of the heart and then lodges in a branch of the pulmonary artery
2. Clients prone to pulmonary embolism are those at risk for deep vein thrombosis, including those who underwent surgery or those with prolonged immobilization, obesity, pregnancy, congestive heart failure, advanced age, or a history of thromboembolism
3. Fat emboli can occur as a complication following a fracture of a long bone and can cause pulmonary emboli
4. Treatment is aimed at prevention through risk factor recognition and elimination

B. Data collection (Box 48-13)
C. Interventions
1. Administer oxygen as prescribed
2. Place the client in the high Fowler's position
3. Monitor lung sounds
4. Maintain bedrest and active and passive range-of-motion exercises as prescribed
5. Encourage the use of incentive spirometry as prescribed
6. Monitor pulse oximetry
7. Prepare for intubation and **mechanical ventilation** for severe hypoxemia

BOX 48-13 Data Collection Findings: Pulmonary Embolism

Blood-tinged sputum
Chest pain
Cough
Cyanosis
Distended neck veins
Dyspnea accompanied by anginal and pleuritic pain, exacerbated by inspiration
Hypotension
Shallow respirations
Tachypnea and tachycardia
Wheezes on auscultation

8. Administer anticoagulation therapy (heparin) intravenously as prescribed
9. Administer warfarin (Coumadin) orally, as prescribed, when heparin infusion is discontinued
10. Closely monitor prothrombin time, international normalized ratio (INR), and partial thromboplastin time
11. Prepare the client for embolectomy, vein ligation, or insertion of an umbrella filter, as prescribed.

XIX. LUNG CANCER AND LARYNGEAL CANCER (Refer to Chapter 42)

XX. CARBON MONOXIDE POISONING (Refer to Chapter 40)

XXI. HISTOPLASMOSIS

A. Description
1. A pulmonary fungal infection caused by spores of *Histoplasma capsulatum*
2. Transmission occurs by the inhalation of spores, which are commonly located in contaminated soil
3. Spores are also usually found in bird droppings

B. Data collection
1. Similar to pneumonia
2. Positive skin test for histoplasmosis
3. Positive agglutination test
4. Splenomegaly and hepatomegaly

C. Interventions
1. Administer oxygen as prescribed
2. Monitor breath sounds
3. Administer antiemetics, antihistamines, antipyretics, and corticosteroids as prescribed
4. Administer fungicidal medications as prescribed
5. Encourage coughing and deep breathing
6. Place the client in the semi-Fowler's position
7. Monitor vital signs
8. Monitor for nephrotoxicity from fungicidal medications
9. Instruct the client to spray the floor area with water before sweeping barn and chicken coops

XXII. SARCOIDOSIS

A. Description
1. The presence of epitheloid cell tubercles in the lung
2. The cause is unknown, but a high titer of Epstein-Barr virus may be identified
3. Viral incidence is highest in blacks and young adults

B. Data collection
1. Night sweats
2. Fever
3. Weight loss
4. Cough
5. Skin nodules
6. Polyarthritis
7. Kveim test: Sarcoid node antigen is injected intradermally and causes a local nodular lesion in about 1 month

C. Interventions
1. Administer corticosteroids to control symptoms
2. Monitor temperature
3. Increase fluid intake
4. Provide frequent periods of rest
5. Encourage small, nutritious meals

XXIII. OCCUPATIONAL LUNG DISEASE

A. Description
1. Caused by exposure to enviromental or occupational fumes, dust, vapors, gases, bacterial or fungal antigens, and allergens; can result in acute reversible effects or chronic lung disease
2. Common disease classifications include occupational **asthmas,** pneumoconiosis (silicosis or coal miner's [black lung] disease), diffuse interstitial fibrosis (asbestosis, talcosis, beryllilosis), or extrinsic allergic alveolitis (farmer's lung, bird fancier's lung, or machine operator's lung)

B. Data collection: Manifestations depend on the type of disease and are respiratory symptoms

C. Interventions
1. Prevention through the use of respiratory protective devices
2. Treatment is based on the symptoms experienced by the client

XXIV. TUBERCULOSIS

A. Description
1. A highly communicable disease caused by *Mycobacterium tuberculosis*
2. *Mycobacterium tuberculosis* is a nonmotile, nonsporulating, acid-fast rod that secretes niacin; when the bacillus reaches a susceptible site, it multiplies freely
3. Because *Mycobacterium tuberculosis* is an aerobic bacterium, it primarily affects the pulmonary system, especially the upper lobes where the oxygen content is greatest, but it can also affect other areas of the body, such as the brain, intestines, peritoneum, kidney, joints, and liver
4. An exudative response causes a nonspecific pneumonitis and the development of granulomas in the lung tissue
5. **Tuberculosis** has an insidious onset, and many clients are not aware of symptoms until the disease is well advanced
6. Improper or noncompliant use of treatment programs may cause the development of mutations in the tubercle bacilli, resulting in a **multidrug-resistant strain (MDRS)**
7. The goal of treatment is to prevent transmission, control symptoms, and prevent progression of the disease

B. Risk factors (Box 48-14)

C. Transmission
1. Transmission of **tuberculosis** is via the airborne route by droplet infection

BOX 48-14 Risk Factors for Tuberculosis

Children younger than 5 years of age
Drinking of unpasteurized milk if the cow is infected
  with bovine tuberculosis
Homeless individuals or those from a lower
  socioeconomic group, minority groups, or refugees
Individuals in constant, frequent contact with an
  untreated or undiagnosed individual
Individuals living in crowded areas, such as long-term
  care facilities, prisons, and mental health facilities
Older clients
Individuals with malnutrition, an infection, or an
  immune dysfunction or human immunodeficiency
  virus infection, or individuals who are
  immunosuppressed as a result of medication therapy
Individuals who abuse alcohol or are intravenous drug
  users

2. When an infected individual coughs, laughs, sneezes, or sings, droplet nuclei containing **tuberculosis** bacteria enter the air and may be inhaled by others
3. Identification of those individuals in close contact with the infected individual is important so that they can be tested and treated as necessary
4. When contacts have been identified, these persons are assessed with a tuberculin skin test and chest x-ray films to determine infection with **tuberculosis**
5. After the infected individual has received **tuberculosis** medication for 2 to 3 weeks, the risk of transmission is reduced greatly

D. Disease progression
1. Droplets enter the lungs, and the bacteria form a tubercle lesion
2. The defense systems of the body encapsulate the tubercle, leaving a scar
3. If encapsulation does not occur, bacteria may enter the lymph system, travel to the lymph nodes, and cause an inflammatory response called granulomatous inflammation
4. Primary lesions form; the primary lesions may become dormant but can be reactivated and become a secondary infection when reexposed to the bacterium
5. In an active phase, **tuberculosis** can cause necrosis and cavitation in the lesions, leading to rupture and the spread of necrotic tissue, as well as damage to various parts of the body

E. Client history
1. Past exposure to **tuberculosis**
2. Client's country of origin and travel to foreign countries in which the incidence of **tuberculosis** is high
3. Recent history of influenza, pneumonia, febrile illness, cough, or foul-smelling sputum production
4. Previous positive tests for tuberculosis

5. Recent **bacille Calmette-Guérin vaccine** (a vaccine containing attenuated tubercle bacilli that may be given to persons in foreign countries or to persons traveling to foreign countries, to produce increased resistance to **tuberculosis**)
6. An individual who has received the **bacille Calmette-Guérin vaccine** will have a positive skin test and should be evaluated for **tuberculosis** with a chest x-ray film

F. Clinical manifestations
1. May be asymptomatic in primary infection
2. Fatigue
3. Lethargy
4. Anorexia
5. Weight loss
6. Low-grade fever
7. Chills
8. Night sweats
9. Persistent cough and the production of mucoid and mucopurulent sputum, which is occasionally streaked with blood
10. Chest tightness and a dull, aching chest pain that may accompany the cough

G. Chest data collection
1. A physical examination of the chest does not provide conclusive evidence of **tuberculosis**.
2. A chest x-ray film is not definitive, but the presence of multinodular infiltrates with calcification in the upper lobes suggests **tuberculosis**
3. If the disease is active, caseation and inflammation may be seen on the chest x-ray film
4. Advanced disease
   a. Dullness with percussion over the involved parenchymal areas, bronchial breath sounds, rhonchi, and crackles indicate advanced disease
   b. Partial obstruction of a bronchus caused by endobronchial disease or compression by lymph nodes may produce localized wheezing and dyspnea

H. Sputum cultures
1. Sputum specimens are obtained for an acid-fast smear
2. A sputum culture identifying *Mycobacterium tuberculosis* confirms the diagnosis
3. After medications are started, sputum samples are obtained again to determine the effectiveness of therapy
4. Most clients have negative cultures after 3 months of treatment

I. Mantoux skin test
1. A positive Mantoux reaction does not mean that active disease is present but indicates exposure to tuberculosis or the presence of inactive (dormant) disease
2. Once the test result is positive, it will be positive in any future tests

3. Purified protein derivative containing 5 tuberculin units is administered intradermally in the forearm

4. An area of induration measuring 10 mm or more in diameter, 48 to 72 hours after injection, indicates that the individual has been exposed to **tuberculosis**

5. For individuals with human immunodeficiency virus infection or who are immunosuppressed, a reaction of 5 mm or greater is considered positive

6. Once an individual's skin test is positive, a chest x-ray film is necessary to rule out active **tuberculosis** or to detect old, healed lesions

J. The hospitalized client

1. The client with active **tuberculosis** is placed with respiratory isolation precautions in a negative-pressure room; to maintain negative pressure, the door of the room must be tightly closed

2. The room should have at least six exchanges of fresh air per hour and should be ventilated to the outside environment if possible

3. The nurse wears a particulate respirator (a special individually fitted mask) when caring for the client and a gown when a possibility exists of contamination of clothing

4. Always thoroughly wash hands before and after caring for the client

5. If the client needs to leave the room for a test or procedure, he or she must wear a mask

6. Respiratory isolation is discontinued when the client is no longer considered infectious

7. After the infected individual has received **tuberculosis** medication for 2 to 3 weeks, the risk of transmission is reduced greatly.

K. Client education (Box 48-15)

L. Medications (Refer to Chapter 49)

PRACTICE QUESTIONS

More questions on the companion CD!

588. A nurse is providing instructions to a hospitalized client with a diagnosis of emphysema about positions that will enhance the effectiveness of breathing during dyspneic periods. Which position will the nurse instruct the client to assume?
    1. Sitting up in bed
    2. Side-lying in bed
    3. Sitting in a recliner chair
    4. Sitting on the side of the bed, leaning on an overbed table

589. A nurse is gathering data on a client with a diagnosis of tuberculosis (TB). The nurse reviews the results of which diagnostic test that will confirm this diagnosis?

BOX 48-15 **Client Education: Tuberculosis**

Provide the client and family with information about tuberculosis and allay concerns about the contagious aspect of the infection.

Instruct the client to follow the medication regimen exactly as prescribed and always to have a supply of the medication on hand.

Advise the client of the side effects of the medication and ways of minimizing them to ensure compliance.

Reassure the client that after 2 to 3 weeks of medication therapy, it is unlikely that the client will infect anyone.

Inform the client to resume activities gradually.

Instruct the client about the need for adequate nutrition and a well-balanced diet to promote healing and to prevent recurrence of the infection.

Instruct the client to increase intake of foods rich in iron, protein, and vitamin C.

Inform the client and family that respiratory isolation is not necessary because family members have already been exposed.

Instruct the client to cover the mouth and nose when coughing or sneezing and to confine used tissues to plastic bags.

Instruct the client and family about thorough handwashing.

Inform the client that a sputum culture is needed every 2-4 weeks once medication therapy is initiated.

Inform the client that when the results of three sputum cultures are negative, the client is no longer considered infectious and usually can return to former employment.

Advise the client to avoid excessive exposure to silicone or dust because these substances can cause further lung damage.

Instruct the client regarding the importance of compliance with treatment, follow-up care, and sputum cultures, as prescribed.

1. Chest x-ray
2. Bronchoscopy
3. Sputum culture
4. Tuberculin skin test

590. Which of the following identifies the route of transmission of tuberculosis (TB)?
    1. Hand to mouth
    2. The enteric route
    3. The airborne route
    4. Blood and body fluids

591. A nurse is caring for a client with emphysema who is receiving oxygen. The nurse checks the oxygen flow rate to ensure that it does not exceed:
    1. 1 L/minute
    2. 2 L/minute
    3. 6 L/minute
    4. 10 L/minute

592. A nurse is instructing a client about pursed lip breathing and the client asks the nurse about its

purpose. The nurse tells the client that the primary purpose of pursed lip breathing is to:

1. Promote oxygen intake
2. Strengthen the diaphragm
3. Strengthen the intercostal muscles
4. Promote carbon dioxide elimination

593. The low-pressure alarm sounds on the ventilator. The nurse checks the client and then attempts to determine the cause of the alarm but is unsuccessful. Which initial action will the nurse take?

1. Administer oxygen
2. Check the client's vital signs
3. Ventilate the client manually
4. Start cardiopulmonary resuscitation (CPR)

594. A nurse is assigned to care for a client following a left pneumonectomy. The nurse would avoid positioning the client:

1. On the side
2. In a low Fowler's position
3. In a semi-Fowler's position
4. With the head of the bed elevated 40 degrees

595. A nurse is caring for a client following pulmonary angiography via catheter insertion into the left groin. The nurse monitors for an allergic reaction to the contrast medium by noting the presence of:

1. Hypothermia
2. Respiratory distress
3. Hematoma in the left groin
4. Discomfort in the left groin

596. A nurse is providing discharge instructions to the client with pulmonary sarcoidosis. The nurse determines that the client understands the information if the client verbalizes which early sign of exacerbation?

1. Fever
2. Fatigue
3. Weight loss
4. Shortness of breath

597. A nurse working on a respiratory nursing unit is caring for several clients with respiratory disorders. The nurse would identify which of the following clients as being at the least risk for developing infection with tuberculosis?

1. An uninsured man who is homeless
2. A woman newly immigrated from Korea
3. A man who is an inspector for the U.S. Postal Service
4. An older woman admitted from a long-term care facility

598. A nurse is reading the results of a Mantoux skin test on a client with no documented health problems. The site has no induration and a 1-mm area of ecchymosis. The nurse interprets that the result is:

1. Positive
2. Negative

3. Uncertain
4. Borderline

599. A nurse is caring for a client who had a Mantoux skin test implantation 48 hours ago on admission to the nursing unit and reads the result of the skin test as positive. Which action by the nurse is the priority?

1. Report the findings
2. Document the finding in the client's record
3. Call the employee health service department
4. Call the radiology department for a chest x-ray

600. A client being discharged from the hospital to home with a diagnosis of tuberculosis (TB) is worried about the possibility of infecting the family and others. The nurse determines that the client would get the most reassurance from the knowledge that:

1. The family does not need therapy, and the client will not be contagious after 1 month of medication therapy
2. The family does not need therapy, and the client will not be contagious after 6 consecutive weeks of medication therapy
3. The family will receive prophylactic therapy, and the client will not be contagious after 1 continuous week of medication therapy
4. The family will be treated prophylactically, and the client will not be contagious after 2 to 3 consecutive weeks of medication therapy

601. A nurse has reinforced discharge teaching with a client who was diagnosed with tuberculosis (TB) and has been on medication for 1½ weeks. The nurse determines that the client has understood the information if the client makes which statement?

1. "I can't shop at the mall for the next 6 months."
2. "I need to continue medication therapy for 2 months."
3. "I can return to work if a sputum culture comes back negative."
4. "I should not be contagious after 2 to 3 weeks of medication therapy."

602. A client with tuberculosis (TB) asks a nurse about precautions to take after discharge from the hospital to prevent infection of others. The nurse develops a response to the client's question based on the understanding that:

1. The disease is transmitted by droplet nuclei
2. The client should maintain enteric precautions only
3. Deep pile carpet should be removed from the home
4. Clothing and sheets should be bleached after each use

603. A nurse is preparing to give a bed bath to an immobilized client with tuberculosis (TB). The nurse should plan to wear which of the following items when performing this care?

1. Surgical mask and gloves
2. Particulate respirator, gown, and gloves
3. Particulate respirator and protective eyewear
4. Surgical mask, gown, and protective eyewear

604. A client with tuberculosis, whose status is being monitored in an ambulatory care clinic, asks the nurse when it is permissible to return to work. The nurse replies that the client may resume employment when:
1. Five sputum cultures are negative
2. Three sputum cultures are negative
3. A sputum culture and a chest x-ray are negative
4. A sputum culture and a Mantoux test are negative

605. A client with acquired immunodeficiency syndrome (AIDS) has histoplasmosis. A nurse checks the client for which sign/symptom?
1. Dyspnea
2. Headache
3. Weight gain
4. Hypothermia

606. A nurse is taking the nursing history of a client with silicosis. The nurse checks whether the client wears which of the following items during periods of exposure to silica particles?
1. Mask
2. Gown
3. Gloves
4. Eye protection

607. A nurse is assisting in planning care for a client scheduled for insertion of a tracheostomy. What equipment would the nurse plan to have at the bedside when the client returns from surgery?
1. Obturator
2. Oral airway
3. Epinephrine
4. Tracheostomy tube with the next larger size

608. A nurse is caring for a client with an endotracheal tube attached to a ventilator. The high-pressure alarm sounds on the ventilator. The nurse prepares to perform which nursing intervention?
1. Suction the client
2. Check for a disconnection
3. Notify the respiratory therapist
4. Evaluate the tube cuff for a leak

609. A nurse is preparing to obtain a sputum specimen from the client. Which nursing action will facilitate obtaining the specimen?

1. Limiting fluids
2. Having the client take three deep breaths
3. Asking the client to obtain the specimen after eating
4. Asking the client to spit into the collection container

610. An emergency room nurse is caring for a client who sustained a blunt injury to the chest wall. Which sign, if noted in the client, would indicate the presence of a pneumothorax?
1. Bradypnea
2. Shortness of breath
3. A low respiratory rate
4. The presence of a barrel chest

611. A nurse is caring for a client hospitalized with acute exacerbation of chronic obstructive pulmonary disease (COPD). Which of the following would the nurse expect to note in evaluating this client?
1. Hypocapnia
2. A hyperinflated chest on x-ray
3. Increased oxygen saturation with exercise
4. A widened diaphragm noted on chest x-ray

ALTERNATE ITEM FORMAT: MULTIPLE RESPONSE

612. The nurse is preparing a list of home care instructions for the client who has been hospitalized and treated for tuberculosis. Choose the instructions that the nurse will include on the list. Select all that apply.
☑ 1. Activities should be resumed gradually
☐ 2. Avoid contact with other individuals, except family members, for at least 6 months
☑ 3. A sputum culture is needed every 2 to 4 weeks once medication therapy is initiated
☑ 4. Respiratory isolation is not necessary because family members have already been exposed
☐ 5. Cover the mouth and nose when coughing or sneezing and confine used tissues to plastic bags
☐ 6. When one sputum culture is negative, the client is no longer considered infectious and can usually return to his or her former employment

ANSWERS

588. **4**
Rationale: Positions that will assist the client with breathing include sitting up and leaning on an overbed table, sitting up and resting with the elbows on the knees, or standing or leaning against the wall. The positions in options 1, 2, and 3 will not enhance the effectiveness of breathing.
Test-Taking Strategy: Use the process of elimination. Eliminate option 2 because side-lying will not promote

appropriate lung expansion. Next, eliminate options 1 and 3 because they are comparable or alike. If you had difficulty with this question, review the positions that will decrease the work of breathing in a client with emphysema.
Level of Cognitive Ability: Application
Client Needs: Physiological Integrity
Integrated Process: Teaching and Learning
Content Area: Adult Health/Respiratory

References: Christensen, B., & Kockrow, E. (2006). *Adult health nursing* (5th ed., p. 454). St. Louis: Mosby.
Linton, A., & Maebius, N. (2007). *Introduction to medical-surgical nursing* (4th ed., p. 555). Philadelphia: Saunders.

589. 3
Rationale: A definitive diagnosis of TB is confirmed through culture and isolation of *Mycobacterium tuberculosis.* A presumptive diagnosis is made on the basis of a tuberculin skin test, a sputum smear that is positive for acid-fast bacteria, a chest x-ray, and histologic evidence of granulomatous disease on biopsy.
Test-Taking Strategy: Use the process of elimination and note the strategic word "confirm" in the question. Confirmation is made by identifying *Mycobacterium tuberculosis.* If you had difficulty with this question, review the diagnostic procedures related to TB.
Level of Cognitive Ability: Application
Client Needs: Physiological Integrity
Integrated Process: Nursing Process/Data Collection
Content Area: Adult Health/Respiratory
Reference: Linton, A., & Maebius, N. (2007). *Introduction to medical-surgical nursing* (4th ed., pp. 562-563). Philadelphia: Saunders.

590. 3
Rationale: Tuberculosis is an infectious disease caused by the bacillus *Mycobacterium tuberculosis* and spread primarily by the airborne route. Options 1, 2, and 4 are incorrect.
Test-Taking Strategy: Use the process of elimination. Recalling that TB is a respiratory disease will direct you to option 3. If you had difficulty with this question, review the transmission of this disease.
Level of Cognitive Ability: Comprehension
Client Needs: Safe and Effective Care Environment
Integrated Process: Nursing Process/Planning
Content Area: Adult Health/Respiratory
Reference: Linton, A., & Maebius, N. (2007). *Introduction to medical-surgical nursing* (4th ed., p. 564). Philadelphia: Saunders.

591. 2
Rationale: Between 1 and 3 L/minute of oxygen by nasal cannula may be required to raise the Pao_2 level to 60 to 80 mm Hg. However, oxygen is used cautiously in the client with emphysema and should not exceed 2 L/minute. Because of the long-standing hypercapnia that occurs in this disorder, the respiratory drive is triggered by low oxygen levels rather than by increased carbon dioxide levels, which is the case in a normal respiratory system.
Test-Taking Strategy: Recalling the physiology associated with emphysema is required to answer this question. Remember that oxygen is used cautiously in the client with emphysema. If you are unfamiliar with this disorder, review this content.
Level of Cognitive Ability: Application
Client Needs: Physiological Integrity
Integrated Process: Nursing Process/Data Collection
Content Area: Adult Health/Respiratory
References: Christensen, B., & Kockrow, E. (2006). *Adult health nursing* (5th ed., p. 452). St. Louis: Mosby.

Linton, A., & Maebius, N. (2007). *Introduction to medical-surgical nursing* (4th ed., p. 556). Philadelphia: Saunders.

592. 4
Rationale: Pursed lip breathing facilitates maximal expiration for clients with obstructive lung disease and promotes carbon dioxide elimination. This type of breathing allows better expiration by increasing airway pressure, which keeps air passages open during exhalation. Options 1, 2, and 3 are not the purposes of this type of breathing.
Test-Taking Strategy: Use the process of elimination. Visualize the use of this breathing technique to assist in answering correctly. Recalling the respiratory conditions in which this type of breathing is helpful will also assist in directing you to option 4. Review the purpose of this breathing technique if you had difficulty with this question.
Level of Cognitive Ability: Application
Client Needs: Physiological Integrity
Integrated Process: Teaching and Learning
Content Area: Adult Health/Respiratory
References: Black, J., & Hawks, J. (2005). *Medical-surgical nursing: Clinical management for positive outcomes* (7th ed., p. 1812). Philadelphia: Saunders.
Linton, A., & Maebius, N. (2007). *Introduction to medical-surgical nursing* (4th ed., p. 522). Philadelphia: Saunders.

593. 3
Rationale: If an alarm is sounding at any time and the nurse cannot quickly ascertain the problem, the client is disconnected from the ventilator and a manual resuscitation device is used to support respirations until the problem can be corrected. There is no reason to begin CPR. Checking vital signs is not the initial action. Although oxygen is helpful, it will not provide ventilation to the client.
Test-Taking Strategy: Use the process of elimination. Read the question carefully and note that the subject relates to adequate ventilation of the client. Focusing on this subject will direct you to option 3. If you are unfamiliar with the management of a client on a ventilator, review this content.
Level of Cognitive Ability: Application
Client Needs: Physiological Integrity
Integrated Process: Nursing Process/Implementation
Content Area: Adult Health/Respiratory
References: Black, J., & Hawks, J. (2005). *Medical-surgical nursing: Clinical management for positive outcomes* (7th ed., p. 1885). Philadelphia: Saunders.
Linton, A., & Maebius, N. (2007). *Introduction to medical-surgical nursing* (4th ed., p. 529). Philadelphia: Saunders.

594. 1
Rationale: Complete lateral positioning should be avoided following pneumonectomy. Because the mediastinum is no longer held in place on both sides by lung tissue, lateral positioning may cause mediastinal shift and compression of the remaining lung.
Test-Taking Strategy: Use the process of elimination and note the strategic word "avoid." This word indicates a negative event query and the need to select the incorrect position. Eliminate options 2, 3, and 4 because they are comparable or alike. If you had difficulty with this question, review care of the client following pneumonectomy.

Level of Cognitive Ability: Application
Client Needs: Physiological Integrity
Integrated Process: Nursing Process/Implementation
Content Area: Adult Health/Respiratory
Reference: Linton, A., & Maebius, N. (2007). *Introduction to medical-surgical nursing* (4th ed., p. 530). Philadelphia: Saunders.

595. **2**
Rationale: Signs of allergic reaction to the contrast medium include localized itching and edema, respiratory distress, stridor, and decreased blood pressure. Hypothermia is an unrelated event. Discomfort is expected. Hematoma formation is a complication of the procedure but does not indicate an allergic reaction.
Test-Taking Strategy: Use the ABCs—airway, breathing, and circulation—and focus on the subject—an allergic reaction. This will direct you to option 2. Review the signs of an allergic reaction to the contrast medium if you had difficulty with this question.
Level of Cognitive Ability: Application
Client Needs: Physiological Integrity
Integrated Process: Nursing Process/Data Collection
Content Area: Adult Health/Respiratory
References: Christensen, B., & Kockrow, E. (2006). *Foundations of nursing* (5th ed., p. 486). St. Louis: Mosby.
Linton, A., & Maebius, N. (2007). *Introduction to medical-surgical nursing* (4th ed., p. 692). Philadelphia: Saunders.

596. **4**
Rationale: Shortness of breath is an early sign of exacerbation of pulmonary sarcoidosis. Others include chest pain, hemoptysis, and pneumothorax. Systemic signs and symptoms that occur later include weakness and fatigue, malaise, fever, and weight loss.
Test-Taking Strategy: Note the strategic word "early" in the question. Because sarcoidosis is a pulmonary problem, eliminate options 1 and 3 first. Choose option 4 over option 2, because the shortness of breath (and impaired ventilation) appears first and would cause the fatigue as a secondary symptom. Review this disorder if you had difficulty with this question.
Level of Cognitive Ability: Analysis
Client Needs: Physiological Integrity
Integrated Process: Teaching and Learning
Content Area: Adult Health/Respiratory
References: Black, J., & Hawks, J. (2005). *Medical-surgical nursing: Clinical management for positive outcomes* (7th ed., p. 1871). Philadelphia: Saunders.
Monahan, F., Sands, J., Marek, J., et al. (2007). *Phipps' medical-surgical nursing: Health and illness perspectives* (8th ed., pp. 642-643). St. Louis: Mosby.

597. **3**
Rationale: People at high risk for acquiring tuberculosis include immigrants from Asia, Africa, Latin America, and Central and South Pacific regions; medically underserved populations (ethnic minorities, homeless); those with human immunodeficiency virus or other immunosuppressive disorders; residents in group settings (long-term care, correctional facilities); and health care workers.

Test-Taking Strategy: Use the process of elimination and note the strategic words "least risk." Begin to answer this question by eliminating options 1 and 2, because immigrants and the medically underserved are more frequently affected by this infection. From the remaining options, note that the postal inspector may or may not come in contact with many people, depending on job description. The client from the long-term care facility, however, lives in a group setting, where a large number of people share a common environment 24 hours a day. Review the risks associated with tuberculosis if you had difficulty with this question.
Level of Cognitive Ability: Analysis
Client Needs: Health Promotion and Maintenance
Integrated Process: Nursing Process/Data Collection
Content Area: Adult Health/Respiratory
References: Black, J., & Hawks, J. (2005). *Medical-surgical nursing: Clinical management for positive outcomes* (7th ed., pp. 1844-1845). Philadelphia: Saunders.
Christensen, B., & Kockrow, E. (2006). *Adult health nursing* (5th ed., pp. 427-428). St. Louis: Mosby.
Linton, A., & Maebius, N. (2007). *Introduction to medical-surgical nursing* (4th ed., p. 562). Philadelphia: Saunders.

598. **2**
Rationale: A positive Mantoux reading has an induration measuring 10 mm or more in diameter in low-risk individuals. A small area of ecchymosis is insignificant and is probably related to injection technique.
Test-Taking Strategy: To answer this question accurately, it is necessary to know that induration is necessary for a positive response. Because the client in this question has no induration, the result is negative. Review Mantoux skin test results if you had difficulty with this question.
Level of Cognitive Ability: Comprehension
Client Needs: Physiological Integrity
Integrated Process: Nursing Process/Data Collection
Content Area: Adult Health/Respiratory
Reference: Christensen, B., & Kockrow, E. (2006). *Adult health nursing* (5th ed., p. 428). St. Louis: Mosby.

599. **1**
Rationale: The nurse who interprets a Mantoux test as positive notifies the physician immediately. The physician would order a chest x-ray to determine whether the client has clinically active tuberculosis (TB) or old, healed lesions. A sputum culture would be done to confirm the diagnosis of active TB. The client is placed on TB precautions prophylactically until a final diagnosis is made. The findings are documented in the client's record, but this action is not the highest priority. Calling the employee health service would be of no benefit to the client.
Test-Taking Strategy: Use the process of elimination and note the strategic word "priority." Because the nurse may not order diagnostic tests, eliminate option 4 first. Similarly, option 3 can be eliminated, because calling the employee health service is of no benefit to the client. From the remaining options, notifying the physician should have a higher priority than the documentation, even though both may be done in the same narrow time period. Review nursing interventions related to Mantoux testing if you had difficulty with this question.

Level of Cognitive Ability: Application
Client Needs: Safe and Effective Care Environment
Integrated Process: Nursing Process/Implementation
Content Area: Adult Health/Respiratory
Reference: Christensen, B., & Kockrow, E. (2006). *Adult health nursing* (5th ed., p. 428). St. Louis: Mosby.

600. 4
Rationale: Family members or others who have been in close contact with a client diagnosed with TB are placed on prophylactic therapy with isoniazid (INH) for 6 to 12 months. The client is usually not contagious after taking medication for 2 to 3 consecutive weeks. However, the client must take the full course of therapy (for 6 months or longer) to prevent reinfection or drug resistant TB.
Test-Taking Strategy: Use the process of elimination. Recalling that the family requires prophylactic therapy allows you to eliminate options 1 and 2. From the remaining options, it is necessary to know that the client is not contagious after 2 to 3 weeks of therapy. Review the concepts related to the prevention of the spread of TB if you had difficulty with this question.
Level of Cognitive Ability: Comprehension
Client Needs: Psychosocial Integrity
Integrated Process: Nursing Process/Planning
Content Area: Adult Health/Respiratory
Reference: Linton, A., & Maebius, N. (2007). *Introduction to medical-surgical nursing* (4th ed., p. 564). Philadelphia: Saunders.

601. 4
Rationale: The client is continued on medication therapy for 6 to 12 months, depending on the situation. The client is generally considered to be not contagious after 2 to 3 weeks of medication therapy. The client is instructed to wear a mask if there will be exposure to crowds, until the medication is effective in preventing transmission. The client is allowed to return to employment when the results of three sputum cultures are negative.
Test-Taking Strategy: Use the process of elimination. Knowing that the medication therapy lasts for at least 6 months helps you eliminate option 2 first. Knowing that three sputum cultures must be negative helps you eliminate option 3 next. From the remaining options, recalling that the client is not contagious after 2 to 3 weeks of therapy helps you choose option 4. If you had difficulty with this question, review the infectious period of TB.
Level of Cognitive Ability: Comprehension
Client Needs: Physiological Integrity
Integrated Process: Nursing Process/Evaluation
Content Area: Adult Health/Respiratory
Reference: Ignatavicius, D., & Workman, M. (2006). *Medical-surgical nursing: Critical thinking for collaborative care* (5th ed., pp. 643-644). Philadelphia: Saunders.

602. 1
Rationale: TB is spread by droplet nuclei or the airborne route. The disease is not carried on objects such as clothing, eating utensils, linens, or furniture. Bleaching of clothing and linens is unnecessary, although the client and family members should use good handwashing technique. It is unnecessary to remove carpeting from the home.
Test-Taking Strategy: Use the process of elimination. Knowing that TB is not carried on inanimate objects helps you eliminate options 3 and 4 first. From the remaining options, recalling that the disease is transmitted by the airborne route will direct you to option 1. If you had difficulty with this question, review the transmission mode of TB.
Level of Cognitive Ability: Comprehension
Client Needs: Safe and Effective Care Environment
Integrated Process: Nursing Process/Planning
Content Area: Adult Health/Respiratory
Reference: Linton, A., & Maebius, N. (2007). *Introduction to medical-surgical nursing* (4th ed., p. 564). Philadelphia: Saunders.

603. 2
Rationale: The nurse who is in contact with a client with TB should wear an individually fitted particulate respirator. The nurse would also wear gloves as per standard precautions. The nurse wears a gown whenever there is a possibility that the clothing could become contaminated, such as when giving a bed bath.
Test-Taking Strategy: Use the process of elimination. Knowing that the nurse should wear a particulate respirator mask helps you eliminate options 1 and 4 first. Recalling standard precautions helps you choose option 2 over option 3. Review care of the client with TB if you had difficulty with this question.
Level of Cognitive Ability: Application
Client Needs: Safe and Effective Care Environment
Integrated Process: Nursing Process/Planning
Content Area: Adult Health/Respiratory
Reference: Christensen, B., & Kockrow, E. (2006). *Foundations of nursing* (5th ed., pp. 292-293). St. Louis: Mosby.

604. 2
Rationale: The client must have sputum cultures tested every 2 to 4 weeks after initiation of antituberculosis medication therapy. The client may return to work when the results of three sputum cultures are negative, because the client is considered noninfectious at that point. The Mantoux test will not revert to negative once it is positive. The chest x-ray may or may not be negative.
Test-Taking Strategy: Use the process of elimination. Knowing that a positive Mantoux test result never reverts to negative helps you eliminate option 4. To discriminate among the remaining options, it is necessary to know that three negative sputum cultures are required. If this question was difficult, review these concepts.
Level of Cognitive Ability: Application
Client Needs: Safe and Effective Care Environment
Integrated Process: Nursing Process/Implementation
Content Area: Adult Health/Respiratory
References: Black, J., & Hawks, J. (2005). *Medical-surgical nursing: Clinical management for positive outcomes* (7th ed., p. 1846). Philadelphia: Saunders.
Ignatavicius, D., & Workman, M. (2006). *Medical-surgical nursing: Critical thinking for collaborative care* (5th ed., p. 644). Philadelphia: Saunders.

605. **1**

Rationale: Histoplasmosis is an opportunistic fungal infection that can occur in the client with AIDS. The infection begins as a respiratory infection and can progress to disseminated infection. Typical signs and symptoms include fever, dyspnea, cough, and weight loss. There may be enlargement of the client's lymph nodes, liver, and spleen as well.

Test-Taking Strategy: Use the process of elimination. Recalling that histoplasmosis is an infectious process helps you eliminate option 4. Because the client has AIDS as well as another infection, weight gain is an unlikely symptom and can be eliminated next. Knowing that histoplasmosis begins as a respiratory infection helps you choose dyspnea over headache as the correct option. Review the signs of histoplasmosis if you had difficulty with this question.

Level of Cognitive Ability: Application
Client Needs: Physiological Integrity
Integrated Process: Nursing Process/Data Collection
Content Area: Adult Health/Respiratory
Reference: Linton, A., & Maebius, N. (2007). *Introduction to medical-surgical nursing* (4th ed., p. 618). Philadelphia: Saunders.

606. **1**

Rationale: Silicosis results from chronic, excessive inhalation of particles of free crystalline silica dust. The client should wear a mask to limit inhalation of this substance, which can cause restrictive lung disease after years of exposure. Options 2, 3, and 4 are not necessary.

Test-Taking Strategy: Use the process of elimination. Recalling that exposure to silica dust causes the illness and that the dust is inhaled into the respiratory tract will direct you to option 1. If you had difficulty with this question, review the protective measures associated with silicosis.

Level of Cognitive Ability: Comprehension
Client Needs: Safe and Effective Care Environment
Integrated Process: Nursing Process/Data Collection
Content Area: Adult Health/Respiratory
Reference: Lewis, S., Heitkemper, M., Dirksen, S., & Bucher, L. (2007). *Medical-surgical nursing: Assessment and management of clinical problems* (7th ed., pp. 577-578). St. Louis: Mosby.

607. **1**

Rationale: A replacement tracheostomy tube of the same size and an obturator is kept at the bedside at all times in case the tracheostomy tube is dislodged. In addition, a curved hemostat that could be used to hold the trachea open if dislodgment occurs should also be kept at the bedside. An oral airway and epinephrine would not be needed.

Test-Taking Strategy: Use the process of elimination. Eliminate option 4 first because a tracheostomy tube of the next larger size would not be appropriate for the client. Next, eliminate option 3 because it is unrelated to the subject of the question. From the remaining options, recall that the airway has been altered because of the tracheostomy, so an oral airway would not be necessary. Remember that a replacement tracheostomy tube, an obturator, and a curved hemostat should be kept at the bedside of a client with a tracheostomy. Review care of the client with a tracheostomy if you had difficulty with this question.

Level of Cognitive Ability: Application
Client Needs: Physiological Integrity
Integrated Process: Nursing Process/Planning
Content Area: Adult Health/Respiratory
Reference: Monahan, F., Sands, J., Marek, J., et al. (2007). *Phipps' medical-surgical nursing: Health and illness perspectives* (8th ed., pp. 616-617). St. Louis: Mosby.

608. **1**

Rationale: When the high-pressure alarm sounds on a ventilator, it is most likely caused by an obstruction. The obstruction can be caused by the client biting on the tube, kinking of the tubing, or mucus plugging requiring suctioning. It is also important to check the tubing for the presence of any water and determine if the client is out of rhythm with breathing with the ventilator. A disconnection or a cuff leak can result in sounding of the low-pressure alarm. The respiratory therapist would be notified if the nurse could not determine the cause of the alarm.

Test-Taking Strategy: Use the process of elimination. Note the strategic words "high-pressure alarm" in the question. Recalling that the high-pressure alarm indicates a possible obstruction will assist in directing you to the correct option. Review nursing interventions related to care of a client on a ventilator if you had difficulty with this question.

Level of Cognitive Ability: Application
Client Needs: Physiological Integrity
Integrated Process: Nursing Process/Implementation
Content Area: Adult Health/Respiratory
References: Black, J., & Hawks, J. (2005). *Medical-surgical nursing: Clinical management for positive outcomes* (7th ed., p. 1887). Philadelphia: Saunders.
Ignatavicius, D., & Workman, M. (2006). *Medical-surgical nursing: Critical thinking for collaborative care* (5th ed., p. 667). Philadelphia: Saunders.

609. **2**

Rationale: To obtain a sputum specimen, the client should brush his or her teeth to reduce mouth contamination. The client should then take three deep breaths and cough into a sputum specimen container. The client should be encouraged to cough and not spit so that sputum can be obtained. Sputum can be thinned by fluids or by a respiratory treatment, such as inhalation of nebulized saline or water. The optimal time to obtain a specimen is on arising in the morning.

Test-Taking Strategy: Use the process of elimination. Option 1 can be eliminated first by recalling that fluids assist in loosening or thinning secretions. Eliminate option 4 because of the word "spit." Spit is very different from saliva. Next, eliminate option 3 because of the words "after eating." Review this procedure if you had difficulty with this question.

Level of Cognitive Ability: Application
Client Needs: Physiological Integrity
Integrated Process: Nursing Process/Implementation
Content Area: Adult Health/Respiratory
References: Christensen, B., & Kockrow, E. (2006). *Adult health nursing* (5th ed., p. 409). St. Louis: Mosby.
Christensen, B., & Kockrow, E. (2006). *Foundations of nursing* (5th ed., p. 513). St. Louis: Mosby.

610. **2**

Rationale: This client has sustained a blunt or a closed chest injury. Basic symptoms of a closed pneumothorax are shortness of breath and chest pain. A larger pneumothorax may present with tachypnea, cyanosis, diminished breath sounds, and subcutaneous emphysema. There may also be hyperresonance on the affected side.

Test-Taking Strategy: Use the process of elimination. Option 4 can be eliminated because a barrel chest is a characteristic finding in a client with chronic obstructive pulmonary disease or emphysema. Next, eliminate options 1 and 3 because they are comparable or alike. Review the signs of pneumothorax if you had difficulty with this question.

Level of Cognitive Ability: Analysis
Client Needs: Physiological Integrity
Integrated Process: Nursing Process/Data Collection
Content Area: Adult Health/Respiratory
Reference: Christensen, B., & Kockrow, E. (2006). *Adult health nursing* (5th ed., p. 441). St. Louis: Mosby.

611. **2**

Rationale: Clinical manifestations of COPD include hypoxemia, hypercapnia, dyspnea on exertion and at rest, oxygen desaturation with exercise, and the use of accessory muscles of respiration. Chest x-ray will reveal a hyperinflated chest and a flattened diaphragm if the disease is advanced.

Test-Taking Strategy: Use the process of elimination. Eliminate option 3 because oxygen desaturation rather than saturation would occur. Next, eliminate option 1 because in the client with COPD, hypercapnia would be noted. From the remaining options, reading carefully will assist in directing you to option 2. If you are unfamiliar with the manifestations associated with COPD, review this content.

Level of Cognitive Ability: Analysis
Client Needs: Physiological Integrity
Integrated Process: Nursing Process/Data Collection
Content Area: Adult Health/Respiratory
Reference: Christensen, B., & Kockrow, E. (2006). *Adult health nursing* (5th ed., p. 452). St. Louis: Mosby.

ALTERNATE ITEM FORMAT: MULTIPLE RESPONSE

612. **1, 3, 4, 5**

Rationale: The nurse should provide the client and family with information about tuberculosis and allay concerns about the contagious aspect of the infection. The client is to follow the medication regimen exactly as prescribed and always to have a supply of the medication on hand. The client is advised of the side effects of the medication and ways of minimizing them to ensure compliance. The client is reassured that, after 2 to 3 weeks of medication therapy, it is unlikely that the client will infect anyone. The client is also informed that activities should be resumed gradually and about the need for adequate nutrition and a well-balanced diet that is rich in iron, protein, and vitamin C to promote healing and prevent recurrence of infection. The client and family are informed that respiratory isolation is not necessary, because family members have already been exposed. The client is instructed about thorough handwashing and to cover the mouth and nose when coughing or sneezing and confine used tissues to plastic bags. The client is informed that a sputum culture is needed every 2 to 4 weeks once medication therapy is initiated and, when the results of three sputum cultures are negative, the client is no longer considered infectious and can usually return to his or her former employment.

Test-Taking Strategy: Knowledge regarding the pathophysiology, transmission, and treatment of tuberculosis is needed to answer this question. Using this knowledge will assist in directing you to the correct options. Review home care instructions for the client with tuberculosis if you had difficulty with this question.

Level of Cognitive Ability: Application
Client Needs: Safe and Effective Care Environment
Integrated Process: Teaching and Learning
Content Area: Adult Health/Respiratory
Reference: Linton, A., & Maebius, N. (2007). *Introduction to medical-surgical nursing* (4th ed., p. 564). Philadelphia: Saunders.

REFERENCES

Black, J., & Hawks, J. (2005). *Medical-surgical nursing: Clinical management for positive outcomes* (7th ed.). Philadelphia: Saunders.

Chernecky, C., & Berger, B. (2008). *Laboratory tests and diagnostic procedures* (5th ed.). Philadelphia: Saunders.

Christensen, B., & Kockrow, E. (2006). *Adult health nursing* (5th ed.). St. Louis: Mosby.

Christensen, B., & Kockrow, E. (2006). *Foundations of nursing* (5th ed.). St. Louis: Mosby.

deWit, S. (2009). *Medical-surgical nursing: concepts & practice* (1st ed.). Philadelphia: Saunders.

Ignatavicius, D., & Workman, M. (2006). *Medical-surgical nursing: Critical thinking for collaborative care* (5th ed.). Philadelphia: Saunders.

Lewis, S., Heitkemper, M., Dirksen, S., & Bucher, L. (2007). *Medical-surgical nursing: Assessment and management of clinical problems* (7th ed.). St. Louis: Mosby.

Linton, A., & Maebius, N. (2007). *Introduction to medical-surgical nursing* (4th ed.). Philadelphia: Saunders.

Monahan, F., Sands, J., Marek, J., Neighbors, M., & Green, C. (2007). *Phipps' Medical-surgical nursing: Health and illness perspectives* (8th ed.). St. Louis: Mosby.

Respiratory Medications

I. BRONCHODILATORS

A. Description

1. Sympathomimetic bronchodilators dilate the airways of the respiratory tree, making air exchange and respiration easier for the client, and relax the smooth muscle of the bronchi (Box 49-1).
2. Xanthine bronchodilators stimulate the central nervous system and respiration, dilate coronary and pulmonary vessels, cause diuresis, and relax smooth muscle (Box 49-2)
3. Bronchodilators are used to treat allergic rhinitis and sinusitis, acute bronchospasm, acute and chronic asthma, bronchitis, **chronic obstructive pulmonary disease,** and **emphysema**
4. Bronchodilators are contraindicated in individuals with hypersensitivity, peptic ulcer disease, severe cardiac disease and cardiac dysrhythmias, hyperthyroidism, or uncontrolled seizure disorders
5. Bronchodilators should be used with caution in clients with hypertension, diabetes mellitus, or narrow-angle glaucoma
6. Theophylline increases the risk of digoxin toxicity and decreases the effects of lithium and phenytoin (Dilantin)
7. If theophylline and a β_2-adrenergic agonist are administered together, cardiac dysrhythmias may result
8. β-Blockers, cimetidine (Tagamet), and erythromycin increase the effects of theophylline
9. Barbiturate and carbamazepine (Tegretol) decrease the effects of theophylline

B. Side effects

1. Palpitations and tachycardia
2. Dysrhythmias
3. Restlessness, nervousness, and tremors
4. Anorexia, nausea, and vomiting
5. Headaches and dizziness
6. Hyperglycemia
7. Decreased clotting time
8. Mouth dryness and throat irritation with inhalers

9. Tolerance and paradoxical bronchoconstriction with inhalers

C. Interventions

1. Assess vital signs
2. Monitor for cardiac dysrhythmias
3. Assess for cough, wheezing, decreased breath sounds, and sputum production
4. Monitor for restlessness and confusion
5. Provide adequate hydration
6. Administer the medication at regular intervals around the clock to maintain a sustained therapeutic level
7. Administer oral medications with or after meals to decrease gastrointestinal irritation
8. Instruct the client not to crush enteric-coated or sustained-release tablets or capsules
9. Instruct the client to avoid caffeinated products such as coffee, tea, cola, and chocolate
10. Instruct the client on the side effects of bronchodilators
11. Instruct the client on how to monitor the pulse and to report any abnormalities to the physician
12. Instruct the client on how to use an inhaler or nebulizer and how to monitor the amount of medication remaining in an inhaler canister; how to use a spacer (a device that enhances the delivery of medication) is also taught

BOX 49-1   Bronchodilators: Sympathomimetics

β_2-Adrenergic Agonists
Inhaled
Albuterol (Proventil HFA)
Bitolterol (Tornalate)
Formoterol (Foradil Aerolizer)
Levalbuterol (Xopenex, Xopenex HFA)
Pirbuterol (Maxair)
Salmeterol (Serevent Diskus)
Oral
Albuterol (Volmax)
Terbutaline (Brethine)
Anticholinergics
Ipratropium inhaled (Atrovent HFA)
Tiotropium, inhaled (Spiriva)

13. Instruct the client to avoid over-the-counter medications
14. Instruct the client to stop smoking, and provide information regarding support resources
15. Instruct the client with diabetes mellitus to monitor blood glucose levels
16. Instruct the client with asthma to wear a Medic-Alert bracelet
17. Monitor for a therapeutic serum theophylline level of 10 to 20 mcg/mL.
18. Note that toxicity is likely to occur when the serum level is greater than 20 mcg/mL
19. Intravenously administered aminophylline or theophylline preparations should be administered slowly and always via an infusion pump

II. GLUCOCORTICOIDS (CORTICOSTEROIDS) (Box 49-3)
A. Glucocorticoids act as anti-inflammatory agents and reduce edema of the airways

BOX 49-2 Bronchodilators: Methylxanthines

Theophylline, oral (Theolair-SR, Theo-24, Uniphyl, and others)

B. Refer to Chapter 45 for information on glucocorticoids

III. USE OF AN INHALER
A. Client instructions for use of a metered-dose inhaler (MDI) (Figure 49-1)
B. If two different inhaled medications are prescribed and one of the medications contains a glucocorticoid (corticosteroid), administer the bronchodilator first and the corticosteroid second
C. Wait 5 minutes following the bronchodilator before inhaling the corticosteroid

BOX 49-3 Glucocorticoids (Corticosteroids)

Inhaled
Beclomethasone dipropionate (QVAR)
Budesonide (Pulmicort Turbohaler, Pulmicort Respules)
Flunisolide (AeroBid)
Fluticasone propionate (Flovent HFA, Flovent Rotadisk, Flovent Diskus)
Mometasone furoate (Asmanex Twisthaler)
Triamcinolone (Azmacort)
Oral
Prednisone
Prednisolone

1. Insert the medicine canister into the inhaler unit and remove the cover from the mouthpiece. Shake the unit gently according to the manufacturer's recommendations.

2. Hold the inhaler ready for inspiration. Exhale slowly. (Do not breathe into the inhaler; that could clog the inhaler valve.)

3. Place the mouthpiece into your mouth and seal it with your lips. Tilt your head slightly back and keep your tongue away from the mouth of the inhaler. (Alternatively, hold the inhaler 1 to 2 inches in front of your mouth and keep your mouth open. With steroids, do not put the inhaler in your mouth. Ineffective use results from medication bouncing off teeth, tongue, or palate.)

4. Press the top of the canister as you breathe in slowly through your mouth. (Failing to coordinate respiration with inhalation will decrease the amount of medication that reaches your lungs.)

5. Remove the inhaler. Hold your breath for 10 seconds, then breathe out slowly through pursed lips.

6. Keep the cap in place between uses to prevent dirt from getting into the inhaler. To clean the inhaler, remove the metal canister and rinse the holder in warm water. Dry the holder thoroughly before using it again.

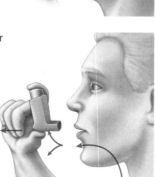

FIG. 49-1 Teaching for self-care: using a metered-dose inhaler. (From Harkreader, H., Hogan, M.A., & Thobaben, M. [2007]. *Fundamentals of nursing: Caring and clinical judgment* (3rd ed.). Philadelphia: Saunders.)

IV. INHALED NONSTEROIDAL ANTIALLERGY AGENTS (Box 49-4)
  A. Description
    1. Antiasthmatic, antiallergic, and mast cell stabilizers inhibit mast cell release after exposure to antigens
    2. These medications are used to treat allergic rhinitis, bronchial asthma, and exercise-induced bronchospasm (Box 49-5)
    3. These medications are contraindicated in clients with known hypersensitivity
    4. Orally administered cromolyn sodium (Intal) is used with caution in clients with impaired hepatic or renal function
  B. Side effects
    1. Cough or bronchospasm following inhalation
    2. Nasal sting or sneezing following inhalation
    3. Unpleasant taste in the mouth
  C. Interventions
    1. Monitor vital signs
    2. Monitor respirations and assess lung sounds for rhonchi or wheezing
    3. Instruct the client to drink a few sips of water before and after inhalation to prevent a cough and an unpleasant taste
    4. Administer oral capsules (cromolyn sodium) at least 30 minutes before meals
    5. Instruct the client not to discontinue the medication abruptly because a rebound asthmatic attack can occur

---

BOX 49-4 Inhaled Nonsteroidal Antiallergy Agents: Mast-Cell Stabilizers

Cromolyn sodium, inhaled (Intal)
Nedocromil, inhaled (Tilade)

BOX 49-5 Treatment for Asthma

Quick-Relief Medications
Bronchodilators
Short-acting inhaled bronchodilators
Anticholinergics
Anti-inflammatory Medications
Systemic glucocorticoids
Long-Term Control Medications
Anti-inflammatory Medications
Inhaled or oral glucocorticoids
Cromolyn (Intal) and nedocromil (Tilade)
Leukotriene modifiers
Omalizumab (xolair)
Bronchodilators
Oral and inhaled bronchodilators
Theophylline

V. LEUKOTRIENE MODIFIERS (Box 49-6)
  A. Description
    1. Used in the prophylaxis and treatment of chronic bronchial asthma (not used for acute asthma episodes)
    2. Inhibit bronchoconstriction caused by specific antigens and reduce airway edema and smooth muscle constriction
    3. Contraindicated in clients with hypersensitivity and in breast-feeding mothers
    4. Should be used with caution in clients with impaired hepatic function
    5. Coadministration of inhaled glucocorticoids increases the risk of upper respiratory infection
  B. Side effects
    1. Headache
    2. Nausea and vomiting
    3. Dyspepsia
    4. Diarrhea
    5. Generalized pain and myalgia
    6. Fever
    7. Dizziness
  C. Interventions
    1. Monitor vital signs
    2. Assess lung sounds for rhonchi and wheezing
    3. Assess liver function laboratory values
    4. Monitor for cyanosis
    5. Instruct the client to take medication 1 hour before or 2 hours after meals
    6. Instruct the client to increase fluid intake
    7. Instruct the client not to discontinue the medication and to take as prescribed even during symptom-free periods

VI. MONOCLONAL ANTIBODIES
  A. Description
    1. Omalizumab (Xolair) is a recombinant DNA-derived humanized IgG murine monoclonal antibody that selectively binds to IgE to limit the release of mediators in the allergic response
    2. Used to treat allergy-related asthma and is administered subcutaneously every 2 to 4 weeks
    3. Dose is titrated based on the serum IgE levels and body weight
    4. Contraindicated in hypersensitivity to the medication
  B. Side effects
    1. Injection site reactions
    2. Viral infections

BOX 49-6 Leukotriene Modifiers

Leukotriene Receptor Antagonists
Montelukast, oral (Singulair)
Zafirlukast, oral (Accolate)
Leukotriene Inhibitor
Zileuton, oral (Zyflo)

3. Upper respiratory infections
4. Sinusitis
5. Headache
6. Pharyngitis
7. Anaphylaxis
8. Malignancies

C. Interventions
1. Assess respiratory rate, rhythm, depth, and auscultate lung fields bilaterally
2. Assess for allergies and/or allergic reaction symptoms such as rash or urticaria
3. Instruct the client that respiratory improvement will not be immediate
4. Instruct the client not to stop taking or decrease the currently prescribed asthma medications unless instructed
5. Avoid live virus vaccines for the duration of treatment
6. Have medications for the treatment of severe hypersensitivity reactions available during initial administration in case anaphylaxis occurs

VII. ANTIHISTAMINES (Box 49-7)

A. Description
1. Antihistamines are called histamine antagonists or H_1 blockers; these medications compete with histamine for receptor sites, thus preventing a histamine response
2. When the H_1 receptor is stimulated, the extravascular smooth muscles, including those lining the nasal cavity, are constricted
3. Antihistamines decrease nasopharyngeal, gastrointestinal, and bronchial secretions by blocking the H_1 receptor
4. Antihistamines are used for the common cold, rhinitis, nausea and vomiting, motion sickness, and urticaria, as well as a sleep aid

---

BOX 49-7 **Antihistamines**

Acrivastine/pseudoephedrine (Semprex-D)
Azelastine hydrochloride (Astelin)
Brompheniramine (BroveX)
Cetirizine hydrochloride (Zyrtec)
Chlorpheniramine maleate (Aller-Chlor, Chlor-Trimeton)
Chlorpheniramine/pseudoephrdrine (Allerest Maximum Strength)
Clemastine fumarate (Tavist)
Desloratidine (Clarinex)
Dexchlorpheniramine maleate (Polaramine)
Dimenhydrinate (Dramamine)
Diphenhydramine (Benadryl)
Doxylamine succinate (Unisom)
Fexofenadine (Allegra)
Fexofenadine/pseudoephedrine (Allegra-D)
Loratadine (Claritin)
Loratadine/pseudoephedrine (Claritin-D)
Triprolidine/pseudoephedrine (Actifed Cold and Allergy)

---

5. Can cause central nervous system (CNS) depression if taken with alcohol, opioids, hypnotics, or barbiturates
6. Should be used with caution in clients with **chronic obstructive pulmonary disease** because of their drying effect
7. Diphenhydramine (Benadryl) has an anticholinergic effect and should be avoided in clients with narrow-angle glaucoma

B. Side effects
1. Drowsiness and fatigue
2. Dizziness
3. Urinary retention
4. Blurred vision
5. Wheezing
6. Constipation
7. Dry mouth
8. Gastrointestinal irritation
9. Hypotension
10. Hearing disturbances
11. Photosensitivity
12. Nervousness and irritability
13. Confusion
14. Nightmares

C. Interventions
1. Monitor vital signs
2. Monitor for signs of urinary dysfunction
3. Administer with food or milk
4. Avoid subcutaneous injection, and administer by intramuscular injection in a large muscle if the intramuscular route is prescribed
5. Instruct the client to avoid hazardous activities, alcohol, and other CNS depressants
6. Instruct the client taking the medication for motion sickness to take the medication 30 minutes before the event and then before meals and at bedtime during the event
7. Instruct the client to suck on hard candy or ice chips in case of dry mouth

VIII. NASAL DECONGESTANTS (Box 49-8)

A. Description
1. Nasal decongestants include adrenergic, anticholinergic, and corticosteroid medications
2. These medications shrink nasal mucosal membranes and reduce fluid secretion
3. Are used for allergic rhinitis, hay fever, and acute coryza (profuse nasal discharge)
4. Are contraindicated or used with extreme caution in clients with hypertension, cardiac disease, hyperthyroidism, or diabetes mellitus
5. Can cause tolerance and rebound nasal congestion (vasodilation) caused by irritation of the nasal mucosa; should not be used for more than 48 hours

B. Side effects
1. Frequent use of decongestants, especially nasal sprays or drops, can result in tolerance and

BOX 49-8 **Nasal Decongestants**

Intranasal Non-Glucocorticosteroids
Naphazoline (Privine)
Oxymetazoline hydrochloride (Afrin)
Phenylephrine hydrochloride (Neo-Synephrine)
Pseudoephedrine hydrochloride (Sudafed)
Tetrahydrozoline (Tyzine)
Xylometazoline (Natru-Vent, Otrivin)
Intranasal Glucosteroids
Beclomethasone dipropionate (Beconase AQ)
Budesonide (Rhinocort Aqua)
Flunisolide (Nasarel)
Fluticasone (Flonase)
Mometasone (Nasonex)
Triamcinolone (Nasacort)

BOX 49-9 **Expectorants and Mucolytic Agents**

Expectorants
Dornase alfa (Pulmozyme)
Guaifenesin (Humibid, Robitussin)
Mucolytic
Acetylcysteine (Mucomyst)

BOX 49-10 **Antitussives**

Opioids
Codeine, codeine phosphate, codeine sulfate
Hydrocodone bitartrate (Hycodan)
Non-Opioids
Diphenhydramine Hydrochloride (Benadryl Cough Syrup, Benadryl)

rebound nasal congestion (vasodilation) caused by irritation of the nasal mucosa
2. Nervousness
3. Restlessness and insomnia
4. Hypertension
5. Hyperglycemia
C. Interventions
1. Assess the client for existing medical disorders
2. Monitor for cardiac dysrhythmias
3. Monitor blood glucose levels
4. Instruct the client to avoid consuming caffeine in large amounts because it can increase restlessness and palpitations
5. Instruct the client on the importance of limiting the use of nasal sprays and drops

IX. EXPECTORANTS AND MUCOLYTIC AGENTS (Box 49-9)
A. Description
1. Expectorants are used to loosen bronchial secretions so that they can be eliminated with coughing; for dry, unproductive cough; and to stimulate bronchial secretions
2. Mucolytic agents thin mucus secretions to help make the cough more productive
3. Mucolytic agents with dextromethorphan should not be used by clients with **chronic obstructive pulmonary disease** because they suppress the cough
4. Acetylcysteine (Mucomyst) can increase airway resistance and should not be used in clients with asthma
B. Side effects
1. Gastrointestinal irritation
2. Rash
3. Oropharyngeal irritation
C. Interventions
1. Instruct the client to take medication with a full glass of water to loosen mucus
2. Instruct the client to maintain an adequate fluid intake

3. Encourage the client to cough and deep breathe
4. Acetylcysteine (Mucomyst), administered by nebulization, should not be mixed with another medication
5. If acetylcysteine is administered with a bronchodilator, the bronchodilator should be administered 5 minutes before the acetylcysteine
6. Monitor for side effects of acetylcysteine, such as nausea and vomiting, stomatitis, and runny nose

X. ANTITUSSIVES (Box 49-10)
A. Description: act on the cough control center in the medulla to suppress the cough reflex and are used for a cough that is nonproductive and irritating
B. Side effects
1. Dizziness, drowsiness, and sedation
2. Gastrointestinal irritation and nausea
3. Dry mouth
4. Constipation
5. Respiratory depression
C. Interventions
1. Instruct the client to notify the physician if the cough lasts longer than 1 week and a fever or rash occurs
2. Encourage the client to take adequate fluids with the medication
3. Encourage the client to sleep with the head of the bed elevated
4. Instruct the client to avoid hazardous activities
5. Note that drug dependency can occur
6. Avoid administration to the client with a head injury or a postoperative cranial surgery client
7. Avoid administration to the client using opioids, sedative hypnotics, barbiturates, or antidepressants because CNS depression can occur
8. Instruct the client to avoid the use of alcohol

BOX 49-11 **Opioid Antagonists**

Nalmefene (Revex)
Naloxone hydrochloride (Narcan)
Naltrexone (ReVia)

XI. OPIOID ANTAGONISTS (Box 49-11)
A. Description
1. An opioid antagonist reverses respiratory depression in opioid overdose
2. Avoid its use in non-opioid respiratory depression
B. Side effects
1. CNS depression
2. Nausea and vomiting
3. Tremors
4. Sweating
5. Increased blood pressure
6. Tachycardia
C. Interventions
1. Assess vital signs, especially respirations
2. For IV administration, the dose is titrated every 2 to 5 minutes as prescribed
3. Have oxygen and resuscitative equipment available during administration

XII. TUBERCULOSIS MEDICATIONS
A. Description
1. **Tuberculosis** medications offer the most effective method for treating the disease and preventing transmission
2. Treatment of identified lesions depends on whether the individual has active disease or has been exposed to the disease
3. Treatment is difficult because the bacterium has a waxy substance on the capsule that makes penetration and destruction difficult
4. The use of a multiple-medication regimen destroys organisms as quickly as possible and minimizes the emergence of medication-resistant organisms
5. Active **tuberculosis** is treated with a combination of medications to which the organism is susceptible
6. Individuals with active **tuberculosis** are treated for 6 to 9 months; however, clients with human immunodeficiency virus (HIV) infection are treated for a longer period
7. After the infected individual has received medication for 2 to 3 weeks, the risk of transmission is reduced greatly
8. Most clients have negative sputum cultures after 3 months of compliance with medication therapy
9. Individuals who have been exposed to active **tuberculosis** are treated with preventive isoniazid (INH) for 9 to 12 months

B. First- or second-line medications
1. First-line medications provide the most effective antituberculosis activity
2. Second-line medications are used in combination with first-line medications but are more toxic
3. Current infecting organisms are proving resistant to standard first-line medications, and the resistant organisms develop because individuals with the disease fail to complete the course of treatment; surviving bacteria adapt to the medication and become resistant
4. Multidrug therapies are instituted because of the resistant organisms.
C. **Multidrug-resistant** strain of **tuberculosis (MDR-TB)**
1. Resistance occurs when a client receiving two medications (first- and second-line medications) discontinues one of the medications
2. The client briefly experiences some response from the single medication but then large numbers of resistant organisms begin to grow
3. The client, infectious again, transmits the drug-resistant organism to other individuals
4. As this event is repeated, an organism develops that is resistant to many of the first-line **tuberculosis** medications

XIII. FIRST-LINE MEDICATIONS FOR TUBERCULOSIS (Box 49-12)
A. Isoniazid (INH, Nydrazid)
1. Description
a. Isoniazid is bactericidal
b. It inhibits the synthesis of mycolic acids and acts to kill actively growing organisms in the extracellular environment
c. It inhibits the growth of dormant organisms in the macrophages and caseating granulomas
d. It is active only during cell division and is used in combination with other antitubercular medications
2. Contraindications and cautions
a. Isoniazid is contraindicated in clients with hypersensitivity or with acute liver disease
b. Use with caution in clients with chronic liver disease, alcoholism, or renal impairment
c. Use with caution in clients taking niacin/nicotinic acid (Nicobid)
d. Use with caution in clients taking hepatotoxic medications because the risk for hepatotoxicity increases
e. Alcohol increases the risk of hepatotoxicity
f. Isoniazid (INH) may increase the risk of toxicity of carbamazepine (Tegretol) and phenytoin (Dilantin)
g. Isoniazid (INH) may decrease ketoconazole (Nizoral) concentrations

BOX 49-12 **First- and Second-Line Medications for Tuberculosis**

First-Line Medications
Ethambutol (Myambutol)
Isoniazid (INH, Nydrazid)
Pyrazinamide (PZA)
Rifampin (Rifadin)
Rifapentine (Priftin)
Rifabutin (Mycobutin)
Second-Line Medications
Amikacin (Amikin)
Capreomycin (Capastat)
Cycloserine (Seromycin)
Ethionamide (Trecator)
Gatifloxacin (Tequin)
Kanamycin (Kantrex)
Levofloxacin (Levaquin)
Moxifloxacin (Avelox)
Para-aminosalicylic acid (Paser)
Streptomycin

3. Side effects
  a. Hypersensitivity reactions
  b. Peripheral neuritis
  c. Neurotoxicity
  d. Hepatotoxicity; elevated liver function test results
  e. Pyridoxine (vitamin B_6) deficiency
  f. Irritation at injection site with intramuscular administration
  g. Nausea and vomiting
  h. Dry mouth
  i. Dizziness
  j. Hyperglycemia
  k. Vision changes
  l. Hepatitis
4. Interventions
  a. Assess for hypersensitivity
  b. Assess for hepatic dysfunction
  c. Assess for sensitivity to niacin/nicotinic acid (Nicobid)
  d. Monitor liver function tests
  e. Monitor for signs of hepatitis, such as anorexia, nausea, vomiting, weakness, fatigue, dark urine, or jaundice; if these symptoms occur, withhold the medication and notify the physician
  f. Monitor for tingling, numbness, or burning of the extremities
  g. Assess mental status
  h. Monitor for visual changes, and notify the physician if they occur
  i. Assess for dizziness and initiate safety precautions
  j. Monitor complete blood count (CBC) and blood glucose levels

  k. Administer isoniazid 1 hour before or 2 hours after a meal because food may delay absorption
  l. Administer isoniazid at least 1 hour before antacids, especially those antacids that contain aluminum
  m. Administer pyridoxine as prescribed to reduce the risk of neurotoxicity
5. Client education
  a. Instruct the client not to skip doses and to take medication for the full length of the prescribed therapy
  b. Instruct the client not to take any other medication without consulting the physician
  c. Advise the client of the importance of follow-up physician visits, vision testing, and laboratory tests
  d. Instruct the client to avoid alcohol
  e. Advise the client to take medication on an empty stomach with 8 oz of water 1 hour before or 2 hours after meals and to avoid taking antacids with the medication
  f. Tell the client to avoid tyramine-containing foods because they may cause a reaction such as red and itching skin, a pounding heartbeat, lightheadedness, a hot or clammy feeling, or a headache; if any of these occur, the client should notify the physician
  g. Instruct the client on the signs of neurotoxicity, hepatitis, and hepatotoxicity
  h. Instruct the client to notify the physician if signs of neurotoxicity, hepatitis or hepatotoxicity, or visual changes occur.
B. Rifampin (Rifadin)
  1. Description
    a. Rifampin inhibits bacterial RNA synthesis
    b. It binds to DNA-dependent RNA polymerase and blocks RNA transcription
    c. It is used with at least one other antitubercular medication
  2. Contraindications and cautions
    a. Rifampin is contraindicated in clients with hypersensitivity
    b. It should be used with caution in clients with hepatic dysfunction or alcoholism
    c. Use of alcohol or hepatotoxic medications may increase the risk of hepatotoxicity
    d. Rifampin decreases the effects of several medications, including oral anticoagulants, oral hypoglycemics, chloramphenicol (Chloromycetin), digoxin (Lanoxin), disopyramide phosphate (Norpace), mexiletine (Mexitil), quinidine polygalacturonate (Cardioquin), tocainide hydrochloride (Tonocard), fluconazole (Diflucan), methadone hydrochloride (Dolophine), phenytoin (Dilantin), and verapamil hydrochloride (Calan)

3. Side effects
   a. Hypersensitivity reaction including fever, chills, shivering, headache, muscle and bone pain, and dyspnea
   b. Heartburn, nausea, vomiting, and diarrhea
   c. Red-orange body secretions
   d. Vision changes
   e. Hepatotoxicity and hepatitis
   f. Increased uric acid levels
   g. Blood dyscrasias
   h. Colitis
4. Interventions
   a. Assess for hypersensitivity
   b. Evaluate CBC, uric acid, and liver function tests
   c. Assess for signs of hepatitis; if they are found, withhold the medication and notify the physician
   d. Monitor stools for signs of colitis
   e. Monitor mental status
   f. Assess for visual changes
5. Client education
   a. Instruct the client not to skip doses and to take medication for the full length of the prescribed therapy
   b. Instruct the client not to take any other medication without consulting the physician
   c. Advise the client of the importance of follow-up physician visits and laboratory tests
   d. Instruct the client to avoid alcohol
   e. Advise the client to take medication on an empty stomach with 8 oz of water 1 hour before or 2 hours after meals and to avoid taking antacids with the medication
   f. Instruct the client that urine, feces, sweat, and tears will be red-orange and that soft contact lenses can become permanently discolored
   g. Instruct the client to notify the physician if jaundice (yellow eyes or skin) develops or if weakness, fatigue, nausea, vomiting, sore throat, fever, or unusual bleeding occurs

C. Ethambutol (Myambutol)
   1. Description
      a. Ethambutol is bacteriostatic
      b. It interferes with cell metabolism and multiplication by inhibiting one or more metabolites in susceptible organism in susceptible organisms
      c. It inhibits bacterial RNA synthesis and is active only during cell division
      d. Ethambutol is slow acting and must be used with other bactericidal agents
   2. Contraindications and cautions
      a. Ethambutol is contraindicated in clients with hypersensitivity or optic neuritis and in children less than 13 years of age.
      b. Use with caution in clients with renal dysfunction, gout, ocular defects, diabetic retinopathy, cataracts, or ocular inflammatory conditions
      c. Use with caution in clients taking neurotoxic medications because the risk for neurotoxicity increases
   3. Side effects
      a. Hypersensitivity reactions
      b. Anorexia, nausea, and vomiting
      c. Dizziness
      d. Malaise
      e. Mental confusion
      f. Joint pain
      g. Dermatitis
      h. Optic neuritis
      i. Peripheral neuritis
      j. Thrombocytopenia
      k. Increased uric acid levels
      l. Anaphylactoid reaction
   4. Interventions
      a. Assess the client for hypersensitivity
      b. Evaluate results of CBC, uric acid, and renal and liver function tests
      c. Obtain baseline visual acuity and color discrimination, especially to green
      d. Monitor for visual changes such as altered color perception and decreased visual acuity; if changes occur, withhold the medication and notify the physician
      e. Administer once every 24 hours and administer with food to decrease gastrointestinal upset
      f. Monitor uric acid concentrations and assess for painful or swollen joints or signs of gout
      g. Monitor I&O and for adequate renal function
      h. Assess mental status
      i. Monitor for dizziness and initiate safety precautions
      j. Assess for peripheral neuritis (numbness, tingling, or burning of the extremities); if it occurs, notify the physician
   5. Client education
      a. Inform the client that he or she can prevent nausea related to the medication by taking the daily dose at bedtime or by taking the prescribed antinausea medications
      b. Instruct the client not to skip doses and to take the medication for the full length of the prescribed therapy
      c. Instruct the client not to take any other medication without consulting the physician
      d. Advise the client of the importance of follow-up physician visits, vision testing, and laboratory tests

e. Instruct the client to notify the physician immediately if any of the following occur: visual problems; a rash; swelling and pain in the joints; or numbness, tingling, or burning in the hands or feet

D. Pyrazinamide (PZA)

1. Description
   a. The exact mechanism of action of pyrazinamide is unknown
   b. Pyrazinamide may be bacteriostatic or bactericidal, depending on its concentration at the infection site and susceptibility of infecting organism
   c. It is used with at least one other antitubercular medication after failure or ineffectiveness of the primary medications occurs

2. Contraindications and cautions
   a. Pyrazinamide is contraindicated in clients with hypersensitivity
   b. Use pyrazinamide with caution in clients with diabetes mellitus, renal impairment, or gout, as well as in children
   c. Pyrazinamide may decrease the effects of allopurinol (Zyloprim), colchicine, probenecid (Benemid), and sulfinpyrazone (Anturane)
   d. Cross-sensitivity is possible with isoniazid (INH), ethionamide (Trecator) or niacin/nicotinic acid (Nicobid)

3. Side effects
   a. Increases liver function and uric acid levels
   b. Arthralgia and myalgia
   c. Photosensitivity
   d. Hepatotoxicity
   e. Thrombocytopenia

4. Interventions
   a. Assess for hypersensitivity
   b. Evaluate CBC, liver function tests, and uric acid levels
   c. Observe for hepatotoxic effects; if they occur, withhold the medication and notify the physician.
   d. Assess for painful or swollen joints
   e. Evaluate blood glucose levels because diabetes mellitus may be difficult to control while the client is taking the medication

5. Client education
   a. Instruct the client to take the medication with food to reduce gastrointestinal distress
   b. Instruct the client to avoid sunlight or ultraviolet light until photosensitivity is determined
   c. Instruct the client to notify the physician if any side effects occur
   d. Instruct the client not to skip doses and to take the medication for the full length of the prescribed therapy

e. Instruct the client not to take any other medication without consulting the physician
f. Advise the client of the importance of follow-up physician visits and laboratory tests

E. Rifabutin (Mycobutin)

1. Description
   a. Inhibits mycobacterial DNA-dependent RNA polymerase and suppresses protein synthesis
   b. Used to prevent disseminated *Mycobacterium avium* complex (MAC) disease in clients with advanced HIV infection
   c. Used to treat active MAC disease and **tuberculosis** in clients with HIV infection

2. Cautions
   a. Can affect blood levels of some medications including oral contraceptives and some medications used to treat HIV infection
   b. A nonhormonal method of birth control should be used instead of an oral contraceptive

3. Side effects
   a. Rash
   b. GI disturbances
   c. Neutropenia
   d. Red-orange body secretions
   e. Uveitis
   f. Myositis
   g. Arthralgia
   h. Hepatitis
   i. Chest pain with dyspnea
   j. Flu-like syndrome

4. Interventions
   a. Assess medication history of the client
   b. Observe for hepatotoxic effects; if they occur, withhold the medication and notify the physician
   c. Assess for painful or swollen joints
   d. Assess for ocular pain or blurred vision

5. Client education
   a. Instruct the client to take the medication without regard to food
   b. Instruct the client to notify the physician if any side effects occur
   c. Instruct the client not to skip doses and to take the medication for the full length of the prescribed therapy
   d. Instruct the client not to take any other medication without consulting the physician
   e. Advise the client of the importance of follow-up physician visits and laboratory tests.

F. Rifapentine (Priftin)

1. Description: used only for pulmonary **tuberculosis**
2. Cautions: can affect blood levels of some medications, including oral contraceptives, warfarin (Coumadin), and some medications used to treat HIV infection

3. Side effects
   a. Red-orange body secretions
   b. Hepatotoxicity
4. Interventions
   a. Assess medication history of the client
   b. Obtain baseline liver function studies throughout therapy
   c. Observe for hepatotoxic effects; if they occur, withhold the medication and notify the physician
5. Client education
   a. Instruct the client to take the medication without regard to food
   b. Instruct the client to notify the physician if any side effects occur
   c. Instruct the client not to skip doses and to take the medication for the full length of the prescribed therapy
   d. Instruct the client not to take any other medication without first onsulting the physician
   e. Advise the client of the importance of follow-up physician visits and laboratory tests

XIV. SECOND-LINE MEDICATIONS FOR TUBERCULOSIS

A. Capreomycin sulfate (Capastat Sulfate)
1. Description
   a. Mechanism of action for capreomycin is unknown
   b. Used to treat MDR-TB when significant resistance to other medications is expected.
   c. Capreomycin must be given intramuscularly
2. Contraindications and cautions
   a. The risk of nephrotoxicity, ototoxicity, and neuromuscular blockade is increased with the use of aminoglycosides or loop diuretics
   b. Use capreomycin with caution in clients with renal insufficiency, acoustic nerve impairment, hepatic disorder, myasthenia gravis, or parkinsonism
   c. Do not administer to clients receiving streptomycin
3. Side effects
   a. Nephrotoxicity
   b. Ototoxicity
   c. Neuromuscular blockade
4. Interventions
   a. Perform baseline audiometric testing
   b. Assess renal, hepatic, and electrolyte levels before administration
   c. Monitor I&O
   d. Reconstituted medication may be stored for 48 hours at room temperature
   e. Administer intramuscularly deep in a large muscle mass

f. Rotate injection sites
g. Observe injection site for redness, excessive bleeding, and inflammation
5. Client education
   a. Instruct the client not to perform tasks that require mental alertness
   b. Instruct the client to report any hearing loss, balance disturbances, respiratory difficulty, weakness, or signs of hypersensitivity reactions

B. Kanamycin (Kantrex) and amikacin (Amikin)
1. Description
   a. Aminoglycoside antibiotics given with at least one other antitubercular medication
   b. These medications are bactericidal because of receptor-binding action, interfering with protein synthesis in susceptible micro-organisms
2. Contraindications and cautions
   a. Contraindicated in clients with hypersensitivity, neuromuscular disorders, or eighth cranial nerve damage.
   b. Used with caution in the older client, in neonates because of renal insufficiency and immaturity, and in young infants because it may cause CNS depression
   c. The risk of toxicity increases if taken with other aminoglycosides or nephrotoxicity- or ototoxicity-producing medications
3. Side effects
   a. Hypersensitivity
   b. Pain and irritation at the injection site
   c. Nephrotoxicity as evidenced by increased blood urea nitrogen and serum creatinine levels
   d. Ototoxicity as evidenced by tinnitus, dizziness, ringing/roaring in the ears, and reduced hearing
   e. Neurotoxicity as evidenced by headache, dizziness, lethargy, tremors, and visual disturbances
   f. Superinfections
4. Interventions
   a. Assess for hypersensitivity
   b. Monitor for ototoxic, neurotoxic, and nephrotoxic reactions
   c. Monitor liver and renal function tests
   d. Obtain baseline audiometric test and repeat every 1 to 2 months because the medication impairs the eighth cranial nerve
   e. Assess acuteness of hearing
   f. Monitor for visual changes
   g. Assess hydration status and maintain adequate hydration during therapy
   h. Monitor I&O
   i. Assess urinalysis
   j. Monitor for superinfection

5. Client education
   a. Instruct the client not to skip doses and to take medication for the full length of the prescribed therapy
   b. Instruct the client not to take any other medication without consulting the physician
   c. Advise the client of the importance of follow-up physician visits and laboratory tests
   d. Instruct the client to notify the physician if hearing loss, changes in vision, or urinary problems occur

C. Ethionamide (Trecator)
   1. Description
      a. Mechanism of action for ethionamide is unknown
      b. Ethionamide is used to treat MDR-TB when significant resistance to other medications is expected
   2. Contraindications and cautions
      a. Ethionamide is contraindicated in clients with hypersensitivity
      b. Use ethionamide with caution in clients with diabetes mellitus or renal dysfunction
   3. Side effects
      a. Anorexia, nausea, and vomiting
      b. Metallic taste in the mouth
      c. Orthostatic hypotension
      d. Jaundice
      e. Mental changes
      f. Peripheral neuritis
      g. Rash
   4. Interventions
      a. Assess liver and renal function tests
      b. Monitor glucose levels in the client with diabetes mellitus
      c. Administer pyridoxine as prescribed to reduce the risk of neurotoxicity
   5. Client education
      a. Instruct the client to take medication with food or meals to minimize gastrointestinal irritation
      b. Instruct the client to change positions slowly
      c. Instruct the client to report signs of a rash, which can progress to exfoliative dermatitis if the medication is not discontinued
      d. Instruct the client to avoid alcohol
      e. Instruct the client to report signs of jaundice and other side effects of the medication if they occur

D. Para-aminosalicylic acid (Paser)
   1. Description
      a. Para-aminosalicylic acid inhibits folic acid metabolism in mycobacteria
      b. It is used to treat MDR-TB when significant resistance to other medications is expected

2. Contraindications and cautions
   a. Contraindicated with hypersensitivity to aminosalicylates, salicylates, or compounds containing para-aminophenyl group
   b. Aminobenzoates block the absorption of aminosalicylate sodium
3. Side effects
   a. Hypersensitivity
   b. Bitter taste in the mouth
   c. Gastrointestinal tract irritation
   d. Exfoliative dermatitis
   e. Blood dyscrasias
   f. Crystalluria
   g. Changes in thyroid function
4. Interventions
   a. Assess for hypersensitivity
   b. Offer clear water to rinse the mouth and chewing gum or hard candy to alleviate the bitter taste
   c. Encourage fluid intake to prevent crystalluria
   d. Monitor I&O
5. Client education
   a. Instruct the client to discard the medication and obtain a new supply if a purplish-brown discoloration occurs
   b. Instruct the client to take the medication with food
   c. Inform the client that urine may turn red on contact with hypochlorite bleach if bleach was used to clean a toilet
   d. Instruct the client not to take aspirin or over-the-counter medications without the physician's approval
   e. Instruct the client to report signs of a blood dyscrasia (e.g., sore throat or mouth, malaise, fatigue, bruising, or bleeding)

E. Cycloserine (Seromycin)
   1. Description
      a. Cycloserine interferes with cell wall biosynthesis
      b. It is used to treat MDR-TB when significant resistance to other medications is expected
   2. Contraindications and cautions
      a. Use of alcohol or ethionamide (Trecator) increases the risk of seizures
      b. Use cycloserine with caution in clients with epilepsy, depression, severe anxiety, psychosis, or renal insufficiency, or in clients who use alcohol
   3. Side effects
      a. Hypersensitivity
      b. CNS reactions
      c. Neurotoxicity
      d. Seizures
      e. Congestive heart failure
      f. Headache

g. Vertigo

h. Altered level of consciousness

i. Irritability, nervousness, and anxiety

j. Confusion

k. Mood changes, depression, or thoughts of suicide

4. Interventions

a. Monitor level of consciousness

b. Monitor for changes in mental status and thought processes

c. Monitor renal and hepatic function tests

d. Monitor serum drug level to avoid the risk of neurotoxicity; peak concentrations, measured 2 hours after dosing, should be 25 to 35 mcg/mL

5. Client education

a. Instruct the client to take the medication after meals to prevent gastrointestinal upset

b. Instruct the client to avoid alcohol

c. Instruct the client to report signs of a rash or signs of CNS toxicity

d. Instruct the client to avoid driving or performing tasks that require alertness until the reaction to the medication has been determined

e. Advise the client of the need for serum drug levels weekly, as prescribed

F. Streptomycin

1. Description

a. Streptomycin is an aminoglycoside antibiotic used with at least one other antitubercular medication

b. It is bactericidal because of receptor-binding action that interferes with protein synthesis in susceptible organisms

2. Contraindications and cautions

a. Streptomycin is contraindicated in clients with hypersensitivity, myasthenia gravis, parkinsonism, or eighth cranial nerve damage

b. Use streptomycin with caution in the older client, in neonates because of renal insufficiency and immaturity, and in young infants because the medication may cause CNS depression

c. The risk of toxicity increases when streptomycin is taken with other aminoglycosides or nephrotoxicity- or ototoxicity-producing medications

3. Side effects (Box 49-13)

a. Hypersensitivity

b. Visual changes

c. Elevated liver and renal function test results

d. Peripheral neuritis such as burning of the face or mouth

4. Interventions

a. Assess for hypersensitivity

b. Monitor liver and renal function tests

c. Monitor for ototoxic, neurotoxic, and nephrotoxic reactions

d. Obtain baseline audiometric test and repeat every l to 2 months because the medication impairs the eighth cranial nerve

e. Assess hearing acuity

f. Monitor for visual changes

g. Assess hydration status and maintain adequate hydration during therapy

h. Monitor I&O

i. Assess urinalysis results

j. Monitor for signs of peripheral neuritis

5. Client education

a. Instruct the client not to skip doses and to take medication for the full length of the prescribed therapy

b. Instruct the client not to take any other medication without consulting the physician

c. Advise the client of the importance of follow-up physician visits and laboratory tests

d. Instruct the client to notify the physician if hearing loss, changes in vision, or urinary problems occur

G. Levofloxacin (Levaquin), moxifloxacin (Avelox), gatifloxacin (Tequin)

1. Fluoroquinolones that are used for a wide variety of infections and are active against *Mycobacterium tuberculosis*

2. Used for infections caused by **multidrug-resistant** organisms

3. Gastrointestinal disturbances are the most common side effect

4. Not recommended for use in children

BOX 49-13 **Side Effects of Streptomycin**

Nephrotoxicity
Changes in urine output
Decreased appetite
Increased thirst
Nausea, vomiting
Neurotoxicity
Muscle numbness
Seizures
Tingling
Twitching
Vestibular Ototoxicity
Clumsiness
Dizziness
Unsteadiness
Auditory Ototoxicity
A full feeling in the ears
Ringing in the ears
Loss of hearing

▲ XV. INFLUENZA MEDICATIONS
▲ A. Vaccines (Box 49-14)
1. Description
   a. The strain of influenza virus differs every year, so annual vaccination is recommended (usually in October or November of each year)
   b. Vaccine is available as inactivated influenza vaccine administered intramuscularly or as a live attenuated influenza vaccine, which is administered nasally
2. Contraindications and cautions
   a. Contraindications of the inactivated vaccine include hypersensitivity, chicken egg allergy, active infection, Guillain-Barré syndrome, active febrile illness, and children less than 6 months of age.
   b. Contraindications of the live attenuated vaccine include age less than 5 years or greater than 50, pregnant women, children or adolescents on long-term aspirin therapy, and those with severe nasal congestion or long-term conditions such as asthma; diabetes mellitus; anemia or blood disorders; or heart, kidney, or lung disease
3. Side effects
   a. Side effects of the inactivated vaccine include localized pain and swelling at the injection site, general body aches and pains, malaise, and fever
   b. Side effects of the attenuated vaccine include runny nose or nasal congestion, cough, headache, and sore throat
4. Interventions
   a. The intramuscular route is recommended for the inactivated vaccine; adults and older children should be vaccinated in the deltoid muscle

b. Monitor for side effects of the vaccine
c. Monitor for hypersensitivity reactions in clients receiving vaccination for the first time
5. Client education
   a. Instruct the client on the importance of an annual vaccination
   b. Instruct the client that the inactivated vaccine contains noninfectious killed viruses and cannot cause influenza
   c. Instruct the client that any respiratory disease unrelated to influenza can occur after the vaccination
   d. Instruct the client who received the attenuated vaccine that the virus may be shed up to 2 days after vaccination
   e. Instruct the client that development of antibodies in adults takes approximately 2 weeks
B. Antiviral medications (Box 49-15) ▲
1. Description
   a. Antiviral medication use during outbreaks of influenza depends on the current strain of influenza.
   b. Diagnosis of influenza should include rapid diagnostic tests because symptoms of infection from other pathogens may cause similar symptoms of influenza infection
   c. Influenza antivirals may also be administered as prophylaxis against infection but should not replace vaccination
2. Contraindication and cautions
   a. Antiviral medications are contraindicated in hypersensitivity
3. Side effects
   a. Common side effects include headache, dizziness, fatigue, nausea, and vomiting
   b. Some side effects depend on the medication (Table 49-1)

BOX 49-14 **Influenza Vaccines**

Inactivated (Intramuscular Administration)
Fluarix
Fluvirin
Fluzone
Live Attenuated (Nasal Administration)
FluMist

BOX 49-15 **Influenza Antiviral Medications**

Amantadine (Symmetrel)
Oseltamivir (Tamiflu)
Rimantadine (Flumadine)
Zanamivir (Relenza)

TABLE 49-1 **Side Effects of Influenza Antiviral Medications**

Antiviral Medication	Side Effects
Amantadine (Symmetrel)	Drowsiness, anxiety, psychosis, depression, hallucinations, tremors, confusion, insomnia, orthostatic hypotension, heart failure, blurred vision, constipation, dry mouth, urinary frequency and retention, leukopenia, photosensitivity, dermatitis
Oseltamivir (Tamiflu)	Insomnia, diarrhea, abdominal pain, cough
Rimantadine (Flumadine)	Depression, hallucinations, tremors, seizures, insomnia, poor concentration, asthenia, gait abnormalities, anxiety, confusion, pallor, palpitations, hypotension, edema, tinnitus, eye pain, constipation, dry mouth, anorexia, abdominal pain, diarrhea, dyspepsia, rash
Zanamivir (Relenza)	Ear, nose, throat infections; diarrhea; nasal symptoms; cough; sinusitis; bronchitis

4. Interventions
   a. Administer within 2 days of onset of the symptoms and continue for entire prescription
   b. Monitor for side effects of specific medications

5. Client education
   a. Teach the client that the medication may not prevent the transmission of influenza to others
   b. Adjust activities if dizziness or fatigue occurs
   c. Instruct the client about management of side effects of various medications
   d. Instruct the client to take medication exactly as prescribed and for the duration of the prescription

XVI. PNEUMOCOCCAL CONJUGATE VACCINE

A. Pneumococcal conjugate vaccine (PCV, Prevnar) is used for the prevention of invasive pneumococcal disease in infants and children
B. Pneumococcal polysaccharide vaccine (PPV, Pneumovax) is used for adults and high-risk children over the age of 2 years
C. Side effects may include erythema, swelling, pain, and tenderness at the injection site; fever; irritability, drowsiness, and reduced appetite
D. Refer to Chapter 38 for additional information about vaccines

PRACTICE QUESTIONS

More questions on the companion CD!

613. A client is receiving acetylcysteine (Mucomyst), 20% solution diluted in 0.9% normal saline by nebulizer. The nurse should have which item available for possible use after giving this medication?
   1. Ambu bag
   2. Intubation tray
   3. Nasogastric tube
   4. Suction equipment

614. A client has an order to take guaifenesin (Humibid) every 4 hours, as needed. The nurse determines that the client understands the most effective use of this medication if the client states that he or she will:
   1. Watch for irritability as a side effect
   2. Take the tablet with a full glass of water
   3. Take an extra dose if the cough is accompanied by fever
   4. Crush the sustained-release tablet if immediate relief is needed

615. A postoperative client has received a dose of naloxone hydrochloride for respiratory depression shortly after transfer to the nursing unit from the postanesthesia care unit. Following

administration of the medication, the nurse checks the client for:
   1. Pupillary changes
   2. Scattered lung wheezes
   3. Sudden increase in pain
   4. Sudden episodes of diarrhea

616. A client has been taking isoniazid (INH) for 2 months. The client complains to a nurse about numbness, paresthesias, and tingling in the extremities. The nurse interprets that the client is experiencing:
   1. Hypercalcemia
   2. Peripheral neuritis
   3. Small blood vessel spasm
   4. Impaired peripheral circulation

617. A client is to begin a 6-month course of therapy with isoniazid (INH). A nurse plans to teach the client to:
   1. Drink alcohol in small amounts only
   2. Report yellow eyes or skin immediately
   3. Increase intake of Swiss or aged cheeses
   4. Avoid vitamin supplements during therapy

618. A client has been started on long-term therapy with rifampin (Rifadin). A nurse teaches the client that the medication:
   1. Should always be taken with food or antacids
   2. Should be double-dosed if one dose is forgotten
   3. Causes orange discoloration of sweat, tears, urine, and feces
   4. May be discontinued independently if symptoms are gone in 3 months

619. A nurse has given a client taking ethambutol (Myambutol) information about the medication. The nurse determines that the client understands the instructions if the client states that he or she will immediately report:
   1. Impaired sense of hearing
   2. Problems with visual acuity
   3. Gastrointestinal (GI) side effects
   4. Orange-red discoloration of body secretions

620. Cycloserine (Seromycin) is added to the medication regimen for a client with tuberculosis. Which of the following would the nurse include in the client-teaching plan regarding this medication?
   1. To take the medication before meals
   2. It is not necessary to call the physician if a skin rash occurs
   3. To return to the clinic weekly for serum drug–level testing
   4. It is not necessary to restrict alcohol intake with this medication

621. A client with tuberculosis is being started on anti-tuberculosis therapy with isoniazid (INH). Before giving the client the first dose, a nurse ensures that which of the following baseline studies has been completed?

1. Electrolyte levels
2. Coagulation times
3. Liver enzyme levels
4. Serum creatinine level

622. A nurse has an order to give a client metaproterenol sulfate (Alupent) (two puffs), and beclomethasone dipropionate (Qvar) (nasal inhalation two puffs), by metered-dose inhaler. The nurse administers the medication by giving the:
    1. Metaproterenol first and then the beclomethasone dipropionate
    2. Beclomethasone dipropionate first and then the metaproterenol
    3. Alternating a single puff of each, beginning with the metaproterenol
    4. Alternating a single puff of each, beginning with the beclomethasone dipropionate

623. A client has begun therapy with theophylline (Theo-24). The nurse tells the client to limit the intake of which of the following while taking this medication?
    1. Oranges and pineapple
    2. Coffee, cola, and chocolate
    3. Oysters, lobster, and shrimp
    4. Cottage cheese, cream cheese, and dairy creamers

624. A client with an order to take theophylline (Theolair-SR) daily has been given medication instructions by the nurse. The nurse determines that the client needs further information about the medication if the client states that he or she will:
    1. Drink at least 2 L fluid per day
    2. Take the daily dose at bedtime
    3. Avoid changing brands of the medication without physician approval

4. Avoid over-the-counter (OTC) cough and cold medications unless approved by the physician

625. A client is taking cetirizine hydrochloride (Zyrtec). The nurse checks for which of the following side effects of this medication?
    1. Diarrhea
    2. Excitability
    3. Drowsiness
    4. Excess salivation

626. A client taking fexofenadine (Allegra) is scheduled for allergy skin testing and tells the nurse in the physician's office that a dose was taken this morning. The nurse determines that:
    1. The client should reschedule the appointment
    2. A lower dose of allergen will need to be injected
    3. A higher dose of allergen will need to be injected
    4. The client should have the skin test read a day later than usual

ALTERNATE ITEM FORMAT: MULTIPLE RESPONSE

627. Rifabutin (Mycobutin) is prescribed for a client with active *Mycobacterium avium* complex (MAC) disease and tuberculosis. The nurse monitors for which side effects of the medication? Select all that apply.
    ☐ 1. Signs of hepatitis
    ☐ 2. Flu-like syndrome
    ☐ 3. Low neutrophil count
    ☐ 4. Vitamin B$_6$ deficiency
    ☐ 5. Ocular pain or blurred vision
    ☐ 6. Tingling and numbness of the fingers

ANSWERS

613. **4**
Rationale: Acetylcysteine can be given orally or by nasogastric tube to treat acetaminophen overdose, or it may be given by inhalation for use as a mucolytic. The nurse administering this medication as a mucolytic should have suction equipment available in case the client cannot manage to clear the increased volume of liquefied secretions.
Test-Taking Strategy: To answer this question, it is necessary to know that acetylcysteine may be given for either acetaminophen overdose or as a mucolytic agent. It is also necessary to know that the inhalation route is only used for mucolytic effects. With this in mind, options 1 and 2 are eliminated because the client does not need resuscitation. Option 3 is eliminated as well, since a nasogastric tube may be used in the client with acetaminophen overdose. If you had difficulty with this question, review the purpose of this medication and the related nursing interventions.
Level of Cognitive Ability: Application
Client Needs: Physiological Integrity

Integrated Process: Nursing Process/Implementation
Content Area: Pharmacology
Reference: Skidmore-Roth, L. (2005). *Mosby's drug guide for nurses* (6th ed., p. 10). St. Louis: Mosby.

614. **2**
Rationale: Guaifenesin is an expectorant. It should be taken with a full glass of water to decrease viscosity of secretions. Sustained-release preparations should not be broken open, crushed, or chewed. The medication may occasionally cause dizziness, headache, or drowsiness as side effects. The client should contact the physician if the cough lasts longer than 1 week or is accompanied by fever, rash, sore throat, or persistent headache.
Test-Taking Strategy: Use the process of elimination. Begin to answer this question by eliminating option 4 first. Sustained-released preparations are not crushed or broken. Option 3 is eliminated next, because fever indicates infection, and an "extra dose" of an expectorant is not helpful in treating infection. From the remaining options, recalling that increased

fluids help liquefy secretions for more effective coughing will direct you to option 2. Review this medication if you had difficulty with this question.
Level of Cognitive Ability: Analysis
Client Needs: Physiological Integrity
Integrated Process: Nursing Process/Evaluation
Content Area: Pharmacology
References: Skidmore-Roth, L. (2008). 2008 *Mosby's nursing drug reference* (21st ed., p. 521). St. Louis: Mosby.
Skidmore-Roth, L. (2005). *Mosby's drug guide for nurses* (6th ed., p. 410). St. Louis: Mosby.

615. **3**
Rationale: Naloxone hydrochloride is an antidote to opioids and may also be given to the postoperative client to treat respiratory depression. When given to the postoperative client for respiratory depression, it may also reverse the effects of analgesics. Therefore, the nurse must check the client for a sudden increase in the level of pain experienced. Options 1, 2, and 4 are not associated with this medication.
Test-Taking Strategy: Use the process of elimination. Recalling that this medication is an antidote to opioid analgesics will assist in directing you to option 3. Remember that this medication will cause sudden pain in the postoperative client or return of pain in the client who received opioid analgesics. If you had difficulty with this question, review this medication.
Level of Cognitive Ability: Application
Client Needs: Physiological Integrity
Integrated Process: Nursing Process/Data Collection
Content Area: Pharmacology
Reference: Skidmore-Roth, L. (2008). 2008 *Mosby's nursing drug reference* (21st ed., pp. 717-718). St. Louis: Mosby.

616. **2**
Rationale: A common side effect of INH is peripheral neuritis. This is manifested by numbness, tingling, and paresthesias in the extremities. This side effect can be minimized by pyridoxine (vitamin B_6) intake. Options 1, 3, and 4 are incorrect.
Test-Taking Strategy: Use the process of elimination. Options 3 and 4 would not cause the symptoms presented in the question, but instead would cause pallor and coolness. From the remaining options, you should know either that peripheral neuritis is a side effect of the medication or that these signs and symptoms do not correlate with hypercalcemia. Review the side effects associated with INH if you had difficulty with this question.
Level of Cognitive Ability: Analysis
Client Needs: Physiological Integrity
Integrated Process: Nursing Process/Data Collection
Content Area: Pharmacology
Reference: Lehne, R. (2007). *Pharmacology for nursing care* (6th ed., p. 1020). Philadelphia: Saunders.

617. **2**
Rationale: INH is hepatotoxic, and therefore the client is taught to report signs and symptoms of hepatitis immediately (which include yellow skin and sclera). For the same reason, alcohol should be avoided during therapy. The client should avoid intake of Swiss cheese, fish such as tuna, and foods containing tyramine because they may cause a reaction

characterized by redness and itching of the skin, flushing, sweating, tachycardia, headache, or lightheadedness. The client can avoid developing peripheral neuritis by increasing the intake of pyridoxine (vitamin B_6) during the course of INH therapy.
Test-Taking Strategy: Use the process of elimination. Alcohol intake is avoided when the client is taking a prescribed medication, so option 1 should be eliminated first. Because the client receiving this medication typically is supplemented with vitamin B_6, option 4 is incorrect and is eliminated next. From the remaining options, recalling that the medication is hepatotoxic will direct you to option 2. If you had difficulty with this question, review this medication.
Level of Cognitive Ability: Application
Client Needs: Physiological Integrity
Integrated Process: Teaching and Learning
Content Area: Pharmacology
Reference: Lehne, R. (2007). *Pharmacology for nursing care* (6th ed., p. 1020). Philadelphia: Saunders.

618. **3**
Rationale: Rifampin should be taken exactly as directed. Doses should not be doubled or skipped. The client should not stop therapy until directed to do so by a physician. The medication should be administered on an empty stomach unless it causes gastrointestinal upset, and then it may be taken with food. Antacids, if prescribed, should be taken at least 1 hour before the medication. Rifampin causes orange-red discoloration of body secretions and will permanently stain soft contact lenses.
Test-Taking Strategy: Use the process of elimination. Use of general medication administration principles will assist in eliminating options 2 and 4. Eliminate option 1 next because of the close-ended word "always." If you had difficulty with this question, review the side effects associated with this medication.
Level of Cognitive Ability: Application
Client Needs: Physiological Integrity
Integrated Process: Teaching and Learning
Content Area: Pharmacology
Reference: Lehne, R. (2007). *Pharmacology for nursing care* (6th ed., p. 1021). Philadelphia: Saunders.

619. **2**
Rationale: Ethambutol causes optic neuritis, which decreases visual acuity and the ability to discriminate between the colors red and green. This poses a potential safety hazard when a client is driving a motor vehicle. The client is taught to report this symptom immediately. The client is also taught to take the medication with food if GI upset occurs. Impaired hearing results from antitubercular therapy with streptomycin. Orange-red discoloration of secretions occurs with rifampin (Rifadin).
Test-Taking Strategy: Use the process of elimination. Option 3 is the least likely symptom to report; rather, it should be managed by taking the medication with food. To select from the other options, it is necessary to know that this medication causes optic neuritis, resulting in difficulty with red-green discrimination. If you had difficulty with this question, review antitubercular medications.
Level of Cognitive Ability: Analysis

Client Needs: Physiological Integrity
Integrated Process: Nursing Process/Evaluation
Content Area: Pharmacology
Reference: Skidmore-Roth, L. (2008). *2008 Mosby's nursing drug reference* (21st ed., p. 441). St. Louis: Mosby.

620. **3**
Rationale: Cycloserine (Seromycin) is an antitubercular medication that requires weekly serum drug level determinations to monitor for the potential of neurotoxicity. Serum drug levels lower than 30 mcg/mL reduce the incidence of neurotoxicity. The medication needs to be taken after meals to prevent gastrointestinal irritation. The client needs to be instructed to notify the physician if a skin rash or signs of central nervous system toxicity are noted. Alcohol needs to be avoided because it increases the risk of seizure activity.
Test-Taking Strategy: Use the process of elimination. Eliminate options 2 and 4 first, using guidelines related to general medication administration principles. From this point, knowing that the medication level needs to be monitored will assist in selecting the correct option. If you had difficulty with this question, review this medication.
Level of Cognitive Ability: Application
Client Needs: Physiological Integrity
Integrated Process: Teaching and Learning
Content Area: Pharmacology
Reference: Lehne, R. (2007). *Pharmacology for nursing care* (6th ed., p. 1028). Philadelphia: Saunders.

621. **3**
Rationale: INH therapy can cause an elevation of hepatic enzyme levels and hepatitis. Therefore, liver enzyme levels are monitored when therapy is initiated and during the first 3 months of therapy. They may be monitored longer in the client who is over age 50 or abuses alcohol.
Test-Taking Strategy: Use the process of elimination. In order to answer this question correctly, it is necessary to know that this medication can be toxic to the liver. Review the adverse effects of the various antituberculosis medications if this is an area that is unfamiliar to you.
Level of Cognitive Ability: Analysis
Client Needs: Physiological Integrity
Integrated Process: Nursing Process/Data Collection
Content Area: Pharmacology
Reference: Lehne, R. (2007). *Pharmacology for nursing care* (6th ed., pp. 1018-1019). Philadelphia: Saunders.

622. **1**
Rationale: Metaproterenol is a bronchodilator. Beclomethasone dipropionate is a glucocorticoid. Bronchodilators are always administered before glucocorticoids when both are to be given on the same time schedule. This allows for widening of the air passages by the bronchodilator, which then makes the glucocorticoid more effective.
Test-Taking Strategy: To answer this question correctly, it is necessary to know two different things. First, you must know that a bronchodilator is always given before a glucocorticoid. This would allow you to eliminate options 3 and 4 because you would not alternate single puffs of the medications. To select between options 1 and 2, it is necessary to know that metaproterenol is a bronchodilator, whereas beclomethasone

is a glucocorticoid. Review these medications if you had difficulty with this question.
Level of Cognitive Ability: Application
Client Needs: Physiological Integrity
Integrated Process: Nursing Process/Implementation
Content Area: Pharmacology
Reference: Kee, J., Hayes, E., & McCuistion, L. (2006). *Pharmacology: A nursing process approach.* (5th ed., p. 595). Philadelphia: Saunders.

623. **2**
Rationale: Theophylline is a xanthine bronchodilator. The nurse teaches the client to limit the intake of xanthine-containing foods while taking this medication. These include coffee, cola, and chocolate.
Test-Taking Strategy: Focus on the name of the medication to determine that theophylline is a xanthine bronchodilator. Recalling which food items are naturally high in xanthines will direct you to option 2. Review the foods naturally high in xanthines if you had difficulty with this question.
Level of Cognitive Ability: Application
Client Needs: Physiological Integrity
Integrated Process: Nursing Process/Implementation
Content Area: Pharmacology
References: Lehne, R. (2007). *Pharmacology for nursing care* (6th ed., p. 882). Philadelphia: Saunders.
Lilley, L., Harrington, S., & Snyder J. (2007). *Pharmacology and the nursing process* (5th ed., p. 263). St. Louis: Mosby.

624. **2**
Rationale: The client taking a single daily dose of theophylline, a xanthine bronchodilator, should take the medication early in the morning. This enables the client to have maximal benefit from the medication during daytime activities. In addition, this medication causes insomnia. The client should take in at least 2 L of fluid per day to decrease viscosity of secretions. The client should check with the physician before changing brands of the medication. The client also checks with the physician before taking OTC cough, cold, or other respiratory preparations because they could cause interactive effects, increasing the side effects of theophylline and causing dysrhythmias.
Test-Taking Strategy: Use the process of elimination. Note the strategic words "needs further information." These words indicate a negative event query and the need to select the incorrect client statement. General principles related to medication therapy will assist in eliminating options 3 and 4. In addition, recalling that option 1 is an important measure to thin secretions will direct you to option 2. Review this medication if you had difficulty with this question.
Level of Cognitive Ability: Analysis
Client Needs: Physiological Integrity
Integrated Process: Teaching and Learning
Content Area: Pharmacology
Reference: Lilley, L., Harrington, S., & Snyder J. (2007). *Pharmacology and the nursing process* (5th ed., p. 263). St. Louis: Mosby.

625. **3**
Rationale: A frequent side effect of cetirizine hydrochloride, an antihistamine, is drowsiness or sedation. Others include

blurred vision, hypertension (and sometimes hypotension), dry mouth, constipation, urinary retention, and sweating.
Test-Taking Strategy: Focus on the name of the medication to determine that this is an antihistamine. Recalling that antihistamines typically cause drowsiness will direct you to option 3. Review the side effects of antihistamines if you had difficulty with this question.
Level of Cognitive Ability: Application
Client Needs: Physiological Integrity
Integrated Process: Nursing Process/Data Collection
Content Area: Pharmacology
Reference: Skidmore-Roth, L. (2008). *2008 Mosby's nursing drug reference* (21st ed., pp. 196-197). St. Louis: Mosby.

626. **1**
Rationale: Fexofenadine is an antihistamine, which provides relief of symptoms caused by allergy. Antihistamines should be discontinued for at least 3 days (72 hours) before allergy skin testing to avoid false-negative readings. This client should have the appointment rescheduled for 3 days after discontinuing the medication.
Test-Taking Strategy: Focus on the name of the medication to determine that this medication is an antihistamine. It is also necessary to know that antihistamines reduce the allergic response. With this in mind, option 2 is eliminated first, because it makes no sense. Options 3 and 4 are also eliminated, because the medication would still interfere with the test results. Review this medication if you had difficulty with this question.
Level of Cognitive Ability: Analysis
Client Needs: Physiological Integrity
Integrated Process: Nursing Process/Planning
Content Area: Pharmacology

References: Chernecky, C., & Berger, B. (2008). *Laboratory tests and diagnostic procedures* (5th ed., p. 1018). Philadelphia: Saunders.
Skidmore-Roth, L. (2008). *2008 Mosby's nursing drug reference* (21st ed., pp. 196-197). St. Louis: Mosby.

ALTERNATE ITEM FORMAT: MULTIPLE RESPONSE
627. **1, 2, 3, 5**
Rationale: Rifabutin (Mycobutin) may be prescribed for a client with active MAC disease and tuberculosis. It inhibits mycobacterial DNA–dependent RNA polymerase and suppresses protein synthesis. Side effects include rash, gastrointestinal disturbances, neutropenia (low neutrophil count), red-orange body secretions, uveitis (blurred vision and eye pain), myositis, arthralgia, hepatitis, chest pain with dyspnea, and flu-like syndrome. Vitamin B_6 deficiency and numbness and tingling in the extremities are associated with the use of isoniazid (INH). Ethambutol (Myambutol) also causes peripheral neuritis.
Test-Taking Strategy: Focus on the name of the medication to assist in answering the question and use the process of elimination. Recalling that vitamin B_6 deficiency and numbness and tingling in the extremities are associated with the use of isoniazid (INH) will assist in answering. Review the side effects associated with rifabutin (Mycobutin) if you had difficulty with this question.
Level of Cognitive Ability: Analysis
Client Needs: Physiological Integrity
Integrated Process: Nursing Process/Data Collection
Content Area: Pharmacology
Reference: Lehne, R. (2007). *Pharmacology for nursing care* (6th ed., p. 1022). Philadelphia: Saunders.

REFERENCES
Chernecky, C., & Berger, B. (2008). *Laboratory tests and diagnostic procedures* (5th ed.). Philadelphia: Saunders.
Kee, J., Hayes, E., & McCuistion, L. (2006). *Pharmacology: A nursing process approach* (5th ed.). Philadelphia: Saunders.
Lehne, R. (2007). *Pharmacology for nursing care* (6th ed.). Philadelphia: Saunders.

Lilley, L., Harrington, S., & Snyder, J. (2007). *Pharmacology and the nursing process* (5th ed.). St. Louis: Mosby.
Skidmore-Roth, L. (2008). *2008 Mosby's nursing drug reference* (21st ed.). St. Louis: Mosby.
Skidmore-Roth, L. (2005). *Mosby's drug guide for nurses* (6th ed.). St. Louis: Mosby.

The Adult Client With a Cardiovascular Disorder

PYRAMID TERMS

arterial anastomosis Ensures that when one of the blood-supplying arteries is damaged, flow is maintained from the other arteries; blood flow to the hands, feet, brain, and other organs is protected by arterial anastomosis

blood pressure (BP) Measures the force exerted by the blood against the walls of the blood vessels; if the BP falls too low, blood flow to the tissues, heart, brain, and other organs becomes inadequate; if the BP becomes too high, the risk of vessel rupture and damage increases

cardiac output The total volume of blood pumped through the heart in 1 minute; the normal cardiac output is 4 to 8 L/minute; cardiac output = stroke volume × heart rate

contractility Refers to the inherent ability of the myocardium to alter contractile force and velocity; sympathetic stimulation increases myocardial contractility, thus increasing stroke volume; conditions that decrease myocardial contractility reduce stroke volume

diastole The phase of the cardiac cycle in which the heart relaxes between contractions; it represents the period when the two ventricles are dilated by the blood flowing into them

diastolic pressure The force of the blood exerted against the artery walls when the heart relaxes or fills

postural (orthostatic) hypotension A blood pressure decrease of more than 10 to 15 mm Hg of the systolic pressure or a decrease of more than 10 mm Hg of the diastolic pressure and a 10% to 20% increase in heart rate; occurs when the client's blood pressure is not adequately maintained when moving from a lying to a sitting or standing position

pulse pressure The difference between the systolic and diastolic pressures; normal pulse pressure is 30 to 40 mm Hg

systole The phase of contraction of the heart, especially of the ventricles, during which blood is forced into the aorta and pulmonary artery

systolic pressure The maximum pressure of blood exerted against the artery walls when the heart contracts

venous pressure The force exerted by the blood against the vein walls; normal venous pressures are highest in the extremities (5 to 14 cm H_2O in the arm), and lowest closest to the heart (6 to 8 cm H_2O in the inferior vena cava)

PYRAMID TO SUCCESS

Pyramid points focus on data collection related to cardiovascular risks, health screening and promotion, complications of the various cardiovascular disorders, emergency implementation measures, and client education. Focus on the findings in angina, myocardial infarction (MI), heart failure and pulmonary edema, hypertension, and arterial and vascular disorders. Focus also on the care of the client following diagnostic treatments and surgical procedures. Note appropriate and therapeutic client positions, particularly with arterial and venous disorders of the extremities. Focus on treatments and medications prescribed for the various cardiovascular disorders and client teaching related to prescribed treatment plans. Be familiar with the components related to cardiac rehabilitation. The Integrated Processes addressed in this unit include Caring, Clinical Problem-Solving Process (Nursing Process), Communication and Documentation, and Teaching and Learning.

CLIENT NEEDS

Safe and Effective Care Environment

Consulting with members of the health care team
Establishing priorities
Initiating cardiovascular consultations and referrals
Maintaining medical and surgical asepsis
Maintaining standard and other precautions
Obtaining informed consent related to treatments and procedures
Upholding client rights

Health Promotion and Maintenance

Discussing alterations in lifestyle
Implementing cardiovascular data collection techniques
Mobilizing appropriate community resources
Promoting cardiac rehabilitation
Providing health screening and health promotion programs
Preventing cardiovascular disease
Teaching related to diet, therapy, exercise, and medications

Psychosocial Integrity

Assisting the client to accept lifestyle changes
Considering religious, spiritual, and cultural influences on health
Discussing grief and loss and end-of-life issues
Discussing situational role changes
Discussing unexpected body-image changes
Identifying coping mechanisms
Identifying fear, anxiety, and denial
Identifying support systems

Physiological Integrity

Assisting with basic care measures
Discussing activity limitations and promoting rest and sleep
Monitoring for complications related to cardiovascular disorders
Monitoring for therapeutic effects of medications
Monitoring of cardiac enzymes, troponin levels, and other laboratory values related to the cardiovascular system
Providing interventions required in emergencies

Providing nonpharmacological and pharmacological comfort interventions
Responding to medical emergencies

REFERENCES

Black, J., & Hawks, J. (2005). *Medical-surgical nursing: Clinical management for positive outcomes* (7th ed.). Philadelphia: Saunders.
Chernecky, C., & Berger, B. (2008). *Laboratory tests and diagnostic procedures* (5th ed.). Philadelphia: Saunders.
Christensen, B., & Kockrow, E. (2006). *Adult health nursing* (5th ed.). St. Louis: Mosby.
Christensen, B., & Kockrow, E. (2006). *Foundations of nursing* (5th ed.). St. Louis: Mosby.
deWit, S. (2009). *Medical-surgical nursing: Concepts & practice.* Philadelphia: Saunders.
Hodgson, B., & Kizior, R. (2008). *Saunders nursing drug handbook 2008.* Philadelphia: Saunders.
Ignatavicius, D., & Workman, M. (2006). *Medical-surgical nursing: Critical thinking for collaborative care* (5th ed.). Philadelphia: Saunders.
Kee, J., Hayes, E., & McCuistion, L. (2006). *Pharmacology: A nursing process approach* (5th ed.). Philadelphia: Saunders.
Lehne, R. (2007). *Pharmacology for nursing care* (6th ed.). Philadelphia: Saunders.
Lewis, S., Heitkemper, M., Dirksen, S., & Bucher, L. (2007). *Medical-surgical nursing: Assessment and management of clinical problems* (7th ed.). St. Louis: Mosby.
Linton, A., & Maebius, N. (2007). *Introduction to medical-surgical nursing* (4th ed.). Philadelphia: Saunders.
McKenry, L., Tessier, E., & Hogan, M. (2006). *Mosby's pharmacology in nursing* (22nd ed.). St. Louis: Mosby.
Monahan, F., Sands, J., Neighbors, M., Marek, J., & Green, C. (2007). *Phipps' medical-surgical nursing: Health and illness perspectives* (8th ed.). St. Louis: Mosby.
National Council of State Boards of Nursing (eds.) (2008). *2008 Detailed Test Plan for the NCLEX-PN® Examination, National Council of State Boards of Nursing,* Chicago: Author.
National Council of State Boards of Nursing, Inc. Web site: http://www.ncsbn.org.
Perry, A., & Potter, P (2006). *Clinical nursing skills & techniques* (6th ed.). St. Louis: Mosby.
Skidmore-Roth, L. (2008). *2008 Mosby's nursing drug reference* (21st ed.). St. Louis: Mosby.

Cardiovascular Disorders

I. ANATOMY AND PHYSIOLOGY

A. Heart and heart wall layers
  1. The heart is located in the left side of the mediastinum
  2. The heart consists of three layers
     a. The epicardium is the outermost layer of the heart
     b. The myocardium is the middle layer and actual contracting muscle of the heart
     c. The endocardium is the innermost layer and lines the inner chambers and heart valves

B. Pericardial sac
  1. Encases and protects the heart from trauma and infection
  2. Has two layers
     a. The parietal pericardium is the tough, fibrous outer membrane that attaches anteriorly to the lower half of the sternum, posteriorly to the thoracic vertebrae, and inferiorly to the diaphragm
     b. The visceral pericardium is the thin, inner layer that closely adheres to the heart
  3. The pericardial space is between the parietal and visceral layers; it holds 5 to 20 mL of pericardial fluid, lubricates the pericardial surfaces, and cushions the heart

C. There are four heart chambers
  1. The right atrium receives deoxygenated blood from the body via the superior and inferior vena cava
  2. The right ventricle receives blood from the right atrium and pumps it to the lungs via the pulmonary artery
  3. The left atrium receives oxygenated blood from the lungs via four pulmonary veins
  4. The left ventricle is the largest and most muscular chamber; it receives oxygenated blood from the lungs via the left atrium and pumps blood into the systemic circulation via the aorta

D. There are four valves in the heart
  1. There are two atrioventricular (AV) valves—the tricuspid and the mitral—that lie between the atria and ventricles

  a. The tricuspid valve is located on the right side of the heart
  b. The bicuspid (mitral) valve is located on the left side of the heart
  c. The AV valves close at the beginning of ventricular contraction and prevent blood from flowing back into the atria from the ventricles; these valves open when the ventricle relaxes
  2. There are two semilunar valves: the pulmonic and the aortic
     a. The pulmonic semilunar valve lies between the right ventricle and the pulmonary artery
     b. The aortic semilunar valve lies between the left ventricle and the aorta
     c. The semilunar valves prevent blood from flowing back into the ventricles during relaxation; they open during ventricular contraction and close when the ventricles begin to relax

E. Sinoatrial (SA) node
  1. The main pacemaker that initiates each heart beat
  2. It is located at the junction of the superior vena cava and the right atrium
  3. The SA node generates electrical impulses at 60 to 100 times per minute and is controlled by the sympathetic and parasympathetic nervous systems

F. AV node
  1. Is located in the lower aspect of the atrial septum
  2. Receives electrical impulses from the SA node
  3. If the SA node fails, the AV node can initiate and sustain a heart rate of 40 to 60 beats/min

G. The bundle of His
  1. A continuation of the AV node and located at the interventricular septum
  2. It branches into the right bundle branch, which extends down the right side of the interventricular septum, and the left bundle branch, which extends into the left ventricle

3. The right and left bundle branches terminate into Purkinje fibers
H. Purkinje fibers
 1. Purkinje fibers are a diffuse network of conducting strands located beneath the ventricular endocardium
 2. These fibers spread the wave of depolarization through the ventricles
 3. Purkinje fibers can act as the pacemaker with a rate between 20 and 40 beats/min when higher pacemakers fail
I. Coronary arteries: supply the capillaries of the myocardium with blood (Box 50-1)
J. Heart sounds
 1. The first heart sound (S1) is heard as the AV valves close and is heard loudest at the apex of the heart
 2. The second heart sound (S2) is heard when the semilunar valves close and is heard loudest at the base of the heart
K. Heart rate (Box 50-2)
 1. The faster the heart rate, the less time the heart has for filling, and the **cardiac output** decreases
 2. An increase in heart rate increases oxygen consumption
L. Autonomic nervous system
 1. Stimulation of sympathetic nerve fibers releases the neurotransmitter norepinephrine, producing an increased heart rate, increased conduction speed through the AV node, increased atrial and ventricular **contractility,** and peripheral vasoconstriction; stimulation occurs when a decrease in pressure is detected
 2. Stimulation of the parasympathetic nerve fibers releases the neurotransmitter acetylcholine, which decreases the heart rate and lessens atrial and ventricular **contractility** and conductivity; stimulation occurs when an increase in pressure is detected

M. **Blood pressure (BP)** control
 1. Baroreceptors, also called pressoreceptors, are located in the walls of the aortic arch and carotid sinuses
 2. Baroreceptors are specialized nerve endings that are affected by changes in the arterial **BP**
 3. Increases in arterial pressure stimulate baroreceptors, and the heart rate and arterial pressure decrease
 4. Decreases in arterial pressure reduce stimulation of the baroreceptors, and vasoconstriction and an increase in heart rate occur
 5. Stretch receptors, located in the vena cava and the right atrium, respond to pressure changes that affect circulatory blood volume
 6. When the **BP** decreases as a result of hypovolemia, a sympathetic response occurs, causing an increased heart rate and blood vessel constriction; when the **BP** increases as a result of hypervolemia, an opposite effect occurs
 7. Antidiuretic hormone (vasopressin) influences **BP** indirectly by regulating vascular volume
 8. Increases in blood volume result in decreased antidiuretic hormone release, increasing diuresis, and decreasing blood volume and thus decreasing **BP**
 9. Decreases in blood volume result in increased antidiuretic hormone release; this promotes an increase in blood volume and thus **BP**
 10. Renin, a potent vasoconstrictor, causes the **BP** to increase
 11. Renin converts angiotensinogen to angiotensin I; angiotensin I is then converted to angiotensin II in the lungs
 12. Angiotensin II stimulates the release of aldosterone, which promotes water and sodium retention by the kidneys; this action increases blood volume and **BP**
N. The vascular system
 1. Arteries are vessels through which the blood passes away from the heart to various parts of the body; they convey highly oxygenated blood from the left side of heart to the tissues
 2. Arterioles control the blood flow into the capillaries
 3. Capillaries allow the exchange of fluid and nutrients between the blood and the interstitial spaces

BOX 50-1 **Coronary Arteries**

Right coronary artery (RCA): Supplies the right atrium and ventricle, the inferior portion of the left ventricle, the posterior septal wall, and the sinoatrial and atrioventricular nodes
Left coronary artery (LCA): Consists of two major branches—the left anterior descending (LAD) and the circumflex arteries
LAD artery: Supplies blood to the anterior wall of the left ventricle, the anterior ventricular septum, and the apex of the left ventricle
Circumflex artery: Supplies blood to the left atrium and the lateral and posterior surfaces of the left ventricle

BOX 50-2 **Heart Rate**

The normal heart rate is 60-100 beats/minute.
Sinus tachycardia is a heart rate higher than 100 beats/minute.
Sinus bradycardia is a heart rate lower than 60 beats/minute.

4. Venules receive blood from the capillary bed and move blood into the veins
5. Veins transport deoxygenated blood from the tissues back to the right heart and then lungs for oxygenation
6. Valves help return blood to the heart against the force of gravity
7. The lymphatics drain the tissues and return the tissue fluid to the blood

II. DIAGNOSTIC TESTS AND PROCEDURES

A. Cardiac enzymes, lactic dehydrogenase (LDH), tropinins, and myoglobin: used to determine the occurrence of myocardial infarction (MI) (refer to Chapter 11)
B. Complete blood count
1. The red blood cell count decreases in rheumatic heart disease and infective endocarditis and increases in conditions characterized by inadequate tissue oxygenation
2. The white blood cell count increases in infectious and inflammatory diseases of the heart and after MI because large numbers of white blood cells are needed to dispose of the necrotic tissue resulting from the infarction
3. An elevated hematocrit can result from vascular volume depletion
4. Decreases in hematocrit and hemoglobin can indicate anemia
C. Blood coagulation factors: An increase in coagulation factors can occur during and after MI, which places the client at greater risk of thrombophlebitis and extension of clots in the coronary arteries
D. Serum lipids: used to assess the risk of developing coronary artery disease (refer to Chapter 11)
E. Electrolytes
1. Potassium
a. Hypokalemia causes increased cardiac electrical instability, ventricular dysrhythmias, and increased risk of digoxin toxicity
b. In hypokalemia, the electrocardiogram would show flattening and inversion of the T wave, the appearance of a U wave, and ST depression
c. Hyperkalemia causes asystole and ventricular dysrhythmias
d. In hyperkalemia, the electrocardiogram may show tall peaked T waves, widened QRS complexes, prolonged PR intervals, or flat P waves
2. Sodium
a. The serum sodium level decreases with the use of diuretics
b. The serum sodium level decreases in heart failure, indicating water excess
F. Calcium
1. Hypocalcemia can cause ventricular dysrhythmias, prolonged ST and QT interval, and cardiac arrest

2. Hypercalcemia can cause a shortened ST segment and widened T wave, AV block, tachycardia or bradycardia, digitalis hypersensitivity, and cardiac arrest
G. Phosphorus level: Phosphorus levels should be interpreted with calcium levels because the kidneys retain or excrete one electrolyte in an inverse relationship to the other
H. Magnesium
1. A low magnesium level can cause ventricular tachycardia (VT) and fibrillation
2. Electrocardiographic changes that may be observed with hypomagnesemia include tall T waves and depressed ST segments
3. A high magnesium level can cause muscle weakness, hypotension, and bradycardia
4. Electrocardiographic changes that may be observed with hypermagnesemia include a prolonged PR interval and widened QRS complex
I. Blood urea nitrogen: The blood urea nitrogen is elevated in heart disorders that adversely affect renal circulation, such as heart failure and cardiogenic shock
J. Blood glucose: An acute cardiac episode can elevate the blood glucose
K. B-type natriuretic peptide (BNP)
1. BNP is released in response to atrial and ventricular stretch; serves as a marker for congestive heart failure
2. BNP levels should be less than 100 pg/mL; the higher the level, the more severe the CHF
L. Chest x-ray film
1. Description
a. Radiography of the chest is done to determine the size, silhouette, and position of the heart
b. Specific pathological changes are difficult to determine via x-ray film, but anatomical changes can be seen
2. Interventions
a. Prepare the client for x-ray film, explaining the purpose and procedure
b. Remove jewelry
M. Electrocardiogram
1. Description: This common noninvasive diagnostic test records the electrical activity of the heart and is useful in detecting cardiac dysrhythmias, detecting location and extent of MI, cardiac hypertrophy, and evaluating the effectiveness of cardiac medications.
2. Interventions
a. Determine the client's ability to lie still; advise the client to lie still, breathe normally, and refrain from talking during the test
b. Reassure the client that an electrical shock will not occur

c. Document any cardiac medications the client is taking

N. Holter monitoring
1. Description
   a. In this noninvasive test, the client wears a Holter monitor and an electrocardiogram tracing is recorded continuously over a period of 24 hours or more while the client performs his activities of daily living
   b. The Holter monitor identifies dysrhythmias if they occur and evaluates the effectiveness of antidysrhythmics or pacemaker therapy
2. Interventions
   a. Instruct the client to resume normal daily activities and to maintain a diary documenting activities and any symptoms that may develop for correlation to the electrocardiograph tracing
   b. Instruct the client to avoid tub baths or showers because they will interfere with the ECG recorder device

O. Echocardiogram
1. Description
   a. This noninvasive procedure is based on the principles of ultrasound and evaluates structural and functional changes in the heart
   b. Heart chamber size is measured, ejection fraction is calculated, and flow gradient across the valves is determined
2. Interventions determine the client's ability to lie still, and advise the client to lie still, breathe normally, and refrain from talking during the test

P. Exercise testing (stress test)
1. Description
   a. This noninvasive test studies the heart during activity and detects and evaluates coronary artery disease
   b. Treadmill testing is the most commonly used mode of stress testing
   c. Stress testing may be used with myocardial radionuclide testing (perfusion imaging), at which point the procedure becomes invasive because a radionuclide must be injected
   d. If the client is unable to tolerate exercise, an intravenous (IV) infusion of dipyridamole (Persantine), dobutamine hydrochloride, or adenosine (Adenocard) is given to dilate the coronary arteries and simulate the effect of exercise
   e. An informed consent is required if a radionuclide is injected
2. Preprocedure interventions
   a. Obtain an informed consent if required
   b. Provide adequate rest the night before the procedure

c. Instruct the client to eat a light meal 1 to 2 hours before the procedure
d. Instruct the client to avoid smoking, alcohol, and caffeine before the procedure
e. Instruct the client to ask the physician about taking prescribed medication on the day of the procedure; theophylline products are usually held 12 hours before the test and calcium channel blockers and β-blockers are usually held for 24 hours.
f. Instruct the client to wear nonconstrictive, comfortable clothing and supportive rubber-soled shoes for the exercise stress test
g. Instruct the client to notify the physician if any chest pain, dizziness, or shortness of breath occurs during the procedure
3. Postprocedure interventions: Instruct the client to avoid taking a hot bath or shower for at least 1 to 2 hours

Q. Digital subtraction angiography
1. Description
   a. This test combines x-ray techniques and a computerized subtraction technique with fluoroscopy for visualization of the cardiovascular system
   b. A contrast medium (dye) is injected
2. Preprocedure interventions
   a. Assess for allergies to seafood, iodine, or radiopaque dyes. If allergic, the client may be premedicated with antihistamines and steroids to prevent a reaction
   b. Obtain informed consent
3. Postprocedure interventions
   a. Monitor vital signs
   b. Assess injection site for bleeding or discomfort

R. Nuclear cardiology
1. Description
   a. Nuclear cardiology is the use of radionuclide techniques and scanning in cardiovascular assessment
   b. The most common tests include technetium pyrophosphate scanning, thallium imaging, and multigated cardiac blood pool imaging
2. Preprocedure interventions
   a. Obtain informed consent
   b. Inform the client that a small amount of radioisotope will be injected and that the radiation exposure and risks are minimal
3. Postprocedure interventions
   a. Assess vital signs
   b. Assess injection site for bleeding or discomfort
   c. Inform the client that fatigue is possible

S. Magnetic resonance imaging (MRI)
 1. Description
  a. This is a noninvasive diagnostic test that produces an image of the heart or great vessels through interaction of magnetic fields, radio waves, and atomic nuclei
  b. It provides information on chamber size and thickness, valve and ventricular function, and blood flow through the great vessesls and coronary arteries
 2. Preprocedure interventions
  a. Evaluate the client for the presence of a pacemaker (contraindication) or other implanted items that present a contraindication to the test
  b. Ensure that the client has removed all metallic objects such as watches, jewelry, clothing with metal fasteners, and metal hair fasteners
  c. Inform the client that they may experience claustraphobia while in the scanner

T. Cardiac catheterization
 1. Description
  a. An invasive test involving insertion of a catheter into the heart and surrounding vessels
  b. Obtains information about the structure and performance of the heart chambers and valves and the coronary circulation
 2. Preprocedure interventions
  a. Obtain informed consent
  b. Assess for allergies to seafood, iodine, or radiopaque dyes; if allergic, the client may be premedicated with antihistamines and corticosteroids to prevent a reaction
  c. Withhold solid food for 6 to 8 hours and liquids for 4 hours as prescribed to prevent vomiting and aspiration during the procedure
  d. Document the client's height and weight because these data will be needed to determine the amount of dye to be administered
  e. Document baseline vital signs and note the quality and presence of peripheral pulses for postprocedure comparison
  f. Inform the client that a local anesthetic will be administered before catheter insertion
  g. Inform the client that he or she may feel fatigued because of the need to lie still and quiet on a hard table for up to 2 hours
  h. Inform the client that he or she may feel a fluttery feeling as the catheter passes through the heart; a flushed, warm feeling when the dye is injected; a desire to cough; and palpitations caused by heart irritability.
  i. If the client is on metformin (Glucophage), plan to withhold the medication 48 hours prior to the test because of risk of acidosis associated with the iodine dye
  j. Prepare the insertion site by shaving and cleaning with an antiseptic solution if prescribed
  k. Administer preprocedure medications such as sedatives if prescribed
  l. Insert an IV line if prescribed
 3. Postprocedure interventions
  a. Monitor vital signs and cardiac rhythm for dysrhythmias at least every 30 minutes for 2 hours initially
  b. Assess for chest pain; if dysrhythmias or chest pain occurs, notify the physician
  c. Monitor peripheral pulses and the color, warmth, and sensation of the extremity distal to the insertion site at least every 30 minutes for 2 hours initially
  d. Notify the physician if the client complains of numbness and tingling; if the extremity becomes cool, pale, or cyanotic; or if loss of the peripheral pulses occurs
  e. Monitor the pressure dressing for bleeding or hematoma formation
  f. Apply a sandbag or compression device to the insertion site to provide additional pressure if prescribed
  g. Monitor for bleeding; if bleeding occurs, apply manual pressure immediately and notify the physician
  h. Monitor for hematoma; if a hematoma develops, notify the physician
  i. Keep extremity extended for 4 to 6 hours, as prescribed, keeping the leg straight to prevent arterial occlusion
  j. Maintain strict bedrest for 6 to 12 hours, as prescribed; however, the client may turn from side to side; do not elevate the head of the bed more than 15 degrees
  k. If the antecubital vessel was used, immobilize the arm with an armboard
  l. Encourage fluid intake, if not contraindicated, to promote renal excretion of the dye and to replace fluid loss caused by the osmotic diuretic effect of the dye
  m. Monitor for nausea, vomiting, rash, or other signs of hypersensitivity to the dye
  n. Do not resume the administration of metformin (Glucophage) until directed by the physician (usually 48 hours after catheterization)

U. Central **venous pressure** (CVP)
 1. Description
  a. The CVP is the pressure within the superior vena cava and reflects the pressure under which blood is returned to the superior vena cava and right atrium

b. The CVP is measured with a central venous line in the superior vena cava and normal pressure is about 3 to 8 mm Hg

c. An elevated CVP measurement indicates an increase in blood volume as a result of sodium and water retention, excessive IV fluids, alterations in fluid balance, or renal failure

d. A decreased CVP measurement indicates a decrease in circulating blood volume and may be due to hemorrhage or severe vasodilation with pooling of blood in the extremities that limits venous return

III. THERAPEUTIC MANAGEMENT

A. Percutaneous transluminal coronary angioplasty (PTCA)
   1. Description (Figure 50-1)
      a. An invasive, nonsurgical technique in which one or more arteries are dilated with a balloon catheter to open the vessel lumen and improve arterial blood flow
      b. PTCA may be used alone for clients with an evolving MI or in combination with medications to achieve reperfusion
      c. The client can experience reocclusion after the procedure, thus the procedure may need to be repeated
      d. Complications can include arterial dissection or rupture, immobilization of plaque fragments, spasm, and acute MI
      e. A firm commitment is needed on the part of the client to stop smoking, adhere to dietary restrictions, lose weight, alter exercise patterns, and discontinue any behaviors that could lead to the progression of artery occlusion

   2. Preprocedure interventions
      a. Maintain NPO status after midnight
      b. Obtain informed consent and allergy assessment to iodine, and hold metformin (Glucophage), as with cardiac catheterization
      c. Prepare the groin area with antiseptic soap and shave per institutional procedure and as prescribed
      d. Assess baseline vital signs and peripheral pulses
      e. Instruct the client that chest pain may occur during balloon inflation and to report it if it does occur

   3. Postprocedure interventions
      a. Monitor vital signs closely
      b. Assess distal pulses in both extremities
      c. Maintain bedrest as prescribed, keeping the limb straight for 6 to 8 hours
      d. Administer anticoagulants such as IV heparin and antiplatelet agents as prescribed to prevent thrombus formation
      e. IV nitroglycerin may be prescribed to prevent coronary artery vasospasm
      f. Encourage fluids if not contraindicated to enhance renal excretion of dye
      g. Instruct the client in the administration of nitrates, calcium channel blockers, antiplatelet agents, and anticoagulants as prescribed
      h. Instruct the client to take acetylsalicylic acid (aspirin) daily permanently if prescribed
      i. Assist the client with planning lifestyle modifications

B. Laser-assisted angioplasty
   1. Description
      a. A laser probe is advanced through a cannula similar to that used for PTCA

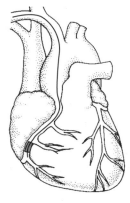 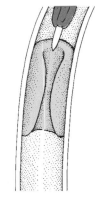 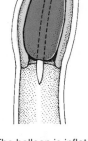 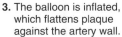

1. The balloon-tipped catheter is positioned in the artery.

2. The uninflated balloon is centered in the obstruction.

3. The balloon is inflated, which flattens plaque against the artery wall.

4. The balloon is removed, and the artery is left unoccluded.

FIG. 50-1 Percutaneous transluminal coronary angioplasty. (From Ignatavicius, D. & Workman, M. [2006]. *Medical-surgical nursing: Critical thinking for collaborative care* [5th ed.]. Philadelphia: Saunders.)

b. Laser-assisted angioplasty is also used for clients with small occlusions in the distal superficial femoral, proximal popliteal, and common iliac arteries, as well as in the coronary arteries

c. Heat from the laser vaporizes the plaque to open the occluded artery

2. Preprocedure and postprocedure interventions

a. Care is similar to that for PTCA

b. Monitor for complications of coronary dissection, acute occlusion, perforation, embolism, and MI

C. Coronary artery stents

1. Description

a. Coronary artery stents are used in conjunction with PTCA to provide a supportive scaffold to eliminate the risk of acute coronary vessel closure and to improve long-term patency of the vessel

b. A balloon catheter bearing the stent is inserted into the coronary artery and positioned at the site of occlusion; ballon inflation deploys the stent

c. When placed in the coronary artery, the stent reopens the blocked artery

2. Preprocedure and postprocedure interventions

a. Care is similar to that for PTCA

b. Acute thrombosis is a major concern following the procedure, and the client is placed on antiplatelet therapy such as clopidogrel (Plavix) and acetylsalicylic acid (aspirin) for several months following the procedure

c. Monitor for complications of the procedure such as stent migration or occlusion, coronary artery dissection, and bleeding resulting from anticoagulation

D. Atherectomy

1. Description

a. Atherectomy removes plaque from a coronary artery by the use of a cutting chamber on the inserted catheter or a rotating blade that pulverizes the plaque

b. Atherectomy is also used to improve blood flow to ischemic limbs in individuals with peripheral arterial disease

2. Preprocedure and postprocedure interventions

a. Care is similar to that for PTCA

b. Monitor for complications of perforation, embolus, and reocclusion

E. Transmyocardial revascularization

1. Used for clients with widespread atherosclerosis involving vessels that are too small and numerous for replacement or balloon catheterization; the procedure is performed through a small chest incision

2. Transmyocardial revascularization uses a high-power laser that creates 20 to 24 channels through the muscle of the left ventricle and blood enters these small channels, providing the affected region of the heart with oxygenated blood

3. The opening on the surface of the heart heals; however, the main channels remain and perfuse the myocardium

F. Arterial revascularization

1. Description

a. Performed to increase arterial blood flow to the affected limb

b. Inflow procedures involve bypassing the arterial occlusion above the superficial femoral arteries

c. Outflow procedures involve bypassing the arterial occlusions at or below the superficial femoral arteries

d. Graft material is sutured above and below the occlusion to facilitate blood flow around the occlusion

2. Preoperative interventions

a. Assess baseline vital signs and peripheral pulses

b. Insert an IV line and urinary catheter as prescribed

c. Maintain a central venous catheter and/or arterial line if inserted

3. Postoperative interventions

a. Assess vital signs

b. Monitor the BP and notify the physician if changes occur

c. Monitor for hypotension, which may indicate hypovolemia

d. Monitor for hypertension, which may place stress on the graft and facilitate clot formation

e. Maintain bedrest for 24 hours as prescribed

f. Instruct the client to keep the affected extremity straight, limit movement, and avoid bending the knee and hip

g. Monitor for warmth, redness, and edema, which are often expected outcomes because of increased blood flow

h. Monitor for graft occlusion, which often occurs within the first 24 hours

i. Assess peripheral pulses and for adverse changes in color and temperature of the extremity

j. Monitor for a sharp increase in pain because pain is frequently the first indicator of postoperative graft occlusion

k. If signs of graft occlusion occur, notify the physician immediately

l. Encourage coughing and deep breathing and the use of incentive spirometry

m. Maintain NPO status, with progression to clear liquids as prescribed

n. Use strict aseptic technique when in contact with the incision
o. Assess the incision for drainage, warmth, or swelling
p. Monitor for excessive bleeding (a small amount of bloody drainage is expected)
q. Monitor the area over the graft for hardness, tenderness, and warmth, which may indicate infection; if this occurs, notify the physician immediately
r. Instruct the client about proper foot care and measures to prevent ulcer formation
s. Instruct the client to take medications as prescribed
t. Instruct the client on how to care for incision
u. Assist the client in modifying lifestyle (such as diet) to prevent further plaque formation

G. Coronary artery bypass graft
1. Description
a. The occluded coronary arteries are bypassed with the client's own venous or arterial blood vessels
b. The saphenous vein, internal mammary artery, or other arteries may be used to bypass lesions in the coronary arteries
c. Coronary artery bypass graft is performed when the client does not respond to medical management of coronary artery disease, when disease progression is evident, or when severe blockage exists
2. Preoperative interventions
a. Familiarize the client and family with the cardiac surgical critical care unit
b. Inform the client to expect a sternal incision, possible arm or leg incision(s), one or two chest tubes, a Foley catheter, and several IV fluid catheters
c. Inform the client that an endotracheal tube will be in place and that he or she will be unable to speak
d. Advise the client that he or she will be on mechanical ventilation and to breathe with—and not fight—the ventilator
e. Instruct the client to inform the nurse of any postoperative pain because pain medication will be available
f. Instruct the client on how to splint the chest incision, cough and deep breathe, use the incentive spirometer, and perform arm and leg exercises
g. Encourage the client and family to discuss anxieties and fears related to surgery
h. Note that prescribed medications may be discontinued preoperatively (usually diuretics 2 to 3 days before surgery, digoxin 12 hours before surgery, and aspirin and anticoagulants 1 week before surgery)

i. Administer medications as prescribed, which may include potassium chloride, antihypertensives, antidysrhythmics, and antibiotics
3. Transfer from the cardiac surgical unit
a. Monitor vital signs, level of consciousness, and peripheral perfusion
b. Monitor for dysrhythmias
c. Auscultate lungs and assess respiratory status
d. Encourage the client to splint the incision, cough and deep breathe, and use the incentive spirometer to raise secretions and prevent atelectasis
e. Monitor temperature and white blood cell count, which indicate infection if elevated after 3 to 4 days
f. Provide adequate fluids and hydration as prescribed to liquefy secretions
g. Assess suture line and chest tube insertion sites for redness, purulent discharge, and signs of infection
h. Assess sternal suture line for instability, which may indicate an infection
i. Guide the client to gradually resume activity
j. Assess the client for tachycardia, **postural (orthostatic) hypotension,** and fatigue before, during, and after activity
k. Discontinue activities if the **BP** drops more than 10 to 20 mm Hg or if the pulse increases more than 10 beats/min
l. Monitor episodes of pain closely
m. See Box 50-3 for home care instructions
H. Heart transplant
1. A donor heart from an individual with a comparable body weight and ABO compatibility is transplanted into a recipient within 6 hours of procurement

BOX 50-3 **Home Care Instructions Following Cardiac Surgery**

Progressively return to activities at home.
Limit pushing or pulling activities for 6 weeks following discharge.
Maintain incisional care and record signs of redness, swelling, or drainage.
Sternotomy incision heals in about 6-8 weeks.
Avoid crossing legs; wear elastic hose as prescribed until edema subsides, and elevate surgical limb when sitting in a chair.
Follow prescribed medications as instructed by the physician.
Follow prescribed dietary measures such as avoiding saturated fat, cholesterol, and salt.
Sexual intercourse can be resumed on the advice of the physician after exercise tolerance is assessed; if the client can walk one block or climb two flights of stairs without symptoms, he or she can resume sexual activity safely.

2. The surgeon removes the diseased heart, leaving the posterior portion of the atria to serve as an anchor for the new heart

3. Because a remnant of the client's atria remains, two unrelated P waves are noted on the electrocardiogram

4. The transplanted heart is denervated and unresponsive to vagal stimulation; because the heart is denervated, clients do not experience angina

5. Symptoms of heart rejection include hypotension, dysrhythmias, weakness, fatigue, and dizziness

6. Endomyocardial biopsies are performed at regular scheduled intervals and whenever rejection is suspected

7. The client requires lifetime immunosuppressive therapy

8. Strict aseptic technique and vigilant handwashing must be maintained when caring for the posttransplant client because of increased risk for infection from immunosuppression

9. The heart rate approximates 100 beats/min and responds slowly to exercise or stress with regard to increases in heart rate, **contractility**, and **cardiac output**.

IV. CARDIAC DYSRHYTHMIAS

A. Normal sinus rhythm (Figure 50-2)
 1. Rhythm originates from the SA node
 2. Atrial and ventricular rhythms are regular at 60 to 100 beats/min

B. Sinus bradycardia
 1. Atrial and ventricular rhythms are regular and rates are less than 60 beats/min
 2. Note that a low heart rate may be normal for some individuals
 3. Treatment may be necessary if the client is symptomatic (signs of decreased **cardiac output**)
 4. Treatment depends on cause and may include holding a medication, oxygen, atropine sulfate, or a pacemaker; notify the registered nurse (RN)

C. Sinus tachycardia
 1. Atrial and ventricular rhythms are regular and rates are 100 to 180 beats/min
 2. Treatment depends on the cause

D. Atrial fibrillation
 1. Multiple rapid impulses from many foci depolarize in the atria in a totally disorganized manner at a rate of 350 to 600 times per minute; the atria quiver, which can lead to the formation of thrombi
 2. No definitive P wave can be observed—only fibrillatory waves before each QRS
 3. Treatment includes oxygen, anticoagulants, cardiac medications, and possible cardioversion; notify the RN

E. Premature ventricular contractions (PVCs) (Box 50-4 and Figure 50-3)
 1. Early ventricular complexes result from increased irritability of the ventricles
 2. Treatment depends on the cause and the RN nurse is notified if PVCs occur

F. Ventricular tachycardia (VT) (Figure 50-4)
 1. VT occurs because of a repetitive firing of an irritable ventricular ectopic focus at a rate of 140 to 250 beats/min or more and can lead to cardiac arrest; notify the RN if VT occurs

BOX 50-4	Premature Ventricular Contractions (PVCs)

Bigeminy: PVC every other heartbeat
Trigeminy: PVC every third heartbeat
Quadrigeminy: PVC every fourth heartbeat
Couplet or pair: Two sequential PVCs
Unifocal: Uniform upward or downward deflection, arising from the same ectopic focus
Multifocal: Different shapes, with the impulse generation from different sites
R-on-T phenomenon: PVC falls on the T wave of the preceding beat and may precipitate ventricular fibrillation

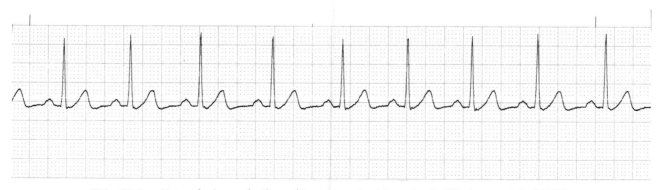

FIG. 50-2 Normal sinus rhythm. (From Ignatavicius, D. & Workman, M. [2006]. *Medical-surgical nursing: Critical thinking for collaborative care* [5th ed.]. Philadelphia: Saunders.)

2. Stable client with sustained VT (with pulse and no signs or symptoms of decreased **cardiac output**) will be treated with oxygen and antidysrhythmics
3. Unstable client with VT (with pulse and signs and symptoms of decreased **cardiac output**) will be treated with oxygen and antidysrhythmics and cough cardiopulmonary resuscitation (CPR) or possible synchronized cardioversion

4. Pulseless client with VT: defibrillation and CPR
G. Ventricular fibrillation (VF) (Figure 50-5)
1. VF is a chaotic rapid rhythm in which the ventricles quiver and there is no **cardiac output**
2. Client lacks a pulse, **BP**, respirations, and heart sounds, and VF is fatal if not successfully terminated within 3 to 5 minutes
3. Treatment includes CPR and immediate defibrillation

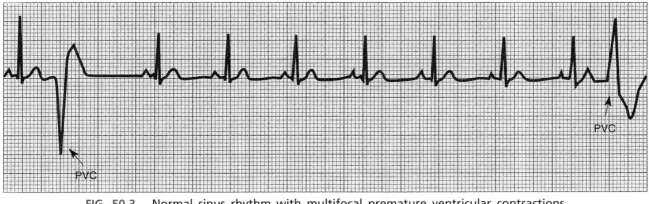

FIG. 50-3 Normal sinus rhythm with multifocal premature ventricular contractions (one negative and the other positive). (From Ignatavicius, D. & Workman, M. [2006]. *Medical-surgical nursing: Critical thinking for collaborative care* [5th ed.]. Philadelphia: Saunders)

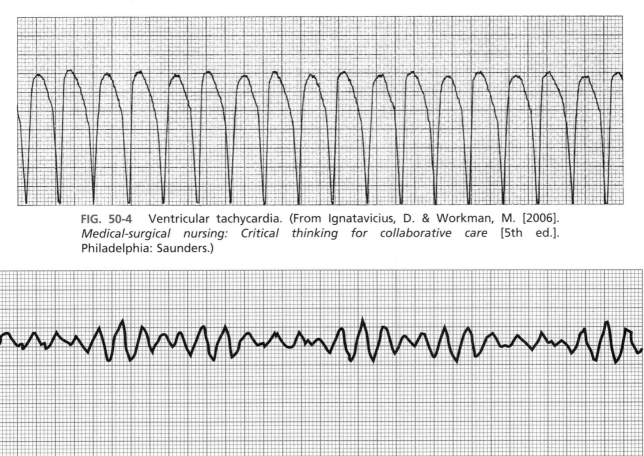

FIG. 50-4 Ventricular tachycardia. (From Ignatavicius, D. & Workman, M. [2006]. *Medical-surgical nursing: Critical thinking for collaborative care* [5th ed.]. Philadelphia: Saunders.)

FIG. 50-5 Ventricular fibrillation. (From Ignatavicius, D. & Workman, M. [2006]. *Medical-surgical nursing: Critical thinking for collaborative care* [5th ed.]. Philadelphia: Saunders.)

V. MANAGEMENT OF DYSRHYTHMIAS
A. Vagal maneuvers
   1. Description: Vagal maneuvers induce vagal stimulation of the cardiac conduction system and are used to terminate supraventricular tachydysrhythmias
   2. Carotid sinus massage
      a. The physician instructs the client to turn the head away from the side to be massaged
      b. The physician massages over one carotid artery for a few seconds to determine if a change in cardiac rhythm occurs
      c. The client should be on a cardiac monitor and an electrocardiogram rhythm strip before, during, and after the procedure should be obtained and documented on the chart
      d. Have a defibrillator and resuscitative equipment available
      e. Monitor vital signs, cardiac rhythm, and level of consciousness following the procedure
   3. Valsalva's maneuver
      a. The physician instructs the client to bear down or induces a gag reflex in the client to stimulate a vagal response
      b. Monitor the heart rate, rhythm, and **BP**
      c. Observe the cardiac monitor for a change in rhythm
      d. Record an electrocardiogram rhythm strip before, during, and after the procedure
      e. Provide an emesis basin if the gag reflex is stimulated, and initiate precautions to prevent aspiration
      f. Have a defibrillator and resuscitative equipment available
B. Cardioversion
   1. Description
      a. Cardioversion is synchronized countershock to convert an undesirable rhythm to a stable rhythm
      b. Cardioversion can be an elective procedure performed by the physician for stable tachydysrhythmias resistant to medical therapies or an emergent procedure for hemodynamically unstable ventricular or supraventricular tachydysrhythmias
      c. A lower amount of energy is used than with defibrillation
      d. Defibrillator is synchronized to the client's R wave to avoid discharging the shock during the vulnerable period (T wave)
      e. If the defibrillator were not synchronized, it could discharge on the T wave and cause VF
   2. Preprocedure interventions
      a. Obtain an informed consent if it is an elective procedure
      b. Administer sedation as prescribed
      c. If it is an elective procedure, hold digoxin (Lanoxin) 48 hours preprocedure as prescribed to prevent postcardioversion ventricular irritability
      d. If it is an elective procedure for atrial fibrillation or atrial flutter, the client should receive anticoagulant therapy for 4 to 6 weeks preprocedure
   3. During the procedure
      a. Ensure that the skin is clean and dry in the area where the electrode paddles will be placed
      b. Stop the oxygen during the procedure to avoid the hazard of fire
      c. Be sure that no one is touching the bed or the client when delivering the countershock
   4. Postprocedure interventions
      a. Priority assessment includes ability of the client to maintain aiway and breathing
      b. Resume oxygen administration as prescribed
      c. Assess vital signs
      d. Assess level of consciousness
      e. Monitor cardiac rhythm
      f. Monitor for indications of successful response such as conversion to sinus rhythm, strong peripheral pulses, an adequate **BP**, and adequate urine output
      g. Assess the skin on the chest for evidence of burns from the edges of the paddles
C. Defibrillation
   1. Description
      a. Defibrillation is an asynchronous countershock used to terminate pulseless VT or VF
      b. Three rapid consecutive shocks are delivered, with the first at an energy of 200 joules (J)
      c. If unsuccessful, the shock is repeated at 200 to 300 J
      d. The third and subsequent shocks will be 360 J
   2. During the procedure
      a. Stop the oxygen during the procedure to avoid the hazard of fire
      b. Be sure that no one is touching the bed or the client when delivering the countershock
D. Use of paddle electrodes
   1. Apply conductive pads
   2. One paddle is placed at the third intercostal space to the right of the sternum; the other is placed at the fifth intercostal space on the left midaxillary line
   3. Apply firm pressure of at least 25 lb to each of the paddles
   4. Be sure that no one is touching the bed or the client when delivering the countershock

E. Automatic external defibrillator
1. An automatic external defibrillator is used by laypersons and emergency medical technicians for prehospital cardiac arrest
2. Place the client on a firm dry surface
3. Stop CPR
4. Ensure that no one is touching the client to avoid motion artifact during rhythm analysis
5. Place the electrode patches in the correct position on the client's chest
6. Press the analyzer button to identify the rhythm, which may take 30 seconds; the machine will advise whether a shock is necessary
7. Shocks are recommended for pulseless VT or VF only
8. If shock is recommended, the shock initially is delivered at an energy of 200 J
9. If unsuccessful, the shock is repeated at 200 to 300 J
10. The third and subsequent shock will be 360 J
11. If unsuccessful, CPR is continued for 1 minute, and then another series of three shocks is delivered, each at 360 J

F. Implantable cardioverter defibrillator (ICD)
1. Description
   a. An ICD monitors cardiac rhythm and detects and terminates episodes of VT and VF
   b. The ICD senses VT or VF and delivers 25 to 30 J up to four times if necessary
   c. An ICD is used in clients with episodes of spontaneous sustained VT or VF unrelated to an MI or in clients whose medication therapy has been unsuccessful in controlling life-threatening dysrhythmias
   d. Transvenous electrode leads are placed in the right atrium and ventricle in contact with the endocardium; leads are used for sensing, pacing, and delivery of cardioversion or defibrillation
   e. The generator is most commonly implanted in the left pectoral region
2. Client education
   a. Instruct the client in the basic functions of the ICD
   b. Teach the client how to perform cough CPR
   c. Know the rate cutoff of the ICD and the number of consecutive shocks that it will deliver
   d. Wear loose-fitting clothing over the ICD generator site
   e. Avoid contact sports to prevent trauma to the ICD generator and lead wires
   f. Report any fever, redness, swelling, or drainage from the insertion site
   g. Report symptoms of fainting, nausea, weakness, blackouts, and rapid pulse rates to the physician
   h. During shock discharge, the client may feel faint or short of breath
   i. Instruct the client to sit or lie down if he or she feels a shock and to notify the physician
   j. Advise the client to maintain a log of the date, time, and activity preceding the shock, the symptoms preceding the shock, and postshock sensations
   k. Instruct the client and family in how to access the emergency medical system
   l. Encourage the family to learn CPR
   m. Instruct the client to avoid electromagnetic fields directly over the ICD since they can inactivate the device
   n. Instruct the client to move away from a magnetic field immediately if beeping tones are heard, and notify the physician
   o. Keep an ICD identification card in the wallet and obtain and wear a Medic-Alert bracelet
   p. Inform all health care providers that an ICD has been inserted; certain diagnostic tests, such as an MRI, and procedures using diathermy or electrocautery interfere with ICD function
   q. Advise the client of restrictions on activites such as driving and operating dangerous equipment

VI. PACEMAKERS
A. Description: a temporary or permanent device that provides electrical stimulation and maintains the heart rate when the client's intrinsic pacemaker fails to provide a perfusing rhythm
B. Settings
1. A synchronous (demand) pacemaker senses the client's rhythm and paces only if the client's intrinsic rate falls below the set pacemaker rate to stimulate depolarization
2. An asynchronous (fixed rate) pacemaker paces at a preset rate regardless of the client's intrinsic rhythm and is used when the client is asystolic or profoundly bradycardic
3. Overdrive pacing suppresses the underlying rhythm in tachydysrhythmias so that the sinus node will regain control of the heart
C. Spikes
1. When a pacing stimulus is delivered to the heart, a spike (straight vertical line) is seen on the monitor or electrocardiogram strip
2. Spikes precede the chamber being paced; a spike preceding a P wave indicates that the atrium is being paced, and a spike preceding the QRS indicates the ventricle is being paced
3. An atrial spike followed by a P wave indicates atrial depolarization, and a ventricular spike followed by a QRS represents ventricular depolarization; this is referred to as "capture"

4. If the electrode is in the atrium, the spike is before the P wave; if the electrode is in the ventricle, the spike is before the QRS complex

D. Temporary pacemakers
  1. Noninvasive transcutaneous pacing
    a. Noninvasive transcutaneous pacing is used as a temporary emergency measure in the profoundly bradycardic or asystolic client until invasive pacing can be initiated
    b. Large electrode pads are placed on the client's chest and back and connected to an external pulse generator
    c. Wash the skin with soap and water before applying electrodes
    d. It is not necessary to shave the hair or apply alcohol or tinctures to the skin
    e. Place the posterior electrode between the spine and left scapula, behind the heart, avoiding placement over bone
    f. Place the anterior electrode between the V_2 and V_5 positions over the heart
    g. Do not place the anterior electrode over female breast tissue; rather, displace breast tissue and place under the breast
    h. Do not take the pulse or **BP** on the left side; the results will not be accurate because of the muscle twitching and electrical current
    i. Ensure that electrodes are in good contact with the skin
    j. If loss of "capture" occurs, assess the skin contact of the electrodes and increase the current until "capture" is regained
    k. Evaluate the client for discomfort from cutaneous and muscle stimulation; adminster analgesics as needed
  2. Invasive transvenous pacing
    a. Pacing lead wire is placed through the antecubital, femoral, jugular, or subclavian vein into the right atrium or right ventricle so that it is in direct contact with the endocardium
    b. Monitor cardiac rhythm continuously
    c. Monitor vital signs
    d. Monitor the pacemaker insertion site
    e. Restrict client movement to prevent lead wire displacement
  3. Invasive epicardial pacing: applied by using a transthoracic approach; the lead wires are threaded loosely on the epicardial surface of the heart after cardiac surgery
  4. Reducing the risk of microshock
    a. Use only inspected and approved equipment
    b. Insulate the exposed portion of wires with plastic or rubber material (fingers of rubber gloves) when wires are not attached to the pulse generator, and cover with nonconductive tape
    c. Ground all electrical equipment using a three-pronged plug
    d. Wear gloves when handling exposed wires
    e. Keep dressings dry

E. Permanent pacemakers
  1. Pulse generator is internal and surgically implanted in a subcutaneous pocket below the clavicle
  2. The leads are passed transvenously via the cephalic or subclavian vein to the endocardium on the right side of the heart; postoperatively, limitation of arm movement on the operative side is required to prevent lead wire dislodgement
  3. Permanent pacemakers may be single chambered, in which the lead wire is placed in the chamber to be paced, or may be dual chambered, with lead wires placed in both the right atrium and ventricle
  4. A permanent pacemaker is programmed when inserted and can be reprogrammed if necessary by noninvasive transmission from an external programmer to the implanted generator
  5. Pacemakers are powered by a lithium battery that has an average life span of 10 years, are nuclear powered with a life span of 20 years or longer, or are designed to be recharged externally
  6. Pacemaker function can be checked in the physician's office or clinic by a pacemaker interrogater/programmer or from home using telephone transmitter devices
  7. The client may be provided with a device that is placed over the pacemaker battery generator with an attachment to the telephone; the heart rate then can be transmitted to the clinic
  8. Provide client teaching as per Box 50-5

VII. **CORONARY ARTERY DISEASE**
A. Description
  1. Coronary artery disease is a narrowing or obstruction of one or more coronary arteries as a result of atherosclerosis, an accumulation of lipid-containing plaque in the arteries (Figure 50-6)
  2. The disease causes decreased perfusion of myocardial tissue and inadequate myocardial oxygen supply, leading to hypertension, angina, dysrhythmias, MI, heart failure, and death
  3. Collateral circulation, more than one artery supplying a muscle with blood, is normally present in the coronary arteries, especially in older persons
  4. The development of collateral circulation takes time and develops when chronic ischemia occurs to meet the metabolic demands; therefore, an occlusion of a coronary artery in a younger individual is more likely to be lethal than in an older individual

BOX 50-5 Pacemakers: Client Education

Instruct the client about the pacemaker, including the programmed rate.

Instruct the client on the signs of battery failure and when to notify the physician.

Instruct the client to report any fever, redness, swelling, or drainage from the insertion site.

Report signs of dizziness, weakness or fatigue, swelling of the ankles or legs, chest pain, or shortness of breath.

Keep a pacemaker identification card in the wallet and obtain and wear a Medic-Alert bracelet.

Instruct the client on how to take the pulse, to take the pulse daily, and to maintain a diary of pulse rates.

Wear loose-fitting clothing over the pulse generator site.

Avoid contact sports.

Inform all health care providers that a pacemaker has been inserted.

Instruct the client to inform airport security that he or she has a pacemaker because the pacemaker may set off the security detector.

Instruct the client that most electrical appliances can be used without any interference with the functioning of the pacemaker; however, advise the client not to operate electrical appliances directly over the pacemaker site.

Avoid transmitter towers and antitheft devices in stores.

Instruct the client that if any unusual feelings occur when near any electrical devices to move 5 to 10 feet away and check the pulse.

Instruct the client about the methods of monitoring the function of the device.

Emphasize the importance of follow-up with the physician.

Use cell phones on the side opposite to the pacemaker.

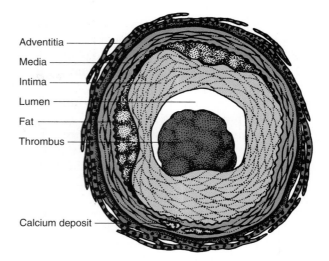

FIG. 50-6 Cross section of an atherosclerotic coronary artery. (From Ignatavicius, D. & Workman, M. [2006]. *Medical-surgical nursing: Critical thinking for collaborative care* [5th ed.]. Philadelphia: Saunders.)

5. Symptoms occur when the coronary artery is occluded to the point that inadequate blood supply to the muscle occurs, causing ischemia

6. Coronary artery narrowing is significant if the lumen diameter of the left main artery is reduced at least 50%, or if any major branch is reduced at least 75%

7. The goal of treatment is to alter the atherosclerotic progression

B. Data collection

1. Possibly normal findings during asymptomatic periods

2. Chest pain

3. Palpitations

4. Dyspnea

5. Syncope

6. Cough or hemoptysis

7. Excessive fatigue

C. Diagnostic studies

1. Electrocardiogram

a. When blood flow is reduced and ischemia occurs, ST segment depression, T wave inversion, or both are noted; the ST segment returns to normal when the blood flow returns

b. With infarction, cell injury results in ST segment elevation, followed by T wave inversion and an abnormal Q wave

2. Cardiac catheterization

a. Cardiac catheterization provides the most definitive source for diagnosis

b. Cardiac catheterization shows the presence of atherosclerotic lesions

3. Blood lipid levels

a. Blood lipid levels may be elevated

b. Cholesterol-lowering medications may be prescribed to reduce the development of atherosclerotic plaques

D. Interventions

1. Instruct the client regarding the purpose of diagnostic medical and surgical procedures and the preprocedure and postprocedure expectations

2. Assist the client to identify risk factors that can be modified

3. Assist the client to set goals to promote lifestyle changes that will reduce the impact of risk factors

4. Assist the client to identify barriers to compliance with the therapeutic plan and to identify methods to overcome barriers

5. Instruct the client regarding a low-calorie, low-sodium, low-cholesterol, and low-fat diet, with an increase in dietary fiber

6. Stress to the client that dietary changes are not temporary and must be maintained for life; teach the client about prescribed medications

7. Provide community resources to the client regarding exercise, smoking reduction, and stress reduction as appropriate

E. Surgical procedures
   1. PTCA to compress the plaque against the walls of the artery and dilate the vessel
   2. Laser angioplasty to vaporize the plaque
   3. Atherectomy to remove the plaque from the artery
   4. Vascular stent to prevent the artery from closing and to prevent restenosis
   5. Coronary artery bypass graft to improve blood flow to the myocardial tissue that is at risk for ischemia or infarction because of the occluded artery
F. Medications
   1. Nitrates to dilate the coronary arteries and to decrease preload and afterload
   2. Calcium channel blockers to dilate coronary arteries and reduce vasospasm
   3. Cholesterol-lowering medications to reduce the development of atherosclerotic plaques
   4. β-Blockers to reduce the **BP** in individuals who are hypertensive

VIII. ANGINA
A. Description
   1. Angina is chest pain resulting from myocardial ischemia caused by inadequate myocardial blood and oxygen supply
   2. Angina is caused by an imbalance between oxygen supply and demand
   3. Causes include obstruction of coronary blood flow because of atherosclerosis, coronary artery spasm, and conditions increasing myocardial oxygen consumption
   4. The goal of treatment is to provide relief of an acute attack, correct the imbalance between myocardial oxygen supply and demand, and prevent the progression of the disease and further attacks to reduce the risk of MI
B. Patterns of angina
   1. Stable angina
      a. Also called exertional angina.
      b. Occurs with activities that involve exertion or emotional stress and is relieved with rest or nitroglycerin
      c. Usually has a stable pattern of onset, duration, severity, and relieving factors

   2. Unstable angina
      a. Also called preinfarction angina
      b. Occurs with an unpredictable degree of exertion or emotion and increases in occurrence, duration, and severity over time
      c. Pain may not be relieved with nitroglycerin
   3. Variant angina
      a. Also called Prinzmetal's or vasospastic angina
      b. Results from coronary artery spasm
      c. May occur at rest
      d. Attacks may be associated with ST segment elevation noted on the electrocardiogram
   4. Intractable angina is a chronic, incapacitating angina that is unresponsive to interventions
   5. Preinfarction angina
      a. Is associated with acute coronary insufficiency
      b. Lasts longer than 15 minutes
      c. Is a symptom of worsening cardiac ischemia
      d. Occurs after an MI, when residual ischemia may cause episodes of angina
C. Data collection
   1. Pain (Table 50-1)
   2. Dyspnea
   3. Pallor
   4. Sweating
   5. Palpitations and tachycardia
   6. Dizziness and faintness
   7. Hypertension
   8. Digestive disturbances
D. Diagnostic studies
   1. Electrocardiogram: Readings are normal during rest, with ST depression and/or T wave inversion during an episode of pain
   2. Stress test: Chest pain or changes in the electrocardiogram or vital signs during testing may indicate ischemia
   3. Cardiac enzymes and troponins: Findings are normal in angina
   4. Cardiac catheterization: Catheterization a definitive diagnosis by providing information about the patency of the coronary arteries
E. Interventions
   1. Immediate management
      a. Assess pain

TABLE 50-1   Characteristics of Pain: Angina and Myocardial Infarction

Angina	Myocardial Infarction
Can develop slowly or quickly.	Occurs without cause, primarily early in the morning
Usually described as mild or moderate pain	Crushing substernal pain
Substernal, crushing, squeezing pain	
May radiate to the shoulders, arms, jaw, neck, and back	May radiate to the jaw, back, and left arm
Usually lasts less than 5 minutes; however, can last up to 15-20 minutes	Lasts 30 minutes or longer
Relieved by nitroglycerin or rest	Is unrelieved by rest or nitroglycerin, and relieved only by opioids

b. Provide bedrest

c. Administer oxygen at 3 L/min by nasal cannula as prescribed

d. Administer nitroglycerin as prescribed to dilate the coronary arteries, reduce the oxygen requirements of the myocardium, and relieve the chest pain

e. Obtain a 12-lead electrocardiogram

f. Provide continuous cardiac monitoring

2. Following the acute episode

a. Instruct the client regarding the purpose of diagnostic medical and surgical procedures and the preprocedure and postprocedure expectations

b. Assist the client to identify angina-precipitating events

c. Instruct the client to stop activity and to rest if chest pain occurs and to take nitroglycerin as prescribed

d. Instruct the client to seek medical attention if pain persists

e. Instruct the client regarding prescribed medications

f. Provide diet instructions to the client, stressing that dietary changes are not temporary and must be maintained for life

g. Assist the client to identify risk factors that can be modified

h. Assist the client to set goals that will promote changes in lifestyle to reduce the impact of risk factors

i. Assist the client to identify barriers to compliance with therapeutic plan and to identify methods to overcome barriers

j. Provide community resources to the client regarding exercise, smoking reduction, and stress reduction

F. Surgical procedures: Refer to the "Coronary Artery Disease" section

G. Medications

1. Refer to the "Coronary Artery Disease" section

2. Antiplatelet therapy may be prescribed and inhibits platelet aggregation and reduces the risk of developing an acute MI

IX. MYOCARDIAL INFARCTION

A. Description

1. MI occurs when myocardial tissue is abruptly and severely deprived of oxygen

2. Ischemia can lead to necrosis of myocardial tissue if blood flow is not restored

3. Infarction does not occur instantly but evolves over several hours

4. Obvious physical changes do not occur in the heart until 6 hours after the infarction, when the infarcted area appears blue and swollen

5. After 48 hours the infarct turns gray with yellow streaks as neutrophils invade the tissue

6. By 8 to 10 days after infarction, granulation tissue forms

7. Over 2 to 3 months, the necrotic area develops into a scar; scar tissue permanently changes the size and shape of the entire left ventricle

8. Not all clients experience the classic symptoms of an MI

9. Women may experience atypical discomfort, shortness of breath, or fatigue

10. An older client may experience shortness of breath, pulmonary edema, dizziness, altered mental status, or dysrhythmia

B. Location of MI

1. Obstruction of the left anterior descending artery results in anterior or septal MI or both

2. Obstruction of the circumflex artery results in posterior wall MI or lateral wall MI

3. Obstruction of the right coronary artery results in inferior wall MI

C. Risk factors

1. Atherosclerosis

2. Coronary artery disease

3. Elevated cholesterol levels

4. Smoking

5. Hypertension

6. Obesity

7. Physical inactivity

8. Impaired glucose tolerance

9. Stress

D. Diagnostic studies

1. Troponin level

a. Level rises within 3 hours

b. Level remains elevated for up to 7 days

2. Total creatine kinase level

a. Level rises within 4 hours after the onset of chest pain

b. Level peaks within 24 hours after damage and death of cardiac tissue

3. CK-MB isoenzyme

a. Peak elevation occurs 18 to 24 hours after the onset of chest pain

b. Level returns to normal 48 to 72 hours later

4. Myoglobin: Level rises within 1 hour after cell death, peaks in 4 to 6 hours, and returns to normal within 24 to 36 hours or less

5. LDH level

a. Level rises 24 hours after MI

b. Level peaks between 48 and 72 hours and falls to normal in 7 days

c. Serum level of LDH_1 isoenzyme rises higher than serum level of LDH_2

6. White blood cell count: An elevated white blood cell count of 10,000 to 20,000 cells/mm^3 appears on the second day following the MI and lasts up to a week

7. Electrocardiogram
   a. Electrocardiogram shows ST segment elevation, T wave inversion, and an abnormal Q wave in leads facing the infarct
   b. Hours to days after the MI, ST and T wave changes will return to normal but the Q wave usually remains permanently
8. Diagnostic tests following the acute stage
   a. Exercise tolerance test or stress test may be prescribed to assess for electrocardiographic changes and ischemia and to evaluate for medical therapy or identify clients who may need invasive therapy
   b. Thallium scans may be prescribed to assess for ischemia or necrotic muscle tissue
   c. Multigated cardiac blood pool imaging scans may be used to evaluate left ventricular function
   d. Cardiac catheterization is performed to determine the extent and location of obstructions of the coronary arteries
E. Data collection
   1. Pain (see Table 50-1)
   2. Nausea and vomiting
   3. Diaphoresis
   4. Dyspnea
   5. Dysrhythmias
   6. Feelings of fear and anxiety
   7. Pallor, cyanosis, and coolness of extremities
F. Complications of MI (Box 50-6)
G. Interventions, acute stage
   1. Obtain a description of the chest discomfort
   2. Assess vital signs
   3. Assess cardiovascular status and maintain cardiac monitoring
   4. Place the client in semi-Fowler's position to enhance comfort and tissue oxygenation
   5. Administer oxygen at 2 to 4 L/min by nasal cannula as prescribed
   6. Establish an IV access route

BOX 50-6 | **Complications of Myocardial Infarction**

Dysrhythmias
Heart failure
Pulmonary edema
Cardiogenic shock
Thrombophlebitis
Pericarditis
Mitral valve insufficiency
Postinfarction angina
Ventricular rupture
Dressler's syndrome (a combination of pericarditis, pericardial effusion, and pleural effusion, which can occur several weeks to several months following a myocardial infarction)

---

7. Administer nitroglycerin as prescribed
8. Morphine sulfate may be prescribed to relieve chest discomfort that is unresponsive to nitroglycerin
9. Obtain a 12-lead electrocardiogram
10. IV nitroglycerin and antidysrhythmics may be prescribed
11. Monitor thrombolytic therapy, which may be prescribed within the first 6 hours of the coronary event
12. Monitor for signs of bleeding if the client is receiving thrombolytic therapy
13. Monitor laboratory values as prescribed
14. Administer β-blockers as prescribed to slow the heart rate and increase myocardial perfusion while reducing the force of myocardial contraction
15. Monitor for complications related to the MI
16. Monitor for cardiac dysrhythmias because tachycardia and PVCs frequently occur in the first few hours after MI
17. Assess distal peripheral pulses and skin temperature because poor **cardiac output** may be identified by cool diaphoretic skin and diminished or absent pulses
18. Monitor intake and output
19. Assess respiratory rate and breath sounds for signs of heart failure, as indicated by the presence of crackles or wheezes or dependent edema
20. Monitor the **BP** closely after the administration of medications; if the **BP** is less than 100 systolic or 25 mm Hg lower than the previous reading, lower the head of the bed and notify the physician
21. Provide reassurance to the client and family
H. Interventions following the acute episode
   1. Maintain bedrest for the first 24 to 36 hours as prescribed
   2. Allow the client to stand to void or use a bedside commode if prescribed
   3. Provide range-of-motion exercises to prevent thrombus formation and maintain muscle strength
   4. Progress to dangling legs at the side of the bed or out of bed to the chair for 30 minutes three times a day as prescribed
   5. Progress to ambulation in the client's room and to the bathroom and then in the hallway three times a day
   6. Monitor for complications
   7. Encourage the client to verbalize feelings regarding the MI
I. Cardiac rehabilitation: Process of actively assisting the client with cardiac disease to achieve and maintain a vital and productive life within the limitations of the heart disease

X. HEART FAILURE

A. Description
   1. Heart failure is the inability of the heart to maintain adequate **cardiac output** to meet the metabolic needs of the body due to impaired pumping ability
   2. Diminshed **cardiac output** results in inadequate peripheral tissue perfusion
   3. Congestion of the lungs and periphery may occur; the client can develop acute pulmonary edema

B. Classification
   1. Acute heart failure occurs suddenly
   2. Chronic heart failure develops over time; however, a client with chronic heart failure can develop an acute episode

C. Types of heart failure
   1. Right ventricular failure/left ventricular failure
      a. Because the two ventricles of the heart represent two separate pumping systems, it is possible for one to fail alone for a short period
      b. Most heart failure begins with left ventricular failure and progresses to failure of both ventricles
      c. Acute pulmonary edema—a medical emergency—results from left ventricular failure
      d. If pulmonary edema is not treated, death will occur from suffocation because the client literally drowns in his or her own fluids
   2. Forward failure/backward failure
      a. In forward failure, an inadequate output of the affected ventricle causes decreased perfusion to vital organs
      b. In backward failure, blood backs up behind the affected ventricle, causing increased pressure in the atrium behind the affected ventricle
   3. Low output/high output
      a. In low-output failure, not enough **cardiac output** is available to meet the demands of the body
      b. High-output failure occurs when a condition causes the heart to work harder to meet the demands of the body
   4. Systolic failure/diastolic failure
      a. Systolic failure leads to problems with contraction and the ejection of blood
      b. Diastolic failure leads to problems with the heart relaxing and filling with blood

D. Compensatory mechanisms
   1. Compensatory mechanisms act to restore **cardiac output** to near-normal levels
   2. Initially these mechanisms increase **cardiac output**; however, they eventually have a damaging effect on pump action
   3. Compensatory mechanisms contribute to an increase in myocardial oxygen consumption, and when this occurs, myocardial reserve is exhausted and clinical manifestations of heart failure develop
   4. Compensatory mechanisms include increased heart rate, improved **stroke volume,** arterial vasoconstriction, sodium and water retention, and myocardial hypertrophy

E. Data collection
   1. Right ventricular failure: Signs of right ventricular failure are evident in the systemic circulation (Table 50-2)
   2. Left ventricular failure: Signs of left ventricular failure are evident in the pulmonary system (see Table 50-2)
   3. Acute pulmonary edema
      a. Severe dyspnea and orthopnea
      b. Pallor
      c. Tachycardia
      d. Expectoration of large amounts of blood-tinged, frothy sputum
      e. Wheezing and crackles on auscultation
      f. Bubbling respirations
      g. Acute anxiety, apprehension, and restlessness
      h. Profuse sweating
      i. Cold, clammy skin
      j. Cyanosis
      k. Nasal flaring
      l. Use of accessory breathing muscles
      m. Tachypnea
      n. Hypocapnia, evidenced by muscle cramps, weakness, dizziness, and paresthesias

TABLE 50-2	Clinical Manifestations of Right-Sided and Left-Sided Heart Failure	
Right-Sided Heart Failure	**Left-Sided Heart Failure**	
Dependent edema (legs and sacrum)	Signs of pulmonary congestion	
Jugular venous distention	Dyspnea	
Abdominal distention	Tachypnea	
Hepatomegaly	Crackles in the lungs	
Splenomegaly	Dry, hacking cough	
Anorexia and nausea	Paroxysmal nocturnal dyspnea	
Weight gain	Increased BP (from fluid volume excess) or decreased BP (from pump failure)	
Nocturnal diuresis		
Swelling of the fingers and hands		
Increased BP (from fluid volume excess) or decreased BP (from pump failure)		

BP, Blood pressure.

F. Immediate management

1. Place the client in high Fowler's position, with the legs in a dependent position, to reduce pulmonary congestion and relieve edema
2. Administer oxygen in high concentrations by mask or cannula as prescribed to improve gas exchange and pulmonary function
3. Prepare for intubation and ventilator support if required; monitor lung sounds for crackles and decreased breath sounds
4. Suction fluids as needed to maintain a patent airway
5. Assess level of consciousness
6. Provide reassurance to the client
7. Monitor vital signs closely, noting tachycardia or pulsus alternans
8. Monitor for hypotension resulting from decreased tissue perfusion or for hypertension resulting from anxiety or history of hypertension
9. Monitor heart rate and monitor for dysrhythmias by using a cardiac monitor
10. Assess for edema in dependent areas and in the sacral, lumbar, and posterior thigh region in the client on bed rest
11. Insert a Foley catheter as prescribed and monitor urine output closely following administration of a diuretic
12. Monitor intake and output (I&O)
13. Avoid the unnecessary IV administration of fluids
14. Morphine sulfate may be prescribed to provide sedation and vasodilation; monitor for respiratory depression or hypotension after administration
15. Diuretics may be prescribed to reduce preload, enhance renal excretion of sodium and water, reduce circulating blood volume, and reduce pulmonary congestion
16. Digoxin (Lanoxin) may be prescribed to increase ventricular **contractility** and improve **cardiac output**
17. Bronchodilators may be prescribed for severe bronchospasm or bronchoconstriction
18. Monitor weight to determine a response to treatment
19. Assess for hepatomegaly and ascites, and measure and record abdominal girth
20. Monitor peripheral pulses
21. Analyze arterial blood gas results and electrolyte values for imbalances; monitor BNP levels
22. Monitor potassium level closely, which may decrease as a result of diuretic therapy, and administer potassium supplements as prescribed to prevent digoxin toxicity

G. Following the acute episode

1. Encourage the client to verbalize feelings about the lifestyle changes required as a result of the heart failure
2. Assist the client to identify precipitating risk factors of heart failure and methods of eliminating these risk factors
3. Instruct the client in the prescribed medication regimen, which may include digoxin (Lanoxin), a diuretic, angiotensin-converting enzyme (ACE) inhibitors, low-dose β-blockers, and vasodilators.
4. Advise the client to notify the physician if side effects occur from the medications
5. Advise the client to avoid over-the-counter medications
6. Instruct the client to contact the physician if he or she is unable to take medications because of illness
7. Instruct the client to avoid large amounts of caffeine, found in coffee, tea, cocoa, chocolate, and some carbonated beverages
8. Instruct the client about the prescribed low-sodium, low-fat, and low-cholesterol diet
9. Provide the client with a list of potassium-rich foods since diuretics can cause hypokalemia (except for potassium-sparing diuretics)
10. Instruct the client regarding fluid restriction, if prescribed, advising the client to spread the fluid out during the day and to suck on hard candy to reduce thirst
11. Instruct the client to balance periods of activity and rest
12. Advise the client to avoid isometric activities, which increase pressure in the heart
13. Instruct the client to monitor daily weight
14. Instruct the client to report signs of fluid retention such as edema or weight gain

XI. CARDIOGENIC SHOCK (Box 50-7)
XII. INFLAMMATORY DISEASES OF THE HEART
A. Pericarditis
1. Description
   a. Pericarditis is an acute or chronic inflammation of the pericardium

---

BOX 50-7 **Cardiogenic Shock**

Failure of the heart to pump adequately, thereby reducing cardiac output and compromising tissue perfusion

Necrosis of more than 40% of the left ventricle, usually as a result of occlusion of major coronary vessels

Goal of treatment: to maintain tissue oxygenation and perfusion and to improve the pumping ability of the heart

b. Chronic pericarditis, a chronic inflammatory thickening of the pericardium, constricts the heart, causing compression

c. The pericardial sac becomes inflamed

d. Pericarditis can result in loss of pericardial elasticity or an accumulation of fluid within the sac

e. Heart failure or cardiac tamponade may result

2. Data collection

a. Precordial pain in the anterior chest that radiates to the left side of the neck, shoulder, or back

b. Pain is grating and is aggravated by breathing (particularly inspiration), coughing, and swallowing

c. Pain that is worse when in the supine position and may be relieved by leaning forward

d. Pericardial friction rub (scratchy, high-pitched sound) heard on auscultation and produced by the rubbing of the inflamed pericardial layers

e. Fever and chills

f. Fatigue and malaise

g. Elevated white blood cell count

h. Electrocardiogram changes with acute pericarditis; ST segment elevation with the onset of inflammation; atrial fibrillation is common

i. Signs of right ventricular failure in clients with chronic constrictive pericarditis

3. Interventions

a. Assess the nature of the pain.

b. Position the client in the high Fowler's position, or upright and leaning forward

c. Administer analgesics, nonsteroidal anti-inflammatory drugs, or corticosteroids for pain as prescribed

d. Auscultate for a pericardial friction rub

e. Check results of blood culture to identify causative organism

f. Administer antibiotics for bacterial infection as prescribed

g. Administer diuretics and digoxin (Lanoxin) as prescribed to the client with chronic constrictive pericarditis; surgical incision of the pericardium (pericardiectomy) may be necessary

h. Monitor for signs of cardiac tamponade, which include pulsus paradoxus, jugular vein distention with clear lung sounds, muffled heart sounds, narrowed **pulse pressure**, tachycardia, and decreased **cardiac output**

i. Notify the physician if signs of cardiac tamponade occur

B. Myocarditis

1. Description: an acute or chronic inflammation of the myocardium as a result of pericarditis, systemic infection, or allergic response

2. Data collection

a. Fever

b. Pericardial friction rub

c. A gallop rhythm

d. A murmur that sounds like fluid passing an obstruction

e. Pulsus alternans

f. Signs of heart failure

g. Fatigue

h. Dyspnea

i. Tachycardia

j. Chest pain

3. Interventions

a. Assist the client to a position of comfort such as sitting up and leaning forward

b. Administer analgesics, salicylates, and non-steroidal anti-inflammatory drugs as prescribed to reduce fever and pain

c. Administer oxygen as prescribed

d. Provide adequate rest periods

e. Limit activities to avoid overexertion and to decrease the workload of the heart

f. Administer digoxin (Lanoxin) as prescribed, and monitor for signs of digoxin toxicity

g. Administer antidysrhythmics as prescribed

h. Administer antibiotics as prescribed to treat the causative organism

i. Monitor for complications, which can include thrombus, heart failure, or cardiomyopathy

C. Endocarditis

1. Description

a. Endocarditis is an inflammation of the inner lining of the heart and valves

b. Occurs primarily in clients who are IV drug abusers, have had valve replacements, or have mitral valve prolapse or other structural defects

c. Ports of entry for the infecting organism include the oral cavity (especially if the client had a dental procedure in the previous 3-6 months), cutaneous invasion, infections, or invasive procedures or surgery

2. Data collection

a. Fever

b. Anorexia

c. Weight loss

d. Fatigue

e. Cardiac murmurs

f. Heart failure

g. Embolic complications from vegetation fragments traveling through the circulation

h. Petechiae

i. Splinter hemorrhages in the nailbeds

j. Osler's nodes (reddish tender lesions) on the pads of the fingers, hands, and toes
k. Janeway's lesions (nontender hemorrhagic lesions) on the fingers, toes, nose, or ear lobes
l. Splenomegaly
m. Clubbing of the fingers
3. Interventions
a. Provide adequate rest balanced with activity to prevent thrombus formation
b. Maintain antiembolism stockings
c. Monitor cardiovascular status
d. Monitor for signs of heart failure
e. Monitor for signs of emboli
f. Monitor for splenic emboli, as evidenced by sudden abdominal pain radiating to the left shoulder, and the presence of rebound abdominal tenderness on palpation
g. Monitor for renal emboli, as evidenced by flank pain radiating to the groin, hematuria, and pyuria
h. Monitor for confusion, aphasia, or dysphasia, which may indicate central nervous system emboli
i. Monitor for pulmonary emboli as evidenced by pleuritic chest pain, dyspnea, and cough
j. Assess skin, mucous membranes, and conjunctiva for petechiae
k. Assess nailbeds for splinter hemorrhages
l. Assess for Osler's nodes on the pads of the fingers, hands, and toes
m. Assess for Janeway's lesions on the fingers, toes, nose, or ear lobes
n. Assess for clubbing of the fingers
o. Evaluate blood culture results
p. Administer antibiotics intravenously as prescribed
q. Plan and arrange for discharge, providing resources required for the continued administration of antibiotics intravenously
4. Client education (Box 50-8)
XIII. **CARDIAC TAMPONADE** (Box 50-9)
XIV. **VALVULAR HEART DISEASE**
A. Description
1. Valvular heart disease occurs when the heart valves cannot fully open (stenosis) or close completely (insufficiency or regurgitation)
2. Valvular heart disease prevents efficient blood flow through the heart
B. Types
1. Mitral stenosis: Valvular tissue thickens and narrows the valve opening, preventing blood flow from the left atrium to left ventricle
2. Mitral insufficiency/regurgitation: Valve is incompetent, preventing complete valve closure during **systole**
3. Mitral valve prolapse: Valve leaflets protrude into the left atrium during **systole**

BOX 50-8 **Home Care Instructions for the Client With Infective Endocarditis**

Teach the client to maintain aseptic technique during set-up and adminstration of IV antibiotics.
Instruct the client to administer IV antibiotics at scheduled times to maintain the blood level.
Instruct the client to monitor IV catheter sites for signs of infection and report immediately to physician.
Instruct the client to record his or her temperature daily for up to 6 weeks and to report fever.
Encourage oral hygiene at least twice a day with a soft toothbrush and rinse well with water after brushing.
Client should avoid use of oral irrigation devices and flossing to avoid bacteremia.
Teach the client to thoroughly cleanse any skin lacerations thoroughly and apply an antibiotic ointment as prescribed.
Client should inform all health care providers of a history of endocarditis and request prophylactic antibiotics prior to every invasive procedure, including dental procedures.
Teach the client to observe for signs and symptoms of embolic phenomena and heart failure.

IV, Intravenous

BOX 50-9 **Cardiac Tamponade**

A pericardial effusion occurs when the space between the parietal and visceral layers of the pericardium fills with fluid.
Pericardial effusion places the client at risk for cardiac tamponade, an accumulation of fluid in the pericardial cavity.
Tamponade restricts ventricular filling, and cardiac output drops; distant, muffled heart sounds are heard
Acute tamponade occurs when a small volume (20-50 mL) of fluid accumulates quickly in the pericardium.

---

4. Aortic stenosis: Valvular tissue thickens and narrows the valve opening, preventing blood flow from the left ventricle into the aorta
5. Aortic insufficiency: Valve is incompetent, preventing complete valve closure during **diastole**
C. Repair procedures
1. Balloon valvuloplasty
a. Balloon valvuloplasty is an invasive, nonsurgical procedure
b. A balloon catheter is passed from the femoral vein through the atrial septum to the mitral valve or through the femoral artery to the aortic valve
c. The balloon is inflated to enlarge the orifice
d. Institute precautions for arterial puncture if appropriate
e. Monitor for bleeding from the catheter insertion site

f. Monitor for signs of systemic emboli

g. Monitor for signs of a regurgitant valve by monitoring cardiac rhythm, heart sounds, and **cardiac output**

2. Mitral annuloplasty: tightening and suturing the malfunctioning valve annulus to eliminate or greatly reduce regurgitation

3. Commissurotomy/valvotomy

a. The procedure is accomplished with cardiopulmonary bypass during open heart surgery

b. The valve is visualized, thrombi are removed from the atria, fused leaflets are incised, and calcium is débrided from the leaflets, thus widening the orifice

D. Valve replacement procedures

1. Mechanical prosthetic valves

a. Prosthetic valves are durable

b. Thromboembolism is a problem following the valve replacement, and lifetime anticoagulant therapy is required

2. Bioprosthetic valves

a. Biological grafts are xenografts (valves from other species): porcine valves (pig), bovine valves (cow), or homografts (human cadavers)

b. The risk of clot formation is small; therefore, long-term anticoagulation is not indicated

3. Preoperative interventions: Consult with the physician regarding discontinuing anticoagulants 72 hours before surgery

4. Postoperative interventions

a. Monitor closely for signs of bleeding

b. Monitor **cardiac output** and for signs of heart failure

c. Administer digoxin (Lanoxin) as prescribed to maintain **cardiac output** and prevent atrial fibrillation

d. Provide client teaching (Box 50-10)

XV. CARDIOMYOPATHY

A. Cardiomyopathy is a subacute or chronic disorder of the heart muscle

B. Treatment is palliative, not curative, and the client needs to deal with numerous lifestyle changes and a shortened life span

C. Types, signs and symptoms, and treatment: Refer to Table 50-3.

XVI. VASCULAR DISORDERS

A. Venous thrombosis

1. Description

a. Thrombus can be associated with an inflammatory process

b. When a thrombus develops, inflammation occurs, thickening the vein wall and leading to embolization

2. Types

a. Thrombophlebitis: A thrombus associated with inflammation

| BOX 50-10 | Client Instructions Following Valve Replacement |

Adequate rest is important, and fatigue is common.

Anticoagulant therapy is necessary if a mechanical prosthetic valve was inserted.

Instruct the client concerning hazards related to anticoagulant therapy and to notify the physician if bleeding or excessive bruising occurs.

Instruct the client concerning the importance of good oral hygiene to reduce the risk of infective endocarditis.

Brush teeth twice daily with a soft toothbrush, followed by oral rinses.

Avoid irrigation devices, electric toothbrushes, and flossing because these activities can cause the gums to bleed, allowing bacteria to enter the mucous membranes and bloodstream.

Monitor incision and report any drainage or redness.

Avoid any dental procedures for 6 months.

Heavy lifting (greater than 10 lb) is to be avoided, and be cautious when in an automobile to prevent injury to the sternal incision.

If a prosthetic valve was inserted, a soft audible clicking sound may be heard.

Instruct the client concerning the importance of prophylactic antibiotics before any invasive procedure and the importance of informing all health care professionals of the valvular disease history.

Obtain and wear a Medic-Alert bracelet.

---

b. Phlebothrombus: A thrombus without inflammation

c. Phlebitis: Vein inflammation associated with invasive procedures such as IV lines

d. Deep vein thrombophlebitis: More serious than a superficial thrombophlebitis because of the risk for pulmonary embolism

3. Risk factors for thrombus formation

a. Venous stasis from varicose veins, heart failure, and immobility

b. Hypercoagulability disorders

c. Injury to the venous wall from IV injections; administration of vessel irritants (chemotherapy, hypertonic solutions)

d. Following surgery, particularly orthopedic and abdominal surgery

e. Pregnancy

f. Ulcerative colitis

g. Use of oral contraceptives

h. Certain malignancies

i. Fractures or other injuries of the pelvis or lower extremities

B. Phlebitis

1. Data collection

a. Red, warm area radiating up the vein of an extremity

b. Pain and soreness

c. Swelling

2. Interventions
   a. Apply warm moist soaks as prescribed to dilate the vein and promote circulation (assess temperature of soak before applying)
   b. Assess for signs of complications such as tissue necrosis, infection, or pulmonary embolus
C. Deep vein thrombophlebitis
   1. Data collection
      a. Calf or groin tenderness or pain with or without swelling
      b. Positive Homans' sign may be noted; false positives are common
      c. Warm skin that is tender to touch

2. Interventions
   a. Provide bedrest as prescribed
   b. Elevate the affected extremity above the level of the heart as prescribed
   c. Avoid using the knee gatch or a pillow under the knees
   d. Do not massage the extremity
   e. Provide thigh-high or knee-high antiembolism stockings as prescribed to reduce venous stasis and to assist in the venous return of blood to the heart
   f. Administer intermittent or continuous warm, moist compresses as prescribed

TABLE 50-3 Pathophysiology, Signs and Symptoms, and Treatment of Cardiomyopathies

| Dilated Cardiomyopathy | Hypertrophic Cardiomyopathy | | Restictive Cardiomyopathy |
	Nonobstructed	Obstructed	
Pathophysiology			
Fibrosis of myocardium and endocardium Dilated chambers Mural wall thrombi prevalent	Hypertrophy of the walls Hypertrophied septum Relatively small chamber size	Same as for nonobstructed except for obstruction of left ventricular outflow tract associated with the hypertrophied septum and mitral valve incompetence	Mimics constrictive pericarditis Fibrosed walls cannot expand or contract Chambers narrowed; emboli common
Signs and Symptoms			
Fatigue and weakness Heart failure (left side) Dysrhytmias or heart block Systemic or pulmonary emboli S_3 and S_4 gallops Moderate to severe cardiomegaly	Dyspnea Angina Fatigue, syncope, palpitations Mild cardiomegaly S_4 gallop Ventricular dysrhythmias Sudden death common Heart failure	Same as for nonobstructed except with mitral regurgitation murmur Atrial fibrillation	Dyspnea and fatigue Heart failure (right sided) Mild to moderate cardiomegaly S_3 and S_4 gallops Heart block Emboli
Treatment			
Symptomatic treatment of heart failure Vasodilators Control of dysrhythmias Surgery: heart transplant	For both: Symptomatic treatment β-Blockers Conversion of artrial fibrillation Surgery: ventriculomyotomy or muscle resection with mitral valve replacement Digoxin, nitrates, and other vasodilators **contraindicated** with the obstructed form		Supportive treatment of symptoms Treatment of hypertension Conversion from dysrhythmias Exercise restrictions Emergency treatment of acute pulmonary edema

From Ignatavicius, D., & Workman, M. (2006). *Medical-surgical nursing: Critical thinking for collaborative care* (5th ed.). Philadelphia: Saunders.

g. Palpate the site gently, monitoring for warmth and edema

h. Measure and record the circumferences of the thighs and calves

i. Monitor for shortness of breath and chest pain, which can indicate pulmonary emboli

j. Administer thrombolytic therapy (tissue plasminogen activator) if prescribed, which must be initiated within 5 days after the onset of symptoms

k. Administer heparin therapy as prescribed to prevent enlargement of the existing clot and prevent the formation of new clots

l. Monitor activated partial thromboplastin time during heparin therapy

m. Administer warfarin (Coumadin) as prescribed following heparin therapy when the symptoms of deep vein thrombophlebitis have resolved

n. Monitor prothrombin time and international normalized ratio during warfarin (Coumadin) therapy

o. Monitor for the hazards and side effects associated with anticoagulant therapy

p. Administer analgesics as prescribed to reduce pain

q. Administer diuretics as prescribed to reduce lower extremity edema

r. Provide client teaching (Box 50-11)

D. Venous insufficiency

1. Description

a. Venous insufficiency results from prolonged venous hypertension, which stretches the veins and damages the valves

b. The resultant edema and venous stasis cause venous stasis ulcers, swelling, and cellulitis

c. Treatment focuses on decreasing edema and promoting venous return from the affected extremity

d. Treatment for venous stasis ulcers focuses on healing the ulcer and preventing stasis and ulcer recurrence

2. Data collection

a. Stasis dermatitis or brown discoloration along the ankles and extending up to the calf

b. Edema

c. Ulcer formation: edges are uneven, ulcer bed is pink, and granulation is present

3. Interventions

a. Instruct the client to wear elastic or compression stockings during the day and evening as prescribed (instruct the client to put on elastic stockings upon awakening before getting out of bed)

b. Advise the client to put on a clean pair of elastic stockings each day and that it will probably be necessary to wear the stockings for the rest of his or her life

c. Instruct the client to avoid prolonged sitting or standing, constrictive clothing, or crossing legs when seated

d. Instruct the client to elevate the legs for 10 to 20 minutes every few hours each day

e. Instruct the client to elevate legs above the level of the heart when in bed

f. Instruct the client in the use of an intermittent sequential pneumatic compression system, if prescribed; instruct the client to apply the compression system twice daily for 1 hour in the morning and evening

g. Advise the client with an open ulcer that the compression system is applied over a dressing

4. Wound care

a. Provide care to the wound as prescribed by the physician

b. Assess the client's ability to care for the wound, and initiate home care resources as necessary

c. If an Unna boot (a dressing constructed of gauze moistened with zinc oxide) is prescribed, the physician will change it weekly

d. The wound is cleansed with normal saline before application of the Unna boot; povidone-iodine (Betadine) and hydrogen peroxide are not used because they destroy granulation tissue

e. The Unna boot is covered with an elastic wrap that hardens to promote venous return and prevent stasis

f. Monitor for signs of arterial occlusion from an Unna boot that may be too tight

g. Keep tape off of the client's skin

BOX 50-11 **Instructions for the Client With Deep Vein Thrombophlebitis**

Instruct the client concerning the hazards of anticoagulation therapy.

Recognize the signs and symptoms of bleeding.

Avoid prolonged sitting or standing, constrictive clothing, or crossing legs when seated.

Elevate the legs for 10-20 minutes every few hours each day.

Plan a progressive walking program.

Inspect the legs for edema, and measure the circumference of the legs.

Wear antiembolism stockings as prescribed.

Avoid smoking.

Avoid any medications unless prescribed by the physician.

Instruct the client concerning the importance of follow-up physician visits and laboratory studies.

Obtain and wear a Medic-Alert bracelet.

h. Occlusive dressings such as polyethylene film or hydrocolloid dressings may be used to cover the ulcer

5. Medications
    a. Apply topical agents to the wound as prescribed to débride the ulcer, eliminate necrotic tissue, and promote healing
    b. When applying topical agents, apply an oil-based agent such as petroleum jelly (Vaseline) on surrounding skin, because débriding agents can injure healthy tissue
    c. Administer antibiotics as prescribed if infection or cellulitis occurs

E. Varicose veins
1. Description
    a. Distended, protruding veins that appear darkened and tortuous are evident
    b. Vein walls weaken and dilate, and valves become incompetent
2. Data collection
    a. Pain in the legs with dull aching after standing
    b. A feeling of fullness in the legs
    c. Ankle edema
3. Trendelenburg's test
    a. Place the client in a supine position with the legs elevated
    b. When the client sits up, if varicosities are present, veins fill from the proxima end; veins normally fill from the distal end
4. Interventions
    a. Assist with Trendelenburg's test
    b. Emphasize the importance of antiembolism stockings as prescribed
    c. Instruct the client to elevate the legs as much as possible
    d. Instruct the client to avoid constrictive clothing and pressure on the legs
    e. Prepare the client for sclerotherapy or vein stripping as prescribed
5. Sclerotherapy
    a. A solution is injected into the vein, followed by the application of a pressure dressing
    b. An incision and drainage of the trapped blood in the sclerosed vein are performed 14 to 21 days after the injection, followed by the application of a pressure dressing for 12 to 18 hours
6. Vein stripping
    a. Varicose veins are removed if they are larger than 4 mm in diameter or if they are in clusters
    b. Preoperatively assist the physician with vein marking
    c. Evaluate pulses as a baseline for comparison postoperatively

d. Maintain elastic (Ace) bandages on the client's legs postoperatively
e. Monitor the groin and leg for bleeding through the elastic bandages
f. Monitor the extremity for edema, warmth, color, and pulses
g. Assess for paresthesias, which could include saphenous nerve damage
h. Elevate the legs above the level of the heart postoperatively
i. Encourage range-of-motion exercises of the legs
j. Instruct the client to avoid leg dangling or chair sitting
k. Instruct the client to elevate the legs when sitting
l. Emphasize the importance of wearing elastic stockings after bandage removal

7. Laser therapy: A laser fiber is used to heat and close the main vessel contributing to the varicosity

XVII. ARTERIAL DISORDERS

A. Peripheral arterial disease
1. Description
    a. A chronic disorder in which partial or total arterial occlusion deprives the lower extremities of oxygen and nutrients
    b. Tissue damage occurs below the level of the arterial occlusion
    c. Atherosclerosis is the most common cause of peripheral arterial disease
2. Data collection
    a. Intermittent claudication (pain in the muscles resulting from an inadequate blood supply)
    b. Rest pain, characterized by numbness, burning, or aching in the distal portion of the lower extremities, which awakens the client at night and is relieved by placing the extremity in a dependent position
    c. Lower back or buttock discomfort
    d. Loss of hair and dry scaly skin on the lower extremities
    e. Thickened toenails
    f. Cold and gray-blue skin in the lower extremities
    g. Elevational pallor and dependent rubor in the lower extremities
    h. Decreased or absent peripheral pulses
    i. Signs of arterial ulcer formation occurring on or between the toes or on the upper aspect of the foot that are characterized as painful
    j. **BP** measurements at the thigh, calf, and ankle are lower than the brachial pressure (normally **BP** readings in the thigh and calf are higher than those in the upper extremities)
3. Interventions
    a. Assess pain

b. Monitor the extremities for color, motion and sensation, and pulses

c. Obtain **BP** measurements

d. Assess for signs of ulcer formation or signs of gangrene

e. Assist in developing an individualized exercise program, which is initiated gradually and slowly increased

f. Encourage prescribed exercise, which will improve arterial flow through the development of collateral circulation

g. Instruct the client to walk to the point of claudication, stop and rest, and then walk a little farther.

h. Because swelling in the extremities prevents arterial blood flow, instruct the client to elevate the feet at rest but to refrain from elevating them above the level of the heart because extreme elevation slows arterial blood flow to the feet

i. In severe cases of peripheral arterial disease, clients with edema may sleep with the affected limb hanging from the bed or sit upright in a chair for comfort

j. Instruct the client with peripheral arterial disease to avoid crossing the legs, which interferes with blood flow

k. Instruct the client to avoid exposure to cold (causes vasoconstriction) to the extremities and to wear socks or insulated shoes for warmth at all times

l. Instruct the client never to apply direct heat to the limb, such as with a heating pad or hot water, because the decreased sensitivity in the limb will cause burning

m. Instruct the client to inspect the skin on the extremities daily and to report any signs of skin breakdown

n. Instruct the client to avoid tobacco and caffeine because of their vasoconstrictive effects

o. Instruct the client in the use of hemorrheologic and antiplatelet medications as prescribed

p. Inform the client of the importance of taking all medications prescribed by the physician

4. Procedures to improve arterial blood flow

a. Percutaneous transluminal angioplasty with or without intravascular stent

b. Laser-assisted angioplasty

c. Atherectomy

d. Bypass surgery: Inflow procedures bypass the occlusion above the superficial femoral arteries and include aortoiliac, aortofemoral, and axillofemoral bypasses; outflow procedures bypass the occlusion at or below the superficial femoral arteries and include femoropopliteal and femorotibial bypasses

B. Raynaud's disease

1. Description

a. Raynaud's disease is vasospasm of the arterioles and arteries of the upper and lower extremities

b. Vasospasm causes constriction of the cutaneous vessels

c. Attacks are intermittent and occur with exposure to cold or stress

d. Primarily affects fingers, toes, ears, and cheeks

2. Data collection

a. Blanching of the extremity, followed by cyanosis during vasoconstriction

b. Reddened tissue when the vasospasm is relieved

c. Numbness, tingling, swelling, and a cold temperature at the affected body part

3. Interventions

a. Monitor pulses

b. Administer vasodilators as prescribed

c. Instruct the client regarding medication therapy

d. Assist the client to identify and avoid precipitating factors such as cold and stress

e. Instruct the client to avoid smoking

f. Instruct the client to wear warm clothing, socks, and gloves in cold weather

g. Advise the client to avoid injuries to fingers and hands

C. Buerger's disease (thromboangiitis obliterans)

1. Description

a. Buerger's disease is an occlusive disease of the median and small arteries and veins

b. The distal upper and lower limbs are affected most commonly

2. Data collection

a. Intermittent claudication

b. Ischemic pain occurring in the digits while at rest

c. Aching pain that is more severe at night

d. Cool, numb, or tingling sensation

e. Diminished pulses in the distal extremities

f. Extremities that are cool and red in the dependent position

g. Development of ulcerations in the extremities

3. Interventions

a. Instruct the client to stop smoking

b. Monitor pulses

c. Instruct the client to avoid injury to the upper and lower extremities

d. Administer vasodilators as prescribed

e. Instruct the client regarding medication therapy

▲ XVIII. AORTIC ANEURYSMS
   A. Description
      1. An aortic aneurysm is an abnormal dilation of the arterial wall caused by localized weakness and stretching in the medial layer or wall of an artery
      2. The aneurysm can be located anywhere along the abdominal aorta
      3. The goal of treatment is to limit the progression of the disease by modifying risk factors, controlling the **BP** to prevent strain on the aneurysm, recognizing symptoms early, and preventing rupture
   B. Types of aortic aneurysm
      1. Fusiform: Diffuse dilation that involves the entire circumference of the arterial segment
      2. Saccular: Distinct localized outpouching of the artery wall
      3. Dissecting: Created when blood separates the layers of the artery wall, forming a cavity between them
      4. False (pseudoaneurysm)
         a. Pseudoaneurysm occurs when the clot and connective tissue are outside the arterial wall
         b. Pseudoaneurysm occurs as a result of vessel injury or trauma to all three layers of the arterial wall
   ▲ C. Data collection
      1. Thoracic aneurysm
         a. Pain extending to neck, shoulders, lower back, or abdomen
         b. Syncope
         c. Dyspnea
         d. Increased pulse
         e. Cyanosis
         f. Weakness
         g. Hoarseness/difficulty swallowing because of pressure from the aneurysm
      2. Abdominal aneurysm
         a. Prominent, pulsating mass in the abdomen, at or above the umbilicus
         b. Systolic bruit over the aorta
         c. Tenderness on deep palpation
         d. Abdominal or lower back pain
   ▲ 3. Rupturing aneurysm
         a. Severe abdominal or back pain
         b. Lumbar pain radiating to the flank and groin
         c. Hypotension
         d. Increased pulse rate
         e. Signs of shock
         f. Hematoma at flank area
      4. Diagnostic tests
         a. Diagnostic tests are done to confirm the presence, size, and location of the aneurysm
         b. Tests include abdominal ultrasound, computed tomography scan, and arteriography

      5. Interventions
         a. Monitor vital signs
         b. Assess risk factors for the arterial disease process
         c. Obtain information regarding back or abdominal pain
         d. Question the client regarding the sensation of pulsation in the abdomen
         e. Inspect the skin for the presence of vascular disease or breakdown
         f. Check peripheral circulation, including pulses, temperature, and color
         g. Observe for signs of rupture
         h. Note any tenderness over the abdomen
         i. Monitor for abdominal distention
      6. Nonsurgical interventions
         a. Modify risk factors
         b. Instruct the client regarding the procedure for monitoring **BP**
         c. Instruct the client on the importance of regular physician visits to follow the size of the aneurysm
         d. Instruct the client to notify the physician immediately if any of the following occur: severe back or abdominal pain or fullness, soreness over the umbilicus, sudden development of discoloration in the extremities, or a persistent elevation of **BP**
         e. Instruct the client with a thoracic aneurysm to report immediately the occurrence of chest or back pain, shortness of breath, difficulty swallowing, or hoarseness
   D. Pharmacological interventions
      1. Administer antihypertensives to maintain the **BP** within normal limits and to prevent strain on the aneurysm
      2. Instruct the client on the purpose of the medications
      3. Instruct the client about the side effects and schedule of the medications
   E. Abdominal aortic aneurysm resection
      1. Description: Surgical resection or excision of the aneurysm; the excised section is replaced with a graft that is sewn end to end
      2. Preoperative interventions
         a. Assess all peripheral pulses as a baseline for postoperative comparison
         b. Instruct the client on coughing and deep-breathing exercises
         c. Administer bowel preparation as prescribed
      3. Postoperative interventions
         a. Monitor vital signs
         b. Monitor peripheral pulses distal to the graft site
         c. Monitor for signs of graft occlusion, including changes in pulses, cool to cold extremities

below the graft, white or blue extremities or flanks, severe pain, or abdominal distention

d. Limit elevation of the head of the bed to 45 degrees to prevent flexion of the graft

e. Monitor for hypovolemia and renal failure resulting from significant blood loss during surgery

f. Monitor urine output hourly, and notify the physician if it is less than 30 to 50 mL/hour

g. Monitor serum creatinine and blood urea nitrogen daily

h. Monitor respiratory status and auscultate breath sounds to identify respiratory complications

i. Encourage turning, coughing, and deep breathing, as well as splinting of the incision

j. Ambulate as prescribed

k. Maintain nasogastric tube to low suction until bowel sounds return

l. Assess for bowel sounds and report their return to the physician

m. Monitor for pain and administer medication as prescribed

n. Assess incision site for bleeding or signs of infection

o. Prepare the client for discharge by providing instructions regarding pain management, wound care, and activity restrictions

p. Instruct the client not to lift objects heavier than 15 to 20 lb for 6 to 12 weeks

q. Advise the client to avoid activities requiring pushing, pulling, or straining

r. Instruct the client not to drive a vehicle until approved by the physician

F. Thoracic aneurysm repair

1. Description

a. A thoracotomy or median sternotomy approach is used to enter the thoracic cavity

b. The aneurysm is exposed and excised, and a graft or prosthesis is sewn onto the aorta

c. Total cardiopulmonary bypass is necessary for excision of aneurysms in the ascending aorta

d. Partial cardiopulmonary bypass is used for clients with an aneurysm in the descending aorta

2. Postoperative interventions

a. Monitor vital signs, neurological, and renal status

b. Monitor for signs of hemorrhage, such as a drop in **BP** and increased pulse rate and respirations, and report to the physician immediately.

c. Monitor chest tubes for an increase in chest drainage, which may indicate bleeding or separation at the graft site

d. Assess sensation and motion of all extremities and notify the physician if deficits occur, which can be due to a lack of blood supply to the spinal cord during surgery

e. Monitor respiratory status and auscultate breath sounds to identify respiratory complications

f. Encourage turning, coughing, and deep breathing while splinting the incision

g. Monitor cardiac status for dysrhythmias

h. Monitor for pain and administer medication as prescribed

i. Assess the incision site for bleeding or signs of infection

j. Prepare the client for discharge by providing instructions regarding pain management, wound care, and activity restrictions

k. Instruct the client not to lift objects heavier than 15 to 20 lb for 6 to 12 weeks

l. Advise the client to avoid activities requiring pushing, pulling, or straining

m. Instruct the client not to drive a vehicle until approved by the physician

XIX. EMBOLECTOMY

A. Embolectomy is removal of an embolus from an artery using a catheter

B. A patch graft may be required to close the artery

C. Postoperative interventions

1. Assess cardiac, respiratory, and neurological status

2. Monitor the affected extremity for color, temperature, and pulse

3. Monitor for complications caused by reperfusion of the artery, such as spasms and swelling of the skeletal muscles

4. Maintain bedrest initially, with the client in a semi-Fowler's position

5. Place a bed cradle on the bed

6. Check incision site for bleeding or hematoma

7. Administer anticoagulants as prescribed

8. Instruct the client to recognize the signs and symptoms of infection and edema

9. Instruct the client to avoid prolonged sitting or crossing the legs when sitting

10. Instruct the client to elevate the legs when sitting

11. Instruct the client to wear antiembolism stockings as prescribed and how to remove and reapply the stockings

12. Instruct the client to ambulate daily

13. Instruct the client about anticoagulant therapy and the hazards associated with anticoagulants

XX. VENA CAVAL FILTER AND LIGATION OF INFERIOR VENA CAVA

A. Vena cava filter: insertion of an intracaval filter (umbrella) that partially occludes the inferior vena cava and traps emboli to prevent pulmonary emboli

B. Ligation: suturing or placing clips on the inferior vena cava to prevent pulmonary emboli; performed via abdominal laparotomy

C. Preoperative interventions: If the client has been taking an anticoagulant, consult with the physician regarding discontinuation of the medication to prevent hemorrhage

▲ D. Postoperative interventions
   1. Maintain a semi-Fowler's position
   2. Avoid hip flexion
   3. Refer to postoperative interventions for embolectomy

▲ XXI. HYPERTENSION
   A. Description
      1. The classification of prehypertension describes an individual with a systolic **BP** between 120 and 139 mm Hg or a **diastolic pressure** between 80 and 89 mm Hg
      2. In an individual over the age of 50, the systolic pressure is a more important value to note than the **diastolic pressure** regarding the need for treatment
      3. Hypertension is a major risk factor for coronary, cerebral, renal, and peripheral vascular disease
      4. The disease is initially asymptomatic
      5. The goals of treatment include reducing the **BP** and preventing or lessening the extent of organ damage (Table 50-4)
      6. Nonpharmacological approaches, such as lifestyle changes, may be prescribed initially; if the **BP** cannot be decreased after a reasonable period (1-3 months), the client may require pharmacological treatment

   ▲ B. Primary or essential hypertension
      1. No known cause
      2. Risk factors
         a. Aging
         b. Family history
         c. Black race, with higher prevalence in males
         d. Obesity
         e. Smoking
         f. Stress
         g. Excessive alcohol
         h. Hyperlipidemia
         i. Increased intake of salt or caffeine

   C. Secondary hypertension
      1. Treatment depends on the cause and the organs involved
      2. Secondary hypertension occurs as a result of other disorders or conditions
      3. Precipitating disorders or conditions
         a. Cardiovascular disorders
         b. Renal disorders
         c. Endocrine system disorders
         d. Pregnancy

TABLE 50-4 **Hypertension**

Organ Involvement	Complications
Eyes	Visual changes
Brain	Stroke
Cardiovascular system	Heart failure
	Heart failure; hypertensive crisis
Kidneys	Renal failure

         e. Medications (such as estrogens, glucocorticoids, and mineralocorticoids)

   D. Data collection
      1. May be asymptomatic
      2. Headache
      3. Visual disturbances
      4. Dizziness
      5. Chest pain
      6. Tinnitus
      7. Flushed face
      8. Epistaxis

   E. Interventions
      1. Goals
         a. One treatment goal is to reduce the **BP**
         b. Another treatment goal is to prevent or lessen the extent of organ damage
      2. Question the client regarding the signs and symptoms indicative of hypertension
      3. Obtain the **BP** two or more times on both arms with the client supine and standing
      4. Compare the **BP** with prior documentation
      5. Determine family history of hypertension
      6. Identify current medication therapy
      7. Obtain weight
      8. Evaluate dietary patterns and sodium intake
      9. Assess for visual changes or retinal damage
      10. Assess for cardiovascular changes such as distended neck veins, increased heart rate, and dysrhythmias
      11. Evaluate chest x-ray film for heart enlargement
      12. Assess neurological system
      13. Evaluate renal function
      14. Evaluate results of diagnostic and laboratory studies

   F. Nonpharmacological interventions
      1. Weight reduction, if necessary, or maintenance of ideal weight
      2. Dietary sodium restriction to 2 g daily as prescribed
      3. Moderate intake of alcohol and caffeine-containing products
      4. Initiation of a regular exercise program
      5. Avoidance of smoking
      6. Relaxation techniques and biofeedback therapy
      7. Elimination of unnecessary medications that may contribute to the hypertension

G. Stepped-care approach
   1. Description
      a. If a pharmacological approach to treating hypertension is required, a single medication is prescribed and monitored for its effectiveness
      b. Medications are added to the treatment regimen until the **BP** is controlled
      c. Refer to Chapter 51 for medications to treat hypertension
   2. Step 1: A single medication is prescribed, which may be a diuretic, β-blocker, calcium-channel blocker, ACE inhibitor, or angiotensin II receptor blocker
   3. Step 2
      a. Step 1 therapy is evaluated after 1 to 3 months
      b. If the response is not adequate, compliance is evaluated
      c. The medication may be increased or a new medication may be prescribed or a second medication may be added to the treatment plan
   4. Step 3
      a. Compliance is evaluated
      b. Further evaluation of Step 2
      c. If a therapeutic response is not adequate, a second medication is substituted or a third medication is added to the treatment plan
   5. Step 4
      a. Compliance is evaluated
      b. Careful assessment of factors limiting the antihypertensive response is performed
      c. A third or fourth medication may be added to the treatment plan
H. See Box 50-12 for client education.
▲ XXII. HYPERTENSIVE CRISIS
A. Description
   1. A hypertensive crisis is any clinical condition requiring immediate reduction in **BP**
   2. A hypertensive crisis is an acute and life-threatening condition
   3. The accelerated hypertension requires emergency treatment because target organ damage (brain, heart, kidneys, retina of the eye) can occur quickly
   4. Death can be caused by stroke, renal failure, or cardiac disease
B. Data collection
   1. An extremely high **BP** and usually the **diastolic pressure** is greater than 120 mm Hg
   2. Headache
   3. Drowsiness and confusion
   4. Blurred vision
   5. Changes in neurological status
   6. Tachycardia and tachypnea
   7. Dyspnea
   8. Cyanosis
   9. Seizures
C. Interventions
   1. Maintain a patent airway
   2. IV antihypertensive medications may be prescribed
   3. Monitor vital signs, assessing the **BP** every 5 minutes
   4. Assess for hypotension during the administration of antihypertensives; place the client in a supine position if hypotension occurs

---

BOX 50-12 **Client Education for Hypertension**

Describe the importance of compliance with the treatment plan.

Describe the disease process, explaining that symptoms usually do not develop until organs have suffered damage.

Initiate and assist the client in planning a regular exercise program, avoiding heavy weight lifting and isometric exercises.

Emphasize the importance of beginning the exercise program gradually.

Encourage the client to express feelings about daily stress.

Assist the client to identify ways to reduce stress.

Teach relaxation techniques.

Instruct the client on how to incorporate relaxation techniques into the daily living pattern.

Instruct the client and family in the technique for monitoring blood pressure.

Instruct the client to maintain a diary of blood pressure readings.

Emphasize the importance of lifelong medication and the need for follow-up treatment.

Instruct the client and family about the dietary restrictions, which may include sodium, fat, calories, and cholesterol.

Instruct the client on how to shop for and prepare low-sodium meals.

Provide a list of products that contain sodium.

Instruct the client to read labels of products to determine sodium content, focusing on substances listed as sodium, NaCl, or MSG (monosodium glutamate).

Instruct the client to bake, roast, or boil foods; avoid salt in preparation of foods; and avoid using salt at the table.

Instruct the client that fresh foods are best to consume and to avoid canned foods.

Instruct the client about the actions, side effects, and scheduling of medications.

Advise the client that if uncomfortable side effects occur to contact the physician and not to stop the medication.

Instruct the client to avoid over-the-counter medications.

Stress the importance of follow-up care.

5. Have emergency medications and resuscitation equipment readily available
6. Maintain bedrest, with the head of the bed elevated at 45 degrees
7. Monitor IV therapy, assessing for fluid overload
8. Monitor I&O
9. Insert a Foley catheter as prescribed
10. Monitor urinary output, and if oliguria or anuria occurs, notify the physician

PRACTICE QUESTIONS

More questions on the companion CD!

628. A postcardiac surgery client has a urine output averaging 20 mL/hr for 2 hours. The client received a single bolus of 500 mL of IV fluid. Urine output for the subsequent hour was 25 mL. Daily laboratory results indicate that the blood urea nitrogen (BUN) level is 45 mg/dL and the serum creatinine level is 2.2 mg/dL. The nurse interprets that the client is at risk for:
    1. Hypovolemia
    2. Acute renal failure
    3. Glomerulonephritis
    4. Urinary tract infection

629. A nurse is preparing to ambulate a postoperative client following cardiac surgery. The nurse plans to do which of the following to enable the client to best tolerate the ambulation?
    1. Provide the client with a walker
    2. Remove the telemetry equipment
    3. Encourage the client to cough and deep breathe
    4. Premedicate the client with an analgesic prior to ambulating

630. A client is wearing a continuous cardiac monitor, which begins to alarm at the nurse's station. The nurse sees no electrocardiographic complexes on the screen. The nurse would first:
    1. Call a code blue
    2. Call the physician
    3. Check the client status and lead placement
    4. Press the recorder button on the ECG console

631. A client with a diagnosis of rapid rate atrial fibrillation asks the nurse why the physician is going to perform carotid massage. The nurse responds that this procedure may stimulate the:
    1. Vagus nerve to slow the heart rate
    2. Vagus nerve to increase the heart rate
    3. Diaphragmatic nerve to slow the heart rate
    4. Diaphragmatic nerve to increase the heart rate

632. A nurse is caring for a client on a cardiac monitor who is alone in a room at the end of the hall. The client has a short burst of ventricular tachycardia (VT) followed by ventricular fibrillation (VF). The client suddenly loses consciousness. The nurse would immediately:
    1. Go to the nurse's station quickly and call a code

2. Run to get a defibrillator from an adjacent nursing unit
3. Call for help and initiate cardiopulmonary resuscitation (CPR)
4. Start oxygen by cannula at 10 L/minute and lower the head of the bed

633. A nurse is monitoring a client following cardioversion. Which of the following observations would be of highest priority to the nurse?
    1. Blood pressure
    2. Status of airway
    3. Oxygen flow rate
    4. Level of consciousness

634. An automatic external defibrillator is available to treat the client who goes into cardiac arrest and is receiving cardiopulmonary resuscitation (CPR). With this device, the nurse checks the cardiac rhythm by:
    1. Holding the defibrillator paddles firmly against the chest
    2. Applying the adhesive patch electrodes to the skin and moving away from the client
    3. Connecting standard electrocardiographic electrodes to a transtelephonic monitoring device
    4. Applying standard electrocardiographic monitoring leads to the client and observing the rhythm

635. The nurse is caring for the client immediately after insertion of a permanent demand pacemaker via the right subclavian vein. The nurse takes care not to dislodge the pacing catheter by:
    1. Limiting movement and abduction of the left arm
    2. Limiting movement and abduction of the right arm
    3. Assisting the client to get out of bed and ambulate with a walker
    4. Having the physical therapist do active range of motion to the right arm

636. A client diagnosed with thrombophlebitis 1 day ago suddenly complains of chest pain and shortness of breath, and the client is visibly anxious. The nurse immediately checks the client for signs and symptoms of:
    1. Pneumonia
    2. Pulmonary edema
    3. Pulmonary embolism
    4. Myocardial infarction

637. A 24-year-old man seeks medical attention for complaints of claudication in the arch of the foot. The nurse also notes superficial thrombophlebitis of the lower leg. The nurse would next check the client for:
    1. Smoking history
    2. Recent exposure to allergens
    3. History of recent insect bites

4. Familial tendency toward peripheral vascular disease

638. A nurse has given instructions to the client with Raynaud's disease about self-management of the disease process. The nurse determines that the client needs further instructions if the client states that:
  1. Smoking cessation is very important
  2. Moving to a warmer climate should help
  3. Sources of caffeine should be eliminated from the diet
  4. Taking nifedipine (Procardia) as prescribed will decrease vessel spasm

639. A client with myocardial infarction suddenly becomes tachycardic, shows signs of air hunger, and begins coughing frothy, pink-tinged sputum. A nurse listens to breath sounds, expecting to hear bilateral:
  1. Rhonchi
  2. Crackles
  3. Wheezes
  4. Diminished breath sounds

640. A nurse is collecting data on a client with a diagnosis of right-sided heart failure. The nurse would expect to note which specific characteristic of this condition?
  1. Dyspnea
  2. Hacking cough
  3. Dependent edema
  4. Crackles on lung auscultation

641. A nurse is checking the neurovascular status of a client who returned to the surgical nursing unit 4 hours ago after undergoing aortoiliac bypass graft. The affected leg is warm, and the nurse notes redness and edema. The pedal pulse is palpable and unchanged from admission. The nurse interprets that the neurovascular status is:
  1. Moderately impaired, and the surgeon should be called
  2. Normal, caused by increased blood flow through the leg
  3. Slightly deteriorating, and should be monitored for another hour
  4. Adequate from an arterial approach, but venous complications are arising

642. A client has an Unna boot applied for treatment of a venous stasis leg ulcer. The nurse notes that the client's toes are mottled and cool, and the client verbalizes some numbness and tingling of the foot. The nurse interprets that the boot:
  1. Has not yet dried
  2. Is controlling leg edema
  3. Is impairing venous return
  4. Has been applied too tightly

643. A client with angina complains that the anginal pain is prolonged and severe and occurs at the same time each day, most often in the morning. On further data collection, the nurse notes that the pain occurs in the absence of precipitating factors. This type of anginal pain is best described as:
  1. Stable angina
  2. Variant angina
  3. Unstable angina
  4. Nonanginal pain

644. A nurse is assisting in monitoring the condition of a client after pericardiocentesis for cardiac tamponade. Which observation would indicate that the procedure was unsuccessful?
  1. Clear breath sounds
  2. Client expressions of relief
  3. Clearly audible heart sounds
  4. Distant and muffled heart sounds

645. A nurse is monitoring a client with an abdominal aortic aneurysm (AAA). Which finding is probably unrelated to the AAA?
  1. Pulsatile abdominal mass
  2. Hyperactive bowel sounds in the area
  3. Systolic bruit over the area of the mass
  4. Subjective sensation of "heart beating" in the abdomen

646. A client arrives in the emergency department after complaining of unrelieved chest pain for 2 days. The pain has subsided slightly but has not disappeared completely. When the nurse approaches the client with a nitroglycerin sublingual tablet, the client states, "I don't need that. My dad takes that for his heart. There's nothing wrong with my heart." Which of the following best describes the client's response?
  1. Angry
  2. Denial
  3. Phobic
  4. Obsessive-compulsive

647. A client is scheduled for a cardiac catheterization using a radiopaque dye. The nurse checks which most critical item before the procedure?
  1. Intake and output
  2. Height and weight
  3. Peripheral pulse rates
  4. Allergy to iodine or shellfish

648. A client is scheduled for a dipyridamole (Persantine) thallium scan. The nurse would check to make sure that the client has not had which of the following before the procedure?
  1. Caffeine
  2. Fatty meal
  3. Excess sugar
  4. Milk products

649. A client with no history of cardiovascular disease presents to the ambulatory clinic with flu-like symptoms. While at the clinic, the client suddenly develops chest pain. Which question would best

help the nurse to discriminate pain caused by a non-cardiac problem?
1. "Can you describe the pain to me?"
2. "Have you ever had this pain before?"
3. "Does the pain get worse when you breathe in?"
4. "Can you rate the pain on a scale of 1 to 10, with 10 being the worst?"

650. A client with myocardial infarction (MI) has been transferred from the coronary care unit (CCU) to the general medical unit with cardiac monitoring via telemetry. The nurse assisting in caring for the client expects to note which type of activity prescribed?
1. Strict bedrest for 24 hours
2. Bathroom privileges and self-care activities
3. Unrestricted activities, because the client is monitored
4. Unsupervised hallway ambulation with distances less than 200 feet

651. A nurse checks the sternotomy incision of a client on the second postoperative day after cardiac surgery. The incision shows some slight "puffiness" along the edges and is non-reddened with no apparent drainage. The client's temperature is 37.2° C (99° F) orally. The white blood cell (WBC) count is 7500/mm^3. The nurse interprets that the incision line:

1. Is slightly edematous but shows no active signs of infection
2. Shows no sign of infection although the WBC count is elevated
3. Shows early signs of infection supported by an elevated WBC count
4. Shows early signs of infection although the temperature is near normal

ALTERNATE ITEM FORMAT: MULTIPLE RESPONSE

652. A nurse in a medical unit is caring for a client with heart failure. The client suddenly develops extreme dyspnea, tachycardia, and lung crackles, and the nurse suspects pulmonary edema. The nurse immediately notifies the registered nurse and expects which interventions to be prescribed?
☐ 1. Administering oxygen
☐ 2. Inserting a Foley catheter
☐ 3. Administering furosemide (Lasix)
☐ 4. Administering morphine sulfate intravenously
☐ 5. Transporting the client to the coronary care unit
☐ 6. Placing the client in a low Fowler's side-lying position

ANSWERS

628. 2
Rationale: The client who undergoes cardiac surgery is at risk for renal injury from poor perfusion, hemolysis, low cardiac output, or vasopressor medication therapy. Renal insult is signaled by a decreased urine output and increased BUN and creatinine levels. The client may need medications to increase renal perfusion and could need peritoneal dialysis or hemodialysis.
Test-Taking Strategy: Use the process of elimination. The question provides no evidence of any infection, so eliminate options 3 and 4 first. Noting that the urine output is inadequate will assist with eliminating option 1. Review laboratory values and postcardiac surgery complications if you had difficulty with this question.
Level of Cognitive Ability: Analysis
Client Needs: Physiological Integrity
Integrated Process: Nursing Process/Data Collection
Content Area: Adult Health/Cardiovascular
References: Linton, A., & Maebius, N. (2007). *Introduction to medical-surgical nursing* (4th ed., p. 274). Philadelphia: Saunders.
Monahan, F., Sands, J., Neighbors, M., Marek, J., & Green, C. (2007). *Phipps' medical-surgical nursing: Health and illness perspectives* (8th ed., pp. 850-851). St. Louis: Mosby.

629. 4
Rationale: The nurse should encourage regular use of pain medication for the first 48 to 72 hours after cardiac surgery,

because analgesia will promote rest, decrease myocardial oxygen consumption caused by pain, and allow better participation in activities such as coughing, deep breathing, and ambulation.
Test-Taking Strategy: Use the process of elimination. The question asks for the best action of the nurse to help a client tolerate ambulation. Coughing and deep breathing will not actively help endurance, so eliminate option 3. Eliminate option 2 because removal of telemetry equipment is contraindicated unless ordered. From the remaining options, noting that the client is postoperative will direct you to option 4. Review postoperative nursing care if you had difficulty with this question.
Level of Cognitive Ability: Application
Client Needs: Physiological Integrity
Integrated Process: Nursing Process/Planning
Content Area: Adult Health/Cardiovascular
Reference: Linton, A., & Maebius, N. (2007). *Introduction to medical-surgical nursing* (4th ed., p. 651). Philadelphia: Saunders.

630. 3
Rationale: Sudden loss of electrocardiographic complexes indicates ventricular asystole or possibly electrode displacement. Assessment of the client and equipment is the first action by the nurse.
Test-Taking Strategy: Use the steps of the nursing process and remember that data collection is the first step. Options 1 and 2 are incorrect because they indicate calling for assistance

prior to collecting data. Option 4 may sound reasonable, but the electrocardiographic monitor automatically starts recording when an alarm sounds. Option 3 is the best option, because you should always check the client directly before taking any action. Review care of a client on a cardiac monitor if you had difficulty with this question.
Level of Cognitive Ability: Application
Client Needs: Physiological Integrity
Integrated Process: Nursing Process/Implementation
Content Area: Adult Health/Cardiovascular
Reference: Christensen, B., & Kockrow, E. (2006). *Adult health nursing* (5th ed., pp. 334-335). St. Louis: Mosby.

631. **1**
Rationale: Carotid sinus massage is one maneuver used for vagal stimulation to decrease a rapid heart rate and possibly terminate a tachydysrhythmia. The other maneuvers are the Valsalva maneuver of inducing the gag reflex and asking the client to strain or bear down. Medication therapy is often needed as an adjunct to keep the rate down or maintain the normal rhythm.
Test-Taking Strategy: Use the process of elimination. Eliminate options 2 and 4 first because these options indicate increasing an already rapid rate. From the remaining options, use knowledge of anatomy and physiology. A rapid-rate dysrhythmia would need to be slowed, which is the function of the vagus nerve. The diaphragmatic nerve affects respiration. If you are unfamiliar with the functions of these nerves, review this content.
Level of Cognitive Ability: Application
Client Needs: Physiological Integrity
Integrated Process: Nursing Process/Implementation
Content Area: Adult Health/Cardiovascular
Reference: Perry, A., & Potter, P. (2006). *Clinical nursing skills & techniques* (6th ed., p. 1369). St. Louis: Mosby.

632. **3**
Rationale: When VF occurs, the nurse remains with the client and initiates CPR until a defibrillator is available and attached to the client. Options 1, 2, and 4 are incorrect.
Test-Taking Strategy: Use the process of elimination. Eliminate options 1 and 2 first because you would never leave the client alone. From the remaining options, lowering the head of bed is appropriate (for resuscitation), but the oxygen by cannula at 10 L/minute is incorrect. Option 3 is the correct option. Review care of the client with VF if you had difficulty with this question.
Level of Cognitive Ability: Application
Client Needs: Physiological Integrity
Integrated Process: Nursing Process/Implementation
Content Area: Adult Health/Cardiovascular
References: Lewis, S., Heitkemper, M., Dirksen, S., & Bucher, L. (2007). *Medical-surgical nursing: Assessment and management of clinical problems* (7th ed., pp. 854-855). St. Louis: Mosby.
Linton, A., & Maebius, N. (2007). *Introduction to medical-surgical nursing* (4th ed., p. 681). Philadelphia: Saunders.

633. **2**
Rationale: Nursing responsibilities after cardioversion include maintenance of a patent airway, oxygen administration,

assessment of vital signs and level of consciousness, and dysrhythmia detection. Airway is the priority.
Test-Taking Strategy: Use the ABCs—airway, breathing, and circulation—to answer the question. This will direct you to option 2. Remember, airway comes first. Review care of the client following cardioversion if you had difficulty with this question.
Level of Cognitive Ability: Analysis
Client Needs: Physiological Integrity
Integrated Process: Nursing Process/Data Collection
Content Area: Delegating/Prioritizing
Reference: deWit, S. (2009). *Medical-surgical nursing: Concepts & practice* (p. 478). Philadelphia: Saunders.

634. **2**
Rationale: The nurse or rescuer puts two large adhesive patch electrodes on the client's chest in the usual defibrillator position. The nurse stops cardiopulmonary resuscitation and orders anyone near the client to move away and not touch the client. The defibrillator then analyzes the rhythm, which may take up to 30 seconds. The machine then indicates if it is necessary to defibrillate. Although automatic external defibrillation can be done transtelephonically, it is done through the use of patch electrodes (not standard electrocardiographic electrodes) that interact via telephone lines to a base station that controls any actual defibrillation. It is not necessary to hold defibrillator paddles against the client's chest with this device.
Test-Taking Strategy: If you are not familiar with this piece of equipment, look first at the word "automatic" in the name. This implies that someone is not as involved in the process as with a conventional defibrillator and thus may help you eliminate option 1. Because standard electrocardiographic monitoring leads are not used (options 3 and 4), you can eliminate these comparable or alike, and incorrect, options. Although automatic external defibrillation can be done transtelephonically, it is done through the use of patch electrodes. Review the use of this device if you had difficulty with this question.
Level of Cognitive Ability: Application
Client Needs: Physiological Integrity
Integrated Process: Nursing Process/Implementation
Content Area: Adult Health/Cardiovascular
References: Lewis, S., Heitkemper, M., Dirksen, S., & Bucher, L. (2007). *Medical-surgical nursing: Assessment and management of clinical problems* (7th ed., pp. 856-857). St. Louis: Mosby.
Linton, A., & Maebius, N. (2007). *Introduction to medical-surgical nursing* (4th ed., p. 228). Philadelphia: Saunders.

635. **2**
Rationale: In the first several hours after insertion of either a permanent or temporary pacemaker, the most common complication is pacing electrode dislodgment. The nurse helps prevent this complication by limiting the client's activities.
Test-Taking Strategy: Use the process of elimination. The question tells you that the pacemaker was inserted on the right side. Therefore, to prevent pacing electrode dislodgment, motion must be limited on that side. Options 3 and 4 involve movement of the right arm. Limiting the movement of the left arm (option 1) is of no benefit to the client. Thus, option 2 is correct. Review care of the client following pacemaker insertion if you had difficulty with this question.

Level of Cognitive Ability: Application
Client Needs: Physiological Integrity
Integrated Process: Nursing Process/Implementation
Content Area: Adult Health/Cardiovascular
Reference: Lewis, S., Heitkemper, M., Dirksen, S., & Bucher, L. (2007). *Medical-surgical nursing: Assessment and management of clinical problems* (7th ed., p. 858). St. Louis: Mosby.

636. 3
Rationale: Pulmonary embolism is a life-threatening complication of deep vein thrombosis and thrombophlebitis. Chest pain is the most common symptom, which is sudden in onset and may be aggravated by breathing. Other signs and symptoms include dyspnea, cough, diaphoresis, and apprehension.
Test-Taking Strategy: Use the process of elimination. This question tests your ability to analyze signs and symptoms of pulmonary embolism in a client at risk. Options 2 and 4 should be eliminated because myocardial infarction and pulmonary edema are cardiac-related problems and are therefore comparable or alike. Eliminate option 1 because pneumonia is an infec-tious process. Review the complications of thrombophlebitis if you had difficulty with this question.
Level of Cognitive Ability: Analysis
Client Needs: Physiological Integrity
Integrated Process: Nursing Process/Data Collection
Content Area: Adult Health/Cardiovascular
Reference: Christensen, B., & Kockrow, E. (2006). *Adult health nursing* (5th ed., p. 389). St. Louis: Mosby.

637. 1
Rationale: The mixture of arterial and venous manifestations (claudication and phlebitis, respectively) in the young male client suggests thromboangiitis obliterans (Buerger's disease). This is a relatively uncommon disorder, characterized by inflammation and thrombosis of smaller arteries and veins. This disorder is typically found in young men who smoke. The cause is unknown but is suspected to have an autoim-mune component.
Test-Taking Strategy: Use the process of elimination. You can first eliminate options 2 and 3 because they would most likely cause local skin reactions. The question asks which item you should check "next." It is often better to assess a modifiable factor before a nonmodifiable one. This will direct you to option 1. Review the causes of Buerger's disease if you had difficulty with this question.
Level of Cognitive Ability: Analysis
Client Needs: Health Promotion and Maintenance
Integrated Process: Nursing Process/Data Collection
Content Area: Adult Health/Cardiovascular
Reference: Linton, A., & Maebius, N. (2007). *Introduction to medical-surgical nursing* (4th ed., pp. 703-704). Philadelphia: Saunders.

638. 2
Rationale: Raynaud's disease responds favorably to the elimination of nicotine and caffeine. Medications such as calcium channel blockers may inhibit vessel spasm and prevent symptoms. Avoiding exposure to cold through a variety of means is very important. However, moving to a warmer climate may

not necessarily be beneficial, because the symptoms could still occur with the use of air conditioning and during periods of cooler weather.
Test-Taking Strategy: Note the strategic words "needs further instructions." These words indicate a negative event query and the need to select the incorrect client statement. All of the options seem reasonable. However, when you analyze each of them, note that relocation is the least favorable of all the options, from the viewpoints of practicality and encountering new environmental concerns. Review treatment measures for this disorder if you had difficulty with this question.
Level of Cognitive Ability: Comprehension
Client Needs: Health Promotion and Maintenance
Integrated Process: Teaching and Learning
Content Area: Adult Health/Cardiovascular
Reference: Linton, A., & Maebius, N. (2007). *Introduction to medical-surgical nursing* (4th ed., p. 704). Philadelphia: Saunders.

639. 2
Rationale: Pulmonary edema is characterized by extreme breathlessness, dyspnea, air hunger, and production of frothy, pink-tinged sputum. Auscultation of the lungs reveals crackles. Wheezes, rhonchi, and diminished breath sounds are not associated with pulmonary edema.
Test-Taking Strategy: Use the process of elimination. Recall that fluid produces sounds that are called crackles. This will assist in eliminating options 1, 3, and 4. If you had difficulty with this question, review the manifestations found in pulmonary edema.
Level of Cognitive Ability: Analysis
Client Needs: Physiological Integrity
Integrated Process: Nursing Process/Data Collection
Content Area: Adult Health/Cardiovascular
Reference: Christensen, B., & Kockrow, E. (2006). *Adult health nursing* (5th ed., p. 360). St. Louis: Mosby.

640. 3
Rationale: Right-sided heart failure is characterized by signs of systemic congestion that occur as a result of right ventricular failure, fluid retention, and pressure buildup in the venous system. Edema develops in the lower legs and ascends to the thighs and abdominal wall. Other characteristics include jugular (neck vein) congestion, enlarged liver and spleen, anorexia and nausea, distended abdomen, swollen hands and fingers, polyuria at night, and weight gain. Left-sided heart failure produces pulmonary signs. These include dyspnea, crackles on lung auscultation, and a hacking cough.
Test-Taking Strategy: Focus on the subject: right-sided heart failure. Eliminate options 1, 2, and 4 because they are comparable or alike and are pulmonary signs. Review the signs of right- and left-sided heart failure if you had difficulty with this question.
Level of Cognitive Ability: Analysis
Client Needs: Physiological Integrity
Integrated Process: Nursing Process/Data Collection
Content Area: Adult Health/Cardiovascular
Reference: Christensen, B., & Kockrow, E. (2006). *Adult health nursing* (5th ed., p. 361). St. Louis: Mosby.

641. 2
Rationale: An expected outcome of surgery is warmth, redness, and edema in the surgical extremity cause by increased blood flow. Options 1, 3, and 4 are incorrect.
Test-Taking Strategy: Use the process of elimination. Option 1 can be eliminated because the pedal pulse is unchanged. Venous complications from immobilization caused by surgery would not be apparent within 4 hours, so eliminate option 4 next. To choose between options 2 and 3, think about the effects of sudden reperfusion in an ischemic limb. There would be redness from new blood flow and edema from the sudden change in pressure in the blood vessels. Thus, option 2 is correct. Review the expected findings following aortoiliac bypass graft if you had difficulty with this question.
Level of Cognitive Ability: Analysis
Client Needs: Physiological Integrity
Integrated Process: Nursing Process/Data Collection
Content Area: Adult Health/Cardiovascular
References: deWit, S. (2009). *Medical-surgical nursing: Concepts & practice* (pp. 444-445). Philadelphia: Saunders.
Lewis, S., Heitkemper, M., Dirksen, S., & Bucher, L. (2007). *Medical-surgical nursing: Assessment and management of clinical problems* (7th ed., p. 898). St. Louis: Mosby.

642. 4
Rationale: An Unna boot that is applied too tightly can cause signs of arterial occlusion. The nurse assesses the circulation in the foot and teaches the client to do the same. Options 1, 2, and 3 are incorrect interpretations.
Test-Taking Strategy: Note that the symptoms described in the question are signs of arterial compromise. Option 4 is the only option that is consistent with this circumstance. Review the signs of arterial compromise if you had difficulty with this question.
Level of Cognitive Ability: Analysis
Client Needs: Physiological Integrity
Integrated Process: Nursing Process/Data Collection
Content Area: Adult Health/Cardiovascular
References: Christensen, B., & Kochrow, E. (2006). *Adult health nursing* (5th ed., pp. 393-394). St. Louis: Mosby.
Monahan, F., Sands, J., Neighbors, M., Marek, J., & Green, C. (2007). *Phipps' medical-surgical nursing: Health and illness perspectives* (8th ed., pp. 893-894). St. Louis: Mosby.

643. 2
Rationale: Stable angina is induced by exercise and relieved by rest or nitroglycerin tablets. Unstable angina occurs at lower and lower levels of activity or at rest, is less predictable, and is often a precursor of myocardial infarction. Variant angina, or Prinzmetal's angina, is prolonged and severe and occurs at the same time each day, most often in the morning.
Test-Taking Strategy: Focus on the data in the question and use knowledge regarding the various types of angina to answer the question. This will assist in eliminating options 1, 3, and 4. Review the characteristics of the various types of angina if you had difficulty with this question.
Level of Cognitive Ability: Comprehension
Client Needs: Physiological Integrity
Integrated Process: Nursing Process/Data Collection

Content Area: Adult Health/Cardiovascular
Reference: Black, J., & Hawks, J. (2005). *Medical-surgical nursing: Clinical management for positive outcomes* (7th ed., p. 1704). Philadelphia: Saunders.

644. 4
Rationale: Following pericardiocentesis, the client usually expresses immediate relief. Heart sounds are no longer muffled or distant. Clear breath sounds and clearly audible heart sounds are positive signs.
Test-Taking Strategy: Note the strategic word "unsuccessful." Successful therapy is measured by the disappearance of the original signs and symptoms of cardiac tamponade. Therefore, look for the option that identifies a sign consistent with continued tamponade. Review signs of cardiac tamponade and the expected effects of pericardiocentesis if you had difficulty with this question.
Level of Cognitive Ability: Analysis
Client Needs: Physiological Integrity
Integrated Process: Nursing Process/Evaluation
Content Area: Adult Health/Cardiovascular
Reference: Chernecky, C., & Berger, B. (2008). *Laboratory tests and diagnostic procedures* (5th ed., pp. 861-863). Philadelphia: Saunders.

645. 2
Rationale: Not all clients with AAA exhibit symptoms. Those who do may describe a feeling of the "heart beating" in the abdomen when supine, or being able to feel the mass throbbing. A pulsatile mass may be palpated in the middle and upper abdomen. A systolic bruit may be auscultated over the mass. Hyperactive bowel sounds are not specifically related to an AAA.
Test-Taking Strategy: Use the process of elimination. Note the strategic word "unrelated." Note that options 1, 3, and 4 are comparable or alike in that they identify a circulatory component. Review the signs of AAA if you had difficulty with this question.
Level of Cognitive Ability: Analysis
Client Needs: Physiological Integrity
Integrated Process: Nursing Process/Data Collection
Content Area: Adult Health/Cardiovascular
Reference: Christensen, B., & Kockrow, E. (2006). *Adult health nursing* (5th ed., pp. 385-386). St. Louis: Mosby.

646. 2
Rationale: Denial is the most common reaction when a client has a myocardial infarction or anginal pain. No angry behavior was identified in the question. Phobias and obsessive-compulsive disorders are mental health diagnoses.
Test-Taking Strategy: Use the process of elimination. Eliminate options 3 and 4 first because these are medical diagnoses. Recalling that denial is the most common reaction when a person has chest pain will direct you to option 2. Review psychosocial responses in the client experiencing chest pain if you had difficulty with this question.
Level of Cognitive Ability: Analysis
Client Needs: Psychosocial Integrity
Integrated Process: Nursing Process/Data Collection
Content Area: Pharmacology

References: Black, J., & Hawks, J. (2005). *Medical-surgical nursing: Clinical management for positive outcomes* (7th ed., p. 526). Philadelphia: Saunders.
Linton, A., & Maebius, N. (2007). *Introduction to medical-surgical nursing* (4th ed., pp. 1240, 1242). Philadelphia: Saunders.

647. 4
Rationale: This procedure requires a signed informed consent, since it involves injection of a radiopaque dye into the blood vessel. The risk of allergic reaction and possible anaphylaxis is serious and must be assessed before the procedure. Although options 1, 2, and 3 may be a component of data collection, they are not the most critical items.
Test-Taking Strategy: Use prioritization skills and note the strategic words "most critical." Recalling the risk of anaphylaxis if an allergy exists will direct you to option 4. Review preprocedure interventions for a cardiac catheterization if you had difficulty with this question.
Level of Cognitive Ability: Application
Client Needs: Physiological Integrity
Integrated Process: Nursing Process/Data Collection
Content Area: Delegating/Prioritizing
Reference: Christensen, B., & Kockrow, E. (2006). *Foundations of nursing* (5th ed., pp. 486, 489). St. Louis: Mosby.

648. 1
Rationale: This test is an alternative to the exercise stress test. Dipyridamole (Persantine) dilates the coronary arteries as exercise would. Before the procedure, any form of caffeine should be withheld, as well as aminophylline or theophylline forms of medication. Aminophylline is the antagonist to dipyridamole.
Test-Taking Strategy: Use the process of elimination and note the strategic words "has not had." Remember, factors that put a strain on the heart, such as nicotine and caffeine, can interfere with cardiac diagnostic test results. Review preprocedure interventions for this test if you had difficulty with this question.
Level of Cognitive Ability: Application
Client Needs: Physiological Integrity
Integrated Process: Nursing Process/Data Collection
Content Area: Adult Health/Cardiovascular
Reference: Chernecky, C., & Berger, B. (2008). *Laboratory tests and diagnostic procedures* (5th ed., p. 606). Philadelphia: Saunders.

649. 3
Rationale: Chest pain is assessed using the standard pain assessment parameters, (characteristics, location, intensity, duration, precipitating and alleviating factors, and associated symptoms). Options 1, 2, and 4 may or may not help determine the origin of pain. Pain of pleuropulmonary origin usually worsens on inspiration.
Test-Taking Strategy: Focus on the subject—a method of discriminating among the causes of pain. The three incorrect options, although appropriate to use in clinical practice, are general assessment questions only. Option 3 will discriminate between a cardiac and noncardiac cause of pain. Review pain data collection techniques if you had difficulty with this question.
Level of Cognitive Ability: Analysis
Client Needs: Physiological Integrity

Integrated Process: Nursing Process/Data Collection
Content Area: Adult Health/Cardiovascular
Reference: deWit, S. (2009). *Medical-surgical nursing: Concepts & practice* (pp. 419, 492). Philadelphia: Saunders.

650. 2
Rationale: Upon transfer from the CCU, the client is allowed self-care activities and bathroom privileges. Supervised ambulation in the hall for brief distances is encouraged, with distances gradually increased (50, 100, 200 feet).
Test-Taking Strategy: Use the process of elimination. Eliminate options 3 and 4 first because they are excessive, given that the client has just transferred from the CCU. Option 1 is not correct, because the client would be doing less activity than in the CCU prior to transfer. Review activity prescriptions for the client with an MI if you had difficulty with this question.
Level of Cognitive Ability: Comprehension
Client Needs: Physiological Integrity
Integrated Process: Nursing Process/Planning
Content Area: Adult Health/Cardiovascular
Reference: Ignatavicius, D., & Workman, M. (2006). *Medical-surgical nursing: Critical thinking for collaborative care.* (5th ed., pp. 851-852). Philadelphia: Saunders.

651. 1
Rationale: Sternotomy incision sites are assessed for signs and symptoms of infection, such as redness, swelling, and induration. An elevated temperature and elevated WBC count after 3 to 4 days usually indicate infection. A WBC count of 7500/mm^3 is within the normal range.
Test-Taking Strategy: Use the process of elimination. Eliminate options 2 and 3 because the WBC count is normal. The lack of drainage and redness helps you choose option 1 over 4. Review the signs of an incisional infection if you had difficulty with this question.
Level of Cognitive Ability: Analysis
Client Needs: Physiological Integrity
Integrated Process: Nursing Process/Data Collection
Content Area: Adult Health/Cardiovascular
References: Black, J., & Hawks, J. (2005). *Medical-surgical nursing: Clinical management for positive outcomes* (7th ed., p. 406). Philadelphia: Saunders.
Christensen, B., & Kockrow, E. (2006). *Foundations of nursing* (5th ed., pp. 320-321). St. Louis: Mosby.
Lewis, S., Heitkemper, M., Dirksen, S., & Bucher, L., (2007). *Medical-surgical nursing: Assessment and management of clinical problems* (7th ed., pp. 808-809). St. Louis: Mosby.

ALTERNATE ITEM FORMAT: MULTIPLE RESPONSE

652. 1, 2, 3, 4
Rationale: Pulmonary edema is a life-threatening event that can result from severe heart failure. In pulmonary edema the left ventricle fails to eject sufficient blood, and pressure increases in the lungs because of the accumulated blood. Oxygen is always prescribed, and the client is placed in a high Fowler's position to ease the work of breathing. Furosemide, a rapid-acting diuretic, will eliminate accumulated fluid. A Foley catheter is inserted to accurately measure

output. Intravenously administered morphine sulfate reduces venous return (preload), decreases anxiety, and reduces the work of breathing. Transporting the client to the coronary care unit is not a priority intervention. In fact, this may not be necessary at all if the client's response to treatment is successful.

Test-Taking Strategy: Note the strategic words "priority interventions" and focus on the client's diagnosis. Recalling the pathophysiology associated with pulmonary edema and using the ABCs—airway, breathing, and circulation—will assist in determining the priority interventions. Review priority interventions for the client with pulmonary edema if you had difficulty with this question.

Level of Cognitive Ability: Analysis
Client Needs: Physiological Integrity
Integrated Process: Nursing Process/Implementation
Content Area: Delegating/Prioritizing
Reference: Christensen, B., & Kockrow, E. (2006). *Adult health nursing* (5th ed., pp. 367-368). St. Louis: Mosby.

REFERENCES

Black, J., & Hawks, J. (2005). *Medical-surgical nursing: Clinical management for positive outcomes* (7th ed.). Philadelphia: Saunders.

Chernecky, C., & Berger, B. (2008). *Laboratory tests and diagnostic procedures* (5th ed.). Philadelphia: Saunders.

Christensen, B., & Kockrow, E. (2006). *Adult health nursing* (5th ed.). St. Louis: Mosby.

Christensen, B., & Kockrow, E. (2006). *Foundations of nursing* (5th ed.). St. Louis: Mosby.

deWit, S. (2009). *Medical-surgical nursing: Concepts & practice.* Philadelphia: Saunders.

Ignatavicius, D., & Workman, M. (2006). *Medical-surgical nursing: Critical thinking for collaborative care* (5th ed.). Philadelphia: Saunders.

Lehne, R. (2007). *Pharmacology for nursing care* (6th ed.). Philadelphia: Saunders.

Lewis, S., Heitkemper, M., Dirksen, S., & Bucher, L. (2007). *Medical-surgical nursing: Assessment and management of clinical problems* (7th ed.). St. Louis: Mosby.

Linton, A., & Maebius, N. (2007). *Introduction to medical-surgical nursing* (4th ed.). Philadelphia: Saunders.

Monahan, F., Sands, J., Neighbors, M., Marek, J., & Green, C. (2007). *Phipps' medical-surgical nursing: Health and illness perspectives* (8th ed.). St. Louis: Mosby.

Perry, A., & Potter, P. (2006). *Clinical nursing skills & techniques* (6th ed.). St. Louis: Mosby.

Cardiovascular Medications

I. ANTICOAGULANTS (Box 51-1)

▲ A. Description
  1. Anticoagulants prevent the extension and formation of clots by inhibiting factors in the clotting cascade and decreasing blood coagulability
  2. Anticoagulants are administered when there is evidence or the likelihood of clot formation: myocardial infarction, unstable angina, atrial fibrillation, deep vein thrombosis, pulmonary embolism, and the presence of mechanical heart valves
  3. Anticoagulants are contraindicated with active bleeding (exception: disseminated intravascular coagulation), bleeding disorders or blood dyscrasias, ulcers, liver and kidney disease, and brain injuries

▲ B. Side effects (Box 51-2)
  1. Hemorrhage
  2. Hematuria
  3. Epistaxis
  4. Ecchymosis
  5. Bleeding gums
  6. Thrombocytopenia
  7. Hypotension

▲ C. Heparin sodium
  1. Description
    a. Heparin prevents thrombin from converting fibrinogen to fibrin
    b. Heparin prevents thromboembolism
    c. The therapeutic dose does not dissolve clots but prevents new thrombus formation

  ▲ 2. Blood levels
    a. The normal activated partial thromboplastin time (aPTT) is 20 to 36 seconds in most laboratories but may be as high as 40 seconds
    b. To maintain a therapeutic level of anticoagulation when the client is receiving a continuous infusion of heparin, the aPTT should be 1.5 to 2.5 times the control value
    c. aPTT therapy should be measured every 4 to 6 hours during initial continuous infusion therapy and then daily

    d. If the aPTT is too long (greater than 80 seconds), the dosage should be lowered
    e. If aPTT is too short (less than 60 seconds), the dosage should be increased
  3. Interventions
    a. Monitor aPTT
    b. Monitor platelet count
    c. Observe for bleeding gums, bruises, nosebleeds, hematuria, hematemesis, occult blood in the stool, and petechiae
    d. When administering heparin subcutaneously, inject into the abdomen with a ⅝-inch needle (25- to 28-gauge) at a 90-degree angle and do not aspirate or rub the injection site
    e. Continous infusions must be run on an infusion pump to ensure precise rate of delivery
    f. Instruct the client regarding measures to prevent bleeding
    g. The antidote to heparin is protamine sulfate ▲

D. Enoxaparin (Lovenox)—Low molecular weight heparin
  1. Description: Enoxaparin has the same mechanism of action and use as heparin but is not interchangeable; has a longer half-life than heparin
  2. Interventions
    a. Administer by subcutaneous injection only to the recumbent client in the anterolateral or posteriorlateral abdominal wall; do not expel the air bubble from the prefilled syringe or aspirate during injection
    b. Monitor the same laboratory values as for heparin and observe for bleeding
    c. The antidote to enoxaparin is protamine sulfate

E. Warfarin sodium (Coumadin) ▲
  1. Description
    a. Warfarin suppresses coagulation by acting as an antagonist of vitamin K by inhibiting four dependent clotting factors (X, IX, VII, and II).

b. Warfarin prolongs clotting time and is monitored by the prothrombin time (PT).

c. It is used for long-term anticoagulation and is used mainly to prevent thromboembolitic conditions such as thrombophlebitis, pulmonary embolism, and embolism formation caused by atrial fibrillation, thrombosis, myocardial infarction, or heart valve damage

2. Blood levels
   a. The normal PT is 9.6 to 11.8 seconds
   b. Warfarin sodium prolongs the PT; therapeutic range is 1.5 to 2 times the control

3. International normalized ratio (INR)
   a. The normal INR is 1.3 to 2.0
   b. The INR is determined by multiplying the observed PT ratio (the ratio of the client's PT to a control PT) by a correction factor specific to a particular thromboplastin preparation used in the testing
   c. The treatment goal is to raise the INR to an appropriate value
   d. An INR of 2 to 3 is appropriate for most clients, although for some clients, the target INR is 3 to 4.5
   e. If the INR is below the recommended range, warfarin sodium should be increased
   f. If the INR is above the recommended range, warfarin sodium should be reduced

---

BOX 51-1 **Anticoagulants**

Oral Anticoagulants
Warfarin sodium (Coumadin)
Parenteral Anticoagulants
Argatroban (Acova)
Bivalirudin (Angiomax)
Dalteparin (Fragmin)
Desirudin (Ipravask)
Enoxaparin (Lovenox)
Fondaparinux (Arixtra)
Heparin sodium
Lepirudin (Refludan)
Tinzaparin (Innohep)

BOX 51-2 **Substances to Avoid With Anticoagulants**

Allopurinol (Zyloprim)
Cimetidine (Tagamet)
Corticosteroids
Green leafy vegetables and foods high in vitamin K
Nonsteroidal anti-inflammatory drugs
Oral hypoglycemic agents
Phenytoin (Dilantin)
Salicylates
Sulfonamides
Ginkgo and ginseng (herbs)

---

4. Interventions
   a. Monitor PT and INR
   b. Observe for bleeding gums, bruises, nosebleeds, hematuria, hematemesis, occult blood in the stool, and petechiae
   c. Instruct the client regarding measures to prevent bleeding
   d. The antidote for warfarin is vitamin K (phytonadione, AquaMEPHYTON)

II. THROMBOLYTIC MEDICATIONS (Box 51-3)
A. Description
   1. Thrombolytic medications activate plasminogen; plasminogen generates plasmin (the enzyme that dissolves clots)
   2. Thrombolytic medications are used early in the course of myocardial infarct (within 4-6 hours of the onset of the infarct) to restore blood flow, limit myocardial damage, preserve left ventricular function, and prevent death
   3. Thrombolytics are also used in arterial thrombosis, deep vein thrombosis, occluded shunts or catheters, and pulmonary emboli.
B. Contraindications
   1. Active internal bleeding
   2. History of hemorrhagic brain attack (stroke)
   3. Intracranial problems, including trauma
   4. Intracranial or intraspinal surgery within the previous 2 months
   5. History of thoracic, pelvic, or abdominal surgery in the previous 10 days
   6. History of hepatic or renal disease
   7. Uncontrolled hypertension
   8. Recently required, prolonged cardiopulmonary resuscitation
   9. Known allergy to the specific product or any of its preservatives
C. Side effects
   1. Bleeding
   2. Dysrhythmias
   3. Fever
   4. Allergic reactions
D. Interventions
   1. Obtain aPTT, PT, fibrinogen level, hematocrit, and platelet count
   2. Monitor vital signs
   3. Assess pulses
   4. Monitor for bleeding
   5. Monitor all excretions for occult blood
   6. Monitor for neurological changes such as lethargy, slurred speech, confusion, and hemiparesis

---

BOX 51-3 **Thrombolytic Medications**

Alteplase (Activase, t-PA)
Reteplase (Retavase)
Streptokinase (Streptase)
Tenecteplase (TNKase)
Urokinase (Abbokinase)

7. Monitor for hypotension and tachycardia
8. Avoid injections if possible
9. Apply direct pressure over a puncture site for 20 to 30 minutes
10. Handle the client as little as possible when moving
11. Instruct the client to use an electric razor for shaving and to brush teeth gently
12. Discontinue the medication if bleeding develops, and notify the physician
13. Antidote
    a. Aminocaproic acid (Amicar) is the antidote for streptokinase
    b. Used only in acute, life-threatening conditions

III. ANTIPLATELET MEDICATIONS (Box 51-4)

A. Description
1. Antiplatelet medications inhibit the aggregation of platelets in the clotting process, thereby prolonging the bleeding time
2. Antiplatelet medications may be used with anticoagulants
3. Used in the prophylaxis of long-term complications following myocardial infarction, coronary revascularization, stents, and brain attacks (stroke)
4. These medications are contraindicated in bleeding disorders and known sensitivity

B. Side effects
1. Gastrointestinal bleeding
2. Bruising
3. Hematuria
4. Tarry stools

C. Interventions
1. Determine sensitivity before administration
2. Monitor vital signs
3. Instruct the client to take medication with food if gastrointestinal upset occurs
4. Monitor bleeding time
5. Monitor for side effects related to bleeding
6. Instruct the client on the use of the medication
7. Instruct the client to monitor for side effects related to bleeding and in the measures to prevent bleeding

---

BOX 51-4   Antiplatelet Medications

Abciximab (ReoPro)
Aspirin (acetylsalicylic acid, A.S.A.)
Cilostazol (Pletal)
Clopidogrel (Plavix)
Dipyridamole (Persantine)
Dipyridamole/Aspirin (Aggrenox)
Eptifibatide (Integrilin)
Ticlopidine (Ticlid)
Tirofiban (Aggrastat)

IV. CARDIAC GLYCOSIDES (Box 51-5)

A. Description
1. Cardiac glycosides inhibit the sodium-potassium pump, thus increasing intracellular calcium, which causes the heart muscle fibers to contract more efficiently
2. Cardiac glycosides produce a positive inotropic action, which increases the force of myocardial contractions
3. Cardiac glycosides produce a negative chronotropic action, which slows the heart rate
4. Cardiac glycosides produce a negative dromotropic action that slows conduction velocity through the AV node
5. The increase in myocardial **contractility** increases cardiac, peripheral, and kidney function by increasing **cardiac output,** decreasing preload, improving blood flow to the periphery and kidneys, decreasing edema, and increasing fluid excretion; as a result, fluid retention in the lungs and extremities is decreased
6. Cardiac glycosides are used for heart failure and cardiogenic shock, atrial tachycardia, atrial fibrillation, and atrial flutter (Figure 51-1)
7. These medications are contraindicated in ventricular dysrhythmias and second- or third-degree heart block and should be used with caution in clients with renal disease, hypothyroidism, and hypokalemia

B. Side effects and toxic effects
1. Anorexia, nausea, vomiting, and diarrhea
2. Headache

BOX 51-5   Cardiac Glycoside

Digoxin (Lanoxicaps, Lanoxin, Digitek)

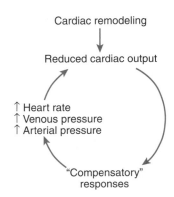

Cardiac remodeling

Reduced cardiac output

↑ Heart rate
↑ Venous pressure
↑ Arterial pressure

"Compensatory" responses

1. Cardiac dilation
2. Activation of the sympathetic nervous system
3. Activation of the renin-angiotensin-aldosterone system
4. Retention of water and increase blood volume

FIG. 51-1   The vicious cycle of maladaptive compensatory responses to a failing heart. (From Lehne, R. [2007]. *Pharmacology for nursing care* [6th ed.]. Philadelphia: Saunders.)

3. Visual disturbances: diplopia, blurred vision, yellow-green halos, and photophobia
4. Drowsiness
5. Bradycardia
6. Fatigue and weakness

C. Interventions
1. Monitor for toxicity as evidenced by anorexia, nausea, vomiting, visual disturbances, confusion, bradycardia, heart block, premature ventricular contractions, and tachydysrhythmias
2. Monitor serum digoxin level, electrolyte levels, and renal function tests
3. Therapeutic digoxin range is 0.5 to 2 ng/mL, and levels above 2 ng/mL are toxic
4. An increased risk of toxicity exists in clients with hypercalcemia, hypokalemia, hypomagnesemia, or hypothyroidism
5. Monitor the potassium level; if hypokalemia occurs (potassium less than 3.5 mEq/L), notify the physician
6. Instruct the client to avoid over-the-counter medications
7. Monitor the client taking a potassium-wasting diuretic or corticosteroids closely for hypokalemia because the hypokalemia can cause digoxin toxicity
8. Note that older clients are more sensitive to digoxin toxicity
9. Advise the client to eat foods high in potassium, such as fresh and dried fruits, fruit juices, vegetables, and potatoes
10. Monitor the apical pulse
11. If the apical pulse rate is less than 60 beats/min, the medication should be held and the physician notified
12. Teach the client how to measure pulse
13. Teach the client to notify the physician if the pulse rate is less than 60 beats/min or greater than 100 beats/min.
14. Teach the client the signs and symptoms of toxicity
15. Antidote: Digoxin immune Fab (Digibind) is used in extreme toxicity

V. ANTIHYPERTENSIVE MEDICATIONS (Box 51-6)
A. Thiazide diuretics (Box 51-7)
1. Description
a. Thiazide diuretics increase sodium and water excretion by inhibiting sodium reabsorption in the distal tubule of the kidney
b. Used for hypertension and peripheral edema
c. Not effective for immediate diuresis
d. Used in clients with normal renal function (contraindicated in clients with renal failure)
e. Use thiazide diuretics with caution in the client taking lithium, because lithium toxicity can occur, and in the client taking digoxin, corticosteroids, or hypoglycemic medications

2. Side effects
a. Hypercalcemia, hyperglycemia, and hyperuricemia
b. Hypokalemia and hyponatremia
c. Hypovolemia
d. Hypotension
e. Headaches
f. Nausea, vomiting
g. Constipation
h. Rashes
i. Photosensitivity
j. Blood dyscrasias
3. Interventions
a. Monitor vital signs
b. Monitor weight
c. Monitor urine output
d. Monitor electrolytes, glucose, calcium, blood urea nitrogen (BUN), creatinine and uric acid levels
e. Check peripheral extremities for edema
f. Instruct the client to take the medication in the morning to avoid nocturia and sleep interruption
g. Instruct the client on how to record the **blood pressure** (BP)
h. Instruct the client to eat foods high in potassium
i. Instruct the client on how to take potassium supplements if prescribed
j. Instruct the client to take medication with food to avoid gastrointestinal upset
k. Instruct the client to change positions slowly to prevent **orthostatic hypotension**
l. Instruct the client to use sunscreen when in direct sunlight because of increased photosensitivity

---

BOX 51-6 **Classifications of Diuretics**

Carbonic anhydrase inhibitors
Loop diuretics
Osmotic diuretics
Potassium-sparing diuretics
Thiazide diuretics

BOX 51-7 **Thiazide and Thiazide-like Diuretics**

Bendroflumethiazide (Naturetin)
Benzthiazide (Exna)
Chlorothiazide (Diuril)
Chlorthalidone (Hygroton, Thalitone)
Hydrochlorothiazide (HydroDIURIL, others)
Hydroflumethazide (Diucardin, Saluron)
Indapamide (Lozol)
Methyclothiazide (Aquatensen, Enduron)
Metolazone (Zaroxolyn)
Polythiazide (Renese)
Quinethazone (Hydromox)
Trichlormethiazide (Metahydrin, Naqua, Diurese)

m. Instruct the client with diabetes mellitus to have the blood glucose checked periodically
B. Loop diuretics (Box 51-8)
  1. Description
    a. Loop diuretics inhibit sodium and chloride reabsorption from the loop of Henle and the distal tubule
    b. Loop diuretics have little effect on the blood glucose; however, they cause depletion of water and electrolytes, increased uric acid levels, and the excretion of calcium
    c. Loop diuretics are more potent than the thiazide diuretics, causing rapid diuresis, thus decreasing vascular fluid volume, **cardiac output,** and **BP**
    d. Used for hypertension, pulmonary edema, edema associated with heart failure, hypercalcemia, and renal disease
    e. Use loop diuretics with caution in the client taking digoxin or lithium and in the client on aminoglycosides, anticoagulants, corticosteroids, or amphotericin B
  2. Side effects
    a. Hypokalemia, hyponatremia, hypocalcemia, and hypomagnesemia
    b. Hypochloremia
    c. Thrombocytopenia
    d. Hyperuricemia
    e. **Orthostatic hypotension**
    f. Skin disturbances
    g. Ototoxicity and deafness
    h. Thiamine deficiency
    i. Dehydration
  3. Interventions
    a. Monitor vital signs
    b. Monitor weight
    c. Monitor urine output
    d. Monitor electrolytes, calcium, magnesium, BUN, creatinine, and uric acid levels
    e. Check the peripheral extremities for edema
    f. Monitor for signs of digoxin or lithium toxicity if the client is on these medications
    g. Instruct the client to take the medication in the morning in order to avoid nocturia and sleep interruption
    h. Instruct the client in how to record the **BP**
    i. Instruct the client to eat foods high in potassium
    j. Instruct the client on how to take potassium supplements if prescribed

BOX 51-8 **Loop Diuretics**

Bumetanide (Bumex)
Ethacrynic acid (Edecrin)
Furosemide (Lasix)
Torsemide (Demadex)

k. Instruct the client to take medication with food to avoid gastrointestinal upset
l. Instruct the client to change positions slowly to prevent **orthostatic hypotension**
m. IV furosemide (Lasix) is administered slowly because hearing loss can occur if injected rapidly
C. Osmotic diuretics
  1. Refer to Chapter 57 for information regarding osmotic diuretics
  2. Refer to Box 51-9 for a list of osmotic diuretics
D. Carbonic anhydrase inhibitors (Box 51-10)
  1. Description
    a. Carbonic anhydrase inhibitors block the action of the enzyme carbonic anhydrase, which is needed to maintain acid-base balance
    b. Inhibition of this enzyme, carbonic anhydrase, causes increased sodium, potassium, and bicarbonate excretion
    c. Metabolic acidosis can occur with prolonged use
    d. Carbonic anhydrase inhibitors are used to decrease intraocular pressure in open-angle (chronic) glaucoma and to produce diuresis, manage epilepsy, and treat high-altitude sickness
    e. Carbonic anhydrase inhibitors are used to treat metabolic alkalosis
    f. Carbonic anhydrase inhibitors are contraindicated in narrow-angle or acute glaucoma
  2. Side effects
    a. Hyperglycemia, hyperuricemia, and hypercalcemia
    b. Hypokalemia
    c. Anorexia, nausea, and vomiting
    d. **Orthostatic hypotension**
    e. Renal calculi
    f. Hemolytic anemia
  3. Interventions
    a. Monitor vital signs
    b. Monitor weight
    c. Monitor urine output
    d. Monitor electrolytes, glucose, calcium, BUN, creatinine, and uric acid levels
    e. Monitor mental status
    f. Instruct the client to monitor for signs of renal calculi

BOX 51-9 **Osmotic Diuretics**

Mannitol (Osmitrol)
Urea (Ureaphil)

BOX 51-10 **Carbonic Anhydrase Inhibitors**

Acetazolamide (Diamox)
Methazolamide (GlaucTabs. Neptazane)

E. Potassium-sparing diuretics (Box 51-11)
1. Description
   a. Potassium-sparing diuretics act on the distal tubule to promote sodium and water excretion and potassium retention
   b. Used for edema and hypertension; to increase urine output; to treat fluid retention and overload associated with heart failure, ascites due to cirrhosis, or nephrotic syndrome; and for diuretic-induced hypokalemia
   c. Potassium-sparing diuretics are contraindicated in severe kidney or hepatic disease or in severe hyperkalemia
   d. Potassium-sparing diuretics should be used with caution in the client with diabetes mellitus, in the client taking antihypertensives or lithium, in the client taking angiotensin-converting enzyme inhibitors because hyperkalemia can result, and in the client taking potassium supplements
2. Side effects
   a. Hyperkalemia
   b. Nausea, vomiting, and diarrhea
   c. Rash
   d. Dizziness and weakness
   e. Headache
   f. Dry mouth
   g. Photosensitivity
   h. Anemia
   i. Thrombocytopenia
3. Interventions
   a. Monitor vital signs
   b. Monitor urine output
   c. Monitor for signs and symptoms of hyperkalemia such as nausea, diarrhea, abdominal cramps, tachycardia followed by bradycardia, tall peaked T wave on the electrocardiogram, or oliguria
   d. Monitor for a potassium level greater than 5.1 mEq/L, which indicates hyperkalemia
   e. Instruct the client to avoid foods high in potassium
   f. Instruct the client to avoid exposure to direct sunlight
   g. Instruct the client to monitor for signs of hyperkalemia
   h. Instruct the client to avoid salt substitutes because they contain potassium

BOX 51-11 **Potassium-Sparing Diuretics**

Amiloride (Midamor)
Amiloride hydrochloride and hydrochlorothiazide (Moduretic)
Spironolactone (Aldactone)
Spironolactone and hydrochlorothiazide (Aldactazide)
Triamterene (Dyrenium)

i. Instruct the client to take with or after meals to decrease gastrointestinal irritation
VI. PERIPHERALLY ACTING α-ADRENERGIC BLOCKERS (Box 51-12)
A. Description
   1. These medications decrease sympathetic vasoconstriction by reducing the effects of norepinephrine at peripheral nerve endings, resulting in vasodilation and decreased **BP**
   2. These medications are used to maintain renal blood flow
   3. These medications are used to treat hypertension
B. Side effects
   1. Orthostatic hypotension
   2. Reflex tachycardia
   3. Sodium and water retention
   4. Gastrointestinal disturbances
   5. Nausea
   6. Drowsiness
   7. Nasal congestion
   8. Edema
   9. Weight gain
C. Interventions
   1. Monitor vital signs
   2. Monitor for fluid retention and edema
   3. Instruct the client to change positions slowly to prevent **orthostatic hypotension**
   4. Instruct the client in how to monitor the **BP**
   5. Instruct the client to monitor for edema
   6. Instruct the client to decrease salt intake
   7. Instruct the client to avoid over-the-counter medications
VII. CENTRALLY ACTING SYMPATHOLYTICS (ADRENERGIC BLOCKERS) (Box 51-13)
A. Description
   1. These medications stimulate α-receptors in the central nervous system to inhibit vasoconstriction, thus reducing peripheral resistance

BOX 51-12 **Peripherally Acting α-Adrenergic Blockers**

Alfuzosin (Uroxatral)
Doxazosin (Cardura)
Phenoxybenzamine (Dibenzyline)
Phentolamine (Regitine)
Prazosin (Minipress)
Tamsulosin (Flomax)
Terazosin (Hytrin)

BOX 51-13 **Centrally Acting Sympatholytics**

Clonidine (Catapres)
Methyldopa (Aldomet)
Guanabenz Acetate

2. Are used to treat hypertension
3. Are contraindicated in impaired liver function

B. Side effects
  1. Sodium and water retention
  2. Drowsiness and dizziness
  3. Dry mouth
  4. Bradycardia
  5. Edema
  6. Impotence
  7. Hypotension
  8. Depression

C. Interventions
  1. Monitor vital signs
  2. Instruct the client not to discontinue medication because abrupt withdrawal can cause severe rebound hypertension
  3. Monitor liver function tests

VIII. ANGIOTENSIN-CONVERTING ENZYME (ACE) INHIBITORS AND ANGIOTENSIN II RECEPTOR BLOCKERS (ARBs) (Box 51-14)
A. Description
  1. ACE inhibitors prevent peripheral vasoconstriction by blocking conversion of angiotensin I to angiotensin II
  2. ARBs prevent peripheral vasoconstriction and secretion of aldosterone, and they block the binding of angiotensin II to type 1 angiotensin II receptors.
  3. These medications are used to treat hypertension and heart failure; ACE inhibitors are administered for their cardioprotective effect after myocardial infarction
  4. Avoid use with potassium supplements and potassium-sparing diuretics

---

BOX 51-14 — Angiotensin-Converting Enzyme Inhibitors and Angiotension Receptor Blockers

Angiotensin-Converting Enzyme Inhibitors
Benazepril (Lotensin)
Captopril (Capoten)
Enalapril, Enalaprilat (Vasotec)
Fosinopril (Monopril)
Lisinopril (Prinivil, Zestril)
Moexipril (Univasc)
Perindopril (Aceon)
Quinapril (Accupril)
Ramipril (Altace)
Trandolapril (Mavik)

Angiotension II Receptor Blockers
Candesartan (Atacand)
Eprosartan (Teveten)
Irbesartan (Avapro)
Losartan (Cozaar)
Olmesartan (Benicar)
Telmisartan (Micardis)
Valsartan (Diovan)

B. Side effects
  1. Nausea, vomiting, and diarrhea
  2. Persistent dry cough (ACE inhibitors only)
  3. Hypotension
  4. Hyperkalemia
  5. Tachycardia
  6. Headache
  7. Dizziness and fatigue
  8. Insomnia
  9. Hypoglycemic reaction in the client with diabetes mellitus
  10. Bruising, petechiae, and bleeding
  11. Diminished taste (ACE inhibitors)

C. Interventions
  1. Monitor vital signs
  2. Monitor protein, albumin, BUN, creatinine, white blood cell count, and potassium level
  3. Monitor for hypoglycemic reactions in the client with diabetes mellitus
  4. Instruct the client to take captopril (Capoten) 20 minutes to 1 hour before a meal
  5. Monitor for bruising, petechiae, or bleeding with captopril
  6. Instruct the client not to discontinue medications because rebound hypertension can occur
  7. Instruct the client not to take over-the-counter medications
  8. Instruct the client on how to take the **BP**
  9. Instruct the client to notify the physician if dizziness occurs and persists.
  10. Inform the client that the taste of food may be diminished during the first month of therapy
  11. Instruct the client to report side effects of angioedema immediately to health care provider

IX. ANTIANGINAL MEDICATIONS (Box 51-15)
A. Nitrates
  1. Description
     a. Nitrates produce vasodilation
     b. Nitrates decrease preload and afterload and reduce myocardial oxygen consumption
     c. Are contraindicated in the client with significant hypotension, increased intracranial pressure, or severe anemia

---

BOX 51-15 — Antianginal Medications (Organic Nitrates)

Amyl nitrate inhalant
Isosorbide dinitrate (Isordil)
Isosorbide mononitrate (Imdur, Monoket)
Nitroglycerin, sublingual (Nitrostat, NitroQuick, Nitrotab)
Nitroglycerin, translingual (Nitrolingual)
Nitroglycerin, transmucosal (Nitrogard)
Nitroglycerin, transdermal patches (Minitran, Nitrodisc, Nitro-Dur, Nitrek, Transderm-Nitro)
Nitroglycerin ointment (Nitro-Bid)

d. Should be used with caution with severe renal or hepatic disease

e. Avoid abrupt withdrawal of long-acting preparations to prevent the rebound effect of severe pain from myocardial ischemia

2. Side effects
   a. Headache
   b. **Orthostatic hypotension**
   c. Dizziness and weakness
   d. Faintness
   e. Nausea and vomiting
   f. Flushing or pallor
   g. Confusion
   h. Rash
   i. Dry mouth
   j. Reflex tachycardia

3. Sublingual medications
   a. Monitor vital signs
   b. Offer sips of water before giving because dryness may inhibit medication absorption
   c. Instruct the client to place under the tongue and leave until fully dissolved
   d. Instruct the client not to swallow the medication
   e. Instruct the client to take one tablet for pain and repeat every 5 minutes for a total of three doses
   f. Instruct the client to seek medical help immediately if pain is not relieved in 15 minutes, following the three doses
   g. Inform the client that a stinging or burning sensation may indicate that the tablet is fresh
   h. Instruct the client to store medication in a dark, tightly closed bottle
   i. Instruct the client to check the expiration date on the medication bottle because expiration may occur within 6 months of obtaining medication
   j. Instruct the client to take acetaminophen (Tylenol) for a headache

4. Translingual medications (spray)
   a. Instruct the client to direct the spray against the oral mucosa
   b. Instruct the client to avoid inhaling the spray

5. Sustained-released medications: Instruct the client to swallow and not to chew or crush the medication

6. Transmucosal-buccal medications
   a. Instruct the client to place the medication between the upper lip and gum or in the buccal area between the cheek and gum
   b. Inform the client that the medication will adhere to the oral mucosa and slowly dissolve

7. Transdermal patch
   a. Instruct the client to apply the patch to a hairless area, using a new patch and a different site each day

   b. As prescribed, instruct the client to remove the patch after 12 to 14 hours, allowing 10 to 12 "patch-free" hours each day to prevent tolerance

8. Topical ointments
   a. Instruct the client to remove the ointment on the skin from the previous dose
   b. Instruct the client to squeeze a ribbon of ointment of the prescribed length onto the applicator paper
   c. Instruct the client to spread the ointment over a 6 × 6–inch area, using the chest, back, abdomen, upper arm, or anterior thigh (avoiding hairy areas), and to cover with a plastic wrap
   d. Instruct the client to rotate sites and to avoid touching the ointment during application

9. Patches and ointments
   a. Wear gloves when applying
   b. Do not apply on the chest in the area of defibrillator-cardioverter paddle placement because skin burns can result if the paddles need to be used

X. β-ADRENERGIC BLOCKERS (Box 51-16)

A. Description
1. β-Adrenergic blockers inhibit response to β-adrenergic stimulation, thus decreasing **cardiac output**
2. β-Adrenergic blockers block the release of the catecholamines, epinephrine, and norepinephrine, thus decreasing the heart rate and **BP**
3. β-Adrenergic blockers decrease the workload of the heart and decrease oxygen demands
4. Are used for angina, dysrhythmias, hypertension, migraine headaches, prevention of myocardial infarction, and glaucoma
5. β-Adrenergic blockers are contraindicated in the client with asthma, bradycardia, heart failure (with exception), severe renal or hepatic disease, hyperthyroidism, or brain attack (stroke); carvedilol, metoprolol and bisoprolol have been approved for use in heart failure once the client has been stabilized with ACE inhibitor and diuretic therapy
6. β-Adrenergic blockers should be used with caution in the client with diabetes mellitus because the medication may mask symptoms of hypoglycemia
7. β-Adrenergic blockers should be used with caution in the client taking antihypertensive medications

B. Side effects
1. Bradycardia
2. Bronchospasm
3. Hypotension
4. Weakness and fatigue

BOX 51-16 β-Adrenergic Blockers

Nonselective (block β₁ and β₂)
Carteolol (Cartrol)
Carvedilol (Coreg)
Labetalol (Trandate)
Nadolol (Corgard)
Penbutolol (Levatol)
Pindolol (Visken)
Propranolol (Inderal)
Sotalol (Betapace)
Timolol (Blocadren)
Cardioselective (block β₁)
Acebutolol (Sectral)
Atenolol (Tenormin)
Betaxolol (Kerlone)
Bisoprolol (Zebeta)
Esmolol (Brevibloc)
Metoprolol (Lopressor, Toprol-XL)

5. Nausea and vomiting
6. Dizziness
7. Hyperglycemia
8. Agranulocytosis
9. Behavioral or psychotic response
10. Depression
11. Nightmares
C. Interventions
 1. Monitor vital signs
 2. Hold the medication if the pulse or **BP** is not within the prescribed parameters
 3. Monitor for signs of heart failure or worsening heart failure
 4. Assess for respiratory distress and for signs of wheezing and dyspnea
 5. Instruct the client to report dizziness, lightheadedness, or nasal congestion
 6. Instruct the client not to stop the medication since rebound hypertension, rebound tachycardia, or an anginal attack can occur
 7. Advise the client taking insulin that the β-blocker can mask early signs of hypoglycemia such as tachycardia and nervousness
 8. Instruct the client taking insulin to monitor the blood glucose level
 9. Instruct the client on how to take pulse and **BP**
 10. Instruct the client to change positions slowly to prevent **orthostatic hypotension**
 11. Instruct the client to avoid over-the-counter cold medications and nasal decongestants

XI. **CALCIUM CHANNEL BLOCKERS** (Box 51-17)
A. Description
 1. Calcium channel blockers decrease cardiac **contractility** (negative inotropic effect by relaxing smooth muscle) and the workload of the heart, thus decreasing the need for oxygen
 2. Calcium channel blockers promote vasodilation of the coronary and peripheral vessels

BOX 51-17 Calcium Channel Blockers

Amlodipine (Norvasc, Amvaz)
Diltiazem (Cardizem, Cartia XT, Dilacor XR, Diltia XT, Tiazac)
Felodipine (Plendil)
Isradipine (DynaCirc)
Nicardipine (Cardene)
Nifedipine (Adalat, Nifedical, Nifediac, Procardia)
Nimodipine (Nimotop)
Nisoldipine (Sular)
Verapamil (Calan, Isoptin, Covera-HS, Verelan)

 3. Are used for angina, dysrhythmias, or hypertension
 4. Should be used with caution in the client with congestive heart failure, bradycardia, or atrioventricular block
B. Side effects
 1. Bradycardia
 2. Hypotension
 3. Reflex tachycardia as a result of hypotension
 4. Headache
 5. Dizziness and lightheadedness
 6. Fatigue
 7. Peripheral edema
 8. Constipation
 9. Flushing of the skin
 10. Changes in liver and kidney function
C. Interventions
 1. Monitor vital signs
 2. Monitor for signs of heart failure
 3. Monitor liver enzyme levels
 4. Monitor kidney function tests
 5. Instruct the client not to discontinue the medication
 6. Instruct the client on how to take a pulse
 7. Instruct the client to notify the physician if dizziness or fainting occurs
 8. Instruct the client not to crush or chew sustained-released tablets

XII. **PERIPHERAL VASODILATORS** (Box 51-18)
A. Description
 1. Peripheral vasodilators decrease peripheral resistance by exerting a direct action on the arteries or on the arteries and the veins
 2. Peripheral vasodilators increase blood flow to the extremities and are used in peripheral vascular disorders of venous and arterial vessels
 3. Peripheral vasodilators are most effective for disorders resulting from vasospasm (Raynaud's disease)
 4. These medications may decrease some of the symptoms of cerebral vascular insufficiency
B. Side effects
 1. Lightheadedness and dizziness
 2. **Orthostatic hypotension**

BOX 51-18 **Peripheral Vasodilators**

α-Adrenergic Blockers
Prazosin (Minipress)
Terazosin (Hytrin)
Calcium Channel Blockers
Diltiazem (Cardizem, Cartia XT, Dilacor XR, Diltia XT,
  Tiazac)
Nifedipine (Procardia)
Nimodipine (Nimotop)
Verapamil (Calan, Isoptin, Covera-HS, Verelan)
Hemorrheologic
Pentoxifylline (Trental) (increases microcirculation and
  tissue perfusion)

BOX 51-19 **Bile Acid Sequestrants**

Cholestyramine (Questran)
Colesevelam (Welchol)
Colestipol (Colestid)

BOX 51-20 **HMG-CoA Reductase Inhibitors**

Atorvastatin (Lipitor)
Fluvastatin (Lescol)
Lovastatin (Mevacor)
Pravastatin (Pravachol)
Rosuvastatin (Crestor)
Simvastatin (Zocor)

3. Tachycardia
4. Palpitations
5. Flushing
6. Gastrointestinal distress

C. Interventions
  1. Monitor vital signs, especially the **BP** and the heart rate
  2. Monitor for **orthostatic hypotension** and tachycardia
  3. Monitor for signs of inadequate blood flow to the extremities such as pallor, coldness of the extremities, and pain
  4. Instruct the client that it may take up to 3 months for a desired therapeutic response
  5. Advise the client not to smoke because smoking increases vasospasm
  6. Instruct the client to avoid aspirin or aspirin-like compounds unless approved by the physician
  7. Instruct the client to take the medication with meals if gastrointestinal disturbances occur
  8. Instruct the client to avoid alcohol because it may cause a hypotensive reaction
  9. Encourage the client to change positions slowly to avoid **orthostatic hypotension**

XIII. ANTILIPEMIC MEDICATIONS
A. Description
  1. Antilipemic medications reduce serum levels of cholesterol, triglycerides, or low-density lipoprotein
  2. When cholesterol, triglycerides, and low-density lipoprotein are elevated, the client is at increased risk for coronary artery disease
  3. In many cases, diet alone will not lower blood lipid levels; therefore, antilipemic medications will be prescribed
B. Bile sequestrants (Box 51-19)
  1. Description
    a. Bind with acids in the intestines, which prevents reabsorption of cholesterol
    b. Should not be used as the only therapy in clients with elevated triglycerides because they may raise triglyceride levels

2. Side effects
  a. Constipation
  b. Gastrointestinal disturbances: heartburn, nausea, belching, and bloating
3. Interventions
  a. Cholestyramine (Questran) comes in a gritty powder that must be mixed thoroughly in juice or water before administration
  b. Monitor the client for early signs of peptic ulcer such as nausea and abdominal discomfort followed by abdominal pain and distention
  c. Instruct the client that the medication must be taken with and followed by sufficient fluids
C. HMG-CoA reductase inhibitors (Box 51-20)
  1. Description
    a. Lovastatin (Mevacor) is highly protein bound and should not be administered with anticoagulants
    b. Lovastatin should not be administered with gemfibrozil (Lopid)
    c. Administer lovastatin with caution to the client taking immunosuppressive medications
  2. Side effects
    a. Nausea
    b. Diarrhea or constipation
    c. Abdominal pain or cramps
    d. Flatulence
    e. Dizziness
    f. Headache
    g. Blurred vision
    h. Rash
    i. Pruritis
    j. Elevated liver enzymes
    k. Gastrointestinal disturbances, headaches, muscle cramps, and fatigue
  3. Interventions
    a. Monitor serum liver enzymes
    b. Instruct the client to receive an annual eye examination because the medication causes cataract formation

Exetimibe (Zetia)
Fenofibrate (Tricor)
Gemfibrozil (Lopid)
Nicotinic acid (Niacin)
Probucol (Lorelco)
Exetimibe/simvastatin (Vytorin)

c. If lovastatin is not effective in lowering the lipid level after 3 months, it should be discontinued
d. Instruct the client to report any unexplained muscular pain to the health care provider immediately
D. Other antilipemic medications (Box 51-21)
1. Description
a. Gemfibrozil should not be taken with anticoagulants because they compete for protein sites; if the client is taking an anticoagulant, the anticoagulant dose should be reduced during antilipemic therapy and the INR should be monitored closely
b. Do not administer gemfibrozil with HMG-CoA reductase inhibitors because it increases the risk for myositis, myalgias, and rhabdomyolysis
2. Interventions
a. Monitor vital signs
b. Monitor liver enzyme levels
c. Monitor serum cholesterol and triglyceride levels
d. Instruct the client to restrict intake of fats, cholesterol, carbohydrates, and alcohol
e. Instruct the client to follow an exercise program
f. Instruct the client that it will take several weeks before the lipid level declines
g. Instruct the client to have annual eye examinations and to report changes in vision
h. Instruct the client with diabetes mellitus who is taking gemfibrozil to monitor blood glucose levels regularly
i. Instruct the client to increase fluid intake
j. Note that nicotinic acid has numerous side effects, which include gastrointestinal disturbances, flushing of the skin, elevated liver enzymes, hyperglycemia, and hyperuricemia
k. Instruct the client that aspirin or nonsteroidal anti-inflammatory drugs taken 30 minutes before may assist in reducing the cutaneous flushing from nicotinic acid
l. Instruct the client to take nicotinic acid with meals to reduce gastrointestinal discomfort

PRACTICE QUESTIONS

More questions on the companion CD!

653. A client has suffered an acute myocardial infarction and is receiving alteplase (tPA). Which of the following is a priority nursing intervention while caring for the client?
1. Monitor for renal failure
2. Monitor psychosocial status
3. Monitor for signs of bleeding
4. Have heparin sodium available
654. A client with a diagnosis of congestive heart failure is seen in the clinic. The client is being treated with a variety of medications, including digoxin (Lanoxin) and furosemide (Lasix). Which findings on data collection would lead the nurse to suspect that the client is hypokalemic?
1. Constipation
2. Intermittent intestinal colic
3. Tingling of fingers and toes
4. Muscle weakness and leg cramps
655. Hydrochlorothiazide (HydroDIURIL) is prescribed for the client. The nurse checks the client's record for documentation of which of the following before administering the medication?
1. Sulfa allergy
2. Hyperkalemia
3. Penicillin allergy
4. History of osteoporosis
656. Cholestyramine resin (Questran) is prescribed for a client with an elevated triglyceride level and a serum cholesterol level of 398 mg/dL. The nurse provides instructions to the client about the medication. Which statement by the client indicates the need for further instructions?
1. "I'll continue to watch my diet and reduce my fats."
2. "Walking a mile each day will help the whole process."
3. "Constipation and bloating might be a problem."
4. "I'll continue my nicotinic acid from the health food store."
657. A nurse is caring for the client with a history of mild heart failure who is receiving diltiazem (Cardizem) for hypertension. The nurse would check the client for:
1. Chest pain and tachycardia
2. Wheezing and shortness of breath
3. Tachycardia and rebound hypertension
4. Lung crackles, weight gain, and peripheral edema
658. A nurse has an order to administer a dose of nitroglycerin ointment (Nitro-Bid) to a client.

The nurse would avoid doing which of the following in preparing the medication for administration?
1. Applying the dose in an even layer
2. Washing off the previous application
3. Using the fingers to spread the ointment
4. Using the manufacturer's applicator papers

659. A 66-year-old client is seen in the clinic complaining of not feeling well. The client is taking several medications for the control of heart disease and hypertension. These medications include atenolol (Tenormin), digoxin (Lanoxin), and chlorothiazide (Diuril). A tentative diagnosis of digoxin toxicity is made. The nurse collects data from the client, knowing that which of the following would support this diagnosis?
1. Dyspnea, edema, and palpitations
2. Chest pain, hypotension, and paresthesia
3. Double vision, loss of appetite, and nausea
4. Constipation, dry mouth, and sleep disorder

660. A 79-year-old client is being treated for congestive heart failure with bumetanide (Bumex). 24 breaths/min. The nurse checks which priority item before administering the medication?
1. Weight
2. Temperature
3. Urine output
4. Blood pressure

661. Atorvastatin (Lipitor) has been prescribed for a client with an elevated cholesterol level. The nurse collects a health history from the client, knowing that the medication is contraindicated in which of the following conditions?
1. Cirrhosis
2. Hypothyroidism
3. Diabetes mellitus
4. Coronary artery disease

662. A nurse provides discharge instructions to a postoperative client taking warfarin sodium (Coumadin). Which statement by the client indicates the need for further teaching?
1. "I will take my pills every day at the same time."
2. "I will be certain to avoid consuming any alcohol."
3. "I will take Ecotrin for my headaches because it is coated."
4. "I have already called my family to pick up a Medic-Alert bracelet."

663. A client taking digoxin (Lanoxin) has a serum potassium level of 3.0 mEq/L and is complaining of anorexia. The physician orders a digoxin level to be obtained to rule out digoxin toxicity.

The nurse checks the results of the test, knowing that the therapeutic serum level for digoxin is which of the following?
1. 1-3 ng/mL
2. 0.5-2 ng/mL
3. 0.3-0.8 ng/mL
4. 0.1-0.5 ng/mL

664. A nurse is caring for a client who is taking propranolol (Inderal). Which data would indicate an adverse reaction associated with this medication?
1. The development of complaints of insomnia
2. The development of audible expiratory wheezes
3. A baseline blood pressure of 150/80 mm Hg followed by a blood pressure of 138/72 mm Hg after two doses of the medication
4. A baseline resting heart rate of 88 beats/min followed by a resting heart rate of 72 beats/min after two doses of the medication

665. Isosorbide mononitrate (Imdur) is prescribed for a client with angina pectoris. The client tells the nurse that the medication is causing a chronic headache. The nurse appropriately suggests that the client:
1. Cut the dose in half
2. Contact the physician
3. Discontinue the medication
4. Take the medication with food

666. Heparin sodium is prescribed for the client. The nurse expects that the physician will order which of the following to monitor for a therapeutic effect of the medication?
1. Hematocrit level
2. Hemoglobin level
3. Prothrombin time (PT)
4. Activated partial thromboplastin time (aPTT)

ALTERNATE ITEM FORMAT: MULTIPLE RESPONSE

667. A client with coronary artery disease complains of substernal chest pain. After assessing the client's heart rate and blood pressure, a nurse administers nitroglycerin, 0.4 mg, sublingually. After 5 minutes, the client states, "My chest still hurts." Select the appropriate actions that the nurse should take. Select all that apply.
☐ 1. Call a code blue
☐ 2. Contact the physician
☐ 3. Contact the client's family
☐ 4. Assess the client's pain level
☐ 5. Check the client's blood pressure
☐ 6. Administer a second nitroglycerin, 0.4 mg, sublingually

ANSWERS

653. 3

Rationale: Alteplase is a thrombolytic. Hemorrhage is a complication of any type of thrombolytic medication. The client should be monitored for bleeding. Monitoring for renal failure and the client's psychosocial status is important; however, they are not the priority. Heparin sodium is given following thrombolytic therapy, but the question is not asking for the associated medications following alteplase therapy.

Test-Taking Strategy: Use the process of elimination and note the strategic word "priority." Use the principles of prioritizing and knowledge regarding this medication to direct you to option 3. In addition, remember that bleeding is a priority. Review this medication if you had difficulty with this question.

Level of Cognitive Ability: Application
Client Needs: Physiological Integrity
Integrated Process: Nursing Process/Implementation
Content Area: Pharmacology
Reference: Lehne, R. (2007). *Pharmacology for nursing care* (6th ed., pp. 603-608). Philadelphia: Saunders.

654. 4

Rationale: Clients on potassium-wasting diuretics are at high risk of hypokalemia. Clinical manifestations of hypokalemia include fatigue, anorexia, nausea, vomiting, muscle weakness, leg cramps, decreased bowel motility, paresthesias, and dysrhythmias. Diarrhea and intestinal colic are signs of hyperkalemia. Tingling of the fingers and toes are signs of hypocalcemia.

Test-Taking Strategy: Knowledge regarding the signs of hypokalemia is required to answer the question. Remember, muscle weakness and leg cramps are associated with hypokalemia. If you had difficulty with this question, review the signs of this electrolyte imbalance.

Level of Cognitive Ability: Comprehension
Client Needs: Physiological Integrity
Integrated Process: Nursing Process/Data Collection
Content Area: Pharmacology
Reference: Christensen, B., & Kockrow, E. (2006). *Foundations of nursing* (5th ed., pp. 672-673). St. Louis: Mosby.

655. 1

Rationale: Thiazide diuretics such as hydrochlorothiazide are sulfa-based medications, and a client with a sulfa allergy is at risk for an allergic reaction. Options 2, 3, and 4 are not associated with the use of this medication.

Test-Taking Strategy: Knowledge of the chemical make-up of thiazide diuretics is necessary to answer this question. Recalling that these medications contain a sulfa ring in their structure will direct you to option 1. Review the contraindications associated with the thiazide diuretics if you had difficulty with this question.

Level of Cognitive Ability: Application
Client Needs: Safe and Effective Care Environment
Integrated Process: Nursing Process/Data Collection
Content Area: Pharmacology
Reference: Kee, J., Hayes, E., & McCuistion, L. (2006). *Pharmacology: A nursing process approach* (5th ed., p. 632). Philadelphia: Saunders.

656. 4

Rationale: Nicotinic acid should not be taken unless prescribed. All lipid-lowering medications can also cause liver abnormalities, so a combination of nicotinic acid and cholestyramine is to be avoided. Constipation and bloating are the two most common side effects. Both walking and the reduction of fats in the diet are therapeutic measures to reduce cholesterol and triglyceride levels.

Test-Taking Strategy: Note the strategic words "need for further instructions." These words indicate a negative event query and the need to select the incorrect client statement. Recalling that over-the-counter medications should be avoided when a client is taking a prescription medication will direct you to option 4. Review client teaching points related to this medication if you had difficulty with this question.

Level of Cognitive Ability: Analysis
Client Needs: Physiological Integrity
Integrated Process: Teaching and Learning
Content Area: Pharmacology
References: Lehne, R. (2007). *Pharmacology for nursing care* (6th ed., p. 563). Philadelphia: Saunders.
Lilley, L., Harrington, S., & Snyder, J. (2007). *Pharmacology and the nursing process* (5th ed., pp. 448-449). St. Louis: Mosby.

657. 4

Rationale: Calcium channel blocking agents, such as diltiazem, are used cautiously in clients with conditions that could be worsened by the medication, such as aortic stenosis, bradycardia, heart failure, acute myocardial infarction, and hypotension. The nurse would assess for signs and symptoms that indicate worsening of these underlying disorders. In this question, the nurse assesses for signs and symptoms indicating heart failure.

Test-Taking Strategy: Focus on the medication name to determine that diltiazem is a calcium channel blocker, and recall that these medications decrease the rate and force of cardiac contraction. This helps you to eliminate options 1 and 3, because bradycardia is expected. Option 2 is eliminated next, because these signs could indicate bronchoconstriction, which does not occur with calcium channel blockers but does occur with some β-adrenergic blockers. Review this medication if you had difficulty with this question.

Level of Cognitive Ability: Analysis
Client Needs: Physiological Integrity
Integrated Process: Nursing Process/Data Collection
Content Area: Adult Health/Cardiovascular
Reference: Skidmore-Roth, L. (2008). *2008 Mosby's nursing drug reference* (21st ed., pp. 367-369). St. Louis: Mosby.

658. 3

Rationale: The ointment is readily absorbed through the skin, so using the fingers will result in the nurse becoming hypotensive. Proper administration of nitroglycerin ointment involves the use of the dose-measuring applicator paper supplied by the manufacturer and application in a thin, uniform even layer to a nonhairy area of the chest, abdomen, anterior thigh, or forearm. The previous dose is removed before applying, and sites are rotated to avoid inflammation.

Test-Taking Strategy: Use the process of elimination and note the strategic word "avoid." This word indicates a negative event query and the need to select the incorrect action. This question tests fundamental principles of medication administration for nitroglycerin ointment. Visualizing each action will direct you to the correct option. Review this medication if you had difficulty with this question.
Level of Cognitive Ability: Application
Client Needs: Physiological Integrity
Integrated Process: Nursing Process/Implementation
Content Area: Adult Health/Cardiovascular
Reference: Lehne, R. (2007). *Pharmacology for nursing care* (6th ed., pp. 577, 583). Philadelphia: Saunders.

659. 3
Rationale: Double vision, loss of appetite, and nausea are signs of digoxin toxicity. Additional signs of digoxin toxicity include bradycardia, visual alterations such as green and yellow vision, seeing spots or halos, confusion, vomiting, diarrhea, decreased libido, and impotence.
Test-Taking Strategy: Knowledge regarding the signs of digoxin toxicity is required to answer the question. Remembering that gastrointestinal and visual disturbances are signs of toxicity will direct you to option 3. If you had difficulty with this question, review the signs of digoxin toxicity.
Level of Cognitive Ability: Analysis
Client Needs: Physiological Integrity
Integrated Process: Nursing Process/Data Collection
Content Area: Pharmacology
Reference: Lehne, R. (2007). *Pharmacology for nursing care* (6th ed., p. 525). Philadelphia: Saunders.

660. 4
Rationale: Hypotension is a common side effect with this medication, and an increased risk exists in an older client. Options 1 and 3 will also require monitoring but are not the priority. The temperature is unrelated to administering this medication.
Test-Taking Strategy: Use the process of elimination and focus on the strategic word "priority." Use the ABCs—airway, breathing, and circulation. Blood pressure reflects circulation. Review the side effects of this medication if you had difficulty with this question.
Level of Cognitive Ability: Application
Client Needs: Physiological Integrity
Integrated Process: Nursing Process/Data Collection
Content Area: Pharmacology
Reference: Skidmore-Roth, L. (2008). *2008 Mosby's nursing drug reference* (21st ed., pp. 199-200). St. Louis: Mosby.

661. 1
Rationale: Atorvastin is an antihyperlipidemic medication. It is contraindicated in pregnancy, lactation, liver disease, biliary cirrhosis or obstruction, and severe renal dysfunction, and in clients who are hypersensitive to the medication. Options 2, 3, and 4 are not contraindications to the use of this medication.
Test-Taking Strategy: Knowledge regarding the contraindications associated with the use of this medication is required to answer this question. Remember, atorvastin is contraindicated in the client with liver disease. Review these contraindications if you had difficulty with this question.

Level of Cognitive Ability: Analysis
Client Needs: Physiological Integrity
Integrated Process: Nursing Process/Data Collection
Content Area: Pharmacology
Reference: Skidmore-Roth, L. (2008). *2008 Mosby's nursing drug reference* (21st ed., pp. 161-162). St. Louis: Mosby.

662. 3
Rationale: Ecotrin is an aspirin-containing product and should be avoided. Alcohol consumption should be avoided when taking warfarin sodium. Taking prescribed medication at the same time increases client compliance. The Medic-Alert bracelet provides health care personnel emergency information.
Test-Taking Strategy: Use the process of elimination. Note the strategic words "need for further teaching." These words indicate a negative event query and the need to select the incorrect client statement. Recalling that warfarin sodium is an anticoagulant and that Ecotrin is an aspirin-containing product will direct you to option 3. Review client teaching points related to warfarin sodium if you had difficulty with this question.
Level of Cognitive Ability: Analysis
Client Needs: Physiological Integrity
Integrated Process: Teaching and Learning
Content Area: Pharmacology
Reference: Skidmore-Roth, L. (2008). *2008 Mosby's nursing drug reference* (21st ed., pp. 1069-1071). St. Louis: Mosby.

663. 2
Rationale: The therapeutic serum digoxin level ranges from 0.5 to 2 ng/mL. Therefore, options 1, 3, and 4 are incorrect.
Test-Taking Strategy: Knowledge of the therapeutic serum digoxin level is necessary to answer the question. Remember the level is 0.5 to 2.0 ng/mL. Review this level if you had difficulty with this question.
Level of Cognitive Ability: Comprehension
Client Needs: Physiological Integrity
Integrated Process: Nursing Process/Data Collection
Content Area: Pharmacology
References: Chernecky, C., & Berger, B. (2008). *Laboratory tests and diagnostic procedures* (5th ed., p. 448). Philadelphia: Saunders.

664. 2
Rationale: Audible expiratory wheezes may indicate a serious adverse reaction: bronchospasm. β-Blockers may induce this reaction particularly in clients with chronic obstructive pulmonary disease or asthma. A normal decrease in blood pressure and heart rate is expected. Insomnia is a frequent mild side effect and should be monitored.
Test-Taking Strategy: Use the process of elimination. Eliminate options 3 and 4 first because these are expected responses from the medication. From the remaining options, noting the strategic words "adverse reaction" will assist in directing you to option 2. Review the adverse effects of this medication if you had difficulty with this question.
Level of Cognitive Ability: Analysis
Client Needs: Physiological Integrity
Integrated Process: Nursing Process/Data Collection

Content Area: Pharmacology
Reference: Lehne, R. (2007). *Pharmacology for nursing care* (6th ed., pp. 169,173). Philadelphia: Saunders.

665. 4
Rationale: Isosorbide mononitrate is an antianginal medication. Headache is a frequent side effect of isosorbide mononitrate and usually disappears during continued therapy. If a headache occurs during therapy, the client should be instructed to take the medication with food or meals. It is not necessary to contact the physician unless the headaches persist with therapy. It is not appropriate to instruct the client to discontinue therapy or adjust the dosages.
Test-Taking Strategy: Use the process of elimination. Eliminate options 1 and 3 first because it is not within the scope of nursing practice to instruct a client to discontinue or adjust dosages. From the remaining options, recalling that the headache can be relieved with the administration of food with the medication will assist in directing you to option 4. Review this medication if you had difficulty with this question.
Level of Cognitive Ability: Application
Client Needs: Physiological Integrity
Integrated Process: Teaching and Learning
Content Area: Pharmacology
References: Lehne, R. (2007). *Pharmacology for nursing care* (6th ed., pp. 575,584). Philadelphia: Saunders.
Lilley, L., Harrington, S., & Snyder, J. (2007). *Pharmacology and the nursing process* (5th ed., p. 364). St. Louis: Mosby.

666. 4
Rationale: The PT will assess for the therapeutic effect of warfarin sodium (Coumadin) and the aPTT will assess the therapeutic effect of heparin sodium. Heparin sodium doses are determined based on these laboratory results. The hemoglobin and hematocrit values assess red blood cell concentrations.
Test-Taking Strategy: Use the process of elimination. Eliminate options 1 and 2 because these laboratory values are unrelated to heparin sodium therapy. From the remaining options, knowledge of the appropriate test for monitoring therapeutic values of both heparin sodium and warfarin sodium is required to answer this question. Review this content if you had difficulty with this question.

Level of Cognitive Ability: Comprehension
Client Needs: Physiological Integrity
Integrated Process: Nursing Process/Data Collection
Content Area: Pharmacology
Reference: Lilley, L., Harrington, S., & Snyder, J. (2007). *Pharmacology and the nursing process* (5th ed., pp. 432-433; 439). St. Louis: Mosby.

ALTERNATE ITEM FORMAT: MULTIPLE RESPONSE

667. 4, 5, 6
Rationale: The usual guideline for administering nitroglycerin tablets for chest pain is to administer one tablet every 5 minutes PRN for chest pain, for a total dose of three tablets. If the client does not obtain relief after taking a third dose of nitroglycerin, the physician is notified. Since the client is still complaining of chest pain, the nurse would administer a second nitroglycerin tablet. The nurse would assess the client's pain level and check the client's blood pressure before administering each nitroglycerin dose. There are no data in the question that indicate the need to call a code blue. In addition, it is not necessary to contact the client's family unless the client has requested this.
Test-Taking Strategy: Focus on the data in the question. Use the steps of the nursing process to determine that assessing the client's pain level and checking the client's blood pressure are appropriate actions. Next, recalling the usual guidelines for administering nitroglycerin tablets will assist in determining that an appropriate action is to administer a second nitroglycerin, 0.4 mg, sublingually. Review care of the client with chest pain and the guidelines for the administration of nitroglycerin if you had difficulty with this question.
Level of Cognitive Ability: Application
Client Needs: Physiological Integrity
Integrated Process: Nursing Process/Implementation
Content Area: Pharmacology
References: Ignatavicius, D. & Workman, M. (2006). *Medical-surgical nursing: Critical thinking for collaborative care* (5th ed., p. 847). Philadelphia: Saunders.
Kee, J., Hayes, E., & McCuistion, L. (2006). *Pharmacology: A nursing process approach.* (5th ed., p. 908). Philadelphia: Saunders.
Linton, A., & Maebius, N. (2007). *Introduction to medical-surgical nursing* (4th ed., p. 642). Philadelphia: Saunders.

REFERENCES

Chernecky, C., & Berger, B. (2008). *Laboratory tests and diagnostic procedures* (5th ed.). Philadelphia: Saunders.

Christensen, B., & Kockrow, E. (2006). *Foundations of nursing* (5th ed.). St. Louis: Mosby.

Ignatavicius, D., & Workman, M. (2006). *Medical-surgical nursing: Critical thinking for collaborative care* (5th ed.). Philadelphia: Saunders.

Kee, J., Hayes, E., & McCuistion, L. (2006). *Pharmacology: A nursing process approach* (5th ed.). Philadelphia: Saunders.

Lehne, R. (2007). *Pharmacology for nursing care* (6th ed.). Philadelphia: Saunders.

Lilley, L., Harrington, S., & Snyder, J. (2007). *Pharmacology and the nursing process* (5th ed.). St. Louis: Mosby.

Linton, A., & Maebius, N. (2007). *Introduction to medical-surgical nursing* (4th ed.). Philadelphia: Saunders.

Skidmore-Roth, L. (2008). *2008 Mosby's nursing drug reference* (21st ed.). St. Louis: Mosby.

The Adult Client With a Renal Disorder

PYRAMID TERMS

acute renal failure (ARF) The sudden loss of kidney function caused by renal cell damage from ischemia or toxic substances; occurs abruptly and can be reversible; leads to hypoperfusion, cell death, and decompensation in renal function; prognosis depends on the cause and the condition of the client; near-normal or normal kidney function may resume gradually

anuria Urine output of less than 100 mL/day

arterial steal syndrome Can develop following the insertion of an arteriovenous (AV) fistula when too much blood is diverted to the vein and arterial perfusion to the hand is compromised

azotemia The retention of nitrogenous waste products in the blood.

chronic renal failure (CRF) The progressive loss and ongoing deterioration in kidney function that occurs slowly over a period of time; irreversible and results in uremia or end-stage renal disease; requires dialysis or kidney transplantation to maintain life

disequilibrium syndrome A rapid change in the composition of the extracellular fluid (ECF) occurs during hemodialysis; solutes are removed from the blood faster than from the cerebrospinal fluid (CSF) and brain; fluid is pulled into the brain, causing cerebral edema

hemodialysis The process of cleansing the client's blood; the diffusion of dissolved particles from one fluid compartment into another across a semipermeable membrane; the client's blood flows through one fluid compartment and the dialysate is in another fluid compartment

internal arteriovenous fistula (AV fistula) Created surgically in which an artery in the arm is anastomosed to a vein, thus creating an opening, or fistula, between a large artery and a large vein; the flow of arterial blood into the venous system causes the vein to become engorged (maturity); maturity is necessary so that the engorged vein can be punctured with a large-bore needle for the dialysis procedure

nephrolithiasis The formation of kidney stones, which are formed in the renal parenchyma

oliguria Urine output of less than 400 mL/day.

peritoneal dialysis The peritoneum is the dialyzing membrane (semipermeable membrane) and substitutes for kidney function during kidney failure; works on the principles of diffusion and osmosis; the dialysis occurs via the transfer of fluid and solute from the bloodstream through the peritoneum

renal failure The loss of kidney function. The types of renal failure include acute and chronic renal failure; the signs and symptoms are caused by the retention of wastes, the retention of fluids, and the inability of the kidneys to regulate electrolytes.

urolithiasis Refers to the formation of urinary stones or calculi; urinary calculi are formed in the ureter

PYRAMID TO SUCCESS

Pyramid points focus on the preprocedure and postprocedure care of the client undergoing diagnostic tests and procedures related to the renal system. Be familiar with renal failure, dialysis procedures such as hemodialysis and continuous ambulatory peritoneal dialysis (CAPD), dialysis access devices, and postoperative care following urinary or renal surgery. Be familiar with urinary diversions, care of the client following prostatectomy, and treatment measures for the client with urinary or renal calculi. In addition, pyramid points address measures that promote urinary elimination, prevent infection, and maintain skin integrity. The Integrated Processes addressed in this unit include Caring, Clinical Problem-Solving Process (Nursing Process), Communication and Documentation, and Teaching and Learning.

CLIENT NEEDS

Safe and Effective Care Environment

Consultating with members of the health care team
Establishing priorities
Identifying the guidelines related to renal organ donation
Maintaining confidentiality related to the renal disorder
Maintaining sepsis related to wound care and dialysis access devices

Obtaining informed consent related to diagnostic and surgical procedures

Preventing injury related to complications associated with the disorder

Maintaining standard and other precautions related to care of the client

Upholding client rights

Health Promotion and Maintenance

Discussing expected body-image changes

Performing data collection techniques specific to the renal system

Providing client instructions regarding care of a urinary diversion, dialysis access device, and dialysis procedures

Providing client instructions regarding postoperative management

Providing client instructions regarding prescribed treatments related to urinary or renal disorder

Providing client instructions regarding the prevention of the recurrence of a urinary and renal disorder

Psychosocial Integrity

Assisting the client to use appropriate coping mechanisms

Discussing body-image disturbances

Discussing the loss of function of a body part that occurs in clients with a renal disorder

Identifying appropriate community resources

Identifying grief and loss and end-of-life issues

Identifying religious and spiritual influences on health

Identifying support systems

Physiological Integrity

Ensuring elimination measures

Informing the client about diagnostic tests and laboratory results

Monitoring for fluid and electrolyte and acid-base disorders

Monitoring for data indicating rejection of renal transplant

Preventing complications arising as a result of dialysis

Providing adequate rest and sleep

Providing preoperative and postoperative care related to renal transplantation

Providing care related to dialysis access devices

Providing care related to hemodialysis and peritoneal dialysis

Providing care to the client following prostatectomy

Providing comfort interventions

Providing pharmacological therapy

Providing treatment measures for the client with urinary or renal calculi or the client with a urinary diversion

Teaching the client about the prescribed nutrition and fluid measures

REFERENCES

Black, J., & Hawks, J. (2005). *Medical-surgical nursing: Clinical management for positive outcomes* (7th ed.). Philadelphia: Saunders.

Chernecky, C., & Berger, B. (2008). *Laboratory tests and diagnostic procedures* (5th ed.). Philadelphia: Saunders.

Christensen, B., & Kockrow, E. (2006). *Adult health nursing* (5th ed.). St. Louis: Mosby.

Christensen, B., & Kockrow, E. (2006). *Foundations of nursing* (5th ed.). St. Louis: Mosby.

deWit, S. (2009). *Medical-surgical nursing: Concepts & practice.* Philadelphia: Saunders.

Hodgson, B., & Kizior, R. (2008). *Saunders nursing drug handbook 2008.* Philadelphia: Saunders.

Ignatavicius, D., & Workman, M. (2006). *Medical-surgical nursing: Critical thinking for collaborative care* (5th ed.). Philadelphia: Saunders.

Kee, J., Hayes, E., & McCuistion, L. (2006). *Pharmacology: A nursing process approach* (5th ed.). Philadelphia: Saunders.

Lehne, R. (2007). *Pharmacology for nursing care* (6th ed.). Philadelphia: Saunders.

Lewis, S., Heitkemper, M., Dirksen, S., & Bucher, L. (2007). *Medical-surgical nursing: Assessment and management of clinical problems* (7th ed.). St. Louis: Mosby.

Linton, A., & Maebius, N. (2007). *Introduction to medical-surgical nursing* (4th ed.). Philadelphia: Saunders.

McKenry, L., Tessier, E., & Hogan, M. (2006). *Mosby's pharmacology in nursing* (22nd ed.). St. Louis: Mosby.

Monahan, F., Sands, J., Neighbors, M., Marek, J., & Green, C. (2007). *Phipps' medical-surgical nursing: Health and illness perspectives* (8th ed.). St. Louis: Mosby.

National Council of State Boards of Nursing (eds.) (2008). *2008 Detailed Test Plan for the NCLEX-PN® Examination, National Council of State Boards of Nursing.* Chicago: Author.

National Council of State Boards of Nursing, Inc. Web site: http://www.ncsbn.org.

Perry, A., & Potter, P. (2006). *Clinical nursing skills & techniques* (6th ed.). St. Louis: Mosby.

Skidmore-Roth, L. (2008). *2008 Mosby's nursing drug reference* (21st ed.). St. Louis: Mosby.

chapter 52

Renal System

I. ANATOMY AND PHYSIOLOGY

A. Kidney anatomy
1. Each person has two kidneys; one is attached to the left abdominal wall and one to the right abdominal wall at the level of the last thoracic and first three lumbar vertebrae.
2. The kidneys are enclosed in the renal capsule
3. The renal cortex is the outer layer of the renal capsule, which contains blood-filtering mechanisms
4. The renal medulla is the inner region, which contains the renal pyramids
5. Together the renal cortex, pyramids, and medulla constitute the parenchyma or functional unit of the kidneys
6. Nephron
   a. The functional unit of the kidney; located within the parenchyma
   b. Composed of glomerulus and tubules
   c. Selectively secretes and reabsorbs ions and filtrates including fluid, wastes, electrolytes, acids, and bases
7. Glomerulus
   a. Each nephron contains tuft of capillaries that filters large plasma protein and blood cells
   b. Blood flows into the glomerular capillaries from the afferent arteriole and flows out of the glomerular capillaries into the efferent arteriole
8. Bowman's capsule
   a. Thin double-walled capsule that surrounds the glomerulus
   b. Fluid and particles from the blood, such as electrolytes, glucose, amino acids, and metabolic waste (glomerular filtrate), are filtered through the glomerular membrane into a fluid-filled space in Bowman's capsule (Bowman's space) and then enters the proximal convoluted tubule (PCT)
9. Tubules
   a. The tubules include the PCT, Henle's loop, and the distal convoluted tubule (DCT)
   b. The PCT receives filtrate from the glomerular capsule and reabsorbs water and electrolytes through active and passive transport
   c. The descending loop of Henle passively reabsorbs water from the filtrate
   d. The ascending loop of Henle passively reabsorbs sodium and chloride from the filtrate and helps to maintain osmolality
   e. The DCT actively and passively removes sodium and water
   f. The filtered fluid is converted to urine in the tubules, and then the urine moves to the pelvis of the kidney
   g. The urine flows from the pelvis of the kidneys through the ureters and empties into the bladder

B. Functions of kidneys
1. Maintain homeostasis of the blood and acid-base balance
2. Excrete end products of body metabolism
3. Control fluid and electrolyte balance
4. Excrete bacterial toxins, water-soluble drugs, and drug metabolites
5. Secrete renin and erythropoietin, which play a role in the function of the parathyroid hormones and vitamin D

C. Urine production
1. As fluid flows through the tubules, water, electrolytes, and solutes are reabsorbed and other solutes such as creatinine, hydrogen ions, and potassium are secreted
2. Water and solutes that are not reabsorbed become urine
3. The process of selective reabsorption determines the amount of water and solutes to be secreted

D. Homeostasis of water
1. The antidiuretic hormone (ADH) is primarily responsible for the reabsorption of water by the kidneys
2. The ADH is produced by the hypothalamus and secreted from the posterior lobe of the pituitary gland

3. Secretion of ADH is stimulated by dehydration or high sodium intake and by a decrease in blood volume
4. The ADH makes the DCTs and collecting duct permeable to water
5. Water is drawn out of the tubules by osmosis and returns to the blood; concentrated urine remains in the tubule to be excreted
6. When ADH is lacking, the client develops diabetes insipidus (DI).
7. Clients with DI produce large amounts of dilute urine; treatment is necessary because the client cannot drink sufficient water to survive

E. Homeostasis of sodium
1. When the amount of sodium increases, extra water is retained to preserve osmotic pressure
2. An increase in sodium and water produces an increase in the blood volume and blood pressure (BP)
3. When BP increases, glomerular filtration increases, and extra water and sodium are lost; blood volume is reduced, returning the BP to normal
4. Reabsorption of sodium in the DCTs is controlled by the renin-angiotensin system
5. Renin, an enzyme, is released from the nephron when the BP or fluid concentration in the DCT is low
6. Renin catalyzes the splitting of angiotensin I from angiotensinogen; angiotensin I converts to angiotensin II as blood flows through the lung
7. Angiotensin II, a potent vasoconstrictor, stimulates the secretion of aldosterone
8. Aldosterone stimulates the DCTs to reabsorb sodium and secrete potassium
9. The additional sodium increases water reabsorption and increases blood volume and BP, returning the BP to normal; the stimulus for the secretion of renin is then removed

F. Homeostasis of potassium
1. Increases in serum potassium stimulate the secretion of aldosterone
2. Aldosterone stimulates the DCTs to secrete potassium; this action returns the serum potassium concentration to normal

G. Homeostasis of acidity (pH)
1. Blood pH is controlled by maintaining the concentration of buffer systems
2. Carbonic acid and sodium bicarbonate form the most important buffers for neutralizing acids in the plasma
3. The concentration of carbonic acid is controlled by the respiratory system
4. The concentration of sodium bicarbonate is controlled by the kidneys
5. Normal arterial pH is 7.35 to 7.45, maintained by keeping the ratio of concentrations of sodium bicarbonate to carbon dioxide constant at 20:1

6. Strong acids are neutralized by sodium bicarbonate to produce carbonic acid and the sodium salts of the strong acid; this process quickly restores the ratio and thus blood pH
7. The carbonic acid dissociates into carbon dioxide and water; because the concentration of carbon dioxide is maintained at a constant level by the respiratory system, the excess carbonic acid is rapidly excreted
8. Sodium combined with the strong acid is actively reabsorbed in the DCTs in exchange for hydrogen or potassium ions; the strong acid is neutralized by ammonia and excreted as ammonia or potassium salts

H. Adrenal glands (Refer to Chapter 44 for information about the adrenal glands)
1. One adrenal gland is on top of each kidney
2. Influence blood pressure and sodium and water retention

I. Bladder
1. The bladder detrusor muscle, composed of smooth muscle, distends during bladder filling and contracts during bladder emptying
2. The ureterovesical sphincter prevents reflux of urine from the bladder to the ureter
3. The total bladder capacity is 1 L; normal adult urine output is 1500 mL/day

J. Prostate gland
1. The prostate gland surrounds the male urethra
2. The prostate gland contains a duct that opens into the prostatic portion of the urethra and secretes the alkaline portion of seminal fluid, which protects passing sperm

K. Risk factors associated with renal disorders (Box 52-1)

II. DIAGNOSTIC TESTS
A. Refer to Chapter 11 and Box 52-2 for information regarding normal values for renal function studies
B. Serum creatinine level
1. Description: A test that measures the amount of creatinine in the serum; creatinine is an end-product from protein and muscle metabolism

---

BOX 52-1 **Risk Factors Associated With Renal Disorders**

Chemical or environmental toxin exposure
Contact sports
Diabetes mellitus
Family history of renal disease
Frequent urinary tract infections
Heart failure
High-sodium diet
Hypertension
Medications
Trauma

2. Analysis
   a. Creatinine level reflects glomerular filtration rate
   b. Renal disease is the only pathological condition that increases the serum creatinine level
   c. Serum creatinine increases only when at least 50% of renal function is lost

C. Blood urea nitrogen (BUN)
   1. Description: A serum test that measures the amount of nitrogenous urea, a by-product of protein metabolism in the liver
   2. Analysis
      a. BUN levels indicate the extent of renal clearance of urea nitrogenous waste products
      b. An elevation does not always mean renal disease is present
      c. Some factors that can elevate the BUN include dehydration, poor renal perfusion, intake of a high-protein diet, infection, stress, corticosteroid use, or gastrointestinal (GI) bleeding
      d. When the BUN and serum creatinine increase at the same rate and the ratio of the BUN/creatinine remains constant, the elevated serum creatinine and BUN levels suggest renal dysfunction

D. Urinalysis
   1. Description: a urine test for evaluation of the renal system and for determining renal disease
   2. Interventions
      a. Wash perineal area and use a clean container for collection
      b. Obtain 10 to 15 mL of the first morning voiding
      c. Refrigerated samples may alter the specific gravity
      d. If the client is menstruating, note this on the laboratory requisition form

E. Specific gravity determination
   1. Description: a urine test that measures the ability of the kidneys to concentrate urine
   2. Interventions
      a. Specific gravity can be measured by a multiple-test dipstick method (most common method), refractometer (an instrument used in the laboratory setting), or urinometer (least accurate method)

b. Factors that interfere with an accurate reading include radiopaque contrast agents, glucose, and proteins
   c. Cold specimens may produce a false high reading
   d. Normal value is 1.016 to 1.022 (may vary depending on the laboratory)
   e. An increase in specific gravity (more concentrated urine) occurs with insufficient fluid intake, decreased renal perfusion, or increased ADH
   f. A decrease in specific gravity (less concentrated urine) occurs with increased fluid intake or DI

F. Urine culture and sensitivity
   1. Description: a urine test that identifies the presence of microorganisms and determines the specific antibiotics to treat the existing microorganism appropriately
   2. Interventions
      a. Clean the perineal area and urinary meatus with a bacteriostatic solution
      b. Collect the midstream sample in a sterile container
      c. Send the collected specimen to the laboratory immediately
      d. Identify any sources of potential contaminants during the collection of the specimen, such as the hands, skin, clothing, hair, or vaginal or rectal secretions
      e. Urine from the client who drank a very large amount of fluids may be too dilute to provide a positive culture

G. Creatinine clearance test
   1. Description
      a. The creatinine clearance test evaluates how well the kidneys remove creatinine from the blood
      b. The test includes obtaining a blood sample and timed urine specimens
      c. Blood is drawn at the start of the test and when the urine specimen collection is complete
      d. The urine specimen for the creatinine clearance is usually collected for 24 hours, but shorter periods (8 or 12 hours) could be prescribed.
   2. Interventions
      a. Encourage fluids before and during the test
      b. Instruct the client to avoid tea, coffee, and, as prescribed, to withhold medications during testing
      c. If the client is taking corticosteroids or thyroid medication, check with the physician regarding the administration of these medications during testing

---

BOX 52-2 **Normal Renal Function Values**

Blood urea nitrogen: 8-25 mg/dL
Serum creatinine: 0.6-1.3 mg/dL
Serum uric acid: 2.5-8.0 mg/dL

d. Instruct the client about the urine collection

e. At the start time, ask the client to void (or empty the tubing and drainage bag if the client has a Foley catheter) and discard that sample

f. Collect all urine for the prescribed time

g. Keep the urine specimen on ice or refrigerated and check with the laboratory regarding adding a preservative to the specimen during collection

h. At the end of the prescribed time, ask the client to empty the bladder (or empty the tubing and drainage bag if the client has a Foley catheter) and add that urine to the collection container

i. Send the labeled urine specimen to the laboratory in a biohazard bag along with the requisition

j. Document specimen collection, time started and completed, and other pertinent data

H. Uric acid test

1. Description: a 24-hour urine collection to diagnose gout and kidney disease

2. Interventions

a. Encourage fluid intake and a regular diet during testing

b. Follow the same procedure for urine collection as with the creatinine clearance test

I. Vanillylmandelic acid test

1. Description

a. The test is a 24-hour urine collection to diagnose pheochromocytoma, a tumor of the adrenal gland

b. The test identifies an assay of urinary catecholamines in the urine

2. Interventions

a. Check with the laboratory regarding medication restrictions

b. Instruct the client to avoid foods such as caffeine, cocoa, vanilla, cheese, gelatin, licorice, and fruits for at least 2 days before and during urine collection and to avoid taking medications for 2 to 3 days before the test, as prescribed

c. Instruct the client to avoid stress and encourage adequate food and fluid intake during the test

d. Follow the same procedure for urine collection as with the creatinine clearance test

J. KUB (kidneys, ureters, and bladder) radiograph

1. Description: an x-ray film of the urinary system and adjacent structures used to detect urinary calculi

2. Interventions: No specific preparation is necessary

K. Bladder ultrasonography (bladder scan)

1. Bladder ultrasonography is a noninvasive method for measuring the volume of urine in the bladder

2. Bladder ultrasonography may be performed for evaluating urinary frequency, inability to urinate, or residual urine (the amount of urine remaining in the bladder after voiding)

L. Computed tomography and magnetic resonance imaging

1. Description: imaging methods that provide cross-sectional views of the kidney and urinary tract

2. Interventions: Refer to Chapter 56

M. Intravenous pyelogram

1. Description: an IV injection of a radiopaque dye is used to visualize and identify abnormalities in the renal system

2. Preprocedure interventions

a. Obtain an informed consent

b. Assess the client for allergies to iodine, seafood, and radiopaque dyes

c. Withhold food and fluids after midnight on the night before the test

d. Administer laxatives if prescribed

e. Inform the client about possible throat irritation, flushing of the face, warmth, or a salty taste during the test

3. Postprocedure interventions

a. Monitor vital signs

b. Instruct the client to drink at least 1 L of fluid unless contraindicated

c. Assess the venipuncture site for bleeding

d. Monitor urinary output

e. Monitor for signs of a possible allergic reaction to the dye used during the test and instruct the client to notify the physician if any signs of an allergic reaction occur

N. Renal angiography

1. Description: an injection of a radiopaque dye through a catheter inserted into the femoral artery to examine the renal blood vessels and renal arterial supply

2. Preprocedure interventions

a. Obtain an informed consent

b. Assess the client for allergies to iodine, seafood, and radiopaque dyes

c. Inform the client about a possible feeling of burning or heat along the vessel when the dye is injected

d. Withhold food and fluids after midnight on the night before the test

e. Instruct the client to void immediately before the procedure

f. Administer enemas if prescribed

g. Shave injection sites as prescribed

h. Assess and mark the peripheral pulses

3. Postprocedure interventions
   a. Assess vital signs and peripheral pulses frequently as prescribed
   b. Maintain bedrest and apply a sandbag or other device that will provide pressure to prevent bleeding, if prescribed, at the insertion site for 4 to 8 hours
   c. Assess the color, temperature, sensation, and movement (CMS) of the toes of the involved extremity with each vital sign check
   d. Inspect the catheter insertion site for bleeding or swelling with each vital sign check
   e. Because the dye may be nephrotoxic, encourage increased fluids unless contraindicated and monitor urinary output

O. Renal scan
   1. Description: an IV injection of a radioisotope for visual imaging of renal blood flow, glomerular filtration, tubular function, and excretion
   2. Preprocedure interventions
      a. Obtain an informed consent
      b. Assess for allergies
      c. Inform the client that the test requires no dietary or activity restrictions
      d. Assist with administering the radioisotope as necessary
      e. Instruct the client to remain motionless during the test
      f. Instruct the client that imaging may be repeated at various intervals before the test is complete
   3. Postprocedure interventions
      a. Encourage fluid intake unless contraindicated
      b. Assess the client for signs of delayed allergic reaction such as itching and hives
      c. The radioactivity is eliminated in 24 hours; wear gloves for excretion precautions
      d. Follow standard precautions when caring for incontinent clients and double-bag client linens per agency policy

P. Cystoscopy and biopsy
   1. Description: the bladder mucosa is examined for inflammation, calculi, or tumors by means of a cystoscope; a biopsy may be obtained
   2. Preprocedure interventions
      a. Obtain an informed consent
      b. If a biopsy is planned, withhold food and fluids after midnight the night before the test
      c. If a cystoscopy alone is planned, no special preparation is necessary, and the procedure may be performed in the physician's office; postprocedure intervention includes increasing fluid intake
   3. Postprocedure interventions following biopsy
      a. Monitor vital signs
      b. Increase fluid intake as prescribed
      c. Monitor intake and output (I&O)
      d. Encourage deep-breathing exercises to relieve bladder spasms
      e. Administer analgesics as prescribed
      f. Administer sitz or tub baths for back and abdominal pain
      g. Note that leg cramps are common because of the lithotomy position maintained during the procedure
      h. Assess the urine for color and consistency
      i. Inform the client that burning on urination, pink-tinged or tea-colored urine, and urinary frequency are common after cystoscopy and resolve in a few days
      j. Monitor for bright red urine or clots, and notify the physician if this occurs

Q. Renal biopsy
   1. Description: insertion of a needle into the kidney to obtain a sample of tissue for examination; usually done percutaneously
   2. Preprocedure interventions
      a. Assess vital signs
      b. Assess baseline coagulation studies; notify the physician if abnormal results are noted
      c. Obtain an informed consent
      d. Withhold food and fluids after midnight the night before the test
   3. Interventions during the procedure: Position the client prone with a pillow under the abdomen and shoulders
   4. Postprocedure interventions
      a. Monitor vital signs, especially for hypotension and tachycardia, which could indicate bleeding
      b. Provide pressure to the biopsy site for 30 minutes
      c. Monitor the hemoglobin and hematocrit levels for decreases, which could indicate bleeding
      d. Place the client in the supine position and on bedrest for 8 hours as prescribed
      e. Check the biopsy site and under the client for bleeding
      f. Encourage fluid intake of 1500 to 2000 mL as prescribed
      g. Observe the urine for gross and microscopic bleeding
      h. Instruct the client to avoid heavy lifting and strenuous activity for 2 weeks

III. ACUTE RENAL FAILURE
A. Description
   1. **Acute renal failure (ARF)** is the rapid loss of kidney function from renal cell damage
   2. Occurs abruptly and can be reversible
   3. Signs and symptoms are primarily caused by the retention of wastes, the retention of fluids, and the inability of the kidneys to regulate electrolytes

BOX 52-3 **Some Potentially Nephrotoxic Substances**

Drugs
Antibiotics/Anti-infectives
- Amphotericin B
- Colistimethate
- Methicillin
- Polymyxin B
- Rifampin
- Sulfonamides
- Tetracycline hydrochloride
- Vancomycin

Aminoglycoside Antibiotics
- Gentamicin
- Kanamycin
- Neomycin
- Netilmicin sulfate
- Tobramycin

Nonsteroidal Anti-inflammatory Drugs (NSAIDs)
- Celecoxib
- Flurbiprofen
- Ibuprofen
- Indomethacin
- Ketorolac
- Meclofenamate
- Meloxicam
- Nabumetone
- Naproxen
- Oxaprozin
- Rofecoxib
- Tolmetin

Antineoplastics
- Cisplatin
- Cyclophosphamide
- Methotrexate

Other Drugs
- Acetaminophen
- Captopril
- Cyclosporine
- Fluorinated anesthetics
- *D*-Penicillamine
- Phenazopyridine hydrochloride
- Quinine

Other Substances
Organic Solvents
- Carbon tetrachloride
- Ethylene glycol

Nondrug Chemical Agents
- Radiographic contrast dye
- Pesticides
- Fungicides
- Myoglobin (from breakdown of skeletal muscle)

Heavy Metals and Ions
- Arsenic
- Bismuth
- Copper sulfate
- Gold salts
- Lead
- Mercuric chloride

From Ignatavicius, D., & Workman, M. (2006). *Medical-surgical nursing: Critical thinking for collaborative care* (5th ed). Philadelphia: Saunders.

4. **ARF** leads to hypoperfusion, cell death, and decompensation of renal function
5. The prognosis depends on the cause and the condition of the client
6. Near-normal or normal kidney function may resume gradually

B. Causes
   1. Prerenal: Outside the kidney; due to intravascular volume depletion, dehydration, decreased cardiac output, decreased peripheral vascular resistance, decreased renovascular blood flow, and prerenal infection or obstruction
   2. Intrarenal: Within the parenchyma of the kidney; due to tubular necrosis, prolonged prerenal ischemia, intrarenal infection or obstruction, and nephrotoxicity (Box 52-3)
   3. Postrenal: Between the kidney and urethral meatus such as bladder neck obstruction, bladder cancer, calculi, and postrenal infection

C. Phases of **ARF** and interventions (Box 52-4)
   1. Onset: Begins with precipitating event
   2. Oliguric phase
      a. Duration of 8 to 15 days; the longer the duration, the less chance of recovery

   b. Sudden decrease in urine output; urine output is less than 400 mL/day
   c. Signs of excess fluid volume: Hypertension, edema, pleural and pericardial effusions, dysrhythmias, congestive heart failure (CHF), and pulmonary edema
   d. Signs of uremia: anorexia, nausea, vomiting, and pruritus
   e. Signs of metabolic acidosis: Kussmaul respirations
   f. Signs of neurological changes: tingling of extremities, drowsiness progressing to disorientation and then coma
   g. Signs of pericarditis: friction rub, chest pain with inspiration, and low-grade fever
   h. Laboratory analysis (see Box 52-4)
   i. Restrict fluid intake; if hypertension is present, daily fluid allowances may be 400 mL to 1000 mL plus the measured urinary output
   j. Administer medications as prescribed such as diuretics (furosemide [Lasix]) to increase renal blood flow and diuresis

BOX 52-4   Acute Renal Failure Phases and Laboratory Findings

Onset
Begins with precipitating event

Oliguric Phase
Elevated blood urea nitrogen and serum creatinine
Decreased urine specific gravity (prerenal causes) or normal (intrarenal causes)
Decreased glomerular filtration rate
Hyperkalemia
Normal or decreased serum sodium
Hypervolemia
Hypocalcemia
Hyperphosphatemia

Diuretic Phase
Gradual decline in blood urea nitrogen and serum creatinine, but still elevated
Low creatinine clearance
Hypokalemia
Hyponatremia
Hypovolemia

Recovery Phase (Convalescent)
Increased glomerular filtration rate
Stabilization or continual decline in blood urea nitrogen and serum creatinine levels toward normal
Complete recovery may take 1-2 years

3. Diuretic phase
   a. Urine output rises slowly, followed by diuresis (4-5 L/day).
   b. Excessive urine output indicates that damaged nephrons are recovering their ability to excrete wastes but not to concentrate urine
   c. Dehydration, hypovolemia, hypotension, and tachycardia can occur
   d. Level of consciousness improves
   e. Laboratory analysis (see Box 52-4)
   f. Administer IV fluids as prescribed, which may contain electrolytes to replace losses
4. Recovery phase (convalescent)
   a. Recovery is a slow process; complete recovery may take 1 to 2 years
   b. Urine volume returns to normal
   c. Memory improves
   d. Strength increases
   e. The older adult is less likely than a younger adult to regain full kidney function
   f. Laboratory analysis (see Box 52-4)
   g. **ARF** can progress to **chronic renal failure**
D. Data collection: Obtain objective and subjective data noted in the phases of ARF (see Box 52-4).
E. Other interventions
   1. Monitor vital signs, especially for signs of hypertension, tachycardia, tachypnea, and an irregular heart rate
   2. Monitor urine and I&O (hourly in **ARF**) and urine color and characteristics

3. Monitor daily weight (same scale, same time of the day), noting that an increase of ½ to 1 lb daily indicates fluid retention
4. Monitor for changes in the BUN, serum creatinine, and serum electrolyte values
5. Monitor for acidosis (may be treated with sodium bicarbonate)
6. Monitor urinalysis for protein, hematuria, casts, and specific gravity
7. Monitor for altered level of consciousness caused by uremia
8. Monitor for signs of infection because the client may not experience an elevated temperature or an increased white blood cell count
9. Monitor the lungs for wheezes and rhonchi and monitor for edema, which can indicate fluid overload
10. Administer prescribed diet, which is usually a moderate-protein (to decrease the workload on the kidneys) and a high-carbohydrate diet
11. Restrict potassium and sodium intake as prescribed based on the electrolyte level
12. Administer medications as prescribed; be alert to the mechanism for metabolism and excretion of all prescribed medications
13. Be alert to nephrotoxic medications, which may be prescribed (see Box 52-3)
14. Be alert to the health care providers' adjustment of medication dosages for **renal failure**
15. Prepare the client for dialysis if prescribed; continuous renal replacement therapy (CRRT) may be used in **ARF** to treat fluid volume overload or rapidly developing **azotemia** and metabolic acidosis
16. Provide emotional support by allowing opportunities for the client to express concerns and fears and by encouraging family interactions
17. Promote consistency in caregivers
18. Also refer to the section in this chapter on special problems in **renal failure** and interventions

IV. **CHRONIC RENAL FAILURE (CRF)**
A. Description
   1. A slow, progressive, irreversible loss in kidney function
   2. Occurs in stages and results in uremia or end-stage renal disease (Box 52-5)
   3. Affects all major body systems and requires dialysis or kidney transplant to maintain life
   4. Hypervolemia can occur because of the kidneys' inability to excrete sodium and water, or hypovolemia can occur because of the kidneys' inability to conserve sodium and water
B. Primary causes
   1. May follow **ARF**
   2. Diabetes mellitus and other metabolic disorders
   3. Hypertension
   4. Chronic urinary obstruction

BOX 52-5   **Stages of Chronic Renal Failure**

Stage I: Diminished Renal Reserve
Renal function reduced
No accumulation of metabolic wastes
Decreased ability to concentrate urine
Nocturia and polyuria
Healthier kidney compensates

Stage II: Renal Insufficiency
Metabolic wastes begin to accumulate
Decreased responsiveness to diuretics
Decreased ability of the healthier kidney
    to compensate
Oliguria and edema

Stage III: End Stage
Excessive accumulation of metabolic wastes
Kidneys unable to maintain homeostasis
Dialysis or other renal replacement therapy
    required

5. Recurrent infections
6. Renal artery occlusion
7. Autoimmune disorders

C. Data collection
   1. Monitor body systems for the manifestations of **chronic renal failure** (Box 52-6)
   2. Monitor psychological changes, which could include emotional lability, withdrawal, depression, anxiety, suicidal behavior, denial, dependence/independence conflict, and changes in body image

D. Interventions
   1. Same as the interventions for **ARF**
   2. Administer prescribed diet, which is usually a moderate protein (to decrease the workload on the kidneys) and a high-carbohydrate, low-potassium, and low-phosphorus diet
   3. Provide oral care to prevent stomatitis and reduce discomfort from mouth sores

BOX 52-6   **Key Features of Chronic Renal Failure**

Neurologic Manifestations
• Lethargy and daytime drowsiness
• Inability to concentrate or decreased attention span
• Seizures
• Coma
• Slurred speed
• Asterixis
• Tremors, twitching, or jerky movements
• Myoclonus
• Ataxia (alteration in gait)
• Paresthesias

Cardiovascular Manifestations
• Cardiomyopathy
• Hypertension
• Peripheral edema
• Heart failure
• Uremic pericarditis
• Pericardial effusion
• Pericardial friction rub
• Cardiac tamponade

Respiratory Manifestations
• Uremic halitosis
• Tachypnea
• Deep sighing, yawning
• Kussmaul respirations
• Uremic pneumonitis
• Shortness of breath
• Pulmonary edema
• Pleural effusion
• Depressed cough reflex
• Crackles

Hematologic Manifestations
• Anemia
• Abnormal bleeding and bruising

Gastrointestinal Manifestations
• Anorexia
• Nausea
• Vomiting
• Metallic taste in mouth
• Changes in taste acuity and sensation
• Uremic colitis (diarrhea)
• Constipation
• Uremic gastritis (possible gastrointestinal bleeding)
• Uremic fetor
• Stomatitis
• Diarrhea

Urinary Manifestations
• Polyuria, nocturia (early)
• Oliguria, anuria (later)
• Proteinuria
• Hematuria
• Diluted, straw-like appearance

Integumentary Manifestations
• Decreased skin turgor
• Yellow-gray pallor
• Dry skin
• Pruritus
• Ecchymosis
• Purpura
• Soft tissue calcifications
• Uremic frost (late, premorbid)

Musculoskeletal Manifestations
• Muscle weakness and cramping
• Bone pain
• Pathologic fractures
• Renal osteodystrophy

Reproductive Manifestations
• Decreased fertility
• Infrequent or absent menses
• Decreased libido
• Impotence

From Ignatavicius, D., & Workman, M. (2006). *Medical-surgical nursing: Critical thinking for collaborative care* (5th ed). Philadelphia: Saunders.

4. Provide skin care to prevent pruritus

5. Teach the client about fluid and dietary restrictions and the importance of daily weights

6. Provide support to promote acceptance of the chronic illness and prepare the client for long-term dialysis and transplantation; note that the client may choose to decline dialysis or transplantation

E. Special problems in **renal failure** and interventions (Box 52-7)

  1. Activity intolerance and insomnia

    a. Fatigue results from anemia and the buildup of wastes from the diseased kidneys

    b. Provide adequate rest periods

    c. Teach the client to plan activities to avoid fatigue

    d. Administer mild central nervous system (CNS) depressants as prescribed to promote rest

  2. Anemia

    a. Anemia results from the decreased secretion of erythropoietin and decreased production of red blood cells as a result of the kidney disease

    b. Monitor for decreased hemoglobin and hematocrit levels

    c. Administer epoetin alfa (Epogen, Procrit) or darbepoetin alfa (Aranesp), or hematopoietics, as prescribed to stimulate the production of red blood cells

    d. Administer folic acid (vitamin B_9) as prescribed

    e. Administer iron orally as prescribed, but not at the same time as phosphate binders

    f. Administer stool softeners as prescribed because of the constipating effects of iron

g. Be alert that oral iron is not well absorbed by the gastrointestinal tract in **chronic renal failure** and causes nausea and vomiting; parenteral iron (iron sucrose [Venofer] or sodium ferric gluconate complex [Ferrlecit]) may be used if iron deficiencies persist despite folic acid or oral iron

h. Administer blood transfusions if prescribed; blood transfusions are prescribed only when necessary (acute blood loss, symptomatic anemia) because they decrease the stimulus to produce red blood cells; note that certain religious beliefs such as Jehovah's Witnesses may refuse blood and blood products

  3. Gastrointestinal bleeding

    a. Urea is broken down by the intestinal bacteria to ammonia; ammonia irritates the gastrointestinal mucosa causing ulceration and bleeding

    b. Monitor for decreasing hemoglobin and hematocrit levels

    c. Monitor stools for occult blood

    d. Instruct the client to use a soft toothbrush

    e. Avoid the administration of acetylsalicylic acid (aspirin) because it is excreted by the kidneys; if administered, aspirin toxicity can occur and prolong the bleeding time

  4. Hyperkalemia

    a. Monitor vital signs for hypertension or hypotension and the apical heart rate; an irregular heart rate could indicate dysrhythmias

    b. Monitor the serum potassium level; a serum potassium level above 6 mEq/L can cause tall peaked T waves, flat P waves, a widened QRS complex, and a prolonged PR interval; decreased cardiac output; heart blocks; fibrillation; or asystole (Figure 52-1)

    c. Place the client on continuous cardiac monitoring because the client is at risk for dysrhythmias

    d. Provide a low-potassium diet, avoiding foods high in potassium (refer to Chapter 9 for a listing of foods that are high in potassium)

    e. Administer electrolyte-binding and electrolyte-excreting medications such as oral or rectal sodium polystyrene sulfonate (Kayexalate) as prescribed to lower the serum potassium level

    f. Administer prescribed medications: 50% dextrose and insulin may be prescribed to shift potassium into the cell; calcium gluconate IV may be prescribed to reduce myocardial irritability from hyperkalemia; and sodium bicarbonate IV may be prescribed to correct acidosis

    g. Administer prescribed loop diuretics to excrete potassium

---

BOX 52-7   **Special Problems in Renal Failure**

Activity intolerance and insomnia
Anemia
Gastrointestinal bleeding
Hyperkalemia
Hypermagnesemia
Hyperphosphatemia
Hypertension
Hypervolemia
Hypocalcemia
Hypovolemia
Infection
Injury
Metabolic acidosis
Muscle cramps
Neurological changes
Ocular irritation
Potential for Injury
Pruritus
Psychosocial problems

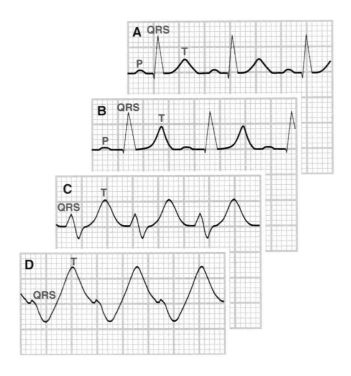

Serum potassium levels

A. normal (3.5-5.1 mEq/L)
B. about 7.0 mEq/L
C. 8.0-9.0 mEq/L
D. >10.0 mEq/L

FIG. 52-1 Cardiac rhythm changes with hyperkalemia. (From Huszar, R.J. [2007]. *Basic dysrhythmias: Interpretation & management* [3rd ed]. St. Louis: Mosby.)

h. Avoid potassium-sparing medications such as spironolactone (Aldactone) and triamterene (Dyrenium) because these medications will increase the potassium level

i. Prepare the client for **peritoneal** or **hemodialysis** as prescribed

5. Hypermagnesemia
   a. Results from decreased renal excretion of magnesium
   b. Monitor cardiac manifestations of bradycardia, peripheral vasodilation, and hypotension
   c. Monitor CNS manifestations of decreased nerve impulse transmission such as drowsiness or lethargy.
   d. Monitor neuromuscular manifestations such as reduced or absent deep tendon reflexes or weak or absent voluntary skeletal muscle contractions
   e. Administer loop diuretics as prescribed such as furosemide (Lasix)
   f. Administer calcium as prescribed for resulting cardiac problems
   g. Avoid medications that contain magnesium such as antacids, laxatives, or enemas

h. During severe elevations, avoid foods that increase magnesium levels (refer to Chapter 9 for a listing of foods that are high in magnesium)

6. Hyperphosphatemia
   a. As the phosphorus level rises, the calcium level drops; this leads to the stimulation of parathyroid hormone, causing bone demineralization
   b. Treatment is aimed at lowering the serum phosphorus levels
   c. Administer phosphate binders such as calcium carbonate (TUMS), calcium acetate (PhosLo), or sevelamer (Renagel) as prescribed with meals to lower serum phosphate levels
   d. Aluminum hydroxide preparations are avoided for use as phosphate binders because they are associated with dementia and osteomalacia
   e. Administer stools softeners and laxatives as prescribed because phosphate binders are constipating
   f. Teach the client about the need to limit the intake of foods high in phosphorus (refer to Chapter 9 for a listing of foods that are high in phosphorus)

7. Hypertension
   a. Caused by failure of the kidneys to maintain BP homeostasis
   b. Monitor vital signs for elevated blood pressure
   c. Maintain fluid and sodium restrictions as prescribed
   d. Administer diuretics and antihypertensives as prescribed
   e. Administer propranolol (Inderal)—a β-adrenergic antagonist—as prescribed; propranolol decreases renin release (renin causes vasoconstriction)

8. Hypervolemia
   a. Monitor vital signs for an elevated blood pressure
   b. Monitor I&O and daily weight for indications of fluid retention
   c. Monitor for periorbital, sacral, and peripheral edema
   d. Monitor the serum electrolytes
   e. Monitor for hypertension and notify the health care provider for sustained elevations
   f. Monitor for signs of CHF and pulmonary edema such as restlessness, heightened anxiety, tachycardia, dyspnea, basilar lung crackles, and blood-tinged sputum; notify the physician immediately if signs occur
   g. Maintain fluid restriction
   h. Avoid the administration of IV fluids

i. Administer diuretics such as furosemide (Lasix) as prescribed

j. Teach the client to maintain a low-sodium diet

k. Teach the client to avoid antacids or cold remedies containing sodium bicarbonate

9. Hypocalcemia

a. Results from the high phosphorus level and the inability of the diseased kidney to activate vitamin D

b. The absence of vitamin D causes poor calcium absorption from the intestinal tract

c. Monitor the serum calcium level

d. Administer calcium supplements as prescribed

e. Administer activated vitamin D as prescribed

f. Refer to Chapter 9 for a listing of foods that are high in calcium

10. Hypovolemia

a. Monitor the vital signs for hypotension and tachycardia

b. Monitor for decreasing I&O and a reduction in the daily weight

c. Monitor for dehydration

d. Monitor electrolytes

e. Provide replacement therapy based on the serum electrolyte results

f. Provide sodium supplements as prescribed, based on the serum electrolyte value

11. Infection

a. The client is at risk for infection because of a suppressed immune system, dialysis access site, and possible malnutrition

b. Monitor for signs of infection

c. Avoid urinary catheters when possible; if used, provide catheter care

d. Provide strict asepsis during urinary catheter insertion and other invasive procedures

e. Instruct the client to avoid fatigue, which decreases body resistance

f. Instruct the client to avoid persons with infections

g. Administer antibiotics as prescribed, monitoring for nephrotoxic effects

12. Metabolic acidosis

a. The kidneys are unable to excrete hydrogen ions or manufacture bicarbonate, resulting in acidosis

b. Administer alkalizers such as sodium bicarbonate as prescribed

c. Note that clients with **chronic renal failure** adjust to low bicarbonate levels and do not become acutely ill

13. Muscle cramps

a. Occur from electrolyte imbalances and the effects of uremia on peripheral nerves

b. Monitor serum electrolytes

c. Administer electrolyte replacements and medications to control muscle cramps as prescribed

d. Administer heat and massage as prescribed

14. Neurological changes

a. The buildup of active particles and fluids causes changes in the brain cells and leads to confusion and impairment in decision-making ability

b. Peripheral neuropathy results from the effects of uremia on peripheral nerves

c. Monitor the level of consciousness and for confusion

15. Ocular irritation

a. Calcium deposits in the conjunctiva cause burning and watering of the eyes

b. Administer medications to control the calcium and phosphate levels as prescribed

c. Administer lubricating eye drops

d. Protect the client from injury

e. Provide a safe and hazard-free environment

f. Use side rails as needed

g. Teach the client to examine areas of decreased sensation for signs of injury

h. Provide a calm and restful environment

i. Provide comfort measures and backrubs

16. Potential for injury

a. The client is at risk for fractures because of alterations in the absorption of calcium and the excretion of phosphate and altered vitamin D metabolism

b. Provide for a safe environment

c. Avoid injury; tissue breakdown causes increased serum potassium levels

17. Pruritus

a. To rid the body of excess wastes, urate crystals are excreted through the skin, causing pruritus

b. The deposit of urate crystals (uremic frost) occurs in advanced stages of **renal failure**

c. Monitor for skin breakdown, rash, and uremic frost

d. Provide meticulous skin care and oral hygiene

e. Avoid the use of soaps

f. Administer antihistamines and antipruritics as prescribed to relieve itching

18. Psychosocial problems

a. Listen to the client's concerns to determine how the client is handling the situation

b. Allow the client time to mourn the loss of kidney function

c. With client permission, include the family members in discussions of the client's concerns

d. Offer information about support groups

e. Provide end-of-life care for the client with end-stage renal disease

V. UREMIC SYNDROME

A. Description
1. The accumulation of nitrogenous waste products in the blood caused by the kidneys' inability to filter out these waste products
2. Uremic syndrome may occur as a result of **acute** or **chronic renal failure**

B. Data collection
1. **Oliguria**
2. The presence of protein, red blood cells, and casts in the urine
3. A urine specific gravity of 1.010
4. Elevated levels of urea, uric acid, potassium, and magnesium in the urine
5. Hypotension or hypertension
6. Alterations in the level of consciousness
7. Electrolyte imbalances
8. Stomatitis
9. Nausea or vomiting from **azotemia**
10. Diarrhea or constipation

C. Interventions
1. Monitor vital signs for hypertension, tachycardia, and an irregular heart rate
2. Monitor serum electrolyte levels
3. Monitor I&O and for **oliguria**
4. Provide a limited, but high-quality, protein diet as prescribed
5. Provide a limited sodium, nitrogen, potassium, and phosphate diet as prescribed
6. Assist the client to cope with body-image disturbances caused by uremic syndrome

VI. HEMODIALYSIS

A. Description
1. The process of cleansing the client's blood
2. Involves the diffusion of dissolved particles from one fluid compartment into another across a semipermeable membrane; the client's blood flows through one fluid compartment, and the dialysate is in another fluid compartment

B. Functions of **hemodialysis**
1. Cleanses the blood of accumulated waste products
2. Removes the by-products of protein metabolism such as urea, creatinine, and uric acid from the blood
3. Removes excess body fluids
4. Maintains or restores the buffer system of the body
5. Maintains or restores electrolyte levels in the body

C. Principles of **hemodialysis**
1. The semipermeable membrane is made of a thin, porous cellophane
2. The pore size of the membrane allows small particles to pass through, such as urea, creatinine, uric acid, and water molecules

3. Proteins, bacteria, and some blood cells are too large to pass through the membrane
4. The client's blood flows into the dialyzer; the movement of substances occurs from the blood to the dialysate
5. Diffusion is the movement of particles from an area of greater concentration to one of lesser concentration
6. Osmosis is the movement of fluids across a semipermeable membrane from an area of lesser concentration of particles to an area of greater concentration
7. Ultrafiltration is the movement of fluid across a semipermeable membrane as a result of an artificially created pressure gradient

D. Dialysate bath
1. Composed of water and major electrolytes
2. Dialysate need not be sterile because bacteria and viruses are too large to pass through the pores of the semipermeable membrane; however, the dialysate must meet specific standards, and water is treated to ensure a safe water supply

E. Interventions
1. Hold antihypertensives and other medications that can affect the blood pressure or result in hypotension until after the dialysis treatment, as prescribed
2. Hold medications that could be removed by dialysis, such as water-soluble vitamins, certain antibiotics, and digoxin (Lanoxin)
3. Monitor vital signs before, during, and after dialysis; the client's temperature may elevate because of slight warming of the blood from the dialysis machine (notify the physician for excessive temperature elevations because this could indicate sepsis; obtain blood cultures as prescribed for excessive temperature elevations)
4. Monitor laboratory values before, during, and after dialysis
5. Assess the client for fluid overload before dialysis and fluid volume deficit after dialysis
6. Weigh the client before and after dialysis to determine fluid loss
7. Assess the patency of the blood access device before, during, and after dialysis
8. Monitor for bleeding; heparin is added to the dialysis bath to prevent clots from forming within the dialyzer or the blood tubing
9. Monitor for hypovolemia and shock during dialysis, which can occur from blood loss or excess fluid and electrolyte removal
10. Provide adequate nutrition; the client may eat before or during dialysis
11. Identify the client's reactions to the treatment and support coping mechanisms; encourage independence and involvement in care

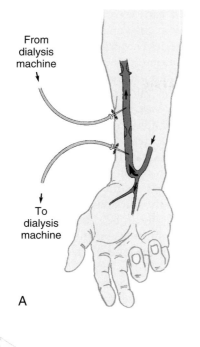

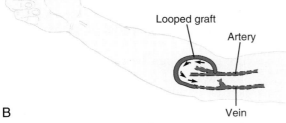

FIG. 52-2 Common means for gaining vascular access for hemodialysis include **A,** arteriovenous fistula and, **B,** arteriovenous graft. (From Monahan, F. Sands, J. Neighbors, M., et al. [2007]. *Phipps' medical-surgical nursing: Health and illness perspectives* [8th ed.]. St. Louis: Mosby.)

VII. ACCESS FOR HEMODIALYSIS

A. Subclavian and femoral catheter (Figure 52-2)
  1. Description
     a. A subclavian (subclavian vein) or femoral (femoral vein) catheter may be inserted for short-term or temporary use in **ARF**
     b. The catheter is used until a fistula or graft matures or develops or may be required when the client's fistula or graft access has failed because of infection or clotting
  2. Interventions
     a. Assess the insertion site for hematoma, bleeding, catheter dislodgement, and infection
     b. These catheters should only be used for dialysis treatments
     c. Maintain an occlusive dressing over the catheter insertion site
  3. Subclavian vein catheter
     a. The catheter is usually filled with heparin and capped to maintain patency between dialysis treatments

  b. The catheter should not be uncapped except for dialysis treatments
  c. The catheter may be left in place for up to 6 weeks if complications do not occur
  4. Femoral vein catheter
     a. The client should not sit up more than 45 degrees or lean forward, or the catheter may kink and occlude
     b. Assess the extremity for circulation, temperature, and pulses
     c. Prevent pulling or disconnecting of the catheter when giving care
     d. Because the groin is not a clean site, meticulous perineal care is required
     e. Use an IV infusion pump or controller with microdrip tubing if a heparin infusion through the catheter to maintain patency is prescribed
B. External arteriovenous shunt (see Figure 52-2)
  1. Description
     a. Two Silastic cannulas are surgically inserted into an artery and a vein in either the forearm or the leg to form an external blood path
     b. The cannulas are connected to form a U shape; blood flows from the client's artery through the shunt into the vein
     c. A tube leading to the membrane compartment of the dialyzer is connected to the arterial cannula
     d. Blood fills the membrane compartment, passes through the dialyzer, and is returned back to the client by way of a tube connected to the venous cannula
     e. When dialysis is complete, the cannulas are clamped and reattached, reforming the U shape
  2. Advantages
     a. The external arteriovenous shunt can be used immediately following its creation
     b. No venipuncture is necessary for dialysis
  3. Disadvantages
     a. Disconnection or dislodgment of the external shunt
     b. Risk of hemorrhage, infection, or clotting
     c. Potential for skin erosion around the catheter site
  4. Interventions
     a. Avoid getting the shunt wet
     b. Wrap a dressing completely around the shunt and keep it dry and intact
     c. Keep cannula clamps at the client's bedside or attached to the arteriovenous dressing for use in the event of accidental disconnection
     d. Teach the client that the shunt extremity should not be used for monitoring BP, drawing blood, placing IV lines, or administering injections

e. Fold back the dressing to expose the shunt tubing and assess for signs of hemorrhage, infection, or clotting

f. Monitor skin integrity around the insertion site

g. Auscultate for a bruit and palpate for a thrill, although a bruit may not be heard with the shunt

h. Notify the physician immediately if signs of clotting, hemorrhage, or infection occur

5. Signs of clotting

a. Fibrin-white flecks noted in the tubing

b. Thrill absent on palpation

c. The absence of a previously heard bruit

d. Coolness of the tubing or extremity

e. Client complaints of a tingling sensation

C. **Internal arteriovenous fistula** (see Figure 52-2)

1. Description

a. The access of choice for the client with **CRF** requiring dialysis

b. The fistula is created surgically by anastomosis of a large artery and a large vein in the arm

c. The flow of arterial blood into the venous system causes the vein to become engorged (matured or developed)

d. Maturity takes about 1 to 2 weeks depending on the client's ability to do hand-flexing exercises such as "ball squeezing," which will help the fistula mature

e. The fistula is required to be mature before it can be used because the engorged vein is punctured with a large-bore needle for the dialysis procedure

f. Subclavian or femoral catheters, **peritoneal dialysis,** or an external arteriovenous shunt can be used for dialysis while the fistula is maturing or developing

2. Advantages

a. Because the fistula is internal, the risk of clotting and bleeding is low

b. The fistula can be used indefinitely

c. Fistulas have a decreased incidence of infection

d. Once healing has occurred, no external dressing is required

e. The fistula allows freedom of movement

3. Disadvantages

a. The fistula cannot be used immediately after insertion

b. Needle insertions through the skin and tissues to the fistula are required for dialysis

c. Infiltration of the needles during dialysis can occur and cause hematomas

d. An aneurysm can form in the fistula

e. **Arterial steal syndrome** can develop (too much blood is diverted to the vein, and arterial perfusion to the hand is compromised)

f. CHF can occur from the increased blood flow in the venous system

D. Internal arteriovenous graft (see Figure 52-2)

1. Description

a. The internal graft is used primarily for chronic dialysis clients who do not have adequate blood vessels for the creation of a fistula

b. An artificial graft made of Gore-Tex or a bovine (cow) carotid artery is used to create an artificial vein for blood flow

c. The procedure involves the anastomosis of the graft to the artery, a tunneling under the skin, and anastomosis to a vein

d. The graft can be used 2 weeks after insertion

e. Complications of the graft include clotting, aneurysms, and infection

2. Advantages

a. Because the graft is internal, the risk of clotting and bleeding is low

b. The graft can be used indefinitely

c. The graft has a decreased incidence of infection

d. Once healing has occurred, no external dressing is required

e. The graft allows freedom of movement

3. Disadvantages

a. The graft cannot be used immediately after insertion

b. Needle insertions through the skin and tissues to the graft are required for dialysis

c. Infiltration of the needles during dialysis can occur and cause hematomas

d. An aneurysm can form in the graft

e. **Arterial steal syndrome** can develop

f. CHF can occur from the increased blood flow in the venous system

E. Interventions for an arteriovenous fistula and arteriovenous graft

1. Teach the client that the shunt extremity should not be used for monitoring blood pressure, drawing blood, placing IV lines, or administering injections

2. Teach the client with an arteriovenous fistula hand-flexing exercises such as "ball squeezing" to promote graft maturity

3. Palpate for a thrill or auscultate for bruit over the fistula or graft

4. Palpate pulses below the fistula or graft, and monitor for hand swelling as an indication of ischemia

5. Note the temperature and capillary refill of the extremity

6. Monitor for clotting

a. Complaints of tingling or discomfort in the extremity

b. Inability to palpate a thrill or auscultate a bruit over the fistula or graft

BOX 52-8 Complications of Hemodialysis

Air embolus	Hepatitis
Disequilibrium syndrome	Hypotension
Electrolyte alterations	Sepsis
Encephalopathy	Shock
Hemorrhage	

7. Monitor for **arterial steal syndrome**
8. Monitor for infection
9. Monitor lung and heart sounds for signs of CHF
10. Notify the physician immediately if signs of clotting, infection, or arterial steal syndrome occur

VIII. **COMPLICATIONS OF HEMODIALYSIS** (Box 52-8)
A. Air embolus
   1. Description
      a. Introduction of air into the circulatory system
      b. Results in cardiopulmonary complications
   2. Data collection
      a. Dyspnea and tachypnea
      b. Chest pain
      c. Hypotension
      d. Reduced oxygen saturation
      e. Cyanosis
      f. Anxiety
      g. Changes in sensorium
   3. Interventions
      a. Stop dialysis
      b. Administer oxygen
      c. Turn the client on the left side, with the head down
      d. Notify the physician (a medical emergency)
B. **Disequilibrium syndrome**
   1. Description
      a. A rapid change in the composition of the extracellular fluid occurs during hemodialysis
      b. Solutes are removed from the blood faster than from the cerebrospinal fluid and brain; fluid is pulled into the brain, causing cerebral edema
   2. Data collection
      a. Nausea and vomiting
      b. Headache
      c. Hypertension
      d. Restlessness and agitation
      e. Muscle cramps
      f. Confusion
      g. Seizures
   3. Interventions
      a. Slow or stop the dialysis
      b. Notify the physician if signs of **disequilibrium syndrome** occur
      c. Reduce environmental stimuli

d. Prepare to administer IV hypertonic saline solution, albumin, or mannitol (Osmitrol) if prescribed
e. Prepare to dialyze the client for a shorter period at reduced flow rates to prevent the occurrence
C. Dialysis encephalopathy
   1. Description: an aluminum toxicity from dialysate water sources containing aluminum or from ingestion of aluminum-containing antacids (phosphate binders)
   2. Data collection
      a. Progressive neurological impairment
      b. Mental cloudiness
      c. Speech disturbances
      d. Dementia
      e. Muscle incoordination
      f. Bone pain
      g. Seizures
   3. Interventions
      a. Monitor for the signs of dialysis encephalopathy and notify the physician signs occur
      b. The administration of aluminum-containing antacids is avoided
      c. Administer aluminum-chelating agents as prescribed so that the aluminum is freed up and dialyzed from the body

IX. **PERITONEAL DIALYSIS**
A. Description
   1. The peritoneum acts as the dialyzing membrane (semipermeable membrane) and substitutes for kidney function during kidney failure
   2. **Peritoneal dialysis (PD)** works on the principles of osmosis, diffusion and ultrafiltration; PD occurs via the transfer of fluid and solute from the bloodstream through the peritoneum
   3. The peritoneal membrane is large and porous, allowing solutes and fluid to move via osmosis from an area of higher concentration in the body to an area of lower concentration in the dialyzing fluid
   4. The peritoneal cavity is rich in capillaries; therefore, it provides a ready access to blood supply
B. Contraindications to **PD**
   1. Peritonitis
   2. Recent abdominal surgery
   3. Abdominal adhesions
   4. Impending renal transplant
C. Access for **PD** (Figure 52-3)
   1. A siliconized rubber catheter such as a Tenckhoff catheter is surgically inserted into the client's peritoneal cavity to allow infusion of dialysis fluid
   2. The preferred insertion site is 3 to 5 cm below the umbilicus; this area is relatively avascular and has less fascial resistance
   3. The catheter is tunneled under the skin, through the fat and muscle tissue to the peritoneum; it is

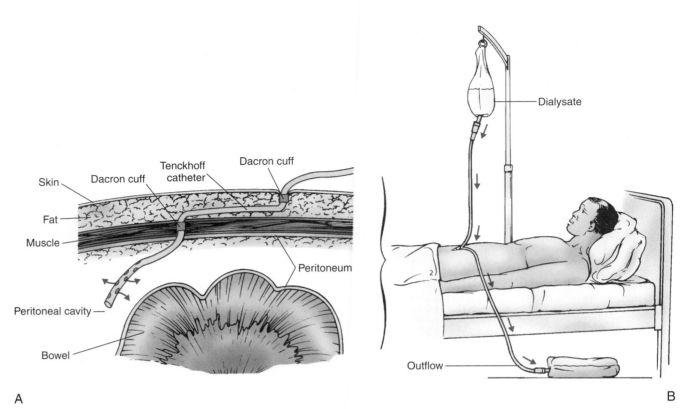

FIG. 52-3 Manual peritoneal dialysis via an implanted abdominal catheter (Tenckhoff catheter). **A,** Implanted abdominal catheter. **B,** Dialysate inflow and outflow through implanted abdominal catheter. (From Ignatavicius, D., & Workman, M. [2006]. *Medical-surgical nursing: Critical thinking for collaborative care* [5th ed.]. Philadelphia: Saunders.)

stabilized with Dacron cuffs in the muscle and under the skin

4. Over a period of 1 to 2 weeks following insertion, fibroblasts and blood vessels grow around the cuffs fixing the catheter in place and providing an extra barrier against dialysate leakage and bacterial invasion

D. Dialysate solution

1. Solution is sterile
2. Solution contains electrolytes and minerals, a specific osmolarity, a specific glucose concentration, and other medication additives as prescribed
3. The higher the glucose concentration, the greater the hypertonicity and the amount of fluid removed during an exchange
4. Increasing the glucose concentration increases the concentration of active particles that cause osmosis, increases the rate of ultrafiltration, and increases the amount of fluid removed
5. If hyperkalemia is not a problem, potassium may be added to each bag of dialysate solution
6. Heparin is added to the dialysate solution to prevent clotting of the catheter
7. Prophylactic antibiotics may be added to the dialysate solution to prevent peritonitis
8. Insulin may be added to the dialysate solution for the client with diabetes mellitus

E. **PD** infusion

1. Description
   a. One infusion (fill), dwell, and drain is considered one exchange
   b. Infection is a concern with **PD**
   c. Fill: the infusion of 1 to 2 L of dialysate as prescribed is infused by gravity into the peritoneal space, which usually takes 10 to 20 minutes
   d. Dwell time: the amount of time that the dialysate solution remains in the peritoneal cavity is prescribed by the physician and can last 20 to 30 minutes to 8 or more hours depending on the type of dialysis used
   e. Drain (outflow): fluid drains out of body by gravity into the drainage bag
2. Interventions before treatment
   a. Monitor vital signs
   b. Obtain weight
   c. Have the client void, if possible
   d. Assess electrolyte and glucose levels
3. Interventions during treatment
   a. Monitor vital signs
   b. Monitor for signs of infection
   c. Monitor for respiratory distress, pain, or discomfort

d. Monitor for signs of pulmonary edema

e. Monitor for hypotension and hypertension

f. Monitor for malaise, nausea, and vomiting

g. Assess the catheter site dressing for wetness or bleeding

h. Monitor dwell time as prescribed by the physician and initiate outflow

i. Do not allow dwell time to extend beyond the physician's order because this increases the risk for hyperglycemia

j. Turn the client from side to side if the outflow is slow to start

k. Monitor outflow, which should be a continuous stream after the clamp is opened

l. Monitor outflow for color and clarity

m. Monitor I&O accurately; if outflow is less than inflow, the difference is equal to the amount absorbed or retained by the client during dialysis and should be counted as intake

F. Types of **PD**

1. Continuous ambulatory **peritoneal dialysis** (CAPD)

   a. Closely resembles renal function because it is a continuous process

   b. Does not require a machine for the procedure

   c. Promotes client independence

   d. The client performs self-dialysis 24 hours a day, 7 days a week

   e. Four dialysis cycles are usually administered in a 24-hour period, including an overnight 8-hour dwell time

   f. Between 1 and 2 L of dialysate are instilled into the abdomen four times daily and allowed to dwell as prescribed

   g. The dialysis bag, attached to the catheter, is folded and carried under the client's clothing until time for outflow

   h. After dwell, the bag is placed lower than the insertion site so that fluid drains by gravity flow

   i. When full, the bag is changed, new dialysate is instilled into the abdomen, and the process continues

2. Automated **PD** (Box 52-9)

   a. Automated dialysis requires a peritoneal cycling machine

   b. Automated dialysis can be done as intermittent **PD,** continuous cycling **PD,** or nightly **PD**

X. COMPLICATIONS OF PERITONEAL DIALYSIS (Box 52-10)

A. Abdominal pain

1. Peritoneal irritation during inflow commonly causes pain during the first few exchanges; the pain usually disappears after 1 to 2 weeks of dialysis treatments

---

BOX 52-9 Types of Automated Peritoneal Dialysis

Continuous Cycling Peritoneal Dialysis

Dialysis requires a peritoneal cycling machine.

Dialysis usually consists of three cycles done at night and one cycle with an 8-hour dwell done in the morning.

The sterile catheter system is opened only for the on-and-off procedures, which reduces the risk of infection.

The client does not need to do exchanges during the day.

Intermittent Peritoneal Dialysis

Dialysis requires a peritoneal cycling machine.

Dialysis is not a continuous procedure.

Dialysis is performed for 10-14 hours, three to four times a week.

Nightly Peritoneal Dialysis

Dialysis is performed 8-12 hours each night with no daytime exchanges or dwells.

BOX 52-10 Complications of Peritoneal Dialysis

Abdominal pain

Bladder or bowel perforation

Insufficient outflow

Leakage around the catheter site

Peritonitis

---

2. Warm the dialysate before administration using a special dialysate warmer pad since the cold temperature of the dialysate can cause discomfort

3. Place a heating pad on the client's abdomen during inflow to relieve discomfort; use a low setting and monitor the client closely

B. Abnormal outflow characteristics indicative of complications

1. Bloody outflow after the first few exchanges indicates vascular complications (the outflow should be clear and colorless after the initial exchanges)

2. Brown outflow indicates bowel perforation

3. Urine-colored outflow indicates bladder perforation

4. Cloudy outflow indicates peritonitis

C. Insufficient outflow

1. The main cause of insufficient outflow is a full colon; encourage a high-fiber diet since constipation can cause inflow and outflow problems and administer stool softeners as prescribed

2. Insufficient outflow may also be caused by catheter migration out of the peritoneal area; if this occurs, notify the physician to reposition the catheter

3. Maintain the drainage bag below the client's abdomen

4. Check for kinks in the tubing
5. Check for fibrin clots in the tubing and milk the tubing to dislodge the clot as prescribed
6. Change the client's outflow position by turning the client to a side-lying position or ambulating the client

D. Leakage around the catheter site
1. Clear fluid that leaks from the catheter exit site will be noted
2. It takes 1 to 2 weeks following insertion of the catheter before fibroblasts and blood vessels grow into the catheter cuffs, fixing it in place and providing an extra barrier against dialysate leakage and bacterial invasion
3. Smaller amounts of dialysate need to be used and it may take up to 2 weeks for the client to tolerate a full 2-L exchange without leaking around the catheter site

E. Peritonitis
1. Monitor for symptoms of peritonitis: fever, cloudy outflow, rebound abdominal tenderness, abdominal pain, general malaise, nausea, and vomiting
2. Cloudy or opaque outflow is an early sign of peritonitis
3. If peritonitis is suspected, obtain a culture of the outflow to determine the infective organism
4. Administer antibiotics as prescribed
5. Avoid infections by maintaining meticulous sterile technique when connecting and disconnecting **PD** solution bags and when caring for the catheter insertion site
6. Prevent the catheter insertion site dressing from becoming wet during care of the client or the dialysis procedure; change the dressing if wet or soiled
7. Follow institutional procedure for connecting and disconnecting **PD** solution bags, which may include scrubbing the connection sites with an antiseptic solution

XI. CONTINUOUS RENAL REPLACEMENT THERAPY (CRRT)
A. Description
1. CRRT provides continuous ultrafiltration of extracellular fluid and clearance of urinary toxins over a period of 8 to 24 hours primarily for clients in **ARF** or critically ill clients with **CRF**
2. Water, electrolytes, and other solutes are removed as the client's blood passes through a hemofilter
3. Because rapid shifts in fluids and electrolytes typically do not occur, hemofiltration is usually well tolerated by critically ill clients.
4. There are five variations of CRRT (Box 52-11), some requiring a **hemodialysis** machine whereas others rely on the client's blood pressure to power the system

---

BOX 52-11 Types of Continuous Renal Replacement Therapy (CRRT)

Continuous venovenous hemofiltration (CVVH)
Continuous arteriovenous hemofiltration (CAVH)
Continuous venovenous hemodialysis (CVVHD)
Continuous arteriovenous hemodialysis (CAVHD)
Slow continuous ultrafiltration (SCUF)

XII. KIDNEY TRANSPLANTATION
A. Description
1. A human kidney from a compatible donor is implanted into a recipient
2. Kidney transplantation is performed for irreversible kidney failure
3. The recipient must take immunosuppressive medications for life
B. Living related donors
1. The most desirable source of kidneys for transplant is living related donors who closely match the client
2. Donors are screened for ABO blood group, tissue-specific antigen, human leukocyte antigen suitability, mixed lymphocyte culture index (histocompatibility), and the presence of any communicable diseases
3. The donor must be in excellent health with two properly functioning kidneys
4. The emotional well-being of the donor is determined
5. Complete understanding on the part of the donor of the donation process and outcome is necessary
C. Cadaver donors
1. Cadaver donors must meet the criteria of brain death
2. Cadaver donors usually need to be under 70 years of age
3. Cadaver donors must have normal renal function
4. No malignant disease outside of the CNS can be present
5. No generalized infection or communicable disease can be present
6. No abdominal or renal trauma can be present
7. The potential donor must be negative for hepatitis B and C antigen and human immunodeficiency virus antibody
8. Once cerebral death has been established for a potential donor, restoration of intravascular volume, weaning from vasopressors, and establishing diuresis are crucial
9. Continuous ventilation, a normal blood pressure, and heart rate are maintained until the kidneys are surgically removed

D. Warm ischemic time
  1. Warm ischemic time is the time elapsed between the cessation of perfusion and cooling of the kidney and the time required for anastomosis of the kidney
  2. Maximal allowable warm ischemic time is 30 to 60 minutes
  3. If the kidney has been cooled, the maximum transplantation time is up to 72 hours
E. Preoperative interventions
  1. Verify histocompatibility tests of identical twin or family member
  2. Administer immunosuppressive medications to the recipient as prescribed for 2 days before the transplantation, if possible
  3. Maintain protective isolation for the recipient
  4. Verify that **hemodialysis** of the recipient was completed 24 hours before the transplant
  5. Ensure that the recipient is free of any infections
  6. Assess renal function studies
  7. Encourage discussion of feelings of the donor and the recipient
  8. Provide psychological support to the live donor or cadaver donor family and the recipient
F. Postoperative interventions for the recipient
  1. Urine output usually begins immediately if the donor was living; it is usually delayed for a few days or more with a cadaver kidney
  2. **Hemodialysis** is performed until adequate kidney function is established
  3. Monitor vital signs, central venous pressure (CVP), and pulse oximetry for signs of complications
  4. Monitor urine output hourly; immediately report a urine output less than 100 mL/hr
  5. Monitor IV fluids closely; for the first 12 to 24 hours, IV fluid volume includes replacement per milliliter of hourly urine output
  6. Administer prescribed diuretics and osmotic agents
  7. Monitor daily weight to evaluate fluid status
  8. Monitor daily laboratory results to evaluate renal function including hematocrit, BUN, serum creatinine levels, and urine for blood and specific gravity
  9. Position the client in the semi-Fowlers position to promote gas exchange, turning from the back to the nonoperative side
  10. Monitor Foley catheter patency; the Foley remains in the bladder for 3 to 5 days to allow for anastomosis healing
  11. Note that urine is pink and bloody initially but gradually returns to normal within several days to weeks
  12. Notify the physician if gross hematuria and clots are noted in the urine

---

BOX 52-12 **Client Instructions Following Kidney Transplant**

Avoid prolonged periods of sitting.
Monitor intake and output.
Recognize the signs and symptoms of infection and rejection.
Use medications as prescribed, and maintain immunosuppressive therapy for life.
Avoid contact sports.
Avoid exposure to persons with infections.
Know the signs and symptoms that require the need to contact the physician.
Ensure follow-up care.

---

  13. Monitor the three-way bladder irrigation, if present, for clots, irrigate only if a physician's order is present
  14. Remove the Foley catheter as soon as possible to prevent infection
  15. Maintain protective isolation precautions, including having the client wear a mask when out of the room, and monitor for infection
  16. Maintain strict aseptic technique with wound care
  17. Monitor for bowel sounds and for the passage of flatus; initiate a diet and oral fluids as prescribed when flatus and bowel sounds return (fluids, sodium, and potassium are usually restricted if the client is oliguric)
  18. Maintain good oral hygiene, monitoring for stomatitis and bacterial and fungal infections
  19. Encourage coughing and deep-breathing exercises
  20. Administer medications as prescribed, which may include antifungal medications, antibiotics, immunosuppressive agents, and corticosteroids
  21. The client is usually ambulated after 24 hours; avoid the sitting position
  22. Assess for organ rejection
  23. Promote live donor and recipient relationship
  24. Monitor both the donor and recipient for depression
  25. Provide the recipient with instructions following the kidney transplant (Box 52-12)
  26. Assist the recipient to cope with the body-image disturbances that occur from long-term use of immunosuppressants
  27. Advise the recipient of available support groups
G. Graft rejection: Except for identical twin donor and recipient, the major postoperative complication is graft rejection
  1. Data collection (Box 52-13)
  2. Hyperacute rejection
    a. Hyperacute rejection occurs immediately after surgery to 48 hours postoperatively
    b. Interventions: removal of rejected kidney

Clinical Signs of Renal Transplant (Graft) Rejection

Fever greater than 100° F (37.7° C)
Pain or tenderness over the grafted kidney
A 2- to 3-lb weight gain in 24 hr
Edema
Hypertension
Malaise
Signs of deteriorating renal function
Elevated BUN and serum creatinine
Decreased creatinine clearance
Elevated white blood cell count
Rejection indicated by ultrasound or biopsy

Causes of Cystitis

Allergens or irritants, such as soaps, sprays, bubble bath, and perfumed sanitary napkins
Bladder distention
Calculus
Hormonal changes, influencing alterations in vaginal flora
Indwelling urethral catheters
Invasive urinary tract procedures
Loss of bactericidal properties of prostatic secretions in the male
Microorganisms
Poor-fitting vaginal diaphragms
Sexual intercourse
Synthetic underwear and pantyhose
Urinary stasis
Use of spermicides
Wet bathing suits

3. Acute rejection
   a. Most common type; occurs within 6 weeks postoperatively but can occur as late as 2 years
   b. Interventions: is potentially reversible with an increase in immunosuppression, or administering high doses of corticosteroids or monoclonal antibodies if corticosteroids are ineffective
4. Chronic rejection
   a. Occurs slowly months to years after transplant and mimics **CRF**
   b. Interventions immunosuppressive medications

XIII. CYSTITIS/URINARY TRACT INFECTIONS (UTI)

A. Description
   1. An inflammation of the bladder from an infection, obstruction of the urethra, or other irritants (Box 52-14)
   2. The most common causative organisms are *Escherichia coli, Enterobacter, Pseudomonas,* and *Serratia*
   3. Cystitis is more common in women because women have a shorter urethra than men and the location of the urethra in the woman is close to the rectum
   4. Sexually active and pregnant women are most vulnerable to cystitis
B. Data collection
   1. Frequency and urgency
   2. Burning on urination
   3. Voiding in small amounts
   4. Inability to void
   5. Incomplete emptying of the bladder
   6. Lower abdominal discomfort or back discomfort
   7. Cloudy, dark, foul-smelling urine
   8. Hematuria
   9. Bladder spasms
   10. Malaise, chills, and fever
   11. Nausea and vomiting

   12. Altered mentation in older adults; frequency and urgency may not be specific symptoms of UTI in older adults because of urinary elimination changes that occur with aging
C. Interventions
   1. Before administering prescribed antibiotics, obtain a urine specimen for culture and sensitivity, if prescribed, to identify bacterial growth ▲
   2. Encourage the client to increase fluids up to 3000 mL/day, especially if the client is taking a sulfonamide; sulfonamides can form crystals in concentrated urine ▲
   3. Administer prescribed medications, which may include analgesics, antiseptics, antispasmodics, antibiotics, and antimicrobials
   4. Maintain an acid urine pH (5.5); instruct the client about foods to consume to maintain acidic urine
   5. Provide heat to the abdomen or sitz baths for complaints of discomfort
   6. Note that if the client is prescribed an aminoglycoside, a sulfonamide, or nitrofurantoin (Macrodantin), the actions of these medications are diminished by acidic urine ▲
   7. Use strict aseptic technique when inserting a urinary catheter ▲
   8. Maintain closed urinary drainage systems for the client with an indwelling catheter and avoid elevating the urinary drainage bag above the level of the bladder ▲
   9. Provide meticulous perineal care for the client with an indwelling catheter ▲
   10. Discourage caffeine products such as coffee, tea, and cola
   11. Client education
       a. Avoid alcohol
       b. Take medications as prescribed

Teaching for Prevention of Cystitis

Use good perineal care, wiping front to back.
Avoid bubble baths, tub baths, and vaginal deodorants or sprays.
Void every 2-3 hours.
Wear cotton pants and avoid wearing tight clothes or pantyhose with slacks.
Avoid sitting in a wet bathing suit for prolonged periods.
If pregnant, void every 2 hours.
If menopausal, use estrogen vaginal creams to restore pH.
Use water-soluble lubricants for intercourse, especially after menopause.
Void and drink a glass of water after intercourse.

  c. Take antibiotics on schedule and complete the entire course of medications as prescribed, which may be 10 to 14 days
  d. Repeat the urine culture following treatment
  e. Prevent recurrence of cystitis (Box 52-15)

XIV. **UROSEPSIS**
A. Description
   1. Urosepsis is a gram-negative bacteremia originating in the urinary tract
   2. The most common responsible organism is *E. coli*
   3. The most common cause is infection from an indwelling urinary catheter or an untreated UTI in a client who is immunocompromised
   4. The major problem is the ability of this bacterium to develop resistant strains
   5. Urosepsis can lead to septic shock if not treated aggressively
B. Data collection: Fever is the most common and earliest manifestation
C. Interventions
   1. Obtain a urine specimen for urine culture and sensitivity before administering antibiotics
   2. Administer IV antibiotics as prescribed, usually until the client has been afebrile for 3 to 5 days
   3. Administer oral antibiotics as prescribed after the 3- to 5-day afebrile period

XV. **URETHRITIS**
A. Description
   1. An inflammation of the urethra commonly associated with sexually transmitted infections and may occur with cystitis
   2. In men, urethritis most often is caused by gonorrhea or chlamydial infection
   3. In women, urethritis is most often caused by feminine hygiene sprays, perfumed toilet paper or sanitary napkins, spermicidal jelly, UTIs, or changes in the vaginal mucosal lining

B. Data collection
   1. Pain or burning on urination
   2. Frequency and urgency
   3. Nocturia
   4. Difficulty voiding
   5. Males may have clear to mucopurulent discharge from the penis
   6. Females may have lower abdominal discomfort
C. Interventions
   1. Encourage fluid intake
   2. Prepare the client for testing to determine if a sexually transmitted infection (STI) is present
   3. Administer antibiotics as prescribed
   4. Instruct the client in the administration of sitz or tub baths
   5. If stricture occurs, prepare the client for dilation of the urethra and instillation of an antiseptic solution
   6. Instruct the female client to avoid the use of perfumed toilet paper or sanitary napkins and feminine hygiene sprays
   7. Instruct the client to avoid intercourse until the symptoms subside or treatment of the STI is complete
   8. Instruct the client on STIs if this is the cause
      a. Prevent STIs by the use of latex condoms or abstinence
      b. All sexual partners during the 30 days before diagnosis with chlamydial infection should be notified, examined, and treated if indicated
      c. Chlamydial infection often coexists with gonorrhea; diagnostic testing is done for both STIs
      d. Treatment for STIs includes antibiotics, as prescribed, to treat the causative organism
      e. The most serious complication of chlamydial infection is sterility
      f. Follow-up culture may be requested in 4 to 7 days to evaluate the effectiveness of medications

XVI. **URETERITIS**
A. Ureteritis
   1. Description: an inflammation of the ureter commonly associated with bacterial or viral infections and pyelonephritis
   2. Data collection
      a. Dysuria
      b. Frequent urination
      c. Clear to mucopurulent penile discharge in males
   3. Interventions
      a. Treatment includes identifying and treating the underlying cause and providing symptomatic relief

b. Administer metronidazole (Flagyl) or clotrimazole (Mycelex) as prescribed for treating trichomonas

c. Administer nystatin (Mycostatin) or fluconazole (Diflucan) as prescribed for treating monilial infections

d. Doxycycline (Vibramycin) or azithromycin (Zithromax) may be prescribed for treating chlamydial infections

XVII. PYELONEPHRITIS

A. Description

1. An inflammation of the renal pelvis and the parenchyma commonly caused by bacterial invasion

2. Acute pyelonephritis often occurs after bacterial contamination of the urethra or following an invasive procedure of the urinary tract

3. Chronic pyelonephritis most commonly occurs following chronic urinary flow obstruction with reflux

4. *E. coli* is the most common bacterial causative organism

B. Acute pyelonephritis

1. Acute pyelonephritis occurs as a new infection or recurs as a relapse of a previous infection

2. It can progress to bacteremia or chronic pyelonephritis

3. Data collection
   a. Fever and chills
   b. Nausea
   c. Flank pain on the affected side
   d. Costovertebral angle tenderness
   e. Headache
   f. Dysuria
   g. Frequency and urgency
   h. Cloudy, bloody, or foul-smelling urine
   i. Increased white blood cells in the urine

C. Chronic pyelonephritis

1. A slow, progressive disease usually associated with recurrent acute attacks

2. Causes contraction of the kidney and dysfunctioning of the nephrons, which are replaced by scar tissue

3. Causes the ureter to become fibrotic and narrowed by strictures

4. Can lead to **renal failure**

5. Data collection
   a. Frequently diagnosed incidentally when a client is being evaluated for hypertension
   b. Poor urine-concentrating ability
   c. Pyuria
   d. **Azotemia**
   e. Proteinuria

D. Interventions

1. Monitor vital signs, especially for elevated temperature

2. Encourage fluid intake up to 3000 mL/day to reduce fever and prevent dehydration

3. Monitor I&O (ensure that output is a minimum of 1500 mL/24 hr)

4. Monitor weight

5. Encourage adequate rest

6. Instruct the client in a high-calorie, low-protein diet

7. Provide warm, moist compresses to the flank area to help relieve pain

8. Encourage the client to take warm baths for pain relief

9. Administer analgesics, antipyretics, antibiotics, urinary antiseptics, and antiemetics as prescribed

10. Monitor for signs of **renal failure**

11. Encourage follow-up urine culture

XVIII. GLOMERULONEPHRITIS (Refer to Chapter 34 for information on this disorder)

XIX. NEPHROTIC SYNDROME (Refer to Chapter 34 for information on this disorder)

XX. POLYCYSTIC KIDNEY DISEASE

A. Description

1. A cystic formation and hypertrophy of the kidneys, which leads to cystic rupture, infection, formation of scar tissue, and damaged nephrons

2. There is no specific treatment to arrest the progress of the destructive cysts

3. The ultimate result of this disease is **renal failure**

B. Types

1. Infantile polycystic disease: an inherited autosomal recessive trait that results in the death of the infant within a few months after birth

2. Adult polycystic disease: an autosomal dominant trait that manifests between 30 and 40 years of age and results in end-stage renal disease

C. Data collection

1. Often asymptomatic before the ages of 30 to 40 years

2. Flank, lumbar, or abdominal pain that worsens with activity and is relieved when lying

3. Fever and chills

4. UTIs

5. Hematuria, proteinuria, and pyuria

6. Calculi

7. Hypertension

8. Palpable abdominal masses and enlarged kidneys

D. Interventions

1. Monitor for gross hematuria, which indicates cyst rupture

2. Increase sodium and water intake because sodium loss rather than retention occurs

3. Provide bedrest if ruptured cysts and bleeding occur
4. Prepare the client for percutaneous cyst puncture for relief of obstruction or for draining an abscess
5. Administer antihypertensives as prescribed
6. Prevent and/or treat urinary tract infections
7. Prepare the client for dialysis or renal transplantation
8. Encourage the client to seek genetic counseling
9. Provide psychological support to the client and family

XXI. **HYDRONEPHROSIS** (Figure. 52-4)
A. Description
  1. The distention of the renal pelvis and calices caused by an obstruction of normal urine flow
  2. The urine becomes trapped proximal to the obstruction
  3. The causes include calculus, tumors, scar tissue, ureter obstructions, and hypertrophy of the prostate
B. Data collection
  1. Hypertension
  2. Headache
  3. Colicky or dull flank pain that radiates to the groin
C. Interventions
  1. Monitor vital signs frequently
  2. Monitor for fluid and electrolyte imbalances, including dehydration after the obstruction is relieved
  3. Monitor for diuresis, which can lead to fluid depletion
  4. Monitor weight daily
  5. Monitor urine for specific gravity, albumin, and glucose
  6. Administer fluid replacement as prescribed
  7. Prepare the client for insertion of a nephrostomy tube or a surgical procedure to relieve the obstruction if prescribed

XXII. **RENAL CALCULI**
A. Description
  1. Calculi are stones that can form anywhere in the urinary tract; however, the most frequent site is the kidneys
  2. Problems resulting from calculi are pain, obstruction, tissue trauma, secondary hemorrhage, and infection
  3. Stone location can be determined through a kidneys, ureters, and bladder film; intravenous pyelogram; computed tomography scan; and renal ultrasonography
  4. A stone analysis will be performed after passage to determine the type of stone and assist in determining treatment
  5. **Urolithiasis** refers to the formation of urinary calculi; these form in the ureters

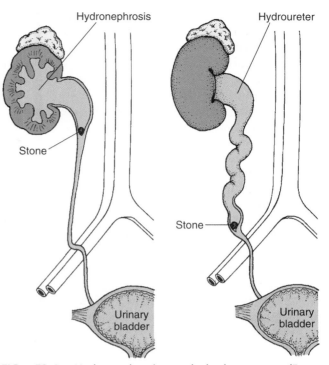

FIG. 52-4 Hydronephrosis and hydroureter. (From Ignatavicius, D., & Workman, M. [2006]. *Medical-surgical nursing: Critical thinking for collaborative care* [5th ed.]. Philadelphia: Saunders.)

  6. **Nephrolithiasis** refers to the formation of kidney calculi; these form in the renal parenchyma
  7. When a calculus occludes the ureter and blocks the flow of urine, the ureter dilates, producing hydroureter (see Figure 52-4)
  8. If the obstruction is not removed, urinary stasis results in infection, impairment of renal function on the side of the blockage, hydronephrosis (see Figure 52-4), and irreversible kidney damage
B. Causes
  1. Family history of stone formation
  2. Diet high in calcium, vitamin D, milk, protein, oxalate, purines, or alkali
  3. Obstruction and urinary stasis
  4. Dehydration
  5. Use of diuretics, which can cause volume depletion
  6. UTIs and prolonged urinary catheterization
  7. Immobilization
  8. Hypercalcemia and hyperparathyroidism
  9. Elevated uric acid level, such as in gout
C. Data collection
  1. Renal colic, which originates in the lumbar region and radiates around the side and down toward the testicle in men and to the bladder in women

2. Ureteral colic, which radiates toward the genitalia and thigh
3. Sudden onset of sharp, severe pain
4. Dull, aching pain in the kidney
5. Nausea and vomiting, pallor, and diaphoresis during acute pain
6. Urinary frequency with alternating retention
7. Signs of a UTI
8. Low-grade fever
9. High numbers of red blood cells, white blood cells, and bacteria in the urinalysis
10. Hematuria

D. Interventions
1. Monitor vital signs, especially the temperature, for signs of infection
2. Monitor I&O
3. Assess for fever, chills, and infection
4. Monitor for nausea, vomiting, and diarrhea
5. Encourage fluid intake up to 3000 mL/day, unless contraindicated, to facilitate the passage of the stone and prevent infection
6. Administer fluids intravenously as prescribed if unable to take fluids orally or in adequate amounts to increase the flow of urine and facilitate the passage of the stone
7. Strain all urine for the presence of stones
8. Send stones to the laboratory for analysis
9. Provide warm baths and heat to the flank area
10. Administer analgesics at regularly scheduled intervals as prescribed to relieve pain
11. Assess the client's response to pain medication
12. Assist the client in performing relaxation techniques to assist in relieving pain
13. Encourage client ambulation if stable to promote the passage of the stone
14. Turn and reposition the immobilized client to promote the passage of the stone
15. Instruct the client in the diet specific to the stone composition if prescribed
16. Prepare the client for surgical procedures if prescribed

E. Stone composition
1. A special diet, such as an alkaline ash or acid ash, may be prescribed, depending on the physician's preference (Boxes 52-16 and 52-17)
2. Calcium phosphate stones
   a. Caused by supersaturation of urine with calcium and phosphate
   b. Diet includes acid-ash foods because calcium stones have an alkaline chemistry
   c. Dietary prescription may include decreasing intake of foods high in calcium and phosphate to reduce urinary calcium content and avoiding excess vitamin D intake to prevent stones from forming

BOX 52-16 Alkaline-Ash Diet

Outcome
Diet increases the pH of the urine.
Diet reduces the acidity of the urine.
Foods To Include
Fruits, except cranberries, plums, and prunes
Milk
Most vegetables
Rhubarb
Small amounts of beef, halibut, veal, trout, and salmon

BOX 52-17 Acid-Ash Diet

Outcome
Diet decreases the pH of the urine.
Diet makes the urine more acidic.
Foods To Include
Bread, cereal, and whole grains
Cheese and eggs
Corn and legumes
Cranberries, prunes, plums, and tomatoes
Meat, fish, oysters, and poultry
Pastries

   d. Medications prescribed for calcium stones may include phosphates, thiazide diuretics, and allopurinol (Zyloprim)
3. Calcium oxalate stones
   a. Caused by supersaturation of urine with calcium and oxalate
   b. Diet includes acid-ash foods because calcium stones have an alkaline chemistry
   c. Dietary prescription may include decreasing the intake of foods high in calcium and avoiding oxalate food sources to reduce urinary oxalate content and stone formation
   d. Oxalate-rich food sources include tea, almonds, cashews, chocolate, cocoa, beans, spinach, and rhubarb
   e. Allopurinol (Zyloprim), pyridoxine (vitamin B_6), or magnesium oxide may be prescribed for clients with oxalate stones
4. Struvite stones
   a. Also called triple phosphate stones; composed of magnesium and ammonium phosphate
   b. Caused by urea-splitting bacteria and tend to form in alkaline urine
   c. Diet includes acid-ash foods and includes limiting high-phosphate foods such as dairy products, red and organ meats, and whole grains to reduce urinary phosphate content

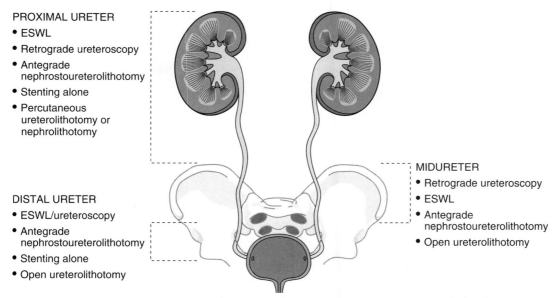

PROXIMAL URETER
- ESWL
- Retrograde ureteroscopy
- Antegrade nephrostoureterolithotomy
- Stenting alone
- Percutaneous ureterolithotomy or nephrolithotomy

DISTAL URETER
- ESWL/ureteroscopy
- Antegrade nephrostoureterolithotomy
- Stenting alone
- Open ureterolithotomy

MIDURETER
- Retrograde ureteroscopy
- ESWL
- Antegrade nephrostoureterolithotomy
- Open ureterolithotomy

FIG. 52-5 Treatment options for ureteral stones. *ESWL,* Extracorporeal shockwave lithotripsy. (From Ignatavicius, D., & Workman, M. [2006]. *Medical-surgical nursing: Critical thinking for collaborative care* [5th ed.]. Philadelphia: Saunders. Modified from Singal, R.K., & Denstedt, J.D. [1997]. Contemporary management of ureteral stones. *Urologic Clinics of North America 24*[1], 59-70.)

d. Treatment includes controlling infection with antibiotics (long-term antibiotic use may be prescribed)

5. Uric acid stones
   a. Caused by excess dietary purine or from gout
   b. Tend to form in acidic urine
   c. Dietary prescription to reduce urinary purine content may include alkaline-ash foods and decreased intake of high purine foods such as organ meats, gravies, red wines, and sardines
   d. Allopurinol (Zyloprim) may be prescribed to lower uric acid levels

6. Cystine stones
   a. Caused by cystine crystal formation and tend to form in acidic urine
   b. Diet includes alkaline-ash foods, and dietary prescription may also include a low intake of methionine, an essential amino acid that forms cystine; the client would be instructed to avoid meat, milk, cheese, and eggs
   c. Dietary measures also focus on encouraging fluid intake up to 3 L/day, unless contraindicated, to help dilute the urine and prevent cystine crystals from forming
   d. Long-term antibiotic use may be prescribed for clients with cystine stones

XXIII. TREATMENT OPTIONS FOR RENAL CALCULI (Figure 52-5)

A. Cystoscopy
   1. Cystoscopy may be done for stones located in the bladder or lower ureter
   2. No incision is made
   3. One or two ureteral catheters are inserted past the stone; the stone may be manipulated and dislodged by the procedure and the catheters may guide the stones mechanically downward as they are removed
   4. The catheters are left in place for 24 hours to drain the urine trapped proximal to the stone and to dilate the ureter
   5. A continuous chemical irrigation may be prescribed to dissolve the stone

B. Extracorporeal shock wave lithotripsy (ESWL)
   1. A noninvasive mechanical procedure for breaking up stones located in the kidney or upper ureter so that they can pass spontaneously or be removed by other methods
   2. No incision is made and no drains are placed; a stent may be placed to promote passing stone fragments
   3. Fluoroscopy is used to visualize the stone, and ultrasonic waves are delivered to the areas of the stone to disintegrate it
   4. The stones are passed in the urine within a few days
   5. Preprocedure: Maintain the client on an NPO status for 8 hours before the procedure
   6. Postprocedure
      a. Monitor vital signs especially for hypotension and tachycardia, which could indicate bleeding
      b. Monitor I&O

c. Monitor for bleeding; hematuria is common after lithotripsy

d. Monitor for pain and signs of urinary obstruction

e. Instruct the client that the ureteral stent placed to promote passage of the stone is usually removed in 1 to 2 weeks

f. Instruct the client to increase fluid intake to flush out the stone fragments

g. Inform the client that ambulation is important

C. Percutaneous lithotripsy

1. Performed for stones in the bladder, ureter, or kidney

2. An invasive procedure in which a guide is inserted under fluoroscopy near the area of the stone; an ultrasonic wave is aimed at the stone to break it into fragments

3. Percutaneous lithotripsy may be performed via cystoscopy or nephroscopy

4. No incision is required for cystoscopy; a small flank incision is needed for nephroscopy

5. The client may possibly have bladder indwelling catheter

6. A nephrostomy tube may be placed to administer chemical irrigations to break up the stone; the nephrostomy tube may remain in place for 1 to 5 days

7. Encourage the client to drink 3000 to 4000 mL of fluid/day after the procedure

8. Monitor for and instruct the client to monitor for complications of infection, hemorrhage, and extravasation of fluid into the retroperitoneal cavity

D. Ureterolithotomy

1. An open surgical procedure is performed if lithotripsy is not effective for removal of a stone in the ureter

2. An incision is made through the lower abdomen or flank and then into the ureter to remove the stone

3. The client may have a Penrose drain, a ureteral stent catheter, and an indwelling bladder catheter

E. Pyelolithotomy and nephrolithotomy

1. Pyelolithotomy is an incision into the renal pelvis to remove a stone; a large flank incision is required and the client may have a Penrose drain and an indwelling bladder catheter

2. Nephrolithotomy is an incision into the kidney made to remove a stone; a large flank incision is required and the client may have a nephrostomy tube and an indwelling bladder catheter

F. Partial or total nephrectomy

1. Performed for extensive kidney damage, renal infection, severe obstruction from stones or tumors, and the prevention of stone recurrence

2. Postoperative interventions

a. The plan of care depends on the incision location and the type of drainage tubes present

b. Monitor the incision, particularly if a Penrose drain is in place, because it will drain large amounts of urine

c. Protect the skin from urinary drainage, changing dressings frequently if necessary

d. Place an ostomy pouch over the Penrose drain to protect the skin if urinary drainage is excessive

e. Monitor the nephrostomy tube, which may be attached to a drainage bag, for a continuous flow of urine

f. Do not irrigate the nephrotomy tube or bladder catheter unless specifically prescribed

g. Monitor the indwelling bladder (Foley) catheter for drainage

h. Encourage fluid intake to ensure a urine output of 2500 to 3000 mL or more/day

i. Measure I&O accurately

j. If a stone was removed, determine its composition from laboratory analysis

XXIV. KIDNEY TUMORS

A. Description

1. Kidney tumors may be benign or malignant, bilateral or unilateral

2. Common sites of metastasis include bone, lungs, liver, spleen, or other kidney

3. The exact cause of renal carcinoma is unknown

B. Data collection for those with advanced disease

1. Dull flank pain

2. Palpable renal mass

3. Painless gross hematuria

C. Radical nephrectomy

1. Description

a. The surgical removal of the entire kidney, adjacent adrenal gland, and renal artery and vein

b. Radiation therapy and possibly chemotherapy may follow radical nephrectomy

c. Before surgery, radiation may be used to embolize (occlude) the arteries supplying the kidney to reduce bleeding during nephrectomy

2. Postoperative interventions

a. Monitor vital signs for signs of bleeding (hypotension and tachycardia)

b. Monitor for abdominal distention, decreases in urinary output, and alterations in level of consciousness as additional signs indicative of bleeding; check the client's bed linens for bleeding

c. Monitor for signs of adrenal insufficiency, which include a large urinary output followed by hypotension and subsequent **oliguria**

d. Administer fluids and packed red blood cells intravenously as prescribed

e. Monitor I&O and daily weight

f. Monitor for a urinary output of 30 to 50 mL/hour to ensure adequate renal function

g. Monitor urine specific gravity

h. Maintain a semi-Fowler's position

i. Monitor for signs of respiratory complications related to surgery; encourage coughing and deep-breathing exercises

j. Monitor for passing of flatus and bowel sounds (lack of flatus and bowel sounds can indicate paralytic ileus)

k. Apply antiembolism stockings as prescribed

l. If a nephrostomy tube is in place, do not irrigate (unless specifically prescribed) or manipulate the tube

m. Administer pain medications as prescribed

XXV. EPIDIDYMITIS

A. Description

1. An acute or chronic inflammation of the epididymis that occurs as a result of a UTI, STI, or prostatitis, or from long-term use of a Foley catheter

2. The infective organism travels upward through the urethra and ejaculatory duct, and along the vas deferens to the epididymis

B. Data collection

1. Scrotal pain

2. Groin pain

3. Swelling in the scrotum and groin

4. Pus and bacteria in the urine

5. Fever and chills

6. Abscess development

C. Interventions

1. Encourage fluid intake

2. Encourage bedrest with the scrotum elevated to prevent traction on the spermatic cord, to facilitate drainage, and to relieve pain

3. Instruct the client in the intermittent application of cold compresses to the scrotum

4. Instruct the client in the use of tub or sitz baths

5. Instruct the client in the administration of antibiotics for self and sexual partner if the cause is chlamydial or gonorrheal infection

6. Instruct the client to avoid lifting and straining and sexual contact until the infection subsides

7. Instruct the client to limit the force of the stream because organisms can be forced into the vas deferens and epididymis from strain or pressure during voiding

8. Teach the client that condom use can help prevent urethritis and epididymitis

9. Teach the client measures to prevent UTI or STI recurrence

XXVI. PROSTATITIS

A. Description

1. An inflammation of the prostate gland commonly caused by an infectious agent (bacterial) or by tissue hyperplasia (abacterial)

2. Bacterial type occurs as a result of the organism reaching the prostate via the urethra, bladder, bloodstream, or lymphatic channels

3. Abacterial type usually occurs following a viral illness or a decrease in sexual activity

B. Data collection

1. Bacterial prostatitis

a. Fever and chills

b. Dysuria

c. Urethral discharge

d. Prostate is tender, indurated, and warm to touch

e. Urethral discharge on palpation of prostate

f. White blood cells found in prostatic secretions

2. Abacterial prostatitis

a. Backache

b. Dysuria

c. Perineal pain

d. Frequency

e. Hematuria

f. Irregularly enlarged, firm, and tender prostate

C. Interventions

1. Encourage adequate fluid intake

2. Instruct the client in the use of tub or sitz baths to promote comfort

3. Administer antibiotics, analgesics, antispasmodics, and stool softeners as prescribed

4. Inform the client of activities to drain the prostate, such as intercourse, masturbation, and prostatic massage

5. Instruct the client to avoid spicy foods, coffee, alcohol, prolonged automobile rides, and sexual intercourse during an acute inflammation

XXVII. BENIGN PROSTATIC HYPERTROPHY OR HYPERPLASIA (BPH)

A. Description

1. A slow enlargement of the prostate gland, with hypertrophy and hyperplasia of normal tissue

2. Enlargement compresses the urethra, resulting in partial or complete obstruction

3. Usually occurs in men older than 50 years

4. Possible causes include stimulation from excessive dihydroxytestosterone, estrogen, or local growth hormone

B. Data collection

1. Diminished size and force of urinary stream (early sign of BPH)

2. Urinary urgency and frequency

3. Nocturia

4. Inability to start (hesitancy) or continue a urinary stream
5. Feelings of incomplete bladder emptying
6. Postvoid dribbling from overflow incontinence (later sign)
7. Urinary retention and bladder distention
8. Hematuria
9. Urinary stasis
10. Dysuria and bladder pain
11. UTIs

C. Interventions
1. Encourage fluid intake of up to 2000 to 3000 mL/day unless contraindicated
2. Prepare for urinary catheterization to drain the bladder and prevent distention
3. Avoid administering medications that cause urinary retention, such as anticholinergics, antihistamines, decongestants, and antidepressants
4. Administer medications as prescribed to shrink the prostate gland and improve urine flow
5. Administer medications as prescribed to relax prostatic smooth muscle and improve urine flow
6. Instruct the client to decrease intake of caffeine and artificial sweeteners and limit spicy or acidic foods
7. Instruct the client to follow a timed voiding schedule
8. Prepare the client for surgery or invasive procedures as prescribed (Box 52-18)

D. Surgical interventions and postoperative care (refer to Chapter 42)

XXVIII. BLADDER CANCER (Refer to Chapter 42)

XXIX. BLADDER TRAUMA

A. Description
1. Occurs following a blunt or penetrating injury to the lower abdomen
2. Penetrating wounds occur as a result of a stabbing, gunshot wound, or other objects piercing the abdominal wall
3. A fractured pelvis that causes bone fragments to puncture the bladder is a common cause of bladder trauma
4. Blunt trauma causes compression of the abdominal wall and the bladder

B. Data collection
1. **Anuria**
2. Hematuria
3. Pain below the level of the umbilicus; can radiate to the shoulders
4. Nausea and vomiting

C. Interventions
1. Monitor vital signs
2. Monitor for hematuria, bleeding, and signs of shock
3. Promote bedrest
4. Monitor pain level

BOX 52-18 | **Surgical and Invasive Procedures for Prostatic Hyperplasia**

Transurethral resection of the prostate (TURP): Removal of benign prostatic tissue surrounding the urethra with use of a resectoscope introduced through the urethra; there is little risk of impotence and is most commonly used for benign prostatic hypertrophy (BPH)

Transurethral incision of the prostate (TUIP): Removal of prostatic tissue through an incision made in the bladder neck

Transurethral microwave thermotherapy: Application of heat to destroy the hypertrophied tissue

Transurethral needle ablation of the prostate (TUNA): Placement of interstitial radiofrequency needles through the urethra and into the lateral lobes of the prostate, causing heat-induced coagulation necrosis of the prostate for treating BPH

Laser prostatectomy: Ablation of the enlarged prostate using laser instead of radiofrequency waves

Transurethral electrovaporization of the prostate: Placement of a special metal instrument that emits a high-frequency electrical current that cuts and vaporizes excess tissue and seals the remaining tissue to prevent bleeding; especially useful for men on anticoagulants and those at risk for complications

Perineal prostatectomy: Removal of prostatic tissue (may be performed for prostatic cancer) low in the pelvic region through an incision between the scrotum and rectum; impotence and incontinence usually result

Retropubic prostatectomy: Removal of hypertrophied prostatic tissue high in the pelvic region through a low abdominal incision; the bladder is not incised

Suprapubic prostatectomy: Removal of prostatic tissue mass through a low midline incision; an incision into the bladder and urethral mucosa to the anterior aspect of the prostate is made

Urethral stents: Application of stents or coils in the urethra where it is narrowed by the prostate

---

5. If blood is seen at the meatus, avoid urinary catheterization until a retrograde urethrogram can be performed
6. Prepare the client for insertion of a suprapubic catheter to aid in urinary drainage if prescribed
7. Prepare the client for surgical repair of the laceration if prescribed

PRACTICE QUESTIONS

🔘 More questions on the companion CD!

668. A nurse is caring for the client with epididymitis. The nurse would avoid using which of the following treatment modalities in the care of the client?
   1. Bedrest
   2. Sitz bath

3. Heating pad
4. Scrotal elevation

669. A client has epididymitis as a complication of urinary tract infection (UTI). The nurse is giving the client instructions to prevent a recurrence. The nurse determines that the client needs further instruction if the client states the intention to:
1. Drink increased amounts of fluids.
2. Limit the force of the stream during voiding.
3. Continue to take antibiotics until all symptoms are gone.
4. Use condoms to eliminate risk from chlamydia and gonorrhea.

670. A nurse is collecting data from a client who has had benign prostatic hyperplasia (BPH) in the past. To determine if the client is currently experiencing exacerbation of BPH, the nurse asks the client about the presence of which early symptom?
1. Nocturia
2. Urinary retention
3. Urge incontinence
4. Decreased force in the stream of urine

671. A client newly diagnosed with chronic renal failure has recently begun hemodialysis. Knowing that the client is at risk for disequilibrium syndrome, the nurse monitors the client during dialysis for:
1. Hypertension, tachycardia, and fever
2. Hypotension, bradycardia, and hypothermia
3. Restlessness, irritability, and generalized weakness
4. Headache, deteriorating level of consciousness, and twitching

672. A client with chronic renal failure has been on dialysis for 3 years. The client is receiving the usual combination of medications for the disease, including aluminum hydroxide as a phosphate-binding agent. The client now has mental cloudiness, dementia, and complaints of bone pain. The nurse interprets that these data are compatible with:
1. Advancing uremia
2. Phosphate overdose
3. Folic acid deficiency
4. Aluminum intoxication

673. A hemodialysis client with a left arm fistula is at risk for arterial steal syndrome. The nurse monitors this client for which manifestation of this disorder?
1. Warmth, redness, and pain in the left hand
2. Aching pain, pallor, and edema of the left arm
3. Edema and purplish discoloration of the left arm
4. Pallor, diminished pulse, and pain in the left hand

674. A nurse is reviewing the medical record of a client with a diagnosis of pyelonephritis.

Which disorder, if noted on the client's record, would the nurse identify as a risk factor for this disorder?
1. Hypoglycemia
2. Diabetes mellitus
3. Coronary artery disease
4. Orthostatic hypotension

675. A nurse is reviewing the client's record and notes that the physician has documented that the client has a renal disorder. On review of the laboratory results, the nurse would most likely expect to note which of the following?
1. Decreased hemoglobin level
2. Decreased red blood cell (RBC) count
3. Decreased white blood cell (WBC) count
4. Elevated blood urea nitrogen (BUN) level

676. A client is scheduled for intravenous pyelography (IVP). Before the test, the priority nursing action would be to:
1. Restrict fluids.
2. Administer a sedative.
3. Determine a history of allergies.
4. Administer an oral preparation of radiopaque dye.

677. Following a renal biopsy, the client complains of pain at the biopsy site, which radiates to the front of the abdomen. Based on this complaint, the nurse further monitors the client for:
1. Bleeding
2. Infection
3. Renal colic
4. Normal, expected pain

678. A nurse is monitoring an 88-year-old woman suspected of having a urinary tract infection (UTI) for signs of the infection. Which of the following would alert the nurse to the possibility of the presence of a UTI?
1. Fever
2. Urgency
3. Confusion
4. Frequency

679. A nurse is performing an admission assessment on a client with a diagnosis of bladder cancer. Which of the following would the nurse most likely expect to note on data collection of this client?
1. Urgency
2. Frequency
3. Hematuria
4. Burning on urination

680. A client with benign prostatic hypertrophy (BPH) undergoes a transurethral resection of the prostate (TURP) and is receiving continuous bladder irrigations postoperatively. The nurse monitors the client for signs of transurethral resection (TUR) syndrome. Which of the

following data would indicate the onset of this syndrome?

1. Tachycardia and diarrhea
2. Bradycardia and confusion
3. Increased urinary output and anemia
4. Decreased urinary output and bladder spasms

681. A client with prostatitis resulting from kidney infection has received instructions on management of the condition at home and prevention of recurrence. The nurse determines that the client understood the instructions if the client has verbalized that he will:
1. Stop antibiotic therapy when pain subsides.
2. Exercise as much as possible to stimulate circulation.
3. Use warm sitz baths and analgesics to increase comfort.
4. Keep fluid intake to a minimum to decrease the need to void.

682. A nurse is assessing the patency of an arteriovenous fistula in the left arm of a client who is receiving hemodialysis for the treatment of chronic renal failure. Which finding indicates that the fistula is patent?
1. Palpation of a thrill over the fistula
2. Presence of a radial pulse in the left wrist
3. Absence of a bruit on auscultation of the fistula
4. Capillary refill less than 3 seconds in the nail beds of the fingers on the left hand

683. A client newly diagnosed with renal failure will be receiving peritoneal dialysis. During the infusion of the dialysate, the client complains of abdominal pain. Which action by the nurse is appropriate?
1. Stop the dialysis.
2. Slow the infusion.
3. Decrease the amount to be infused.
4. Explain that the pain will subside after the first few exchanges.

684. The nurse is instructing a client with diabetes mellitus about peritoneal dialysis. The nurse tells the client that it is important to maintain the dwell time for the dialysis at the prescribed time because of the risk of:
1. Infection
2. Fluid overload
3. Hyperglycemia
4. Disequilibrium syndrome

685. A client is diagnosed with polycystic kidney disease and the nurse provides information to the client about the treatment plan. The nurse determines that the client needs additional information if the client states that which of the following is a component of the treatment plan?
1. Sodium restriction
2. Genetic counseling
3. Increased water intake
4. Antihypertensive medications

686. The client with chronic renal failure who is scheduled for hemodialysis this morning is due to receive a daily dose of enalapril (Vasotec). The nurse should plan to administer this medication:
1. During dialysis
2. Just prior to dialysis
3. The day after dialysis
4. On return from dialysis

687. A nurse is caring for the client who had a renal biopsy. Which intervention would the nurse avoid in the care of the client after this procedure?
1. Administering pain medication as prescribed
2. Encouraging fluids to at least 3 L in the first 24 hours
3. Testing serial urine samples with dipsticks for occult blood
4. Ambulating the client in the room and hall for short distances

688. A female client is admitted to the emergency room following a fall from a horse. The physician orders insertion of a Foley catheter. The nurse notes blood at the urinary meatus while preparing for the procedure. The nurse should:
1. Notify the physician.
2. Use a smaller catheter.
3. Administer pain medication before inserting the catheter.
4. Use extra povidone-iodine solution in cleansing the meatus.

689. A male client has a tentative diagnosis of urethritis. The nurse collects data from the client, knowing that which of the following are manifestations of the disorder?
1. Hematuria and pyuria
2. Dysuria and proteinuria
3. Dysuria and penile discharge
4. Hematuria and penile discharge

690. A male client who is hospitalized is diagnosed with urethritis caused by chlamydial infection. The nursing assistant assigned to the client asks the nurse what measures are necessary to prevent contraction of the infection during care. The nurse tells the assistant that:
1. Enteric precautions should be instituted for the client.
2. Gloves and mask should be used when in the client's room.
3. Contact isolation should be initiated, because the disease is highly contagious.
4. Standard precautions are sufficient, because the infection is transmitted sexually.

691. A nurse is caring for a client with epididymitis. The nurse anticipates noting which of the following findings on data collection?
1. Diarrhea, groin pain, and scrotal edema
2. Fever, diarrhea, groin pain, and ecchymosis

3. Fever, nausea and vomiting, and painful scrotal edema

4. Nausea, vomiting, and scrotal edema with ecchymosis

ALTERNATE ITEM FORMAT: MULTIPLE RESPONSE

692. The nurse monitoring a client receiving peritoneal dialysis notes that the client's outflow is less than the inflow. Select all nurse actions in this situation.

☐ **1.** Contact the physician.
☐ **2.** Check the level of the drainage bag.
☑ **3.** Reposition the client to his or her side.
☑ **4.** Place the client in good body alignment.
☐ **5.** Check the peritoneal dialysis system for kinks.
☐ **6.** Increase the flow rate of the peritoneal dialysis solution.

ANSWERS

668. **3**

Rationale: Common interventions used in the treatment of epididymitis include bedrest, elevation of the scrotum, ice packs, sitz baths, analgesics, and antibiotics. A heating pad would not be used because direct application of heat could increase blood flow to the area and increase the swelling.

Test-Taking Strategy: Note the strategic word "avoid." Eliminate options 1 and 4 because they are obviously the most helpful in the care of the client. Note that both remaining options address the application of heat to the client. A sitz bath provides heat that is moist and soothing. Knowing that direct heat may increase inflammation with tissue that is already at risk will guide you to option 3 as the item to avoid. Review care of the client with epididymitis if you had difficulty with this question.

Level of Cognitive Ability: Application
Client Needs: Physiological Integrity
Integrated Process: Nursing Process/Implementation
Content Area: Adult Health/Renal
Reference: Christensen, B., & Kockrow, E. (2006). *Adult health nursing* (5th ed., p. 617). St. Louis: Mosby.

669. **3**

Rationale: The client who experiences epididymitis from UTI should increase intake of fluids to flush the urinary system. Because organisms can be forced into the vas deferens and epididymis from strain or pressure during voiding, the client should limit the force of the stream. Condom use can help prevent urethritis and epididymitis from sexually transmitted infections. Antibiotics are always taken until the full course of therapy is completed.

Test-Taking Strategy: Note the strategic words "needs further instruction." These words indicate a negative event query and the need to select the incorrect client statement. Because option 1 is consistent with good practices in the prevention of UTI, this option can be eliminated first. From the remaining options, it is necessary to know that the force of stream should be limited to prevent backflow into the epididymis, and that condoms are helpful in preventing this disorder from occurring as a complication of a sexually transmitted infection. Remember that antibiotics are not stopped when symptoms subside but must be taken until the full course of therapy is completed. Review care of the client with epididymitis if you had difficulty with this question.

Level of Cognitive Ability: Comprehension
Client Needs: Health Promotion and Maintenance
Integrated Process: Teaching and Learning
Content Area: Adult Health/Renal
Reference: Monahan, F., Sands, J., Marek, J., Neighbors, M., Marek, J, & Green, C. (2007). *Phipps' medical-surgical nursing: Health and illness perspectives* (8th ed., p. 1722). St. Louis: Mosby.

670. **4**

Rationale: Decreased force in the stream of urine is an early sign of BPH. The stream later becomes weak and dribbling. The client may then develop hematuria, frequency, urgency, urge incontinence, and nocturia. If untreated, complete obstruction and urinary retention can occur.

Test-Taking Strategy: Note the strategic words "early symptom." Option 2 identifies the most severe symptom and therefore is eliminated first. From the remaining options, focusing on the strategic words and recalling the pathophysiology related to BPH will direct you to option 4. Review the signs of benign prostatic hypertrophy if you had difficulty with this question.

Level of Cognitive Ability: Comprehension
Client Needs: Physiological Integrity
Integrated Process: Nursing Process/Data Collection
Content Area: Adult Health/Renal
Reference: Linton, A., & Maebius, N. (2007). *Introduction to medical-surgical nursing* (4th ed., p. 1088). Philadelphia: Saunders.

671. **4**

Rationale: Disequilibrium syndrome is characterized by headache, mental confusion, decreasing level of consciousness, nausea, vomiting, twitching, and possible seizure activity. It is caused by rapid removal of solutes from the body during hemodialysis. At the same time, the blood-brain barrier interferes with the efficient removal of wastes from brain tissue. As a result, water goes into cerebral cells because of the osmotic gradient, causing brain swelling and onset of symptoms. It most often occurs in clients who are new to dialysis and is prevented by dialyzing for shorter times or at reduced blood flow rates.

Test-Taking Strategy: Use the process of elimination. Noting the relation between the words "disequilibrium syndrome" and the signs in option 4 will direct you to this option. Review this syndrome if you had difficulty with this question.

Level of Cognitive Ability: Application
Client Needs: Physiological Integrity
Integrated Process: Nursing Process/Data Collection
Content Area: Adult Health/Renal
Reference: Linton, A., & Maebius, N. (2007). *Introduction to medical-surgical nursing* (4th ed., p. 872). Philadelphia: Saunders.

672. **4**

Rationale: Aluminum intoxication may occur when there is accumulation of aluminum, an ingredient in many phosphate-binding antacids. It results in mental cloudiness, dementia, and bone pain from infiltration of the bone with aluminum. This condition was formerly known as dialysis dementia. It may be treated with aluminum-chelating agents, which make aluminum available to be dialyzed from the body. It can be prevented by avoiding or limiting the use of phosphate-binding agents that contain aluminum.

Test-Taking Strategy: Use the process of elimination. Note the relation between the medication name in the question and option 4. Review the signs of aluminum intoxication if you had difficulty with this question.

Level of Cognitive Ability: Analysis

Client Needs: Physiological Integrity

Integrated Process: Nursing Process/Data Collection

Content Area: Adult Health/Renal

Reference: Monahan, F., Sands, J., Neighbors, M., Marek, J, & Green, C. (2007). *Phipps' medical-surgical nursing: Health and illness perspectives* (8th ed., p. 1018). St. Louis: Mosby.

673. **4**

Rationale: Arterial steal syndrome results from vascular insufficiency after creation of a fistula. The client exhibits pallor and diminished pulse distal to the fistula and complains of pain distal to the fistula, which is caused by tissue ischemia. Warmth, redness, and pain would more likely characterize a problem with infection. Options 2 and 3 are not characteristics of steal syndrome.

Test-Taking Strategy: Use the process of elimination. Recalling that arterial steal syndrome results from vascular insufficiency will direct you to option 4. Review these signs if you had difficulty with this question.

Level of Cognitive Ability: Analysis

Client Needs: Physiological Integrity

Integrated Process: Nursing Process/Data Collection

Content Area: Adult Health/Renal

Reference: Lewis, S., Heitkemper, M., Dirksen, S., & Bucher, L. (2007). *Medical-surgical nursing: Assessment and management of clinical problems* (7th ed., p. 1221). St. Louis: Mosby.

674. **2**

Rationale: Risk factors associated with pyelonephritis include diabetes mellitus, hypertension, chronic renal calculi, chronic cystitis, structural abnormalities of the urinary tract, presence of urinary stones, and indwelling or frequent urinary catheterization.

Test-Taking Strategy: Use the process of elimination. Eliminate options 1 and 4 first as least likely being associated as risk factors. From the remaining options, remember that diabetes mellitus can cause renal complications. This will direct you to the correct option. Review these risk factors if you had difficulty with this question.

Level of Cognitive Ability: Analysis

Client Needs: Health Promotion and Maintenance

Integrated Process: Nursing Process/Data Collection

Content Area: Adult Health/Renal

Reference: Ignatavicius, D., & Workman, M. (2006). *Medical-surgical nursing: Critical thinking for collaborative care* (5th ed., p. 1712). Philadelphia: Saunders.

675. **4**

Rationale: BUN testing is a frequently used laboratory test to determine renal function. The BUN level starts to rise when the glomerular filtration rate falls below 40% to 60%. A decreased hemoglobin and RBC count may be noted if bleeding from the urinary tract occurs or if erythropoietic function by the kidney is impaired. An increased WBC is most likely to be noted in renal disease.

Test-Taking Strategy: Use the process of elimination. Focus on the client's diagnosis and note the strategic words "most likely expect to note." Eliminate option 3 first because it is unassociated with the renal system. Although options 1 and 2 may be noted in some renal disorders, option 4 is the most likely laboratory finding. Remember, the BUN level is a frequently used laboratory test to determine renal function. Review the laboratory tests to determine renal function if you had difficulty with this question.

Level of Cognitive Ability: Analysis

Client Needs: Physiological Integrity

Integrated Process: Nursing Process/Data Collection

Content Area: Adult Health/Renal

Reference: Linton, A., & Maebius, N. (2007). *Introduction to medical-surgical nursing* (4th ed., p. 842). Philadelphia: Saunders.

676. **3**

Rationale: An iodine-based dye may be used during the IVP and can cause allergic reactions such as itching, hives, rash, tight feeling in the throat, shortness of breath, and bronchospasm. Assessing for allergies is the priority. Options 1, 2, and 4 are unnecessary.

Test-Taking Strategy: Note the strategic word " priority," and use the nursing process as a guide. Options 1, 2, and 4 address implementation. Option 3 is the only option that addresses data collection. Review this test if you had difficulty with this question.

Level of Cognitive Ability: Application

Client Needs: Physiological Integrity

Integrated Process: Nursing Process/Implementation

Content Area: Adult Health/Renal

Reference: Chernecky, C., & Berger, B. (2008). *Laboratory tests and diagnostic procedures* (5th ed., p. 682). Philadelphia: Saunders.

677. **1**

Rationale: If pain originates at the biopsy site and begins to radiate to the flank area and around the front of the abdomen, bleeding should be suspected. Hypotension, a decreasing hematocrit, and gross or microscopic hematuria would also indicate bleeding. Signs of infection would not appear immediately following a biopsy. Pain of this nature is not normal. There are no data to support the presence of renal colic.

Test-Taking Strategy: Use the process of elimination. Focusing on the data in the question will assist in eliminating options 3 and 4. Recalling that signs of infection may not appear immediately following biopsy will assist in directing you to option 1 from the remaining options. Review the complications following renal biopsy if you had difficulty with this question.

Level of Cognitive Ability: Analysis

Client Needs: Physiological Integrity

Integrated Process: Nursing Process/Data Collection
Content Area: Adult Health/Renal
Reference: Pagana, K., & Pagana, T. (2005). *Mosby's diagnostic and laboratory test reference* (7th ed., p. 794). St. Louis: Mosby.

678. 3
Rationale: In an older client, the only symptom of a UTI may be something as vague as increasing mental confusion or frequent unexplained falls. Frequency and urgency may commonly occur in an older client, and fever can be associated with a variety of conditions.
Test-Taking Strategy: Use the process of elimination. Note the client's age in the question. Eliminate options 2 and 4 because they may commonly occur in an older client. Eliminate option 1 next, because fever can be associated with a variety of conditions. Review the clinical manifestations of UTI that occur in the older client if you had difficulty with this question.
Level of Cognitive Ability: Comprehension
Client Needs: Physiological Integrity
Integrated Process: Nursing Process/Data Collection
Content Area: Adult Health/Renal
References: Lewis, S., Heitkemper, M., Dirksen, S., & Bucher, L. (2007). *Medical-surgical nursing: Assessment and management of clinical problems* (7th ed., p. 1160). St. Louis: Mosby. Wold, G. (2008). *Basic geriatric nursing* (4th ed., p. 54). St. Louis: Mosby.

679. 3
Rationale: Gross, painless hematuria is most frequently the first manifestation of bladder cancer. As the disease progresses, the client may experience burning, frequency, and urgency.
Test-Taking Strategy: Use the process of elimination and focus on the subject—a manifestation of bladder cancer. Eliminate options 1, 2, and 4 because they are common signs of a urinary tract infection. Review the specific manifestations associated with bladder cancer if you had difficulty with this question.
Level of Cognitive Ability: Comprehension
Client Needs: Physiological Integrity
Integrated Process: Nursing Process/Data Collection
Content Area: Adult Health/Renal
Reference: Linton, A., & Maebius, N. (2007). *Introduction to medical-surgical nursing* (4th ed., p. 865). Philadelphia: Saunders.

680. 2
Rationale: TUR syndrome is caused by increased absorption of nonelectrolyte irrigating fluid used during surgery. The client may show signs of cerebral edema and increased intracranial pressure such as increased blood pressure, bradycardia, confusion, disorientation, muscle twitching, visual disturbances, and nausea and vomiting.
Test-Taking Strategy: Knowledge regarding TUR syndrome is required to answer this question. Recalling that increased intracranial pressure is the concern will direct you to option 2. Review this disorder if you had difficulty with this question.
Level of Cognitive Ability: Analysis
Client Needs: Physiological Integrity
Integrated Process: Nursing Process/Data Collection

Content Area: Adult Health/Renal
Reference: Ignatavicius, D., & Workman, M. (2006). *Medical-surgical nursing: Critical thinking for collaborative care* (5th ed., pp. 1862-1863). Philadelphia: Saunders.

681. 3
Rationale: Treatment of prostatitis includes medication with antibiotics, analgesics, and stool softeners. The client is also taught to rest, increase fluid intake, and use sitz baths for comfort. Antimicrobial therapy is always continued until the prescription is completely finished.
Test-Taking Strategy: Use the process of elimination. Eliminate option 1 first, because stopping medication therapy before the end of the course is contraindicated. Option 4 is also eliminated, since fluid intake should be increased. From the remaining options, it is necessary to understand that sitz baths provide comfort and that rest is helpful in the healing process. Knowledge of either of these concepts will direct you to option 3. Review the measures to prevent prostatitis if you had difficulty with this question.
Level of Cognitive Ability: Analysis
Client Needs: Physiological Integrity
Integrated Process: Nursing Process/Evaluation
Content Area: Adult Health/Renal
Reference: Christensen, B., & Kockrow, E. (2006). *Adult health nursing* (5th ed., p. 487). St. Louis: Mosby.

682. 1
Rationale: The nurse assesses the patency of the fistula by palpating for the presence of a thrill or auscultating for a bruit. The presence of a thrill and bruit indicates patency of the fistula. Although the presence of a radial pulse in the left wrist and capillary refill less than 3 seconds in the nail beds of the fingers on the left hand are normal findings, they do not assess fistula patency.
Test-Taking Strategy: Use the process of elimination. Eliminate options 2 and 4 first because they are comparable or alike and assess for adequate circulation in the distal portion of the extremity (not the fistula). From the remaining options, focusing on the subject—patency—and noting the word "absence" in option 3 will assist in eliminating this option. Review the expected findings when assessing an arteriovenous fistula if you had difficulty with this question.
Level of Cognitive Ability: Analysis
Client Needs: Physiological Integrity
Integrated Process: Nursing Process/Data Collection
Content Area: Adult Health/Renal
Reference: Ignatavicius, D., & Workman, M. (2006). *Medical-surgical nursing: Critical thinking for collaborative care* (5th ed., p. 1753). Philadelphia: Saunders.

683. 4
Rationale: Pain during the inflow of dialysate is common during the first few exchanges because of peritoneal irritation; however, it disappears after a week or two. The infusion amount should not be decreased, and the infusion should not be slowed or stopped.
Test-Taking Strategy: Use the process of elimination. Eliminate options 1, 2, and 3 because they are comparable or alike actions. Review the complications associated with

peritoneal dialysis and the appropriate nursing actions if you had difficulty with this question.
Level of Cognitive Ability: Application
Client Needs: Physiological Integrity
Integrated Process: Nursing Process/Implementation
Content Area: Adult Health/Renal
Reference: Ignatavicius, D., & Workman, M. (2006). *Medical-surgical nursing: Critical thinking for collaborative care.* (5th ed., pp. 1758-1759). Philadelphia: Saunders.

684. **3**
Rationale: An extended dwell time increases the risk of hyperglycemia in the client with diabetes mellitus as a result of absorption of glucose from the dialysate and electrolyte changes. Diabetic clients may require extra insulin when receiving peritoneal dialysis. Options 1, 2, and 4 are not associated with dwell time.
Test-Taking Strategy: Use the process of elimination. Noting the client's diagnosis and recalling that the dialysate solution contains glucose will direct you to option 3. Review the complications associated with peritoneal dialysis if you had difficulty with this question.
Level of Cognitive Ability: Application
Client Needs: Physiological Integrity
Integrated Process: Teaching and Learning
Content Area: Adult Health/Renal
Reference: Black, J., & Hawks, J. (2005). *Medical-surgical nursing: Clinical management for positive outcomes* (7th ed., p. 956). Philadelphia: Saunders.

685. **1**
Rationale: Individuals with polycystic kidney disease seem to waste rather than retain sodium. Thus, they need an increased sodium and water intake. Aggressive control of hypertension is essential. Genetic counseling is advisable because of the hereditary nature of the disease.
Test-Taking Strategy: Note the strategic words "needs additional information." These words indicate a negative event query and the need to select the incorrect client statement. Recalling that sodium is wasted in polycystic kidney disease will direct you to option 1. Review the manifestations associated with this disease if you had difficulty with this question.
Level of Cognitive Ability: Analysis
Client Needs: Physiological Integrity
Integrated Process: Teaching and Learning
Content Area: Adult Health/Renal
Reference: Ignatavicius, D., & Workman, M. (2006). *Medical-surgical nursing: Critical thinking for collaborative care* (5th ed., pp. 1709, 1711). Philadelphia: Saunders.

686. **4**
Rationale: Antihypertensive medications such as enalapril are given to the client following hemodialysis. This prevents the client from becoming hypotensive during dialysis and from having the medication removed from the bloodstream by dialysis. There is no rationale for waiting a full day to resume the medication. This would lead to ineffective control of the blood pressure.
Test-Taking Strategy: Use the process of elimination. Begin to answer this question by thinking about the effects of an antihypertensive medication on blood pressure when fluid is

being removed from the body. Because hypotension is much more likely to occur in this circumstance, eliminate options 1 and 2. Eliminate option 3 because this action would lead to ineffective blood pressure control. Review preprocedure hemodialysis measures if you had difficulty with this question.
Level of Cognitive Ability: Application
Client Needs: Physiological Integrity
Integrated Process: Nursing Process/Planning
Content Area: Adult Health/Renal
Reference: Ignatavicius, D., & Workman, M. (2006). *Medical-surgical nursing: Critical thinking for collaborative care* (5th ed., p. 1756). Philadelphia: Saunders.

687. **4**
Rationale: After renal biopsy, the nurse ensures that the client remains in bed for at least 24 hours. Vital signs and puncture site assessments are done frequently during this time. Encouraging fluids is done to reduce possible clot formation in the kidney and urinary tract. A Hematest is done on serial urine samples with urine dipsticks to evaluate bleeding. Analgesics are often needed to manage the renal colic pain that some clients feel after this procedure.
Test-Taking Strategy: Begin to answer this question by recalling that pain and bleeding are potential concerns after this procedure. This will help eliminate options 1 and 3. From the remaining options, you need to recall that encouraging fluids will reduce clotting, whereas ambulation could initiate or enhance bleeding. Review care of the client following a renal biopsy if you had difficulty with this question.
Level of Cognitive Ability: Application
Client Needs: Physiological Integrity
Integrated Process: Nursing Process/Implementation
Content Area: Adult Health/Renal
Reference: Pagana, K., & Pagana, T. (2005). *Mosby's diagnostic and laboratory test reference* (7th ed., p. 794). St. Louis: Mosby.

688. **1**
Rationale: The presence of blood at the urinary meatus may indicate urethral trauma or disruption. The nurse notifies the physician, knowing that the client should not be catheterized until the cause of the bleeding is determined by diagnostic testing.
Test-Taking Strategy: Focus on the data in the question, that the client experienced a traumatic injury. This will direct you to option 1. Review this procedure and the indications of urethral trauma if you had difficulty with this question.
Level of Cognitive Ability: Application
Client Needs: Physiological Integrity
Integrated Process: Nursing Process/Implementation
Content Area: Adult Health/Renal
Reference: Monahan, F., Sands, J., Neighbors, M., Marek, J, & Green, C. (2007). *Phipps' medical-surgical nursing: health and illness perspectives* (8th ed., pp. 990-992). St. Louis: Mosby.

689. **3**
Rationale: Urethritis in the male client often results from chlamydial infection and is characterized by dysuria, which is accompanied by a clear to mucopurulent discharge. Hematuria and proteinuria are not characteristics.

Test-Taking Strategy: Use the process of elimination. Begin to answer this question by eliminating options 1 and 4. Urethritis is generally accompanied by dysuria in the male client. Knowing that the problem originates in the urethra, not the kidney, you would then eliminate the option with proteinuria, which indicates a problem with kidney function. This leaves option 3 as the correct option. The male client with urethritis has dysuria and discharge from the penis. Review the signs of urethritis if you had difficulty with this question.
Level of Cognitive Ability: Comprehension
Client Needs: Physiological Integrity
Integrated Process: Nursing Process/Data Collection
Content Area: Adult Health/Renal
Reference: Linton, A., & Maebius, N. (2007). *Introduction to medical-surgical nursing* (4th ed., p. 849). Philadelphia: Saunders.

690. **4**
Rationale: Chlamydia is a sexually transmitted infection, and is frequently called non-gonococcal urethritis in the male client. It requires no special precautions. Caregivers cannot acquire the disease during administration of care, and following standard precautions is the only measure that needs to be used.
Test-Taking Strategy: A basic knowledge of infection control and disease transmission guides you to select option 4 as correct. Also, note that option 4 is the umbrella option. If this question was difficult, review transmission of this disorder and standard precautions.
Level of Cognitive Ability: Application
Client Needs: Safe and Effective Care Environment
Integrated Process: Teaching and Learning
Content Area: Adult Health/Renal
Reference: deWit, S. (2009). *Medical-surgical nursing: Concepts & practice* (pp. 120, 1002). Philadelphia: Saunders.

691. **3**
Rationale: Typical signs and symptoms of epididymitis include scrotal pain and edema, which are often accompanied by fever, nausea and vomiting, and chills. It is most often caused by infection, although sometimes it can be caused by trauma. Diarrhea and ecchymosis are not characteristics.
Test-Taking Strategy: Use the process of elimination. Any disorder that ends in "-itis" results from inflammation or infection. Therefore, an expected finding would be elevated temperature. With this in mind, you can eliminate options 1 and 4 because they do not contain fever as part of the option. From the remaining options, recalling that ecchymosis results from bleeding, which is not part of this clinical picture, directs you to option 3. Review the signs of this infection if you had difficulty with this question.
Level of Cognitive Ability: Comprehension
Client Needs: Physiological Integrity
Integrated Process: Nursing Process/Data Collection
Content Area: Adult Health/Renal
Reference: Linton, A., & Maebius, N. (2007). *Introduction to medical-surgical nursing* (4th ed., p. 1087). Philadelphia: Saunders.

ALTERNATE ITEM FORMAT: MULTIPLE RESPONSE

692. **Answer: 2, 3, 4, 5**
Rationale: If outflow drainage is inadequate, the nurse attempts to stimulate outflow by changing the client's position. Turning the client to the other side or making sure that the client is in good body alignment may assist with outflow drainage. The drainage bag needs to be lower than the client's abdomen to enhance gravity drainage. The connecting tubing and the peritoneal dialysis system is also checked for kinks or twisting, and the clamps on the system are checked to ensure that they are open. There is no reason to contact the physician. Increasing the flow rate is an inappropriate action and is unassociated with the amount of outflow solution.
Test-Taking Strategy: Use the principles related to gravity flow and preventing obstruction to flow to answer this question. This will assist in determining the correct interventions. Review the nursing interventions related to insufficient flow of dialysate if you had difficulty with this question.
Level of Cognitive Ability: Application
Client Needs: Physiological Integrity
Integrated Process: Nursing Process/Implementation
Content Area: Adult Health/Renal
Reference: Ignatavicius, D., & Workman, M. (2006). *Medical-surgical nursing: Critical thinking for collaborative care* (5th ed., p. 1759). Philadelphia: Saunders.

REFERENCES

Black, J., & Hawks, J. (2005). *Medical-surgical nursing: Clinical management for positive outcomes* (7th ed.). Philadelphia: Saunders.

Chernecky, C., & Berger, B. (2008). *Laboratory tests and diagnostic procedures* (5th ed.). Philadelphia: Saunders.

Christensen, B., & Kockrow, E. (2006). *Adult health nursing* (5th ed.). St. Louis: Mosby.

Christensen, B., & Kockrow, E. (2006). *Foundations of nursing* (5th ed.). St. Louis: Mosby.

deWit, S. (2009). *Medical-surgical nursing: Concepts & practice.* Philadelphia: Saunders.

Ignatavicius, D., & Workman, M. (2006). *Medical-surgical nursing: Critical thinking for collaborative care* (5th ed.). Philadelphia: Saunders.

Lewis, S., Heitkemper, M., Dirksen, S., & Bucher, L. (2007). *Medical-surgical nursing: Assessment and management of clinical problems* (7th ed.). St. Louis: Mosby.

Linton, A., & Maebius, N. (2007). *Introduction to medical-surgical nursing* (4th ed.). Philadelphia: Saunders.

Monahan, F., Sands, J., Neighbors, J., Marek, J., & Green, C., (2007). *Phipps' medical-surgical nursing: Health and illness perspectives* (8th ed.). St. Louis: Mosby.

Nix, S. (2005). *Williams' basic nutrition and diet therapy* (11th ed.). St. Louis: Mosby.

Pagana, K., & Pagana, T. (2005). *Mosby's diagnostic and laboratory test reference* (7th ed.). St. Louis: Mosby.

Schlenker, E., & Long, S. (2007). *Williams' essentials of nutrition & diet therapy* (9th ed.). St. Louis: Mosby.

Wold, G. (2008). *Basic geriatric nursing* (4th ed.). St. Louis: Mosby.

CHAPTER

53

Renal Medications

I. URINARY TRACT ANTISEPTICS

A. Description

1. Inhibit the growth of bacteria in the urine
2. Act as disinfectants within the urinary tract. (Figure 53-1 and Box 53-1)
3. Used to treat acute cystitis or urinary tract infections (UTIs)
4. Do not achieve effective antibacterial concentrations in blood or tissues and therefore cannot be used for infections outside the urinary tract

B. Side effects and nursing considerations

1. Cinoxacin (Cinobac)
   a. Side effects are similar to those of nalidixic acid.
   b. Dosage should be reduced in clients with renal impairment; failure to do so could result in accumulation of the medication to toxic levels

2. Methenamine (Mandelamine, Hiprex, Urex)
   a. Used to treat chronic UTIs, but not recommended for acute infections
   b. Administer after meals and at bedtime to minimize gastric distress
   c. Chronic high-dose therapy can cause bladder irritation
   d. Methenamine can cause crystalluria and should not be used in clients with renal impairment
   e. Decomposition of medication generates ammonia; thus, it should not be used for clients with liver dysfunction
   f. Methenamine requires acidic urine with a pH of 5.5 or less
   g. Increasing fluids reduces antibacterial effects by diluting the medication and raising urine pH
   h. Methenamine should not be combined with sulfonamides because of the risk of crystalluria and urinary tract injury
   i. Clients taking this medication should avoid alkalinizing agents including over-the-counter (OTC) antacids contaning sodium bicarbonate or sodium carbonate

3. Nalidixic acid (NegGram)
   a. Gastrointestinal side effects include anorexia, nausea, vomiting, and diarrhea
   b. Skin side effects include rash and photosensitivity
   c. CNS side effects include visual disturbances and insomnia
   d. Nalidixic acid may produce intracranial hypertension in pediatric clients and should not be administered to children under 3 months of age
   e. When nalidixic acid is used for more than 2 weeks, complete blood cell counts and liver function tests should be performed
   f. Nalidixic acid can intensify the effects of orally administered anticoagulants
   g. Nalidixic acid is contraindicated in clients with a history of convulsive disorders

4. Nitrofurantoin (Furadantin, Macrodantin, Macrobid)
   a. Gastrointestinal side effects include anorexia, nausea, vomiting, and diarrhea; administration with milk or meals minimizes gastrointestinal distress
   b. Pulmonary reactions include dyspnea, chest pain, chills, fever, cough, and alveolar infiltrates; these resolve in 2 to 4 days after cessation of treatment
   c. Hematological side effects include agranulocytosis, leukopenia, thrombocytopenia, and megaloblastic anemia
   d. Peripheral neuropathy side effects include muscle weakness, tingling sensations, and numbness
   e. Neurological side effects include headache, vertigo, drowsiness, and nystagmus
   f. Allergic reactions include anaphylaxis, hives, rash, and tingling sensations around the mouth
   g. Nitrofurantoin may produce a harmless brown color in the urine
   h. Nitrofurantoin is contraindicated in clients with renal impairment

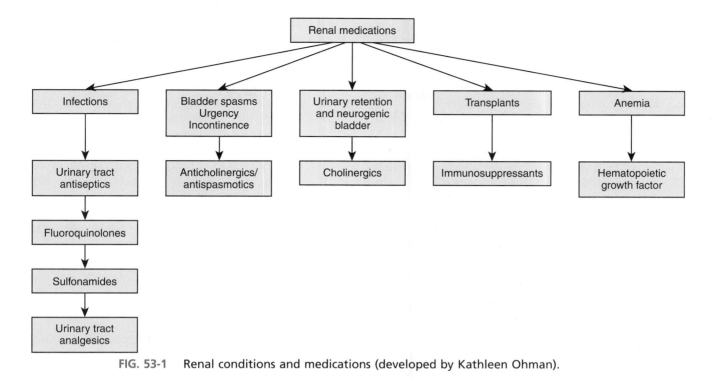

FIG. 53-1 Renal conditions and medications (developed by Kathleen Ohman).

BOX 53-1 Urinary Tract Antiseptics

Cinoxacin (Cinobac)
Methenamine (Mandelamine, Hiprex, Urex)
Nalidixic acid (NegGram)
Nitrofurantoin (Furadantin, Macrodantin, Macrobid)

BOX 53-2 Fluoroquinolones

Ciprofloxacin (Cipro)
Enoxacin (Penetrex)
Gatifloxacin (Tequin)
Gemifloxacin (Factive)
Levofloxacin (Levaquin)
Lomefloxacin (Maxaquin)
Moxifloxacin (Avelox)
Norfloxacin (Noroxin)
Ofloxacin (Floxin)
Sparfloxacin (Zagam)
Trovafloxacin (Trovan)

    i. Instruct the client to monitor the expected side effects and signs warranting physician notification, and to avoid taking nitrofurantoin with antacids

II. FLUOROQUINOLONES (Box 53-2)

A. Description: suppress bacterial growth by inhibiting an enzyme necessary for DNA synthesis and are active against a broad spectrum of microbes

B. Side effects and nursing considerations
  1. Significant side effects include dizziness, drowsiness, gastric distress, diarrhea, vaginitis (trovafloxacin), nausea, and vomiting
  2. Adverse effects include psychoses, hallucinations, confusion, tremors, hypersensitivity, and interstitial nephritis
  3. Fluoroquinolones should be used with caution in clients with hepatic, renal, or central nervous system disorders
  4. Monitor client for side effects or signs of adverse reactions
  5. Administer fluoroquinolones with a full glass of water and ensure that the client maintains a urine output of at least 1200 to 1500 mL daily to minimize the occurrence of crystalluria
  6. Enoxacin (Penetrex) and norfloxacin (Noroxin) are to be taken on an empty stomach
  7. Ciprofloxacin (Cipro), lomefloxacin (Maxaquin), and ofloxacin (Floxin) may be taken with or without food
  8. Intravenously administered ciprofloxacin (Cipro) and ofloxacin (Floxin) are infused slowly over 60 minutes to minimize discomfort and vein irritation
  9. Advise the client to report dizziness, lightheadedness, visual disturbances, increased light sensitivity, and feelings of depression because these signs could indicate central nervous system toxicity
  10. Inform the client of signs of hepatic and renal toxicity and the importance of reporting these signs to the physician

III. SULFONAMIDES (Box 53-3)
   A. Description: suppress bacterial growth by inhibiting the synthesis of folic acid, are active against a broad spectrum of microbes, and are used primarily to treat acute UTIs
   B. Side effects and nursing considerations
      1. Hypersensitivity reactions include rash, fever, and photosensitivity
      2. Stevens-Johnson syndrome, the most severe hypersensitivity response, produces symptoms that include widespread lesions of the skin and mucous membranes, fever, malaise, and toxemia
      3. Sulfonamides should be discontinued if a rash is noted; the physician is notified if a rash appears
      4. Sulfonamides can cause hemolytic anemia, agranulocytosis, leukopenia, and thrombocytopenia; instruct the client to notify the physician if sore throat or fever occurs
      5. Administer sulfonamides with caution in clients with renal impairment
      6. Sulfonamides are contraindicated if hypersensitivity exists to sulfonamides, sulfonylureas, or thiazide or loop diuretics
      7. Sulfonamides are contraindicated in infants under 2 months of age and in pregnant women or mothers who are breast-feeding
      8. Sulfonamides can potentiate the effects of warfarin sodium (Coumadin), phenytoin (Dilantin), and orally administered hypoglycemics such as tolbutamide (Orinase); when combined with sulfonamides, these medications may require a reduction in dosage
      9. Instruct the client to take the medication on an empty stomach with a full glass of water
      10. Instruct the client to complete the entire course of antibiotics as prescribed
      11. Instruct the client to avoid prolonged exposure to sunlight, wear protective clothing, and apply a sunscreen to exposed skin
      12. Adults should maintain a daily urine output of 1200 mL by consuming 8 to 10 glasses of water each day to minimize the risk of renal damage from the medication
      13. Inform the client that some combination medications of sulfonamides can cause the urine to turn dark brown or red
      14. The combination sulfonamide, trimethoprim (TMP)-sulfamethoxazole (SMZ) (Bactrim, Cotrim, Septra), is more effective than either medication alone since it inhibits the sequential steps in bacterial folic acid synthesis
      15. TMP/SMZ is used cautiously with clients experiencing impaired kidney function, folate deficiency, severe allergy, or bronchial asthma
      16. IV dose of TMP/SMZ is administered over 60 to 90 minutes and is not mixed with other medications

IV. URINARY TRACT ANALGESIC (Box 53-4)
   A. Description
      1. Phenazopyridine hydrochloride is a urinary tract analgesic to treat pain from urinary tract irritation or infection
      2. A urinary tract analgesic is administered with an antibiotic because the analgesic only treats pain, not the infection
   B. Side effects
      1. Nausea
      2. Headache
      3. Vertigo
   C. Nursing considerations
      1. Instruct the client that the urine will turn red or orange and stain clothing
      2. A urinary tract analgesic is contraindicated in clients with renal or hepatic disease
      3. The medication interferes with accurate urine testing for glucose or ketones

V. ANTICHOLINERGICS/ANTISPASMODICS (Box 53-5)
   A. Description
      1. Oxybutynin chloride (Ditropan) relaxes smooth muscles of the urinary tract
      2. Propantheline bromide (Pro-Banthine) is used to decrease bladder muscle spasms
      3. Tolterodine tartrate (Detrol, Detrol LA) reduces urinary incontinence, urgency, and frequency by controlling bladder contractions

---

BOX 53-3 Sulfonamides

Sulfadiazine
Sulfamethizole
Sulfamethoxazole
Sulfisoxazole
Trimethoprim (Proloprim, Trimpex)
Trimethoprim (TMP)-sulfamethoxazole (SMZ) (Bactrim, Cotrim, Septra)
Azo-Sulfisoxazole

BOX 53-4 Urinary Tract Analgesic

Phenazopyridine hydrochloride (Pyridium, Azo-Standard, Phenazo, Pyridiate, Urogesic)

BOX 53-5 Anticholinergics/Antispasmodics

Oxybutynin chloride (Ditropan, Ditropan XL)
Propantheline bromide (Pro-Banthine)
Tolterodine tartrate (Detrol, Detrol LA)

B. Side effects
1. Anorexia, nausea, vomiting, and dry mouth
2. Blurred vision
3. Confusion in older clients
4. Constipation
5. Decreased sweating
6. Dizziness
7. Drowsiness
8. Dry eyes
9. Gastric distress
10. Headache
11. Tachycardia
12. Urinary retention

C. Nursing considerations
1. Extended-release capsules should not be split, chewed, or crushed
2. Tolterodine tartrate (Detrol LA) should be used cautiously in clients with narrow-angle glaucoma
3. Do not administer oxybutynin to clients with known hypersensitivity, gastrointestinal or genitourinary obstruction, glaucoma, severe colitis, or myasthenia gravis
4. Do not administer propantheline bromide to clients with narrow-angle glaucoma, obstructive uropathy, gastrointestinal disease, or ulcerative colitis
5. Instruct the client to avoid hazardous activities because of the side effects of dizziness and drowsiness
6. Monitor intake and output (I&O)
7. Provide gum or hard candy for dry mouth
8. Monitor for signs of toxicity (central nervous system stimulation) such as hypotension, hypertension, confusion, tachycardia, flushed or red face, signs of respiratory depression, nervousness, restlessness, hallucinations, and irritability

VI. **CHOLINERGIC** (Box 53-6)
A. Description: bethanechol chloride (Urecholine) is a cholinergic used to increase bladder tone and function and to treat nonobstructive urinary retention and neurogenic bladder

B. Side effects
1. Headache
2. Hypotension
3. Flushing and sweating
4. Increased salivation
5. Abdominal cramps
6. Nausea and vomiting
7. Diarrhea
8. Urinary urgency

9. Bronchoconstriction
10. Transient complete heart block

C. Nursing considerations
1. Do not administer if the client has a urinary stricture or obstruction
2. Administer on an empty stomach, 1 hour before or 2 hours after meals to lessen nausea and vomiting
3. Never administer by the intramuscular or IV route
4. Monitor I&O
5. Monitor for increased bladder tone and function
6. Monitor for cholinergic overdose (excessive salivation, sweating, involuntary urination and defecation, bradycardia, and severy hypotension)
7. Have atropine sulfate (antidote) readily available for IV or subcutaneous administration

VII. **MEDICATIONS FOR PREVENTION OF ORGAN REJECTION** (Box 53-7)
A. Medications include immunosuppressants, corticosteroids, cytotoxic medications, and antibodies
B. Cyclosporine (Sandimmune, Gengraf, Neoral)
1. Cyclosporine inhibits calcineurin and acts on T-cells to suppress the production of interleukin-2, gamma-interferon, and other cytokines
2. Cyclosporine is used to prevent rejection of allogenic kidney, liver, and heart transplants
3. Prednisone (Deltasone) is usually administered concurrently
4. Oral administration of cyclosporine is preferred; IV administration is reserved for clients who cannot take the medication orally
5. Blood levels of the medication should be measured periodically
6. The most common adverse effects are nephrotoxicity, infection, hypertension, tremor, and hirsutism

---

BOX 53-6 **Cholinergic**

Bethanechol chloride (Urecholine)

BOX 53-7 **Preventing Organ Rejection**

Immunosuppressants
Cyclosporine (Sandimmune, Gengraf, Neoral)
Tacrolimus (Prograf)
Sirolimus (Rapamune)
Glucocorticoid
Prednisone (Deltasone)
Cytotoxic Medications
Azathioprine (Imuran)
Mycophenolate mofetil (CellCept)
Antibodies
Basiliximab (Simulect)
Daclizumab (Zenapax)
Lymphocyte Immune Globulin (Atgam)
Muromonab-CD3 (Orthoclone OKT3)

7. Assure the client that hirsutism is reversible; instruct on the use of a depilatory
8. Other adverse effects include neurotoxicity, gastrointestinal effects, hyperkalemia, and hyperglycemia
9. The risk of infection and lymphomas is increased with the use of cyclosporine
10. Cyclosporine is contraindicated in the presence of hypersensitivity, pregnancy and breast-feeding, recent inoculation with live virus vaccines, and recent contact with an active infection such as chickenpox or herpes zoster
11. Cyclosporine is embryotoxic, and women of childbearing age should use a mechanical form of contraception and avoid oral contraceptives
12. The client should be informed about the possibility of renal and liver damage and the need for periodic blood urea nitrogen, serum creatinine, liver function tests, coagulation factors, serum potassium, and blood glucose levels
13. The client should be instructed to monitor for early signs of infection and to report these signs immediately
14. Instruct the client to dispense the oral liquid medication into a glass container by using a specially calibrated pipette, mix well, and drink immediately; rinse the glass container with diluent and drink it to ensure ingestion of the complete dose; dry the outside of the pipette and return to its cover for storage
15. To promote palatablity, instruct the client to mix the medication with milk, chocolate milk, or orange juice just before administration
16. Consuming grapefruit juice is prohibited because it raises cyclosporine levels and increases the risk of toxicity
17. Ketoconazole (Nizoral), erythromycin, and amphotericin B (Fungizone) can elevate cyclosporine levels
18. Phenytoin (Dilantin), phenobarbital, rifampin (Rifadin), and trimethoprim-sulfamethoxazole can decrease cyclosporine levels
19. Renal damage can be intensified by the concurrent use of other nephrotoxic medications

C. Sirolimus (Rapamune)
1. Sirolimus is used for the prevention of renal transplant rejection by inhibiting the response of helper T- and B-cells to cytokinesis
2. It is used with cyclosporine and corticosteroids
3. Increases the risk of infection, increases the risk of renal injury, increases the risk of lymphocele (a complication of renal transplant surgery), and raises cholesterol and triglyceride levels
4. Side effects include rash, acne, anemia, thrombocytopenia, joint pain, diarrhea, and hypokalemia

D. Tacrolimus (Prograf)
1. Tacrolimus inhibits calcineurin and thereby prevents T-cells from producing interleukin-2, gamma-interferon, and other cytokines
2. Tacrolimus is more effective than cyclosporine but is more toxic
3. Adverse effects are similar to those of cyclosporine and include nephrotoxicity, infection, hypertension, tremor, hirsutism, neurotoxicity, gastrointestinal effects, hyperkalemia, and hyperglycemia
4. Tacrolimus should be used cautiously in immunosuppressed clients and those with renal, hepatic, or pancreatic impairments
5. Tacrolimus is contraindicated for clients hypersensitive to cyclosporine
6. Concurrent use of glucocorticoids is recommended
7. Monitor blood glucose levels and administer prescribed insulin or oral hypoglycemics

E. Prednisone (Deltasone)
1. Prednisone is a glucocorticoid that prevents proliferation of T-cytotoxic cells, thus suppressing inflammatory responses
2. Hyperglycemia and hypokalemia can occur with prednisone use; monitor glucose and serum potassium levels.
3. Refer to Chapter 45 for additional information about prednisone

F. Azathioprine (Imuran)
1. Suppresses cell-mediated and humoral immune responses by inhibiting the proliferation of B- and T-cells
2. Is used as an adjunct to cyclosporine and glucocorticoids to help suppress transplant rejection
3. Can cause neutropenia and thrombocytopenia from bone marrow suppression
4. Is contraindicated in pregnancy and is associated with an increased incidence of neoplasms
5. Monitor hematocrit, white blood cell count, platelet count, liver enzymes, and coagulation factors

G. Mycophenolate mofetil (CellCept)
1. Mycophenolate mofentil causes selective inhibition of B- and T-cell proliferation
2. It is used along with cyclosporine and glucocorticoids for prophylaxis against organ rejection
3. Major adverse effects include diarrhea, severe neutropenia, vomiting, and sepsis
4. Mycophenolate mofetil is associated with an increased risk of infection and malignancies
5. Absorption is decreased by the use of magnesium and aluminum antacids and by cholestyramine (Questran, Prevalite)
6. It is contraindicated in pregnancy and while breast-feeding

7. Instruct the client to take the medication on an empty stomach and not to open or crush capsules
8. Instruct the client to contact the physician for unusual bleeding or bruising, sore throat, mouth sores, abdominal pain, or fever

H. Daclizumab (Zenapax) and basiliximab (Simulect)
1. Daclizumab (Zenapax) and basiliximab (Simulect) bind to interleukin-2 receptors on lymphocytes, resulting in diminished cell-mediated immune reactions
2. Are used along with other immunosuppressants such as cyclosporine and glucocorticoids to prevent acute rejection of transplanted kidneys
3. Are administered intravenously
4. Are contraindicated in the client with an allergy to protein
5. Daclizumab (Zenapax)
   a. Initial dose is administered within 24 hours before transplantation
   b. Side effects include chest pain, gastrointestinal distress, edema, shortness of breath, pain in the joints, and slow wound healing
6. Basiliximab (Simulect)
   a. Initial dose is administered within 2 hours before transplantation
   b. Side effects are similar to those for daclizumab; in addition, headache, insomnia, dizziness, and tremors can occur

I. Lymphocyte Immune Globulin (Atgam)
1. Lymphocyte Immune Globulin causes a decrease in the number and activity of thymus-derived lymphocytes and is used to suppress organ rejection following renal, liver, bone marrow, and heart transplants
2. Before the first infusion, the client should receive an intradermal skin test to test for hypersensitivity
3. Because this product is made using equine and human blood components, it may carry a risk of transmitting infectious agents, such as viruses
4. Monitor the platelet count and report if below 100,000/mm^3
5. Arrange for outpatient referral to repeat infusions after discharge

J. Muromonab-CD3 (Orthoclone OKT3)
1. Blocks all T-cell functions and is used to prevent acute allograft rejection of kidney transplants
2. Adverse reactions include fever, chills, dyspnea, chest pain, and nausea and vomiting
3. Is administered intravenously; the client is pretreated with IV glucocorticoid

VIII. HEMATOPOIETIC GROWTH FACTORS (Box 53-8)
A. Erythropoietic growth factors
1. Stimulate the production of red blood cells
2. Used to treat anemia of **chronic renal failure,** chemotherapy-induced anemia, anemia caused

---

BOX 53-8 Hematopoietic Growth Factors

Erythropoietic Growth Factors
Epoetin alfa (Epogen, Procrit)
Darbepoetin alfa (Aranesp)
Leukopoietic Growth Factors
Filgrastim (Neupogen)
Pegfilgrastim (Neulasta)
Sargramostim (Leukine)
Thrombopoietic Growth Factor
Oprelvekin (Neumega)

---

by zidovudine (AZT), and anemia in clients requiring surgery
3. Initial effects can be seen within 1 to 2 weeks, and the hematocrit reaches normal levels (30% to 33%) in 2 to 3 months
4. Major side effect: hypertension
5. Other effects can include heart failure, thrombotic effects such as stroke or myocardial infarction, and cardiac arrest

B. Leukopoietic growth factors
1. Stimulate the production of white blood cells (leukocytes)
2. Used for clients undergoing myelosuppressive chemotherapy or bone marrow transplant and those with severe chronic neutropenia.
3. Can cause bone pain, leukocytosis, elevation of plasma uric acid, lactate dehydrogenase, and alkaline phosphatase; long-term therapy has caused splenomegaly

C. Thrombopoietic growth factor
1. Stimulates the production of platelets
2. Used for clients undergoing myelosuppressive chemotherapy to minimize thrombocytopenia and to decrease the need for platelet transfusions
3. Adverse effects include fluid retention, cardiac dysrhythmias, conjunctival infection, visual blurring, and papilledema

PRACTICE QUESTIONS

More questions on the companion CD!

693. Oxybutynin chloride (Ditropan) is prescribed for the client with neurogenic bladder. The nurse monitors the client, knowing that which of the following would indicate a possible toxic effect related to this medication?
   1. Pallor
   2. Drowsiness
   3. Bradycardia
   4. Restlessness
694. Following kidney transplant, cyclosporine (Sandimmune) is prescribed for the client. Which of the following laboratory results

indicates an adverse effect from the use of this medication?
1. Decreased creatinine level
2. Decreased hemoglobin level
3. Decreased white blood cell (WBC) count
4. Elevated blood urea nitrogen (BUN) level

695. A nurse is providing dietary instructions to a client who has been prescribed cyclosporine (Sandimmune). Which of the following food items would the nurse instruct the client to avoid?
1. Red meats
2. Orange juice
3. Grapefruit juice
4. Green leafy vegetables

696. A nurse is monitoring a client receiving cyclosporine (Sandimmune). Which of the following indicates to the nurse that the client is experiencing an adverse effect from this medication?
1. Nausea
2. Tremor
3. Alopecia
4. Hypotension

697. A nurse is reviewing the laboratory results documented in the record of a client receiving tacrolimus (Prograf). Which of the following indicates to the nurse that the client is experiencing an adverse effect of the medication?
1. Potassium level, 3.8 mEq/L
2. Blood glucose level, 200 mg/dL
3. Platelet count, 300,000 cells/mm^3
4. White blood cell (WBC) count, 6000/mm^3

698. Mycophenolate mofetil (CellCept) is prescribed for a client as prophylaxis for organ rejection following allogneic renal transplant. Which of the following instructions does the nurse provide regarding administration of this medication?
1. Administer following meals
2. Contact the physician if a sore throat occurs
3. Take the medication with a magnesium type antacid
4. Open the capsule and mix with food for administration

699. A client with chronic renal failure (CRF) is receiving epoetin alfa (Epogen). The nurse is reviewing the laboratory results and notes that which of the following results indicates a therapeutic effect of the medication?
1. Hematocrit level, 32%
2. Platelet count, 400,000 cells/mm^3
3. White blood cell (WBC) count, 6000/mm^3
4. Blood urea nitrogen (BUN) level, 15 mg/dL

700. A nurse is monitoring the client receiving epoetin alfa (Epogen) for adverse effects of the medication. The nurse notes that which of the following indicates an adverse effect?
1. Depression
2. Bradycardia
3. Hypotension
4. Hypertension

701. A nurse is administering 5 mg of bethanechol chloride (Urecholine) subcutaneously to a client with urinary retention. Which of the following would the nurse prepare to have readily available when administering this medication?
1. Vitamin K
2. Mucomyst
3. Atropine sulfate
4. Protamine sulfate

702. Laboratory analysis of urine for culture and sensitivity reveals a gram-negative bacterial infection. Nalidixic acid (NegGram) is prescribed for the client. The nurse questions the prescription if the client has which of the following disorders?
1. Seizure disorder
2. Diabetes mellitus
3. Peptic ulcer disease
4. Coronary artery disease

703. A client receiving nitrofurantoin (Macrodantin) calls the physician's office complaining of side effects related to the medication. Which side effect indicates the need to stop treatment with this medication?
1. Nausea
2. Diarrhea
3. Anorexia
4. Cough and chest pain

704. Trimethoprim-sulfamethoxazole (Bactrim) is prescribed for the client. The nurse tells the client to report which of the following symptoms if it develops during the course of this medication therapy?
1. Nausea
2. Diarrhea
3. Headache
4. Sore throat

705. Phenazopyridine hydrochloride (Pyridium) is prescribed for the client for symptomatic relief of pain resulting from a lower urinary tract infection (UTI). The nurse tells the client:
1. To take the medication on an empty stomach
2. To discontinue the medication if a headache occurs
3. To take the medication at bedtime on an empty stomach
4. That a reddish-orange discoloration of the urine may occur

706. Bethanechol chloride (Urecholine) is prescribed for the client with urinary retention. The nurse reviews the client's record, knowing that which of the following preexisting disorders would be a contraindication to the administration of this medication?
1. Gastric atony
2. Urinary strictures
3. Neurogenic atony
4. Gastroesophageal reflux

ALTERNATE ITEM FORMAT: CHART/EXHIBIT

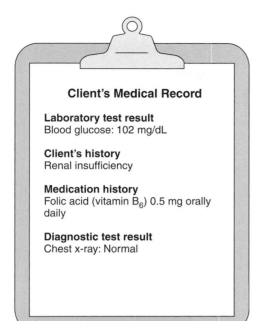

Client's Medical Record

Laboratory test result
Blood glucose: 102 mg/dL

Client's history
Renal insufficiency

Medication history
Folic acid (vitamin B$_6$) 0.5 mg orally daily

Diagnostic test result
Chest x-ray: Normal

707. Cinoxacin (Cinobac), a urinary antiseptic, is prescribed for the client. The nurse reviews the client's medical record and would contact the physician regarding which documented finding to verify the prescription?
    1. Client's history
    2. Medication history
    3. Diagnostic test result
    4. Laboratory test results

ANSWERS

693. 4
Rationale: Toxicity produces central nervous system excitation, such as nervousness, restlessness, hallucinations, and irritability. Other signs of toxicity include either hypotension or hypertension, confusion, tachycardia, flushed or red face, and signs of respiratory depression. Drowsiness is a frequent side effect of the medication but does not indicate toxicity.
Test-Taking Strategy: Knowledge regarding the manifestations related to toxicity is required to answer this question. Remember, central nervous system excitation is a sign of toxicity. Review this medication if you had difficulty with this question.
Level of Cognitive Ability: Analysis
Client Needs: Physiological Integrity
Integrated Process: Nursing Process/Data Collection
Content Area: Pharmacology
Reference: Skidmore-Roth, L. (2008). *2008 Mosby's nursing drug reference* (21st ed., pp. 772-773). St. Louis: Mosby.

694. 4
Rationale: Nephrotoxicity can occur from the use of Cyclosporine. Nephrotoxicity is evaluated by monitoring for elevated BUN and serum creatinine levels. Cyclosporine does not depress the bone marrow.
Test-Taking Strategy: Use the process of elimination. Eliminate options 2 and 3 first because they are unrelated to renal function. Next, eliminate option 1 because the creatinine level would be elevated, not decreased. Option 4 is the only option that indicates an increased level of a renal function test. Review these adverse effects if you had difficulty with this question.
Level of Cognitive Ability: Analysis
Client Needs: Physiological Integrity
Integrated Process: Nursing Process/Data Collection

Content Area: Pharmacology
Reference: Lehne, R. (2007). *Pharmacology for nursing care* (6th ed., pp. 796, 801). Philadelphia: Saunders.

695. 3
Rationale: A compound present in grapefruit juice inhibits the metabolism of cyclosporine. As a result, consuming grapefruit juice can raise cyclosporine levels by 50% to 100%, thereby greatly increasing the risk of toxicity. Options 1, 2, and 4 do not need to be avoided.
Test-Taking Strategy: Note the strategic word "avoid." Knowledge regarding substances that inhibit the metabolism of cyclosporine is required to answer this question. Remember, grapefruit juice inhibits the metabolism of cyclosporine. Review this medication if you had difficulty with this question.
Level of Cognitive Ability: Application
Client Needs: Physiological Integrity
Integrated Process: Teaching and Learning
Content Area: Pharmacology
Reference: Lehne, R. (2007). *Pharmacology for nursing care* (6th ed., pp. 796, 801). Philadelphia: Saunders.

696. 2
Rationale: The most common adverse effects of cyclosporine are nephrotoxicity, infection, hypertension, tremor, and hirsutism. Of these, nephrotoxicity and infection are the most serious.
Test-Taking Strategy: Knowledge regarding the adverse effects associated with cyclosporine is required to answer this question. Remember that tremor is an indication of an adverse effect. Review these effects if you had difficulty with this question.
Level of Cognitive Ability: Analysis
Client Needs: Physiological Integrity
Integrated Process: Nursing Process/Data Collection

Content Area: Pharmacology
Reference: Lehne, R. (2007). *Pharmacology for nursing care* (6th ed., pp. 796, 801). Philadelphia: Saunders.

697. 2
Rationale: Nephrotoxicity is a major concern with this medication. Other common reactions include neurotoxicity evidenced by headache, tremor, and insomnia; gastrointestinal effects (such as diarrhea, nausea, and vomiting); hypertension; hyperkalemia; and hyperglycemia.
Test-Taking Strategy: Use the process of elimination, noting that options 1, 3, and 4 represent normal values. Option 2 is the only abnormal value reflecting an elevation. Review these normal laboratory values if you had difficulty with this question.
Level of Cognitive Ability: Analysis
Client Needs: Physiological Integrity
Integrated Process: Nursing Process/Data Collection
Content Area: Pharmacology
Reference: Skidmore-Roth, L. (2008). *2008 Mosby's nursing drug reference* (21st ed., pp. 940-941). St. Louis: Mosby.

698. 2
Rationale: Mycophenolate mofetil should be administered on an empty stomach. The capsules should not be opened or crushed. The client should contact the physician if unusual bleeding or bruising, sore throat, mouth sores, abdominal pain, or fever occurs. Antacids containing magnesium and aluminum may decrease the absorption of the medication and therefore should not be taken with the medication. The medication is given in combination with corticosteroids and cyclosporine.
Test-Taking Strategy: Knowledge regarding the teaching points associated with the administration of this medication is required to answer this question. Recalling that neutropenia can occur with this medication will direct you to option 2. Review this medication if you had difficulty with this question.
Level of Cognitive Ability: Application
Client Needs: Physiological Integrity
Integrated Process: Teaching and Learning
Content Area: Pharmacology
Reference: Skidmore-Roth, L. (2008). *2008 Mosby's nursing drug reference* (21st ed., pp. 708-709). St. Louis: Mosby.

699. 1
Rationale: Epoetin alfa is used to reverse anemia associated with CRF. A therapeutic effect is seen when the hematocrit is between 30% and 33%.
Test-Taking Strategy: Use the process of elimination. Relate the name of the medication, "Epogen," to the potential action or effect. The only laboratory test that would reflect the effect of this medication is identified in option 1. Review the therapeutic effect of this medication if you had difficulty with this question.
Level of Cognitive Ability: Analysis
Client Needs: Physiological Integrity
Integrated Process: Nursing Process/Evaluation
Content Area: Pharmacology
References: Chernecky, C., & Berger, B. (2008). *Laboratory tests and diagnostic procedures* (5th ed., pp. 615-616). Philadelphia: Saunders.

Kee, J., Hayes, E., & McCuistion, L. (2006). *Pharmacology: A nursing process approach* (5th ed., p. 559). Philadelphia: Saunders.
Skidmore-Roth, L. (2008). *2008 Mosby's nursing drug reference* (21st ed., p. 418). St. Louis: Mosby.

700. 4
Rationale: Epoetin alfa is generally well tolerated. The most significant adverse effect is hypertension. Occasionally, a tachycardia may occur as a side effect. It may also cause an improved sense of well-being, which is a positive effect.
Test-Taking Strategy: Knowledge regarding the significant adverse effect associated with epoetin alfa is required to answer this question. Noting that options 3 and 4 identify opposite conditions will assist in answering the question. Remember, hypertension is an adverse effect. Review this medication if you had difficulty with this question.
Level of Cognitive Ability: Analysis
Client Needs: Physiological Integrity
Integrated Process: Nursing Process/Data Collection
Content Area: Pharmacology
Reference: Lehne, R. (2007). *Pharmacology for nursing care* (6th ed., p. 638). Philadelphia: Saunders.

701. 3
Rationale: Cholinergic overdose can occur with bethanechol. The antidote is atropine sulfate administered subcutaneously or intravenously, which should be readily available for use should overdose occur. Protamine sulfate is the antidote for heparin. Vitamin K is the antidote for Coumadin. Mucomyst is the antidote for acetaminophen (Tylenol) overdose.
Test-Taking Strategy: Knowledge regarding the antidotes for certain medication overdoses is required to answer this question. Remember the antidote for this medication is atropine sulfate. Review these antidotes if you had difficulty with this question.
Level of Cognitive Ability: Application
Client Needs: Physiological Integrity
Integrated Process: Nursing Process/Implementation
Content Area: Pharmacology
Reference: Skidmore-Roth, L. (2008). *2008 Mosby's nursing drug reference* (21st ed., p. 182). St. Louis: Mosby.

702. 1
Rationale: Nalidixic acid is used for acute and chronic urinary tract infections, especially gram-negative bacterial infections. The medication is contraindicated in clients with a history of seizures. It is used with caution in clients with liver or renal disorders. Options 2, 3, and 4 are not contraindicated
Test-Taking Strategy: Knowledge regarding the contraindications associated with this medication is required to answer the question. Remember, nalidixic acid is contraindicated in clients with a history of seizures. Review this medication if you had difficulty with this question.
Level of Cognitive Ability: Application
Client Needs: Safe and Effective Care Environment
Integrated Process: Nursing Process/Implementation
Content Area: Pharmacology
Reference: Lehne, R. (2007). *Pharmacology for nursing care* (6th ed., p.1013). Philadelphia: Saunders.

703. 4
Rationale: Gastrointestinal effects are the most frequent adverse reactions to this medication and can be minimized by administering the medication with milk or meals. Pulmonary reactions, manifested as dyspnea, chest pain, chills, fever, cough, and the presence of alveolar infiltrates on the x-ray, would indicate the need to stop the treatment. These symptoms resolve in 2 to 4 days following discontinuation of this medication.
Test-Taking Strategy: Use the process of elimination. Eliminate options 1, 2, and 3 because they are gastrointestinal-related side effects. Also, use the ABCs—airway, breathing, and circulation—to direct you to option 4. Review this medication if you had difficulty with this question.
Level of Cognitive Ability: Analysis
Client Needs: Physiological Integrity
Integrated Process: Nursing Process/Data Collection
Content Area: Pharmacology
Reference: Lehne, R. (2007). *Pharmacology for nursing care* (6th ed., p. 1012). Philadelphia: Saunders.

704. 4
Rationale: Clients taking trimethoprim-sulfamethoxazole should be informed about early signs of blood disorders that can occur from this medication. These signs include sore throat, fever, or pallor, and the client should be instructed to notify the physician if these symptoms occur. The other options do not require physician notification.
Test-Taking Strategy: Focus on the subject—the symptoms to report. Recalling that this medication can cause blood dyscrasias will direct you to option 4. Review this medication if you had difficulty with this question.
Level of Cognitive Ability: Application
Client Needs: Physiological Integrity
Integrated Process: Nursing Process/Implementation
Content Area: Pharmacology
Reference: Kee, J., Hayes, E., & McCuistion, L. (2006). *Pharmacology: A nursing process approach* (5th ed., pp. 456, 458). Philadelphia: Saunders.

705. 4
Rationale: The client should be instructed that a reddish-orange discoloration of urine may occur. The client should also be instructed that this discoloration can stain fabric. The medication should be taken after meals to reduce the possibility of gastrointestinal upset. A headache is an occasional side effect of the medication and does not warrant discontinuation of the medication.
Test-Taking Strategy: Use the process of elimination. Eliminate options 1 and 3 first because they are comparable or alike. From the remaining options, eliminate option 2 because the nurse would not advise the client to discontinue

this medication. Review this medication if you had difficulty with this question.
Level of Cognitive Ability: Application
Client Needs: Health Promotion and Maintenance
Integrated Process: Nursing Process/Implementation
Content Area: Pharmacology
Reference: Skidmore-Roth, L. (2008). *2008 Mosby's nursing drug reference* (21st ed., p. 811). St. Louis: Mosby.

706. 2
Rationale: Urecholine can be hazardous to clients with urinary tract obstruction or weakness of the bladder wall. The medication has the ability to contract the bladder and thereby increase pressure within the urinary tract. Elevation of pressure within the urinary tract could rupture the bladder in clients with these conditions. Options 1, 2, and 4 are not contraindicated.
Test-Taking Strategy: Focus on the data in the question. Noting that the medication is used for urinary retention will assist in directing you to option 2. Review this medication if you had difficulty with this question.
Level of Cognitive Ability: Analysis
Client Needs: Physiological Integrity
Integrated Process: Nursing Process/Data Collection
Content Area: Pharmacology
Reference: Skidmore-Roth, L. (2008). *2008 Mosby's nursing drug reference* (21st ed., pp. 181-182). St. Louis: Mosby.

ALTERNATE ITEM FORMAT: CHART/EXHIBIT
707. 1
Rationale: Cinoxacin should be administered with caution in clients with renal impairment. The dosage should be reduced, and failure to do so could result in accumulation of cinoxacin to toxic levels. Therefore, the nurse would verify the prescription with the physician if the client had a documented history of renal insufficiency. The laboratory test result and diagnostic test result are normal findings. Folic acid (vitamin B_6) may be prescribed for a client with renal insufficiency to prevent anemia.
Test-Taking Strategy: Focus on the subject: the need to contact the physician. Eliminate options 3 and 4 because the laboratory test result and diagnostic test result are normal findings. From the remaining options, note the disorder in the client's history. This will direct you to option 1. Review the contraindications associated with this medication if you had difficulty with this question.
Level of Cognitive Ability: Analysis
Client Needs: Physiological Integrity
Integrated Process: Nursing Process/Data Collection
Content Area: Pharmacology
Reference: Lehne, R. (2007). *Pharmacology for nursing care* (6th ed., p. 1013). Philadelphia: Saunders.

REFERENCES

Chernecky, C., & Berger, B. (2008). *Laboratory tests and diagnostic procedures* (5th ed.). Philadelphia: Saunders.

Hodgson, B., & Kizior, R. (2008). *Saunders nursing drug handbook 2008*. Philadelphia: Saunders.

Kee, J., Hayes, E., & McCuistion, L. (2006). *Pharmacology: A nursing process approach* (5th ed.). Philadelphia: Saunders.

Lehne, R. (2007). *Pharmacology for nursing care* (6th ed.). Philadelphia: Saunders.

Skidmore-Roth, L. (2008). *2008 Mosby's nursing drug reference* (21st ed.). St. Louis: Mosby.

The Adult Client With an Eye or Ear Disorder

PYRAMID TERMS

accommodation Process by which a clear visual image is maintained as the gaze is shifted from a distant to a near point

astigmatism A condition that results from an uneven curvature of the cornea or lens in which light rays do not focus on a single point on the retina

cataract An opacity of the lens that distorts the image projected onto the retina and that can progress to blindness

conductive hearing loss A mechanical dysfunction or blockage of sound waves to the inner ear fibers because of external ear or middle ear disorders; the blockage can be caused by impacted cerumen, foreign bodies, pus, or serum in the middle ear; disorders can often be corrected with no damage to hearing or minimal permanent hearing loss

cycloplegia The paralysis of the ciliary muscles by medications that block muscarinic receptors; cycloplegia causes blurred vision because the shape of the lens can no longer be adjusted to near vision.

fenestration Removal of the stapes with a small hole drilled in the footplate and connection of a prosthesis between the incus and footplate; sounds cause the prosthesis to vibrate in the same manner as did the stapes

glaucoma Increased intraocular pressure as a result of inadequate drainage of aqueous humor from the canal of Schlemm or from overproduction of aqueous humor; the condition damages the optic nerve and can result in blindness

hyperopia Farsightedness; objects converge to a point behind the retina; vision beyond 20 feet is normal, but near vision is poor; correction is done by a convex lens

legally blind The best visual acuity with corrective lenses in the better eye of 20/200 or less, or visual acuity of less than 20 degrees of the visual field in the better eye

macular degeneration A blurred central vision caused by progressive degeneration of the center of the retina; condition may be atrophic or age related, or dry or exudative (wet).

Meniere's syndrome A syndrome also called endolymphatic hydrops that refers to dilation of the endolymphatic system by overproduction or decreased reabsorption of endolymphatic fluid; the syndrome is characterized by tinnitus, unilateral sensorineural hearing loss, and vertigo

miosis A constricted and fixed pupil achieved primarily by stimulation of the muscarinic receptors of the sphincter muscles; occurs with the use of pilocarpine drops when treating glaucoma, when using opioids, or when there is brain damage of the pons

miotics Medications that cause contraction of the pupil

mydriasis A dilated pupil achieved by blockage of the muscarinic receptors of the sphincter muscles or by stimulation of the α receptors of the dilator muscles; enlarged pupils occur with stimulation of the sympathetic nervous system, use of dilating drops, acute glaucoma, or past or recent trauma

mydriatics Medications that dilate the pupil

myopia Nearsightedness; rays coming from an object are focused in front of the retina; near vision is normal, but distant vision is defective; a biconcave lens is used for correction

otosclerosis Disease of the labyrinthine capsule of the middle ear that results in a bony overgrowth of tissue surrounding the ossicles; causes the development of irregular areas of new bone formation and causes fixation of the bones; stapes fixation leads to a conductive hearing loss

presbycusis Gradual nerve degeneration associated with aging and is a common cause of sensorineural hearing loss

retinal detachment Separation of the layers of the retina because of the accumulation of fluid between them or because both retinal layers elevate away from the choroid as a result of a tumor; partial separation becomes complete if untreated; when detachment becomes complete, blindness occurs

sensorineural hearing loss A pathological process of the inner ear or of the sensory fibers that lead to the cerebral cortex; such hearing loss is often permanent, and measures must be taken to reduce further damage or to attempt to amplify sound as a means of improving hearing to some degree

PYRAMID TO SUCCESS

Pyramid points focus on nursing interventions for clients with impairment in sight or hearing and on the nursing care related to disorders such as cataracts, glaucoma, and retinal detachment. Pyramid points also focus on emergency interventions for eye and ear disorders and injuries. Review nursing care related to organ donation for the donor and recipient. Pyramid points also focus on client instructions related to medication administration, sensory perceptual alterations and safety issues, and available support systems. The Integrated Processes addressed in this unit include Caring, Clinical Problem-Solving Process (Nursing Process), Communication and Documentation, and Teaching and Learning.

▲ CLIENT NEEDS

Safe and Effective Care Environment

Caring for the recipient of a tissue (corneal) donation
Consulting with members of the health care team
Establishing priorities
Maintaining asepsis with procedures and treatments
Maintaining standard and other precautions
Obtaining informed consent for invasive procedures
Preventing accidents that can occur as a result of sensory impairments
Upholding client rights

Health Promotion and Maintenance

Discussing changes that occur with the aging process
Discussing expected body-image changes and self-care deficits
Implementing measures for the prevention and early detection of health problems and diseases related to the eye and the ear
Performing data dollection techniques for eye and ear disorders
Providing home care instructions following procedures related to the eye and ear
Providing instructions regarding the administration of eye and ear medications
Providing instructions regarding activity limitations or postoperative activities
Teaching the importance of compliance to the prescribed therapy

Psychosocial Integrity

Assessing the client's ability to cope with feelings of isolation, fear, or anxiety regarding a possible change in vision and/or hearing status, and loss of independence
Discussing role changes

Identifying family support systems
Informing the client about available community resources
Monitoring for sensory perceptual alterations
Using appropriate communication techniques for impaired vision and hearing

Physiological Integrity

Monitoring for complications related to procedures
Monitoring for expected responses to therapy
Providing care to assistive devices such as glasses, contact lenses, and hearing aids
Taking action in medical emergencies

REFERENCES

Black, J., & Hawks, J. (2005). *Medical-surgical nursing: Clinical management for positive outcomes* (7th ed.). Philadelphia: Saunders.

Chernecky, C., & Berger, B. (2008). *Laboratory tests and diagnostic procedures* (5th ed.). Philadelphia: Saunders.

Christensen, B., & Kockrow, E. (2006). *Adult health nursing* (5th ed.). St. Louis: Mosby.

Christensen, B., & Kockrow, E. (2006). *Foundations of nursing* (5th ed.). St. Louis: Mosby.

deWit, S. (2009). *Medical-surgical nursing: Concepts & practice.* Philadelphia: Saunders.

Hodgson, B., & Kizior, R. (2008). *Saunders nursing drug handbook 2008.* Philadelphia: Saunders.

Ignatavicius, D., & Workman, M. (2006). *Medical-surgical nursing: Critical thinking for collaborative care* (5th ed.). Philadelphia: Saunders.

Kee, J., Hayes, E., & McCuistion, L. (2006). *Pharmacology: A nursing process approach* (5th ed.). Philadelphia: Saunders.

Lehne, R. (2007). *Pharmacology for nursing care* (6th ed.). Philadelphia: Saunders.

Lewis, S., Heitkemper, M., Dirksen, S., & Bucher, L. (2007). *Medical-surgical nursing: Assessment and management of clinical problems* (7th ed.). St. Louis: Mosby.

Linton, A., & Maebius, N. (2007). *Introduction to medical-surgical nursing* (4th ed.). Philadelphia: Saunders.

McKenry, L., Tessier, E., & Hogan, M. (2006). *Mosby's pharmacology in nursing* (22nd ed.). St. Louis: Mosby.

Monahan, F., Sands, J., Neighbors, M., Marek, J., & Green, C. (2007). *Phipps' medical-surgical nursing: Health and illness perspectives* (8th ed.). St. Louis: Mosby.

National Council of State Boards of Nursing (eds.) (2008). *2008 Detailed Test Plan for the NCLEX-PN® Examination, National Council of State Boards of Nursing.* Chicago: Author.

National Council of State Boards of Nursing. Inc. Web site: http://www.ncsbn.org.

Perry, A., & Potter, P. (2006). *Clinical nursing skills & techniques* (6th ed.). St. Louis: Mosby.

Skidmore-Roth, L. (2008). *2008 Mosby's nursing drug reference* (21st ed.). St. Louis: Mosby.

The Eye and the Ear

I. ANATOMY AND PHYSIOLOGY OF THE EYE

A. The eye
   1. Is 1 inch in diameter and is located in the anterior portion of the orbit
   2. The orbit is the bony structure of the skull that surrounds the eye and offers protection to the eye

B. Layers of the eye
   1. External layer
      a. The fibrous coat that supports the eye
      b. Contains the sclera, which is an opaque white tissue
      c. Contains the cornea, which is a dense transparent layer
   2. Middle layer
      a. The second layer of the eyeball
      b. Is vascular and heavily pigmented
      c. Consists of the choroid, the ciliary body, and the iris
      d. The choroid is the dark brown membrane located between the sclera and the retina that has dark pigmentation to prevent light from reflecting internally
      e. The choroid lines most of the sclera and is attached to the retina but can detach easily from the sclera
      f. The choroid contains many blood vessels and supplies nutrients to the retina
      g. The ciliary body connects the choroid with the iris and secretes aqueous humor that helps give the eye its shape; the muscles of the ciliary body control the thickness of the lens
      h. The iris is the colored portion of the eye, is located in front of the lens, and has a central circular opening called the pupil; the pupil controls the amount of light admitted into the retina (darkness produces dilation and light produces constriction)
   3. Internal layer
      a. Consists of the retina, a thin, delicate structure in which the fibers of the optic nerve are distributed
      b. The retina is bordered externally by the choroid and sclera and internally by the vitreous
      c. The retina is the visual receptive layer of the eye in which light waves are changed into nerve impulses and contains blood vessels and photoreceptors called rods and cones

C. Vitreous body
   1. Contains a gelatinous substance that occupies the vitreous chamber, which is the space between the lens and the retina
   2. The vitreous body transmits light and gives shape to the posterior eye

D. Vitreous: a gel-like substance that maintains the shape of the eye and provides additional physical support to the retina

E. Rods and cones
   1. Rods are responsible for peripheral vision and function at reduced levels of illumination
   2. Cones function at bright levels of illumination and are responsible for color vision and central vision

F. Optic disc
   1. The optic disc is a creamy pink to white depressed area in the retina
   2. The optic nerve enters and exits the eyeball at this area
   3. This area is called the blind spot because it contains only nerve fibers, lacks photoreceptor cells, and is insensitive to light

G. Macula lutea
   1. A small, oval, yellowish-pink area located lateral and temporal to the optic disc
   2. The central depressed part of the macula is the fovea centralis, the area of sharpest and keenest vision, where most acute vision occurs

H. Aqueous humor
   1. The aqueous humor is a clear watery fluid that fills the anterior and posterior chambers of the eye
   2. The aqueous humor is produced by the ciliary processes, and the fluid drains into the canal of Schlemm

3. The anterior chamber lies between the cornea and the iris
4. The posterior chamber lies between the iris and the lens

I. Canal of Schlemm: a passageway that extends completely around the eye that permits fluid to drain out of the eye into the systemic circulation so that a constant intraocular pressure is maintained

J. Lens
   1. A transparent convex structure behind the iris and in front of the vitreous body
   2. The lens bends rays of light so that the light falls on the retina
   3. The curve of the lens changes to focus on near or distant objects

K. Conjunctiva: the thin transparent mucous membrane of the eye that lines the posterior surface of each eyelid and is located over the sclera

L. Lacrimal gland
   1. The lacrimal gland produces tears
   2. Tears are drained through the punctum into the lacrimal duct and sac

M. Eye muscles
   1. Muscles do not work independently but work with the muscle that produces the opposite movement
   2. Rectus muscles exert their pull when the eye turns temporally
   3. Oblique muscles exert their pull when the eye turns nasally

N. Nerves
   1. Cranial nerve II: optic nerve (nerve of sight)
   2. Cranial nerve III: oculomotor
   3. Cranial nerve IV: trochlear
   4. Cranial nerve VI: abducens

O. Blood vessels
   1. The ophthalmic artery is the major artery supplying the structures in the eye
   2. The ophthalmic veins drain the blood from the eye

II. ASSESSMENT OF VISION (Box 54-1)
A. Acuity
   1. Visual acuity tests measure the client's distance and near vision
   2. Snellen's chart or "eye chart"
      a. The chart is a simple tool to measure distance vision

---

BOX 54-1 **Assessment of Vision**

Color vision
Confrontational test
Extraocular muscle function
Ophthalmoscopy
Snellen's chart

---

b. The client stands 20 feet from the chart and covers one eye and uses the other eye to read the line that appears most clearly
c. If the client is able to do this accurately, the client reads the next lower line
d. This sequence is repeated until the client is unable to identify correctly more than half of the characters on the line
e. The procedure is repeated for the other eye; then both eyes together may be tested
f. The findings are recorded as a comparison between what the client can read at 20 feet and the distance at which an individual with normal vision can read the same line
g. A result of 20/50 means that the client is able to read at 20 feet from the chart what a healthy eye can read at 50 feet
h. Clients who wear corrective lenses other than for reading should have their vision tested with the lens in place

B. Confrontational test
   1. The confrontational test is performed to examine visual fields or peripheral vision
   2. The examiner and the client sit facing each other
   3. The client is asked to look directly into the eyes of the examiner throughout the test
   4. The examiner covers his or her right eye while the client covers his or her left eye (the client covers the eye directly opposite to the examiner's covered eye)
   5. The examiner moves a finger from a nonvisible area into the client's line of vision
   6. The examiner and client should see the object at approximately the same time
   7. When the client sees the object coming into the line of vision, the client informs the examiner
   8. The procedure is repeated on the opposite eye
   9. The test assumes that the examiner has normal peripheral vision

C. Extraocular muscle function
   1. The six muscles that attach the eyeball to its orbit and serve to direct the eye to points of interest are tested
   2. Six cardinal positions of gaze include the following
      a. Client's right (lateral position)
      b. Upward and right (temporal position)
      c. Down and right
      d. Client's left (lateral position)
      e. Upward and left (temporal position)
      f. Down and left
   3. Client holds head still and is asked to move eyes and to follow a small object
   4. The examiner monitors for any parallel movements of the eye or for nystagmus, an involuntary rhythmic rapid twitching of the eyeballs.

D. Color vision
1. Tests for color vision involve picking numbers or letters out of a complex and colorful picture
2. Ishihara chart
   a. The Ishihara chart consists of numbers that are composed of colored dots located within a circle of colored dots
   b. The client is asked to read the numbers on the chart
   c. Each eye is tested separately
   d. Reading the numbers correctly indicates normal color vision
   e. The test is sensitive for the diagnosis of red/green blindness but is not effective for the detection of the discrimination of blue

▲ E. Pupils
1. The pupils are round and of equal size
2. Increasing light causes pupillary constriction
3. Decreasing light causes pupillary dilation
4. Constriction of both pupils is a normal response to direct light
5. The client is asked to look straight ahead while the examiner quickly brings a beam of light (flashlight) in from the side and directs it onto the eye
6. The constriction of the eye is a direct response to the shining of a light into that eye; constriction of the opposite eye is known as a consensual response

F. Sclera and cornea
1. Normal sclera color is white
▲ 2. A yellow sclera may indicate jaundice or systemic problems
▲ 3. In a dark-skinned person, the sclera may normally appear yellow; pigmented dots may be present
4. The cornea is transparent, smooth, shiny, and bright
5. Cloudy areas or specks on the cornea may be the result of an accident or eye injury

▲ G. Ophthalmoscopy
1. The ophthalmoscope is an instrument used to examine the external structures and the interior of the eye
2. The room is darkened so that the pupil will dilate
3. The instrument is held with the right hand when examining the right eye and with the left hand when examining the left eye
4. The client is asked to look straight ahead at an object on the wall
5. The examiner should approach the client's eye from about 12 to 15 inches away and 15 degrees lateral to the client's line of vision
6. As the instrument is directed at the pupil, a red glare (red reflex) is seen in the pupil

7. The red reflex is the reflection of light on the vascular retina
8. Absence of the red reflex may indicate opacity of the lens
9. The retina, optic disc, optic vessels, fundus, and macula can be examined

III. DIAGNOSTIC TESTS FOR THE EYE (Box 54-2)
A. Fluorescein angiography
1. Description
   a. A detailed imaging and recording of ocular circulation by a series of photographs after the administration of a dye
   b. This test is useful for assessing problems with retinal circulation, such as those that occur in diabetic retinopathy, retinal bleeding, and **macular degeneration,** or to rule out intraocular tumors
2. Preprocedure interventions
   a. Assess the client for allergies and previous reactions to dyes
   b. Obtain informed consent
   c. A mydriatic medication, which causes pupil dilation, is instilled into the eye 1 hour before the test
   d. The dye is injected into a vein of the client's arm
   e. Inform the client that the dye may cause the skin to appear yellow for several hours after the test and is eliminated gradually through the urine
   f. The client may experience nausea, vomiting, sneezing, paresthesia of the tongue, or pain at the injection site
   g. If hives appear, orally or intramuscularly administered antihistamines such as diphenhydramine (Benadryl) are given as prescribed
3. Postprocedure interventions
   a. Encourage rest
   b. Encourage fluid intake to assist in eliminating the dye from the client's system
   c. Remind the client that the yellow skin appearance will disappear
   d. Inform the client that the urine will appear bright green until the dye is excreted
   e. Advise the client to avoid direct sunlight for a few hours after the test and to wear sunglasses if staying inside is not possible

---

BOX 54-2   **Diagnostic Tests for the Eye**

Computed tomography
Corneal staining
Fluorescein angiography
Slit lamp
Tonometry

f. Inform the client that the photophobia will continue until pupil size returns to normal

B. Computed tomography
  1. Description
     a. The test is performed to examine the eyes, the bony structures around the eye, and the extraocular muscles
     b. A beam of x-rays scans the skull and orbits of the eye
     c. A cross-sectional image is formed by the use of a computer
     d. Contrast material may be used unless eye trauma is suspected
  2. Interventions
     a. No special client preparation or follow-up care is required
     b. Instruct the client that he or she will be positioned in a confined space and will need to keep his or her head still during the procedure

▲ C. Slit lamp
  1. Description
     a. A slit lamp allows examination of the anterior ocular structures under microscopic magnification
     b. The client leans on a chin rest to stabilize the head while a narrowed beam of light is aimed so that it illuminates only a narrow segment of the eye
  2. Interventions
     a. Explain the procedure the client
     b. Advise the client about the brightness of the light and the need to look forward at a point over the examiner's ear

▲ D. Corneal staining
  1. Description
     a. A topical dye is instilled into the conjuctival sac to outline irregularities of the corneal surface that are not easily visible
     b. The eye is viewed through a blue filter, and a bright green color indicates areas of a nonintact corneal epithelium
  2. Interventions
     a. If the client wears contact lenses, the lenses must be removed
     b. The client is instructed to blink after the dye has been applied to distribute the dye evenly across the cornea

▲ E. Tonometry
  1. Description
     a. The test is used primarily to assess for an increase of intraocular pressure and potential **glaucoma**
     b. Normal intraocular pressure is 10 to 21 mm Hg; intraocular pressure varies throughout the day and is normally higher in the morning (always document the time of intraocular pressure measurement)
  2. Noncontact tonometry measurement
     a. No direct contact with the client's cornea is needed and no topical eye anesthetic is needed
     b. A puff of air is directed at the cornea to indent the cornea, which can be unpleasant and may startle the client
     c. It is a less accurate method of measurement compared with contact tonometry measurement
  3. Contact tonometry measurement
     a. Requires a topical anesthetic
     b. A flattened cone is brought in contact with the cornea, and the amount of pressure needed to flatten the cornea is measured
     c. The client must be instructed to avoid rubbing the eye following the examination if the eye has been anesthetized because the potential for scratching the cornea exists

IV. DISORDERS OF THE EYE
A. Risk factors related to eye disorders (Box 54-3)
B. Refractive errors
  1. Description
     a. Refraction is the bending of light rays; any problem associated with either eye length or refraction can lead to refractive errors
     b. **Myopia** (nearsightedness): refractive ability of the eye is too strong for the eye length; images are bent and fall in front of, not on, the retina
     c. **Hyperopia** (farsightedness): refractive ability of the eye is too weak; images are focused behind the retina
     d. Presbyopia: loss of lens elasticity caused by aging; less able to focus the eye for close work and images fall behind the retina
     e. **Astigmatism**: occurs because of the irregular curvature of the cornea; image does not focus on the retina
  2. Data collection
     a. Refractive errors are diagnosed through a process called refraction
     b. The client views an eye chart while various lenses of different strengths are systematically placed in front of the eye and is asked

---

BOX 54-3 **Risk Factors of Eye Disorders**

Aging process
Congenital
Diabetes mellitus
Hereditary
Medications
Trauma

whether each lens sharpens or worsens the vision

3. Non-surgical interventions: eyeglasses or contact lenses
4. Surgical interventions
   a. Radial keratotomy: incisions are made through the peripheral cornea to flatten the cornea, which allows the image to be focused closer to the retina; used to treat **myopia**
   b. Photorefractive keratotomy: a laser beam is used to remove small portions of the corneal surface to reshape the cornea to focus an image properly on the retina; used to treat **myopia** and **astigmatism**
   c. Laser in-situ keratomileusis (LASIK): the superficial layers of the cornea are lifted as a flap, a laser reshapes the deeper corneal layers, then the corneal flap is replaced; used to treat **hyperopia, myopia,** and **astigmatism**
   d. Intrastromal corneal rings (Intacs): the shape of the cornea is changed by placing a flexible ring in the outer edges of the cornea; used to treat **myopia**

C. **Legally blind**
   1. Description: the best visual acuity with corrective lenses in the better eye of 20/200 or less or visual acuity of less than 20 degrees of the visual field in the better eye
   2. Interventions
      a. When speaking to the client who has limited sight or is blind, the nurse uses a normal tone of voice
      b. Alert the client when approaching
      c. Orient the client to the environment
      d. Use a focal point and provide further orientation to the environment from that focal point
      e. Allow the client to touch objects in the room
      f. Use the clock placement of foods on the meal tray to orient the client
      g. Promote independence as much as possible
      h. Provide radios, televisions, and clocks that give the time orally, or provide a braille watch
      i. When ambulating, allow the client to grasp the nurse's arm at the elbow; the nurse keeps his or her arm close to the body so that the client can detect the direction of movement
      j. Instruct the client to remain one step behind the nurse when ambulating
      k. Instruct the client in the use of the cane used for the blind client, which is differentiated from other canes by its straight shape and white color with red tip
      l. Instruct the client that the cane is held in the dominant hand several inches off the floor
      m. Instruct the client that the cane sweeps the ground where the client's foot will be placed next to determine the presence of obstacles

D. Cataracts (Figure 54-1)
   1. Description
      a. A **cataract** is an opacity of the lens that distorts the image projected onto the retina and that can progress to blindness
      b. Causes include the aging process (senile cataracts), heredity (congenital cataracts), and injury (traumatic cataracts); cataracts can also result from another eye disease (secondary cataracts).
      c. Intervention is indicated when visual acuity has been reduced to a level that the client finds to be unacceptable or adversely affects lifestyle
   2. Data collection
      a. Blurred vision and decreased color perception are early signs
      b. Diplopia, reduced visual acuity, absence of the red reflex, and the presence of a white pupil are late signs
      c. Pain or eye redness is associated with age-related **cataract** formation
      d. Loss of vision is gradual
   3. Interventions
      a. Surgical removal of the lens, one eye at a time, is performed
      b. With extracapsular extraction, the lens is lifted out without removing the lens capsule; the procedure may be performed by phacoemulsification, in which the lens is broken up by ultrasonic vibrations and is extracted

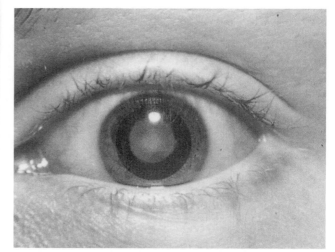

FIG. 54-1 The cloudy appearance of a lens affected by cataract. (From Black, J., & Hawks, J. [2005]. *Medical-surgical nursing: Clinical management for positive outcomes* [7th ed.]. Philadelphia: Saunders. Courtesy of Opthalmic Photography at the University of Michigan W.K. Kellogg Eye Center, Ann Arbor, MI.)

c. With intracapsular extraction, the lens and capsule are removed completely

d. A partial iridectomy may be performed with the lens extraction to prevent acute secondary **glaucoma**

e. A lens implantation may be performed at the time of the surgical procedure

4. Preoperative interventions

a. Instruct the client regarding the postoperative measures to prevent or decrease intraocular pressure

b. Stress to the client that care after surgery requires instillation of different types of eye drops several times a day for 2 to 4 weeks

c. Administer eye medications preoperatively, including **mydriatics** and cycloplegics as prescribed

5. Postoperative interventions

a. Elevate the head of the bed 30 to 45 degrees

b. Turn the client to the back or nonoperative side

c. Provide an eye patch as prescribed; orient the client to the environment

d. Position the client's personal belongings to the nonoperative side

e. Use side rails for safety

f. Assist with ambulation

6. Client education (Box 54-4)

E. **Glaucoma**

1. Description

a. A group of ocular diseases resulting in increased intraocular pressure

---

BOX 54-4 Client Education Following Cataract Surgery

Avoid eye straining.

Avoid rubbing or placing pressure on the eyes.

Avoid rapid movements, straining, sneezing, coughing, bending, vomiting, or lifting objects of more than 5 lb.

Take measures to prevent constipation.

Follow instructions for dressing changes and prescribed eye drops and medications.

Wipe excess drainage or tearing with a sterile wet cotton ball from the inner to the outward canthus.

Use an eye shield at bedtime.

If a lens implant is not performed, accomodation is affected and glasses must be worn at all times.

Cataract glasses act as magnifying glasses and replace central vision only.

Because cataract glasses magnify, objects will appear closer; therefore, the client needs to accommodate, judge distance, and climb stairs carefully.

Contact lenses provide sharp visual acuity, but dexterity is needed to insert them.

Contact the physician for any decrease in vision, severe eye pain, or increase in eye discharge.

---

b. Intraocular pressure is the fluid (aqueous humor) pressure within the eye (normal intraocular pressure is 10 to 21 mm Hg)

c. Increased intraocular pressure results from inadequate drainage of aqueous humor from the canal of Schlemm or overproduction of aqueous humor

d. The condition damages the optic nerve and can result in blindness

e. The gradual loss of visual fields may go unnoticed because central vision is unaffected

2. Types

a. Acute closed- or narrow-angle **glaucoma** results from obstruction to outflow to aqueous humor

b. Chronic closed-angle **glaucoma** follows an untreated attack of acute closed-angle **glaucoma**

c. Chronic open-angle **glaucoma** results from overproduction or obstruction to the outflow of aqueous humor

d. Acute **glaucoma** is a rapid onset of intraocular pressure greater than 50 to 70 mm Hg

e. Chronic **glaucoma** is a slow, progressive, gradual onset of intraocular pressure greater than 30 to 50 mm Hg

3. Data collection

a. Early signs include diminished **accommodation** and increased intraocular pressure

b. Late signs include loss of peripheral vision, decreased visual acuity not correctable with glasses, and halos around lights; headache or eye pain occurs with acute closed-angle **glaucoma**

4. Interventions for acute **glaucoma**

a. Treat acute **glaucoma** as a medical emergency

b. Administer medications as prescribed to lower intraocular pressure

c. Prepare the client for peripheral iridectomy, which allows aqueous humor to flow from the posterior to the anterior chamber

5. Interventions for chronic **glaucoma**

a. Instruct the client on the importance of medications (**miotics**) to constrict the pupils, carbonic anhydrase inhibitors to decrease the production of aqueous humor, and β-blockers to decrease the production of aqueous humor and intraocular pressure

b. Instruct the client on the need for lifelong medication use

c. Instruct the client to wear a Medic-Alert bracelet

d. Instruct the client to avoid anticholinergic medications

e. Instruct the client to report eye pain, halos around the eyes, and changes in vision to the physician

f. Instruct the client that when maximal medical therapy has failed to halt the progression of visual field loss and optic nerve damage, surgery will be recommended

g. Prepare the client for trabeculoplasty as prescribed to facilitate aqueous humor drainage

h. Prepare the client for trabeculectomy as prescribed, which allows drainage of aqueous humor into the conjunctival spaces by the creation of an opening

F. **Retinal detachment**

1. Description
   a. Detachment or separation of the retina from the epithelium
   b. **Retinal detachment** occurs when the layers of the retina separate because of the accumulation of fluid between them, or when both retinal layers elevate away from the choroid as a result of a tumor
   c. Partial detachment becomes complete if untreated
   d. When detachment becomes complete, blindness occurs

2. Data collection
   a. Flashes of light
   b. Floaters or black spots (signs of bleeding)
   c. Increase in blurred vision
   d. Sense of a curtain being drawn over the eye
   e. Loss of a portion of the visual field

3. Immediate interventions
   a. Provide bedrest
   b. Cover both eyes with patches as prescribed to prevent further detachment
   c. Speak to the client before approaching
   d. Position the client's head as prescribed
   e. Protect the client from injury
   f. Avoid jerky head movements
   g. Minimize eye stress
   h. Prepare the client for a surgical procedure as prescribed

4. Surgical procedures
   a. Draining fluid from the subretinal space so that the retina can return to the normal position
   b. Sealing retinal breaks by cryosurgery, a cold probe applied to the sclera, to stimulate an inflammatory response leading to adhesions
   c. Diathermy, the use of an electrode needle and heat through the sclera, to stimulate an inflammatory response
   d. Laser therapy, to stimulate an inflammatory response and to seal small retinal tears before the detachment occurs

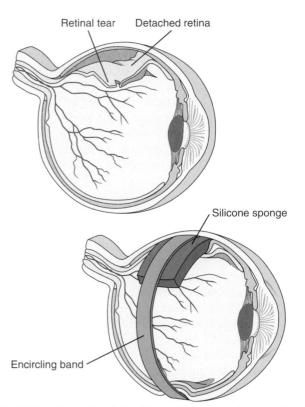

FIG. 54-2 The scleral buckling procedure for repair of retinal detachment. (From Ignatavicius, D., & Workman, M. [2006]. *Medical surgical nursing: Critical thinking for collaborative care* [5th ed.]. Philadelphia: Saunders.)

   e. Scleral buckling, to hold the choroid and retina together with a splint until scar tissue forms and closes the tear (Figure 54-2)
   f. Insertion of gas or silicone oil to promote reattachment; these agents float against the retina to hold it in place until healing occurs

5. Postoperative interventions
   a. Maintain eye patches as prescribed
   b. Monitor for hemorrhage
   c. Prevent nausea and vomiting and monitor for restlessness, which can cause hemorrhage
   d. Monitor for sudden, sharp eye pain (notify the physician)
   e. Encourage deep breathing but avoid coughing
   f. Provide bedrest for 1 to 2 days as prescribed
   g. Position the client as prescribed (positioning depends on the location of the detachment)
   h. Administer eye medications as prescribed
   i. Assist the client with activities of daily living
   j. Avoid sudden head movements or anything that increases intraocular pressure
   k. Instruct the client to limit reading for 3 to 5 weeks
   l. Instruct the client to avoid squinting, straining and constipation, lifting heavy objects, and bending from the waist

m. Instruct the client to wear dark glasses during the day and an eye patch at night

n. Encourage follow-up care because of the danger of recurrence or occurrence in the other eye

G. Macular degeneration

1. A deterioration of the macula, the area of central vision

2. Can be atrophic (age related or dry) or exudative (wet)

3. Age-related: caused by gradual blocking of retinal capillaries leading to an ischemic and necrotic macula; rods and cones photoreceptors die

4. Exudative: serous detachment of pigment epithelium in the macula occurs and fluid and blood collect under the macula, resulting in scar formation and visual distortion

5. Interventions are aimed at maximinzing the remaining vision

6. Data collection
   a. A decline in central vision
   b. Blurred vision and distortion

7. Interventions
   a. Initiate strategies to assist in maximizing remaining vision and maintaining independence
   b. Provide referrals to comminity organizations
   c. Laser therapy or photodynamic therapy may be prescribed to seal the leaking blood vessels in or near the macula

H. Ocular melanoma

1. Most common malignant eye tumor in adults

2. Tumor usually found in the uveal tract and can spread easily because of rich blood supply

3. Data collection
   a. Tumor can be discovered during routine examination
   b. If macular area is invaded, blurring of vision occurs
   c. Increased intraocular pressure is present if the canal of Schlemm is invaded
   d. Change of iris color is noted if the tumor invades the iris
   e. Ultrasonography may be performed to detect the tumor size and location

4. Interventions
   a. Enucleation: the entire eyeball is removed surgically and a ball implant is inserted to provide a base for socket prosthesis
   b. Radiation via a radioactive plaque that is sutured to the sclera; the radioactive plaque remains in place until the prescribed radiation dose is delivered

I. Enucleation and exenteration

1. Description
   a. Enucleation is the removal of the entire eyeball

BOX 54-5 Types of Eye Injuries

Chemical burn
Contusion
Foreign body
Hyphema
Penetrating object

---

   b. Exenteration is the removal of the eyeball and surrounding tissues and bone
   c. The procedures are performed for the removal of ocular tumors
   d. After the eye is removed, a ball implant is inserted to provide a firm base for socket prosthesis and to facilitate the best cosmetic result
   e. A prosthesis is fitted about 1 month after surgery

2. Preoperative interventions
   a. Provide emotional support to the client
   b. Encourage the client to verbalize feelings related to loss

3. Postoperative interventions
   a. Monitor vital signs
   b. Assess a pressure patch or dressing as prescribed
   c. Report changes in vital signs or the presence of bright red drainage on the pressure patch or dressing

J. Hyphema (Box 54-5)

1. Description
   a. The presence of blood in the anterior chamber that cccurs as a result of an injury
   b. The condition usually resolves in 5 to 7 days

2. Interventions
   a. Encourage rest with the client in the semi-Fowler's position
   b. Avoid sudden eye movements for 3 to 5 days to decrease the likelihood of bleeding
   c. Administer cycloplegic eye drops as prescribed to relax the eye muscles and place the eye at rest
   d. Instruct the client in the use of eye shields or eye patches as prescribed
   e. Instruct the client to restrict reading and limit watching television

K. Contusions (see Box 54-5)

1. Description
   a. Bleeding into the soft tissue as a result of an injury
   b. A contusion causes a black eye, and the discoloration disappears in about 10 days
   c. Pain, photophobia, edema, and diplopia may occur

2. Interventions
   a. Place ice on the eye immediately
   b. Instruct the client to receive a thorough eye examination
L. Foreign bodies (see Box 54-5)
   1. Description: an object such as dust or dirt that enters the eye and causes irritation
   2. Interventions
      a. Have the client look upward, expose the lower lid, wet a cotton-tipped applicator with sterile normal saline, and gently twist the swab over the particle, and remove it
      b. If the particle cannot be seen, have the client look downward, place a cotton applicator horizontally on the outer surface of the upper eye lid, grasp the lashes, and pull the upper lid outward and over the cotton applicator; if the particle is seen, gently twist a swab over it to remove
M. Penetrating objects (see Box 54-5)
   1. Description: an injury that occurs to the eye in which an object penetrates the eye
   2. Interventions
      a. Never remove the object since it may be holding ocular structures in place; the object must be removed by the physician
      b. Cover the object with a cup
      c. Do not allow the client to bend over or lie flat
      d. Do not place pressure on the eye
      e. Client is to be seen by a physician immediately
      f. X-rays and computed tomography (CT) scans of the orbit are usually performed
      g. Magnetic resonance imaging (MRI) is contraindicated because of the possibility of metal-containing projectile movement during the procedure
N. Chemical burns (see Box 54-5)
   1. Description: an eye injury in which a caustic substance enters the eye
   2. Interventions
      a. Treatment should begin immediately
      b. Flush the eyes at the scene of the injury with water for at least 15 to 20 minutes
      c. At the scene of the injury, obtain a sample of the chemical involved
      d. At the emergency department, the eye is irrigated with normal saline solution or an ophthalmic irrigation solution for at least 10 minutes
      e. The solution is directed across the cornea and toward the lateral canthus
      f. Prepare for visual acuity assessment
      g. Apply an antibiotic ointment as prescribed
      h. Cover the eye with a patch as prescribed

O. Eye (tissue) donation
   1. Donor eyes
      a. Donor eyes are obtained from cadavers
      b. Donor eyes must be enucleated soon after death because of rapid endothelial cell death
      c. Donor eyes must be stored in a preserving solution
      d. Storage, handling, and coordination of donor tissue with surgeons are provided by a network of state eye bank associations across the country
   2. Care to the deceased client as a potential eye donor
      a. Discuss the option of eye donation with the physician and family
      b. Raise the head of the bed 30 degrees
      c. Instill antibiotic eye drops as prescribed
      d. Close the eyes and apply a sterile gauze and a small ice pack to the closed eyes
   3. Preoperative care to the recipient of the cornea
      a. Recipient may be told of the tissue (cornea) availability only several hours to 1 day before the surgery
      b. Assist in alleviating client anxiety
      c. Assess the recipient's eye for signs of infection
      d. Report the presence of any redness, watery or purulent drainage, or edema around the recipient's eye to the physician
      e. Instill antibiotic drops into the recipient's eye as prescribed to reduce the number of microorganisms
      f. Administer fluids and medications intravenously as prescribed
   4. Postoperative care to the recipient
      a. Eye is covered with a pressure patch and protective shield that is left in place for 1 day
      b. Do not remove or change the dressing without a physician's order
      c. Monitor vital signs
      d. Monitor level of consciousness
      e. Assess the eye dressing
      f. Position the client with the head elevated and on the nonoperative side to reduce intraocular pressure
      g. Orient the client frequently
      h. Monitor for complications of bleeding, wound leakage, infection, and tissue rejection
      i. Instruct the client on how to apply a patch and eye shield
      j. Instruct the client to wear the eye shield at night for 1 month and whenever around small children or pets
      k. Advise the client not to rub the eye
   5. Graft rejection (Box 54-6)
      a. Rejection can occur at any time
      b. Inform the client of the signs of rejection

BOX 54-6 **Signs of Graft Rejection following Corneal Transplant:** *RSVP*

*R*edness
*S*welling
*V*isual acuity decreased
*P*ain

---

c. Signs include redness, swelling, decreased vision, and pain (RSVP)
d. The eye is treated with topical corticosteroids

V. ANATOMY AND PHYSIOLOGY OF THE EAR

A. Functions
   1. Hearing
   2. Maintenance of balance
B. External ear (pinna)
   1. The external ear is embedded in the temporal bone bilaterally at the level of the eyes
   2. The external ear extends from the auricle through the external canal to the tympanic membrane or eardrum
   3. The external ear includes the mastoid process, which is the bony ridge located over the temporal bone
C. Middle ear
   1. The middle ear consists of the medial side of the tympanic membrane
   2. The middle ear contains three bony ossicles
      a. Malleus
      b. Incus
      c. Stapes
   3. Functions of the middle ear
      a. Conduct sound vibrations from the outer ear to the central hearing apparatus in the inner ear
      b. Protect the inner ear by reducing the amplitude of loud sounds
      c. The eustachean tube allows equalization of air pressure on each side of the tympanic membrane so that the membrane does not rupture
D. Inner ear
   1. The inner ear contains the semicircular canals, the cochlea, and the distal end of the eighth cranial nerve
   2. The semicircular canals contain fluid and hair cells connected to sensory nerve fibers of the vestibular portion of the eighth cranial nerve
   3. The inner ear maintains sense of balance or equilibrium
   4. The cochlea is the spiral-shaped organ of hearing
   5. The organ of Corti (within the cochlea) is the receptor and organ of hearing

---

BOX 54-7   **Assessment of Hearing**

Otoscopic Examination
Tuning Fork Tests
Rinne tuning fork test
Weber tuning fork test
Vestibular Assessment
Gaze nystagmus evaluation
Hallpike's maneuver
Test for falling
Test for past pointing
Tests for Hearing
Voice test
Watch test

---

   6. Eighth cranial nerve
      a. The cochlear branch of the nerve transmits neuroimpulses from the cochlea to the brain where they are interpreted as sound
      b. The vestibular branch maintains balance and equilibrium
E. Hearing and equilibrium
   1. The external ear conducts sound waves to the middle ear
   2. The middle ear, also called the tympanic cavity, conducts sound waves to the inner ear
   3. The middle ear is filled with air, which is kept at atmospheric pressure by the opening of the eustachian tube
   4. The inner ear contains sensory receptors for sound and for equilibrium
   5. The receptors in the inner ear transmit sound waves and changes in body position to the nerve impulses

VI. ASSESSMENT OF THE EAR (Box 54-7)

A. Otoscopic examination
   1. The speculum is never introduced blindly into the external canal because of the risk of perforating the tympanic membrane
   2. The client's head is tilted slightly away and the otoscope is held upside down as if it were a large pen, since this permits the examiner's hand to lay against the client's head for support
   3. Pull the pinna up and back to straighten the external canal in an adult
   4. Visualize the external canal while slowly inserting the speculum
   5. The normal external canal is pink and intact without lesions and with various amounts of cerumen and fine little hairs
   6. Assess the tympanic membrane for intactness; the normal tympanic membrane is intact, without perforations, and should be free from lesions
   7. The tympanic membrane is transparent, opaque, pearly gray, and slightly concave

B. Auditory assessment
 1. Sound is transmitted by air conduction and bone conduction
 2. Air conduction takes two to three times longer than bone conduction
 3. Hearing loss is categorized as conductive, sensorineural, and mixed conductive and sensorineural
 4. **Conductive hearing loss** is due to any physical obstruction to the transmission of sound waves.
 5. **Sensorineural hearing loss** is due to a defect in the cochlea, in the eighth cranial nerve, or in the brain itself
 6. A mixed **conductives/ensorineural hearing loss** results in profound hearing loss
C. Voice test
 1. Ask the client to block one external canal
 2. The examiner stands 1 to 2 feet away and whispers a statement
 3. The client is asked to repeat the whispered statement
 4. Each ear is tested separately
D. Watch test
 1. A ticking watch is used to test for high frequency sounds
 2. The examiner holds a ticking watch about 5 inches from each ear and asks the client if the ticking is heard
E. Tuning fork tests
 1. Weber tuning fork test
  a. Place the vibrating tuning fork stem in the middle of the client's head, at the midline of the forehead, or above the upper lip over the teeth
  b. Hold the fork by the stem only
  c. The client is asked whether the sound is heard equally in both ears or whether the sound is louder in one ear
  d. Normal test result is hearing the sound equally in both ears
  e. If the client hears the sound louder in one ear, the term *lateralization* is applied to the side hearing the loudest
  f. Such a finding may indicate that the client has a **conductive hearing loss** in the ear to which the sound is lateralized or that **sensorineural hearing loss** has occurred in the opposite ear
 2. Rinne tuning fork test
  a. The test compares the client's hearing by air conduction and bone conduction
  b. Air conduction is two to three times longer than bone conduction
  c. The vibrating tuning fork stem is placed on the client's mastoid process and the client is asked to indicate when he or she no longer hears the sound

  d. The examiner quickly brings the tuning fork in front of the pinna without touching the client and asks the client to indicate if he or she still hears the sound
  e. The client normally continues to hear the sound two times longer in front of the pinna; such results are a positive Rinne test
  f. The examiner records the duration of both phases—bone conduction followed by air conduction—and compares the times
  g. If the client is unable to hear the sound through the ear in front of the pinna, the client may have a **conductive hearing loss** on the side tested; in this situation, the bone conduction is greater than the air conduction (negative Rinne test)
  h. Both the Rinne test and the Weber tuning fork test are limited in distinguishing between **conductive** and **sensorineural hearing losses**
F. Vestibular assessment
 1. Test for falling
  a. The examiner asks the client to stand with feet together, arms hanging loosely at the side, and eyes closed.
  b. The client normally remains erect with only slight swaying
  c. A significant sway is a positive Romberg's sign
 2. Test for past pointing
  a. The client sits in front of the examiner
  b. The client closes his or her eyes and extends the arms in front, pointing both index fingers at the examiner
  c. The examiner holds and touches his or her own extended index fingers under the extended index fingers of the client to give the client a point of reference
  d. The client is instructed to raise both arms and then lower them, attempting to return to the examiner's extended index fingers
  e. The normal test response is that the client can easily return to the point of reference
  f. The client with a vestibular function problem lacks a normal sense of position and is unable to return the extended fingers to the point of reference; instead, the fingers deviate to the right or the left of the reference point
 3. Gaze nystagmus evaluation
  a. The client's eyes are examined as the client looks straight ahead, 30 degrees to each side, upward and downward
  b. Any spontaneous nystagmus—an involuntary, rhythmic, rapid twitching of the eyeballs—represents a problem with the vestibular system

4. Hallpike's maneuver
   a. Assesses for positional vertigo or induced dizziness
   b. The client assumes a supine position
   c. The head is rotated to one side for 1 minute
   d. A positive test results in nystagmus after 5 to 10 seconds

VII. **DIAGNOSTIC TESTS FOR THE EAR** (Box 54-8)
A. Tomography
   1. Description
      a. Tomography may be performed with or without contrast medium
      b. Tomography assesses the mastoid, middle ear, and inner ear structures
      c. Multiple radiographs of the head are obtained
      d. Tomography is especially helpful in the diagnosis of acoustic tumors
   2. Interventions
      a. All jewelry is removed
      b. Lead eye shields are used to cover the cornea to diminish the radiation dose to the eyes
      c. The client must remain still in a supine position
      d. No follow-up care is required
▲ B. Audiometry
   1. Description
      a. Audiometry measures hearing acuity
      b. Audiometry uses two types: pure tone audiometry and speech audiometry
      c. Pure tone audiometry is used to identify problems with hearing, speech, music, and other sounds in the environment
      d. In speech audiometry, the client's ability to hear spoken words is measured
      e. After testing, audiogram patterns are depicted on a graph to determine the type and level of the hearing loss
   2. Interventions
      a. Inform the client regarding the procedure
      b. Instruct the client to identify the sounds as they are heard
C. Electronystagmography (ENG)
   1. Description
      a. ENG is a vestibular test that evaluates spontaneous and induced eye movements known as nystagmus
      b. ENG is used to distinguish between normal nystagmus and medication-induced nystagmus or nystagmus caused by a lesion in the central or peripheral vestibular pathway

c. ENG records changing electrical fields with the movement of the eye, as monitored by electrodes placed on the skin around the eye
   2. Interventions
      a. The client is instructed to remain NPO for 3 hours before testing and to avoid caffeine-containing beverages for 24 to 48 hours before the test
      b. Unnecessary medications are omitted for 24 hours before testing
      c. Instruct the client that this is a long and tiring procedure
      d. The client should bring prescription eyeglasses to the examination
      e. The client sits and is instructed to gaze at lights, focus on a moving pattern, focus on a moving point, and then close the eyes
      f. While sitting in a chair, the client may be rotated to provide information about vestibular function
      g. In addition, the client's ears are irrigated with cool and warm water, which may cause nausea and vomiting
      h. Following the procedure, the client begins taking clear fluids slowly and cautiously since nausea and vomiting may occur
      i. Assistance with ambulation may also be necessary following the procedure

VIII. **DISORDERS OF THE EAR**
A. Risk factors related to ear disorders (Box 54-9) ▲
B. **Conductive hearing loss**
   1. Description
      a. **Conductive hearing loss** occurs when sound waves are blocked to the inner ear fibers because of external ear or middle ear disorders
      b. Disorders can often be corrected with no damage to hearing or with minimal permanent hearing loss
   2. Causes
      a. Any inflammatory process or obstruction of the external or middle ear
      b. Tumors
      c. **Otosclerosis**
      d. A buildup of scar tissue on the ossicles from previous middle ear surgery

---

BOX 54-8 Diagnostic Tests for the Ear

Audiometry
Electronystagmography
Tomography

BOX 54-9 Risk Factors of Ear Disorders

Aging process
Infection
Medications
Ototoxicity
Trauma
Tumors

BOX 54-10 Signs of Hearing Loss

Frequently asking others to repeat statements
Straining to hear
Turning head or leaning forward to favor one ear
Shouting in conversation
Ringing in the ears
Failing to respond when not looking in the direction of the sound
Answering questions incorrectly
Raising the volume of the television or radio
Avoiding large groups
Better understanding of speech when in small groups
Withdrawing from social interactions

BOX 54-11 Facilitation of Communication

Using written words if the client is able to see, read, and write
Providing plenty of light in the room
Getting the attention of the client before beginning to speak
Facing the client when speaking
Talking in a room without distracting noises
Moving close to the client and speaking slowly and clearly
Keeping hands and other objects away from the mouth when talking to the client
Talking in normal volume and lower pitch, since shouting is not helpful and higher frequencies are less easily heard
Rephrasing sentences and repeating information
Validating with the client the understanding of statements made by asking the client to repeat what was said
Using lip-reading
Encouraging the client to wear glasses when talking to someone to improve vision for lip reading
Using sign language, which combines speech with hand movements that signify letters, words, or phrases
Using telephone amplifiers
Using flashing lights that are activated by ringing of the telephone or doorbell
Using specially trained dogs that help the client to be aware of sound and to alert the client to potential dangers

C. **Sensorineural hearing loss**
  1. Description
     a. **Sensorineural hearing loss** is a pathological process of the inner ear or of the sensory fibers that lead to the cerebral cortex
     b. **Sensorineural hearing loss** is often permanent, and measures must be taken to reduce further damage or to attempt to amplify sound as a means of improving hearing to some degree
  2. Causes
     a. Damage to the inner ear structures
     b. Damage to the eighth cranial nerve
     c. Prolonged exposure to loud noise
     d. Medications
     e. Trauma
     f. Inherited disorders
     g. Metabolic and circulatory disorders
     h. Infections
     i. Surgery
     j. **Meniere's syndrome**
     k. Diabetes mellitus
     l. Myxedema
D. Mixed hearing loss
  1. Mixed hearing loss also is known as **conductive-sensorineural hearing loss**
  2. Client has **sensorineural** and **conductive hearing loss**
E. Signs of hearing loss and facilitating communication (Boxes 54-10 and 54-11)
F. Cochlear implantation (Figure 54-3)
  1. Cochlear implants are used for **sensorineural hearing loss**
  2. A small computer converts sound waves into electrical impulses
  3. Electrodes are placed by the internal ear with a computer device attached to the external ear
  4. Electronic impulses directly stimulate nerve fibers
G. Hearing aids
  1. Hearing aids are used for the client with **conductive hearing loss**

  2. Hearing aids can help the client with **sensorineural hearing loss**, although they are not as effective
  3. A difficulty that exists in the use of hearing aids is the amplification of background noise and of voices
  4. Client education (Box 54-12)
H. **Presbycusis**
  1. Description
     a. **Presbycusis** is a **sensorineural hearing loss** associated with aging
     b. **Presbycusis** leads to degeneration or atrophy of the ganglion cells in the cochlea and a loss of elasticity of the basilar membranes
     c. **Presbycusis** leads to compromise of the vascular supply to the inner ear with changes in several areas of the ear structure
  2. Data collection
     a. Hearing loss is gradual and bilateral
     b. Client states that he or she has no problem with hearing but cannot understand what the words are
     c. Client thinks that the speaker is mumbling

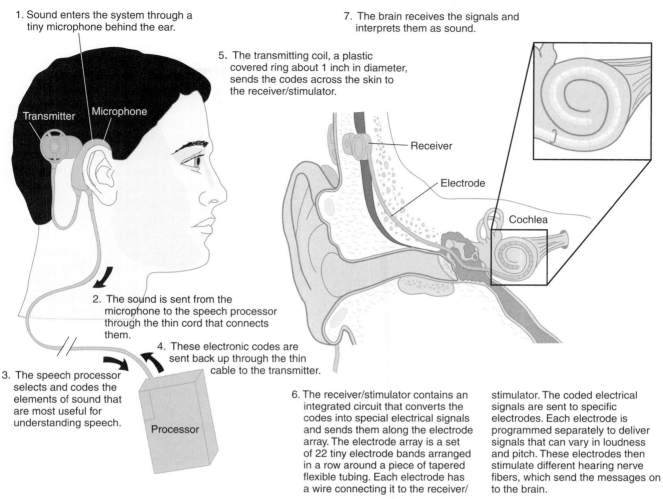

1. Sound enters the system through a tiny microphone behind the ear.

Transmitter   Microphone

5. The transmitting coil, a plastic covered ring about 1 inch in diameter, sends the codes across the skin to the receiver/stimulator.

7. The brain receives the signals and interprets them as sound.

Receiver

Electrode

Cochlea

2. The sound is sent from the microphone to the speech processor through the thin cord that connects them.

4. These electronic codes are sent back up through the thin cable to the transmitter.

3. The speech processor selects and codes the elements of sound that are most useful for understanding speech.

Processor

6. The receiver/stimulator contains an integrated circuit that converts the codes into special electrical signals and sends them along the electrode array. The electrode array is a set of 22 tiny electrode bands arranged in a row around a piece of tapered flexible tubing. Each electrode has a wire connecting it to the receiver/ stimulator. The coded electrical signals are sent to specific electrodes. Each electrode is programmed separately to deliver signals that can vary in loudness and pitch. These electrodes then stimulate different hearing nerve fibers, which send the messages on to the brain.

FIG. 54-3   Cochlear implant to restore hearing. (From Black, J., & Hawks, J. [2009]. *Medical-surgical nursing: Clinical management for positive outcomes* [8th ed.]. Philadelphia: Saunders.)

I. External otitis
  1. Description
     a. External otitis is an infective inflammatory or allergic response involving the structure of the external auditory canal or the auricles
     b. An irritating or infective agent comes in contact with the epithelial layer of the external ear
     c. Contact leads to an allergic response or signs and symptoms of an infection
     d. The skin becomes red, swollen, and tender to touch on movement
     e. The extensive swelling of the canal can lead to **conductive hearing loss** because of obstruction
     f. External otitis is more common in children, is termed "swimmer's ear," and occurs more often in hot, humid environments
     g. Prevention includes the elimination of irritating or infecting agents

BOX 54-12   **Client Education Regarding a Hearing Aid**

Encourage the client to begin using the hearing aid slowly to adjust to the device.

Adjust the volume to the minimal hearing level to prevent feedback squeaking.

Teach the client to concentrate on the sounds that are to be heard and to filter out background noise.

Instruct the client to clean the ear mold with mild soap and water.

Avoid excessive wetting of the hearing aid, and try to keep the hearing aid dry.

Clean the ear cannula of the hearing aid with a toothpick or pipe cleaner.

Turn off the hearing aid before removing from the ear to prevent squealing feedback; remove the battery when not in use.

Keep extra batteries on hand.

Keep the hearing aid in a safe place.

Prevent hair sprays, oils, or other hair and face products from coming in contact with the receiver of the hearing aid.

2. Data collection
   a. Pain
   b. Itching
   c. Plugged feeling in the ear
   d. Redness and edema
   e. Exudate
   f. Hearing loss
3. Interventions
   a. Apply heat locally for 20 minutes three times a day
   b. Encourage rest to assist in reducing pain
   c. Administer antibiotics or corticosteroids as prescribed
   d. Administer analgesics such as aspirin or acetaminophen (Tylenol) for the pain as prescribed
   e. Instruct the client that the ears should be kept clean and dry
   f. Instruct the client to use earplugs for swimming
   g. Instruct the client that cotton-tipped applicators should not be used to dry ears because their use can lead to trauma to the canal
   h. Instruct the client that irritating agents such as hair products or headphones should be discontinued
J. Otitis media: Refer to Chapter 31
   1. Myringotomy
      a. Refer to Chapter 31
      b. Client education (Box 54-13)
K. Chronic otitis media
   1. Description
      a. Chronic otitis media is a chronic infective, inflammatory, or allergic response involving the structure of the middle ear

---

BOX 54-13 **Client Education Following Myringotomy**

Avoid strenuous activities.
Avoid rapid head movements, bouncing, or bending.
Avoid straining on bowel movement.
Avoid drinking through a straw.
Avoid traveling by air.
Avoid forceful coughing.
Avoid contact with persons with colds.
Avoid washing hair, showering, or getting the head wet for 1 week as prescribed.
Instruct the client that if he or she needs to blow the nose, to blow one side at a time with the mouth open.
Instruct the client to keep ears dry by keeping a ball of cotton coated with petroleum jelly in the ear and to change the cotton ball daily.
Instruct the client to report excessive ear drainage to the physician.

---

b. Surgical treatment is necessary to restore hearing
c. The type of surgery can vary and includes a simple reconstruction of the tympanic membrane, a myringoplasty, or replacement of the ossicles within the middle ear
d. A tympanoplasty, a reconstruction of the middle ear, may be attempted to improve **conductive hearing loss**
2. Preoperative interventions
   a. Administer antibiotic drops as prescribed
   b. Clean the ear of debris as prescribed; irrigate the ear with a solution as prescribed to restore the normal pH of the ear
   c. Instruct the client to avoid persons with upper respiratory infections
   d. Instruct the client to obtain adequate rest, eat a balanced diet, and drink adequate fluids
   e. Instruct the client in deep breathing and coughing; forceful coughing, which increases pressure in the middle ear, is to be avoided postoperatively
3. Postoperative interventions
   a. Inform the client that initial hearing after surgery is diminished because of the packing in the ear canal and that hearing improvement will occur after the packing is removed
   b. Keep the dressing clean and dry
   c. Keep the client flat with the operative ear up for at least 12 hours as prescribed
   d. Administer antibiotics as prescribed
   e. Instruct the client that the client may return to work in about 3 weeks postoperatively as prescribed
L. Mastoiditis
   1. Description
      a. Mastoiditis may be acute or chronic and results from untreated or inadequately treated chronic or acute otitis media
      b. The pain is not relieved by myringotomy
   2. Data collection
      a. Swelling behind the ear and pain with minimal movement of the head
      b. Cellulitis on the skin or external scalp over the mastoid process
      c. A reddened, dull, thick, immobile tympanic membrane with or without perforation
      d. Tender and enlarged postauricular lymph nodes
      e. Low-grade fever
      f. Malaise
      g. Anorexia
   3. Interventions
      a. Prepare the client for surgical removal of infected material

b. Monitor for complications

c. Simple or modified radical mastoidectomy with tympanoplasty is the most common treatment

d. Once tissue that is infected is removed, the tympanoplasty is performed to reconstruct the ossicles and the tympanic membranes in an attempt to restore normal hearing

4. Complications

a. Damage to the abducens and facial cranial nerves

b. Damage exhibited by inability to look laterally (cranial nerve VI, abducens) and a drooping of the mouth on the affected side (cranial nerve VII, facial)

c. Meningitis

d. Brain abscess

e. Chronic purulent otitis media

f. Wound infections

g. Vertigo, if the infection spreads into the labyrinth

5. Postoperative interventions

a. Monitor for dizziness

b. Monitor for signs of meningitis as evidenced by a stiff neck and vomiting

c. Prepare for a wound dressing change 24 hours postoperatively

d. Monitor the surgical incision for edema, drainage, and redness

e. Position the client flat with the operative side up

f. Restrict the client to bed with bedside commode privileges for 24 hours as prescribed

g. Assist the client with getting out of bed to prevent falling or injuries from dizziness

h. With reconstruction of the ossicles via a graft, take precautions to prevent dislodging of the graft

M. **Otosclerosis**

1. Description

a. **Otosclerosis** is a disease of the labyrinthine capsule of the middle ear that results in a bony overgrowth of the tissue surrounding the ossicles

b. **Otosclerosis** causes the development of irregular areas of new bone formation and causes the fixation of the bones

c. Stapes fixation leads to a **conductive hearing loss**

d. If the disease involves the inner ear, **sensorineural hearing loss** is present

e. Bilateral involvement is not uncommon, although hearing loss may be worse in one ear

f. The cause is unknown, although it is thought to have a familial tendency

g. Nonsurgical intervention promotes the improvement of hearing through amplification

h. Surgical intervention involves removal of the bony growth that is causing the hearing loss

i. A partial stapedectomy or complete stapedectomy with prosthesis (**fenestration**) may be performed surgically

2. Data collection

a. Slowly progressing **conductive hearing loss**

b. Bilateral hearing loss

c. A ringing or roaring type of constant tinnitus

d. Loud sounds heard in the ear when chewing

e. Pinkish discoloration (Schwartze's sign) of the tympanic membrane, which indicates vascular changes within the ear

f. Negative Rinne test

g. Weber test that shows lateralization of sound to the ear with the most **conductive hearing loss**

N. **Fenestration**

1. Description

a. **Fenestration** is removal of the stapes with a small hole drilled in the footplate, and a prosthesis is connected between the incus and footplate

b. Sounds cause the prosthesis to vibrate in the same manner as did the stapes

c. Complications include complete hearing loss, prolonged vertigo, infection, or facial nerve damage

2. Preoperative interventions

a. Instruct the client on measures to prevent middle ear or external ear infections

b. Instruct the client to avoid excessive nose blowing

c. Instruct the client not to clean the ear canal with cotton-tipped applicators and to avoid trauma or injury to the ear canal

3. Postoperative interventions

a. Inform the client that hearing is initially worse after the surgical procedure because of swelling and that no noticeable improvement in hearing may occur for as long as 6 weeks

b. Inform the client that the Gelfoam ear packing interferes with hearing but is used to decrease bleeding

c. Assist with ambulating during the first 1 to 2 days after surgery

d. Provide side rails when the client is in bed

e. Administer antibiotics, antivertiginous, and pain medications as prescribed

f. Assess for facial nerve damage, weakness, changes in tactile sensation, changes in taste sensation, vertigo, nausea, and vomiting

g. Instruct the client to move the head slowly when changing positions to prevent vertigo

h. Instruct the client to avoid persons with upper respiratory tract infections

i. Instruct the client to avoid showering and getting the head and wound wet

j. Instruct the client to avoid using small objects (cotton-tipped applicators) to clean the external ear canal

k. Instruct the client to avoid rapid, extreme changes in pressure caused by quick head movements, sneezing, nose blowing, straining, and changes in altitude

l. Instruct the client to avoid changes in middle ear pressure since they could dislodge the graft or prosthesis

O. Labyrinthitis

1. Description: infection of the labyrinth that occurs as a complication of acute or chronic otitis media

2. May result from growth of a cholesteatoma—benign overgrowth of squamous cell epithelium

3. Data collection

a. Hearing loss that may be permanent on the affected side

b. Tinnitus

c. Spontaneous nystagmus to the affected side

d. Vertigo

e. Nausea and vomiting

4. Interventions

a. Monitor for signs of meningitis, the most common complication, as evidenced by headache, stiff neck, and lethargy

b. Administer systemic antibiotics as prescribed

c. Advise the client to rest in bed in a darkened room

d. Administer antiemetics and antivertiginous medications as prescribed

e. Instruct the client that the vertigo subsides as the inflammation resolves

f. Instruct the client that balance problems that persist may require gait training through physical therapy

P. **Meniere's syndrome**

1. Description

a. **Meniere's syndrome** is also called endolymphatic hydrops and refers to dilation of the endolymphatic system by overproduction or decreased reabsorption of endolymphatic fluid

b. The syndrome is characterized by tinnitus, unilateral **sensorineural hearing loss,** and vertigo

c. Symptoms occur in attacks and last for several days, and the client becomes totally incapacitated during the attacks

d. Initial hearing loss is reversible but as the frequency of attacks continues, hearing loss becomes permanent

e. Repeated damage to the cochlea caused by increased fluid pressure leads to the permanent hearing loss

2. Causes

a. Any factor that increases endolymphatic secretion in the labyrinth

b. Viral and bacterial infections

c. Allergic reactions

d. Biochemical disturbances

e. Vascular disturbance producing changes in the microcirculation in the labyrinth

f. Long-term stress may be a possible contributing factor

3. Data collection

a. Feelings of fullness in the ear

b. Tinnitus, as a continuous low-pitched roar or humming sound, that is present much of the time but worsens just before and during severe attacks

c. Hearing loss that is worse during an attack

d. Vertigo, as periods of whirling, that might cause the client to fall to the ground

e. Vertigo that is so intense that even while lying down, the client holds the bed or ground in an attempt to prevent the whirling

f. Nausea and vomiting

g. Nystagmus

h. Severe headaches

4. Nonsurgical interventions

a. Prevent injury during vertigo attacks

b. Provide bedrest in a quiet environment

c. Provide assistance with walking

d. Instruct the client to move the head slowly to prevent worsening of the vertigo

e. Initiate sodium and fluid restrictions as prescribed

f. Instruct the client to stop smoking

g. Administer nicotinic acid (niacin) as prescribed for its vasodilatory effect

h. Administer antihistamines as prescribed, which will reduce the production of histamine and the inflammation

i. Administer antiemetics as prescribed

j. Administer tranquilizers and sedatives as prescribed to calm the client and allow the client to rest and to control vertigo, nausea, and vomiting

k. Mild diuretics may be prescribed to decrease endolymph volume

5. Surgical interventions

a. Surgery is performed when medical therapy is ineffective and the functional level of the client has decreased significantly

b. Endolymphatic drainage and insertion of a shunt may be performed early in the course of the disease to assist with the drainage of excess fluids

c. A resection of the vestibular nerve or total removal of the labyrinth or a labyrinthectomy may be performed

6. Postoperative interventions

a. Assess packing and dressing on the ear

b. Speak to the client on the side of the unaffected ear

c. Perform neurological assessments

d. Maintain side rails

e. Assist with ambulating

f. Encourage the client to use a bedside commode rather than ambulating to the bathroom

g. Administer antivertiginous and antiemetic medications as prescribed

Q. Acoustic neuroma

1. Description

a. Acoustic neuroma is a benign tumor of the vestibular or acoustic nerve

b. The tumor may cause damage to hearing and to facial movements and sensations

c. Treatment includes surgical removal of the tumor via craniotomy

d. Care is taken to preserve the function of the facial nerve

e. The tumor rarely recurs after surgical removal

f. Postoperative nursing care is similar to postoperative craniotomy care

2. Data collection

a. Symptoms usually begin with tinnitus and progress to gradual **sensorineural hearing loss**

b. As the tumor enlarges, damage to adjacent cranial nerves occurs

R. Trauma

1. Description

a. The tympanic membrane has a limited stretching ability and gives way under high pressure

b. Foreign objects placed in the external canal may exert pressure on the tympanic membrane and cause perforation

c. If the object continues through the canal, the bony structure of the stapes, incus, and malleus may be damaged

d. A blunt injury to the basal skull and ear can damage the middle ear structures through fractures extending to the middle ear

e. Excessive nose blowing and rapid changes of pressure that occur with nonpressurized air flights can increase pressure in the middle ear

f. Depending on the damage to the ossicles, hearing loss may or may not return

2. Interventions

a. Tympanic membrane perforations usually heal within 24 hours

b. Surgical reconstruction of the ossicles and tympanic membrane through tympanoplasty or myringoplasty may be performed to improve hearing

S. Cerumen and foreign bodies

1. Description

a. Cerumen or wax is the most common cause of impacted canals

b. Foreign bodies can include vegetables, beads, pencil erasers, insects, or other objects

2. Data collection

a. Sensation of fullness in the ear with or without hearing loss

b. Pain, itching, or bleeding

3. Cerumen

a. Removal of wax by irrigation may be a slow process

b. Irrigation is contraindicated in clients with a history of tympanic membrane perforation or otitis media

c. To soften cerumen, add three drops of glycerin or mineral oil to the ear at bedtime, and three drops of hydrogen peroxide twice a day as prescribed

d. After several days, irrigate the ear

e. The maximal amount of solution that should be used for irrigation is 50 to 70 mL

4. Foreign bodies

a. With a foreign object of vegetable matter, irrigation is used with care because this material expands with hydration

b. Insects are killed before removal, unless they can be coaxed out by flashlight or a humming noise

c. Mineral oil or diluted alcohol is instilled to suffocate the insect, which then is removed using ear forceps

d. Use a small ear forceps to remove the object and avoid pushing the object farther into the canal and damaging the tympanic membrane

PRACTICE QUESTIONS

More questions on the companion CD!

708. A client is diagnosed with glaucoma. Which data gathered by the nurse indicate a risk factor associated with glaucoma?
     1. Cardiovascular disease
     2. A history of migraine headaches
     3. Frequent urinary tract infections
     4. Frequent upper respiratory infections

709. A nurse is assisting in developing a teaching plan for the client with glaucoma. Which instruction would the nurse suggest to include in the plan of care?
     1. Decrease the amount of salt in the diet.
     2. Decrease fluid intake to control the intraocular pressure.
     3. Avoid reading the newspaper and watching the television.
     4. Eye medications will need to be administered for the rest of your life.

710. A nurse is assigned to care for a client with a detached retina. Which finding would the nurse expect to be documented in the client's record?
     1. Blurred vision
     2. Pain in the effected eye
     3. A yellow discoloration of the sclera
     4. A sense of a curtain falling across the field of vision

711. A nurse is assigned to care for a client with a diagnosis of detached retina. Which finding would indicate that bleeding has occurred as a result of retinal detachment?
     1. Total loss of vision
     2. A reddened conjunctiva
     3. A sudden sharp pain in the eye
     4. Complaints of a burst of black spots or floaters

712. A client arrives in the emergency department following an automobile crash. The client's forehead hit the steering wheel and a hyphema has been diagnosed. The nurse would prepare to position the client:
     1. Flat on bedrest
     2. On bedrest in a semi-Fowler's position
     3. In lateral position on the unaffected side
     4. In the lateral position on the affected side

713. A client sustains a contusion of the eyeball following a traumatic injury with a blunt object. The nurse takes which action immediately?
     1. Notifies the physician
     2. Applies ice to the affected eye
     3. Irrigates the eye with cool water
     4. Accompanies the client to the emergency dapartment

714. A client sustains a chemical eye injury from a splash of battery acid. The nurse prepares the client for which immediate measure?
     1. Assessing visual acuity
     2. Covering the eye with a pressure patch
     3. Swabbing the eye with antibiotic ointment
     4. Irrigating the eye with sterile normal saline

715. A nurse is caring for a client following enucleation and notes the presence of bright red drainage on the dressing. The nurse takes which appropriate action?
     1. Reports the finding
     2. Documents the finding
     3. Continues to monitor vital signs
     4. Marks the drainage on the dressing and monitors for any increase in bleeding

716. A nurse is preparing to administer ear drops to an adult client. The nurse administers the ear drops by:
     1. Pulling the pinna up and back
     2. Pulling the earlobe down and back
     3. Tilting the client's head forward and down
     4. Instructing the client to stand and lean to one side

717. A nurse is caring for a client who is hearing-impaired and takes which approach to facilitate communication?
     1. Speaks loudly
     2. Speaks frequently
     3. Speaks in a normal tone
     4. Speaks directly into the impaired ear

718. A client arrives at the emergency dapartment with a foreign body in the left ear that has been determined to be an insect. Which intervention would the nurse anticipate to be prescribed initially?
     1. Irrigation of the ear
     2. Instillation of diluted alcohol
     3. Instillation of antibiotic ear drops
     4. Instillation of corticosteroid ointment

719. A nurse notes that the physician has documented a diagnosis of presbycusis on the client's chart. The nurse understands that this condition is accurately described as:
     1. Tinnitus that occurs with aging
     2. Nystagmus that occurs with aging
     3. A conductive hearing loss that occurs with aging
     4. A sensorineural hearing loss that occurs with aging

720. A client with Meniere's disease is experiencing severe vertigo. The nurse instructs the client to do which of the following to assist in controlling the vertigo?
     1. Increase sodium in the diet.
     2. Lie still and watch television.
     3. Avoid sudden head movements.
     4. Increase fluid intake to 3000 mL/day.

721. A nurse is assigned to care for a client hospitalized with Meniere's disease. The nurse expects that which of the following would most likely be prescribed for the client?
     1. Low-fat diet
     2. Low-sodium diet

3. Low-cholesterol diet
4. Low-carbohydrate diet

722. A nurse is reviewing the record of a client with mastoiditis. The nurse would expect to note which of the following documented regarding the results of the otoscopic examination?
1. A pink tympanic membrane
2. A pearl-colored tympanic membrane
3. A transparent and clear tympanic membrane
4. A red, dull, thick, and immobile tympanic membrane

723. A client is diagnosed with a disorder involving the inner ear. The nurse caring for the client understands that which of the following is the common client complaint associated with a disorder involving the inner ear?
1. Pruritus
2. Tinnitus
3. Hearing loss
4. Burning in the ear

724. A nurse is reviewing the health care record of a client with a diagnosis of otosclerosis. The nurse would expect to note documentation of which early symptom of this disorder?
1. Vertigo
2. Headache
3. Blurred vision
4. Ringing in the ears

725. A nurse provides discharge instructions to the client who was hospitalized for an acute attack of Meniere's disease. Which statement, if made by the client, indicates a need for further instructions?
1. "I need to take a vasodilator."
2. "It is not necessary to restrict salt in my diet."
3. "I need to take the antihistamine as prescribed."
4. "I need to take the diuretics to decrease the fluid in the ear."

726. A nurse is providing instructions to a client regarding the use of a hearing aid. Which statement by the client indicates a need for further instructions?
1. "I should keep an extra battery available at all times."
2. "I should not wear the hearing aid during an ear infection."
3. "I should turn the hearing aid off after removing it from my ear."
4. "I should wash the ear mold frequently with mild soap and water."

727. Tonometry is performed on the client with a suspected diagnosis of glaucoma. The nurse reviews the test results as documented in the client's chart and understands that normal intraocular pressure is:
1. 2 to 7 mm Hg
2. 10 to 21 mm Hg

3. 22 to 30 mm Hg
4. 31 to 35 mm Hg

728. A nurse is assisting in developing a plan of care for the client scheduled for cataract surgery. The nurse makes suggestions regarding the plan, knowing that which problem is specifically associated with this type of surgery?
1. Anxiety
2. Self-care deficit
3. Imbalanced nutrition
4. Sensory perceptual alteration

729. A nurse is reviewing the health record of a client diagnosed with a cataract. The chief clinical manifestation that the nurse would expect to note in the early stages of cataract formation is:
1. Eye pain
2. Diplopia
3. Floating spots
4. Blurred vision

730. A nurse is assigned to care for a client following a cataract extraction. The nurse plans to position the client:
1. Prone
2. Supine
3. On the operative side
4. On the nonoperative side

731. During the early postoperative stage, the cataract extraction client complains of nausea and severe eye pain over the operative site. The nurse takes which action?
1. Reports the client's complaints
2. Reassures the client that this is normal
3. Turns the client on his or her operative side
4. Administers the ordered pain medication and antiemetic

ALTERNATE ITEM FORMAT: MULTIPLE RESPONSE

732. The nurse is preparing a teaching plan for a client who is undergoing cataract extraction with intraocular implant. Which home care measures will the nurse include in the plan?
☑ 1. To avoid activities that require bending over
☐ 2. To contact the surgeon if eye scratchiness occurs
☑ 3. To place an eye shield on the surgical eye at bedtime
☐ 4. That episodes of sudden severe pain in the eye is expected
☐ 5. To contact the surgeon if a decrease in visual acuity occurs
☐ 6. To take acetaminophen (Tylenol) for minor eye discomfort

ANSWERS

708. 1

Rationale: Hypertension, cardiovascular disease, diabetes mellitus, and obesity are associated with the development of glaucoma. Smoking, ingestion of caffeine or large amounts alcohol, illicit drugs, corticosteroids, altered hormone levels, posture, and eye movements may cause varying transient increases in intraocular pressure.

Test-Taking Strategy: Use knowledge regarding the risk factors associated with glaucoma to answer this question. Remember, cardiovascular disease is associated with the development of glaucoma. If you had difficulty with this question, review the risk factors associated with this disorder.

Level of Cognitive Ability: Comprehension
Client Needs: Health Promotion and Maintenance
Integrated Process: Nursing Process/Data Collection
Content Area: Adult Health/Eye
Reference: Ignatavicius, D., & Workman, M. (2006). *Medical-surgical nursing: Critical thinking for collaborative care* (5th ed., pp. 1096-1097). Philadelphia: Saunders.

709. 4

Rationale: The administration of eye drops is a critical component of the treatment plan for the client with glaucoma. The client needs to be instructed that medications will need to be taken for the rest of his or her life. Limiting fluids and reducing salt will not decrease intraocular pressure. Option 3 is not necessary.

Test-Taking Strategy: Use the process of elimination. Knowing that medications are an integral component of the treatment plan will assist in directing you to the correct option. Review the treatment associated with the care of the client with glaucoma if you had difficulty with this question.

Level of Cognitive Ability: Application
Client Needs: Health Promotion and Maintenance
Integrated Process: Nursing Process/Planning
Content Area: Adult Health/Eye
Reference: Christensen, B., & Kockrow, E. (2006). *Adult health nursing* (5th ed., p. 662). St. Louis: Mosby.

710. 4

Rationale: A characteristic clinical manifestation of retinal detachment described by clients is the feeling that a shadow or curtain is falling across the field of vision. There is no pain associated with detachment of the retina. A retinal detachment is an ophthalmic emergency and even more so if visual acuity is still normal. Options 1 and 3 are not specifically associated with a detached retina.

Test-Taking Strategy: Use the process of elimination. Remember that a characteristic clinical manifestation is the feeling that a shadow or curtain is falling across the field of vision. Retinal detachment can occur suddenly and is an ophthalmic emergency. Review the clinical manifestations associated with this condition if you had difficulty with this question.

Level of Cognitive Ability: Comprehension
Client Needs: Physiological Integrity
Integrated Process: Nursing Process/Data Collection
Content Area: Adult Health/Eye
Reference: Christensen, B., & Kockrow, E. (2006). *Adult health nursing* (5th ed., p. 656). St. Louis: Mosby.

711. 4

Rationale: Complaints of a sudden burst of black spots or floaters indicate that bleeding has occurred as a result of the detachment. Options 1, 2, and 3 are not specifically associated with bleeding as a result of detached retina.

Test-Taking Strategy: Use the process of elimination. Hemorrhage is a serious complication associated with retinal detachment. Remember, complaints of a sudden burst of black spots or floaters indicate that bleeding has occurred as a result of the detachment. Review the clinical manifestations associated with the complications of a detached retina if you had difficulty with this question.

Level of Cognitive Ability: Analysis
Client Needs: Physiological Integrity
Integrated Process: Nursing Process/Data Collection
Content Area: Adult Health/Eye
References: Christensen, B., & Kockrow, E. (2006). *Adult health nursing* (5th ed., p. 657). St. Louis: Mosby.
Linton, A., & Maebius, N. (2007). *Introduction to medical-surgical nursing* (4th ed., p. 1183). Philadelphia: Saunders.

712. 2

Rationale: A hyphema is the presence of blood in the anterior chamber. It is produced when a force is sufficient to break the integrity of the blood vessels in the eye. It can be caused by direct injury, such as penetrating injury from a BB pellet, or indirectly, such as from striking the forehead on a steering wheel during an accident. The client is treated by bedrest in a semi-Fowler's position to assist gravity in keeping the hyphema away from the optical center of the cornea.

Test-Taking Strategy: Use the process of elimination. Eliminate options 1, 3, and 4 because they are comparable or alike. Placing the client flat will produce an increase in pressure at the injured site. Review care of the client with hyphema if you had difficulty with this question.

Level of Cognitive Ability: Application
Client Needs: Physiological Integrity
Integrated Process: Nursing Process/Implementation
Content Area: Adult Health/Eye
References: Jarvis, C. (2008). *Physical examination & health assessment* (5th ed., p. 339). Philadelphia: Saunders.
Linton, A., & Maebius, N. (2007). *Introduction to medical-surgical nursing* (4th ed., p. 439). Philadelphia: Saunders.

713. 2

Rationale: Treatment for a contusion begins at the time of injury. Ice is applied immediately. The client should receive a thorough eye examination to rule out the presence of other eye injuries. Eye irrigation is not indicated in a contusion. Options 1 and 4 will delay immediate treatment. Following the application of ice, the physician would be notified.

Test-Taking Strategy: Use the process of elimination, noting the strategic word "immediately." Noting that the client sustained a contusion to the eye will direct you to option 2. Review immediate treatment of an eye contusion if you had difficulty with this question.

Level of Cognitive Ability: Application
Client Needs: Physiological Integrity
Integrated Process: Nursing Process/Implementation
Content Area: Adult Health/Eye

Reference: Christensen, B., & Kockrow, E. (2006). *Adult health nursing* (5th ed., p. 178). St. Louis: Mosby.

714. 4

Rationale: Emergency care following a chemical burn to the eye includes irrigating the eye immediately with sterile normal saline or ocular irrigating solution. The irrigation should be maintained for at least 10 minutes. Following this emergency treatment, visual acuity is assessed. Options 2 and 3 are not immediate measures.
Test-Taking Strategy: Use the process of elimination. Read the question carefully, noting the type of injury to the eye. The question asks about emergency care; therefore, in this type of injury, it is necessary to irrigate the eye first. Review this content if you had difficulty with this question.
Level of Cognitive Ability: Application
Client Needs: Physiological Integrity
Integrated Process: Nursing Process/Implementation
Content Area: Adult Health/Eye
References: deWit, S. (2009). *Medical-surgical nursing: Concepts & practice* (p. 641). St. Louis: Saunders.
Linton, A., & Maebius, N. (2007). *Introduction to medical-surgical nursing* (4th ed., p. 233). Philadelphia: Saunders.

715. 1

Rationale: If the nurse notes the presence of bright red drainage on the dressing, it must be reported to the registered nurse, because this can indicate hemorrhage. Options 2, 3, and 4 will delay necessary treatment.
Test-Taking Strategy: Note the strategic words "bright red." Bright red drainage indicates active bleeding. The registered nurse needs to be notified if this type of drainage occurs. Review postoperative complications associated with an enucleation if you had difficulty with this question.
Level of Cognitive Ability: Application
Client Needs: Physiological Integrity
Integrated Process: Nursing Process/Implementation
Content Area: Adult Health/Eye
Reference: Linton, A., & Maebius, N. (2007). *Introduction to medical-surgical nursing* (4th ed., p. 1185). Philadelphia: Saunders.

716. 1

Rationale: The nurse tilts the client's head slightly away and pulls the pinna up and back. Asking the client to stand and lean to one side is inappropriate and unsafe.
Test-Taking Strategy: Use the process of elimination, noting that the question addresses an adult client. Use basic knowledge regarding the administration of ear medications in selecting the correct option. In the adult, the pinna is pulled up and back. Review this procedure if you had difficulty with this question.
Level of Cognitive Ability: Application
Client Needs: Physiological Integrity
Integrated Process: Nursing Process/Implementation
Content Area: Adult Health/Ear
Reference: Linton, A., & Maebius, N. (2007). *Introduction to medical-surgical nursing* (4th ed., p. 1193). Philadelphia: Saunders.

717. 3

Rationale: It is important to speak in a normal tone to the client with impaired hearing and to avoid shouting. The nurse should talk directly to the client while facing the client and speak clearly. If the client does not seem to understand what is said, the nurse should express it differently. Moving closer to the client and toward the better ear may facilitate communication, but it is important to avoid talking directly into the impaired ear.
Test-Taking Strategy: Knowledge regarding effective communication techniques for the hearing impaired is required to answer this question. Thinking about the effect of each action identified in the options will direct you to option 3. If you had difficulty with this question, review these techniques.
Level of Cognitive Ability: Application
Client Needs: Psychosocial Integrity
Integrated Process: Communication and Documentation
Content Area: Adult Health/Ear
Reference: Christensen, B., & Kockrow, E. (2006). *Adult health nursing* (5th ed., p. 668). St. Louis: Mosby.

718. 2

Rationale: Insects are killed before removal unless they can be coaxed out by a flashlight or a humming noise. Mineral oil or diluted alcohol is instilled into the ear to suffocate the insect, which is then removed by using ear forceps. When the foreign object is vegetable matter, irrigation is not used since this material expands with hydration and the impaction becomes worse. Options 1, 3, and 4 may be prescribed after the initial treatment if necessary and if inflammation or infection is a concern.
Test-Taking Strategy: Use the process of elimination and knowledge regarding care of the client with a foreign body in the ear to answer this question. Remember, insects are killed before removal with mineral oil or diluted alcohol. If you had difficulty with this question, review the treatment for this occurrence.
Level of Cognitive Ability: Comprehension
Client Needs: Physiological Integrity
Integrated Process: Nursing Process/Planning
Content Area: Adult Health/Ear
Reference: Linton, A., & Maebius, N. (2007). *Introduction to medical-surgical nursing* (4th ed., p. 1199). Philadelphia: Saunders.

719. 4

Rationale: Presbycusis is a type of hearing loss that occurs with aging. It is a gradual sensorineural loss caused by nerve degeneration in the inner ear or auditory nerve. Options 1, 2, and 3 are not accurate descriptions.
Test-Taking Strategy: Knowledge regarding the description of presbycusis is required to answer this question. Remember presbycusis is a sensorineural hearing loss that occurs with aging. If you are unfamiliar with this condition, review this age-related disorder.
Level of Cognitive Ability: Comprehension
Client Needs: Physiological Integrity
Integrated Process: Nursing Process/Data Collection
Content Area: Adult Health/Ear
Reference: Linton, A., & Maebius, N. (2007). *Introduction to medical-surgical nursing* (4th ed., p. 1205). Philadelphia: Saunders.

720. 3

Rationale: The nurse instructs the client to make slow head movements to prevent worsening of the vertigo. Dietary changes such as salt and fluid restrictions that reduce the amount of endolymphatic fluid are sometimes prescribed. Watching television can increase the vertigo.

Test-Taking Strategy: Identify the subject of the question. The subject is severe vertigo. Note the relation between severe vertigo and the correct option, avoiding sudden head movements. If you had difficulty with this question, review measures that will reduce vertigo in the client with Meniere's disease.

Level of Cognitive Ability: Application
Client Needs: Physiological Integrity
Integrated Process: Nursing Process/Implementation
Content Area: Adult Health/Ear
Reference: Linton, A., & Maebius, N. (2007). *Introduction to medical-surgical nursing* (4th ed., p. 1203). Philadelphia: Saunders.

721. 2

Rationale: Dietary changes such as salt and fluid restrictions that reduce the amount of endolymphatic fluid are sometimes prescribed. Options 1, 3, and 4 are not specific dietary prescriptions for this condition.

Test-Taking Strategy: Use the process of elimination. Recalling the pathophysiology related to Meniere's disease will direct you to option 2. Review the pathophysiology related to this condition and the treatment if you had difficulty with this question.

Level of Cognitive Ability: Comprehension
Client Needs: Physiological Integrity
Integrated Process: Nursing Process/Planning
Content Area: Adult Health/Ear
Reference: Linton, A., & Maebius, N. (2007). *Introduction to medical-surgical nursing* (4th ed., p. 1203). Philadelphia: Saunders.

722. 4

Rationale: Otoscopic examination in a client with mastoiditis reveals a red, dull, thick, and immobile tympanic membrane with or without perforation. Postauricular lymph nodes are tender and enlarged. Clients also have a low-grade fever, malaise, anorexia, swelling behind the ear, and pain with minimal movement of the head. Options 1, 2, and 3 are not findings that would be noted in an otoscopic examination in the client with mastoiditis.

Test-Taking Strategy: Focus on the name of the disorder: mastoiditis. Recalling that "-itis" indicates inflammation or infection will direct you to option 4. If you had difficulty with this question, review these findings.

Level of Cognitive Ability: Comprehension
Client Needs: Physiological Integrity
Integrated Process: Nursing Process/Data Collection
Content Area: Adult Health/Ear
References: Christensen, B., & Kockrow, E. (2006). *Adult health nursing* (5th ed., p. 671). St. Louis: Mosby.
Linton, A., & Maebius, N. (2007). *Introduction to medical-surgical nursing* (4th ed., pp. 1200-1201). Philadelphia: Saunders.

723. 2

Rationale: Tinnitus is the most common complaint of clients with otologic disorders, especially disorders involving the inner ear. Symptoms of tinnitus range from mild ringing in the ear that can go unnoticed during the day to a loud roaring in the ear that can interfere with the client's thinking process and attention span. Hearing loss may or may not occur. Options 1 and 4 are not specifically associated with inner ear problems.

Test-Taking Strategy: Use the process of elimination. Recalling the functions of the inner ear will direct you to the correct option. Review inner ear problems and the associated findings if you had difficulty with this question.

Level of Cognitive Ability: Comprehension
Client Needs: Physiological Integrity
Integrated Process: Nursing Process/Data Collection
Content Area: Adult Health/Ear
References: Christensen, B., & Kockrow, E. (2006). *Adult health nursing* (5th ed., p. 671). St. Louis: Mosby.
Linton, A., & Maebius, N. (2007). *Introduction to medical-surgical nursing* (4th ed., pp. 1202-1203). Philadelphia: Saunders.

724. 4

Rationale: Otosclerosis involves the formation of spongy bone in the capsule of the labyrinth of the ear, often causing the auditory ossicles to become fixed and less able to vibrate when sound enters the ear. An early symptom is ringing in the ears, but the most noticeable symptom is progressive hearing loss. Options 1, 2, and 3 are not associated with this condition.

Test-Taking Strategy: Use the process of elimination and note the strategic word "early." Recalling that this disorder involves the ear will assist in eliminating options 2 and 3. Focusing on the strategic word will assist in directing you to option 4 from the remaining options. If you had difficulty with this question, review this disorder.

Level of Cognitive Ability: Comprehension
Client Needs: Physiological Integrity
Integrated Process: Nursing Process/Data Collection
Content Area: Adult Health/Ear
Reference: Christensen, B., & Kockrow, E. (2006). *Adult health nursing* (5th ed., p. 675). St. Louis: Mosby.

725. 2

Rationale: Management during remission includes diuretics to decrease the fluid and thereby decrease pressure in the endolymphatic system. Antihistamines, vasodilators, and diuretics may be prescribed for the client. A low-salt diet is prescribed for the client to reduce fluids. The major goal of treatment is to preserve the client's hearing; careful medical management helps achieve this in most clients with Meniere's disease.

Test-Taking Strategy: Note the strategic words "need for further instructions." These words indicate a negative event query and the need to select the incorrect client statement. Recalling that Meniere's disease occurs as a result of a disturbance in the fluid of the endolymphatic system will direct you to option 2. If you are unfamiliar with the management of this disorder during remission, review this content.

Level of Cognitive Ability: Comprehension

Client Needs: Health Promotion and Maintenance
Integrated Process: Teaching an Learning
Content Area: Adult Health/Ear
Reference: Christensen, B., & Kockrow, E. (2006). *Adult health nursing* (5th ed., p. 676). St. Louis: Mosby.

726. 3
Rationale: Nurses should have a basic knowledge of the care of a hearing aid to assist the client in its use. The client should be instructed to turn the hearing aid off before removing it from the ear to prevent squealing feedback. The hearing aid should be turned off when not in use, and the client should keep an extra battery available at all times. The client should wash the ear mold frequently with mild soap and water, using a pipe cleaner to cleanse the cannula. The client should not wear the hearing aid during an ear infection.
Test-Taking Strategy: Use the process of elimination and note the strategic words "need for further instructions." These words indicate a negative event query and the need to select the incorrect client statement. Recalling the causes of squealing feedback will direct you to the correct option. If you had difficulty with this question, review the use of the hearing aid.
Level of Cognitive Ability: Comprehension
Client Needs: Health Promotion and Maintenance
Integrated Process: Teaching and Learning
Content Area: Adult Health/Ear
Reference: deWit, S. (2009). *Medical-surgical nursing: Concepts & practice.* (p. 632). St. Louis: Saunders.

727. 2
Rationale: Tonometry is the method of measuring intraocular fluid pressure using a calibrated instrument that indents or flattens the corneal apex. Pressures between 10 and 21 mm Hg are considered within the normal range.
Test-Taking Strategy: Knowledge regarding the normal intraocular pressure is required to answer this question. Remember, pressures between 10 and 21 mm Hg are considered within the normal range. Review this normal value if you had difficulty with this question.
Level of Cognitive Ability: Comprehension
Client Needs: Physiological Integrity
Integrated Process: Nursing Process/Data Collection
Content Area: Adult Health/Eye
Reference: Linton, A., & Maebius, N. (2007). *Introduction to medical-surgical nursing* (4th ed., pp. 1162-1163). Philadelphia: Saunders.

728. 4
Rationale: The most specific associated problem for the client scheduled for cataract surgery is sensory perceptual alteration (visual) related to lens extraction and replacement. Options 2 and 3 may also be concerns but would occur as a result of a sensory perceptual alteration. Option 1 can occur with any type of surgical procedure.
Test-Taking Strategy: Use the process of elimination, focusing on the type of surgery. Remember, disorders of the eye or ear relate to sensory perceptual alterations. Review the problems associated with these disorders if you had difficulty with this question.
Level of Cognitive Ability: Comprehension
Client Needs: Psychosocial Integrity

Integrated Process: Nursing Process/Planning
Content Area: Adult Health/Eye
Reference: Linton, A., & Maebius, N. (2007). *Introduction to medical-surgical nursing* (4th ed., pp. 1176-1177). Philadelphia: Saunders.

729. 4
Rationale: A gradual, painless blurring of central vision is the chief clinical manifestation of a cataract. Early symptoms include slightly blurred vision and a decrease in color perception. Options 1, 2, and 3 are not specifically associated with a cataract.
Test-Taking Strategy: Note the strategic word "chief." Recall the pathophysiology related to cataract development. As a cataract develops, the lens of the eye becomes opaque. This description will assist in directing you to the correct option. If you had difficulty with this question, review the signs associated with cataract development.
Level of Cognitive Ability: Comprehension
Client Needs: Physiological Integrity
Integrated Process: Nursing Process/Data Collection
Content Area: Adult Health/Eye
Reference: Linton, A., & Maebius, N. (2007). *Introduction to medical-surgical nursing* (4th ed., p. 1176). Philadelphia: Saunders.

730. 4
Rationale: Postoperatively, cataract extraction clients should be positioned on their backs in a semi-Fowler's position or on the nonoperative side to prevent edema in the surgical site. Options 1, 2, and 3 are incorrect positions and will cause swelling at the surgical site.
Test-Taking Strategy: Use the process of elimination. Remember, edema at the surgical site can occur following the trauma of surgery. Think about the principles of gravity and the prevention of the accumulation of fluid around the surgical site. This will assist in directing you to the correct option. If you had difficulty with this question, review postoperative care of a client following cataract surgery.
Level of Cognitive Ability: Application
Client Needs: Physiological Integrity
Integrated Process: Nursing Process/Planning
Content Area: Adult Health/Eye
Reference: Linton, A., & Maebius, N. (2007). *Introduction to medical-surgical nursing* (4th ed., p. 1178). Philadelphia: Saunders.

731. 1
Rationale: Severe pain or pain accompanied by nausea is an indicator of increased intraocular pressure and should be reported to the physician immediately. Options 2, 3, and 4 are incorrect.
Test-Taking Strategy: Note the strategic word "severe." Eliminate option 2 because this is not a normal condition. The client should not be turned to the operative side; therefore, eliminate option 3. From the remaining options, noting the strategic word will direct you to the correct option. If you had difficulty with this question, review the postoperative complications of cataract surgery requiring notification of the registered nurse and the physician.
Level of Cognitive Ability: Application

Client Needs: Physiological Integrity
Integrated Process: Nursing Process/Implementation
Content Area: Adult Health/Eye
Reference: Linton, A., & Maebius, N. (2007). *Introduction to medical-surgical nursing* (4th ed., p. 1178). Philadelphia: Saunders.

ALTERNATE ITEM FORMAT: MULTIPLE RESPONSE

732. **1, 3, 5, 6**
Rationale: Following eye surgery, some scratchiness and mild eye discomfort may occur in the operative eye and is usually relieved by mild analgesics. If the eye pain becomes severe, the client should notify the surgeon because this may indicate hemorrhage, infection, or increased intraocular pressure. The nurse would also instruct the client to notify the surgeon of purulent drainage, increased redness, or any decrease in visual acuity. The client is instructed to place an eye shield over the operative eye at bedtime to protect the eye from injury during sleep and to avoid activities that increase intraocular pressure such as bending over.
Test-Taking Strategy: Note that the client has had eye surgery. Recalling that the eye needs to be protected and that a concern is increased intraocular pressure will assist in determining the home care measures to be included in the plan. Review these measures if you had difficulty with this question.
Level of Cognitive Ability: Application
Client Needs: Physiological Integrity
Integrated Process: Teaching and Learning
Content Area: Adult health/Eye
Reference: deWit, S. (2009). *Medical-surgical nursing: Concepts & practice* (pp. 643-644). St. Louis: Saunders.

REFERENCES

deWit, S. (2009). *Medical-surgical nursing: Concepts & practice.* St. Louis: Saunders.
Christensen, B., & Kockrow, E. (2006). *Adult health nursing* (5th ed.). St. Louis: Mosby.
Ignatavicius, D., & Workman, M. (2006). *Medical-surgical nursing: Critical thinking for collaborative care* (5th ed.). Philadelphia: Saunders.
Jarvis, C. (2008). *Physical examination & health assessment* (5th ed.). Philadelphia: Saunders.
Linton, A., & Maebius, N. (2007). *Introduction to medical-surgical nursing* (4th ed.). Philadelphia: Saunders.
Monahan, F., Sands, J., Neighbors, M., Marek, J., & Green, C. (2007). *Phipps' medical-surgical nursing: Health and illness perspectives* (8th ed.). St. Louis: Mosby.

Ophthalmic and Otic Medications

I. OPHTHALMIC MEDICATION ADMINISTRATION

A. Guidelines for the use of eye medications

1. Eye medications are usually in the form of drops or ointments
2. Since the timing of medication administration is critical, administer medications at frequent, precise intervals; separate the instillation by 3 to 5 minutes if two medications must be administered at the same time
3. To prevent overflow of medication into the nasal and pharyngeal passages, thus reducing systemic absorption, instruct the client to apply pressure over the inner canthus next to the nose for 30 to 60 seconds following administration of the medication; instruct the client to close the eye gently to help distribute the medication
4. If both an eye drop and an eye ointment are scheduled to be administered at the same time, administer the eye drop first
5. Wash hands and don gloves before administering eye medications to avoid contaminating the eye or medication dropper or applicator
6. Use a separate bottle or tube of medication for each client to avoid accidental cross-contamination
7. Place the prescribed dose of eye medication in the lower conjunctival sac, never directly onto the cornea
8. Avoid touching any part of the eye with the dropper or applicator
9. Administer glucocorticoid preparations before other medications
10. Monitor the pulse of the client receiving an ophthalmic β-blocker, and instruct the client to do the same; if the pulse is less than 50 to 60 beats/minute (adult), withhold the next dose of eye medication and notify the physician
11. Instruct the client how to instill medication correctly and supervise instillation until the client can do it safely
12. Instruct the client to read the medication labels carefully to ensure administration of the correct medication and correct strength
13. Remind the client to keep these medications out of the reach of children
14. Instruct the client to avoid driving or operating hazardous equipment if vision is blurred
15. Inform the client that he or she may be unable to drive home after eye examinations when medications to dilate the pupil (**mydriatics**) or medications to paralyze the ciliary muscle (cycloplegics) are used
16. If photophobia occurs, instruct the client to wear sunglasses and avoid bright lights
17. Instruct the client to administer a missed dose of the eye medication as soon as it is remembered, unless the next dose is scheduled to be administered in 1 to 2 hours
18. Inform the client with **glaucoma** that the disorder cannot be cured, only controlled
19. Reinforce the importance of using medications to treat **glaucoma** as prescribed and not to discontinue these medications without consulting the physician
20. Inform the client that medications used to treat **glaucoma** may cause pain and blurred vision, especially when therapy is begun
21. Instruct the client to report the development of any eye irritation
22. Inform the client using eye gel to store the gel at room temperature or in the refrigerator but not to freeze it
23. Instruct the client to discard unused eye gel kept at room temperature as recommended by the physician and/or pharmacist
24. Inform the client that soft contact lenses may absorb certain eye medications and that preservatives in eye medications may discolor the contact lenses
25. Advise the client wearing contact lenses to question the physician carefully about special precautions to observe with eye medications
26. In infants, inform the parents that atropine sulfate eye drops may contribute to abdominal distention

27. Instruct the parents to keep a record of the infant's bowel movements if atropine sulfate eye drops are being administered
28. Auscultate bowel sounds of the infant or child receiving atropine sulfate eye drops

B. Instillation of eye medications
1. Drops
   a. Wash hands
   b. Put on gloves
   c. Check the name, strength, and expiration date of the medication
   d. Instruct the client to tilt the head backward, open the eyes, and look up
   e. Pull the lower lid down against the cheekbone
   f. Hold the bottle like a pencil with the tip downward
   g. Holding the bottle, gently rest the wrist of the hand on the client's cheek
   h. Squeeze the bottle gently to allow the drop to fall into the conjunctival sac
   i. Instruct the client to close the eyes gently and not to squeeze the eyes shut
   j. Wait 3 to 5 minutes before instilling another drop, if more than one drop is prescribed, promote maximal absorption of medication
   k. Do not allow the medication bottle, dropper, or applicator to come in contact with the eyelid or conjunctival sac
   l. To prevent systemic absorption of the medication, apply gentle pressure with a clean tissue to the client's nasolacrimal duct for 30 to 60 seconds
2. Ointments
   a. Instruct the client to lie down or tilt the head backward and look up
   b. Hold the ointment tube near, but not touching, the eye or eyelashes
   c. Squeeze a thin ribbon of ointment along the lining of the lower conjunctival sac from the inner to the outer canthus
   d. Instruct the client to close the eyes gently, rolling the eyeball in all directions, which increases contact area of medication to the eye
   e. Instruct the client that vision may be blurred by the ointment
   f. If possible, apply ointment just before bedtime

II. MYDRIATIC/CYCLOPLEGIC AND ANTICHOLINERGIC MEDICATIONS (Box 55-1)
A. Description (Figure 55-1)
1. **Mydriatics** and cycloplegics dilate the pupils (**mydriasis**) and relax the ciliary muscles (**cycloplegia**)
2. Anticholinergics block responses of the sphincter muscle in the ciliary body, producing **mydriasis** and **cycloplegia**
3. These medications are used preoperatively or for eye examinations to produce **mydriasis**

4. These medications are contraindicated in clients with **glaucoma** because of the risk of increased intraocular pressure
5. **Mydriatics** are contraindicated in cardiac dysrhythmias and cerebral atherosclerosis and should be used with caution in the older client and in clients with prostatic hypertrophy, diabetes mellitus, or parkinsonism

B. Side effects and toxicities
1. Tachycardia
2. Photophobia
3. Conjunctivitis
4. Dermatitis
5. Elevated blood pressure

C. Atropine toxicity
1. Dry mouth
2. Blurred vision
3. Photophobia
4. Tachycardia
5. Fever
6. Urinary retention
7. Constipation
8. Headache and brow pain
9. Confusion
10. Hallucinations and delirium
11. Coma
12. Worsening of narrow-angle **glaucoma**

D. Systemic reactions of anticholinergics
1. Dry mouth and skin

BOX 55-1   Mydriatic/Cycloplegic Medications

Atropine (Atropisol, Isopto Atropine, Atropine Care)
Cyclopentolate (AK-Pentolate, Cyclogyl, Pentolair)
Homatropine (Isopto Homatropine)
Scopolamine (Isopto hyoscine)
Tropicamide (Mydriacyl, Tropicacyl, Opticyl)

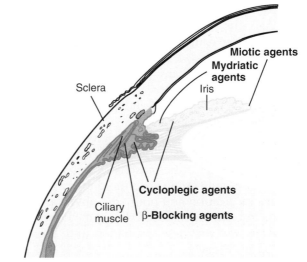

FIG. 55-1 Sites of action of mydriatic, β-blocking, cycloplegic, and miotic agents. (From Black, J., & Hawks, J. [2005]. *Medical-surgical nursing: Clinical management for positive outcomes* [7th ed.]. Philadelphia: Saunders.)

2. Fever
3. Thirst
4. Confusion
5. Hyperactivity
E. Interventions
1. Monitor for allergic response
2. Assess for risk of injury
3. Assess for constipation and urinary retention
4. Instruct the client that a burning sensation may occur on instillation
5. Instruct the client not to drive or perform hazardous activities for 24 hours after instillation of the medication unless otherwise directed by the physician
6. Instruct the client to wear sunglasses until the effects of the medication wear off
7. Instruct the client to notify the physician if blurring of vision, loss of sight, difficulty breathing, sweating, or flushing occurs
8. Instruct the client to report eye pain to the physician
F. α-Adrenergic blocker
1. Medication: dapiprazole hydrochloride (Rev-Eyes)
2. Use: to counteract **mydriasis**
III. ANTI-INFECTIVE EYE MEDICATIONS (Box 55-2)
A. Description: anti-infective medications kill or inhibit the growth of bacteria, fungi, and viruses
B. Side effects
1. Superinfection
2. Global irritation
C. Interventions
1. Assess for risk of injury
2. Instruct the client on how to apply the eye medication; remind the client to clean exudates from the eyes before administering drops
3. Reinforce the importance of completing the prescribed medication regimen
4. Instruct the client to wash hands thoroughly and frequently
5. Advise the client to notify the physician if improvement does not occur

IV. ANTI-INFLAMMATORY EYE MEDICATIONS (Box 55-3)
A. Description
1. Anti-inflammatory medications control inflammation, thereby reducing vision loss and scarring
2. Antiinflammatory medications are used for uveitis, allergic conditions, and inflammation of the conjunctiva, cornea, and lids
B. Side effects
1. **Cataracts**
2. Increased intraocular pressure
3. Impaired healing
4. Masking signs and symptoms of infection
C. Interventions
1. Interventions are the same as for anti-infective medications
2. Note that dexamethasone (Maxidex) should not be used for eye abrasions and wounds
V. TOPICAL ANESTHETICS FOR THE EYE (Box 55-4)
A. Description
1. Topical anesthetics produce corneal anesthesia
2. Topical anesthetics are used for anesthesia for eye examinations and surgery or to remove foreign bodies from the eye
3. Do not use discolored solution, and store the bottle tightly closed
B. Side effects
1. Temporary stinging or burning of the eye
2. Temporary loss of corneal reflex
C. Interventions
1. Assess for risk of injury

BOX 55-2 Anti-Infective Eye Medications

Antibacterial
Chloramphenicol (Chloromycetin powder)
Erythromycin (Ilotycin)
Aminoglycosides
Gentamicin sulfate (Garamycin, Genoptic)
Tobramycin (Tobrex)
Antifungal
Natamycin (Natacyn)
Antiviral
Idoxuridine
Trifluridine (Viroptic)
Sulfonamides
Sulfacetamide (Bleph-10, Sodium Sulamyd)

BOX 55-3 Anti-Inflammatory Eye Medications

Antiallergic Agents
Cromolyn sodium (Crolom, Opticrom)
Ketotifen fumarate (Zaditor)
Levocabastine (Livostin)
Lodoxamide (Alomide)
Nedocromil sodium (Alocril)
Pemirolast potassium (Alamast)
Corticosteroids
Dexamethasone (Maxidex)
Fluorometholone (FML-S Ophthalmic Suspension)
Medrysone (HMS)
Prednisolone (Pred-G, Pred-Forte)
Nonsteroidal Anti-Inflammatory Agents
Cyclosporine (Restasis)
Diclofenac (Voltaren)
Flurbiprofen sodium (Ocufen)
Ketorolac tromethamine (Acular)

BOX 55-4 Topical Anesthetics for the Eye

Proparacaine hydrochloride (Ophthetic)
Tetracaine hydrochloride (Pontocaine)

2. Note that the medications should not be given to the client for home use and are not to be self-administered by the client
3. Instruct the client not to rub or touch the eye while it is anesthetized
4. Note that the blink reflex is lost temporarily and that the corneal epithelium needs to be protected
5. Provide an eye patch to protect the eye from injury until the corneal reflex returns

VI. EYE LUBRICANTS (Box 55-5)
A. Description
1. Eye lubricants replace tears or add moisture to the eyes
2. Eye lubricants moisten contact lenses or an artificial eye and protect the eyes during surgery or diagnostic procedures
3. Eye lubricants are used for keratitis, during anesthesia, or in a disorder that results in unconsciousness or decreased blinking
B. Side effects
1. Burning on instillation
2. Discomfort or pain on instillation
C. Interventions
1. Inform the client that burning may occur on instillation
2. Be alert to allergic responses to the preservatives in the lubricants

VII. MIOTICS (Box 55-6; see Figure 55-1)
A. Description
1. **Miotics** reduce intraocular pressure by constricting the pupil and contracting the ciliary muscle, thereby increasing the blood flow to the retina and decreasing retinal damage and loss of vision
2. **Miotics** open the anterior chamber angle and increase the outflow of aqueous humor
3. Miotic cholinergic medications reduce intraocular pressure by mimicking the action of acetylcholine
4. Miotic acetylcholine inhibitors reduce intraocular pressure by inhibiting the action of cholinesterase
5. **Miotics** are used for chronic open-angle **glaucoma** or acute and chronic closed-angle **glaucoma**

BOX 55-5 Eye Lubricants

Hydroxypropyl methylcellulose (Lacril, Isopto Plain)
Petroleum-based ointment (Artificial Tears)
Polyvinyl alcohol (Liquifilm Tears)

BOX 55-6 Miotics

Carbachol (Carboptic)
Echothiophate
Pilocarpine hydrochloride (Isopto Carpine)

---

6. **Miotics** are used to achieve **miosis** during eye surgery
7. **Miotics** are contraindicated in clients with retinal detachment, adhesions between the iris and lens, or inflammatory diseases
8. Use **miotics** with caution in clients with asthma, hypertension, corneal abrasion, hyperthyroidism, coronary vascular disease, urinary tract obstruction, gastrointestinal obstruction, ulcer disease, parkinsonism, and bradycardia
B. Side effects
1. Myopia
2. Headache
3. Eye pain
4. Decreased vision in poor light
5. Local irritation
6. Systemic effects
   a. Flushing
   b. Diaphoresis
   c. Gastrointestinal upset and diarrhea
   d. Frequent urination
   e. Increased salivation
   f. Muscle weakness
   g. Respiratory difficulty
7. Toxicity
   a. Vertigo and syncope
   b. Bradycardia
   c. Hypotension
   d. Cardiac dysrhythmias
   e. Tremors
   f. Seizures
C. Interventions
1. Assess vital signs
2. Assess for risk of injury
3. Assess the client for the degree of diminished vision
4. Monitor for side effects and toxic effects
5. Monitor for postural hypotension, and instruct the client to change positions slowly
6. Assess breath sounds for wheezes and rhonchi because cholinergic medications can cause bronchospasm and an increase in bronchial secretions
7. Maintain oral hygiene because of the increase in salivation
8. Have atropine sulfate available as an antidote for pilocarpine
9. Instruct the client or family regarding the correct administration of eye medications
10. Instruct the client not to stop the medication suddenly
11. Instruct the client to avoid activities such as driving while vision is impaired
12. Instruct the client with **glaucoma** to read labels on over-the-counter medications and to avoid atropine-like medications because atropine will increase intraocular pressure

VIII. OCUSERT SYSTEM (Ocusert Pilo-20, Ocusert Pilo-40)

A. Description
1. Ocusert is a thin eye wafer (disk) impregnated with a time-release dose of pilocarpine
2. Ocusert is devised to overcome the frequent application of pilocarpine
3. Ocusert is placed in the upper or lower cul-de-sac of the eye
4. The pilocarpine is released over 1 week
5. The disk is replaced every 7 days
6. Drawbacks of its use include sudden leakage of pilocarpine, migration of the system over the cornea, and unnoticed loss of the system

B. Interventions
1. Assess the client's ability to insert the medication disk
2. Store the medication in the refrigerator
3. Instruct the client to discard damaged or contaminated disks
4. Inform the client that temporary stinging is expected but to notify the physician if blurred vision or brow pain occurs
5. Instruct the client to check for the presence of the disk in the conjunctival sac daily at bedtime and on arising
6. Because vision may change in the first few hours after the eye system is inserted, instruct the client to replace the disk at bedtime

IX. β-ADRENERGIC BLOCKER EYE MEDICATIONS (Box 55-7)

A. Description (see Figure 55-1)
1. These medications reduce intraocular pressure by decreasing sympathetic impulses and decreasing aqueous humor production without affecting accommodation or pupil size
2. These medications are used to treat chronic open-angle **glaucoma**
3. These medications are contraindicated in the client with asthma or chronic obstructive pulmonary disease because systemic absorption can cause increased airway resistance
4. Use these medications with caution in the client receiving oral β-blockers

B. Side effects
1. Ocular irritation
2. Visual disturbances

3. Bradycardia
4. Hypotension
5. Bronchospasm

C. Interventions
1. Monitor vital signs, especially blood pressure and pulse, before administering the medication
2. If the pulse is 60 beats/minute or less or if the systolic blood pressure is less than 90 mm Hg, withhold the medication and contact the physician
3. Monitor for shortness of breath
4. Assess for risk of injury
5. Monitor intake and output (I&O)
6. Instruct the client to notify the physician if shortness of breath occurs
7. Instruct the client not to discontinue the medication abruptly
8. Instruct the client to change positions slowly because of the potential for orthostatic hypotension
9. Instruct the client to avoid hazardous activities
10. Instruct the client to avoid over-the-counter medications without the physician's approval
11. Instruct clients with diabetes mellitus using β-adrenergic blockers to monitor blood glucose levels frequently

D. Adrenergic medications (Box 55-8)
1. Adrenergic medications decrease the production of aqueous humor and lead to a decrease in intraocular pressure
2. Adrenergic medications may be used to treat **glaucoma**

X. CARBONIC ANHYDRASE INHIBITORS (Box 55-9)

A. Description
1. Carbonic anhydrase inhibitors interfere with the production of carbonic acid, which leads to decreased aqueous humor formation and decreased intraocular pressure
2. These medications are used for long-term treatment of open-angle **glaucoma**
3. These medications are contraindicated in the client allergic to sulfonamides
4. Use with caution for clients with severe renal or liver disease

---

BOX 55-7 β-Adrenergic Blocker Eye Medications

Betaxolol hydrochloride (Betoptic)
Carteolol hydrochloride (Ocupress)
Levobetaxolol
Levobunolol hydrochloride (Betagan)
Metipranolol (Optipranolol)
Timolol maleate (Timoptic)

BOX 55-8 Adrenergic Medications

Hydroxyamphetamine (Paredrine)
Naphazoline (Allerest)
Oxymetazoline (OcuClear)
Tetrahydrozoline (Murine Plus, Visine)

BOX 55-9 Carbonic Anhydrase Inhibitors: Eye Medications

Acetazolamide (Diamox)
Brinzolamide (Azopt)
Dorzolamide hydrochloride (Trusopt)

BOX 55-10   **Osmotic Medications for the Eye**

Glycerin (Osmoglyn)
Mannitol (Osmitrol)

B. Side effects
 1. Appetite loss
 2. Gastrointestinal upset
 3. Paresthesias in the fingers, toes, and face
 4. Polyuria
 5. Hypokalemia
 6. Renal calculi
 7. Photosensitivity
 8. Lethargy and drowsiness
 9. Depression
C. Interventions
 1. Monitor vital signs
 2. Assess visual acuity
 3. Assess for risk of injury
 4. Monitor I&O
 5. Monitor weight
 6. Maintain oral hygiene
 7. Monitor for side effects such as lethargy, anorexia, drowsiness, polyuria, nausea, and vomiting
 8. Monitor electrolytes for hypokalemia
 9. Increase fluid intake unless contraindicated
 10. Advise the client to avoid prolonged exposure to sunlight
 11. Encourage the use of artificial tears for dry eyes
 12. Instruct the client not to discontinue the medication abruptly
 13. Instruct the client to avoid hazardous activities while vision is impaired
 14. Teach the client not to wear contact lenses during or within 15 minutes of instilling these medications

XI. OSMOTIC MEDICATIONS (Box 55-10)
A. Description
 1. Osmotic medications lower intraocular pressure
 2. Osmotic medications are used in emergency treatment of acute closed-angle **glaucoma**
 3. Osmotic medications are used preoperatively and postoperatively to decrease vitreous humor volume
B. Side effects
 1. Headache
 2. Nausea, vomiting, diarrhea, and dehydration
 3. Disorientation
 4. Electrolyte imbalances
C. Interventions
 1. Assess vital signs
 2. Assess visual acuity
 3. Assess for risk of injury
 4. Monitor I&O
 5. Monitor weight
 6. Monitor for electrolyte imbalances
 7. Increase fluid intake unless contraindicated
 8. Monitor for changes in level of orientation

BOX 55-11   **Medications That Affect Hearing**

Antibiotics
Amikacin (Amikin)
Chloramphenicol (Chloromycetin, Chloroptic)
Erythromycin (ERYC, Ery-Tab, PCE Dispertabs, Ilotycin)
Gentamicin (Garamycin)
Streptomycin sulfate
Tobramycin sulfate (Nebcin)
Vancomycin (Vancocin)
Diuretics
Acetazolamide (Diamox)
Ethacrynic acid (Edecrin)
Furosemide (Lasix)
Others
Cisplatin (Platinol)
Nitrogen mustard
Quinine
Quinidine

XII. OTIC MEDICATION ADMINISTRATION
  (Box 55-11)
A. Instillation of ear drops
 1. In an adult, pull the pinna up and back to straighten the external canal to instill ear drops
 2. Tilt the client's head in the opposite direction of the affected ear and apply the drops into the ear
 3. With the head tilted, gently move the head back and forth five times
 4. Pull the pinna down and back for infants and children younger than 3 years of age, and up and back for older children
B. Irrigation of the ear
 1. Irrigation of the ear needs to be prescribed by the physician
 2. Ensure direct visualization of the tympanic membrane
 3. Warm irrigating solution to 98° F since solutions that are not close to the client's body temperature will cause ear injury, nausea, and vertigo
 4. Irrigation must be done gently to avoid damage to the eardrum
 5. When irrigating, do not direct irrigation solution directly toward the eardrum
 6. If a perforation of the eardrum is suspected, do not perform irrigation
XIII. ANTI-INFECTIVE EAR MEDICATIONS
  (Box 55-12)
A. Description
 1. Anti-infective medications kill or inhibit the growth of bacteria and are used for otitis media or otitis externa
 2. Anti-infective medications are contraindicated if a prior hypersensitivity exists
B. Side effects: overgrowth of nonsusceptible organisms

BOX 55-12 **Anti-infective Ear Medications**

Acetic acid and aluminum acetate (Otic Domeboro)
Amoxicillin (Amoxil)
Ampicillin trihydrate (Principen)
Cefaclor (Ceclor)
Chloramphenicol (Chloromycetin Otic)
Clarithromycin (Biaxin)
Clindamycin hydrochloride (Cleocin)
Erythromycin (Ilotycin)
Gentamicin sulfate otic solution (Garamycin)
Loracarbef (Lorabid)
Penicillin V potassium (Veetids)
Trimethoprim and sulfamethoxazole (Bactrim, Cotrim, and Septra)

BOX 55-13 **Antihistamines and Decongestants**

Cetirizine (Zyrtec)
Chlorpheniramine (Chlor-Trimeton)
Clemastine (Tavist)
Naphazoline hydrochloride (Allerest, Albalon)

C. Interventions
   1. Monitor vital signs
   2. Assess for allergies
   3. Assess for pain
   4. Monitor for nephrotoxicity
   5. Instruct the client to report dizziness, fatigue, fever, or sore throat, which may indicate a superimposed infection
   6. Instruct the client to complete the entire course of the medication
   7. Instruct the client to keep ear canals dry
XIV. ANTIHISTAMINES AND DECONGESTANTS (Box 55-13)
A. Description
   1. These medications produce vasoconstriction
   2. These medications stimulate the receptors of the respiratory mucosa
   3. These medications reduce respiratory tissue hyperemia and edema to open obstructed eustachian tubes
   4. These medications are used for acute otitis media
B. Side effects
   1. Drowsiness
   2. Blurred vision
   3. Dry mucous membranes
C. Interventions
   1. Inform the client that drowsiness, blurred vision, and a dry mouth may occur
   2. Instruct the client to increase fluid intake unless contraindicated and to suck on hard candy to alleviate the dry mouth
   3. Instruct the client to avoid hazardous activities if drowsiness occurs

BOX 55-14 **Ceruminolytic Medications**

Boric acid (Ear-Dry)
Carbamide peroxide (Debrox)
Trolamine polypeptide oleate—condensate (Cerumenex)

XV. LOCAL ANESTHETICS
A. Description
   1. Local anesthetics block nerve conduction at or near the application site to control pain
   2. Local anesthetics are used for pain associated with ear infections
B. Medication: benzocaine (Tympagesic)
C. Side effects
   1. Allergic reaction
   2. Irritation
D. Interventions
   1. Monitor for effectiveness if used for pain relief
   2. Assess for irritation or allergic reaction
XVI. CERUMINOLYTIC MEDICATIONS (Box 55-14)
A. Description
   1. Ceruminolytic medications emulsify and loosen cerumen deposits
   2. Ceruminolytic medications are used to loosen and remove impacted wax from the ear canal
B. Side effects
   1. Irritation
   2. Redness or swelling of the ear canal
C. Interventions
   1. Instruct the client not to use drops more often than prescribed
   2. Moisten a cotton plug with medication before insertion
   3. Keep the container tightly closed and away from moisture
   4. Avoid touching the ear with the dropper
   5. Thirty minutes after instillation, gently irrigate the ear as prescribed with warm water using a soft rubber bulb ear syringe
   6. Irrigation may be done with hydrogen peroxide solution as prescribed to flush cerumen deposits out of the ear canal
   7. For a chronic cerumen impaction, one to two drops of mineral oil will soften the wax
   8. Instruct the client to notify the physician if redness, pain, or swelling persists

PRACTICE QUESTIONS

More questions on the companion CD!

733. A miotic medication has been prescribed for the client with glaucoma and the client asks the nurse about the purpose of the medication. The nurse tells the client that:
   1. "The medication will help dilate the eye to prevent pressure from occurring."

2. "The medication will relax the muscles of the eye and prevent blurred vision."

3. "The medication will help block the responses that are sent to the muscles in the eye."

4. "The medication will lower the pressure in your eye and increase the blood flow to the retina."

734. Pilocarpine hydrochloride (Isopto Carpine) is prescribed for the client with glaucoma. Which medication does the nurse plan to have available in the event of systemic toxicity?
1. Atropine sulfate
2. Timolol maleate (Timoptic)
3. Metipranolol (Optipranolol)
4. Carteolol hydrochloride (Ocupress)

735. Betaxolol hydrochloride (Betoptic) eye drops have been prescribed for the client with glaucoma. Which nursing action is appropriate related to monitoring for the side effects of this medication?
1. Monitor temperature
2. Monitor blood pressure
3. Monitor peripheral pulses
4. Monitor urine for glucose and acetone

736. A nurse is assisting the physician with an ear irrigation on an assigned client. The nurse would plan to:
1. Cool the irrigating solution to 85° F (29.4° C)
2. Warm the irrigating solution to 98° F (36.6° C)
3. Position the client with the affected side up following the irrigation
4. Ask the client to turn his or her head so that the ear to be irrigated is facing upward

737. In preparation for cataract surgery, the nurse is to administer cyclopentolate hydrochloride (Cyclogyl) eye drops. The nurse administers the medication knowing that the purpose of the medication is to:
1. Produce miosis of the operative eye
2. Dilate the pupil of the operative eye
3. Provide lubrication to the operative eye
4. Constrict the pupil of the operative eye

738. A nurse is providing instructions to the client regarding the administration of the prescribed eye drops. Which of the following statements by the client indicates a need for further instructions?
1. "I can lie down, pull up on the upper lid, and place the drop in the lower lid."
2. "I can lie down, pull down on the lower lid, and place the drop in the lower lid."
3. "I can tilt my head back, pull down on the lower lid, and place the drop in the lower lid."

4. "I can lie on my side opposite to the eye in which I am going to place the drop, put the drop in the corner of the lid nearest my nose, and then slowly turn to my other side while blinking."

739. To minimize the systemic effects that eye drops can produce, the nurse plans to instruct the client to:
1. Eat before instilling the drops.
2. Swallow several times after instilling the drops.
3. Blink vigorously to encourage tearing after instilling the drops.
4. Occlude the nasolacrimal duct with a finger for several minutes after instilling the drops.

740. A client is receiving brinzolamide (Azopt) and timolol maleate (Timoptic) eye drops. When instructing the client on the administration of the eye drops, the nurse plans to tell the client to:
1. Wait 3 minutes between the instillation of each medication.
2. Administer the brinzolamide first, followed by the timolol maleate.
3. Administer the timolol maleate first, followed by the brinzolamide.
4. Administer brinzolamide in the morning and the timolol maleate in the evening.

741. A licensed practical nurse (LPN) is assigned to care for a client with glaucoma. The LPN reviews the client's medication record and would notify the registered nurse (RN) if which medication was noted on the client's record?
1. Carbachol (Carboptic)
2. Atropine sulfate (Isopto Atropine)
3. Pilocarpine hydrochloride (Isopto Carpine)
4. Pilocarpine (Ocusert Pilo-20, Ocusert Pilo-40)

ALTERNATE ITEM FORMAT: MULTIPLE RESPONSE

742. The nurse is preparing to administer eye drops. Select the interventions that the nurse takes to administer the drops. Select all that apply.
□ 1. Wash hands.
□ 2. Put on gloves.
□ 3. Place the drop in the conjunctival sac.
□ 4. Pull the lower lid down against the cheek bone.
□ 5. Instruct the client to squeeze the eyes shut after instilling the eye drop.
□ 6. Instruct the client to tilt the head forward, open the eyes, and look down.

ANSWERS

733. **4**

Rationale: Miotics are used to lower the intraocular pressure, thereby increasing blood flow to the retina and decreasing retinal damage and loss of vision. Options 1, 2, and 3 all describe actions related to mydriatic medications, which primarily dilate the pupils and relax the ciliary muscles.

Test-Taking Strategy: Use the process of elimination. Note that the client has glaucoma. This should provide you with the clue to direct you to the correct option. Remember,

prevention of increased intraocular pressure is the goal in clients with glaucoma. Review this type of medication if you had difficulty with this question.
Level of Cognitive Ability: Application
Client Needs: Physiological Integrity
Integrated Process: Nursing Process/Implementation
Content Area: Adult Health/Eye
Reference: Kee, J., Hayes, E., & McCuistion, L. (2006). *Pharmacology: A nursing process approach* (5th ed., pp. 728-729). Philadelphia: Saunders.

734. 1
Rationale: Systemic absorption of pilocarpine hydrochloride can produce toxicity and includes manifestations of vertigo, bradycardia, tremors, hypotension, and seizures. Atropine sulfate must be available in the event of systemic toxicity. Pindolol, timolol maleate, and carteolol hydrochloride are β-blockers.
Test-Taking Strategy: Note that options 2, 3, and 4 are comparable or alike and are β-blockers. Also remember that atropine sulfate is the antidote for systemic reactions that occur with pilocarpine hydrochloride. Review antidotes if you had difficulty with this question.
Level of Cognitive Ability: Application
Client Needs: Physiological Integrity
Integrated Process: Nursing Process/Planning
Content Area: Adult Health/Eye
Reference: Kee, J., Hayes, E., & McCuistion, L. (2006). *Pharmacology: A nursing process approach* (5th ed., pp. 286, 288). Philadelphia: Saunders.

735. 2
Rationale: This medication is an antiglaucoma medication and a β-adrenergic blocker. Hypotension manifested as dizziness, nausea, diaphoresis, headache, and fatigue are systemic effects of the medication. The nurse would monitor the client's blood pressure. Options 1, 3, and 4 are not related to side effects associated with this medication.
Test-Taking Strategy: Focus on the name of the medication and recall that medication names that end with the letters "-lol" are β-blockers. Also, use the ABCs—airway, breathing, and circulation. Although option 3 is also related to circulation monitoring, the blood pressure is the umbrella option. Review the side effects of this medication if you had difficulty with this question.
Level of Cognitive Ability: Application
Client Needs: Physiological Integrity
Integrated Process: Nursing Process/Implementation
Content Area: Adult Health/Eye
Reference: McKenry, L., Tessier, E., & Hogan, M. (2006). *Mosby's pharmacology in nursing* (22nd ed., p. 798). St. Louis: Mosby.

736. 2
Rationale: Irrigation solutions that are not close to the client's body temperature can be uncomfortable and may cause injury, nausea, and vertigo. The client is positioned so that the ear to be irrigated is facing downward; this allows gravity to assist in the removal of the ear wax and solution. Following the irrigation, the client is to lie on the affected side for a period of time to finish the drainage of the irrigating solution.
Test-Taking Strategy: Use the process of elimination. Visualizing the procedure will assist in eliminating options

3 and 4. Recalling that the irrigating solution should be close to body temperature will assist in eliminating option 1. Review this procedure if you had difficulty with this question.
Level of Cognitive Ability: Application
Client Needs: Physiological Integrity
Integrated Process: Nursing Process/Planning
Content Area: Adult Health/Ear
Reference: Fultz, J., & Sturt, P. (2005). *Emergency nursing reference* (3rd ed., pp. 820-822). St. Louis: Mosby.

737. 2
Rationale: Cyclopentolate is a rapidly acting mydriatic (dilates) and cycloplegic medication. It is effective in 25 to 75 minutes, and accommodation returns in 6 to 24 hours. Cyclopentolate is used for preoperative mydriasis. Options 1, 3, and 4 are not actions of this medication.
Test-Taking Strategy: Use the process of elimination. Options 1 and 4 are comparable or alike because miosis refers to the constricted pupil. Note that the question identifies a client being prepared for cataract surgery. The pupil would need to be dilated for the surgical procedure. Review the action and purpose of this medication if you had difficulty with this question.
Level of Cognitive Ability: Comprehension
Client Needs: Physiological Integrity
Integrated Process: Nursing Process/Implementation
Content Area: Adult Health/Eye
Reference: Lehne, R. (2007). *Pharmacology for nursing care* (6th ed., p. 1196). Philadelphia: Saunders.

738. 1
Rationale: The client can either lie down or sit with the head tilted back. The lower lid should be pulled downward with the thumb or fingers. The client holds the bottle like a pencil, with the tip downward, and squeezes the bottle gently, allowing one drop to fall into the sac. The client gently closes the eye. An alternative method for clients who blink very easily is to place the client in the supine position with the head turned to one side. The eye to receive the eye drops should be uppermost. With the eye closed, drop the prescribed dose on the inner canthus of the eye. Have the client turn from side to midline and to the other side while blinking. The eye drops will move via gravity and surface tension into the conjunctival sac.
Test-Taking Strategy: Note the strategic words "a need for further instructions." These words indicate a negative event query and the need to select the incorrect client statement. Knowing that the client places drops into the eye by pulling down on the lower lid will direct you to the correct option. Review the procedure for the administration of eye medications if you had difficulty with this question.
Level of Cognitive Ability: Comprehension
Client Needs: Physiological Integrity
Integrated Process: Teaching and Learning
Content Area: Adult Health/Eye
References: Kee, J., Hayes, E., & McCuistion, L. (2006). *Pharmacology: A nursing process approach* (5th ed., pp. 34-35). Philadelphia: Saunders.
Lilley, L., Harrington, S., & Snyder, J. (2007). *Pharmacology and the nursing process* (5th ed., p. 122). St. Louis: Mosby.

739. 4

Rationale: Applying pressure on the nasolacrimal duct prevents systemic absorption of the medication. Options 1, 2, and 3 will not prevent this.

Test-Taking Strategy: Use the process of elimination. Eliminate options 1 and 2 because eating and swallowing are comparable or alike and are unrelated to the systemic absorption of an eye medication. Blinking vigorously to produce tearing may result in the loss of the administered medication. Review this procedure if you had difficulty with this question.

Level of Cognitive Ability: Application
Client Needs: Physiological Integrity
Integrated Process: Teaching and Learning
Content Area: Adult Health/Eye
Reference: Linton, A., & Maebius, N. (2007). *Introduction to medical-surgical nursing* (4th ed., p. 1165). Philadelphia: Saunders.

740. 1

Rationale: When two or more medications are to be administered, the client should wait 3 to 5 minutes between instillations. Options 2, 3, and 4 are incorrect.

Test-Taking Strategy: Use the process of elimination and focus on the subject—the administration of two different prescribed eye drops. Note that option 1 is different from the other options and provides specific information related to the question. Also, remember that when two or more medications are to be administered, the client should wait 3 to 5 minutes between instillations. Review the administration of eye medications if you had difficulty with this question.

Level of Cognitive Ability: Application
Client Needs: Physiological Integrity
Integrated Process: Teaching and Learning
Content Area: Adult Health/Eye
Reference: Kee, J., Hayes, E., & McCuistion, L. (2006). *Pharmacology: A nursing process approach* (5th ed., pp. 34, 73-75). Philadelphia: Saunders.

741. 2

Rationale: Atropine sulfate is a mydriatic and cycloplegic medication, and its use is contraindicated in clients with glaucoma. Mydriatic medications dilate the pupil and can cause an increase in intraocular pressure in the eye. Options 1, 3, and 4 are miotic agents used in the treatment of glaucoma.

Test-Taking Strategy: Focus on the classifications of the medications identified in the options to assist you in answering the question. Remember that my"d"riatics "d"ilate, and these medications are contraindicated in glaucoma. Review these medications if you had difficulty with this question.

Level of Cognitive Ability: Analysis
Client Needs: Safe and Effective Care Environment
Integrated Process: Nursing Process/Implementation
Content Area: Adult Health/Eye
Reference: Kee, J., Hayes, E., & McCuistion, L. (2006). *Pharmacology: A nursing process approach* (5th ed., p. 734). Philadelphia: Saunders.

ALTERNATE ITEM FORMAT: MULTIPLE RESPONSE

742. **1, 2, 3, 4**

Rationale: To administer eye medications, the nurse would wash hands and put on gloves. The client is instructed to tilt the head backward, open the eyes, and look up. The nurse pulls the lower lid down against the cheekbone and holds the bottle like a pencil with the tip downward. Holding the bottle, the nurse gently rests the wrist of the hand on the client's cheek and squeezes the bottle gently to allow the drop to fall into the conjunctival sac. The client is instructed to close the eyes gently and not to squeeze the eyes shut to prevent the loss of medication.

Test-Taking Strategy: Use guidelines related to standard precautions and visualize this procedure. This will assist in determining the correct interventions. If you are unfamiliar with the procedure for administering eye medications, review these guidelines.

Level of Cognitive Ability: Application
Client Needs: Physiological Integrity
Integrated Process: Nursing Process/Implementation
Content Area: Adult Health/Eye
References: deWit, S. (2009). *Medical-surgical nursing: Concepts & practice* (p. 648). St. Louis: Saunders.
Perry, A., & Potter, P. (2006). *Clinical nursing skills & techniques* (6th ed., pp. 654-656). St. Louis: Mosby.

REFERENCES

deWit, S. (2009). *Medical-surgical nursing: Concepts & practice.* St. Louis: Saunders.
Fultz, J., & Sturt, P. (2005). *Emergency nursing reference* (3rd ed.). St. Louis: Mosby.
Kee, J., Hayes, E., & McCuistion, L. (2006). *Pharmacology: A nursing process approach* (5th ed.). Philadelphia: Saunders.
Lehne, R. (2007). *Pharmacology for nursing care* (6th ed.). Philadelphia: Saunders.
Lilley, L., Harrington, S., & Snyder, J. (2007). *Pharmacology and the nursing process* (5th ed.). St. Louis: Mosby.
Linton, A., & Maebius, N. (2007). *Introduction to medical-surgical nursing* (4th ed.). Philadelphia: Saunders.
McKenry, L., Tessier, E., & Hogan, M. (2006). *Mosby's pharmacology in nursing* (22nd ed. p. 798). St. Louis: Mosby.
Perry, A., & Potter, P. (2006). *Clinical nursing skills & techniques* (6th ed.). St. Louis: Mosby.

The Adult Client With a Neurological Disorder

PYRAMID TERMS

agnosia The inability to use an object correctly

apraxia The inability to carry out a purposeful activity

autonomic dysreflexia Also known as hyperreflexia; characterized by paroxysmal hypertension, bradycardia, excessive sweating, facial flushing, nasal congestion, pilomotor responses, and headache; occurs with spinal lesions above T6 after the period of spinal shock is complete; causes include visceral distention from a distended bladder or impacted rectum; the syndrome is a neurological emergency and must be treated immediately to prevent a hypertensive stroke

Babinski's reflex Dorsiflexion of the ankle and great toe with fanning of the other toes elicited by firmly stroking the lateral aspect of the sole of the foot; indicates a disruption of the pyramidal tract

Brudzinski's sign Flexion of the head that causes flexion of both thighs at the hips and knee flexion and indicates meningeal irritation

decerebrate posturing Stiff extension of one or both arms and possibly the legs that indicates a brainstem lesion

decorticate posturing Flexure of one or both arms on the chest and possibly stiff extension of the legs that indicates a nonfunctioning cortex

flaccid posturing No motor response display in any extremity

Glasgow Coma Scale A method of assessing a client's neurological condition; a scoring system based on a scale of 1 to 15 points; a score of less than 8 indicates that coma is present; eye-opening is the most important indicator

halo traction Insertion of pins or screws into the client's skull and application of a circular fixation device and halo jacket or cast; used to immobilize the cervical spine

hemianopsia Blindness in half of the visual field

homonymous hemianopsia Blindness in the same visual field of both eyes

increased intracranial pressure An increase in intracranial pressure caused by trauma, hemorrhage, growths or tumors, hydrocephalus, edema, or inflammation; can impede circulation to the brain and absorption of cerebrospinal fluid and can affect the functioning of nerve cells and lead to brainstem compression and death

Kernig's sign Flexure of the thigh and knee to right angles, and when they are extended it causes spasm of the hamstring and pain; indicates meningeal irritation

nuchal rigidity Stiff neck; flexion of the neck onto the chest causes intense pain

skull tongs Tongs inserted into the outer aspect of the client's skull, just above the ears, with application of traction; some types include Gardner-Wells, Barton, and Crutchfield tongs

spinal shock Also known as neurogenic shock; a sudden depression of reflex activity in the spinal cord below the level of injury (areflexia) that occurs within the first hour of injury and lasts days to months; the muscles become completely paralyzed and flaccid, and reflexes are absent

Tensilon test Test performed to diagnose myasthenia gravis and to differentiate between myasthenic crisis and cholinergic crisis

unconscious client A state of depressed cerebral functioning with unresponsiveness to sensory and motor function; causes include head trauma, cerebral toxins, shock, hemorrhage, tumor, and infections

unilateral neglect Also known as neglect syndrome; an inability to recognize a physical impairment that occurs most commonly in clients who have had a right cerebral stroke

PYRAMID TO SUCCESS

Pyramid points related to neurological disorders focus on safety issues; care of the unconscious client; monitoring for increased intracranial pressure; monitoring level of consciousness; positioning clients; nursing interventions during a seizure, head injury, brain attack (stroke), spinal cord injury, Parkinson's disease, and meningitis; and care of the client with myasthenia gravis. Altered body image and psychosocial issues that occur as a result of the neurological disorder are also a focus of the Pyramid to Success. The Integrated Processes addressed in this unit include Caring, Clinical Problem-Solving Process (Nursing Process), Communication and Documentation, and Teaching and Learning.

▲ CLIENT NEEDS

Safe and Effective Care Environment

Acting as a client advocate

Consulting with members of the health care team

Ensuring advance directives are in the client's medical record

Establishing priorities

Initiating referrals to appropriate services

Maintaining asepsis with procedures and treatments

Maintaining confidentiality

Maintaining standard and other precautions

Obtaining informed consent for invasive procedures

Preventing accidents that can occur as a result of neurological deficits

Upholding client rights

Health Promotion and Maintenance

Discussing expected and unexpected body-image changes resulting from neurological deficits

Performing neurological data collection techniques

Preventing and detecting health problems associated with neurological deficits

Providing home care instructions regarding care related to the neurological disorder

Teaching about the importance of prescribed therapy

Psychosocial Integrity

Acknowledging end-of-life issues and grief and loss issues

Assessing the ability to cope with feelings of isolation and loss of independence

Considering the cultural, religious, and spiritual influences of the client when planning care

Identifying sensory and perceptual alterations

Identifying support systems and encouraging the use of community resources

Mobilizing coping mechanisms

Physiological Integrity

Administering pharmacological therapy

Monitoring for alterations in body systems

Monitoring for complications related to procedures

Monitoring for fluid and electrolyte imbalances

Providing assistive devices for mobility

Providing emergency care

Providing measures to promote comfort

Promoting normal elimination patterns

Promoting self-care measures

REFERENCES

Black, J., & Hawks, J. (2005). *Medical-surgical nursing: Clinical management for positive outcomes* (7th ed.). Philadelphia: Saunders.

Chernecky, C., & Berger, B. (2008). *Laboratory tests and diagnostic procedures* (5th ed.). Philadelphia: Saunders.

Christensen, B., & Kockrow, E. (2006). *Adult health nursing* (5th ed.). St. Louis: Mosby.

Christensen, B., & Kockrow, E. (2006). *Foundations of nursing* (5th ed.). St. Louis: Mosby.

deWit, S. (2009). *Medical-surgical nursing: Concepts & practice.* Philadelphia: Saunders.

Hodgson, B., & Kizior, R. (2008). *Saunders nursing drug handbook 2008.* Philadelphia: Saunders.

Ignatavicius, D., & Workman, M. (2006). *Medical-surgical nursing: Critical thinking for collaborative care* (5th ed.). Philadelphia: Saunders.

Kee, J., Hayes, E., & McCuistion, L. (2006). *Pharmacology: A nursing process approach* (5th ed.). Philadelphia: Saunders.

Lehne, R. (2007). *Pharmacology for nursing care* (6th ed.). Philadelphia: Saunders.

Lewis, S., Heitkemper, M., Dirksen, S., & Bucher, L. (2007). *Medical-surgical nursing: Assessment and management of clinical problems* (7th ed.). St. Louis: Mosby.

Linton, A., & Maebius, N. (2007). *Introduction to medical-surgical nursing* (4th ed.). Philadelphia: Saunders.

McKenry, L., Tessier, E., & Hogan, M. (2006). *Mosby's pharmacology in nursing* (22nd ed.). St. Louis: Mosby.

Monahan, F., Sands, J., Neighbors, M., Marek, J., & Green, C. (2007). *Phipps' medical-surgical nursing: Health and illness perspectives* (8th ed.). St. Louis: Mosby.

National Council of State Boards of Nursing (eds.) (2008). *2008 Detailed Test Plan for the NCLEX-PN® Examination,* National Council of State Boards of Nursing, Chicago: Author.

National Council of State Boards of Nursing, Inc. Web site: http://www.ncsbn.org.

Perry, A., & Potter, P. (2006). *Clinical nursing skills & techniques* (6th ed.). St. Louis: Mosby.

Skidmore-Roth, L. (2008). *2008 Mosby's nursing drug reference* (21st ed.). St. Louis: Mosby.

Neurological System

I. ANATOMY AND PHYSIOLOGY OF THE BRAIN AND SPINAL CORD

A. Cerebrum
   1. The cerebrum consists of the right and left hemispheres
   2. Each hemisphere receives sensory information from the opposite side of the body and controls the skeletal muscles of the opposite side
   3. The cerebrum governs sensory and motor activity and thought and learning

B. Cerebral cortex (Box 56-1)
   1. The cerebral cortex is the outer gray layer and it is divided into five lobes
   2. It is responsible for the conscious activities of the cerebrum

C. Basal ganglia: cell bodies in white matter that assist the cerebral cortex in producing smooth voluntary movements

D. Diencephalon
   1. Thalamus
      a. Relays sensory impulses to the cortex
      b. Provides a pain gate
      c. Is part of the reticular activating system
   2. Hypothalamus
      a. Regulates autonomic responses of the sympathetic and parasympathetic nervous systems
      b. Regulates the stress response, sleep, appetite, body temperature, fluid balance, and emotions
      c. Is responsible for the production of hormones secreted by the pituitary gland and the hypothalamus

E. Brainstem
   1. Midbrain
      a. Responsible for motor coordination
      b. Contains the visual reflex and auditory relay centers
   2. Pons: contains the respiratory centers and regulates breathing
   3. Medulla oblongata
      a. Contains all afferent and efferent tracts and contains cardiac, respiratory, vomiting, and vasomotor centers
      b. Controls heart rate, respiration, blood vessel diameter, sneezing, swallowing, vomiting, and coughing

F. Cerebellum: coordinates smooth muscle movement, posture, equilibrium, and muscle tone

G. Spinal cord
   1. Provides neuron and synapse networks to produce involuntary responses to sensory stimulation
   2. Controls body movement and regulates visceral function
   3. Carries sensory information to and motor information from the brain
   4. Extends from the first cervical to the second lumbar vertebra
   5. Is protected by the meninges, cerebrospinal fluid (CSF), and adipose tissue
   6. Horns
      a. Inner column of gray matter contains two anterior and two posterior horns
      b. Posterior horns connect with afferent (sensory) nerve fibers
      c. Anterior horns contain efferent (motor) nerve fibers
   7. Nerve tracts
      a. White matter contains the nerve tract
      b. Ascending tracts (sensory pathway)
      c. Descending tract (motor pathway)

H. Meninges
   1. Dura mater is the tough and fibrous membrane
   2. Arachnoid membrane is the delicate membrane and contains subarachnoid fluid
   3. Pia mater is the vascular membrane
   4. Subarachnoid space is formed by the arachnoid membrane and the pia mater

I. Cerebrospinal fluid (CSF)
   1. Secreted in the ventricles and circulates in the subarachnoid space and through the ventricles to the subarachnoid layer of the meninges, where it is reabsorbed
   2. Acts as a protective cushion and aids in the exchange of nutrients and wastes
   3. Normal pressure is 50 to 175 mm H_2O

BOX 56-1   Cerebral Cortex

Frontal Lobe
Broca's area for speech
Morals, emotions, reasoning and judgments,
    concentration, and abstraction
Parietal Lobe
Interpretation of taste, pain, touch, temperature, and
    pressure
Spatial perception
Temporal Lobe
Auditory center
Wernicke's area for sensory and speech
Occipital Lobe
Visual area
Limbic Lobe
Emotional and visceral patterns for survival
Learning and memory

    4. Normal volume is 125 to 150 mL
J. Ventricles
    1. Four ventricles
    2. The ventricles communicate between the subarachnoid spaces and produce and circulate CSF
K. Blood supply
    1. Right and left internal carotids
    2. Right and left vertebral arteries
    3. These arteries supply the brain via an anastamosis at the base of the brain called the circle of Willis
L. Neurotransmitters
    1. Acetylcholine
    2. Norepinephrine
    3. Dopamine
    4. Serotonin
    5. Amino acids
    6. Polypeptides
M. Neurons
    1. The neuron consists of cell body, axons, and dendrites
    2. The cell body contains the nucleus
    3. Neurons carrying impulses to the central nervous system (CNS) are called sensory neurons
    4. Neurons carrying impulses away from the CNS are called motor neurons
    5. Synapse is the chemical transmission of impulses from one neuron to another
N. Axons and dendrites
    1. The axon conducts impulses from the cell body
    2. The dendrites receive stimuli from the body and transmit them to the axon
    3. The neurons are protected and insulated by Schwann cells
    4. The Schwann cell sheath is called the neurilemma
    5. Neurons do not reproduce after the neonatal period

    6. If an axon or dendrite is damaged, it will die and be replaced slowly only if the neurilemma is intact and the cell body has not died
O. Spinal nerves
    1. Human beings have 31 pairs of spinal nerves
    2. Mixed nerve fibers are formed by the joining of the anterior motor and posterior sensory roots
    3. Posterior roots contain afferent (sensory) nerve fibers
    4. Anterior roots contain efferent (motor) nerve fibers
P. Autonomic nervous system
    1. Sympathetic (adrenergic) fibers dilate pupils, increase heart rate and rhythm, contract blood vessels, and relax smooth muscles of the bronchi
    2. Parasympathetic (cholinergic) fibers produce the opposite effect

II. DIAGNOSTIC TESTS

A. Skull and spinal radiography
    1. Description
       a. Radiographs of the skull reveal the size and shape of the skull bones, suture separation in infants, fractures or bony defects, erosion, or calcification
       b. Spinal radiographs identify fractures, dislocation, compression, curvature, erosion, narrowed spinal cord, and degenerative processes
    2. Preprocedure interventions
       a. Provide nursing support for the confused, combative, or ventilator-dependent client
       b. Maintain immobilization of the neck if a spinal fracture is suspected
       c. Remove metal items from body parts
       d. If the client has thick and heavy hair, this should be documented because it may affect interpretation of the x-ray film
    3. Postprocedure intervention: Maintain immobilization until results are known
B. Computed tomography (CT) scan
    1. Description
       a. CT is a type of brain scanning that may or may not require an injection of a dye
       b. It is used to detect intracranial bleeding, space-occupying lesions, cerebral edema, infarctions, hydrocephalus, cerebral atrophy, and shifts of brain structures
    2. Preprocedure interventions
       a. Obtain an informed consent if a dye is used
       b. Assess for allergies to iodine, contrast dyes, or shellfish if a dye is used
       c. Instruct the client on the need to lie still and flat during the test
       d. Instruct the client to hold his or her breath when requested
       e. Initiate an IV line if prescribed
       f. Remove objects from the head, such as wigs, barrettes, earrings, and hairpins

g. Assess for claustrophobia

h. Inform the client of possible mechanical noises as the scanning occurs

i. Inform the client that there may be a hot, flushed sensation and a metallic taste in the mouth when the dye is injected

j. Note that some clients may be given the dye even if they report an allergy and are treated with an antihistamine and corticosteroids before the injection to reduce the severity of a reaction

3. Postprocedure interventions

a. Provide replacement fluids because diuresis from the dye is expected

b. Monitor for an allergic reaction to the dye

c. Assess dye injection site for bleeding or hematoma, and monitor the extremity for color, warmth, and the presence of distal pulses

C. Magnetic resonance imaging (MRI)

1. Description

a. MRI is a noninvasive procedure that identifies types of tissues, tumors, and vascular abnormalities

b. It is similar to the CT scan but provides more detailed pictures

2. Preprocedure interventions

a. Remove all metal objects from the client

b. Determine whether the client has a pacemaker, implanted defibrillator, or other metal implants such as a hip prosthesis or vascular clips because these clients cannot have this test performed

c. Remove IV fluid pumps during the test

d. Provide precautions for the client who is attached to pulse oximeter since it can cause a burn during testing if coiled around the body or a body part

e. Provide an assessment of the client with claustrophobia

f. Administer medication as prescribed for the client with claustrophobia

g. Determine if a contrast agent is to be used, and follow the prescription related to the administration of food, fluids, and medications

h. Instruct the client that he or she will need to remain still during the procedure

3. Postprocedure interventions

a. Client may resume normal activities

b. Expect diuresis if a contrast agent was used

D. Lumbar puncture

1. Description

a. The insertion of a spinal needle through the L3-L4 interspace into the lumbar subarachnoid space to obtain CSF, measure CSF fluid or pressure, or instill air, dye, or medications

b. The test is contraindicated in clients with increased intracranial pressure (ICP) because the procedure will cause a rapid decrease in

pressure within the CSF around the spinal cord, leading to brain herniation

2. Preprocedure interventions

a. Obtain an informed consent

b. Have the client empty the bladder

3. Interventions during the procedure

a. Position the client in a lateral recumbent position and have the client draw the knees up to the abdomen and the chin onto the chest

b. Assist with the collection of specimens (label the specimens in sequence)

c. Maintain strict asepsis

4. Postprocedure interventions

a. Monitor vital signs and neurological signs that may indicate leakage of CSF

b. Position the client flat as prescribed

c. Encourage fluids to replace CSF obtained from the specimen collection or from leakage

d. Monitor intake and output (I&O)

E. Myelogram

1. Description: injection of dye or air into the subarachnoid space to detect abnormalities of the spinal cord and vertebrae

2. Preprocedure interventions

a. Obtain an informed consent

b. Provide hydration for at least 12 hours before the test

c. Assess for allergies to contrast agents, iodine, or shellfish

d. If the client is taking a phenothiazine, hold the medication since this medication lowers the seizure threshold

e. Premedicate for sedation as prescribed

3. Postprocedure interventions

a. Assess vital signs and neurological condition frequently as prescribed

b. Bedrest for 6 to 8 hours; the head position varies according to the dye used because the head is usually elevated if an oil-based or water-soluble contrast agent is used and usually positioned lower than the trunk if air-contrast is used

c. Administer analgesics for headache or backache as prescribed

d. Encourage fluids to help excrete the contrast material

e. Monitor I&O to ensure adequate fluid intake and adequate urine output of at least 30 mL/hour; this ensures excretion of contrast material

F. Cerebral angiography

1. Description: injection of a contrast material through the femoral artery into the carotid arteries to visualize the cerebral arteries and assess for lesions

2. Preprocedure interventions

a. Obtain an informed consent

b. Assess the client for allergies to iodine and shellfish

c. Encourage hydration for 2 days before the test

d. Maintain the client on NPO status 4 to 6 hours before the test as prescribed

e. Obtain a baseline neurological assessment

f. Mark the peripheral pulses

g. Remove metal items from the hair

h. Administer premedication as prescribed

3. Postprocedure interventions

a. Monitor neurological status and vital signs frequently until stable

b. Monitor for swelling in the neck and for difficulty swallowing, and notify the physician if these symptoms occur

c. Maintain bedrest for 12 hours as prescribed

d. Elevate the head of the bed 15 to 30 degrees only if prescribed

e. Keep the bed flat if the femoral artery is used, as prescribed

f. Assess peripheral pulses

g. Apply sandbags or another device to immobilize the limb and a pressure dressing to the injection site to decrease bleeding, as prescribed

h. Place ice on the puncture site as prescribed

i. Encourage fluid intake

G. Electroencephalography

1. Description: a graphic recording of the electrical activity of the superficial layers of the cerebral cortex

2. Preprocedure interventions

a. Wash the client's hair

b. Inform the client that electrodes are attached to the head and that electricity does not enter the head

c. Withhold stimulants, such as coffee, tea, and caffeine beverages; antidepressants; tranquilizers; and possibly anticonvulsants for 24 to 48 hours before the test as prescribed

d. Allow the client to have breakfast if prescribed

e. Premedicate for sedation as prescribed

3. Postprocedure interventions

a. Wash the client's hair

b. Maintain side rails and safety precautions, if the client was sedated

H. Caloric testing (oculovestibular reflex)

1. Description: caloric testing provides information about the function of the vestibular portion of the eighth cranial nerve and aids in the diagnosis of cerebellum and brainstem lesions

2. Procedure

a. Patency of the external auditory canal is confirmed

b. The client is positioned supine with the head of the bed elevated 30 degrees

c. Water that is warmer or cooler than body temperature is infused into the ear

d. A normal response is the onset of vertigo and nystagmus (involuntary eye movements) within 20 to 30 seconds

e. Absent or dysconjugate eye movements indicate brainstem damage

III. NEUROLOGICAL DATA COLLECTION

A. Risk factors

1. Trauma

2. Hemorrhage

3. Tumors

4. Infection

5. Toxicity

6. Metabolic disorders

7. Hypoxic conditions

8. Hypertension

9. Cigarette smoking

10. Stress

11. Aging process

12. Chemicals, either ingestion or environmental exposure

B. Testing the cranial nerves

1. Cranial nerve I (olfactory): sensory, smell

a. Have the client close the eyes and occlude one nostril with finger

b. Ask the client to identify nonirritating odors such as coffee, tea, cloves, toothpaste, orange, and peppermint

c. Repeat the test on the other nostril

2. Cranial nerve II (optic): sensory, vision

a. Assess visual acuity with Snellen's chart or newspaper, or ask the client to count how many fingers the examiner is holding up

b. Check visual fields by confrontation

1. Have the client sit directly in front of you and stare at your nose

2. Slowly move your finger from the periphery toward the center until the client says it can be seen

c. Check color vision by asking the client to name the colors of several nearby objects

3. Cranial nerve III (oculomotor); cranial nerve IV (trochlear); cranial nerve VI (abducens)

a. The motor functions of these nerves overlap; therefore, they need to be tested together

b. First, inspect the eyelids for ptosis (drooping); then assess ocular movements and note any eye deviation

c. Test the pupils for size, regularity, equality, direct and consensual light reflexes, and accommodation; may be documented as PERRLA (pupils equal, round, reactive to light and accommodation) (Figure 56-1)

d. Test extraocular movements (EOMs) by the cardinal positions of gaze (Figure 56-2)

e. Test for nystagmus by assessing downward and inward eye movements
4. Cranial nerve V (trigeminal): sensory and motor
   a. Test assesses sensation to the cornea, nasal and oral mucosa, facial skin, and mastication
   b. To test motor function, ask the client to close his or her jaws tightly and then try to separate the clenched jaw
   c. If decreased level of consciousness (LOC) is present, test the corneal reflex by lightly touching the client's cornea with a cotton wisp
   d. Check sensory function by asking the client to close the eyes; then lightly touch the forehead, cheeks, and chin, noting whether the client can feel the touch equally on both sides
5. Cranial nerve VII (facial): sensory and motor
   a. Test taste perception on the anterior two thirds of the tongue
   b. Place sugar, salt, or vinegar on the front of the tongue with an applicator, and have the client identify these substances by their tastes
   c. Have the client show the teeth
   d. Attempt to close the client's eyes against resistance, and ask the client to puff out the cheeks
6. Cranial nerve VIII (acoustic): sensory
   a. The ability to hear tests the cochlear portion

b. The sense of equilibrium tests the vestibular portion
   c. Check the client's ability to hear a watch ticking or a whisper
   d. Observe the client's balance, and observe for swaying when walking or standing
7. Cranial nerve IX (glossopharyngeal): sensory and motor
   a. Test assesses swallowing ability
   b. Test assesses sensation to the pharyngeal soft palate and tonsillar mucosa and taste perception on the posterior third of the tongue and salivation
8. Cranial nerve X (vagus): sensory and motor
   a. Test assesses swallowing and phonation, sensation to the exterior ear's posterior wall, and sensation behind the ear
   b. Test assesses sensation to the thoracic and abdominal viscera
9. Cranial nerve IX (glossopharyngeal); cranial nerve X (vagus)
   a. Have the client identify a taste at the back of the tongue
   b. Inspect the soft palate and observe for symmetrical elevation when the client says "aah"
   c. Touch the posterior pharyngeal wall with a tongue depressor to elicit a gag reflex
10. Cranial nerve XI (spinal accessory): motor
   a. Test assesses uvula and soft palate movement and sternocleidomastoid and trapezius muscles
   b. Test assesses upper portion of the trapezius muscle, which governs shoulder movement and neck rotation
   c. Palpate and inspect the sternocleidomastoid muscle as the client pushes the chin against the examiner's hand
   d. Palpate and inspect the trapezius muscle as the client shrugs the shoulders against the examiner's resistance
11. Cranial nerve XII (hypoglossal): motor
   a. Test assesses tongue movements involved in swallowing and speech
   b. Observe the tongue for asymmetry, atrophy, deviation to one side, and fasciculations

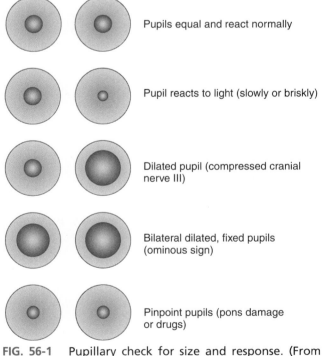

FIG. 56-1 Pupillary check for size and response. (From Lewis, S., Heitkemper, M., & Dirksen, S. [2007]. *Medical-surgical nursing: Assessment and management of clinical problems* [7th ed.]. St. Louis: Mosby.)

Pupils equal and react normally

Pupil reacts to light (slowly or briskly)

Dilated pupil (compressed cranial nerve III)

Bilateral dilated, fixed pupils (ominous sign)

Pinpoint pupils (pons damage or drugs)

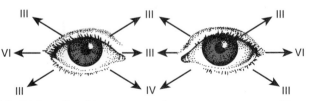

FIG. 56-2 Checking extraocular eye movements. (From Ignatavicius, D., and Workman, M. [2006]. *Medical-surgical nursing: Critical thinking for collaborative care* [5th ed. pupils]. Philadelphia: Saunders.)

BOX 56-2 **Data Collection: Respirations**

Cheyne-Stokes
Rhythmic with periods of apnea
Can indicate a metabolic dysfunction or dysfunction in the cerebral hemisphere or basal ganglia
Neurogenic Hyperventilation
Regular rapid and deep sustained respirations
Indicates a dysfunction in the low midbrain and middle pons
Apneustic
Irregular respirations with pauses at the end of inspiration and expiration
Indicates a dysfunction in the middle or caudal pons
Ataxic
Totally irregular in rhythm and depth
Indicates a dysfunction in the medulla
Cluster
Clusters of breaths with irregularly spaced pauses
Indicates a dysfunction in the medulla and pons

BOX 56-3 **Data Collection: Reflexes**

Babinski's Reflex
Dorsiflexion of the ankle and great toe with fanning of the other toes when firmly stroking the lateral aspect of the sole of the foot
Indicates a disruption of the pyramidal tract
Corneal Reflex
Loss of the blink reflex
Indicates a dysfunction of cranial nerve V
Gag Reflex
Loss of the gag reflex
Indicates a dysfunction of cranial nerves IX and X

  c. Ask the client to push the tongue against a tongue depressor, and then have the client move the tongue rapidly in and out and from side to side
  d. Ask the client to say "light, tight, dynamite" and observe that the sounds of letters *l, t, d,* and *n* are clear and distinct
C. Data collection: level of alertness (becomes increasingly invasive as the client is less responsive)
  1. Speak to the client
  2. Lightly touch the client
  3. Painful stimuli (sternal rub, supraorbital pressure, trapezius squeeze)
D. Data collection: LOC
  1. LOC is the most sensitive indicator of changes in neurological status
  2. Assess client behavior to determine LOC, such as confusion, delirium, unconsciousness, stupor, and coma
E. Vital signs: Monitor for blood pressure or pulse changes, which may indicate increased ICP
F. Respirations (Box 56-2)
G. Temperature
  1. An elevated temperature increases the metabolic rate of the brain
  2. An elevation in temperature may indicate a dysfunction of the hypothalamus or brainstem
  3. A slow rise in temperature may indicate infection
H. Pupils (see Figure 56-1)
  1. Size
  2. Equality
  3. Reactions to light: described as brisk, slow, or fixed
  4. Unusual eye movements
  5. Unilateral pupil dilation indicates compression of the third cranial nerve

  6. Midposition fixed pupil indicates midbrain injury
  7. Pinpoint fixed pupil indicates pontine damage
I. Motor function
  1. Muscle tone, including strength and equality
  2. Voluntary and involuntary movements
  3. Purposeful and nonpurposeful movements
J. Posturing (refer to Figure 30-1)
  1. Posturing indicates a deterioration of the condition
  2. Flexor (**decorticate posturing**)
    a. Client flexes one or both arms on the chest and may extend the legs stiffly
    b. Flexor posturing indicates a nonfunctioning cortex
  3. Extensor (**decerebrate posturing**)
    a. Client stiffly extends one or both arms and possibly the legs
    b. Extensor posturing indicates a brainstem lesion
  4. **Flaccid posturing**: client displays no motor response in any extremity
K. Reflexes (Box 56-3)
L. Meningeal irritation (Box 56-4)
M. Autonomic system
  1. Sympathetic functions/adrenergic responses
    a. Increased pulse and blood pressure
    b. Dilated pupils
    c. Decreased peristalsis
    d. Increased perspiration
  2. Parasympathetic function/cholinergic responses
    a. Decreased pulse and blood pressure
    b. Constricted pupils
    c. Increased salivation
    d. Increased peristalsis
    e. Dilated blood vessels
    f. Bladder contraction
N. Sensory function
  1. Touch
  2. Pressure
  3. Pain
  4. Bladder control
  5. Bowel control

BOX 56-4 Data Collection: Meningeal Irritation

General Findings
Irritability
Nuchal rigidity
Severe, unrelenting headaches
Generalized muscle aches and pains
Nausea and vomiting
Fever and chills
Tachycardia
Pupil Reaction and Eye Movements
Photophobia
Nystagmus
Abnormal eye movement
Brudzinski's Sign
Flexion of the head causes flexion of both thighs at the
   hips and knee flexion
Kernig's Sign
Flexion of the thigh and knee to right angles and when
   the limbs are extended, it causes spasm of the
   hamstring and pain
Motor Response
Hemiparesis, hemiplegia, and decreased muscle tone
Cranial nerve dysfunction, especially cranial nerves III, IV,
   VI, VII, and VIII
Memory Changes
Short attention span
Personality and behavioral changes
Bewilderment

BOX 56-5 Glasgow Coma Scale

Score
The highest possible score is 15 points
Motor Response Points
Obeys a simple response = 6
Localizes painful stimuli = 5
Normal flexion (withdrawal) = 4
Abnormal flexion (decorticate posturing) = 3
Extensor response (decerebrate posturing) = 2
No motor response to pain = 1
Verbal Response Points
Oriented = 5
Confused conversation = 4
Inappropriate words = 3
Responds with incomprehensible sounds = 2
No verbal response = 1
Eye-Opening Points
Spontaneous = 4
In response to sound = 3
In response to pain = 2
No response even to painful stimuli = 1

Modified from Ignatavicius, D. & Workman, M. (2006). *Medical-surgical nursing: Critical thinking for collaborative care* (5th ed.). Philadelphia: Saunders.

O. **Glasgow Coma Scale** (Box 56-5)
   1. The scale is a method of assessing a client's neurological condition
   2. The scoring system is based on a scale of 1 to 15 points
   3. A score of less than 8 indicates coma is present
   4. Eye opening is the most important indicator

IV. **THE UNCONSCIOUS CLIENT**
A. Description
   1. The **unconscious client** is in a state of depressed cerebral functioning with unresponsiveness to sensory and motor function
   2. Some of the causes include head trauma, cerebral toxins, shock, hemorrhage, tumor, and infection
B. Data collection
   1. Unarousable
   2. Primitive or no response to painful stimuli
   3. Altered respirations
   4. Decreased cranial nerve and reflex activity
C. Interventions (Box 56-6)

V. **INCREASED INTRACRANIAL PRESSURE (ICP)**
A. Description
   1. An increase in ICP may be caused by trauma, hemorrhage, growths or tumors, hydrocephalus, edema, or inflammation
   2. Increased ICP can impede circulation to the brain, impede the absorption of CSF, affect the functioning of nerve cells, and lead to brainstem compression and death

B. Data collection
   1. Altered LOC, which is the most sensitive and earliest indication of increasing ICP
   2. Headache
   3. Abnormal respirations (see Box 56-2)
   4. Rise in blood pressure with widening pulse pressure
   5. Slowing of pulse
   6. Elevated temperature
   7. Vomiting
   8. Pupil changes
   9. Late signs of increased ICP including increased systolic blood pressure, widened pulse pressure, and slowed heart rate
   10. Other late signs include changes in motor function from weakness to hemiplegia, a positive **Babinski's reflex, decorticate** or **decerebrate posturing,** and seizures
C. Interventions
   1. Elevate the head of the bed 30 to 40 degrees as prescribed
   2. Avoid Trendelenburg's position
   3. Prevent flexion of the neck and hips
   4. Monitor respiratory status and prevent hypoxia
   5. Avoid the administration of morphine sulfate to prevent the occurrence of hypoxia
   6. Maintain mechanical ventilation as prescribed; maintaining the $Paco_2$ at 30 to 35 mm Hg will result in vasoconstriction of the cerebral blood vessels, decreased blood flow, and therefore decreased ICP
   7. Maintain body temperature
   8. Prevent shivering, which can increase ICP

BOX 56-6 Care of the Unconscious Client

Assess patency of the airway and keep airway and emergency equipment at the bedside.

Monitor blood pressure, pulse, and heart sounds.

Assess respiratory and circulatory status.

Maintain a patent airway and ventilation since a high CO_2 level increases intracranial pressure.

Assess lung sounds for the accumulation of secretions.

Suction fluids from the airway as needed.

Assess neurological status, including level of consciousness, pupillary reactions, and motor and sensory function, using the Glasgow Coma Scale.

Place the client in a semi-Fowler's position.

Change position of the client every 2 hours, avoiding injury when turning.

Avoid Trendelenburg's position.

Use side rails at all times.

Assess for edema.

Monitor for dehydration.

Monitor intake and output and daily weight.

Maintain NPO status until consciousness returns.

Maintain nutrition as prescribed, and monitor fluid and electrolyte balance.

Check the gag and swallow reflex before resuming a diet, and begin the diet with ice chips and fluids when the client becomes alert.

Provide intravenous or enteral feedings as prescribed.

Assess bowel sounds.

Monitor elimination patterns.

Monitor for constipation, impaction, and paralytic ileus.

Maintain urinary output to prevent stasis, infection, and calculus formation.

Monitor the status of skin integrity.

Initiate measures to prevent skin breakdown.

Provide frequent mouth care.

Remove dentures and contact lenses.

Assess the eyes for the presence of a corneal reflex and irritation, and instill artificial tears or cover the eyes with eye patches.

Monitor drainage from the ears or nose for the presence of cerebrospinal fluid.

Assume that the unconscious client can hear.

Avoid restraints.

Do not leave the client unattended if unstable.

Initiate seizure precautions if necessary.

Provide range-of-motion exercises to prevent contractures.

Use a footboard or high-top sneakers to prevent foot drop.

Use splints to prevent wrist deformities.

Initiate physical therapy as appropriate.

BOX 56-7 Medications for Intracranial Pressure

Anticonvulsants

Anticonvulsants may be given prophylactically to prevent seizures.

Seizures increase metabolic requirements and cerebral blood flow and volume, thus increasing intracranial pressure.

Antipyretics and Muscle Relaxants

Temperature reduction decreases metabolism, cerebral blood flow, and thus intracranial pressure.

Antipyretics prevent temperature elevations.

Muscle relaxants prevent shivering.

Blood Pressure Medication

Blood pressure medication may be required to maintain cerebral perfusion at a normal level.

Notify the physician if the blood pressure range is less than 100 or greater than 150 mm Hg systolic.

Corticosteroids

Corticosteroids stabilize the cell membrane and reduce the leakiness in the blood-brain barrier.

Corticosteroids decrease cerebral edema.

A histamine blocker may be administered to counteract the excess gastric secretion that occurs with the corticosteroid.

Clients must be withdrawn slowly from corticosteroid therapy to reduce the risk of adrenal crisis.

Intravenous Fluids

Fluids are administered intravenously via an infusion pump to control the amount administered.

Monitor fluid administration closely because rapid administration can lead to fluid overload and worsen cerebral edema, thus increasing intracranial pressure.

Mannitol (Osmitrol)

Mannitol is a hyperosmotic agent that increases intravascular pressure by drawing fluid from the interstitial spaces and from the brain cells.

Monitor renal function.

Diuresis is expected.

D. Medications (Box 56-7)

E. Surgical intervention (Box 56-8)

VI. HYPERTHERMIA

A. Description

   1. A temperature greater than 105° F, which increases the cerebral metabolism and increases the risk of hypoxia

   2. The causes include infection, heat stroke, exposure to high environmental temperatures, and dysfunction of the thermoregulatory center

B. Data collection

   1. Temperature greater than 105° F

   2. Shivering

   3. Nausea and vomiting

C. Interventions

   1. Maintain a patent airway

   2. Initiate seizure precautions

   3. Monitor I&O and assess the skin and mucous membranes for signs of dehydration

   9. Decrease environmental stimuli

  10. Monitor electrolyte levels and acid-base balance

  11. Monitor I&O

  12. Limit fluid intake to 1200 mL/day

  13. Instruct the client to avoid straining activities, such as coughing and sneezing

  14. Instruct the client to avoid Valsalva's maneuver

| BOX 56-8 | Surgical Intervention for Intracranial Pressure: Ventriculoperitoneal Shunt |

Description
Ventriculoperitoneal shunt directs cerebrospinal fluid from the ventricles into the peritoneum.
Postprocedure Interventions
Position the client supine and turn from the back to the nonoperative side.
Monitor for signs of increasing intracranial pressure resulting from shunt failure.
Monitor for signs of infection.

| BOX 56-9 | Medications to Prevent Shivering |

Dantrolene Sodium (Dantrium)
Dantrium, given intravenously, relaxes skeletal muscle to reduce shivering.
Chlorpromazine Hydrochloride (Thorazine)
Chlorpromazine depresses thermoregulation in the hypothalamus and reduces peripheral vasoconstriction, muscle tone, and shivering.
Meperidine Hydrochloride (Demerol)
Meperidine relaxes the smooth muscle and reduces shivering.

4. Monitor lung sounds
5. Monitor for dysrhythmias
6. Assess peripheral pulses for systemic blood flow
7. Induce normothermia with fluids, cool baths, fans, or a hypothermia blanket
D. Inducement of normothermia
1. Prevent shivering, which will increase ICP and oxygen consumption
2. Administer medications as prescribed to prevent shivering
3. Monitor neurological status
4. Monitor for infection and respiratory complications since hypothermia may mask the signs of infection
5. Monitor for cardiac dysrhythmias
6. Monitor I&O
7. Prevent trauma to the skin and tissues
8. Apply lotion to the skin frequently
9. Inspect for frostbite
E. Medications to prevent shivering (Box 56-9)

VII. HEAD INJURY
A. Description
1. Head injury is trauma to the skull resulting in mild to extensive damage to the brain
2. Immediate complications include cerebral bleeding, hematomas, uncontrolled increased ICP, infections, and seizures
3. Changes in personality or behavior, cranial nerve deficits, and any other residual deficits depend on the area of the brain damage and the extent of the damage
B. Types of head injuries (Box 56-10)
1. Open
a. Scalp lacerations
b. Fractures in the skull
c. Interruption of the dura mater
2. Closed
a. Concussions
b. Contusions
c. Fractures
C. Hematoma
1. Description: hematoma can occur as a result of a subarachnoid hemorrhage or an intracerebral hemorrhage

2. Data collection
a. Findings depend on the injury
b. Clinical manifestations usually result from increased ICP
c. Changing neurological signs in the client
d. Changes in LOC
e. Airway and breathing pattern changes
f. Vital signs changes reflecting increasing ICP
g. Headache, nausea, and vomiting
h. Visual disturbances, pupillary changes, and papilledema
i. **Nuchal rigidity** (not tested until spinal cord injury is ruled out)
j. CSF drainage from the ears or nose: When the drainage is placed on a white, sterile background, such as a gauze pad, it can be distinguished from other fluids by the presence of concentric rings (yellowish stain surrounded by bloody fluid); also, CSF tests positive for glucose when tested by a strip test
k. Weakness and paralysis
l. Posturing
m. Decreased sensation or absence of feeling
n. Reflex activity changes
o. Seizure activity
3. Interventions
a. Monitor respiratory status and maintain a patent airway since increased CO_2 levels increase cerebral edema
b. Monitor neurological status and vital signs, including temperature
c. Monitor for increased ICP
d. Maintain head elevation to reduce venous pressure
e. Prevent neck flexion
f. Initiate normothermia measures for increased temperature
g. Assess cranial nerve function, reflexes, and motor and sensory function
h. Initiate seizure precautions
i. Monitor for pain and restlessness
j. Morphine sulfate may be prescribed to decrease agitation and control restlessness caused by pain for the head-injured client

BOX 56-10 **Types of Head Injuries**

Concussion
Concussion is a jarring of the brain within the skull with temporary loss of consciousness.
Contusion
Contusion is a bruising of brain tissue.
Contusion may occur with subdural or extradural collections of blood.
Skull Fractures
Linear
Depressed
Compound
Comminuted
Epidural Hematoma
As the most serious type of hematoma, epidural hematoma forms rapidly and results from arterial bleeding.
Epidural hematoma forms between the dura and the skull from a tear in the meningeal artery.
Epidural hematoma is a surgical emergency.
Subdural Hematoma
Subdural hematoma forms slowly and results from a venous bleed.
Subdural hematoma occurs under the dura as a result of tears in the veins crossing the subdural space.
Intracerebral Hemorrhage
Multiple hemorrhages occur around a contused area.
Subarachnoid Hemorrhage
Bleeding occurs directly into the brain, the ventricles, or the subarachnoid space

on a ventilator; administer with caution since it is a respiratory depressant and may increase ICP
  - k. Monitor for drainage from the nose or ears because this fluid may be CSF
  - l. Do not attempt to clean the nose, suction, or allow the client to blow the nose if drainage occurs
  - m. Do not clean the ear if drainage is noted, but apply a loose, dry sterile dressing
  - n. Check drainage for the presence of CSF
  - o. Notify the physician if drainage from the ears or nose is noted and if the drainage tests positive for CSF
  - p. Instruct the client to avoid coughing because this increases ICP
  - q. Monitor for signs of infection
  - r. Prevent complications of immobility
- D. Craniotomy
  1. Description
    - a. A surgical procedure that involves an incision through the cranium to remove accumulated blood or a tumor
    - b. Complications of the procedure include increased ICP from cerebral edema, hemorrhage, or obstruction of normal flow of CSF
    - c. Additional complications include hematomas, hypovolemic shock, hydrocephalus,

respiratory and neurogenic complications, pulmonary edema, and wound infections
    - d. Complications related to fluid and electrolyte imbalances include diabetes insipidus and inappropriate secretion of antidiuretic hormone
  2. Preoperative interventions
    - a. Explain the procedure to the client and family
    - b. Ensure that an informed consent has been obtained
    - c. Prepare to shave the client's head as prescribed (usually done in the operating room) and cover the head with appropriate covering
    - d. Stabilize the client before surgery
  3. Postoperative interventions (Box 56-11)
  4. Postoperative positioning (Box 56-12)

VIII. SPINAL CORD INJURY
- A. Description
  1. Trauma to the spinal cord causes partial or complete disruption of the nerve tracts and neurons
  2. The injury can involve contusion, laceration, or compression of the cord
  3. Spinal cord edema develops, and necrosis of the spinal cord can develop as a result of compromised capillary circulation and venous return
  4. Loss of motor function, sensation, reflex activity, and bowel and bladder control may result
  5. The most common causes include motor vehicle accidents, falls, sporting and industrial accidents, and gunshot or stab wounds
  6. Complications related to the injury include respiratory failure, **autonomic dysreflexia, spinal shock,** further cord damage, and death.
- B. Most frequently involved vertebrae
  1. Cervical 5, 6, and 7
  2. Thoracic 12
  3. Lumbar 1
- C. Transection of the cord
  1. Complete transection of the cord. The spinal cord is severed completely, with total loss of sensation, movement, and reflex activity below the level of injury
  2. Partial transection of the cord
    - a. The spinal cord is damaged or severed partially
    - b. The symptoms depend on the extent and location of the damage
    - c. If the cord has not suffered irreparable damage, early treatment is needed to prevent partial damage from developing into total and permanent damage
- D. Types of injuries (Figure 56-3)
  1. Central cord syndrome
    - a. Central cord syndrome cccurs from a lesion in the central portion of the spinal cord
    - b. Loss of motor function is more pronounced in the upper extremities, and varying degrees and patterns of sensation remain intact

BOX 56-11	Nursing Care Following Craniotomy

Monitor vital signs and neurological status every 30 minutes to 1 hour.

Monitor for increased intracranial pressure.

Monitor for decreased level of consciousness, motor weakness or paralysis, aphasia, visual changes, and personality changes.

Maintain mechanical ventilation and slight hyperventilation for the first 24 to 48 hours as prescribed to prevent increased intracranial pressure.

Assess the physician's orders regarding client positioning.

Avoid extreme hip or neck flexion, and maintain the head in a midline neutral position.

Provide a quiet environment.

Monitor the head dressing frequently for signs of drainage.

Mark any area of drainage at least once each nursing shift for baseline comparison.

Monitor the Hemovac or Jackson-Pratt drain, which may be in place for 24 hours.

Maintain suction on the Hemovac or Jackson-Pratt drain.

Measure drainage from the Hemovac or Jackson-Pratt drain every 8 hours, and record the amount and color.

Notify the physician if drainage is greater than the normal of 30 to 50 mL per shift.

Notify the physician immediately of excessive amounts of drainage or a saturated head dressing.

Record strict measurement of hourly intake and output.

Maintain fluid restriction at 1500 mL/day as prescribed.

Monitor electrolyte values.

Monitor for dysrhythmias, which may occur as a result of fluid and electrolyte imbalance.

Apply ice packs or cool compresses as prescribed; expect periorbital edema and ecchymosis of one or both eyes, which is not an unusual occurrence.

Provide range-of-motion exercises every 8 hours.

Place antiembolism stockings on the client as prescribed.

Administer anticonvulsants, antacids, corticosteroids, and antibiotics as prescribed.

Administer analgesics such as codeine sulfate and acetaminophen (Tylenol) as prescribed for pain.

BOX 56-12	Client Positioning Following Craniotomy

Positions prescribed following craniotomy vary with the type of surgery and the specific postoperative physician's orders.

Always check the physician's orders regarding client positioning.

Incorrect positioning may cause serious and possibly fatal complications.

Removal of a Bone Flap for Decompression

To facilitate brain expansion, the client should be turned from the back to the nonoperative side, but not to the side of the operation.

Posterior Fossa Surgery

To protect the operative site from pressure and to minimize tension on the suture line, position the client on the side, with a pillow under the head for support and not on the back.

Infratentorial Surgery

Supratentorial surgery involves surgery below the tentorium of the brain.

The physician may order a flat position without head elevation or may order the head of the bed to be elevated at 30 to 45 degrees.

Do not elevate the head of the bed in the acute phase of care following surgery without a physician's order.

Supratentorial Surgery

Supratentorial surgery involves surgery above the tentorium of the brain.

The physician may order the head of the bed to be elevated at 30 degrees to promote venous outflow through the jugular veins.

Do not lower the head of the bed in the acute phase of care following surgery without a physician's order.

2. Anterior cord syndrome
   a. Anterior cord syndrome is caused by damage to the anterior portion of the gray and white matter of the spinal cord
   b. Motor function, pain, and temperature sensation are lost below the level of injury; however, the sensations of position, vibration, and touch remain intact
3. Posterior cord syndrome
   a. Posterior cord syndrome is caused by damage to the posterior portion of the gray and white matter of the spinal cord
   b. Motor function remains intact, but the client experiences a loss of vibratory sense, crude touch, and position sensation
4. Brown-Séquard's syndrome
   a. Brown-Séquard's syndrome results from penetrating injuries that cause hemisection of the spinal cord or injuries that affect half of the cord
   b. Motor function, vibration, proprioception, and deep touch sensations are lost on the same side of the body (ipsilateral) as the lesion or cord damage
   c. On the opposite side of the body (contralateral) from the lesion or cord damage, the sensations of pain, temperature, and light touch are affected
5. Conus medullaris syndrome
   a. Conus medullaris syndrome follows damage to the lumbar nerve roots and conus medullaris in the spinal cord
   b. Client experiences bowel and bladder areflexia and flaccid lower extremities
   c. If damage is limited to the upper sacral segments of the spinal cord, bulbospongiosus penile (erection) and micturition reflexes will remain

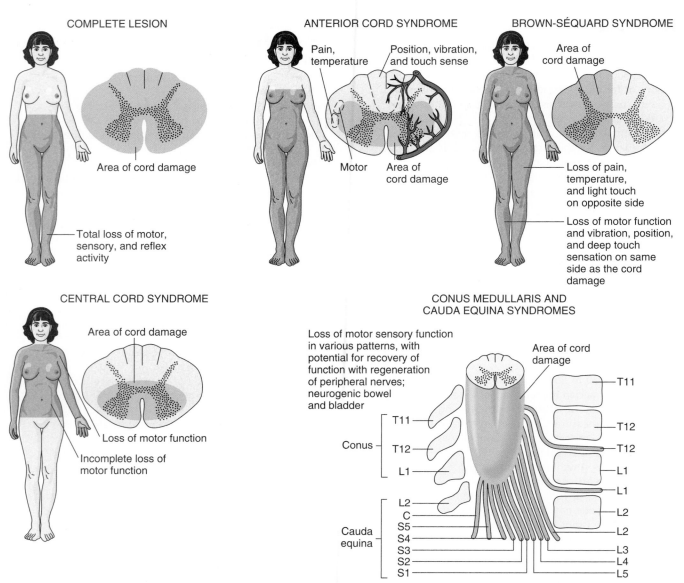

FIG. 56-3   Common spinal cord syndromes. (From Ignatavicius, D., and Workman, M. [2006]. *Medical-surgical nursing: Critcal thinking for collaborative care* [5th ed.]. Philadelphia: Saunders.)

6. Cauda equina syndrome
    a. Cauda equina syndrome occurs from injury to the lumbosacral nerve roots below the conus medullaris
    b. The client experiences areflexia of the bowel, bladder, and lower reflexes
E. Data collection: spinal cord injuries (Box 56-13)
    1. Dependent on the level of the cord injury
    2. The level of spinal cord injury: the lowest spinal cord segment with intact motor and sensory function
    3. Respiratory status changes
    4. Motor and sensory changes below the level of injury
    5. Total sensory loss and motor paralysis below the level of injury
    6. Loss of reflexes below the level of injury

BOX 56-13   Effects of the Spinal Cord Injury

Quadriplegia
Injury occurring between C1 and C8
Paralysis involving all four extremities
Paraplegia
Injury occurring between T1 and L4
Paralysis involving only the lower extremities

---

    7. Loss of bladder and bowel control
    8. Urinary retention and bladder distention
    9. Presence of sweat, which does not occur on paralyzed areas
F. Cervical injuries
    1. Injury at C2 to C3 is usually fatal
    2. C4 is the major innervation to the diaphragm by the phrenic nerve

3. Involvement above C4 causes respiratory difficulty and paralysis of all four extremities
4. Client may have movement in the shoulder if the injury is at C5 or below

G. Thoracic level injuries
1. Loss of movement of the chest, trunk, bowel, bladder, and legs may occur, depending on the level of injury
2. Leg paralysis (paraplegia) may occur
3. **Autonomic dysreflexia** with lesions or injuries above T6 and in cervical lesions may occur
4. Visceral distention from a noxious stimulus such as a distended bladder or impacted rectum may cause reactions such as sweating, bradycardia, hypertension, nasal stuffiness, and goose flesh

H. Lumbar and sacral level injuries
1. Loss of movement and sensation of the lower extremities may occur
2. S2 and S3 center on micturation; therefore, below this level, the bladder will contract but not empty (neurogenic bladder)
3. Injury above S2 in males allows them to have an erection, but they are unable to ejaculate because of sympathetic nerve damage
4. Injury between S2 and S4 damages the sympathetic and parasympathetic response, preventing erection or ejaculation

I. Emergency interventions
1. Emergency management is critical because improper movement can cause further damage and loss of neurological function
2. Assess the respiratory pattern and maintain a patent airway
3. Always suspect spinal cord injury until this injury is ruled out
4. Immobilize the client on a spinal backboard with the head in a neutral position to prevent an incomplete injury from becoming complete
5. Prevent head flexion, rotation, or extension
6. During immobilization, maintain traction and alignment on the head by placing hands on either side of the head by the ears
7. Maintain an extended position
8. Logroll the client
9. No part of the body should be twisted or turned, and the client is not allowed to assume a sitting position
10. In the emergency department, a client who has sustained a severe cervical fracture should be placed immediately in skeletal traction via **skull tongs** or **halo traction** to immobilize the cervical spine and reduce the fracture and dislocation

J. Interventions during hospitalization
1. Respiratory system
   a. Assess respiratory status since paralysis of the intercostal and abdominal muscles occurs with C4 injuries
   b. Monitor arterial blood gases and maintain mechanical ventilation if prescribed to prevent respiratory arrest, especially with cervical injuries
   c. Encourage deep breathing and the use of an incentive spirometer
   d. Monitor for signs of infection, particularly pneumonia
2. Cardiovascular system
   a. Monitor for cardiac dysrhythmias
   b. Assess for signs of hemorrhage or bleeding around the fracture site
   c. Assess for signs of shock, such as hypotension, tachycardia, and a weak and thready pulse
   d. Assess the lower extremities for deep vein thrombosis
   e. Measure circumferences of the calf and thigh to identify increases in size
   f. Apply thigh-high antiembolism stockings as prescribed
   g. Remove antiembolism stockings daily to assess the skin
   h. Monitor for orthostatic hypotension when repositioning the client
3. Neuromuscular system
   a. Assess neurological status
   b. Assess motor and sensory status to determine the level of injury
   c. Assess motor ability by testing the client's ability to squeeze hands, spread the fingers, move the toes, and turn the feet
   d. Assess for absent sensation hyposensation, or hypersensation by pinching the skin or pricking it with a pin, starting at the shoulders and working down the extremities
   e. Monitor for signs of **autonomic dysreflexia** and **spinal shock**
   f. Immobilize the client to promote healing and prevent further injury
   g. Assess pain
   h. Initiate measures to reduce pain
   i. Administer analgesics as prescribed
   j. Monitor for complications of immobility
   k. Prepare the client for decompression laminectomy, spinal fusion, or insertion of instrumentation or rods if prescribed
   l. Collaborate with the physical therapist and occupational therapist to determine appropriate exercise techniques, to assess the need for hand and wrist splints, and to develop an appropriate plan to prevent footdrop
4. Gastrointestinal system
   a. Assess abdomen for distention and hemorrhage
   b. Monitor bowel sounds and assess for paralytic ileus

c. Prevent bowel retention
d. Initiate a bowel control program as appropriate
e. Maintain adequate nutrition and a high-fiber diet
5. Renal system
a. Prevent urinary retention
b. Initiate a bladder control program as appropriate
c. Maintain fluid and electrolyte balance
d. Maintain adequate fluid intake of 2000 mL/day
e. Monitor for urinary tract infection and calculi
6. Integumentary system
a. Assess skin integrity
b. Turn the client every 2 hours
7. Psychosocial integrity
a. Assess psychosocial status
b. Encourage the client to express feelings of anger and depression
c. Discuss the sexual concerns of the client
d. Promote self-care, setting realistic goals based on the client's potential functional level
e. Encourage contact with appropriate community resources
K. **Spinal shock**
1. Description
a. **Spinal shock** is also known as neurogenic shock
b. A sudden depression of reflex activity in the spinal cord occurs below the level of injury (areflexia)
c. **Spinal shock** occurs within the first hour of injury and can last days to months
d. The muscles become completely paralyzed and flaccid, and reflexes are absent
e. **Spinal shock** ends when the reflexes are regained
2. Data collection (Box 56-14)
3. Interventions
a. Monitor for signs of **spinal shock** following a spinal cord injury
b. Monitor for hypotension and bradycardia
c. Monitor for reflex activity
d. Assess bowel sounds
e. Monitor for bowel and urinary retention
f. Provide supportive measures as prescribed, based on the presence of symptoms
g. Monitor for the return of reflexes
L. **Autonomic dysreflexia**
1. Description
a. **Autonomic dysreflexia** is also known as autonomic hyperreflexia
b. **Autonomic dysreflexia** generally occurs after the period of **spinal shock** is resolved and occurs with lesions or injuries above T6 and in cervical lesions

---

| BOX 56-14 | **Spinal Shock and Autonomic Dysreflexia** |

Spinal Shock
Flaccid paralysis
Loss of reflex activity below the level of injury
Bradycardia
Paralytic ileus
Hypotension
Autonomic Dysreflexia
Sudden onset of severe, throbbing headache
Severe hypertension
Flushing above the level of the lesion
Pale extremities below the level of injury
Nasal stuffiness
Nausea
Dilated pupils or blurred vision
Sweating
Piloerection (goose bumps)
Restlessness and a feeling of apprehension

---

c. It is commonly caused by visceral distention from a distended bladder or impacted rectum
d. It is a neurological emergency and must be treated immediately to prevent a hypertensive stroke
2. Data collection (see Box 56-14)
3. Interventions
a. Notify the registered nurse and physician if signs of **autonomic dysreflexia** occur
b. Assess for the potential cause and remove the stimulus
c. Raise the head of the bed to a high Fowler's position
d. Loosen tight clothing
e. Monitor vital signs, particularly the blood pressure, every 15 minutes
f. Assess for bladder distention, and prepare for urinary catheterization
g. If a urinary catheter is present, check for kinks in the tubing and for drainage
h. Assess for a fecal impaction and disimpact immediately
i. Assess the environment to ensure it is not too cool or too drafty
j. Administer antihypertensives as prescribed
M. Cervical spine traction for cervical injuries
1. Description
a. Skeletal traction is used to stabilize fractures or dislocations of the cervical or upper thoracic spine
b. Two types of equipment used for cervical traction are **skull** (cervical) **tongs** and **halo traction** (halo fixation device)
2. **Skull tongs**
a. **Skull tongs** are inserted into the outer aspect of the client's skull, and traction is applied

b. Weights are attached to the tongs, and the client is used as countertraction

c. Monitor neurological status of the client

d. Determine the amount of weight prescribed to be added to the traction

e. Ensure that weights hang securely and freely at all times

f. Ensure that the ropes for the traction remain within the pulley

g. Maintain body alignment and maintain care of the client on a special bed (such as a Roto-Rest bed, Stryker, or Foster frame) as prescribed

h. Turn the client every 2 hours

i. Assess insertion site of the tongs for infection

j. Provide sterile pin site care as prescribed

3. **Halo traction**

a. **Halo traction** is a static traction device that consists of a headpiece with four pins—two anterior and two posterior—inserted into the client's skull

b. The metal halo ring may be attached to a vest (jacket) or cast when the spine is stable, allowing increased client mobility

c. Monitor the client's neurological status for changes in movement or decreased strength

d. Never move or turn the client by holding or pulling on the **halo traction** device

e. Assess tightness of the jacket by ensuring that one finger can be placed under the jacket

f. Assess skin integrity to ensure that the jacket or cast is not causing pressure

g. Provide sterile pin site care as prescribed

4. Client education for **halo traction** device (Box 56-15)

5. Initiate interventions in support of the client's self image

6. Teach the client and family pin care, care of the vest, and signs and symptoms of infection to report to his or her health care provider

N. Interventions for thoracic and lumbar/sacral injuries

1. Bedrest

2. Immobilization with a body cast if prescribed

3. Assess for respiratory impairment and for paralytic ileus, as possible complications of the body cast

4. Use of a brace or corset when the client is out of bed

O. Surgical interventions for thoracic and lumbar/sacral injuries

1. Decompressive laminectomy

a. Removal of one or more laminae

b. Allows for cord expansion from edema and is performed if conventional methods fail to prevent neurological deterioration

---

BOX 56-15 **Client Education for a Halo Fixation Device**

Notify the physician if the halo vest (jacket) or ring bolts loosen.

Use fleece or foam inserts to relieve pressure points.

Keep the vest lining dry.

Clean the pin site daily.

Notify the physician if redness, swelling, drainage, open areas, pain, tenderness, or a clicking sound occurs from the pin site.

A sponge bath or tub bath is allowed; showers are prohibited.

Assess the skin under the vest daily for breakdown, using a flashlight.

Do not use any products other than shampoo on the hair.

When shampooing the hair, cover the vest with plastic.

When getting out of bed, roll onto the side and push on the mattress with the arms.

Never use the metal frame for turning or lifting.

Use a rolled towel or pillowcase between the back of the neck and the bed or next to the cheek when lying on the side, and raise the head of the bed to increase sleep comfort.

Adapt clothing to fit over the halo device.

Eat foods high in protein and calcium to promote bone healing.

Have the correct-size wrench available at all times for an emergency.

If cardiopulmonary resuscitation is required, the anterior portion of the vest will be loosened and the posterior portion will remain in place to provide stability.

---

2. Spinal fusion

a. Spinal fusion is used for thoracic spinal injuries

b. Bone is grafted between the vertebrae for support and to strengthen the back

3. Postoperative interventions

a. Monitor for respiratory impairment

b. Monitor vital signs, motor function, sensation, and circulatory status in the lower extremities

c. Encourage breathing exercises

d. Assess for signs of fluid and electrolyte imbalance

e. Observe for complications of immobility

f. Keep the client in a flat position as prescribed

g. Provide cast care if the client is in a full body cast

h. Turn and reposition frequently by logrolling side to back to side, using turning sheets and pillows between the legs to maintain alignment

i. Administer pain medication as prescribed

j. Maintain an NPO status until the client is passing flatus

k. Monitor bowel sounds

l. Provide the use of a fracture bedpan

m. Monitor I&O

n. Maintain nutritional status

P. Medications

1. Dexamethasone (Decadron)

a. Used for its anti-inflammatory and edema-reducing effects

b. May interfere with healing

2. Dextran: a plasma expander used to increase capillary blood flow within the spinal cord and to prevent or treat hypotension

3. Dantrolene (Dantrium)/Baclofen (Lioresal): these medications are used for clients with upper motor neuron injuries to control muscle spasticity

IX. CEREBRAL ANEURYSM

A. Description

1. A dilation of the walls of a weakened cerebral artery

2. Aneurysm can lead to rupture

B. Data collection

1. Headache and pain

2. Irritability

3. Diplopia

4. Blurred vision

5. Tinnitus

6. Hemiparesis

7. **Nuchal rigidity**

8. Seizures

C. Interventions

1. Maintain a patent airway (suction only with a physician's order)

2. Administer oxygen as prescribed

3. Monitor vital signs and for hypertension or dysrhythmias

4. Avoid taking temperatures via the rectum

5. Initiate aneurysm precautions (Box 56-16)

X. SEIZURES

A. Description

1. Seizures are an abnormal, sudden, excessive discharge of electrical activity within the brain

2. Epilepsy is a disorder characterized by chronic seizure activity and indicates brain or CNS irritation

3. Causes include genetic factors, trauma, tumors, circulatory or metabolic disorders, toxicity, and infections

4. Status epilepticus involves a rapid succession of epileptic spasms without intervals of consciousness; it is a potential complication that can occur with any type of seizure, and brain damage may result

B. Types of seizures (Box 56-17)

1. Generalized seizures

2. Partial seizures

C. Data collection

1. Seizure history

2. Type of seizure

3. Occurrences before, during, and after the seizure

4. Prodromal signs, such as mood changes, irritability, and insomnia

5. Aura: a sensation that warns the client of the impending seizure

6. Loss of motor activity or bowel and bladder function or loss of consciousness during the seizure

7. Occurrences during the postictal state, such as headache, loss of consciousness, sleepiness, and impaired speech or thinking

D. Interventions

1. Note the time and duration of the seizure

2. Assess behavior at the onset of the seizure: if the client experienced an aura, if a change in facial expression occurred, or if a sound or cry occurred from the client

3. If the client is standing, place the client on the floor and protect the head and body

4. Support the ABCs—airway, breathing, and circulation

5. Maintain a patent airway (do not force the jaws open or place anything in the client's mouth)

6. Administer oxygen

7. Prepare to suction secretions from the airway

8. Turn the client to the side, to allow secretions to drain, while maintaining the airway

---

BOX 56-16 **Aneurysm Precautions**

Maintain bedrest in a semi-Fowler's or side-lying position.

Maintain a darkened room (subdued lighting and no direct, bright, artificial lights) without stimulation (a private room is optimal).

Provide a quiet environment (avoid activities or startling noises); telephone in the room is not usually allowed.

Reading, watching television, and listening to music are permitted, provided they do not overstimulate the client.

Limit visitors.

Maintain fluid restrictions.

Provide diet as ordered; avoid stimulants in the diet.

Prevent any activities that initiate the Valsalva maneuver (straining at stooling, coughing); provide stool softeners to prevent straining.

Administer care gently (e.g., the bath, back rub, range of motion).

Limit invasive procedures.

Maintain normothermia.

Prevent hypertension.

Provide sedation.

Provide pain control.

Administer prophylactic anticonvulsant medications.

Provide deep vein thrombosis (DVT) prophylaxis as prescribed.

9. Prevent injury during the seizure
10. Remain with the client
11. Do not restrain the client
12. Loosen restrictive clothing
13. Note the type, character, and progression of the movements during the seizure
14. Monitor for incontinence
15. Administer IV medications as prescribed to stop the seizure
16. Document the characteristics of the seizure
17. Provide privacy, if possible
18. Monitor behavior following the seizure, such as the state of consciousness, motor ability, and speech ability
19. Instruct the client about the importance of life-long medication and the need for follow-up medication blood levels
20. Instruct the client to avoid alcohol, excessive stress, fatigue, and strobe lights

21. Encourage the client to contact available community resources, such as the Epilepsy Foundation of America
22. Encourage the client to wear a Medic-Alert bracelet

XI. **STROKE (BRAIN ATTACK)**
  A. Description
    1. A stroke or brain attack, formerly known as a cerebrovascular accident (CVA), is a sudden focal neurological deficit caused by cerebrovascular disease
    2. A stroke is a syndrome in which the cerebral circulation is interrupted, causing neurological deficits
    3. Cerebral anoxia lasting longer than 10 minutes causes cerebral infarction with irreversible change
    4. Cerebral edema and congestion cause further dysfunction
    5. Diagnosis is determined by CT scan, electro-encephalogram, cerebral arteriography, and MRI
    6. The permanent disability cannot be determined until the cerebral edema subsides
    7. The order in which function may return is facial, swallowing, lower limb, speech, and arms
    8. Carotid endarterectomy is a surgical intervention used in stroke management and is targeted at stroke prevention, especially in clients with symptomatic carotid stenosis
  B. Causes
    1. Thrombosis
    2. Embolism
    3. Hemorrhage from rupture of a vessel
    4. Transient ischemic attack
  C. Risk factors
    1. Atherosclerosis
    2. Hypertension
    3. Anticoagulation therapy
    4. Diabetes mellitus
    5. Stress
    6. Obesity
    7. Oral contraceptives
  D. Data collection (Boxes 56-18 and 56-19; Figure 56-4)
    1. Findings depend on the area of the brain affected

BOX 56-17 **Types of Seizures**

Generalized Seizures
Tonic-Clonic
Tonic-clonic seizures may begin with an aura.
The tonic phase involves the stiffening or rigidity of the muscles of the arms and legs and usually lasts 10 to 20 seconds, followed by loss of consciousness.
The clonic phase consists of hyperventilation and jerking of the extremities and usually lasts about 30 seconds.
Full recovery from the seizure may take several hours.
Absence
Brief seizure lasts seconds, and the individual may or may not lose consciousness.
No loss or change in muscle tone occurs.
Seizures may occur several times during a day.
The victim appears to be daydreaming.
This type of seizure is more common in children.
Myoclonic
Myoclonic seizures present as a brief generalized jerking or stiffening of extremities.
The victim may fall to the ground from the seizure.
Atonic or Akinetic (Drop Attacks)
An atonic seizure is a sudden momentary loss of muscle tone.
The victim may fall to the ground as a result of the seizure.
Partial Seizures
Simple Partial
The simple partial seizure produces sensory symptoms accompanied by motor symptoms that are localized or confined to a specific area.
The client remains conscious and may report an aura.
Complex Partial
The complex partial seizure is a psychomotor seizure.
The area of the brain most involved is the temporal lobe.
The seizure is characterized by periods of altered behavior of which the client is not aware.
The client loses consciousness for a few seconds.

BOX 56-18 **Neurological Data Collection: Stroke**

Changes in level of consciousness
Signs of increasing intracranial pressure
Assessment of cranial nerves V, VII, IX, X, and XII
  Cranial nerve V: difficulty with chewing
  Cranial nerve VII: facial paralysis or paresis
  Cranial nerves IX and X: dysphagia
  Cranial nerve IX: absent gag reflex
  Cranial nerve XII: impaired tongue movement

BOX 56-19 **Data Collection Findings: Stroke**

Agnosia
Inability to use an object correctly
Apraxia
Inability to carry out a purposeful activity
Hemianopsia
Blindness in half of the visual field
Homonymous Hemianopsia
Blindness in the same visual field of both eyes
Neglect Syndrome (Unilateral Neglect)
Client unaware of the existence of his or her paralyzed
    side
Proprioception Alterations
Altered position sense that places the client at increased
    risk of injury
Pyramid Point
With visual problems, the client must turn the head to
    scan the complete range of vision.

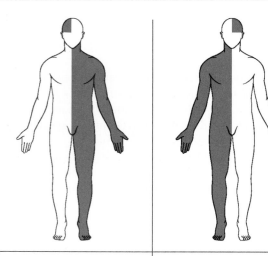

Right-brain damage (stroke on right side of the brain)	**Left-brain damage** (stroke on left side of the brain)
• Paralyzed left side: hemiplegia	• Paralyzed right side: hemiplegia
• Left-sided neglect	• Impaired speech/language aphasias
• Spatial-perceptual deficits	
• Tends to deny or minimize problems	• Impaired right/left discrimination
• Rapid performance, short attention span	• Slow performance, cautious
• Impulsive, safety problems	• Aware of deficits: depression, anxiety
• Impaired judgment	• Impaired comprehension related to language, math
• Impaired time concepts	

FIG. 56-4 Manifestations of right brain and left brain stroke. (From Lewis, S., Heitkemper, M., & Dirksen, S. [2007]. *Medical-surgical nursing: Assessment and management of clinical problems* [7th ed.]. St. Louis: Mosby.)

2. Lesions in the cerebral hemisphere result in manifestations on the contralateral side, which is the side of the body opposite the stroke
3. Airway patency is always a priority
4. Pulse (may be slow and bounding)

5. Respirations (Cheyne-Stokes)
6. Blood pressure (hypertension)
7. Headache, nausea, and vomiting
8. Facial drooping
9. **Nuchal rigidity**
10. Visual changes
11. Ataxia
12. Dysarthria
13. Dysphagia
14. Speech changes
15. Decreased sensation to pressure, heat, and cold
16. Bowel and bladder dysfunctions
17. Paralysis
E. Aphasia
    1. Expressive
        a. Damage occurs in Broca's area of the frontal brain
        b. Client understands what is said but is unable to communicate verbally
    2. Receptive
        a. Injury involves Wernicke's area in the temporoparietal area
        b. Client is unable to understand the spoken and often the written word
    3. Global or mixed: language dysfunction occurs in expression and reception
    4. Interventions for aphasia
        a. Provide repetitive directions
        b. Break tasks down to one step at a time
        c. Repeat names of objects frequently used
        d. Allow time for the client to communicate
        e. Use a picture board, communication board, or computerized technologies
F. Interventions during the acute phase of stroke
    1. Maintain a patent airway and administer oxygen as prescribed
    2. Monitor vital signs
    3. Maintain a blood pressure of 150/100 mm Hg or as prescribed to maintain cerebral perfusion
    4. Suction secretions as prescribed, but never suction nasally and for longer than 10 seconds to prevent increasing ICP
    5. Monitor for increasing ICP because the client is at most risk during the first 72 hours following the stroke
    6. Position the client on the side, with the head of the bed elevated 15 to 30 degrees as prescribed
    7. Monitor LOC, pupillary response, motor and sensory response, cranial nerve function, and reflexes
    8. Maintain a quiet environment, and provide minimal handling of the client to prevent further bleeding
    9. Insert a Foley catheter as prescribed
    10. Monitor prescribed IV fluids closely
    11. Maintain fluid and electrolyte balance

12. Prepare to administer anticoagulants, antiplatelets, diuretics, antihypertensives, and anticonvulsants as prescribed
13. Establish a form of communication

G. Interventions in the postacute phase of a stroke
1. Continue with interventions from the acute phase
2. Position the client 2 hours on the unaffected side, 20 minutes on the affected side
3. Position the client in the prone position if prescribed, for 30 minutes three times daily
4. Provide skin, mouth, and eye care
5. Perform passive range-of-motion exercises to prevent contractures
6. Place antiembolism stockings on client
7. Measure thighs and calves for an increase in size
8. Monitor gag reflex and ability to swallow
9. Provide sips of fluids and slowly advance diet to foods that are easy to chew and swallow
10. Provide soft and semisoft foods and flavored, cool or warm, thickened fluids rather than thin liquids because the stroke client is better able to tolerate these types of food; speech therapists may do swallow studies to recommend consistency of food and fluids
11. When the client is eating, position the client sitting in a chair, or sitting up in bed, with the head and neck positioned slightly forward and flexed
12. Place food in the back of the mouth on the unaffected side to prevent trapping of food in the affected cheek

H. Interventions in the chronic phase of stroke
1. Neglect syndrome
   a. Client is unaware of the existence of his or her paralyzed side (**unilateral neglect**), which places the client at risk for injury
   b. Teach the client to touch and use both sides of the body
2. **Hemianopsia**
   a. Client has blindness in half of the visual field
   b. **Homonymous hemianopsia** is blindness in the same visual field of both eyes
   c. Encourage the client to turn the head to scan the complete range of vision; otherwise, the client does not see half of the visual field
3. Approach the client from the unaffected side
4. Place the client's personal objects within the visual field
5. Provide eye care for visual deficits
6. Place a patch over the affected eye if the client has diplopia
7. Increase mobility as tolerated
8. Encourage fluid intake and a high-fiber diet
9. Administer stool softeners as prescribed
10. Encourage the client to express feelings

11. Encourage independence in activities of daily living
12. Assess the need for assistive devices such as a cane, walker, splints, or braces
13. Teach transfer technique from bed to chair and chair to bed
14. Provide gait training
15. Initiate physical and occupational therapy
16. Refer client to a speech and language pathologist as prescribed
17. Encourage the client and family to contact available community resources

XII. MULTIPLE SCLEROSIS
A. Description
1. Multiple sclerosis is a chronic, progressive, noncontagious, degenerative disease of the CNS characterized by demyelinization of the neurons
2. It usually occurs between the ages of 20 and 40 and consists of periods of remissions and exacerbations
3. The causes are unknown, but the disease is thought to be a result of an autoimmune response or viral infection
4. Precipitating factors include pregnancy, fatigue, stress, infection, and trauma
5. Electroencephalogram findings are abnormal
6. A lumbar puncture indicates increased gammaglobulin, but the serum globulin level is normal
B. Data collection
1. Fatigue and weakness
2. Ataxia and vertigo
3. Tremors and spasticity of the lower extremities
4. Parasthesias
5. Blurred vision, diplopia, and transient blindness
6. Nystagmus
7. Dysphasia
8. Decreased perception to pain, touch, and temperature
9. Bladder and bowel disturbances, including urgency, frequency, retention, and incontinence
10. Abnormal reflexes, including hyperreflexia, absent reflexes, and a positive **Babinski's reflex**
11. Emotional changes such as apathy, euphoria, irritability, and depression
12. Memory changes and confusion
C. Interventions
1. Provide bedrest during exacerbation
2. Protect the client from injury by providing safety measures
3. Place an eye patch on the eye for diplopia
4. Monitor for potential complications such as urinary tract infections, calculi, pressure ulcers, respiratory tract infections, and contractures
5. Promote regular elimination by bladder and bowel training
6. Encourage independence
7. Assist the client to establish a regular exercise and rest program

8. Instruct the client to balance moderate activity with rest periods
9. Assess the need for and provide assistive devices
10. Initiate physical and speech therapy
11. Instruct the client to avoid fatigue, stress, infection, overheating, and chilling
12. Instruct the client to increase fluid intake and eat a balanced diet, including low-fat, high-fiber foods and foods high in potassium
13. Instruct the client on safety measures related to sensory loss, such as regulating the temperature of bath water and avoiding heating pads
14. Instruct the client on safety measures related to motor loss, such as avoiding the use of scatter rugs and using assistive devices
15. Instruct the client in the self-administration of prescribed medications (Box 56-20)
16. Provide information about the National Multiple Sclerosis Society

XIII. MYASTHENIA GRAVIS
A. Description
1. Myasthenia gravis is a neuromuscular disease that is characterized by considerable weakness and abnormal fatigue of the voluntary muscles
2. A defect in the transmission of nerve impulses at the myoneural junction occurs
3. Causes include insufficient secretion of acetylcholine, excessive secretion of cholinesterase, and unresponsiveness of the muscle fibers to acetylcholine
B. Data collection
1. Weakness and fatigue

BOX 56-20 Medications Used With Multiple Sclerosis

Baclofen (Lioresal), Dantrolene (Dantrium), or Diazepam (Valium)
Used to lessen muscle spasticity
Bethanechol
Used to prevent urinary retention
Carbamazepine (Tegretol)
Used to treat paresthesia
Corticosteroids
Used to reduce edema and the inflammatory response
Used to decrease the length of time the client's symptoms are exacerbated and to improve the degree of recovery
Immunosuppressive Medications
Used to treat chronic progressive multiple sclerosis to stabilize the disease process
Oxybutynin Chloride (Ditropan)
Used to increase bladder capacity, decrease bladder spasms, and control urge incontinence and frequency
Propranolol (Inderal) and Clonazepam (Klonopin)
Used to treat cerebellar ataxia

---

2. Difficulty chewing
3. Dysphagia
4. Ptosis
5. Diplopia
6. Weak, hoarse voice
7. Difficulty breathing
8. Diminished breath sounds
9. Respiratory paralysis and failure
C. Interventions
1. Monitor respiratory status and ability to cough and deep breathe adequately
2. Monitor for respiratory failure
3. Maintain suctioning and emergency equipment at the bedside
4. Monitor vital signs
5. Monitor speech and swallowing abilities to prevent aspiration
6. Encourage the client to sit up when eating
7. Assess muscle status
8. Instruct the client to conserve strength
9. Plan short activities that coincide with times of maximal muscle strength
10. Monitor for myasthenic and cholinergic crises
11. Administer anticholinesterase medications as prescribed
12. Instruct the client to avoid stress, infection, fatigue, and over-the-counter medications
13. Instruct the client to wear a Medic-Alert bracelet
14. Inform the client about services from the Myasthenia Gravis Foundation
D. Anticholinesterase medications
1. Action: increase levels of acetycholine at the myoneural junction
2. Medications
a. Neostigmine bromide (Prostigmin)
b. Pyridostigmine bromide (Mestinon)
c. Edrophonium chloride (Tensilon)
3. Side effects
a. Sweating
b. Salivation
c. Nausea
d. Diarrhea and abdominal cramps
e. Bradycardia
f. Hypotension
4. Interventions
a. Administer medications on time
b. Administer medication 30 minutes before meals with milk and crackers to reduce gastrointestinal upset
c. Monitor and record muscle strength
d. Note that excessive doses lead to cholinergic crisis
e. Have the antidote (atropine sulfate) available
E. Myasthenic crisis
1. Description
a. Myasthenic crisis is an acute exacerbation of the disease

b. The crisis is caused by a rapid, unrecognized progression of the disease; an inadequate amount of medication; infection; fatigue; or stress

2. Data collection
   a. Increased pulse, respirations, and blood pressure
   b. Respiratory distress and cyanosis
   c. Bowel and bladder incontinence
   d. Decreased urine output
   e. Absent cough and swallow reflex

3. Interventions
   a. Assess for signs of myasthenic crisis
   b. Increase anticholinesterase medication, as prescribed

F. Cholinergic crisis
1. Description
   a. Cholinergic crisis results in depolarization of the motor end plates
   b. The crisis is caused by overmedication with anticholinesterase

2. Data collection
   a. Abdominal cramps
   b. Nausea, vomiting, and diarrhea
   c. Blurred vision
   d. Pallor
   e. Facial muscle twitching
   f. Hypotension
   g. Pupillary miosis

3. Interventions
   a. Hold anticholinesterase medication
   b. Prepare to administer the antidote, atropine sulfate, if prescribed

G. **Tensilon test**
1. Description: The **Tensilon test** is performed to diagnose myasthenia gravis and to differentiate between myasthenic crisis and cholinergic crisis

2. To diagnose myasthenia gravis
   a. Edrophonium (Tensilon) injection is administered to the client
   b. Positive for myasthenia gravis: The client shows improvement in muscle strength after the administration of Tensilon
   c. Negative for myasthenia gravis: client shows no improvement in muscle strength, and strength may even deteriorate after injection of Tensilon

3. To differentiate crisis
   a. Myasthenic crisis: Tensilon is administered, and if strength improves, the client needs more medication
   b. Cholinergic crisis: Tensilon is administered, and if the client's weakness is more severe, then the client is overmedicated; administer atropine sulfate, which is the the antidote, as prescribed

XIV. PARKINSON'S DISEASE

A. Description
1. Parkinson's disease is a degenerative disease caused by the depletion of dopamine, which interferes with the inhibition of excitatory impulses, resulting in a dysfunction of the extrapyramidal system
2. It is a slow, progressive disease that results in a crippling disability
3. The debilitation can result in falls, self-care deficits, failure of body systems, and depression
4. Mental deterioration occurs late in the progression of disease

B. Data collection
1. Bradykinesia, abnormal slowness of movement, and sluggishness of physical and mental responses
2. Akinesia
3. Monotonous speech
4. Handwriting that becomes progressively smaller
5. Tremors in hands and fingers at rest (pill rolling)
6. Tremors increasing when fatigued and decreasing with purposeful activity or sleep
7. Rigidity with jerky movements
8. Restlessness and pacing
9. Blank facial expression—mask-like facies
10. Drooling
11. Difficulty swallowing and speaking
12. Loss of coordination and balance
13. Shuffling steps, stooped position, and propulsive gait

C. Interventions
1. Assess neurological status
2. Assess ability to swallow and chew
3. Provide a high-calorie, high-protein, high-fiber soft diet with small, frequent feedings
4. Increase fluid intake to 2000 mL/day
5. Monitor for constipation
6. Promote independence along with safety measures
7. Avoid rushing the client with activities
8. Assist with ambulation and provide assistive devices
9. Instruct the client to rock back and forth to initiate movement
10. Instruct the client to wear low-heeled shoes
11. Encourage the client to lift his or her feet when walking and to avoid prolonged sitting
12. Provide a firm mattress, and position the client prone, without a pillow, to facilitate proper posture
13. Instruct in proper posture by teaching the client to hold the hands behind the back to keep the spine and neck erect
14. Promote physical therapy and rehabilitation

15. Administer anticholinergic medications as prescribed to treat tremors and rigidity and to inhibit the action of acetylcholine
16. Administer antiparkinsonian medications to increase the level of dopamine in the CNS
17. Instruct the client to avoid foods high in vitamin B_6 because they block the effects of antiparkinsonian medications
18. Instruct the client to avoid monoamine oxidase inhibitors because they will precipitate hypertensive crisis
19. Refer to Chapter 57 regarding medication to treat Parkinson's disease

XV. TRIGEMINAL NEURALGIA
A. Description
   1. Trigeminal neuralgia is a sensory disorder of the trigeminal or cranial nerve V
   2. It results in severe, recurrent, sharp, facial pain along the trigeminal nerve
B. Data collection
   1. Client has severe pain on the lips, gums, or nose, or across the cheeks
   2. Situations that stimulate symptoms include cold, washing the face, chewing, or food or fluids of extreme temperatures
C. Interventions
   1. Instruct the client to avoid hot or cold foods and fluids
   2. Provide small feedings of liquid and soft foods
   3. Instruct the client to chew food on the unaffected side
   4. Administer medications as prescribed (Box 56-21)
D. Surgical interventions
   1. Microvascular decompression: surgical relocation of the artery that compresses the trigeminal nerve as it enters the pons may relieve pain without compromising facial sensation
   2. Radiofrequency wave forms: Creates lesions that provide relief from pain without compromising touch or motor function
   3. Rhizotomy: Resection of the root of the nerve to relieve pain
   4. Glycerol injection: destroys the myelinated fibers of the trigeminal nerve (may take up to 3 weeks for pain relief to occur)

BOX 56-21	**Medications to Treat Trigeminal Neuralgia**

Baclofen (Lioresal)
Carbamazepine (Tegretol)
Gabapentin (Neurontin)
Phenytoin (Dilantin)

XVI. BELL'S PALSY (FACIAL PARALYSIS)
A. Description
   1. Bell's palsy is caused by a lower motor neuron lesion of cranial nerve VII that may result from infection, trauma, hemorrhage, meningitis, or a tumor
   2. It results in paralysis of one side of the face
   3. Recovery usually occurs in a few weeks without residual effects
B. Data collection
   1. Flaccid facial muscles
   2. Inability to raise the eyebrows, frown, smile, close the eyelids, or puff out the cheeks
   3. Upward movement of the eye when attempting to close the eyelid
   4. Loss of taste
C. Interventions
   1. Encourage the client to do facial exercises in order to prevent the loss of muscle tone (a face sling may be prescribed to prevent stretching of weak muscles)
   2. Protect the eyes from dryness and prevent injury
   3. Promote frequent oral care
   4. Instruct the client to chew on the unaffected side

XVII. GUILLAIN-BARRÉ SYNDROME
A. Description
   1. Guillain-Barré syndrome is an acute infectious neuronitis of the cranial and peripheral nerves
   2. The immune system overreacts to the infection and destroys the myelin sheath
   3. The syndrome is usually preceded by a mild upper respiratory infection or gastroenteritis
   4. Recovery is a slow process and can take years
   5. The major concern is difficulty breathing
B. Data collection
   1. Paresthesias
   2. Weakness of lower extremities
   3. Gradual progressive weakness of the upper extremities and facial muscles
   4. Possible progression to respiratory failure
   5. Cardiac dysrhythmias
   6. CSF that reveals an elevated protein level
   7. Abnormal electroencephalogram
C. Interventions
   1. Direct care toward the treatment of symptoms
   2. Monitor respiratory status
   3. Provide respiratory treatments
   4. Prepare to initiate respiratory support
   5. Monitor cardiac status
   6. Assess for complications of immobility
   7. Provide the client and family with support

XVIII. AMYOTROPHIC LATERAL SCLEROSIS
A. Description
   1. Amyotrophic lateral sclerosis is also known as Lou Gehrig's disease

2. It is a progressive degenerative disease involving the motor system
3. The sensory and autonomic systems are not involved, and mental status changes do not result from the disease
4. The cause of the disease may be related to an excess of glutamate, a chemical responsible for relaying messages between the motor neurons
5. As the disease progresses, muscle weakness and atrophy develop until a flaccid quadriplegia develops
6. Eventually the respiratory muscles become affected, leading to respiratory compromise, pneumonia, and death
7. No cure is known, and the treatment is symptomatic

B. Data collection
1. Fatigue (including while talking)
2. Respiratory distress
3. Muscle weakness and atrophy
4. Tongue atrophy
5. Dysphagia
6. Weakness of the hands and arms
7. Fasciculations of the face
8. Nasal quality of speech
9. Dysarthria

C. Interventions
1. Care is directed toward the treatment of symptoms
2. Monitor respiratory status
3. Provide respiratory treatments
4. Prepare to initiate respiratory support
5. Assess for complications of immobility
6. Provide the client and family with support

XIX. ENCEPHALITIS

A. Description
1. Encephalitis is an inflammation of the brain parenchyma and often the meninges
2. It affects the cerebrum, the brainstem, and the cerebellum
3. It is most often caused by a viral agent, although bacteria, fungi, or parasites may also be involved
4. Viral encephalitis is almost always preceded by a viral infection

B. Transmission
1. Arboviruses can be transmitted to human beings through the bite of an infected mosquito or tick
2. Echovirus, coxsackievirus, poliovirus, herpes zoster, and viruses that cause mumps and chickenpox are common enteroviruses associated with encephalitis
3. Herpes simplex type 1 virus can cause viral encephalitis
4. The organism that causes amebic meningoencephalitis can enter the nasal mucosa of persons swimming in warm freshwater ponds and lakes

C. Data collection
1. Presence of cold sores, lesions, or ulcerations of the oral cavity
2. History of insect bites and swimming in freshwater
3. Exposure to infectious diseases
4. Travel to areas where the disease is prevalent
5. Fever
6. Nausea and vomiting
7. **Nuchal rigidity**
8. Changes in LOC and mental status
9. Signs of increased ICP
10. Motor dysfunction and focal neurological deficits

D. Interventions
1. Monitor vital and neurological signs
2. Assess LOC using the **Glasgow Coma Scale**
3. Assess for mental status changes and personality and behavior changes
4. Assess for signs of increased ICP
5. Assess for the presence of **nuchal rigidity** and a positive **Kernig's sign** or **Brudzinski's sign**, indicating meningeal irritation
6. Assist the client to turn, cough, and deep breathe frequently
7. Elevate the head of the bed 30 to 45 degrees
8. Assess for muscle and neurological deficits
9. Administer acyclovir (Zovirax) as prescribed (medication of choice for herpes encephalitis)
10. Initiate rehabilitation as needed for motor dysfunction or neurological deficits

XX. WEST NILE VIRUS

A. Description
1. West Nile virus is a potentially serious illness that affects the CNS
2. The virus is contracted primarily by the bite of an infected mosquito (mosquitoes become carriers when they feed on infected birds)
3. Symptoms typically develop between 3 and 14 days after being bitten by the infected mosquito
4. Neurological effects can be permanent

B. Data collection
1. Many individuals will not experience any symptoms
2. Mild symptoms include fever, headache and body aches, nausea, vomiting, swollen glands, or a rash on the chest, stomach, or back
3. Severe symptoms include a high fever, headache, neck stiffness, stupor, disorientation, tremors, muscle weakness, vision loss, numbness, paralysis, seizures, or coma

C. Interventions are supportive; there is no specific treatment for the virus

D. Prevention
1. Use insect repellents containing DEET (*N,N*-diethyl-meta-toluamide) when outdoors

and wear long sleeves and pants and light-colored clothing

2. Stay indoors at dusk and dawn when mosquitoes are most active

3. Ensure that mosquito breeding sites are eliminated, such as standing water and water in bird baths, and keep wading pools empty and on their sides when not in use

▲ XXI. MENINGITIS

A. Description

1. Meningitis is inflammation of the arachnoid and pia mater of the brain and spinal cord

2. It is caused by bacterial and viral organisms, although fungal and protozoal meningitis also occurs

3. Predisposing factors include skull fractures, brain or spinal surgery, sinus or upper respiratory infections, the use of nasal sprays, and individuals with a compromised immune system

4. CSF is analyzed to determine the diagnosis and the type of meningitis

B. Transmission

1. Transmission is by direct contact, including droplet spread

2. Transmission occurs in areas of high-population density, crowded living areas such as college dormitories, and prisons

▲ C. Data collection (see Box 56-4)

1. Mild lethargy; photophobia

2. Deterioration in the level of consciousness

3. Signs of meningeal irritation such as **nuchal rigidity** and positive **Kernig's sign** and **Brudzinski's sign**

4. Red, macular rash with meningococcal meningitis

5. Abdominal and chest pain with viral meningitis

▲ D. Interventions

1. Monitor vital signs and neurological signs

2. Assess for signs of increasing ICP

3. Initiate seizure precautions

4. Monitor for seizure activity

5. Monitor for signs of meningeal irritation

6. Perform cranial nerve assessment

7. Assess peripheral vascular status (septic emboli may block circulation)

8. Maintain isolation precautions as necessary with bacterial meningitis

9. Maintain urine and stool precautions with viral meningitis

10. Maintain respiratory isolation for the client with pneumococcal meningitis

11. Elevate the head of the bed 30 degrees, and avoid neck flexion and extreme hip flexion

12. Prevent stimulation and restrict visitors

13. Administer analgesics as prescribed

14. Administer antibiotics as prescribed

PRACTICE QUESTIONS

More questions on the companion CD!

743. A client is having a lumbar puncture (LP) performed. The nurse would place the client in which position for the procedure?
1. Supine, in semi-Fowler's
2. Prone, in slight Trendelenburg's
3. Prone, with a pillow under the abdomen
4. Side-lying, with legs pulled up and head bent down onto the chest

744. A client has just undergone computerized tomography (CT) scanning with a contrast medium. The nurse determines that the client understands postprocedure care if the client verbalizes that he or she will:
1. Drink extra fluids for the day.
2. Hold medications for at least 4 hours.
3. Eat lightly for the remainder of the day.
4. Rest quietly for the remainder of the day.

745. A nurse is caring for a client with increased intracranial pressure (ICP). The nurse would monitor for which of the following trends in vital signs that would occur if ICP is rising?
1. Increasing temperature, decreasing pulse, decreasing respirations, increasing blood pressure (BP)
2. Decreasing temperature, decreasing pulse, increasing respirations, decreasing BP
3. Decreasing temperature, increasing pulse, decreasing respirations, increasing BP
4. Increasing temperature, increasing pulse, increasing respirations, decreasing BP

746. A nurse is positioning the client with increased intracranial pressure (ICP). Which position would the nurse avoid?
1. Head midline
2. Head turned to the side
3. Neck in neutral position
4. Head of bed elevated 30 to 45 degrees

747. A client recovering from a head injury is arousable and participating in care. The nurse determines that the client understands measures to prevent elevations in intracranial pressure (ICP) if the nurse observes the client doing which of the following activities?
1. Blowing the nose
2. Isometric exercises
3. Coughing vigorously
4. Exhaling during repositioning

748. A client has clear fluid leaking from the nose following a basilar skull fracture. The nurse determines that this is cerebrospinal fluid (CSF) if the fluid:
1. Is grossly bloody in appearance and has a pH of 6

2. Clumps together on the dressing and has a pH of 7

3. Is clear in appearance and tests negative for glucose

4. Separates into concentric rings and tests positive for glucose

749. A client is admitted to the hospital for observation with a probable minor head injury after an automobile crash. The nurse would plan on leaving the cervical collar in place until:
1. The family comes to visit.
2. The physician makes rounds.
3. The nurse needs to do physical care.
4. The result of spinal x-rays is known.

750. A client was seen and treated in the emergency department for treatment of a concussion. The nurse determines that the family needs further discharge instructions if they say to bring the client back to the emergency department if which of the following occurs?
1. Vomiting
2. Minor headache
3. Difficulty speaking
4. Difficulty awakening

751. A nurse is caring for a client who has undergone craniotomy with a supratentorial incision. The nurse would plan to place the client in which position postoperatively?
1. Head of bed flat, head and neck midline
2. Head of bed flat, head turned to the nonoperative side
3. Head of bed elevated 30 to 45 degrees, head and neck midline
4. Head of bed elevated 30 to 45 degrees, head turned to the operative side

752. A client with a cervical spine injury has Crutchfield tongs applied in the emergency department. The nurse would avoid which of the following when planning care for this client?
1. Using a Stryker frame bed
2. Removing the weights to reposition the client
3. Assessing the integrity of the weights and pulleys
4. Comparing the amount of ordered traction with the amount in use

753. A nurse has provided discharge instructions to a client with an application of a halo device. The nurse determines that the client needs further clarification of the instructions if the client states that he or she will:
1. Use a straw for drinking.
2. Drive only during the daytime.
3. Use caution, because the device alters balance.
4. Wash the skin daily under the lamb's wool liner of the vest.

754. A nurse is caring for the client who has suffered spinal cord injury. The nurse further monitors the client for signs of autonomic dysreflexia and suspects this complication if which of the following is noted?
1. Sudden tachycardia
2. Pallor of the face and neck
3. Severe, throbbing headache
4. Severe and sudden hypotension

755. A client with spinal cord injury is prone to experiencing autonomic dysreflexia. The nurse would avoid which measure to minimize the risk of recurrence?
1. Strict adherence to a bowel retraining program
2. Keeping the linen wrinkle-free under the client
3. Avoiding unnecessary pressure on the lower limbs
4. Limiting bladder catheterization to once every 12 hours

756. A client with spinal cord injury suddenly experiences an episode of autonomic dysreflexia. After checking vital signs, the nurse immediately:
1. Raises the head of the bed and removes the noxious stimulus
2. Lowers the head of the bed and removes the noxious stimulus
3. Lowers the head of the bed and administers an antihypertensive agent
4. Removes the noxious stimulus and administers an antihypertensive agent

757. A nurse is caring for a client with an intracranial aneurysm who was previously alert. Which finding would be an early indication that the level of consciousness (LOC) is deteriorating?
1. Drowsiness
2. Clear speech
3. Ptosis of the left eyelid
4. Frequent spontaneous speech

758. A nurse is planning to put aneurysm precautions in place for the client with a cerebral aneurysm. Which item would be included as part of the precautions?
1. Limiting cigarettes to three per day
2. Allowing out-of-bed activities as tolerated
3. Maintaining the head of the bed at 15 degrees
4. Allowing one cup of caffeinated coffee per day

759. A nurse is caring for a client who begins to experience seizure activity while in bed. Which action by the nurse would be contraindicated?
1. Restraining the client's limbs
2. Loosening restrictive clothing
3. Removing the pillow and raising the padded side rails
4. Positioning the client to the side, if possible, with head flexed forward

760. A nurse is planning care for the client with hemiparesis of the right arm and leg. The nurse incorporates in the care plan placement of objects:
1. Within the client's reach, on the right side

2. Within the client's reach, on the left side
3. Just out of the client's reach, on the left side
4. Just out of the client's reach, on the right side

761. A nurse has instructed the family of a brain attack (stroke) client who has homonymous hemianopsia about measures to help the client overcome the deficit. The nurse determines that the family understands the measures to use if they state that they will:
1. Place objects in the client's impaired field of vision.
2. Discourage the client from wearing own eyeglasses.
3. Approach the client from the impaired field of vision.
4. Remind the client to turn the head to scan the lost visual field.

762. A family of a spinal cord–injured client rushes to the nursing station, saying that the client needs immediate help. On entering the room, the nurse notes that the client is diaphoretic, with a flushed face and neck, and complains of a severe headache. The pulse is 40 beats/minute and the blood pressure (BP) is 230/100 mm Hg. The nurse acts quickly, knowing that the client is experiencing:
1. Spinal shock
2. Pulmonary embolism
3. Autonomic dysreflexia
4. Malignant hyperthermia

763. A client has experienced an episode of myasthenic crisis. The nurse collects data to determine whether the client has precipitating factors such as:
1. Too little exercise
2. Omitted doses of medication
3. Increased doses of medication
4. Increased intake of fatty foods

764. A client with Parkinson's disease is embarrassed about the symptoms of the disorder and is bored and lonely. The nurse would plan which approach as therapeutic in assisting the client to cope with the disease?
1. Assist the client with ADLs as much as possible.
2. Plan only a few activities for the client during the day.

3. Cluster activities at the end of the day when the client is most bored.
4. Encourage and praise perseverance in exercising and performing activities of daily living (ADLs).

765. A nurse has given suggestions to the client with trigeminal neuralgia about strategies to minimize episodes of pain. The nurse determines that the client needs additional information if the client made which of the following statements?
1. "I will wash my face with cotton pads."
2. "I'll have to start chewing on the unaffected side."
3. "I should rinse my mouth if toothbrushing is painful."
4. "I will try to eat my food either very warm or very cold."

766. A client has an impairment of cranial nerve II. Specific to this impairment, the nurse would plan to do which of the following to ensure client safety?
1. Speak loudly to the client.
2. Test the temperature of the shower water.
3. Check the temperature of the food on the dietary tray.
4. Provide a clear path for ambulation without obstacles.

ALTERNATE ITEM FORMAT: PRIORITIZING (ORDERED RESPONSE)

767. The client with a spinal cord injury suddenly experiences an episode of autonomic dysreflexia. After checking the client's vital signs, number the nurses's actions in order of priority, with the first selected action being of highest priority and the last selected action of lowest priority. (Number 1 is the first priority action and number 6 is the last priority action.)
___ Contact the physician.
___ Raise the head of the bed.
___ Check for bladder distention.
___ Loosen tight clothing on the client.
___ Administer an antihypertensive medication.
___ Document the occurrence, treatment, and response.

744. 1
Rationale: After CT scanning, the client may resume all usual activities. The client should be encouraged to take in extra fluids to replace those lost with diuresis from the contrast dye. Options 2, 3, and 4 are unnecessary.
Test-Taking Strategy: Use the process of elimination. Recalling that there is no special aftercare following this procedure and noting the words "contrast medium" in the question will direct you to option 1. Review the procedure related to CT scanning if you had difficulty with this question.
Level of Cognitive Ability: Comprehension
Client Needs: Physiological Integrity
Integrated Process: Nursing Process/Evaluation
Content Area: Adult Health/Neurological
Reference: Pagana, K., & Pagana, T. (2005). *Mosby's diagnostic and laboratory test reference* (7th ed., p. 299). St. Louis: Mosby.

745. 1
Rationale: A change in vital signs may be a late sign of increased ICP. Trends include increasing temperature and blood pressure and decreasing pulse and respirations. Respiratory irregularities may also arise.
Test-Taking Strategy: Use the process of elimination. This question looks complex but can be answered logically. If you remember that temperature rises, you are able to eliminate options 2 and 3. If you know that the client becomes bradycardic, or know that the BP rises, you are able to select the correct option. Review the signs of increased ICP if you had difficulty with this question.
Level of Cognitive Ability: Analysis
Client Needs: Physiological Integrity
Integrated Process: Nursing Process/Data Collection
Content Area: Adult Health/Neurological
Reference: Linton, A., & Maebius, N. (2007). *Introduction to medical-surgical nursing* (4th ed., p. 433). Philadelphia: Saunders.

746. 2
Rationale: The head of the client with increased ICP should be positioned so that the head is in a neutral, midline position. The nurse should avoid flexing or extending the neck or turning the head side to side. The head of the bed should be raised to 30 to 45 degrees. Use of proper positions promotes venous drainage from the cranium to keep ICP down.
Test-Taking Strategy: Note the strategic word "avoid." This word indicates a negative event query and the need to select the incorrect position. This would be one that interferes with arterial circulation to the brain or with venous drainage from the brain. The only position that meets one of those criteria is option 2. Review client positioning with ICP if you had difficulty with this question.
Level of Cognitive Ability: Application
Client Needs: Physiological Integrity
Integrated Process: Nursing Process/Implementation
Content Area: Adult Health/Neurological
Reference: Linton, A., & Maebius, N. (2007). *Introduction to medical-surgical nursing* (4th ed., p. 434). Philadelphia: Saunders.

747. 4
Rationale: Activities that increase intrathoracic and intraabdominal pressures cause indirect elevation of the ICP. Some of these activities include isometric exercises, Valsalva maneuver, coughing, sneezing, and blowing the nose. Exhaling during activities such as repositioning or pulling up in bed opens the glottis, which prevents intrathoracic pressure from rising.
Test-Taking Strategy: Use the process of elimination. Evaluate each option in terms of the tension it puts on the body to help you eliminate each of the incorrect options. Review the measures that will reduce or prevent increased intracranial pressure if you had difficulty with this question.
Level of Cognitive Ability: Comprehension
Client Needs: Physiological Integrity
Integrated Process: Nursing Process/Evaluation
Content Area: Adult Health/Neurological
Reference: Linton, A., & Maebius, N. (2007). *Introduction to medical-surgical nursing* (4th ed., p. 439). Philadelphia: Saunders.

748. 4
Rationale: Leakage of CSF from the ears or nose may accompany basilar skull fracture. It can be distinguished from other body fluids because the drainage will separate into bloody and yellow concentric rings on dressing material, which is known as the halo sign. It also tests positive for glucose. Options 1, 2, and 3 are not characteristics of CSF.
Test-Taking Strategy: Use the process of elimination. Recalling that CSF contains glucose, whereas other secretions such as mucus do not, will direct you to option 4. Also, remember that CSF separates into rings. Review testing for CSF fluid if you had difficulty with this question.
Level of Cognitive Ability: Analysis
Client Needs: Physiological Integrity
Integrated Process: Nursing Process/Evaluation
Content Area: Adult Health/Neurological
Reference: Christensen, B., & Kockrow, E. (2006). *Adult health nursing* (5th ed., p. 742). St. Louis: Mosby.

749. 4
Rationale: There is a significant association between cervical spine injury and head injury. For this reason, the nurse leaves any form of spinal immobilization in place until lateral cervical spine x-rays rule out fracture or other damage.
Test-Taking Strategy: Focus on the data in the question and note the client's injury. Remember that the reason for spinal immobilization is to protect the spine from movement, which could cause further damage if the cervical spine were injured. If x-ray results are negative, there is no reason to leave the collar in place. Review emergency care of the client with a suspected cervical injury if this question was difficult.
Level of Cognitive Ability: Application
Client Needs: Physiological Integrity
Integrated Process: Nursing Process/Implementation
Content Area: Adult Health/Neurological
Reference: Christensen, B., & Kockrow, E. (2006). *Adult health nursing* (5th ed., p. 746). St. Louis: Mosby.

750. 2
Rationale: A concussion after head injury is a temporary loss of consciousness (from a few seconds to a few minutes) without evidence of structural damage. After concussion, the family is taught to monitor the client and call the physician

or return the client to the emergency department if certain signs and symptoms are noted. These include confusion, difficulty awakening or speaking, one-sided weakness, vomiting, or severe headache. Minor headache is expected.
Test-Taking Strategy: Note the strategic words "needs further discharge instructions." These words indicate a negative event query and the need to select the incorrect family statement. Noting the word "minor" in option 2 will direct you to this option. Review care of the client with a concussion if you had difficulty with this question.
Level of Cognitive Ability: Analysis
Client Needs: Physiological Integrity
Integrated Process: Teaching and Learning
Content Area: Adult Health/Neurological
Reference: Christensen, B., & Kockrow, E. (2006). *Adult health nursing* (5th ed., p. 743). St. Louis: Mosby.

751. 3
Rationale: Following supratentorial surgery, the head of the bed is kept at a 30- to 45-degree angle. The head and neck should not be angled either anteriorly or laterally, but rather should be kept in a neutral (midline) position. This will promote venous return through the jugular veins, which will help prevent a rise in intracranial pressure.
Test-Taking Strategy: This question tests knowledge of differences in positioning the craniotomy client with an infratentorial versus supratentorial incision. If you remember that with "supra-" one should "keep the head up," and with "infra-" one should "keep the head down," options 1 and 2 can be eliminated. Knowing how to position the head for optimal venous drainage helps you select option 3 over option 4. Review client positioning following craniotomy if you had difficulty with this question.
Level of Cognitive Ability: Application
Client Needs: Physiological Integrity
Integrated Process: Nursing Process/Planning
Content Area: Adult Health/Neurological
Reference: Christensen, B., & Kockrow, E. (2006). *Adult health nursing* (5th ed., p. 705). St. Louis: Mosby.

752. 2
Rationale: Crutchfield tongs are applied after drilling holes in the client's skull under local anesthesia. Weights are attached to the tongs, which exert pulling pressure on the longitudinal axis of the cervical spine. Serial x-rays of the cervical spine are taken, with weights being added gradually until radiography reveals that the vertebral column is realigned. Weights then may be gradually reduced to a point that maintains alignment. The client with Crutchfield tongs is placed on a Stryker frame or RotoRest bed. The nurse ensures that weights hang freely and the amount of weight matches the current order. The nurse also inspects the integrity and position of the ropes and pulleys. The nurse does not remove the weights to administer care.
Test-Taking Strategy: Note the strategic word "avoid." This word indicates a negative event query and the need to select the item that would be contraindicated. Recalling the basics of traction and recalling that weights are not removed will direct you to option 2. Review nursing care related to the client with cervical tongs if you had difficulty with this question.
Level of Cognitive Ability: Application

Client Needs: Physiological Integrity
Integrated Process: Nursing Process/Planning
Content Area: Adult Health/Neurological
Reference: deWit, S. (2009). *Medical-surgical nursing: Concepts & practice* (p. 552). St. Louis: Saunders.

753. 2
Rationale: The halo device alters balance and can cause fatigue because of its weight. The client should cleanse the skin daily under the vest or the device to protect the skin from ulceration and should use powder or lotions sparingly or not at all. The wool liner should be changed if odor becomes a problem. The client should have food cut into small pieces to facilitate chewing and use a straw for drinking. Pin care is done as instructed. The client should not drive because the device impairs the range of vision.
Test-Taking Strategy: Note the strategic words "needs further clarification." These words indicate a negative event query and the need to select the incorrect client statement. Recall that a halo device is used to allow mobility for the client who needs continuous cervical traction; it maintains the head and spine in a neutral position. With this in mind, it will be easy to select option 2 as the correct answer as stated. The inability to turn the head without turning the torso would contraindicate driving. Review client-teaching points related to a halo device if you had difficulty with this question.
Level of Cognitive Ability: Comprehension
Client Needs: Safe and Effective Care Environment
Integrated Process: Teaching and Learning
Content Area: Adult Health/Neurological
Reference: Lewis, S., Heitkemper, M., Dirksen, S., & Bucher, L. (2007). *Medical-surgical nursing: Assessment and management of clinical problems* (7th ed., p. 1606). St. Louis: Mosby.

754. 3
Rationale: The client with spinal cord injury above the level of T7 is at risk for autonomic dysreflexia. It is characterized by severe, throbbing headache, flushing of the face and neck, bradycardia, and sudden severe hypertension. Other signs include nasal stuffiness, blurred vision, nausea, and sweating. It is a life-threatening syndrome triggered by a noxious stimulus below the level of the injury.
Test-Taking Strategy: Use the process of elimination. To answer this question correctly, it is necessary to know what causes autonomic dysreflexia. Remember, it results from the sudden exaggerated response of the sympathetic nervous system to a noxious stimulus. A massive sympathetic nervous system response causes severe hypertension. This would account for the throbbing headache (the correct answer) and cause flushing of the face and neck. Baroreceptors sense the sudden hypertension, causing a reflex bradycardia. Also, remember that the pulse and blood pressure changes with autonomic dysreflexia are actually the opposite of what would occur with hypovolemic shock. Review the signs of autonomic dysreflexia if you had difficulty with this question.
Level of Cognitive Ability: Analysis
Client Needs: Physiological Integrity
Integrated Process: Nursing Process/Data Collection
Content Area: Adult Health/Neurological
Reference: Christensen, B., & Kockrow, E. (2006). *Adult health nursing* (5th ed., pp. 743, 745). St. Louis: Mosby.

755. 4
Rationale: The most frequent cause of autonomic dysreflexia is a distended bladder. Straight catheterization should be performed every 4 to 6 hours, and Foley catheters should be checked frequently for kinks in the tubing. Constipation and fecal impaction are other causes, so maintaining bowel regularity is important. Other causes include stimulation of the skin from tactile, thermal, or painful stimuli. The nurse administers care to minimize risk in these areas.
Test-Taking Strategy: Note the strategic word "avoid." Remember that autonomic dysreflexia is caused by noxious stimuli to the bowel, bladder, or skin. With this in mind, you can eliminate each of the incorrect options. Review the measures to minimize the risk of autonomic dysreflexia if you had difficulty with this question.
Level of Cognitive Ability: Application
Client Needs: Physiological Integrity
Integrated Process: Nursing Process/Implementation
Content Area: Adult Health/Neurological
References: deWit, S. (2009). *Medical-surgical nursing: Concepts & practice* (p. 554). St. Louis: Saunders.
Linton, A., & Maebius, N. (2007). *Introduction to medical-surgical nursing* (4th ed., p. 494). Philadelphia: Saunders.

756. 1
Rationale: Key nursing actions are to sit the client up in bed, remove the noxious stimulus, and bring the blood pressure under control with antihypertensive medication per protocol. The nurse can also clearly label the client's chart identifying the risk for autonomic dysreflexia. Client and family should be taught to recognize, and later manage, the signs and symptoms of this syndrome.
Test-Taking Strategy: Note the strategic word "immediately" in the question. This is a clue that the first item in each option must be the first action. If you know to raise the head of the client's bed first (to try to minimize cerebral hypertension), then this eliminates each of the incorrect options. Review immediate nursing interventions for the client experiencing autonomic dysreflexia if you had difficulty with this question.
Level of Cognitive Ability: Application
Client Needs: Physiological Integrity
Integrated Process: Nursing Process/Implementation
Content Area: Adult Health/Neurological
Reference: Linton, A., & Maebius, N. (2007). *Introduction to medical-surgical nursing* (4th ed., p. 503). Philadelphia: Saunders.

757. 1
Rationale: Ptosis of the eyelid is due to pressure on and dysfunction of cranial nerve III and does not relate to LOC. Early changes in LOC relate to alertness and verbal responsiveness. Less frequent speech, slight slurring of speech, and mild drowsiness are early signs of decreasing LOC.
Test-Taking Strategy: Use the process of elimination. Recalling that LOC includes orientation, awareness, and verbal responsiveness will direct you to option 1. Review the early signs of decreasing LOC if you had difficulty with this question.
Level of Cognitive Ability: Analysis
Client Needs: Physiological Integrity
Integrated Process: Nursing Process/Data Collection
Content Area: Adult Health/Neurological

Reference: Linton, A., & Maebius, N. (2007). *Introduction to medical-surgical nursing* (4th ed., pp. 421-422, 433). Philadelphia: Saunders.

758. 3
Rationale: Aneurysm precautions include placing the client on bedrest with the head of the bed elevated in a quiet setting. Lights are kept dim to minimize environmental stimulation. Any activity that increases blood pressure (BP) or impedes venous return from the brain is prohibited, such as pushing, pulling, sneezing, coughing, or straining. The nurse provides all physical care to minimize increases in BP. For the same reason, visitors, radio, television, and reading materials are prohibited or limited. Stimulants such as caffeine and nicotine are prohibited; decaffeinated coffee or tea may be given.
Test-Taking Strategy: Use the process of elimination. Recall that a global principle in aneurysm precautions is to limit the amount of stimulation (in any form) that the client receives, and to prevent increased intracranial pressure. This will direct you to option 3. Review aneurysm precautions if you had difficulty with this question.
Level of Cognitive Ability: Application
Client Needs: Physiological Integrity
Integrated Process: Nursing Process/Implementation
Content Area: Adult Health/Neurological
Reference: Monahan, F., Sands, J., Neighbors, M., Marek, J., & Green, C. (2007). *Phipps' medical-surgical nursing: Health and illness perspectives* (8th ed., p. 1441). St. Louis: Mosby.

759. 1
Rationale: Nursing actions during a seizure include providing privacy, loosening restrictive clothing, removing the pillow and raising the padded side rails in bed, and placing the client on one side with the head flexed forward, if possible, to allow the tongue to fall forward and facilitate drainage. The limbs are never restrained, because the strong muscle contractions could cause the client harm. If the client is not in bed when seizure activity begins, the nurse lowers the client to the floor, if possible, protects the head against injury, and moves furniture that may injure the client.
Test-Taking Strategy: Note the strategic word "contraindicated." This word indicates a negative event query and the need to select the harmful action. No harm can come to the client from any of the options except for restraining the limbs. Remember to avoid restraints. Review care of a client during a seizure if you had difficulty with this question.
Level of Cognitive Ability: Application
Client Needs: Physiological Integrity
Integrated Process: Nursing Process/Implementation
Content Area: Adult Health/Neurological
Reference: deWit, S. (2009). *Medical-surgical nursing: Concepts & practice* (p. 567). St. Louis: Saunders.

760. 2
Rationale: Hemiparesis is a weakness of the face, arm, and leg on one side. The client with one-sided hemiparesis benefits from having objects placed on the unaffected side and within reach. Other helpful activities with hemiparesis include range-of-motion exercises to the affected side and muscle-strengthening exercises to the unaffected side.

Test-Taking Strategy: Focus on the client's diagnosis. Begin by eliminating options 3 and 4 since they are hazardous to the client. This question also tests your ability to distinguish between hemiparesis and unilateral neglect. The client with hemiparesis has weakness on one side, and therefore objects should be placed on the stronger side. With unilateral neglect, objects are placed on the affected side to train the client to attend to that part of the environment. Knowing this, you would select option 2 as the correct answer. Review care of the client with hemiparesis if you had difficulty with this question.
Level of Cognitive Ability: Application
Client Needs: Safe and Effective Care Environment
Integrated Process: Nursing Process/Planning
Content Area: Adult Health/Neurological
Reference: deWit, S. (2009). *Medical-surgical nursing: Concepts & practice* (pp. 529;532). St. Louis: Saunders.

761. **4**
Rationale: Homonymous hemianopsia is loss of half of the visual field. The client with homonymous hemianopsia should have objects placed in the intact field of vision, and the nurse should approach the client from the intact side. The nurse instructs the client to scan the environment to overcome the visual deficit and performs client teaching from within the intact field of vision. The nurse encourages the use of personal eyeglasses, if they are available.
Test-Taking Strategy: To answer this question accurately, you need to be able to distinguish between homonymous hemianopsia and unilateral neglect. Clients are approached differently with these two deficits. Remember that the similarity is that the client must be taught to scan the environment, which is the answer to this question. Review care of the client with homonymous hemianopsia if you had difficulty with this question.
Level of Cognitive Ability: Analysis
Client Needs: Physiological Integrity
Integrated Process: Nursing Process/Evaluation
Content Area: Adult Health/Neurological
Reference: Linton, A., & Maebius, N. (2007). *Introduction to medical-surgical nursing* (4th ed., p. 481). Philadelphia: Saunders.

762. **3**
Rationale: The client with spinal cord injury above the level of T7 is at risk for autonomic dysreflexia. It is characterized by severe, throbbing headache; flushing of the face and neck; bradycardia; and sudden severe hypertension. Other signs include nasal stuffiness, blurred vision, nausea, and sweating. It is a life-threatening syndrome triggered by a noxious stimulus below the level of the injury.
Test-Taking Strategy: Use the process of elimination. Begin to answer this question by eliminating options 1 and 2. The client in spinal shock would be hypotensive (not hypertensive), and the client's clinical picture does not match pulmonary embolism. (It may also be useful to know that autonomic dysreflexia does not occur until spinal shock resolves.) Eliminate option 4 because malignant hyperthermia occurs with anesthesia. Review the signs of autonomic dysreflexia if you had difficulty with this question.
Level of Cognitive Ability: Analysis

Client Needs: Physiological Integrity
Integrated Process: Nursing Process/Data Collection
Content Area: Adult Health/Neurological
Reference: Linton, A., & Maebius, N. (2007). *Introduction to medical-surgical nursing* (4th ed., p. 502). Philadelphia: Saunders.

763. **2**
Rationale: Myasthenic crisis is often caused by undermedication and responds to administration of cholinergic medications such as neostigmine (Prostigmin) and pyridostigmine (Mestinon). Cholinergic crisis (the opposite problem) is caused by excess medication and responds to withholding of medications. Too little exercise and fatty food intake are incorrect options. Overexertion and overeating could trigger myasthenic crisis.
Test-Taking Strategy: Focus on the client's diagnosis and recall that myasthenic crisis is treated with medication. Remember, undermedication is a cause of myasthenic crisis. Review the causes of this type of crisis if you are unfamiliar with them.
Level of Cognitive Ability: Analysis
Client Needs: Physiological Integrity
Integrated Process: Nursing Process/Data Collection
Content Area: Adult Health/Neurological
Reference: deWit, S. (2009). *Medical-surgical nursing: Concepts & practice* (p. 607). St. Louis: Saunders.

764. **4**
Rationale: The client with Parkinson's disease tends to become withdrawn and depressed and therefore should become an active participant in his or her own care to prevent this. Activities should be planned throughout the day to inhibit daytime sleeping and boredom. The nurse gives the client encouragement and praises the client for perseverance. Activities such as exercise helps prevent progression of the disease, and self-care improves self-esteem.
Test-Taking Strategy: Use the process of elimination. Eliminate option 2 because of the close-ended word "only." Option 1 is well-intentioned but is not therapeutic in helping the client cope with the disease and therefore promotes dependence. From the remaining options, eliminate option 3 because it will promote fatigue. Review care of the client with Parkinson's disease if you had difficulty with this question.
Level of Cognitive Ability: Application
Client Needs: Psychosocial Integrity
Integrated Process: Nursing Process/Planning
Content Area: Adult Health/Neurological
Reference: Linton, A., & Maebius, N. (2007). *Introduction to medical-surgical nursing* (4th ed., p. 449). Philadelphia: Saunders.

765. **4**
Rationale: Facial pain can be minimized by using cotton pads to wash the face, using room temperature water. The client should chew on the unaffected side of the mouth, eat a soft diet, and take in foods and beverages at room temperature. If toothbrushing triggers pain, sometimes an oral rinse after meals is helpful instead.
Test-Taking Strategy: Note the strategic words "needs additional information." These words indicate a negative event query and the need to select the incorrect client statement.

Recalling that the pain of trigeminal neuralgia is triggered by mechanical or thermal stimuli will direct you to the correct option. Remember, very hot or cold foods are likely to trigger the pain, not relieve it. Review these client teaching points if you had difficulty with this question.
Level of Cognitive Ability: Comprehension
Client Needs: Physiological Integrity
Integrated Process: Teaching and Learning
Content Area: Adult Health/Neurological
References: Christensen, B., & Kockrow, E. (2006). *Adult health nursing* (5th ed., p. 734). St. Louis: Mosby.

766. **4**
Rationale: Cranial nerve II is the optic nerve, which governs vision. The nurse can provide safety for the visually impaired client by clearing the path of obstacles when ambulating. Testing the shower water temperature would be useful if there were impairment of peripheral nerves. Speaking loudly may help overcome a deficit of cranial nerve VIII (vestibulocochlear). Cranial nerves VII (facial) and IX (glossopharyngeal) control taste from the anterior two thirds and posterior one third of the tongue, respectively.
Test-Taking Strategy: Focus on the subject, impairment of cranial nerves. Recalling that cranial nerve II is the optic nerve will direct you to option 4. Review these cranial nerves if you had difficulty with this question.
Level of Cognitive Ability: Application
Client Needs: Safe and Effective Care Environment
Integrated Process: Nursing Process/Planning
Content Area: Adult Health/Neurological
References: Christensen, B., & Kockrow, E. (2006). *Adult health nursing* (5th ed., pp. 689-690). St. Louis: Mosby.
deWit, S. (2009). *Medical-surgical nursing: Concepts & practice* (p. 516). St. Louis: Saunders.

ALTERNATE ITEM FORMAT: PRIORITIZING (ORDERED RESPONSE)
767. **4, 1, 3, 2, 5, 6**

Rationale: Autonomic dysreflexia is characterized by severe hypertension, bradycardia, severe headache, nasal stuffiness, and flushing. The cause is a noxious stimulus, most often a distended bladder or constipation. Autonomic dysreflexia is a neurological emergency and must be treated promptly to prevent a hypertensive stroke. Immediate nursing actions are to sit the client up in bed in a high-Fowler's position and to remove the noxious stimulus. The nurse would loosen any tight clothing and then check for bladder distention. If the client has a Foley catheter, the nurse would check for kinks in the tubing. The nurse would also check for a fecal impaction and disimpact the client if necessary. The physician is contacted especially if these actions do not relieve the signs and symptoms. Antihypertensive medication may be prescribed by the physician to minimize cerebral hypertension. Finally, the nurse documents the occurrence, treatment, and client response.
Test-Taking Strategy: Recalling that this syndrome causes severe hypertension will assist you in determining that elevating the head of the bed is the first action. Next, recalling that the syndrome is caused by a noxious stimulus will assist you in determining that loosening tight clothing and checking for bladder distention would be the next actions. Because loosening any tight clothing would take less time than checking for bladder distention, this action would be taken next. Antihypertensives require a physician's order; therefore, calling the physician would be the next action. Review immediate nursing interventions for the client experiencing autonomic dysreflexia if you had difficulty with this question.
Level of Cognitive Ability: Application
Client Needs: Physiological Integrity
Integrated Process: Nursing Process/Implementation
Content Area: Adult Health/Neurological
References: Black, J., & Hawks, J. (2005). *Medical-surgical nursing: Clinical management for positive outcomes* (7th ed., pp. 2215, 2229). Philadelphia: Saunders.
Linton, A., & Maebius, N. (2007). *Introduction to medical-surgical nursing* (4th ed., p. 502). Philadelphia: Saunders.

REFERENCES

Black, J., & Hawks, J. (2005). *Medical-surgical nursing: Clinical management for positive outcomes* (7th ed.). Philadelphia: Saunders.

Chernecky, C., & Berger, B. (2008). *Laboratory tests and diagnostic procedures* (5th ed.). Philadelphia: Saunders.

Christensen, B., & Kockrow, E. (2006). *Adult health nursing* (5th ed.). St. Louis: Mosby.

deWit, S. (2009). *Medical-surgical nursing: Concepts & practice.* St. Louis: Saunders.

Ignatavicius, D., & Workman, M. (2006). *Medical-surgical nursing: Critical thinking for collaborative care* (5th ed.). Philadelphia: Saunders.

Lehne, R. (2007). *Pharmacology for nursing care* (6th ed.). Philadelphia: Saunders.

Lewis, S., Heitkemper, M., Dirksen, S., & Bucher, L. (2007). *Medical-surgical nursing: Assessment and management of clinical problems* (7th ed.). St. Louis: Mosby.

Linton, A., & Maebius, N. (2007). *Introduction to medical-surgical nursing* (4th ed.). Philadelphia: Saunders.

McKenry, L., Tessier, E., & Hogan, M. (2006). *Mosby's pharmacology in nursing* (22nd ed.). St. Louis: Mosby.

Monahan, F., Sands, J., Neighbors, M., Marek, J., & Green, C. (2007). *Phipps' medical-surgical nursing: Health and illness perspectives* (8th ed.). St. Louis: Mosby.

Pagana, K., & Pagana, T. (2005). *Mosby's diagnostic and laboratory test reference* (7th ed.). St. Louis: Mosby.

Perry, A., & Potter, P. (2006). *Clinical nursing skills & techniques* (6th ed.). St. Louis: Mosby.

Neurological Medications

I. ANTIMYASTHENIC MEDICATIONS

A. Description

1. Antimyasthenic, also called anticholinesterase, medications relieve muscle weakness associated with myasthenia gravis by blocking acetylcholine breakdown at the neuromuscular junction
2. Antimyasthenic medications are used to treat or diagnose myasthenia gravis or to distinguish cholinergic crisis from myasthenic crisis
3. Neostigmine bromide (Prostigmin), pyridostigmine (Mestinon), and ambenonium chloride (Mytelase) are used to control myasthenic symptoms
4. Edrophonium chloride (Tensilon) is used to diagnose myasthenia gravis and to distinguish cholinergic crisis from myasthenic crisis

B. Medications (Box 57-1)

C. Side effects: cholinergic crisis (Box 57-2)

D. Interventions

1. Assess neuromuscular status, including reflexes, muscle strength, and gait
2. Monitor the client for signs and symptoms of medication overdose (cholinergic crisis) and underdose (myasthenic crisis)
3. Instruct the client to take medications on time to maintain therapeutic blood level, thus preventing weakness because weakness can impair the client's ability to breathe and swallow
4. Instruct the client to take the medication with a small amount of food to prevent gastrointestinal symptoms
5. Instruct the client to eat 45 minutes to an hour after taking medications to decrease the risk for aspiration
6. Instruct the client to wear a Medic-Alert bracelet
7. Note that antimyasthenic therapy is lifelong therapy
8. Evaluate for medication effectiveness, which is based on the improvement of neuromuscular symptoms or strength without cholinergic signs and symptoms
9. When administering edrophonium chloride (Tensilon), have emergency resuscitation equipment on hand and atropine sulfate available for cholinergic crisis

E. Tensilon test

1. Edrophonium (Tensilon) is injected intravenously
2. The **Tensilon test** can cause bronchospasm, laryngospasm, hypotension, bradycardia, and cardiac arrest
3. Atropine sulfate is the antidote for overdose
4. Diagnosis of myasthenia gravis: Most myasthenic clients will show a significant improvement in muscle tone within 30 to 60 seconds after injection, and the muscle improvement lasts 4 to 5 minutes
5. The **Tensilon test** is used to diagnose cholinergic crisis (overdose with anticholinesterase) or myasthenic crisis (undermedication)
    a. In cholinergic crisis, muscle tone does not improve after the administration of Tensilon, and muscle twitching may be noted around the eyes and face
    b. A Tensilon injection makes the client in cholinergic crisis temporarily worse (negative **Tensilon test**)
    c. A Tensilon injection temporarily improves the condition when the client is in myasthenic crisis (positive **Tensilon test**)

II. ANTIPARKINSONIAN MEDICATIONS

A. Description

1. Antiparkinsonian medications restore the balance of the neurotransmitters acetylcholine and dopamine in the central nervous system (CNS), decreasing the signs and symptoms of Parkinson's disease to maximize the client's functional abilities
2. These medications include the dopaminergics, which stimulate the dopamine receptors, and the anticholinergics, which block the cholinergic receptors
3. Antiparkinsonian medications are used for drug-induced parkinsonism, in which neuroleptic agents block dopamine receptors in the CNS, leading to functional loss of dopamine activity

BOX 57-1 **Antimyasthenic Medications**

Ambenonium chloride (Mytelase)
Edrophonium chloride (Tensilon, Enlon, Reversol)
Neostigmine bromide (Prostigmin)
Pyridostigmine (Mestinon)

BOX 57-2 **Signs of Cholinergic Crisis**

Abdominal cramps
Nausea, vomiting, and diarrhea
Pupillary miosis
Hypotension and dizziness
Increased bronchial secretions
Increased tearing and salivation
Increased perspiration
Increased bronchial secretions
Bronchospasm, wheezing, and bradycardia

BOX 57-3 **Medications to Treat Parkinson's Disease**

Medications Affecting the Amount of Dopamine
Amantadine (Symmetrel)
Bromocriptine (Parlodel)
Carbidopa-levodopa (Sinemet)
Levodopa (Larodopa, Dopar)
Pergolide mesylate
Pramipexole (Mirapex)
Ropinirole (Requip)
Selegiline hydrochloride (Carbex, Eldepryl)
Anticholinergics
Benztropine mesylate (Cogentin)
Biperiden hydrochloride (Akineton)
Procyclidine hydrochloride (Kemadrin)
Trihexyphenidyl hydrochloride (Artane)
Cathechol *O*-methyltransferase (COMT) inhibitors
Entacapone (Comtan)
Tolcapone (Tasmar)

4. Antiparkinsonian medications are used for Parkinson's disease, in which dopamine-containing neurons in the basal ganglia are destroyed or deficient, which causes loss of fine motor control

B. Dopaminergic medications
1. Description
   a. Dopaminergic medications stimulate the dopamine receptors and increase the amount of dopamine available in the CNS or enhance neurotransmission of dopamine
   b. Dopaminergic medications are contraindicated in clients with cardiac, renal, or psychiatric disorders
   c. Levodopa taken with a monoamine oxidase inhibitor antidepressant can cause a hypertensive crisis
2. Medications (Box 57-3 and Figure 57-1)
3. Side effects
   a. Dyskinesia
   b. Involuntary body movements
   c. Chest pain
   d. Nausea and vomiting
   e. Urinary retention
   f. Constipation
   g. Sleep disturbances—either insomnia or periods of sedation
   h. Orthostatic hypotension and dizziness
   i. Confusion
   j. Mood changes, especially depression
   k. Hallucinations
   l. Dry mouth
4. Interventions
   a. Assess vital signs
   b. Assess for risk of injury
   c. Instruct the client to take the medication with food if nausea or vomiting occur

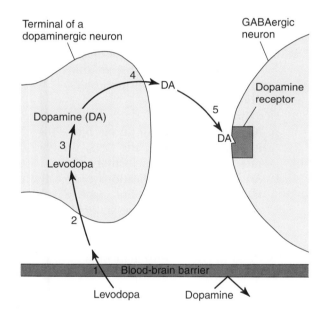

FIG. 57-1 Steps leading to alteration of central nervous system function by levodopa. To produce its beneficial effects in Parkinson's disease (PD), levodopa must be (1) transported across the blood-brain barrier; (2) taken up by dopaminergic nerve terminals in the striatum; (3) converted into dopamine (DA); (4) released into the synaptic space; and (5) bound to DA receptors on striatal GABAergic neurons, causing them to fire at a slower rate. Note that DA itself is unable to cross the blood-brain barrier, and hence cannot be used to treat PD. (From Lehne, R. [2007]. *Pharmacology for nursing care* [6th ed.]. Philadelphia: Saunders.)

   d. Assess for signs and symptoms of parkinsonism such as rigidity, tremors, akinesia, and bradykinesia; a stooped forward posture; shuffling gait; and masked facies.

e. Monitor for signs of dyskinesia

f. Instruct the client to report side effects and symptoms of dyskinesia

g. Monitor the client for improvement in signs and symptoms of parkinsonism without the development of severe side effects from the medications

h. Instruct the client to change positions slowly to minimize orthostatic hypotension

i. Instruct the client not to discontinue the medication abruptly

j. Instruct the client to avoid alcohol

k. Inform the client that urine or perspiration may be discolored and that this is harmless but may stain clothing

l. Advise the client with diabetes mellitus that glucose testing should not be done through urine testing because the results will not be reliable

m. Instruct the client taking carbidopa-levodopa (Sinemet) to eat low-protein foods because high-protein diets interfere with medication transport to the CNS

n. When administering levodopa, instruct the client to avoid excessive vitamin B_6 intake to prevent medication reactions

C. Anticholinergic medications

1. Description

a. Anticholinergic medications block the cholinergic receptors in the CNS, thereby suppressing acetylcholine activity

b. Anticholinergic medications reduce the tremors and drooling but have a minimal effect on the bradykinesia, rigidity, or balance abnormalities

c. Anticholinergic medications are contraindicated in clients with glaucoma

d. The client with chronic obstructive lung disease can develop dry, thick mucous secretions

2. Medications (see Box 57-3)

3. Side effects

a. Blurred vision

b. Dryness of the nose, mouth, throat, and respiratory secretions

c. Increased pulse rate, palpitations, and arrhythmias

d. Constipation

e. Urinary retention

f. Restlessness, confusion, depression, and hallucinations

g. Photophobia

4. Interventions

a. Monitor vital signs

b. Assess for risk of injury

c. Assess for signs and symptoms of parkinsonism such as rigidity, tremors, akinesia, and

bradykinesia; a stooped forward posture; shuffling gait; and masked facies

d. Monitor the client for improvement in signs and symptoms

e. Assess the client's bowel and urinary function, and monitor for urinary retention, constipation, and paralytic ileus

f. Monitor for involuntary movements

g. Encourage the client to avoid alcohol, smoking, caffeine, and aspirin to decrease gastric acidity

h. Instruct the client to consult with the physician before taking any nonprescription medications

i. Instruct the client to minimize dry mouth by increasing fluid intake and by using ice chips, hard candy, or gum

j. Instruct the client to prevent constipation by increasing fluids and fiber in the diet

k. Instruct the client to use sunglasses in direct sunlight because of possible photophobia

l. Instruct the client to have routine eye examinations to assess for intraocular pressure

III. ANTICONVULSANT MEDICATIONS

A. Description

1. Anticonvulsant medications are used to depress abnormal neuronal discharges and prevent the spread of seizures to adjacent neurons

2. Anticonvulsant medications should be used with caution in clients taking anticoagulants, aspirin, sulfonamides, cimetidine (Tagamet), and antipsychotic drugs

3. Absorption is decreased with the use of antacids, calcium preparations, and antineoplastic medications

B. Interventions for clients on anticonvulsants

1. Initiate seizure precautions

2. Monitor urinary output

3. Monitor liver and renal function tests and medication blood serum levels (Table 57-1)

4. Monitor for signs of medication toxicity, which would include CNS depression, ataxia, nausea, vomiting, drowsiness, dizziness, restlessness, and visual disturbances

TABLE 57-1	Anticonvulsant Medications
Medication	**Therapeutic Serum Range**
Amobarbital (Amytal)	1-5 mcg/mL
Carbamazepine (Tegretol)	3-14 mcg/mL
Clonazepam (Klonopin)	20-80 ng/mL
Ethosuximide (Zarontin)	40-100 mcg/mL
Ethotoin (Peganone)	10-50 mcg/mL
Lorazepam (Ativan)	50-240 ng/mL
Mephobarbital (Mebaral)	15-40 mcg/mL
Phenobarbital (Luminal)	15-40 mcg/mL
Phenytoin (Dilantin)	10-20 mcg/mL

5. If a seizure occurs, assess seizure activity, including location and duration
6. Protect the client from hazards in the environment during a seizure

C. Client education (Box 57-4)

D. Hydantoins (Box 57-5)
1. Hydantoins are used to treat partial and generalized tonic-clonic seizures
2. Phenytoin (Dilantin) is also used to treat dysrhythmias
3. Phenytoin decreases the effectiveness of some birth control pills and can have teratogenic effects if taken during pregnancy
4. Side effects
    a. Gingival hyperplasia (reddened gums that bleed easily)
    b. Slurred speech
    c. Confusion
    d. Sedation and drowsiness
    e. Nausea and vomiting
    f. Blurred vision and nystagmus
    g. Headaches
    h. Blood dyscrasias: decreased platelet count and decreased white blood cell count
    i. Elevated blood glucose

BOX 57-4 **Client Education: Anticonvulsants**

Take the prescribed medication in the prescribed dose and frequency.
Take anticonvulsants with food to decrease gastrointestinal irritation, but avoid milk and antacids, which impair absorption.
If taking liquid medication, shake well before ingesting.
Do not discontinue the medications.
Avoid alcohol.
Avoid over-the-counter medications.
Wear a Medic-Alert bracelet.
Use caution when driving or performing activities that require alertness.
Maintain good oral hygiene and use a soft toothbrush.
Maintain preventive dental checkups.
Maintain follow-up health care visits with periodic blood studies related to determining toxicity.
Monitor serum glucose levels (diabetes mellitus).
Urine may be a harmless pink-red or red-brown in color.
Report symptoms of sore throat, bruising, and nosebleeds, which may indicate a blood dyscrasia.
Inform the physician if adverse reactions occur, such as gingivitis, nystagmus, slurred speech, rash, or dizziness.

BOX 57-5 **Hydantoins**

Ethotoin (Peganone)
Fosphenytoin (Cerebyx)
Phenytoin (Dilantin)

---

j. Alopecia or hirsutism
k. Rash or pruritus
5. Interventions
    a. Oral tube feedings may interfere with the absorption of orally administered phenytoin and diminish the effectiveness of the medication; therefore, feedings should be scheduled as far as possible from the phenytoin administration
    b. Monitor therapeutic serum levels to assess for toxicity
    c. Monitor for signs of toxicity
    d. When administering phenytoin intravenously, dilute in normal saline because dextrose causes the medication to precipitate
    e. IV phenytoin is administered slowly (no faster than 25 to 50 mg/minute), otherwise hypotension and cardiac dysrhythmias can occur
    f. Assess for ataxia (staggering gait)
    g. Instruct the client to consult with the physician before taking other medications to ensure compatibility with anticonvulsants

E. Barbiturates (Box 57-6)
1. Barbiturates are used for tonic-clonic seizures and acute episodes of seizures caused by status epilepticus
2. Barbiturates may also be used as adjuncts to anesthesia
3. Side effects
    a. Sedation, ataxia, and dizziness, during initial treatment
    b. Mood changes
    c. Hypotension
    d. Respiratory depression
    e. Tolerance to the medication

F. Benzodiazepines (Box 57-7)
1. Benzodiazepines are used to treat absence seizures
2. Diazepam (Valium) is used to treat status epilepticus, anxiety, and skeletal muscle spasms
3. Clorazepate (Tranxene) is used as adjunctive therapy for partial seizures

---

BOX 57-6 **Barbiturates**

Amobarbital (Amytal)
Mephobarbital (Mebaral)
Phenobarbital (Luminal)

BOX 57-7 **Benzodiazepines**

Clonazepam (Klonopin)
Clorazepate (Tranxene)
Diazepam (Valium)
Lorazepam (Ativan)

4. Side effects
  a. Sedation, drowsiness, dizziness, and blurred vision
  b. Bradycardia if administered rapidly by the IV route
  c. Medication tolerance and drug dependency
  d. Blood dyscrasias: decreased platelet count and decreased white blood cell count
  e. Hepatotoxicity
G. Succinimides (Box 57-8)
  1. Succinimides are used to treat absence seizures
  2. Side effects
    a. Anorexia, nausea, and vomiting
    b. Blood dyscrasias
H. Oxazolidinediones (Box 57-9)
  1. Oxazolidinediones are used for absence seizures
  2. Side effects
    a. Sedation, drowsiness, and fatigue
    b. Headache
    c. Photophobia
    d. Blood dyscrasias
I. Valproates (Box 57-10)
  1. Valproates are used to treat tonic-clonic, partial, myoclonic, and psychomotor seizures
  2. Side effects
    a. Transient nausea, vomiting, and indigestion
    b. Sedation, drowsiness, and dizziness
    c. Pancreatitis
    d. Blood dyscrasias: decreased platelet count and decreased white blood cell count
    e. Hepatotoxicity
J. Iminostilbenes
  1. Iminostilbenes are used to treat seizure disorders that have not responded to other anticonvulsants (Box 57-11)
  2. Iminostilbenes are used to treat trigeminal neuralgia
  3. Side effects
    a. Drowsiness
    b. Dizziness

c. Nausea and vomiting
d. Constipation or diarrhea
e. Rash
f. Visual abnormalities
g. Dry mouth
h. Headache

IV. CENTRAL NERVOUS SYSTEM STIMULANTS
A. Description
  1. Amphetamines and caffeine stimulate the cerebral cortex of the brain (Box 57-12)
  2. Amphetamines have high potential for abuse
  3. Analeptics and caffeine act on the brainstem and medulla to stimulate respiration
  4. Anorexiants act on the cerebral cortex and hypothalamus to suppress appetite (Box 57-13)
  5. CNS stimulants are used to treat narcolepsy and attention deficit hyperactivity disorders
  6. CNS stimulants are used as adjunctive therapy for exogenous obesity
  7. Other CNS stimulants (Box 57-14)
B. Side effects
  1. Irritability
  2. Restlessness
  3. Tremors
  4. Insomnia
  5. Heart palpitations
  6. Tachycardia and dysrhythmias
  7. Hypertension
  8. Dry mouth
  9. Anorexia and weight loss
  10. Abdominal cramping
  11. Diarrhea or constipation
  12. Hepatic failure
  13. Psychoses
  14. Impotence
  15. Dependence and tolerance

BOX 57-8   Succinimides

Ethosuximide (Zarontin)
Methsuximide (Celontin)

BOX 57-9   Oxazolidinediones

Paramethadione (Paradione)
Trimethadione (Troxidone)

BOX 57-10   Valproates

Valproic acid (Depakene, Depacon)
Divalproex sodium (Depakote)

BOX 57-11   Other Anticonvulsants

Carbamazepine (Tegretol)
Gabapentin (Neurontin)
Lamotrigine (Lamictal)
Levetiracetam (Keppra)
Oxycarbazepine (Trileptal)
Pregabalin (Lyrica)
Tiagabine (Gabitril Filmtabs)
Topiramate (Topamax)
Zonisamide (Zonegran)
Vigabatrin (Sabril)

BOX 57-12   Amphetamines

Amphetamine Sulfate
Amphetamine/dextroamphetamine (Adderall)
Dextroamphetamine sulfate (Dexedrine)
Methylphenidate hydrochloride (Ritalin)

C. Interventions
1. Monitor vital signs
2. Assess mental status
3. Document the degree of inattention, impulsivity, hyperactivity, or periods of sleepiness
4. Assess height, weight, and growth of the child
5. Monitor complete blood count and white blood cell and platelet counts before and during therapy
6. Monitor for side effects
7. Monitor sleep patterns
8. Monitor for withdrawal symptoms such as nausea, vomiting, weakness, and headache
9. Instruct the client to take the medication before meals
10. Instruct the client to avoid foods and beverages containing caffeine to prevent additional stimulation
11. Instruct the client not to chew or crush long-acting forms of the medications
12. Instruct the client to read labels on over-the-counter products since many contain caffeine
13. Instruct the client to avoid alcohol
14. Instruct the client not to discontinue the medication abruptly
15. Instruct the client to take the last daily dose of the CNS stimulant at least 6 hours before bedtime to prevent insomnia
16. Monitor for drug dependence and abuse with amphetamines
17. If a child is taking a CNS stimulant, instruct the parents to notify the school nurse
18. Monitor for calming effects of CNS stimulants within 3 to 4 weeks on children with attention deficit hyperactivity disorder
19. Monitor growth in the child on long-term therapy with methylphenidate hydrochloride (Ritalin) or other medication to treat attention deficit hyperactivity disorder

---

BOX 57-13 Anorexiants

Benzphetamine hydrochloride (Didrex)
Diethylpropion hydrochloride (Tenuate)
Orlistat (Xenical)
Phendimetrazine (Bontril, Melfiat)
Phentermine hydrochloride (Adipex-P Ionamin)
Sibutramine (Meridia)

BOX 57-14 Other Central Nervous System Stimulants

Aminophylline
Caffeine
Doxapram (Dopram)
Theophylline

V. NON-OPIOID ANALGESICS (Box 57-15)
A. Nonsteroidal anti-inflammatory drugs (NSAIDs)
1. Description
a. NSAIDs are aspirin and aspirin-like medications that inhibit the synthesis of prostaglandins
b. The medications act as an analgesic to relieve pain, as an antipyretic to reduce body temperature, and as an anticoagulant to inhibit platelet aggregation
c. NSAIDs are used to relieve inflammation and pain and to treat rheumatoid arthritis, bursitis, tendinitis, osteoarthritis, and acute gout
d. NSAIDs are contraindicated in clients with hypersensitivity or liver or renal disease
e. Children with flu symptoms or a viral infection should not take aspirin because of the risk of Reye's syndrome
f. Clients taking anticoagulants should not take aspirin or NSAIDs
g. Aspirin and an NSAID should not be taken together because aspirin decreases the blood level and the effectiveness of the NSAID and can increase the risk of bleeding

---

BOX 57-15 Non-Opioid Analgesics

Acetominophen
Acetaminophen (Tylenol)
Aspirin
Aspirin (acetylsalicylic acid) (A.S.A., Aspergum, Bayer, Ecotrin)
Aspirin (acetylsalicylic acid), buffered (Alka-Seltzer, Bufferin)
Nonsteroidal Anti-inflammatory Drugs
Fenoprofen (Nalfon)
Flurbiprofen (Ansaid)
Ibuprofen (Motrin, Advil)
Ketoprofen (Orudis, Oruvail)
Naproxen (Advil, Anaprox, Naprosyn, Aleve, Naprelan)
Oxaprozin (Daypro)
Cyclo-oxygenase-2 Inhibitors (Cox-2 Inhibitors)
Celecoxib (Celebrex)
Other Nonsteroidal Anti-inflammatory Drugs
Diclofenac (Voltaren)
Diflunisal (Dolobid)
Etodolac (Lodine)
Indomethacin (Indocin)
Ketorolac
Meclofenamate
Mefenamic acid (Ponstan)
Moloxicam (Mobic)
Nabumetone (Relafen)
Piroxicam (Feldene)
Sulindac (Clinoril)
Tolmetin (Tolectin)

BOX 57-16	Side Effects of Aspirin and Nonsteroidal Anti-inflammatory Drugs

Aspirin
Allergic reactions (anaphylaxis, laryngeal edema)
Bleeding (anemia, hemolysis, increased bleeding time)
Dizziness
Drowsiness
Flushing
Gastrointestinal symptoms (distress, heartburn, nausea, vomiting)
Headaches
Decreased renal function
Tinnitus
Visual changes
Nonsteroidal Anti-inflammatory Drugs
Arrhythmias
Blood dyscrasias
Cardiovascular thrombotic events
Dizziness
Gastric irritation
Hepatotoxicity
Hypotension
Pruritus
Decreased renal function
Sodium and water retention
Tinnitus

h. NSAIDs can increase the effects of warfarin (Coumadin), sulfonamides, cephalosporins, and phenytoin (Dilantin)
i. Hypoglycemia can result if ibuprofen (Motrin) is taken with insulin or an oral hypoglycemic medication
j. A high risk of toxicity exists if ibuprofen is taken concurrently with calcium blockers
2. Side effects (Box 57-16)
3. Interventions
a. Assess client for allergies
b. Obtain a medication history on the client
c. Assess for history of gastric upset or bleeding or liver or renal disease
d. Assess the client for gastrointestinal upset during medication administration
e. Monitor for edema
f. Monitor serum salicylate (aspirin) level when the client is taking high doses
g. Monitor for signs of bleeding such as tarry stools, bleeding gums, petechiae, ecchymosis, and purpura
h. Instruct the client to take the medication with water, milk, or food
i. Enteric-coated form or buffered form of aspirin can be taken to decrease gastric distress
j. Instruct the client that enteric-coated tablets cannot be crushed or broken

k. Advise the client to inform other health care professionals if he or she is taking high doses of aspirin
l. Note that aspirin should be discontinued 3 to 7 days before surgery to reduce the risk of bleeding
m. Instruct the client to avoid alcoholic beverages
B. Acetaminophen (Tylenol)
1. Description
a. Acetaminophen inhibits prostaglandin synthesis
b. Acetaminophen is used to decrease pain and fever
c. Acetaminophen is contraindicated in hepatic or renal disease, alcoholism, and hypersensitivity
2. Side effects
a. Anorexia, nausea, and vomiting
b. Rash
c. Hypoglycemia
d. Oliguria
e. Hepatotoxicity
3. Interventions
a. Monitor vital signs
b. Assess the client for history of liver and renal dysfunction, alcoholism, and malnutrition
c. Monitor for hepatic damage, which includes nausea, vomiting, diarrhea, and abdominal pain
d. Monitor liver enzyme tests
e. Instruct the client that self-medication should not be used longer than 10 days for an adult and 5 days for a child
f. Note that the antidote for acetaminophen is acetylcysteine (Mucomyst)
g. Evaluate for the effectiveness of the medication
VI. OPIOID ANALGESICS
A. Description
1. Opioid analgesics suppress pain impulses but can suppress respiration and coughing by acting on the respiratory and cough center in the medulla of the brainstem
2. Opioid analgesics can produce euphoria and sedation and can cause physical dependence
3. Opioid analgesics are used for relief of mild, moderate, or severe pain
B. Medications (Box 57-17)
1. Codeine sulfate
a. Codeine sulfate is also an effective cough suppressant at low doses
b. Codeine sulfate can cause constipation
2. Hydromorphone hydrochloride (Dilaudid)
a. Hydromorphone can decrease respiration
b. Hydromorphone can cause constipation

BOX 57-17 Opioid Analgesics

Buprenorphine hydrochloride (Buprenex)
Butorphanol tartrate (Stadol)
Codeine sulfate, codeine phosphate
Fentanyl (Duragesic, Sublimaze)
Hydrocodone (Hycodan)
Hydromorphone hydrochloride (Dilaudid)
Levorphanol tartrate (Levo-Dromoran)
Meperidine hydrochloride (Demerol)
Methadone hydrochloride (Dolophine, Methadone)
Morphine sulfate (Duramorph, MS Contin, Kadian, Oramorph)
Nalbuphine hydrochloride (Nubain)
Oxycodone (Roxicodone, OxyContin)
Oxycodone hydrochloride with acetaminophen (Percocet)
Oxycodone with aspirin (Percodan)
Oxymorphone hydrochloride (Numorphan)
Pentazocine (Talwin)
Propoxyphene napsylate (Darvon-N)
Remifentanil (Ultiva)
Sufentanil (Sufenta)
Tramadol (Ultram)

3. Meperidine hydrochloride (Demerol)
   a. Meperidine can cause hypotension, dizziness, or urinary retention
   b. Meperidine is used for acute pain and as a preoperative medication
   c. Meperidine can increase intracranial pressure in head injuries
   d. Meperidine is contraindicated in clients with head injuries and **increased intracranial pressure,** respiratory disorders, hypotension, shock, and severe hepatic and renal disease, as well as in clients taking monoamine oxidase inhibitors
   e. Meperidine should not be taken with alcohol or sedative hypnotics because it may increase the CNS depression
4. Morphine sulfate
   a. Morphine can cause respiratory depression, orthostatic hypotension, and constipation
   b. Morphine may cause nausea and vomiting because of increased vestibular sensitivity
   c. Morphine is used for acute pain caused by myocardial infarction or cancer, for dyspnea caused by pulmonary edema, and for surgery; it can also be used as a preoperative medication
   d. Morphine is contraindicated in severe respiratory disorders, head injuries, **increased intracranial pressure,** severe renal, hepatic, or pulmonary disease, or seizure activity
   e. Morphine is used with caution in clients with shock or blood loss

5. Oxycodone with aspirin (Percodan)
   a. Percodan should not be taken by a client allergic to aspirin
   b. Percodan can cause gastric irritation and should be taken with food or plenty of liquids
6. Propoxyphene hydrochloride (Darvon) and propoxyphene napsylate (Darvon-N)
   a. Darvon compound contains aspirin and should not be taken by a client allergic to aspirin
   b. Darvocet-N contains acetaminophen
7. Nalbuphine hydrochloride (Nubain) is preferable for treating the pain of a myocardial infarction since it reduces the oxygen needs of the heart without reducing blood pressure
8. Methadone hydrochloride (Dolophine, Methadone)
   a. Dilute doses of oral concentrate with at least 90 mL of water
   b. Dilute dispersible tablets in at least 120 mL of water, orange juice, or acidic fruit beverage
   c. Methadone is used as a replacement medication for opiate dependence or to facilitate withdrawal
9. Hydrocodone (Hycodan) is frequently used for cough suppression
C. Interventions for opioid analgesics
   1. Monitor vital signs
   2. Assess the client thoroughly before administering pain medication
   3. Initiate nursing measures such as massage, distraction, deep breathing and relaxation exercises, the application of heat or cold as prescribed, and providing care and comfort before administering the opioid analgesic
   4. Administer medications 30 to 60 minutes before painful activities
   5. Monitor respiratory rate, and if the rate is less than 12 breaths/minute in an adult, withhold the medication unless ventilatory support is being provided
   6. Monitor pulse, and if bradycardia develops, hold the dose and notify the physician
   7. Monitor blood pressure for hypotension
   8. Auscultate breath sounds because opioid analgesics suppress the cough reflex
   9. Encourage activities such as turning, deep breathing, and incentive spirometry to prevent atelectasis and pneumonia
   10. Monitor level of consciousness
   11. Initiate safety precautions such as side rails, a night light, and supervised ambulation
   12. Monitor I&O
   13. Assess for urinary retention
   14. Instruct the client to take oral doses with milk or a snack to reduce gastric irritation

15. Instruct the client to avoid alcohol
16. Instruct the client to avoid activities that require alertness
17. Assess bowel function for constipation, abdominal distention, and decreased peristalsis
18. Evaluate the effectiveness of medication
19. Have the opioid antagonist, oxygen, and resuscitation equipment available

D. Morphine sulfate
  1. Side effects
     a. Respiratory depression
     b. Orthostatic hypotension
     c. Urinary retention
     d. Nausea and vomiting
     e. Constipation
     f. Sedation, confusion, and hallucinations
     g. Cough suppression
     h. Miosis
  2. Interventions
     a. Have naxolone available for overdose
     b. Assess vital signs and level of consciousness
     c. Compare rate and depth of respirations to baseline
     d. Withhold the medication if the respiratory rate is less than 12 breaths/minute; respirations of less than 10 breaths/minute can indicate respiratory distress
     e. Monitor urinary output, which should be at least 30 mL/hour
     f. Monitor bowel sounds for decreased peristalsis since constipation can occur
     g. Monitor for pupil changes since pinpoint pupils can indicate morphine overdose
     h. Avoid alcohol or CNS depressants since they can cause respiratory depression
     i. Instruct the client to report dizziness or difficulty breathing
     j. If taking sustained-release morphine, may need short-acting opioid doses for breakthrough pain
     k. Explain to client and family how and when to administer morphine and how to care for infusion equipment

E. Meperidine hydrochloride (Demerol)
  1. Side effects
     a. Respiratory depression
     b. Hypotension and dizziness
     c. Tachycardia
     d. Drowsiness and confusion
     e. Constipation
     f. Urinary retention
     g. Nausea and vomiting
     h. Seizures
     i. Tremors
  2. Interventions
     a. Monitor vital signs

BOX 57-18 **Opioid Antagonists**

Nalmefene (Revex)
Naloxone hydrochloride (Narcan)
Naltrexone (ReVia)

BOX 57-19 **Osmotic Diuretics**

Mannitol (Osmitrol)
Urea (Ureaphil)

---

     b. Monitor for respiratory depression and hypotension
     c. Have naloxone available for overdose
     d. Monitor for urinary retention
     e. Monitor bowel sounds and for constipation

VII. **OPIOID ANTAGONISTS** (Box 57-18)
A. Opioid antagonists are used to treat respiratory depression from opioid overdose
B. Interventions
  1. Monitor blood pressure, pulse, and respiratory rate every 5 minutes initially, tapering to every 15 minutes, and then every 30 minutes until the client is stable
  2. Place the client on a cardiac monitor and monitor cardiac rhythm
  3. Auscultate breath sounds
  4. Have resuscitation equipment available
  5. Do not leave the client unattended
  6. Monitor the client closely for several hours because when the effects of the antagonist wears off, the client may again display signs of opioid overdose

VIII. **OSMOTIC DIURETICS** (Box 57-19)
A. Description
  1. Osmotic diuretics increase osmotic pressure of the glomerular filtrate, inhibiting reabsorption of water and electrolytes
  2. Osmotic diuretics are used for oliguria and to prevent renal failure, to decrease intracranial pressure, and to decrease intraocular pressure in narrow-angle glaucoma
  3. Mannitol is used with chemotherapy to induce diuresis
B. Side effects
  1. Fluid and electrolyte imbalances
  2. Pulmonary edema from the rapid shifts of fluid
  3. Nausea and vomiting
  4. Headache
  5. Tachycardia from the rapid fluid loss
  6. Hyponatremia and dehydration
C. Interventions
  1. Monitor vital signs
  2. Monitor weight

3. Monitor urine output
4. Monitor electrolytes levels
5. Monitor lungs and heart sounds for signs of pulmonary edema
6. Monitor for signs of dehydration
7. Monitor neurological status
8. Monitor for increased intraocular pressure
9. Assess for signs of decreasing intracranial pressure if appropriate
10. Change the client's position slowly to prevent orthostatic hypotension
11. If crystallization in a vial of mannitol is noted, the medication is not used and is returned to the pharmacy

PRACTICE QUESTIONS

More questions on the companion CD!

768. A client with myasthenia gravis is suspected of having cholinergic crisis. Which of the following would indicate that this crisis exists?
    1. Ataxia
    2. Mouth sores
    3. Hypotension
    4. Hypertension

769. A client with myasthenia gravis is receiving pyridostigmine (Mestinon). The nurse monitors for signs and symptoms of cholinergic crisis caused by overdose of the medication. The nurse checks the medication supply to ensure that which medication is available for administration if a cholinergic crisis occurs?
    1. Vitamin K
    2. Atropine sulfate
    3. Protamine sulfate
    4. Acetylcysteine (Mucomyst)

770. A client with myasthenia gravis becomes increasingly weaker. The physician prepares to identify whether the client is reacting to an overdose of the medication (cholinergic crisis) or to increasing severity of the disease (myasthenic crisis). An injection of edrophonium (Tensilon) is administered. Which of the following would indicate that the client is in cholinergic crisis?
    1. No change in the condition
    2. Complaints of muscle spasms
    3. An improvement of the weakness
    4. A temporary worsening of the condition

771. Levodopa (Dopar) is prescribed for a client with Parkinson's disease, and the nurse monitors the client for adverse reactions to the medication. Which of the following would indicate that the client is experiencing an adverse reaction?
    1. Pruritus
    2. Tachycardia

    3. Hypertension
    4. Impaired voluntary movements

772. Phenytoin (Dilantin), 100 mg PO three times daily, has been prescribed for a client for seizure control. The nurse provides instructions regarding the medication to the client. Which statement by the client would indicate an understanding of the instructions?
    1. "I will use a soft toothbrush to brush my teeth."
    2. "It's all right to break the capsules to make it easier for me to swallow them."
    3. "If I forget to take my medication, I can wait until the next dose and eliminate that dose."
    4. "If my throat becomes sore, it's a normal effect of the medication and it's nothing to be concerned about."

773. A client is taking phenytoin (Dilantin) for seizure control and a sample for a serum drug level is drawn. Which of the following would indicate a therapeutic serum drug range?
    1. 5 to 10 mcg/mL
    2. 10 to 20 mcg/mL
    3. 20 to 30 mcg/mL
    4. 30 to 40 mcg/mL

774. Ibuprofen (Motrin) is prescribed for a client. The nurse tells the client to take the medication:
    1. With 8 oz of milk
    2. In the morning after arising
    3. 60 minutes before breakfast
    4. At bedtime on an empty stomach

775. A nurse is caring for a client who is taking phenytoin (Dilantin) for control of seizures. During data collection, the nurse notes that the client is taking birth control pills. Which of the following information should the nurse provide to the client?
    1. Pregnancy should be avoided while taking phenytoin (Dilantin).
    2. The client may stop taking the phenytoin (Dilantin) if it is causing severe gastrointestinal effects.
    3. The potential for decreased effectiveness of the birth control pills exists while taking phenytoin (Dilantin).
    4. The increased risk of thrombophlebitis exists while taking phenytoin (Dilantin) and birth control pills together.

776. A client with trigeminal neuralgia is being treated with carbamazepine (Tegretol). Which laboratory result would indicate that the client is experiencing an adverse reaction to the medication?
    1. Sodium level, 140 mEq/L
    2. Uric acid level, 5.0 mg/dL
    3. White blood cell count, 3000 cells/mm^3
    4. Blood urea nitrogen (BUN) level, 15 mg/dL

777. A nurse is caring for a client receiving morphine sulfate subcutaneously for pain. Because morphine sulfate has been prescribed for this client, which nursing action would be included in the plan of care?
    1. Encourage fluid intake.
    2. Monitor the client's temperature.
    3. Maintain the client in a supine position.
    4. Encourage the client to cough and deep breath.

778. Meperidine hydrochloride (Demerol) is prescribed for the client with pain. Which of the following would the nurse monitor for as a side effect of this medication?
    1. Diarrhea
    2. Bradycardia
    3. Hypertension
    4. Urinary retention

779. A nurse is caring for a client with severe back pain, and codeine sulfate has been prescribed for the client. Which of the following would the nurse include in the plan of care while the client is taking this medication?
    1. Restrict fluid intake.
    2. Monitor bowel activity.
    3. Monitor for hypertension.
    4. Monitor peripheral pulses.

780. Carbamazepine (Tegretol) is prescribed for a client with a diagnosis of psychomotor seizures. The nurse reviews the client's health history, knowing that this medication is contraindicated if which of the following disorders is present?
    1. Headaches
    2. Liver disease
    3. Hypothyroidism
    4. Diabetes mellitus

781. A client with trigeminal neuralgia tells the nurse that acetaminophen (Tylenol) is taken on a frequent daily basis for relief of generalized discomfort. The nurse reviews the client's laboratory results and determines that which of the following indicates toxicity associated with the medication?
    1. Sodium of 140 mEq/L
    2. Prothrombin time of 12 seconds
    3. Platelet count of 400,000 cells/mm^3
    4. A direct bilirubin level of 2 mg/dL

ALTERNATE ITEM FORMAT: MULTIPLE RESPONSE

782. A client is receiving meperidine hydrochloride (Demerol) for pain. Select the side effects of this medication. Select all that apply.
    ☐ 1. Diarrhea
    ☐ 2. Tremors
    ☐ 3. Drowsiness
    ☐ 4. Hypotension
    ☐ 5. Urinary frequency
    ☐ 6. Increased respiratory rate

ANSWERS

768. 4
Rationale: Cholinergic crisis occurs as a result of an overdose of medication. Indications of cholinergic crisis include gastrointestinal disturbances, nausea, vomiting, diarrhea, abdominal cramps, increased salivation and tearing, miosis, hypertension, sweating, and increased bronchial secretions.
Test-Taking Strategy: Use the process of elimination. Note that options 3 and 4 identify opposite effects. This indicates that one of them may be the correct option. Remember, hypertension occurs with cholinergic crisis. Review both cholinergic and myasthenic crisis if you had difficulty with this question.
Level of Cognitive Ability: Analysis
Client Needs: Physiological Integrity
Integrated Process: Nursing Process/Data Collection
Content Area: Pharmacology
Reference: Kee, J., Hayes, E., & McCuistion, L. (2006). *Pharmacology: A nursing process approach* (5th ed., pp. 365-366). Philadelphia: Saunders.

769. 2
Rationale: The antidote for cholinergic crisis is atropine sulfate. Vitamin K is the antidote for warfarin (Coumadin). Protamine sulfate is the antidote for heparin, and acetylcysteine (Mucomyst) is the antidote for acetaminophen (Tylenol).
Test-Taking Strategy: Knowledge regarding antidotes for various medications is needed to answer this question. Remember that atropine sulfate is the antidote for cholinergic crisis. Review antidotes if you had difficulty with this question.

Level of Cognitive Ability: Application
Client Needs: Physiological Integrity
Integrated Process: Nursing Process/Implementation
Content Area: Pharmacology
Reference: Kee, J., Hayes, E., & McCuistion, L. (2006). *Pharmacology: A nursing process approach* (5th ed., p. 366). Philadelphia: Saunders.

770. 4
Rationale: An edrophonium (Tensilon) injection makes the client in cholinergic crisis temporarily worse. This is known as a negative Tensilon test. An improvement of weakness would occur if the client were experiencing myasthenia gravis. Options 1 and 2 would not occur in either crisis.
Test-Taking Strategy: Focus on the data in the question. Noting the words "overdose of the medication (cholinergic crisis)" will direct you to option 4. It makes sense that administering additional medication will worsen the condition. Review this diagnostic test and the differences between cholinergic and myasthenic crisis if you had difficulty with this question.
Level of Cognitive Ability: Analysis
Client Needs: Physiological Integrity
Integrated Process: Nursing Process/Evaluation
Content Area: Pharmacology
References: Chernecky, C., & Berger, B. (2008). *Laboratory tests and diagnostic procedures* (5th ed., pp. 1053-1056). Philadelphia: Saunders.

Kee, J., Hayes, E., & McCuistion, L. (2006). *Pharmacology: A nursing process approach* (5th ed., p. 366). Philadelphia: Saunders.

771. 4

Rationale: Dyskinesia and impaired voluntary movement may occur with high levodopa dosages. Nausea, anorexia, dizziness, orthostatic hypotension, bradycardia, and akinesia (the temporary muscle weakness that lasts 1 minute to 1 hour, also known as the "on-off phenomenon") are frequent side effects of the medication.

Test-Taking Strategy: Use the process of elimination. Options 2 and 3 are cardiac-related options, so these options can be eliminated first. Note that the question asks for an adverse reaction; therefore, select option 4 over option 1 as the correct answer. Review the adverse effects of carbidopa and levodopa if you had difficulty with this question.

Level of Cognitive Ability: Analysis
Client Needs: Physiological Integrity
Integrated Process: Nursing Process/Data Collection
Content Area: Pharmacology
Reference: Skidmore-Roth, L. (2008). *2008 Mosby's nursing drug reference* (21st ed., pp. 607-608). St. Louis: Mosby.

772. 1

Rationale: Phenytoin (Dilantin) is an anticonvulsant. Gingival hyperplasia, bleeding, swelling, and tenderness of the gums can occur with the use of this medication. The client needs to be taught good oral hygiene, gum massage, and the need for regular dentist visits. The client should not skip medication doses, because this could precipitate a seizure. Capsules should not be chewed or broken and they must be swallowed. The client needs to be instructed to report a sore throat, fever, glandular swelling, or any skin reaction, because this indicates hematological toxicity.

Test-Taking Strategy: Use the process of elimination. Note the strategic words "an understanding of the instructions." Eliminate option 3 because the client needs to be encouraged to take medications on time. Also, eliminate option 4 because the client needs to report these symptoms to the physician. From the remaining options, recalling that capsules should not be broken will direct you to option 1. Review the side effects related to phenytoin (Dilantin) if you had difficulty with this question.

Level of Cognitive Ability: Analysis
Client Needs: Physiological Integrity
Integrated Process: Nursing Process/Evaluation
Content Area: Pharmacology
Reference: Skidmore-Roth, L. (2008). *2008 Mosby's nursing drug reference* (21st ed., p. 818). St. Louis: Mosby.

773. 2

Rationale: The therapeutic serum drug level range for phenytoin (Dilantin) is 10 to 20 mcg/mL. Therefore, options 1, 3, and 4 are incorrect.

Test-Taking Strategy: Knowledge regarding the therapeutic serum range of this medication is required to answer the question. A helpful hint may be to remember that the theophylline therapeutic range and the acetaminophen (Tylenol) therapeutic range are the same as the phenytoin (Dilantin) therapeutic range. Remembering this may assist you when answering questions related to any of these three medications. Review this therapeutic level if you had difficulty with this question.

Level of Cognitive Ability: Comprehension
Client Needs: Physiological Integrity
Integrated Process: Nursing Process/Data Collection
Content Area: Pharmacology
Reference: Pagana, K., & Pagana, T. (2005). *Mosby's diagnostic and laboratory test reference* (7th ed., pp. 894-895). St. Louis: Mosby.

774. 1

Rationale: Ibuprofen (Motrin) is a nonsteroidal anti-inflammatory drug (NSAID). NSAIDs should be given with milk or food to prevent gastrointestinal irritation. Options 2, 3, and 4 are incorrect.

Test-Taking Strategy: Use the process of elimination. Note that options 2, 3, and 4 are comparable or alike. Each of these options indicates administering the medication without food. Remember, NSAIDs can cause gastric irritation. Review this medication if you had difficulty with this question.

Level of Cognitive Ability: Application
Client Needs: Physiological Integrity
Integrated Process: Teaching and Learning
Content Area: Pharmacology
Reference: Lilley, L., Harrington, S., & Snyder, J. (2007). *Pharmacology and the nursing process* (5th ed., p. 689). St. Louis: Mosby.

775. 3

Rationale: Phenytoin (Dilantin) enhances the rate of estrogen metabolism, which can decrease the effectiveness of some birth control pills. Options 1, 2, are 4 are not accurate.

Test-Taking Strategy: Use the process of elimination. Option 4 would cause anxiety in the client. A client should not be instructed to stop anticonvulsant medication. Pregnancy does not need to be "avoided." Review medication interactions related to phenytoin (Dilantin) if you had difficulty with this question.

Level of Cognitive Ability: Application
Client Needs: Health Promotion and Maintenance
Integrated Process: Nursing Process/Implementation
Content Area: Pharmacology
Reference: Lehne, R. (2007). *Pharmacology for nursing care* (6th ed., pp. 222, 234). Philadelphia: Saunders.

776. 3

Rationale: Adverse effects of carbamazepine (Tegretol) appear as blood dyscrasias, including aplastic anemia, agranulocytosis, thrombocytopenia, leukopenia, cardiovascular disturbances, thrombophlebitis, dysrhythmias, and dermatological effects. Options 1, 2, and 4 identify normal laboratory values.

Test-Taking Strategy: Use the process of elimination. If you are familiar with normal laboratory values, you will note that the only option that indicates an abnormal value is option 3. Review the signs of adverse reactions related to this medication if you had difficulty with this question.

Level of Cognitive Ability: Comprehension
Client Needs: Physiological Integrity
Integrated Process: Nursing Process/Data Collection
Content Area: Pharmacology

Reference: Lehne, R. (2007). *Pharmacology for nursing care* (6th ed., p. 223). Philadelphia: Saunders.

777. 4
Rationale: Morphine sulfate suppresses the cough reflex. Clients need to be encouraged to cough and deep breathe to prevent pneumonia. Options 1, 2, and 3 are not specifically associated with this medication.
Test-Taking Strategy: Use the process of elimination. Recalling that morphine sulfate suppresses the cough reflex and the respiratory reflex will direct you to the correct option. In addition, use the ABCs—airway, breathing, and circulation—to direct you to option 4. Review this medication if you had difficulty with this question.
Level of Cognitive Ability: Application
Client Needs: Physiological Integrity
Integrated Process: Nursing Process/Planning
Content Area: Pharmacology
Reference: McKenry, L., Tessier, E., & Hogan, M. (2006). *Mosby's pharmacology in nursing* (22nd ed., p. 261). St. Louis: Mosby.

778. 4
Rationale: Side effects of this medication include respiratory depression, orthostatic hypotension, tachycardia, drowsiness and mental clouding, constipation, and urinary retention.
Test-Taking Strategy: Knowledge regarding side effects associated with opioid analgesics will assist you in answering the question. Remember, a side effect of meperidine is urinary retention. If you had difficulty with this question, review this medication.
Level of Cognitive Ability: Analysis
Client Needs: Physiological Integrity
Integrated Process: Nursing Process/Data Collection
Content Area: Pharmacology
Reference: Skidmore-Roth, L. (2008). *2008 Mosby's nursing drug reference* (21st ed., p. 650). St. Louis: Mosby.

779. 2
Rationale: While the client is taking codeine sulfate, the nurse would monitor vital signs and monitor for hypotension. The nurse should also increase fluid intake, palpate the bladder for urinary retention, auscultate bowel sounds, and monitor the pattern of daily bowel activity and stool consistency. The nurse should monitor respiratory status and initiate breathing and coughing exercises. In addition, the nurse monitors the effectiveness of the pain medication.
Test-Taking Strategy: Use the process of elimination. Recalling that codeine sulfate can cause constipation will direct you to option 2. If you had difficulty with this question, review nursing measures related to the administration of codeine sulfate.
Level of Cognitive Ability: Application
Client Needs: Physiological Integrity
Integrated Process: Nursing Process/Planning
Content Area: Pharmacology
Reference: Skidmore-Roth, L. (2008). *2008 Mosby's nursing drug reference* (21st ed., p. 299). St. Louis: Mosby.

780. 2
Rationale: Carbamazepine (Tegretol) is contraindicated in liver disease, and liver function tests are routinely prescribed for baseline purposes and are monitored during therapy. It is also contraindicated if the client has a history of blood dyscrasias. It is not contraindicated in the conditions noted in options 1, 3, and 4.
Test-Taking Strategy: Knowledge regarding the contraindications associated with carbamazepine (Tegretol) is required to answer this question. Remember, carbamazepine (Tegretol) is contraindicated in liver disease. Review this medication if you are unfamiliar with it.
Level of Cognitive Ability: Analysis
Client Needs: Physiological Integrity
Integrated Process: Nursing Process/Data Collection
Content Area: Pharmacology
Reference: Lehne, R. (2007). *Pharmacology for nursing care* (6th ed., p. 234). Philadelphia: Saunders.

781. 4
Rationale: In adults, overdose of acetaminophen (Tylenol) causes liver damage. Option 4 is an indicator of liver function and is the only option that indicates an abnormal laboratory value. The normal direct bilirubin is 0 to 0.4 mg/dL. The normal platelet count is 150,000 to 400,000 cells/mm^3. The normal prothrombin time is 10 to 13 seconds. The normal sodium level is 135 to 145 mEq/L.
Test-Taking Strategy: Knowledge that acetaminophen (Tylenol) causes liver damage and knowledge of the normal laboratory results will be helpful in answering this question. Reviewing the laboratory values in the options will direct you to option 4, the only abnormal value. Also, of all the options, the bilirubin is the laboratory value most directly related to liver function. Review the indicators of toxicity if you had difficulty with this question.
Level of Cognitive Ability: Analysis
Client Needs: Physiological Integrity
Integrated Process: Nursing Process/Data Collection
Content Area: Pharmacology
Reference: Skidmore-Roth, L. (2008). *2008 Mosby's nursing drug reference* (21st ed., p. 77). St. Louis: Mosby.

ALTERNATE ITEM FORMAT: MULTIPLE RESPONSE
782. 2, 3, 4
Rationale: Meperidine hydrochloride is an opioid analgesic. Side effects include respiratory depression, drowsiness, hypotension, constipation, urinary retention, nausea, vomiting, and tremors.
Test-Taking Strategy: Focus on the name of the medication. Recalling that this medication is an opioid analgesic and recalling the effects of an opioid analgesic will assist in identifying the side effects. Review the side effects of this medication if you had difficulty with this question.
Level of Cognitive Ability: Analysis
Client Needs: Physiological Integrity
Integrated Process: Nursing Process/Data Collection
Content Area: Pharmacology
References: Lehne, R. (2007). *Pharmacology for nursing care* (6th ed., p. 279). Philadelphia: Saunders.
Skidmore-Roth, L. (2005). *Mosby's 2005 drug consult for nurses* (p. 812). St. Louis: Mosby.

REFERENCES

Chernecky, C., & Berger, B. (2008). *Laboratory tests and diagnostic procedures* (5th ed.). Philadelphia: Saunders.

Gahart, B., & Nazareno, A. (2006). *Intravenous medications* (22nd ed.). St. Louis: Mosby.

Kee, J., Hayes, E., & McCuistion, L. (2006). *Pharmacology: A nursing process approach* (5th ed.). Philadelphia: Saunders.

Lehne, R. (2007). *Pharmacology for nursing care* (6th ed.). Philadelphia: Saunders.

Lilley, L., Harrington, S., & Snyder, J. (2007). *Pharmacology and the nursing process* (5th ed.). St. Louis: Mosby.

McKenry, L., Tessier, E., & Hogan, M. (2006). *Mosby's pharmacology in nursing* (22nd ed.). St. Louis: Mosby.

Pagana, K., & Pagana, T. (2005). *Mosby's diagnostic and laboratory test reference* (7th ed.). St. Louis: Mosby.

Skidmore-Roth, L. (2008). *2008 Mosby's nursing drug reference* (21st ed.). St. Louis: Mosby.

The Adult Client With a Musculoskeletal Disorder

PYRAMID TERMS

casts Stiff dressing or casting, made of plaster of Paris or synthetic material, to stabilize a part or parts of the body until healing occurs

compartment syndrome Condition in which pressure increases in a confined anatomical space that leads to decreased blood flow, ischemia, and dysfunction of these tissues; initial ischemia with pain, pallor, paresthesia, muscle weakness, and loss of pulses may progress to necrosis and permanent muscle cellular dysfunction

external fixation Stabilization of a fracture by the use of an external frame, with multiple pins applied through the bone

fat embolism Sudden dislodgement of that is freed into the circulation where it can lodge in a blood vessel and obstruct blood flow to tissue that is distal to the obstruction

internal fixation Stabilization of a fracture that involves the application of screws, plates, pins, or nails to hold the fragments in alignment

reduction Correction or realignment of a bone fracture or joint dislocation

traction Exertion of a pulling force to a fractured bone or dislocated joint to establish and maintain correct alignment for healing and to decrease muscle spasms and pain

▲ PYRAMID TO SUCCESS

The Pyramid to Success focuses on the emergency care for a client who sustains a fracture or other musculoskeletal injury, monitoring for complications related to fractures, and interventions if complications occur. Nursing care related to casts and traction is emphasized. Skill related to instructing the client on the use of an assistive device such as a cane, walker, or crutches is a pyramid point. Pyramid points also include postoperative care following hip surgery or amputation, as well as

care of the client with rheumatoid arthritis or osteoporosis. Focus on the points related to the psychosocial effects as a result of the musculoskeletal disorder, such as unexpected body-image changes, and the appropriate and available support services needed for the client. The Integrated Processes addressed in this unit include Caring, Clinical Problem-Solving Process (Nursing Process), Communication and Documentation, and Teaching and Learning.

CLIENT NEEDS

Safe and Effective Care Environment

Establishing priorities
Handling hazardous and infectious materials safely
Maintaining asepsis related to wounds
Maintaining confidentiality regarding the disorder and plan of care
Maintaining standard and other precautions
Preventing accidents and injuries
Providing a dietary consultation
Providing informed consent for diagnostic treatments and surgical procedures
Providing physical therapy and occupational therapy referrals
Upholding client rights

Health Promotion and Maintenance

Discussing expected body-image changes
Performing physical assessment related to the musculoskeletal system
Promoting health related to diet and activity
Preventing diseases that occur as a result of the aging process
Providing home care instructions regarding care related to the musculoskeletal disorder
Reinforcing the importance of prescribed therapy

Psychosocial Integrity

Assessing available support systems and use of community resources

Assessing the client's ability to cope with feelings of isolation and loss of independence

Considering cultural, religious, and spiritual influences

Discussing grief and loss related to mobility limitations and restrictions

Discussing situational role changes as a result of the musculoskeletal disorder

Identifying unexpected body-image changes as a result of injury or disease

Identifying sensory and perceptual alterations

Mobilizing coping mechanisms

Physiological Integrity

Identifying complications of a fracture

Identifying complications related to procedures or injuries

Providing care related to casts and traction

Promoting normal elimination patterns

Promoting self-care measures

Providing emergency care for a fracture or other injury

Providing measures to promote comfort

Teaching about the use of assistive devices for mobility such as canes, walkers, and crutches

Teaching pharmacological therapy

REFERENCES

Black, J., & Hawks, J. (2005). *Medical-surgical nursing: Clinical management for positive outcomes* (7th ed.). Philadelphia: Saunders.

Chernecky, C., & Berger, B. (2008). *Laboratory tests and diagnostic procedures* (5th ed.). Philadelphia: Saunders.

Christensen, B., & Kockrow, E. (2006). *Adult health nursing* (5th ed.). St. Louis: Mosby.

Christensen, B., & Kockrow, E. (2006). *Foundations of nursing* (5th ed.). St. Louis: Mosby.

deWit, S. (2009). *Medical-surgical nursing: Concepts & practice.* Philadelphia: Saunders.

Hodgson, B., & Kizior, R. (2008). *Saunders nursing drug handbook 2008.* Philadelphia: Saunders.

Ignatavicius, D., & Workman, M. (2006). *Medical-surgical nursing: Critical thinking for collaborative care* (5th ed.). Philadelphia: Saunders.

Kee, J., Hayes, E., & McCuistion, L. (2006). *Pharmacology: A nursing process approach* (5th ed.). Philadelphia: Saunders.

Lehne, R. (2007). *Pharmacology for nursing care* (6th ed.). Philadelphia: Saunders.

Lewis, S., Heitkemper, M., Dirksen, S., & Bucher, L. (2007). *Medical-surgical nursing: Assessment and management of clinical problems* (7th ed.). St. Louis: Mosby.

Linton, A., & Maebius, N. (2007). *Introduction to medical-surgical nursing* (4th ed.). Philadelphia: Saunders.

McKenry, L., Tessier, E., & Hogan, M. (2006). *Mosby's pharmacology in nursing* (22nd ed.). St. Louis: Mosby.

Monahan, F., Sands, J., Neighbors, M., Marek, J., & Green, C. (2007). *Phipps' medical-surgical nursing: Health and illness perspectives* (8th ed.). St. Louis: Mosby.

National Council of State Boards of Nursing, *2008 Detailed Test Plan for the NCLEX-PN® Examination,* National Council of State Boards of Nursing. Chicago: Author.

National Council of State Boards of Nursing, Inc. Web site: http://www.ncsbn.org.

Perry, A., & Potter, P. (2006). *Clinical nursing skills & techniques* (6th ed.). St. Louis: Mosby.

Skidmore-Roth, L. (2008). *2008 Mosby's nursing drug reference* (21st ed.). St. Louis: Mosby.

Musculoskeletal System

I. ANATOMY AND PHYSIOLOGY

A. Skeleton
1. Axial portion
   a. Cranium
   b. Vertebrae
   c. Ribs
2. Appendicular portion
   a. Limbs
   b. Shoulders
   c. Hips

B. Types of bones (Box 58-1)
1. Spongy bone
   a. Spongy bone is located in the ends of long bones and the center of flat and irregular bones
   b. Spongy bone can withstand forces applied in many directions
2. Dense (compact) bone
   a. Dense bone covers spongy bone
   b. Forms a cylinder around a central marrow cavity
   c. Can withstand force predominantly in one direction
3. Characteristics of the bones
   a. Support and protect structures of the body
   b. Provide attachments for muscles, tendons, and ligaments
   c. Contain tissue in the central cavities, which aids in the formation of blood cells
   d. Assist in regulating calcium and phosphate concentrations
4. Bone growth
   a. The length of bone growth results from the ossification of the epiphyseal cartilage at the ends of bones, and bone growth stops between the ages of 18 and 25 years
   b. The width of bone growth results from the activity of osteoblasts and occurs throughout life but does slow down with aging
   c. As aging occurs, bone resorption accelerates, decreasing bone mass and predisposing the client to injury

C. Types of joints (Table 58-1)
1. Characteristics of the joints
   a. Allow the movement between bones
   b. Are formed where two bones join
   c. Surfaces are covered with cartilage
   d. Are enclosed in a capsule
   e. Contain a cavity filled with synovial fluid
   f. Ligaments hold the bone and joint in the correct position
   g. Articulation is the meeting point of two or more bones
2. Synovial fluid
   a. Is found in the joint capsule
   b. Is formed by the synovial membrane, which lines the joint capsule
   c. Lubricates the cartilage
   d. Provides a cushion against shocks

D. Muscles
1. Characteristics of muscles
   a. Are made up of bundles of muscle fibers
   b. Provide the force to move bones
   c. Assist in maintaining posture
   d. Assist with heat production
2. The process of contraction and relaxation
   a. Muscle contraction and relaxation require large amounts of adenosine triphosphate
   b. Contraction also requires calcium, which functions as a catalyst
   c. Acetylcholine released by the motor end plate of the motor neuron initiates an action potential
   d. Acetylcholine is then destroyed by acetylcholinesterase
   e. Calcium is required to contract muscle fibers and acts as a catalyst for the enzyme needed for the sliding-together action of actin and myosin
   f. Following contraction, adenosine triphosphate transports calcium out to allow actin and myosin to separate and to allow the muscle to relax

BOX 58-1	Types of Bones

Long
Short
Flat
Irregular

TABLE 58-1	Types of Joints

Type	Description
Amphiarthrosis	Cartilaginous joints
	Slightly movable joints
Condyloid	Freely movable joints
	Allow frictionless, painless movement
Diarthrosis	Synovial joints
	Ball-and-socket joints
Synarthrosis	Fibrous or fixed joints
	No movement associated with these joints

3. Skeletal muscles
   a. Skeletal muscles are attached to two bones and cross at least one joint
   b. The point of origin is the point of attachment on the bone closest to the trunk
   c. The point of insertion is the point of attachment on the bone farthest from the trunk
   d. Skeletal muscles act in groups
   e. Prime movers contract to produce movement
   f. Antagonists relax
   g. Synergists contract to stabilize body movement
   h. Nerves activate and control the muscles
E. Bone Healing
   1. Description: bone union or healing is the process that occurs after the integrity of a bone is interrupted
   2. Three stages
      a. The fracture causes soft tissue edema and bleeding because of the vascularity of the bone, and this blood solidifies into a hematoma over 48 to 72 hours
      b. After injury, the blood supply is interrupted, leading to ischemia and necrosis of the bone around the injury site
      c. Dead cells promote migration of osteoblasts and fibroblasts to the area, and healing starts with the formation of fibrocartilage
      d. Bone union begins as a callus forms with vascular and cellular proliferation surrounding the fracture site; this loose fibrous tissue or "callus" changes into bone over the next 3 to 6 months

BOX 58-2	Risk Factors Associated With Musculoskeletal Disorders

Autoimmune disorders
Calcium deficiency
Degenerative conditions
Falls
Hyperuricemia
Infection
Medications
Metabolic disorders
Neoplastic disorders
Obesity
Postmenopausal states
Trauma and injury

   e. Remodeling occurs as the excess bone tissue of the callus resorbs as time passes and weight-bearing activities are gradually increased; the time required for complete healing varies and is related to variables such as age, bone type, trauma severity, infection, and blood supply
II. RISK FACTORS ASSOCIATED WITH MUSCULOSKELETAL DISORDERS (Box 58-2)
III. DIAGNOSTIC TESTS
A. Radiographs (x-rays)
   1. Description: radiography is a commonly used procedure to diagnose disorders of the musculoskeletal system
   2. Interventions
      a. Handle injured areas carefully and support extremities above and below the joint
      b. Administer analgesics as prescribed before the procedure, particularly if the client is in pain
      c. Remove any radiopaque objects, such as jewelry
      d. Shield client's testes, ovaries, or pregnant abdomen (may be contraindicated in pregnancy)
      e. Instruct the client to lie still during a radiograph
      f. Inform the client that exposure to radiation is minimal and not dangerous
      g. Wear a lead apron if staying in the room with the client
B. Arthrocentesis
   1. Description: arthrocentesis is used to diagnose joint inflammation and infection
      a. Arthrocentesis involves aspirating synovial fluid, blood, or pus via a needle inserted into a joint cavity
      b. Medication, such as corticosteroids, may be instilled into the joint if necessary to alleviate inflammation

2. Interventions
   a. Obtain an informed consent
   b. Apply an elastic compression bandage post-procedure as prescribed
   c. Use ice to decrease pain and swelling
   d. Pain may worsen after aspirating fluid from the joint
   e. Pain can continue up to 2 days after administration of corticosteroids into a joint
   f. Instruct the client to rest the joint for 8 to 24 hours postprocedure
   g. Instruct the client to notify the physician if a fever or swelling of the joint occurs

C. Arthrography
   1. Description: arthrography is used in unexplained joint pain or inflammation
      a. Arthrography is a radiographic examination of the soft tissues of the joint structures and is used to diagnose trauma to the joint capsule or ligaments
      b. A local anesthetic is used for the procedure
      c. A contrast medium or air is injected into the joint cavity, and the joint is moved through range of motion as a series of x-ray films are taken
   2. Interventions
      a. Instruct the client to fast from food and fluids for 8 hours before the procedure as prescribed
      b. Assess the client for allergies to iodine or shellfish before the procedure
      c. Obtain an informed consent
      d. Inform the client of the need to remain as still as possible, except when asked to reposition
      e. Minimize the use of the joint for 12 hours after the procedure
      f. Instruct the client that the joint may be edematous and tender for 1 to 2 days after the procedure and may be treated with ice packs and analgesics as prescribed
      g. Instruct the client to notify the physician if edema and tenderness last longer than 2 days
      h. If knee arthrography was performed, an elastic compression wrap over the knee may be prescribed for 3 to 4 days and ice applied to decrease pain and swelling
      i. If air was used for injection, crepitus may be felt in the joint for up to 2 days

D. Arthroscopy
   1. Description: arthroscopy is used to diagnose acute and chronic disorders of the joint.
      a. Arthroscopy provides an endoscopic examination of various joints
      b. Articular cartilage abnormalities can be assessed, loose bodies can be removed, and the cartilage can be trimmed

c. A biopsy may be performed during the procedure
   2. Interventions
      a. Instruct the client to fast for 8 to 12 hours before the procedure
      b. Obtain an informed consent
      c. Administer pain medication as prescribed postprocedure
      d. Assess the neurovascular status of the affected extremity
      e. An elastic compression bandage should be worn for 2 to 4 days as prescribed post-procedure
      f. Instruct the client that walking without weight bearing is usually permitted after sensation returns but to limit activity for 1 to 4 days as prescribed post-procedure
      g. Instruct the client to elevate the extremity as often as possible for 2 days following the procedure and to place ice on the site to minimize swelling
      h. Reinforce instructions regarding the use of crutches, which may be used for 5 to 7 days postprocedure for walking
      i. Advise the client to notify the physician if fever or increased knee pain occurs or if edema continues for more than 3 days postprocedure

E. Bone mineral density measurements
   1. Dual energy x-ray absorptiometry
      a. Measures bone mass of the spine, other bones, and the total body
      b. Radiation exposure is minimal
      c. Used to diagnose metabolic bone disease and to monitor changes in bone density with treatment
      d. Inform the client that the procedure is painless
      e. All metallic objects are removed before test
   2. Quantitative ultrasound
      a. Quantitative ultrasound evaluates strength, density, and elasticity of various bones using ultrasound rather than radiation
      b. Inform the client that the procedure is painless

F. Bone scan
   1. Description: a bone scan is used to identify, evaluate, and stage bone cancer before and after treatment
      a. Radioisotope is injected intravenously and will collect in areas that indicate abnormal bone metabolism and some fractures, if they exist
      b. The isotope is excreted in the urine and feces within 48 hours and is not harmful to others

2. Interventions
   a. Hold fluids for 4 hours before the procedure
   b. Obtain an informed consent
   c. Remove all jewelry and metal objects
   d. Following the injection of the radioisotope, the client must drink 32 oz of water (if not contraindicated) to promote renal filtering of the excess isotope
   e. From 1 to 3 hours after the injection, have the client void to clear excess isotope from the bladder before the scanning procedure is completed
   f. Inform the client of the need to lie supine during the procedure and that the procedure is not painful
   g. No special precautions are required after the procedure because a minimal amount of radioactivity exists in the radioisotope
   h. Monitor the injection site for redness and swelling
   i. Encourage oral fluid intake after the procedure

G. Bone or muscle biopsy
   1. Description: biopsy may be performed during surgery or through aspiration or punch or needle biopsy
   2. Interventions
      a. Obtain an informed consent
      b. Monitor for bleeding, swelling, hematoma, or severe pain
      c. Elevate the site for 24 hours following the procedure to reduce edema
      d. Apply ice packs as prescribed following the procedure to prevent the development of a hematoma and to decrease site discomfort
      e. Monitor for signs of infection following the procedure
      f. Inform the client that mild to moderate discomfort is normal following the procedure

H. Electromyography (EMG)
   1. Description: An EMG is used to evaluate muscle weakness
      a. Electromyography measures electrical potential associated with skeletal muscle contractions
      b. Needles are inserted into the muscle, and recordings of muscular electrical activity are traced on recording paper through an oscilloscope
   2. Interventions
      a. Obtain an informed consent
      b. Instruct the client that the needle insertion is uncomfortable
      c. Instruct the client not to take any stimulants or sedatives for 24 hours before the procedure

   d. Inform the client that slight bruising may occur at the needle insertion sites
   e. Mild analgesics can be used for the pain

I. Myelography (refer to Chapter 56)

IV. INJURIES
A. Strains
   1. Strains are an excessive stretching of a muscle or tendon
   2. Management involves cold and heat applications, exercise with activity limitations, anti-inflammatory medications, and muscle relaxants
   3. Surgical repair may be required for a severe strain (ruptured muscle or tendon)

B. Sprains
   1. Sprains are an excessive stretching of a ligament, usually caused by a twisting motion, such as in a fall or step on an uneven surface
   2. Sprains are characterized by pain and swelling
   3. Management involves rest, ice, a compression bandage, and elevation in order to reduce swelling and provide joint support
   4. Casting may be required for moderate sprains to allow the tear to heal
   5. Surgery may be necessary for severe ligament damage

C. Rotator cuff injuries
   1. Musculotendinous or rotator cuff of the shoulder sustains a tear, usually as a result of trauma
   2. Injury is characterized by shoulder pain and the inability to maintain abduction of the arm at the shoulder (drop arm test)
   3. Management involves nonsteroidal anti-inflammatory drugs (NSAIDs), physical therapy, sling support, and ice/heat applications
   4. Surgery may be required if medical management is unsuccessful or for those who have a complete tear

V. FRACTURES
A. Description: a fracture is a break in the continuity of the bone caused by trauma, twisting as a result of muscle spasm or indirect loss of leverage, or bone decalcification and disease that result in osteopenia
B. Types of fractures (Box 58-3)
C. Data collection: fracture of an extremity
   1. Pain or tenderness over the involved area
   2. Decrease or loss of muscular strength or function
   3. Obvious deformity of affected area
   4. Crepitation, erythema, edema, or bruising
   5. Muscle spasm and neurovascular impairment
D. Initial care of a fracture of an extremity
   1. Immobilize affected extremity with cast or splint
   2. If a compound (open) fracture exists, splint the extremity and cover the wound with a sterile dressing

BOX 58-3 Types of Fractures

Closed or simple: Skin over the fractured area remains intact

Comminuted: The bone is splintered or crushed, with three or more fragments

Complete: The bone is separated completely by a break into two parts

Compression: A fractured bone is compressed by other bone

Depressed: Bone fragments are driven inward

Greenstick: One side of the bone is broken and the other is bent; these fractures occur most commonly in children

Impacted: A part of the fractured bone is driven into another bone

Incomplete: The bone is partially broken

Oblique: The break extends in an oblique direction

Open or compound: The bone is exposed to air through a break in the skin, and soft tissue injury and infection are common

Pathological: The fracture results from weakening of the bone structure by pathological processes such as neoplasia or osteomalacia; also called spontaneous fracture

Spiral: The break partially encircles bone

Transverse: The bone is fractured straight across

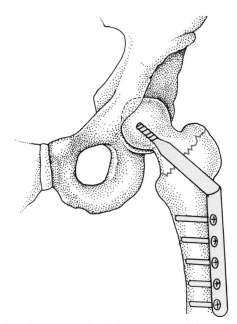

FIG. 58-1 A compression hip screw used for open reduction with internal fixation. (From Ignatavicius, D., & Workman, M. [2006]. *Medical-surgical nursing: Critical thinking for collaborative care* [5th ed.]. Philadelphia: Saunders.)

BOX 58-4 Interventions for a Fracture

Reduction
Fixation
Traction
Casts

3. Assess neurovascular status of the extremity
4. Interventions for a fracture (Box 58-4)
E. **Reduction** restores the bone to proper alignment
  1. Closed **reduction** is a nonsurgical intervention that is performed by manual manipulation
    a. Closed **reduction** may be performed under local or general anesthesia
    b. A cast may be applied following **reduction**
  2. Open **reduction** involves a surgical intervention
    a. Fracture may be treated with **internal fixation** devices
    b. The client may be placed in **traction** or a cast following the procedure
F. Fixation
  1. **Internal fixation** follows an open **reduction** (Figure 58-1)
    a. **Internal fixation** involves the application of screws, plates, pins, or intramedullary rods to hold the fragments in alignment
    b. **Internal fixation** may involve the removal of damaged bone and replacement with a prosthesis

    c. **Internal fixation** provides immediate bone strength
  2. **External fixation** is the use of an external frame to stabilize a fracture by attaching skeletal pins through bone fragments to a rigid external support
    a. **External fixation** provides more freedom of movement than with **traction**.
    b. Monitor pin stability and provide pin care to decrease infection risks
    c. Risk of infection exists with both fixation methods
    d. **External fixation** is commonly used when massive tissue trauma is present
G. **Traction** (Figure 58-2)
  1. Description
    a. **Traction** is the exertion of a pulling force applied in two directions to reduce and immobilize a fracture
    b. **Traction** provides proper bone alignment and reduces muscle spasms
  2. Interventions
    a. Maintain proper body alignment
    b. Ensure that the weights hang freely and do not touch the floor
    c. Do not remove or lift the weights without a physician's order
    d. Ensure that pulleys are not obstructed and that ropes in the pulleys move freely
    e. Place knots in the ropes to prevent slipping
    f. Check the ropes for fraying

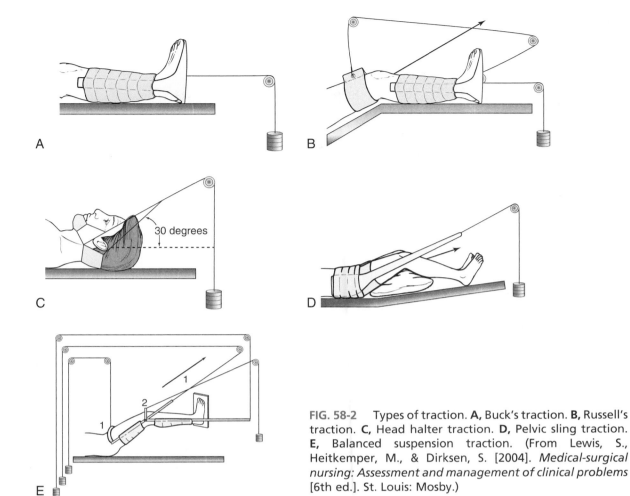

FIG. 58-2   Types of traction. **A,** Buck's traction. **B,** Russell's traction. **C,** Head halter traction. **D,** Pelvic sling traction. **E,** Balanced suspension traction. (From Lewis, S., Heitkemper, M., & Dirksen, S. [2004]. *Medical-surgical nursing: Assessment and management of clinical problems* [6th ed.]. St. Louis: Mosby.)

H. Skeletal **traction** (Figure 58-3)
   1. Description: **traction** is applied mechanically to the bone with pins, wires, or tongs
   2. Interventions
      a. Monitor color, motion, and sensation of the affected extremity
      b. Monitor the insertion sites for redness, swelling, drainage, or increased pain
      c. Provide insertion site care as prescribed
   3. Cervical tongs and a halo fixation device (refer to Chapter 56 regarding care of the client with these types of devices)
I. Skin **traction** (Box 58-5)
   1. Description: Skin **traction** is applied by using elastic bandages or adhesive
   2. Cervical skin **traction** relieves muscle spasms and compression in the upper extremities and neck (see Figure 58-2)
      a. Cervical skin **traction** uses a head halter and a chin pad to attach the **traction**
      b. Use powder to protect the ears from friction rub
      c. Position the client with the head of the bed elevated 30 to 40 degrees, and attach the weights to a pulley system over the head of the bed

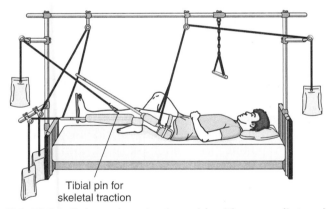

Tibial pin for skeletal traction

FIG. 58-3   Balanced suspension with a Thomas splint and Pearson attachment. The apparatus can be used alone or, as in this case, with skeletal traction. (From Monahan, F. Sands, J. Neighbors, M., Marek, J., & Green, C. [2007]. *Phipps' medical-surgical nursing: Concepts and clinical practice* [8th ed.]. St. Louis: Mosby.)

BOX 58-5   **Types of Skin Traction**

Buck's traction	Pelvic traction
Cervical traction	Russell's traction

3. Buck's (extension) skin **traction** is used to alleviate muscle spasms and immobilize a lower limb by maintaining a straight pull on the limb with the use of weights (see Figure 58-2)
   a. A boot appliance is applied to attach to the **traction**
   b. Weight is attached to a pulley; allow the weights to hang freely over the edge of bed
   c. Not more than 8 to 10 lb of weight should be applied
   d. Elevate the foot of the bed to provide the **traction**
4. Russell's skin **traction** (refer to Chapter 36 regarding information related to these types of **traction**)
5. Pelvic skin (sling) **traction** is used to relieve low back, hip, or leg pain or to reduce muscle spasm (see Figure 58-2).
   a. Apply the **traction** snugly over the pelvis and iliac crest and attach to the weights
   b. Use measures as prescribed to prevent the client from slipping down in bed
J. Balanced suspension **traction** (see Figure 58-2 and 58-3)
   1. Description
      a. Balanced suspension **traction** is used with skin or skeletal **traction**
      b. It is used to approximate fractures of the femur, tibia, or fibula
      c. Balanced suspension **traction** is produced by a counterforce other than client
   2. Interventions
      a. Position the client in a low Fowler's position on either the side or the back
      b. Maintain a 20-degree angle from the thigh to the bed
      c. Protect the skin from breakdown
      d. Provide pin care if pins are used with the skeletal **traction**
      e. Clean the pin sites with sterile normal saline and hydrogen peroxide or povidone-iodine (Betadine) as prescribed or per agency policy
K. Dunlop's **traction**
   1. Description: horizontal **traction** is used to align fractures of the humerus; vertical **traction** maintains the forearm in proper alignment
   2. Interventions: nursing care is similar to that for Buck's skin **traction**
L. **Casts**
   1. Description: plaster or fiberglass **casts** are used to immobilize bones and joints into correct alignment after a fracture or injury
   2. Interventions
      a. Keep the **cast** and extremity elevated
      b. Allow a wet **cast** 24 to 72 hours to dry (synthetic **casts** dry in 20 minutes)

c. Handle a wet **cast** with the palms of the hands until dry
d. Turn the extremity every 1 to 2 hours, unless contraindicated to allow air circulation and promote drying of the **cast**
e. Cool setting on a hair dryer can be used to dry a plaster **cast** (heat cannot be used on a plaster **cast** because the **cast** heats up and burns the skin)
f. Monitor the extremity for circulatory impairment such as pain, swelling, discoloration, tingling, numbness, coolness, or diminished pulse
g. Notify the physician immediately if circulatory compromise occurs
h. Prepare for bivalving or cutting the **cast** if circulatory impairment occurs
i. Petal the **cast**; maintain smooth edges around the **cast** to prevent crumbling of the **cast** material
j. Monitor for signs of infection such as temperature, hot spots on the **cast,** foul odor or changes in pain
k. If an open draining area exists on the affected extremity, the physician will make a cutout portion of the **cast** or a window
l. Instruct the client not to stick objects inside the **cast**
m. Teach the client to keep the **cast** clean and dry
n. Instruct the client on isometric exercises to prevent muscle atrophy

VI. COMPLICATIONS OF FRACTURES (Box 58-6)
A. **Fat embolism**
   1. Description: a **fat embolism** originates in the bone marrow and occurs after a fracture when a fat globule is released into the blood stream
      a. Clients with long bone fractures are at the greatest risk for the development of **fat embolism**
      b. **Fat embolism** can occur within the first 48 to 72 hours following the injury
   2. Data collection: findings often suggest pulmonary embolism
      a. Restlessness, hypoxemia, or mental status changes
      b. Tachycardia and hypotension
      c. Dyspnea and tachypnea
      d. Petechial rash over the upper chest and neck

BOX 58-6 Complications of Fractures

Fat embolism
Compartment syndrome
Infection and osteomyelitis
Avascular necrosis
Pulmonary embolism

3. Interventions
   a. Notify the physician immediately while initiating emergency care
   b. Treat symptoms as prescribed to prevent respiratory failure and death
   c. Corticosteroids may be given to reduce pulmonary injury
B. **Compartment syndrome**
   1. Description
      a. Tough fascia surrounds muscle groups forming compartments from which arteries, veins, and nerves enter and exit opposite ends
      b. **Compartment syndrome** occurs when pressure increases within one or more compartments, leading to decreased blood flow, tissue ischemia, and neurovascular impairment
      c. Within 4 to 6 hours after the onset of **compartment syndrome,** neurovascular damage is irreversible if not treated
   2. Data collection
      a. Unrelieved or increased pain in the limb
      b. Tissue that is distal to the involved area becomes pale, dusky, or edematous
      c. Pain with passive movement and joint dysfunction
      d. Pulselessness and loss of sensation (paresthesia)
   3. Interventions
      a. Notify the physician immediately and prepare to assist physician
      b. If severe, assist the physician with fasciotomy to relieve pressure and restore tissue perfusion
      c. Loosen tight dressings or bivalve restrictive **cast** as prescribed
C. Infection and osteomyelitis
   1. Description: infection and osteomyelitis (inflammatory response in bone tissue) can be caused by the introduction of organisms into bones initially leading to localized bone infection
   2. Data collection
      a. Tachycardia and fever (usually above 101° F)
      b. Erythema and pain in the area surrounding the infection
      c. Leukocytosis and elevated erythrocyte sedimentation rate (ESR)
   3. Interventions
      a. Physician notification
      b. Initiation of aggressive, long-term IV antibiotic therapy
      c. Hyperbaric oxygen therapy to promote client healing
      d. Surgery for resistant osteomyelitis with sequestrectomy and/or bone grafts

D. Avascular necrosis
   1. Description: occurs when a fracture interrupts the blood supply to a section of bone, leading to bone death
   2. Data collection
      a. Pain
      b. Decreased sensation
   3. Interventions
      a. Notify the physician if pain or numbness occurs
      b. Prepare the client for removal of necrotic tissue since it serves as a focus for infection
E. Pulmonary embolism
   1. Description: caused by the movement of foreign particles (blood clot, fat, or air) into the pulmonary circulation
   2. Data collection
      a. Restlessness and apprehension
      b. Sudden onset of dyspnea and chest pain
      c. Cough, hemoptysis, hypoxemia, or crackles
   3. Interventions
      a. Notify the physician if signs of emboli are present
      b. Administer oxygen and IV anticoagulant therapy if prescribed
VII. CRUTCH WALKING
A. Description
   1. An accurate measurement of the client for crutches is important because an incorrect measurement could damage the brachial plexus
   2. The distance between the axillae and the arm pieces on the crutches should be two to three fingerwidths in the axilla space
   3. The elbows should be slightly flexed, 20 to 30 degrees, when the client is walking
   4. When ambulating with the client, stand on the affected side
   5. Instruct the client never to rest the axilla on the axillary bars
   6. Instruct the client to look up and outward when ambulating and to place the crutches 6 to 10 inches diagonally in front of the foot
   7. Instruct the client to stop ambulation if numbness or tingling in the hands or arms occurs
B. Crutch gaits (Table 58-2)
C. Assisting the client with crutches to sit and stand
   1. Place the unaffected leg against the front of the chair
   2. Move the crutches to the affected side, and grasp the arm of the chair with the hand on the unaffected side
   3. Flex the knee of the unaffected leg to lower self into the chair while placing the affected leg straight out in front
   4. Reverse the steps to move from a sitting to a standing position

TABLE 58-2 **Crutch Gaits**

Type of Gait	Use	Procedure
Two-point gait	Used with partial weight-bearing limitations and with bilateral lower extremity prostheses	The crutch on one side and the opposite foot are advanced at the same time
Three-point gait	Used for partial weight bearing or no weight bearing on the affected leg; requires that the client have strength and balance	Both crutches and the foot of the affected extremity are advanced together, followed by the foot of the unaffected extremity
Four-point gait	Used if weight bearing is allowed and one foot can be placed in front of the other	The right crutch is advanced, then the left foot, then the left crutch, then the right foot
Swing-to gait	Used when there is adequate muscle power and balance in the arms and legs	Both crutches are advanced together, then both legs are lifted and placed down on a spot behind the crutches; the feet and crutches form a tripod
Swing-through gait	Used when there is adequate muscle power and balance in the arms and legs	Both crutches are advanced together, then both legs are lifted through and beyond the crutches and placed down again at a point in front of the crutches

Modified from Linton, A. & Maebius, N. (2003). *Introduction to medical-surgical nursing* (3rd ed.). Philadelphia: Saunders.

D. Going up and down stairs
 1. Up the stairs
  a. The client moves the unaffected leg up first
  b. The client moves the affected leg and the crutches up
 2. Down the stairs
  a. The client moves the crutches and the affected leg down
  b. The client moves the unaffected leg down

VIII. CANES AND WALKERS
A. Description: canes and walkers are made of a lightweight material with a rubber tip at the bottom
B. Interventions
 1. Stand at the affected side of the client when ambulating
 2. The handle should be at the level of the client's greater trochanter
 3. The client's elbow should be flexed at a 15- to 30-degree angle
 4. Instruct the client to hold the cane 4 to 6 inches to the side of the foot
 5. Instruct the client to hold the cane in the hand on the unaffected side so that the cane and weaker leg can work together with each step
 6. Instruct the client to move the cane at the same time as the affected leg
 7. Instruct the client to inspect the rubber tips regularly for worn places
C. Hemicanes or quadripod canes
 1. Hemicanes or quadripod canes are used for clients who have the use of only one upper extremity
 2. Hemicanes provide more security than a quadripod cane; however, both types provide more security than a single-tipped cane

3. Position the cane at the client's unaffected side, with the straight, nonangled side adjacent to the body
4. Position the cane 6 inches from client's side, with the handgrips level with the greater trochanter
D. Walker
 1. Stand adjacent to the client on the affected side
 2. Instruct the client to put all four points of the walker flat on the floor before putting weight on the handpieces
 3. Instruct the client to move the walker forward and to walk into it

IX. FRACTURED HIP
A. Types
 1. Intracapsular (femoral head is broken within the joint capsule)
  a. Femoral head and neck receives decreased blood supply and heals slowly
  b. Skin **traction** is applied preoperatively to reduce fracture and immobilize bone
  c. Treatment includes a total hip replacement or open **reduction internal fixation** (ORIF) with femoral head replacement.
  d. To prevent hip displacement postoperatively, avoid extreme hip flexion
 2. Extracapsular (fracture is outside the joint capsule)
  a. Fracture can occur at the greater trochanter or can be an intertrochanteric fracture
  b. Trochanteric fracture is outside the joint
  c. Preoperative treatment includes balanced suspension **traction** or skin **traction** to relieve muscle spasms and reduce pain
  d. Avoid extreme hip flexion to prevent joint displacement
  e. Surgical treatment includes ORIF with nail plate, screws, pins, or wires

B. Postoperative interventions
1. Maintain leg and hip in proper alignment and prevent internal or external rotation
2. Turn the client to the unaffected side; turn to affected side only if prescribed by physician.
3. Elevate the head of the bed 30 to 45 degrees for meals only
4. Assist the client to ambulate with weight bearing as prescribed by the physician
5. Avoid weight bearing on the affected leg as prescribed; instruct the client on the use of a walker to avoid weight bearing
6. Weight bearing is often restricted after an ORIF and unrestricted after total hip arthroplasty (THA) (always refer to physician's orders)
7. Keep the operative leg extended, supported, and elevated when getting client out of bed
8. Avoid hip flexion greater than 90 degrees and avoid low chairs when out of bed
9. Monitor for wound infection or hemorrhage
10. Perform neurovascular assessment of affected extremity: check color, pulses, capillary refill, movement, and sensation
11. Maintain the compression of the Hemovac or Jackson-Pratt drain to facilitate wound drainage
12. Monitor and record drainage amount, which decreases consistently about 80 mL every 8 hours until 48 hours postoperatively
13. Postoperative blood salvage may be done to collect, filter, and reinfuse salvaged blood into client
14. Use antiembolism stockings or sequential compression stockings and encourage the client to flex and extend the feet to reduce the risk of deep vein thrombosis (DVT)
15. Instruct the client to avoid crossing the legs and activities that require bending over
16. Physical therapy will be instituted postoperatively with progressive ambulation as prescribed by the physician

X. TOTAL KNEE REPLACEMENT
A. Description: total knee replacement is the implantation of a device to substitute for the femoral condyles and the tibial joint surfaces
B. Postoperative interventions
1. Monitor surgical incision for drainage and infection
2. Maintain the Hemovac or Jackson-Pratt drain if in place
3. Begin continuous passive motion 24 to 48 hours postoperatively as prescribed to exercise the knee and provide moderate flexion and extension
4. Administer analgesics before continuous passive motion to decrease pain
5. The leg should not be dangled to prevent dislocation

6. Prepare the client for out-of-bed activities as prescribed
7. Avoid weight bearing and instruct the client in crutch walking
8. Postoperative blood salvage may be done to collect, filter, and reinfuse salvaged blood into client may be prescribed

XI. JOINT DISLOCATION AND SUBLUXATION
A. Dislocation: injury of the ligaments surrounding a joint that leads to displacement or separation of the articular surfaces of the joint
B. Subluxation: incomplete displacement of joint surfaces when forces disrupt the soft tissue that surrounds the joints
C. Data collection
1. Asymmetry of the contour of affected body parts
2. Pain, tenderness, dysfunction, and swelling
3. Complications include neurovascular compromise, avascular necrosis, and open joint injuries
4. X-rays are completed to determine joint shifting
D. Interventions
1. Focus of treatment includes pain relief, joint support, and joint protection
2. Immediate treatment is done to reduce the dislocation and realign the dislocated joint
3. Open or closed **reduction** is done with a postprocedural joint immobilization
4. IV conscious sedation, local, or general anesthesia is used during joint manipulation
5. Initial activity restriction is followed by gentle range of motion and a gradual return of activities to normal levels while supporting the affected joint.
6. A weakened joint is prone to recurrent dislocation and may require extended activity restriction

XII. HERNIATION: INTERVERTEBRAL DISK
A. Description: nucleus of the disk protrudes into the annulus, causing nerve compression
B. Cervical disk herniation occurs at C5-C6 and C6-C7 interspaces
1. Cervical disk herniation causes pain radiation to shoulders, arms, hands, scapula, and pectoral muscles
2. Motor and sensory deficits can include paresthesia, numbness, and weakness of the upper extremities
3. Interventions
a. Use conservative management unless client develops signs of neurological deterioration
b. Advocate bedrest to decrease pressure, inflammation, and pain
c. Immobilize the cervical area with cervical collar, **traction,** or brace
d. Apply heat to reduce muscle spasms; apply ice to reduce inflammation and swelling

e. Maintain the head and spine in alignment
f. Instruct the client in the use of analgesics, sedatives, anti-inflammatory agents, and corticosteroids as prescribed
g. Prepare the client for a corticosteroid injection into the epidural space if prescribed
h. Assist and instruct client in the use of cervical collar or cervical **traction** as prescribed
4. Cervical collar is used for cervical disk herniation
   a. A cervical collar limits neck movement and holds the head in a neutral or slightly flexed position
   b. The cervical collar may be worn intermittently or 24 hours a day
   c. Inspect skin under the collar for irritation
   d. When prescribed and after pain decreases, exercises are prescribed to strengthen the muscles
5. Client education related to cervical disk conditions
   a. Avoid flexing, extending, and rotating neck
   b. Avoid prone position, and maintain neck, spine, and hips in neutral position while sleeping
   c. Minimize long periods of sitting
   d. Instruct the client regarding medications such as analgesics, sedatives, anti-inflammatory agents, and corticosteroids
C. Lumbar disk herniation most often occurs at L4-L5 or L5-S1 interspaces
1. Herniation produces muscle weakness, sensory deficits, and diminished tendon reflexes
2. The client experiences pain and muscle spasms in the lower back, with radiation of the pain into one hip and down the leg (sciatica)
3. Pain is relieved by bedrest and aggravated by movement, lifting, straining, and coughing
4. Interventions
   a. Conservative management is indicated unless neurological deterioration or bowel and bladder dysfunction occurs
   b. Apply moist heat to decrease muscle spasms and apply ice to decrease inflammation
   c. Instruct the client to sleep on the side, with the knees and hips flexed, and place a pillow between the legs
   d. Apply pelvic **traction** as prescribed to relieve muscle spasms and decrease pain
   e. Begin progressive ambulation as inflammation, edema, and pain subside
5. Client education related to lumbar disk conditions
   a. Instruct the client in the use of prescribed medications such as analgesics, muscle relaxants, anti-inflammatory agents, or corticosteroids

BOX 58-7 Types of Disk Surgery

Diskectomy: Removal of herniated disk tissue and related matter
Diskectomy with fusion: Fusion of vertebrae with bone graft
Laminectomy: Excision of part of the vertbrae (lamina) to remove the disk
Laminotomy: Division of the lamina of a vertebra

   b. Instruct the client about application techniques for corsets or braces to maintain immobilization and proper spine alignment
   c. Instruct the client on correct posture while sitting, standing, walking, and working
   d. Instruct the client on the correct technique to use when lifting objects such as bending knees, maintaining a straight back, and avoiding lifting objects above the elbow
   e. Instruct in weight control program as prescribed
   f. Instruct the client in an exercise program to strengthen back and abdominal muscles as prescribed
D. Disk surgery is used when spinal cord compression is suspected or client symptoms do not respond to conservative treatment (Box 58-7)
1. Preoperative interventions
   a. Routine preoperative instructions related to postoperative care
   b. Instruct the client about logrolling and range-of-motion exercises
2. Postoperative interventions: cervical disk
   a. Monitor for respiratory difficulty from inflammation or hematoma
   b. Encourage coughing, deep breathing, and early ambulation as prescribed
   c. Monitor for hoarseness and inability to cough effectively since this may indicate laryngeal nerve damage
   d. Use throat sprays or lozenges for sore throat, avoiding anesthetic lozenges that may numb the throat and increase choking risks
   e. Monitor the surgical wound for infection, swelling, redness, drainage, or pain
   f. Provide a soft diet if the client complains of dysphagia
   g. Monitor for sudden return of radicular pain, which may indicate cervical spine instability
3. Postoperative interventions: lumbar disk
   a. Monitor for wound hemorrhage
   b. Monitor lower extremities for sensation, movement, color, temperature, and paresthesia
   c. Monitor for urinary retention, paralytic ileus, and constipation, which can result from

decreased movement, opioid administration, or spinal cord compression

    d. Prevent constipation by encouraging a high-fiber diet, increased fluid intake, and stool softeners, as prescribed

    e. Administer opioids and sedatives as prescribed to relieve pain and anxiety.

    f. Assist and instruct the client to apply a prescribed back brace or corset with cotton underwear to prevent skin irritation

4. Postoperative lumbar disk positioning concerns

    a. In the immediate postoperative period, the client may be expected to lie supine or have other activity restrictions depending on specific surgical intervention

    b. Instruct the client on correct logrolling techniques to turn and to use when getting out of bed

    c. Instruct the client to avoid spinal flexion or twisting and that the spine should be kept aligned

    d. Instruct the client to minimize sitting, which may place a strain on the surgical site

    e. When the client is lying supine, place a pillow under the neck and slightly flex the knees

    f. Avoid extreme hip flexion when lying on side

XIII. AMPUTATION OF A LOWER EXTREMITY (Figure 58-4)

A. Description: amputation is the surgical removal of a limb or part of the limb

B. Postoperative interventions

1. Monitor vital signs
2. Monitor for infection and hemorrhage
3. Mark bleeding and drainage on the dressing if it occurs
4. Keep a tourniquet at the bedside
5. Observe for and prevent contractures, which can result from prolonged residual limb elevation
6. Monitor for signs of infection, necrosis, and neuroma
7. Evaluate for phantom limb sensation and pain; explain sensation and pain to the client, and medicate the client as prescribed
8. First 24 hours: elevate the foot of the bed to reduce edema, then keep the bed flat to prevent hip flexion contractures, if prescribed by the physician
9. After 24 to 48 hours postoperatively, position the client prone to stretch the muscles and prevent hip flexion contractures, if prescribed
10. Do not elevate the residual limb on a pillow, which also prevents hip flexion contractures
11. Maintain surgical application of dressing, elastic compression wrap, or elastic stump (residual

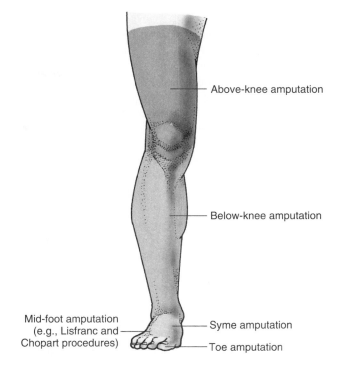

FIG. 58-4 Common levels of lower-extremity amputation. (From Ignatavicius, D., & Workman, M. [2006]. *Medical-surgical nursing: Critical thinking for collaborative care* [5th ed.]. Philadelphia: Saunders.)

limb) shrinker, as prescribed, to reduce swelling, minimize pain, and mold the residual limb in preparation for prosthesis

12. Wash the residual limb with mild soap and water and dry completely
13. Massage the skin toward the suture line to mobilize scar and prevent its adherence to underlying bone
14. Prepare for the prosthesis and instruct the client in progressive resistive techniques by gently pushing the residual limb against pillows and progressing to firmer surfaces
15. Encourage verbalization regarding loss of the body part, and assist the client to identify coping mechanisms to deal with the loss

C. Interventions for below-the-knee amputation

1. Prevent edema
2. Do not allow the residual limb to hang over the edge of the bed
3. Discourage long periods of sitting to lessen complications of knee flexion

D. Interventions for above-the-knee amputation

1. Prevent internal or external rotation of the limb
2. Place a sandbag, rolled towel, or trochanter roll along the outside of the thigh to prevent external rotation

E. Rehabilitation
1. Instruct the client in crutch walking
2. Prepare the residual limb for a prosthesis
3. Prepare the client for fitting of the residual limb for a prosthesis
4. Instruct the client in exercises to maintain range of motion and upper body strengthening
5. Provide psychosocial support to the client

XIV. RHEUMATOID ARTHRITIS
A. Description
1. Rheumatoid arthritis is a chronic systemic inflammatory disease (immune complex–disorder); the cause may be related to a combination of environmental and genetic factors
2. Rheumatoid arthritis leads to destruction of connective tissue and synovial membrane within the joints
3. Rheumatoid arthritis weakens the joint, leading to dislocation, and permanent deformity of the joint
4. Formation of pannus occurs at the junction of synovial tissue and articular cartilage and projects into the joint cavity, causing necrosis
5. Exacerbations of disease manifestations occur during periods of physical or emotional stress and fatigue
6. Risk factors include exposure to infectious agents
7. Vasculitis can impede blood flow, leading to organ or organ system malfunction and failure because of tissue ischemia

B. Data collection
1. Inflammation, tenderness, and stiffness of the joints
2. Moderate to severe pain with morning stiffness lasting longer than 30 minutes
3. Joint deformities, muscle atrophy, and decreased range of motion in affected joints
4. Spongy, soft feeling in the joints
5. Low-grade temperature, fatigue, and weakness
6. Anorexia, weight loss, and anemia
7. Elevated sedimentation rate and positive rheumatoid factor
8. Radiographic study showing joint deterioration
9. Synovial tissue biopsy reveals inflammation

C. Rheumatoid factor
1. A blood test used to diagnose rheumatoid arthritis
2. Values
a. Nonreactive: 0 to 39 international units/mL
b. Weakly reactive: 40 to 79 international units/mL
c. Reactive: greater than 80 international units/mL

D. Pain: a combination of pharmacological therapies including NSAIDs, disease-modifying antirheumatic drugs (DMARDs), and glucocorticoids

E. Physical mobility
1. Preserve joint function
2. Provide range-of-motion exercises to maintain joint motion and muscle strengthening
3. Balance rest and activity
4. Splints may be used during acute inflammation to prevent deformity
5. Prevent flexion contractures
6. Apply heat or cold therapy to joints as prescribed
7. Apply paraffin baths and massage as prescribed
8. Encourage consistency with exercise program
9. Instruct the client to stop exercise if pain increases
10. Exercise only to the point of pain
11. Avoid weight bearing on inflamed joints

F. Self-care (Box 58-8)
1. Assess the need for assistive devices such as raised toilet seats, self-rising chairs, wheelchairs, and scooters to facilitate mobility
2. Collaborate with an occupational therapist or health care provider to obtain assistive or adaptive devices
3. Instruct the client in alternative strategies for providing activities of daily living

G. Fatigue
1. Identify factors that may contribute to fatigue
2. Monitor for signs of anemia, and administer iron, folic acid, and vitamins as prescribed
3. Monitor for medication-related blood loss by testing the stool for occult blood
4. Instruct the client in measures to conserve energy, such as pacing activities and obtaining assistance when possible

H. Disturbed body image
1. Assess the client's reaction to the body change
2. Encourage the client to verbalize feelings

BOX 58-8 Client Education for Rheumatoid Arthritis and Degenerative Joint Disease

Assist the client to identify and correct safety hazards in the home.
Instruct the client on the correct use of assistive or adaptive devices.
Instruct the client in energy conservation measures.
Review the prescribed exercise program.
Instruct the client to sit in a chair with a high, straight back.
Instruct the client to use only a small pillow when lying down.
Instruct the client on measures to protect the joints.
Instruct the client regarding prescribed medications.
Stress the importance of follow-up visits with the health care provider.

3. Assist the client with self-care activities and grooming
4. Encourage the client to wear street clothes

I. Surgical interventions
   1. Synovectomy: surgical removal of the synovia to help maintain joint function
   2. Arthrodesis: bony fusion of a joint to regain some mobility
   3. Joint replacement (arthroplasty): surgical replacement of diseased joints with artificial joints, which is performed to restore motion to a joint and function to the muscles, ligaments, and other soft tissue structures that control a joint

XV. OSTEOARTHRITIS (DEGENERATIVE JOINT DISEASE)

A. Description
   1. Osteoarthritis is progressive degeneration of the joints as a result of wear and tear
   2. It causes the formation of bony buildup and the loss of articular cartilage in peripheral and axial joints
   3. Osteoarthritis affects the weight-bearing joints and joints that receive the greatest stress, such as the hips, knees, and lower vertebral column and hands
   4. The cause is unknown but contributing factors may include trauma, fractures, infections, obesity, or job-related repetitive stress activities

B. Data collection
   1. Client experiences joint pain that diminishes after rest and intensifies after activity, noted early in the disease process
   2. As the disease progresses, pain occurs with slight motion or even at rest
   3. Symptoms are aggravated by temperature change and climate humidity
   4. Presence of Heberden's nodes or Bouchard's nodes
   5. Joint swelling, crepitus, and limited range of motion
   6. Difficulty getting up after prolonged sitting
   7. Skeletal muscle disuse atrophy
   8. Inability to perform activities of daily living
   9. Compression of the spine as manifested by radiating pain, stiffness, and muscle spasms in one or both extremities

C. Pain
   1. Administer NSAIDs, muscle relaxants, and other medications as prescribed
   2. Prepare the client for corticosteroid injections into joints as prescribed
   3. Position the joints in function position and avoid flexion of knees and hips
   4. Immobilize the affected joint with a splint or brace until inflammation subsides
   5. Avoid large pillows under the head or knees

6. Provide a bed or foot cradle to keep linen off the feet
7. Instruct the client on the importance of moist heat, hot packs or compresses, and paraffin dips as prescribed
8. Apply cold applications as prescribed when the joint is acutely inflamed
9. Encourage adequate rest, recommending 10 hours of sleep at night and a 1- to 2-hour nap in the afternoon

D. Nutrition
   1. Encourage a well-balanced diet
   2. Maintain weight within normal range to decrease stress on the joints

E. Physical mobility
   1. Instruct the client to balance activity with rest while participating in an exercise program that limits stressing affected joints
   2. Instruct the client that exercises should be active rather than passive and to stop exercise if pain occurs
   3. Instruct the client to limit exercise when joint inflammation is severe

F. Surgical management
   1. Osteotomy: the bone is resected to correct joint deformity, promote realignment, and reduce joint stress
   2. Total joint replacement or arthroplasy
      a. Total joint replacement is performed when all measures of pain relief have failed
      b. Hips and knees are replaced most commonly
      c. Total joint replacement is contraindicated in the presence of infection, advanced osteoporosis, or severe joint inflammation

XVI. OSTEOPOROSIS

A. Description
   1. Osteoporosis is an age-related metabolic disease
   2. Bone demineralizes, losing calcium and phosphorous salts, leading to fragile bones and subsequent fractures
   3. Bone resorption accelerates as bone formation slows
   4. Osteoporosis occurs most commonly in the wrist, hip, and vertebral column
   5. Osteoporosis can occur postmenopausally or as a result of a metabolic disorder or calcium deficiency
   6. Client may be asymptomatic until the bones become fragile and a minor injury or movement causes a fracture
   7. Primary osteoporosis
      a. Most often occurs in postmenopausal women
      b. Risk factors include decreased calcium intake, deficient estrogen, and limited exercise

BOX 58-9 **Risk Factors for Osteoporosis**

Cigarette smoking
Early menopause
Excessive use of alcohol
Family history
Female gender
Increasing age
Insufficient intake of calcium
Sedentary lifestyle
Thin, small frame
White (European descent) or Asian race

8. Secondary osteoporosis
   a. Causes include prolonged therapy with corticosteroids, thyroid-reducing medications, aluminum-containing antacid, or anticonvulsants
   b. Associated with immobility, alcoholism, malnutrition, or malabsorption
9. Risk factors (Box 58-9)

B. Data collection
1. Possibly asymptomatic
2. Back pain can occur after lifting, bending, or stooping
3. Back pain that increases with palpation
4. Pelvic or hip pain, especially with weight bearing
5. Problems with balance
6. Decline in height from vertebral compression
7. Kyphosis of the dorsal spine also known as "dowager's hump"
8. Pathological fractures
9. Degeneration of lower thorax and lumber vertebrae on radiographic studies

C. Interventions
1. Assess risk for and prevent injury in client's personal environment
   a. Assist client to identify and correct hazards in his or her environment
   b. Position household items and furniture for an unobstructed walkway
   c. Use side rails to prevent falls
   d. Instruct in the use of assistive devices such as a cane or walker
   e. Encourage use of firm mattress
2. Provide personal care to client to reduce injuries
   a. Move the client gently when turning and repositioning
   b. Assist with ambulation if client is unsteady
   c. Provide gentle range-of-motion exercises
   d. Apply a back brace as prescribed during an acute phase to immobilize the spine and provide spinal column support
3. Provide client instructions to promote optimal level of health and function
   a. Instruct the client in the use of good body mechanics
   b. Instruct the client in exercises to strengthen abdominal and back muscles to improve posture and provide support for the spine
   c. Instruct the client to avoid activities that can cause vertebral compression
   d. Instruct the client to eat a diet high in protein, calcium, vitamins C and D, and iron
   e. Instruct the client to avoid alcohol and coffee
   f. Instruct the client to maintain an adequate fluid intake to prevent renal calculi
4. Administer medication to promote bone strength and decrease pain
   a. Administer calcium, vitamin D, and phosphorus as prescribed for bone metabolism
   b. Administer calcitonin as prescribed to inhibit bone loss
   c. Administer estrogen or androgens to decrease the rate of bone resorption as prescribed
   d. Administer analgesics, muscle relaxants, and anti-inflammatory medications as prescribed

XVII. GOUT

A. Description
1. Gout is a systemic disease in which urate crystals deposit in joints and other body tissues
2. Gout leads to abnormal amounts of uric acid in the body
3. Primary gout results from a disorder of purine metabolism
4. Secondary gout involves excessive uric acid in the blood that is caused by another disease

B. Phases
1. Asymptomatic: client has no symptoms but serum uric acid is elevated
2. Acute: client has excruciating pain and inflammation of one or more small joints, especially the great toe
3. Intermittent: client has intermittent periods without symptoms between acute attacks
4. Chronic: results from repeated episodes of acute gout
   a. Chronic gout results in deposits of urate crystals under the skin
   b. Chronic gout results in deposits of urate crystals within major organs such as kidneys, leading to organ dysfunction

C. Data collection
1. Swelling and inflammation of the joints, leading to excruciating pain
2. Tophi: hard, irregular-shaped nodules in the skin containing chalky deposits of sodium urate
3. Low-grade fever, malaise, and headache
4. Pruritis from urate crystals in the skin
5. Presence of renal stones from elevated uric acid levels

D. Interventions
1. Provide a low-purine diet as prescribed; foods such as organ meats, wines, and aged cheese should be avoided
2. Encourage a high fluid intake of 2000 mL to prevent stone formation
3. Encourage weight-reduction diet if required
4. Instruct the client to avoid alcohol and starvation diets since they may precipitate a gout attack
5. Increase urinary pH (above 6) by eating alkaline ash foods such as milk and other dairy products
6. Provide bedrest during the acute attacks with affected extremity elevated
7. Monitor joint range-of-motion ability and for swelling and inflammation
8. Position the joint in mild flexion during acute attack
9. Protect the affected joint from excessive movement or direct contact with sheets or blankets
10. Provide heat or cold for local treatments to the affected joint as prescribed
11. Administer medications such as analgesics, anti-inflammatory medications, and uricosuric agents as prescribed

PRACTICE QUESTIONS

More questions on the companion CD!

783. A nurse is one of several people who witness a vehicle hit a pedestrian at a fairly low speed on a small street. The individual is dazed and tries to get up, and the leg appears fractured. The nurse would plan to:
1. Try to manually reduce the fracture.
2. Assist the person to get up and walk to the sidewalk.
3. Leave the person for a few moments to call an ambulance.
4. Stay with the person and encourage the person to remain still.

784. A nurse witnesses a client sustain a fall and suspects that the client's leg may be fractured. Which action is the priority?
1. Take a set of vital signs.
2. Call the radiology department.
3. Immobilize the leg before moving the client.
4. Reassure the client that everything will be fine.

785. A client with a hip fracture asks the nurse why Buck's extension traction is being applied before surgery. The nurse's response is based on the understanding that Buck's extension traction primarily:
1. Allows bony healing to begin before surgery
2. Provides rigid immobilization of the fracture site

3. Lengthens the fractured leg to prevent severing of blood vessels
4. Provides comfort by reducing muscle spasms and provides fracture immobilization

786. A nurse is evaluating the pin sites of a client in skeletal traction. The nurse would be least concerned with which finding?
1. Inflammation
2. Serous drainage
3. Pain at a pin site
4. Purulent drainage

787. A nurse is caring for the client who has had skeletal traction applied to the left leg. The client is complaining of severe left leg pain. Which action should the nurse take first?
1. Provide pin care.
2. Call the physician immediately.
3. Check the client's alignment in bed.
4. Medicate the client with an analgesic.

788. A nurse has provided instructions regarding specific leg exercises for the client immobilized in right skeletal lower leg traction. The nurse determines that the client needs further instruction if the nurse observes the client:
1. Pulling up on the trapeze
2. Flexing and extending the feet
3. Doing quadriceps-setting and gluteal-setting exercises
4. Performing active range of motion (ROM) to the right ankle and knee

789. A nurse is checking the casted extremity of a client. The nurse would check for which of the following signs and symptoms indicative of infection?
1. Dependent edema
2. Diminished distal pulse
3. Presence of a "hot spot" on the cast
4. Coolness and pallor of the extremity

790. A client has sustained a closed fracture and has just had a cast applied to the affected arm. The client is complaining of intense pain. The nurse has elevated the limb, applied an ice bag, and administered an analgesic, which was ineffective in relieving the pain. The nurse interprets that this pain may be caused by:
1. Infection under the cast
2. The anxiety of the client
3. Impaired tissue perfusion
4. The newness of the fracture

791. A nurse is assigned to care for a client with multiple trauma who is admitted to the hospital. The client has a leg fracture, and a plaster cast has been applied. In positioning the casted leg, the nurse should:
1. Keep the leg in a level position.
2. Elevate the leg for 3 hours, and put it flat for 1 hour.

3. Keep the leg level for 3 hours, and elevate it for 1 hour.
4. Elevate the leg on pillows continuously for 24 to 48 hours.

792. A client is complaining of skin irritation from the edges of a cast applied the previous day. The nurse should plan for which of the following actions?
1. Massaging the skin at the rim of the cast
2. Petaling the cast edges with adhesive tape
3. Using a rough file to smooth the cast edges
4. Applying lotion to the skin at the rim of the cast

793. A client is being discharged home after application of a plaster leg cast. The nurse determines that the client understands proper care of the cast if the client states that he or she will:
1. Avoid getting the cast wet.
2. Cover the casted leg with warm blankets.
3. Use the fingertips to lift and move the leg.
4. Use a padded coat hanger end to scratch under the cast.

794. A nurse is planning to provide instructions to the client about how to stand on crutches. In the written instructions, the nurse plans to tell the client to place the crutches:
1. 3 inches to the front and side of the client's toes
2. 8 inches to the front and side of the client's toes
3. 20 inches to the front and side of the client's toes
4. 15 inches to the front and side of the client's toes

795. A nurse is evaluating the client's use of a cane for left-sided weakness. The nurse would intervene and correct the client if the nurse observed that the client:
1. Holds the cane on the right side
2. Moves the cane when the right leg is moved
3. Leans on the cane when the right leg swings through
4. Keeps the cane 6 inches out to the side of the right foot

796. A nurse is caring for a client with fresh application of a plaster leg cast. The nurse plans to prevent the development of compartment syndrome by:
1. Elevating the limb and applying ice to the affected leg
2. Elevating the limb and covering the limb with bath blankets
3. Keeping the leg horizontal and applying ice to the affected leg
4. Placing the leg in a slightly dependent position and applying ice

797. A client with diabetes mellitus has had a right below-knee amputation. The nurse would be especially vigilant in monitoring for which of the following because of the client's history of diabetes mellitus?
1. Hemorrhage
2. Edema of residual limb
3. Slight redness of incision
4. Separation of wound edges

798. A client is admitted to the nursing unit after a left below-knee amputation following a crush injury to the foot and lower leg. The client tells the nurse, "I think I'm going crazy. I can feel my left foot itching." The nurse interprets the client's statement to be:
1. A normal response, and indicates the presence of phantom limb pain
2. A normal response, and indicates the presence of phantom limb sensation
3. An abnormal response, and indicates that the client is in denial about the limb loss
4. An abnormal response, and indicates that the client needs more psychological support

799. A nurse has provided instructions to client with a herniated lumbar disk about proper body mechanics and other items pertinent to low back care. The nurse determines that the client needs further instructions if the client verbalizes that he or she will:
1. Increase fiber and fluids in the diet
2. Bend at the knees to pick up objects
3. Strengthen the back muscles by swimming or walking
4. Get out of bed by sitting straight up and swinging legs over the side of the bed

800. A client with a left arm fracture exhibits loss of sensation in the left fingers, pallor, slow refill, and diminished left radial pulse. The nurse should take which of the following actions?
1. Administer an analgesic.
2. Notify the registered nurse.
3. Check the circulation again in 30 minutes.
4. Provide range-of-motion exercises to the fingers of the left hand.

801. A client is complaining of pain underneath a cast in the area of a bony prominence. The nurse interprets that this client may need to have:
1. The cast bivalved
2. A window cut in the cast
3. The cast replaced with an air splint
4. Extra padding put over this area of the cast

802. A nursing instructor asks a nursing student about the risk factors associated with osteoporosis. The instructor tells the student that she needs to read and learn about this disorder if the student states that which of the following is an associated risk factor?
1. Postmenopausal age
2. Family history of osteoporosis

3. High-calcium diet consumption
4. Long-term use of corticosteroids

803. A nurse is providing instructions to a client with osteoporosis regarding appropriate food items to include in the diet. The nurse tells the client that which food item would provide the least amount of calcium?
   1. Pork
   2. Seafood
   3. Sardines
   4. Plain yogurt

804. A nurse is caring for a client with osteoarthritis. The nurse collects data, knowing that which of the following is a clinical manifestation associated with the disorder?
   1. Morning stiffness
   2. Positive rheumatoid factor
   3. An elevated sedimentation rate
   4. Dull aching pain in the affected joints

805. A client is treated in the physician's office after a fall, which sprained the ankle. Radiography has ruled out fracture. Before sending the client home, the nurse would plan to teach the client about which item that is to be avoided in the next 24 hours?
   1. Resting the foot
   2. Application of an Ace wrap
   3. Application of a heating pad
   4. Elevating the ankle on a pillow while sitting or lying down

806. A nurse has provided instructions to the client returning home after arthroscopy of the knee. The nurse determines that the client understands the instructions if the client states that he or she will:
   1. Resume regular exercise the following day.
   2. Stay off the leg entirely for the rest of the day.
   3. Refrain from eating food for the remainder of the day.
   4. Report fever or site inflammation to the physician.

ALTERNATE ITEM FORMAT: MULTIPLE RESPONSE

807. A nurse is preparing a list of cast care instructions for a client who just had a plaster cast applied to his right forearm. Select all instructions that the nurse includes on the list.
   ☐ 1. Keep the cast and extremity elevated.
   ☐ 2. The cast needs to be kept clean and dry.
   ☐ 3. Allow the wet cast 24 to 72 hours to dry.
   ☐ 4. Expect tingling and numbness in the extremity.
   ☐ 5. Use a hair dryer set on a warm to hot setting to dry the cast.
   ☐ 6. Use a soft padded object that will fit under the cast to scratch the skin under the cast.

ANSWERS

783. **4**
Rationale: With a suspected fracture, the client is not moved unless it is dangerous to remain in that spot. The nurse should remain with the client and have someone else call for emergency help. A fracture is not reduced at the scene. Before moving the client, the site of the fracture is immobilized to prevent further injury.
Test-Taking Strategy: Use the process of elimination. Eliminate options 1 and 2 first because these actions could result in further injury to the client. From the remaining options, the most prudent action would be for the nurse to remain with the client and have someone else call for emergency assistance. Review immediate care of the client with a fracture if you had difficulty with this question.
Level of Cognitive Ability: Application
Client Needs: Physiological Integrity
Integrated Process: Nursing Process/Implementation
Content Area: Adult Health/Musculoskeletal
Reference: Lewis, S., Heitkemper, M., Dirksen, S., & Bucher, L. (2007). *Medical-surgical nursing: Assessment and management of clinical problems* (7th ed., p. 1642). St. Louis: Mosby.

784. **3**
Rationale: When a fracture is suspected, it is imperative that the area is splinted before the client is moved. Emergency help should be called if the client is not hospitalized; a physician is called for the hospitalized client. The nurse should remain

with the client and provide realistic reassurance. The nurse does not prescribe radiology tests.
Test-Taking Strategy: Note the strategic word "priority." Eliminate option 2 because the nurse does not order x-rays. Option 4 is eliminated next, because the nurse never tells a client that "everything will be fine." From the remaining options, focus on the data in the question. Immobilizing the limb is imperative for the client's safety, which makes it a better choice than taking vital signs. Review care of the client when a fracture is suspected if you had difficulty with this question.
Level of Cognitive Ability: Application
Client Needs: Physiological Integrity
Integrated Process: Nursing Process/Implementation
Content Area: Adult Health/Musculoskeletal
Reference: deWit, S. (2009). *Medical-surgical nursing: Concepts & practice* (p. 786). St. Louis: Saunders.

785. **4**
Rationale: Buck's extension traction is a type of skin traction often applied after hip fracture, before the fracture is reduced in surgery. It reduces muscle spasms and helps immobilize the fracture. It does not lengthen the leg for the purpose of preventing blood vessel severance. It also does not allow for bony healing to begin.
Test-Taking Strategy: Use the process of elimination. Recalling the purpose of traction will assist in eliminating options 1 and 3. From the remaining options, eliminate option 2 because of

the words "rigid immobilization." Review this type of traction if you had difficulty with this question.
Level of Cognitive Ability: Application
Client Needs: Physiological Integrity
Integrated Process: Nursing Process/Implementation
Content Area: Adult Health/Musculoskeletal
Reference: Christensen, B., & Kockrow, E. (2006). *Adult health nursing* (5th ed., p. 173). St. Louis: Mosby.

786. **2**
Rationale: A small amount of serous oozing is expected at pin insertion sites. Signs of infection such as inflammation, purulent drainage, and pain at the pin site are not expected findings and should be reported.
Test-Taking Strategy: Note the strategic words "least concerned with." Options 1 and 4 indicate infection and are eliminated. To select between options 2 and 3, look at them carefully. The complaint of pain is at "a pin site" only. It gives no indication that the pain is related to the fracture or muscle spasm. Because serous drainage is an expected finding, you would select this over the complaint of pain. Review care of the client in skeletal traction if you had difficulty with this question.
Level of Cognitive Ability: Analysis
Client Needs: Physiological Integrity
Integrated Process: Nursing Process/Evaluation
Content Area: Adult Health/Musculoskeletal
Reference: Christensen, B., & Kockrow, E. (2006). *Adult health nursing* (5th ed., p. 175). St. Louis: Mosby.

787. **3**
Rationale: A client who complains of severe pain may need realignment or may have had traction weights ordered that are too heavy. The nurse realigns the client and, if ineffective, calls the physician. Severe leg pain, once traction has been established, indicates a problem. Medicating the client should be done after trying to determine and treat the cause. Providing pin care is unrelated to the problem as described.
Test-Taking Strategy: Note the strategic word "first." Use the steps of the nursing process. Option 3 is the only option that addresses data collection. Review care of the client in skeletal traction if you had difficulty with this question.
Level of Cognitive Ability: Application
Client Needs: Physiological Integrity
Integrated Process: Nursing Process/Implementation
Content Area: Adult Health/Musculoskeletal
Reference: deWit, S. (2009). *Medical-surgical nursing: Concepts & practice* (p. 793). St. Louis: Saunders.

788. **4**
Rationale: Exercise is indicated within therapeutic limits for the client in skeletal traction to maintain muscle strength and ROM. The client may pull up on the trapeze, perform active ROM with uninvolved joints, and do isometric muscle-setting exercises (e.g., quadriceps- and gluteal-setting exercises). The client may also flex and extend his or her feet.
Test-Taking Strategy: Note the strategic words "needs further instruction." These words indicate a negative event query and the need to select the incorrect client action. Options 1 and 3 are most easily identified as correct actions and are therefore eliminated as possible answers. To select between options 2

and 4, imagine the lines of pull on the fracture site with the movements described. Although flexing and extending the feet does not disrupt the line of pull from the traction, performing active ROM to the affected knee and ankle does. Review care of the client in traction if you had difficulty with this question.
Level of Cognitive Ability: Comprehension
Client Needs: Physiological Integrity
Integrated Process: Teaching and Learning
Content Area: Adult Health/Musculoskeletal
References: Linton, A., & Maebius, N. (2007). *Introduction to medical-surgical nursing* (4th ed., p. 928). Philadelphia: Saunders.
Monahan, F., Sands, J., Neighbors, M., Marek, J., & Green, C. (2007). *Phipps' medical-surgical nursing: Health and illness perspectives* (8th ed., p. 1537). St. Louis: Mosby.

789. **3**
Rationale: Signs and symptoms of infection under a casted area include odor or purulent drainage from the cast, or the presence of "hot spots," which are areas of the cast that are warmer than others. The physician should be notified if any of these occur. Signs of impaired circulation in the distal limb include coolness and pallor of the skin, diminished arterial pulse, and edema.
Test-Taking Strategy: Begin to answer this question by thinking of what you would expect to find with infection: redness, swelling, heat, and purulent drainage. With these in mind, options 2 and 4 can be eliminated. To select between options 1 and 3, "dependent edema" is not necessarily indicative of infection; swelling would be continuous. The "hot spot" on the cast could signify infection underneath that area. Review the complications of a cast if you had difficulty with this question.
Level of Cognitive Ability: Application
Client Needs: Physiological Integrity
Integrated Process: Nursing Process/Data Collection
Content Area: Adult Health/Musculoskeletal
Reference: Ignatavicius, D., & Workman, M. (2006). *Medical-surgical nursing: Critical thinking for collaborative care* (5th ed., p. 1200). Philadelphia: Saunders.

790. **3**
Rationale: Most pain associated with fractures can be minimized with rest, elevation, application of cold, and administration of analgesics. Pain that is not relieved from these measures should be reported to the physician since it may be the result of impaired tissue perfusion, tissue breakdown, or necrosis. Because this is a new closed fracture and cast, infection would not have had time to set in.
Test-Taking Strategy: Use the process of elimination. Options 2 and 4 can be eliminated first, based on the description in the question. Because the fracture and cast are so new, it is extremely unlikely that infection could have set in. The most likely option is impaired tissue perfusion, because pain from ischemia is not relieved by comfort measures and analgesics. Review the complications of a cast if you had difficulty with this question.
Level of Cognitive Ability: Analysis
Client Needs: Physiological Integrity
Integrated Process: Nursing Process/Data Collection

Content Area: Adult Health/Musculoskeletal
References: Black, J., & Hawks, J. (2005). *Medical-surgical nursing: Clinical management for positive outcomes* (7th ed., pp. 633;644). Philadelphia: Saunders.
Linton, A., & Maebius, N. (2007). *Introduction to medical-surgical nursing* (4th ed., p. 925). Philadelphia: Saunders.

791. 4
Rationale: A casted extremity is elevated continuously for the first 24 to 48 hours to minimize swelling and to promote venous drainage.
Test-Taking Strategy: Use the process of elimination. Recall that edema sets in after fracture and can be aggravated by casting. For this reason, options 1 and 3 are the least helpful and can be eliminated first. There is no useful purpose for the timing in option 2. Review care of the client with a cast if you had difficulty with this question.
Level of Cognitive Ability: Application
Client Needs: Physiological Integrity
Integrated Process: Nursing Process/Implementation
Content Area: Adult Health/Musculoskeletal
Reference: Christensen, B., & Kockrow, E. (2006). *Adult health nursing* (5th ed., p. 172). St. Louis: Mosby.

792. 2
Rationale: The edges of the cast can be petaled with tape to minimize skin irritation. If a client has a cast applied and returns home, the client can be taught to do the same.
Test-Taking Strategy: Use the process of elimination. Options 1 and 4 are comparable or alike, and neither helps to get rid of the cause of the irritation, so they are eliminated first. Imagine the use of a "rough file"; it would create plaster chips and dust, which could go underneath the cast. Review cast petaling if you had difficulty with this question.
Level of Cognitive Ability: Application
Client Needs: Physiological Integrity
Integrated Process: Nursing Process/Planning
Content Area: Adult Health/Musculoskeletal
References: Linton, A., & Maebius, N. (2007). *Introduction to medical-surgical nursing* (4th ed., p. 920). Philadelphia: Saunders.
Monahan, F., Sands, J., Neighbors, M., Marek, J., & Green, C. (2007). *Phipps' Medical-surgical nursing: Health and illness perspectives* (8th ed., p. 1536). St. Louis: Mosby.

793. 1
Rationale: A plaster cast must remain dry to keep its strength. The cast should be handled using the palms of the hands, not the fingertips, until fully dry. Air should circulate freely around the cast to help it dry; the cast also gives off heat as it dries. The client should never scratch under the cast; a cool hair dryer may be used to eliminate itching.
Test-Taking Strategy: Knowledge of cast care is needed to answer this question. Knowing that a wet cast can be dented with the fingertips, causing pressure underneath, helps you eliminate option 3 first. Knowing that the cast needs to dry helps you eliminate option 2 next. Option 4 is dangerous to skin integrity and is also eliminated. Plaster casts, once they have dried after application, should not become wet. Review home care instructions for a client with a cast if you had difficulty with this question.

Level of Cognitive Ability: Comprehension
Client Needs: Physiological Integrity
Integrated Process: Nursing Process/Evaluation
Content Area: Adult Health/Musculoskeletal
Reference: Linton, A., & Maebius, N. (2007). *Introduction to medical-surgical nursing* (4th ed., p. 922). Philadelphia: Saunders.

794. 2
Rationale: The classic tripod position is taught to the client before giving instructions on gait. The crutches are placed anywhere from 6 to 10 inches in front and to the side of the client, depending on the client's body size. This provides a wide enough base of support to the client and improves balance.
Test-Taking Strategy: Use the process of elimination and visualize each position. Three inches and 20 inches seem excessively short and long, respectively. These options can be eliminated first. Of the remaining options, 8 inches seems more in keeping with the normal length of a stride than 15 inches. Review crutch walking if you had difficulty with this question.
Level of Cognitive Ability: Application
Client Needs: Safe and Effective Care Environment
Integrated Process: Nursing Process/Planning
Content Area: Adult Health/Musculoskeletal
Reference: Linton, A., & Maebius, N. (2007). *Introduction to medical-surgical nursing* (4th ed., pp. 923-924). Philadelphia: Saunders.

795. 2
Rationale: The cane is held on the stronger side to minimize stress on the affected extremity and provide a wide base of support. The cane is held 6 inches lateral to the fifth great toe. The cane is moved forward with the affected leg. The client leans on the cane for added support while the stronger side swings through.
Test-Taking Strategy: Note the strategic word "intervenes." This word indicates a negative event query and the need to select the incorrect client action. Knowing that the cane is held on the stronger side helps you eliminate options 1 and 4 first. To select from the remaining options, recall that the client moves the cane with the weaker leg and leans on it for support when the stronger leg swings through. Review client instructions for cane walking if you had difficulty with this question.
Level of Cognitive Ability: Comprehension
Client Needs: Safe and Effective Care Environment
Integrated Process: Teaching and Learning
Content Area: Adult Health/Musculoskeletal
References: Ignatavicius, D., & Workman, M. (2006). *Medical-surgical nursing: Critical thinking for collaborative care* (5th ed., p. 1204). Philadelphia: Saunders.
Perry, A., & Potter, P. (2006). *Clinical nursing skills & techniques* (6th ed., p.296). St. Louis: Mosby.

796. 1
Rationale: Compartment syndrome is prevented by controlling edema. This is achieved most optimally with elevation and application of ice.
Test-Taking Strategy: Use the process of elimination. Recalling that edema is controlled or prevented with limb elevation

helps you eliminate options 3 and 4 first. From the remaining options, think about the effects of ice versus bath blankets. Ice will further control edema, but bath blankets will produce heat and prevent air circulation needed for the cast to dry. Review measures to prevent compartment syndrome if you had difficulty with this question.
Level of Cognitive Ability: Application
Client Needs: Physiological Integrity
Integrated Process: Nursing Process/Planning
Content Area: Adult Health/Musculoskeletal
Reference: Christensen, B., & Kockrow, E. (2006). *Adult health nursing* (5th ed., pp. 164-165). St. Louis: Mosby.

797. **4**
Rationale: Clients with diabetes mellitus are more prone to wound infection and delayed wound healing because of the disease. Postoperative residual limb edema and hemorrhage are complications in the immediate postoperative period that apply to any client with an amputation. Slight redness of the incision is considered normal, as long as it is dry and intact.
Test-Taking Strategy: The question guides you to look for complications that are primarily the result of the co-existing condition of diabetes mellitus. Recalling that diabetes mellitus increases the client's risk of developing infection and delayed wound healing helps eliminate options 1 and 2 first. From the remaining options, select option 4 because separation of wound edges is a more serious problem than a slight redness to the incision line, which is considered normal. Review the complications of an amputation if you had difficulty with this question.
Level of Cognitive Ability: Comprehension
Client Needs: Physiological Integrity
Integrated Process: Nursing Process/Data Collection
Content Area: Adult Health/Musculoskeletal
References: deWit, S. (2009). *Medical-surgical nursing: Concepts & practice* (p. 930). St. Louis: Saunders.
Lewis, S., Heitkemper, M., Dirksen, S., & Bucher, L. (2007). *Medical-surgical nursing: Assessment and management of clinical problems* (7th ed., p. 1659). St. Louis: Mosby.

798. **2**
Rationale: Phantom limb sensations are felt in the area of the amputated limb. These can include itching, warmth, and cold. The sensations are caused by intact peripheral nerves in the area amputated. Whenever possible, clients should be prepared for these sensations. The client may also feel painful sensations in the amputated limb, called phantom limb pain. The origin of the pain is less well understood, but the client should also be prepared for this, whenever possible.
Test-Taking Strategy: Use the process of elimination. Knowing that sensation and pain may be felt in the residual limb helps you eliminate options 3 and 4 first, because the sensations are not abnormal responses. From the remaining options, select option 2 because the client has described an itching sensation but has not complained of pain in the residual limb. Review the expected findings following amputation if you had difficulty with this question.
Level of Cognitive Ability: Analysis
Client Needs: Psychosocial Integrity
Integrated Process: Nursing Process/Evaluation
Content Area: Adult Health/Musculoskeletal

Reference: Linton, A., & Maebius, N. (2007). *Introduction to medical-surgical nursing* (4th ed., p. 937). Philadelphia: Saunders.

799. **4**
Rationale: Clients are taught to get out of bed by sliding near the edge of the mattress. The client then rolls onto one side and pushes up from the bed using one or both arms. The back is kept straight and the legs are swung over the side. Increasing fluids and dietary fiber helps prevent straining at stool, thereby preventing increases in intraspinal pressure. Walking and swimming are excellent exercises for strengthening lower back muscles. Proper body mechanics includes bending at the knees, not the waist, to lift objects.
Test-Taking Strategy: Note the strategic words "needs further instructions." These words indicate a negative event query and the need to select the incorrect client statement. Options 2 and 3 are examples of interventions that are indicated and are eliminated first. Clients with low back pain should avoid situations that increase intraspinal pressure; option 1 prevents increases in intraspinal pressure. Option 4 causes an increase in intraspinal pressure if you think of the body mechanics involved in getting out of bed this way. Review the principles of proper body mechanics if you had difficulty with this question.
Level of Cognitive Ability: Comprehension
Client Needs: Physiological Integrity
Integrated Process: Teaching and Learning
Content Area: Adult Health/Musculoskeletal
Reference: deWit, S. (2009). *Medical-surgical nursing: Concepts & practice* (p. 559). St. Louis: Saunders.

800. **2**
Rationale: The client with pallor, slow capillary refill, weakened or lost pulse, and absence of sensation or motion to the distal limb may have arterial damage from a lacerated, contused, thrombosed, or severed artery. These signs can occur with constriction from a tight cast as well. Regardless of the cause, the nurse notifies the registered nurse immediately, who will contact the physician. Emergency intervention is needed, which could include removal of the constricting bandage, fracture reduction, or surgery to repair the area.
Test-Taking Strategy: Use the process of elimination. Recall that these signs indicate insufficient arterial circulation and can lead to irreversible ischemia and damage. Because of this, eliminate options 1 and 4 first as not being helpful. Rechecking the circulation in 30 minutes loses valuable time for action to restore the impaired circulation, so eliminate option 3. The registered nurse should be notified immediately. Review the complications of a fracture if you had difficulty with this question.
Level of Cognitive Ability: Application
Client Needs: Physiological Integrity
Integrated Process: Nursing Process/Implementation
Content Area: Adult Health/Musculoskeletal
Reference: deWit, S. (2009). *Medical-surgical nursing: Concepts & practice* (pp. 794-765). St. Louis: Saunders.

801. **2**
Rationale: A window may be cut in a dried cast to relieve pressure, monitor pulses, relieve discomfort, or

remove drains. Bivalving the cast involves splitting the cast along both sides to allow space for swelling, facilitate taking x-rays, or make a half-cast for use as an intermittent splint. Padding is not placed on top of a cast. The use of an air splint is not indicated.
Test-Taking Strategy: Note the strategic words "bony prominence." Wherever there is a bony prominence, there is a risk of pressure and skin breakdown. If the pressure area is under a cast, the cast must be removed in that area to relieve the pressure. Therefore, options 1 and 3 can be eliminated. Because extra padding over the area of the cast does no good either, option 4 can be eliminated next. This leaves putting a window in the cast as the correct answer. This will relieve the pressure in that one area without disrupting the cast. Review the complications of a cast and the treatments for complications if you had difficulty with this question.
Level of Cognitive Ability: Analysis
Client Needs: Physiological Integrity
Integrated Process: Nursing Process/Evaluation
Content Area: Adult Health/Musculoskeletal
Reference: Christensen, B., & Kockrow, E. (2006). *Adult health nursing* (5th ed., p. 171). St. Louis: Mosby.

802. **3**
Rationale: Risk factors associated with osteoporosis include a diet that is deficient in calcium. Options 1, 2, and 4 include risk factors associated with osteoporosis. Additional risk factors include being sedentary, cigarette smoking, excessive alcohol consumption, chronic illness, and long-term use of anticonvulsants and furosemide (Lasix).
Test-Taking Strategy: Note the strategic words "needs to read and learn about this disorder." These words indicate a negative event query and the need to select the incorrect student statement. Remember, risk factors associated with osteoporosis include a diet that is deficient in calcium. Review these risk factors if you are not familiar with them.
Level of Cognitive Ability: Comprehension
Client Needs: Health Promotion and Maintenance
Integrated Process: Teaching and Learning
Content Area: Adult Health/Musculoskeletal
References: Christensen, B., & Kockrow, E. (2006). *Foundations of nursing* (5th ed., p. 1106). St. Louis: Mosby.
Linton, A., & Maebius, N. (2007). *Introduction to medical-surgical nursing* (4th ed., p. 904). Philadelphia: Saunders.

803. **1**
Rationale: Foods high in calcium include plain yogurt, dairy products, seafood, sardines, green vegetables, calcium-fortified orange juice, and cereal. Of the items listed in the options, option 1 would contain the least amount of calcium.
Test-Taking Strategy: Note the strategic words "least amount of calcium." Recalling the foods that are high and low in calcium will direct you to option 1. Review foods high in calcium if you had difficulty with this question.
Level of Cognitive Ability: Application
Client Needs: Health Promotion and Maintenance
Integrated Process: Teaching and Learning
Content Area: Adult Health/Musculoskeletal
References: Linton, A., & Maebius, N. (2007). *Introduction to medical-surgical nursing* (4th ed., p. 906). Philadelphia: Saunders.

Schlenker, E. & Long, S. (2007). *Williams' essentials of nutrition & diet therapy* (9th ed., pp. 151-152). St. Louis: Mosby.

804. **4**
Rationale: The stiffness and joint pain that occur in osteoarthritis diminish after rest and intensify after activity, and they may be aggravated by cold, damp weather. No specific laboratory findings are useful in diagnosing osteoarthritis. Dull, aching pain occurs in the affected joints and, unlike rheumatoid arthritis, systemic manifestations are absent and joint involvement is not symmetrical. Morning stiffness, an elevated sedimentation rate, and a positive rheumatoid factor occur in rheumatoid arthritis.
Test-Taking Strategy: Use the process of elimination and knowledge about the differences between osteoarthritis and rheumatoid arthritis. Remember, dull, aching pain occurs in the affected joints in osteoarthritis. Review the characteristics of osteoarthritis if you had difficulty with the question.
Level of Cognitive Ability: Analysis
Client Needs: Physiological Integrity
Integrated Process: Nursing Process/Data Collection
Content Area: Adult Health/Musculoskeletal
Reference: Linton, A., & Maebius, N. (2007). *Introduction to medical-surgical nursing* (4th ed., p. 893). Philadelphia: Saunders.

805. **3**
Rationale: Soft tissue injuries such as sprains are treated by RICE (rest, ice, compression, elevation) for the first 24 hours after the injury. Ice is applied intermittently for 20 to 30 minutes at a time. Heat is not used in the first 24 hours because it could increase venous congestion, which would increase edema and pain.
Test-Taking Strategy: Note the strategic word "avoided." This word indicates a negative event query and the need to select the incorrect intervention. It is likely that sprains should be rested and elevated, so options 1 and 4 are eliminated. Use of an Ace wrap is also helpful in reducing the pain and swelling, so eliminate option 2. By the process of elimination, heat is the item to avoid in the first 24 hours. Review the measures to treat a sprain if you had difficulty with this question.
Level of Cognitive Ability: Application
Client Needs: Physiological Integrity
Integrated Process: Nursing Process/Planning
Content Area: Adult Health/Musculoskeletal
Reference: Linton, A., & Maebius, N. (2007). *Introduction to medical-surgical nursing* (4th ed., p. 231). Philadelphia: Saunders.

806. **4**
Rationale: After arthroscopy, the client can usually walk carefully on the leg once sensation has returned. The client is instructed to avoid strenuous exercise for at least a few days. The client may resume the usual diet. Signs and symptoms of infection should be reported to the physician.
Test-Taking Strategy: Note the strategic words "understands the instructions." Remember, the client is always taught the signs and symptoms of infection to report to the physician. Review home care instructions following arthroscopy if you had difficulty with this question.

Level of Cognitive Ability: Comprehension
Client Needs: Physiological Integrity
Integrated Process: Nursing Process/Evaluation
Content Area: Adult Health/Musculoskeletal
Reference: deWit, S. (2009). *Medical-surgical nursing: Concepts & practice* (p. 770). St. Louis: Saunders.

ALTERNATE ITEM FORMAT: MULTIPLE RESPONSE

807. **1, 2, 3**
Rationale: A plaster cast takes 24 to 72 hours to dry (synthetic casts dry in 20 minutes). The cast and extremity may be elevated to reduce edema. However, some authors report that this may impede circulation to the affected limb. A wet cast is handled with the palms of the hand until it is dry, and the extremity is turned (unless contraindicated) so that all sides of the wet cast will dry. A cool setting on the hair dryer can be used to dry a plaster cast (heat cannot be used on a plaster cast because the cast heats up and burns the skin). The cast needs to be kept clean and dry, and the client is instructed not to stick anything under the cast because of the risk of breaking skin integrity. The client is instructed to monitor the extremity for circulatory impairment such as pain, swelling, discoloration, tingling, numbness, coolness, or diminished pulse. The physician is notified immediately if circulatory impairment occurs.
Test-Taking Strategy: Focus on the subject—a plaster cast. Recalling that edema occurs following a fracture and recalling the complications associated with a cast will assist you in answering the question. Review cast care instructions if you had difficulty with this question.
Level of Cognitive Ability: Application
Client Needs: Physiological Integrity
Integrated Process: Teaching and Learning
Content Area: Adult Health/Musculoskeletal
References: deWit, S. (2009). *Medical-surgical nursing: Concepts & practice* (p. 788). St. Louis: Saunders.
Linton, A., & Maebius, N. (2007). *Introduction to medical-surgical nursing* (4th ed., p. 920). Philadelphia: Saunders.

REFERENCES

Black, J., & Hawks, J. (2005). *Medical-surgical nursing: Clinical management for positive outcomes* (7th ed.). Philadelphia: Saunders.

Chernecky, C., & Berger, B. (2008). *Laboratory tests and diagnostic procedures* (5th ed.). Philadelphia: Saunders.

Christensen, B., & Kockrow, E. (2006). *Adult health nursing* (5th ed.). St. Louis: Mosby.

Christensen, B., & Kockrow, E. (2006). *Foundations of nursing* (5th ed.). St. Louis: Mosby.

deWit, S. (2009). *Medical-surgical nursing: Concepts & practice*. St. Louis: Saunders.

Ignatavicius, D., & Workman, M. (2006). *Medical-surgical nursing: Critical thinking for collaborative care* (5th ed.). Philadelphia: Saunders.

Jarvis, C. (2008). *Physical examination & health assessment* (5th ed.). Philadelphia: Saunders.

Lewis, S., Heitkemper, M., Dirksen, S., & Bucher, L. (2007). *Medical-surgical nursing: Assessment and management of clinical problems* (7th ed.). St. Louis: Mosby.

Linton, A., & Maebius, N. (2007). *Introduction to medical-surgical nursing* (4th ed.). Philadelphia: Saunders.

Monahan, F., Sands, J., Neighbors, M., Marek, J., & Green, C. (2007). *Phipps' medical-surgical nursing: Health and illness perspectives* (8th ed.). St. Louis: Mosby.

Pagana, K., & Pagana, T. (2005). *Mosby's diagnostic and laboratory test reference* (7th ed.). St. Louis: Mosby.

Perry, A., & Potter, P. (2006). *Clinical nursing skills & techniques* (6th ed.). St. Louis: Mosby.

Schlenker, E., & Long, S. (2007). *Williams' essentials of nutrition & diet therapy* (9th ed.). St. Louis: Mosby.

CHAPTER 59

Musculoskeletal Medications

I. SKELETAL MUSCLE RELAXANTS (Box 59-1)
A. Description
1. Skeletal muscle relaxants act directly on the neuromuscular junction or act indirectly on the central nervous system (CNS)
2. Centrally acting muscle relaxants depress neuron activity in the spinal cord or brain
3. Peripherally acting muscle relaxants act directly on the skeletal muscles interfering with calcium release from muscle tubules, thus preventing the fibers from contracting
4. Skeletal muscle relaxants are used to prevent or relieve muscle spasms, to treat spasticity associated with spinal cord disease or lesions, for acute painful musculoskeletal conditions, and for chronic debilitating disorders such as multiple sclerosis, brain attacks (stroke), or cerebral palsy
5. Skeletal muscle relaxants are contraindicated in clients with severe liver, renal, or heart disease; these medications are often metabolized in the liver or excreted from the kidney
6. Skeletal muscle relaxants should not be taken with CNS depressants, such as barbiturates, opioids and alcohol; sedatives; hypnotics; or tricyclic antidepressants

B. Side effects
1. Dizziness and hypotension
2. Drowsiness and muscle weakness
3. Dry mouth
4. Gastrointestinal upset
5. Photosensitivity
6. Liver toxicity

C. Interventions
1. Obtain a medical history
2. Monitor vital signs
3. Monitor for CNS side effects
4. Assess for risk of injury
5. Assess involved joints and muscles for pain and mobility
6. Monitor liver function tests since hepatotoxicity can occur
7. Monitor renal function studies

8. Instruct the client to take the medication with food to decrease gastrointestinal upset
9. Instruct the client to report side effects
10. Instruct the client to avoid alcohol and CNS depressants
11. Instruct the client to avoid activities requiring alertness such as driving or operating equipment

D. Nursing considerations
1. Baclofen (Lioresal)
   a. Baclofen causes CNS effects such as drowsiness, dizziness, weakness, and fatigue and nausea; constipation; and urinary retention
   b. Administer with caution in the client with renal or hepatic dysfunction or a seizure disorder
   c. Baclofen can be administered by the physician through intrathecal infusion using an implantable pump or direct intrathecal administration over 1 minute
   d. Instruct the client with an implantable pump to maintain medication refill appointments to prevent the pump from emptying and experiencing sudden withdrawal symptoms (which could be life threatening)
2. Carisoprodol (Soma)
   a. Advise the client to take the medication with food to prevent gastrointestinal upset
   b. Instruct the client to report any rash or hypersensitivity to the physician
3. Chlorzoxazone (Paraflex, Parafon Forte, Remular-S)
   a. Monitor the client for hypersensitivity reactions such as urticaria, redness or itching, and possibly angioedema
   b. Chlorzoxazone may cause malaise and may cause the urine to turn orange or red
   c. Can cause hepatitis and hepatic necrosis
4. Cyclobenzaprine (Flexeril)
   a. Cyclobenzaprine is contraindicated in clients who have received monoamine oxidase inhibitors (MAOIs) within 14 days of initiation of cyclobenzaprine therapy, and in clients with cardiac disorders

877

BOX 59-1 **Skeletal Muscle Relaxants**

Baclofen (Lioresal)
Carisoprodol (Soma)
Chlorphenesin carbamate (Maolate)
Chlorzoxazone (Paraflex, Parafon Forte, Remular-S)
Cyclobenzaprine (Flexeril)
Dantrolene (Dantrium)
Diazepam (Valium)
Metaxalone (Skelaxin)
Methocarbamol (Robaxin)
Orphenadrine (Norflex)
Tizanidine (Zanaflex)

BOX 59-2 **Antigout Medications**

Allopurinol (Zyloprim)
Colchicine
Probenecid
Sulfinpyrazone (Anturane)

---

b. Cyclobenzaprine has significant anticholinergic (atropine-like) effects and should be used with caution in clients with a history of urinary retention, angle-closure glaucoma, or increased intraocular pressure
c. Cyclobenzaprine should be used only for short-term (2-3 weeks) therapy
5. Dantrolene (Dantrium)
a. Dantrolene acts directly on skeletal muscles to relieve spasticity
b. Liver damage is the most serious adverse effect
c. Liver function tests should be monitored before the initiation of treatment and during treatment
d. Dantrolene can cause gastrointestinal bleeding, urinary frequency, impotence, photosensitivity, rash, and muscle weakness
e. Instruct the client to wear protective clothing when in the sun
f. Instruct the client to notify the physician if rash, bloody or tarry stools, or yellow discoloration of the skin or eyes occurs
6. Diazepam (Valium)
a. Acts in the CNS to suppress spasticity; does not affect skeletal muscle directly
b. Sedation is a common side effect
7. Methocarbamol (Robaxin)
a. The parenteral form is contraindicated in clients with renal impairment
b. The parenteral form can cause hypotension, bradycardia, anaphylaxis, and seizures, especially when the medication is given too rapidly
c. Monitor IV site for extravasation, which can result in thrombophlebitis and tissue sloughing
d. Methocarbamol may cause the urine to turn brown, black, or green
e. Inform the client to notify the physician if blurred vision, nasal congestion, urticaria, or rash occurs
8. Tizanidine (Zanaflex) and metaxalone (Skelaxin): can cause liver damage

9. Orphenadrine (Norflex) has significant anticholinergic (atropine-like) effects and should be used with caution in clients with a history of urinary retention, angle-closure glaucoma, or increased intraocular pressure
II. ANTIGOUT MEDICATIONS (Box 59-2)
A. Description
1. Antigout medications reduce uric acid production and increase uric acid excretion (uricosuric) to prevent or relieve gout or to manage hyperuricemia
2. Nonsteroidal anti-inflammatory drugs (NSAIDs) are used for their anti-inflammatory effects and to relieve pain during an acute gouty attack (refer to Chapter 57 for information on NSAIDs)
3. Glucocorticoids may be prescribed to reduce inflammation during an acute gouty attack (refer to Chapter 45 for information on glucocorticoids)
4. Antigout medications should be used cautiously in clients with gastrointestinal, renal, cardiac, or hepatic disease
B. Side effects
1. Headaches
2. Nausea, vomiting, and diarrhea
3. Blood dyscrasias, such as bone marrow depression
4. Flushed skin and skin rash
5. Uric acid kidney stones
6. Sore gums
7. Metallic taste
C. Interventions
1. Assess serum uric acid levels
2. Monitor intake and output (I&O)
3. Maintain a fluid intake of at least 2000 to 3000 mL/day to avoid kidney stones
4. Monitor complete blood cell count and renal and liver function studies
5. Instruct the client to avoid alcohol and caffeine because these products can increase uric acid levels
6. Encourage the client to comply with therapy to prevent elevated uric acid levels, which can trigger a gout attack
7. Instruct the client to avoid foods high in purine as prescribed, such as wine, alcohol, organ meats, sardines, salmon, scallops, and gravy

8. Instruct the client to take the medication with food to decrease gastric irritation
9. Instruct the client to report side effects to the physician
10. Advise the client to minimize exposure to sunlight and have a yearly eye examination because visual changes can occur from prolonged use of allopurinol
11. Caution the client not to take aspirin with these medications because this could trigger a gout attack
12. Concurrent use of aspirin causes elevated uric acid levels; instruct the client to take acetaminophen (Tylenol)
D. Nursing considerations
1. Allopurinol (Zyloprim)
a. Can increase the effect of warfarin (Coumadin) and oral hypoglycemic agents
b. Instruct the client not to take large doses of vitamin C while taking allopurinol (Zyloprim) since kidney stones may occur
c. Hypersensitivity syndrome (rare) can occur, characterized by rash, fever, eosinophilia, and dysfunction of the liver and kidneys (medication is stopped and the physician is notified)
2. Colchicine
a. Used with caution in the older client, in the debilitated client, and in clients with cardiac, renal, and gastrointestinal disease
b. If gastrointestinal symptoms (nausea, vomiting, diarrhea, and abdominal pain) occur, the medication is stopped and the physician is notified
3. Probenecid
a. Mild gastrointestinal effects can occur and can be reduced by taking the medication with food
b. Aspirin and other salicylates interfere with the uricosuric action of the medication
4. Sulfinpyrazone (Anturane)
a. Contraindicated in clients with active ulcer disease and used with caution in clients with a history of ulcer disease
b. Salicylates counteract the uricosuric action of the medication
c. Inhibits hepatic metabolism of tolbutamide (Orinase), causing hypoglycemia, and of warfarin (Coumadin), causing bleeding tendencies
III. ANTIARTHRITIC MEDICATIONS (Box 59-3)
A. Description (Figure 59-1)
1. Rheumatoid arthritis occurs as inflammation progresses into the synovia, cartilage, and bone; if this inflammation is not controlled, it will lead to joint destruction, thus affecting client mobility and comfort

---

BOX 59-3   Antiarthritic Medications

Anakinra (Kineret)
Adalimumab (Humira)
Auranofin (Ridaura)
Aurothioglucose (Solganal)
Azathioprine (Imuran)
Cyclosporine (Neoral)
Etanercept (Enbrel)
Gold sodium thiomalate (Aurolate, Myochrysine)
Hydroxychloroquine sulfate (Plaquenil)
Infliximab (Remicade)
Leflunomide (Arava)
Methotrexate (Rheumatrex, Trexall)
Penicillamine (Cuprimine)
Sulfasalazine (Azulfidine)

---

2. The focus of treatment is early diagnosis and aggressive treatment in order to preserve joint function
3. Medication therapy includes NSAIDs, glucocorticoids, and disease-modifying antirheumatic drugs (DMARDs)
4. Gold salts: use of gold salts has decreased, but its purpose is to reduce the progression of joint damage caused from the arthritic processes; gold toxicity, which includes pruritis, rash, metallic taste, stomatitis, and diarrhea, can occur, and if toxicity occurs, dimercaprol (BAL in oil) may be prescribed to enhance gold excretion
B. NSAIDs: may be prescribed for their anti-inflammatory and analgesic effects (refer to Chapter 57 for information on NSAIDs)
C. Glucocorticoids: may be prescribed for their anti-inflammatory effects (refer to Chapter 45 for information on glucocorticoids).
D. Disease-modifying antirheumatic drugs (DMARDs)
1. Description
a. DMARDs are effective antirheumatic medications used to slow the degenerative effects of the disorder
b. DMARDs are usually prescribed secondary to NSAIDs in most arthritic treatment but are often the first choice in the treatment of severe arthritis
2. Common side effects of DMARDs include infection; injection site inflammation and pain, ecchymosis, and edema; pancytopenia and infection; fatigue, headache, nausea, vomiting, and flu-like symptoms; and allergic response
3. Interventions
a. Instruct the client to monitor for signs of infection and report signs to the physician
b. Monitor the injection site for signs of irritation, pain, inflammation, and swelling

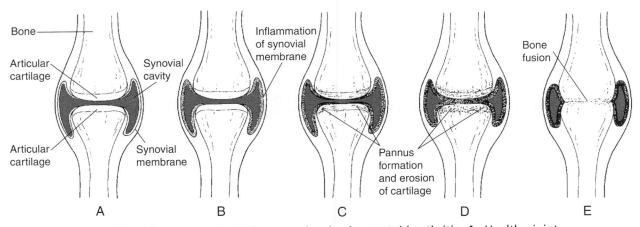

FIG. 59-1 Progressive joint degeneration in rheumatoid arthritis. **A,** Healthy joint. **B,** Inflammation of synovial membrane. **C,** Onset of pannus formation and cartilage erosion. **D,** Pannus formation progresses and cartilage deteriorates further. **E,** Complete destruction of joint cavity together with fusion of articulating bone. (From Lehne, R. [2007]. *Pharmacology for nursing care* [6th ed.]. Philadelphia: Saunders.)

   c. Instruct the client to consult with the physician before receiving live vaccines and to avoid exposure to infections

   d. Inform the client about the importance of laboratory tests for neutrophil counts, white blood cell counts, and platelet counts before initiation of treatment and during treatment

4. Anakinra (Kineret): injection site reactions are common (pruritus, erythema, rash, pain)

5. Adalimumab (Humira)
   a. Injection site reactions are common
   b. Has been associated with neurological injury (numbness, tingling, dizziness, disturbed vision, weakness in the legs)

6. Auranofin (Ridaura): an oral gold preparation

7. Gold sodium thiomalate (Aurolate, Myochrysine) and aurothioglucose (Solganal): intramuscular gold preparations

8. Azathioprine (Imuran): immunosuppressive and anti-inflammatory actions; toxicities include hepatitis and blood dyscrasias

9. Cyclosporine (Neoral): immunosuppressive actions; can cause nephrotoxicity

10. Etanercept (Enbrel)
   a. Injection site reactions are common
   b. Poses a risk for heart failure and has been associated with CNS demyelinating disorders and hematologic disorders

11. Hydroxychloroquine sulfate (Plaquenil): associated with retinal damage; inform the client to contact the physician if visual disturbances occur

12. Leflunomide (Arava): side effects include diarrhea, respiratory infection, reversible alopecia, rash, and nausea; is hepatotoxic

13. Methotrexate (Rheumatrex, Trexall): can cause hepatic fibrosis, bone marrow suppression, gastrointestinal ulceration, and pneumonitis

14. Penicillamine (Cuprimine): can cause bone marrow suppression and autoimmune disorders

15. Infliximab (Remicade): can cause infusion reactions (fever, chills, pruritus, urticaria, chest pain); is hepatotoxic

16. Sulfasalazine (Azulfidine) can cause gastrointestinal reactions, dermatological reactions, bone marrow suppression, hepatitis

IV. MEDICATIONS TO PREVENT AND TREAT OSTEOPOROSIS

A. Description

1. Osteoporosis is characterized by low bone mass and increased bone fragility

2. Calcium and vitamin D supplementation can reduce the risk of osteoporosis; calcium maximizes bone growth early in life and maintains bone integrity later in life and vitamin D ensures calcium absorption (refer to Chapter 45 for information on calcium and vitamin D supplements)

3. Treatment is aimed at reducing the occurrence of fractures by maintaining or increasing bone strength

4. Medications that decrease bone resorption (antiresorptive) and medications that promote bone formation are used

5. Antiresorptive medications include raloxifene (Evista), calcitonin, and bisphosphonates; bisphosphonates include alendronate (Fosamax), risedronate (Actonel), and ibandronate (Boniva)

6. Teriparatide (Forteo) promotes bone growth

B. Interventions
   1. Salmon calcitonin (Miacalcin, Calcimar, Osteocalcin)
      a. Calcitonin is secreted by the thyroid gland and inhibits osteoclastic bone resorption
      b. Instruct the client how to administer the intranasal or subcutaneous form, depending on the route prescribed
      c. Intranasal route: examine the nares for irritation; alternate nostrils for doses
      d. When calcitonin is taken, it is important to monitor for hypocalcemia
   2. Bisphosphonates (Box 59-4)
      a. Bisphosphonates inhibit osteoclast-mediated bone resorption, thereby increasing total bone mass
      b. Biphosphonates include alendronate (Fosamax), risedronate (Actonel), and ibandronate (Boniva)
      c. Contraindicated for clients with esophageal disorders that can impede swallowing and for clients who cannot sit or stand for at least 30 minutes (60 minutes with ibandronate [Boniva]
      d. Must be administered in the morning before eating or drinking with a full glass of water; the client must then remain sitting or standing for at least 30 minutes (60 minutes with ibandronate [Boniva])
      e. After taking the medication, the client is instructed to postpone ingesting anything for at least 30 minutes (60 minutes with ibandronate [Boniva])
      f. Adverse effects include esophagitis, muscle pain, and ocular problems; the client is instructed to contact the physician if adverse effects occur
   3. Raloxifene (Evista)
      a. An antiresorptive medication (non-bisphosphonate)
      b. Contraindicated in clients who have a history of venous thrombotic events
      c. Needs to be discontinued 72 hours prior to prolonged immobilization periods (such as with periods of extended bedrest)
      d. Instruct the client to avoid extended periods of restricted activity (such as with traveling)
   4. Teriparatide (Forteo)
      a. Teriparatide stimulates new bone formation, thus increasing bone mass
      b. Teriparatide is a portion of the human parathyroid hormone and works by increasing the action of osteoblasts
      c. Reserved for use in clients at high risk for fractures
      d. Has been associated with the development of bone cancer

---

BOX 59-4 Medications Used to Prevent or Treat Osteoporosis

Calcium and vitamin D
Alendronate (Fosamax)
Ibandronate (Boniva)
Raloxifene (Evista)
Risedronate (Actonel)
Salmon calcitonin (Miacalcin, Calcimar, Osteocalcin)
Teriparatide (Forteo)

PRACTICE QUESTIONS

More questions on the companion CD!

808. Baclofen (Lioresal) is prescribed for the client with multiple sclerosis. The nurse assists in planning care, knowing that the primary therapeutic effect of this medication is which of the following?
   1. Increased muscle tone
   2. Decreased muscle spasms
   3. Increased range of motion
   4. Decreased local pain and tenderness

809. A nurse is monitoring a client receiving baclofen (Lioresal) for side effects related to the medication. Which of the following would indicate that the client is experiencing a side effect?
   1. Polyuria
   2. Diarrhea
   3. Drowsiness
   4. Muscular excitability

810. A nurse is providing discharge instructions to a client receiving baclofen (Lioresal). Which of the following would the nurse include in the instructions?
   1. Restrict fluid intake.
   2. Avoid the use of alcohol.
   3. Notify the physician if fatigue occurs.
   4. Stop the medication if diarrhea occurs.

811. A client with acute muscle spasms has been taking baclofen (Lioresal). The client calls the clinic nurse because of continuous feelings of weakness and fatigue and asks the nurse about discontinuing the medication. The nurse should make which appropriate response to the client?
   1. "You should never stop the medication."
   2. "It is best that you taper the dose if you intend to stop the medication."
   3. "It is alright to stop the medication if you think that you can tolerate the muscle spasms."
   4. "Weakness and fatigue commonly occur and will diminish with continued medication use."

812. Dantrolene sodium (Dantrium) is prescribed for a client experiencing flexor spasms, and the client asks the nurse about the action of the medication. The nurse responds, knowing that the

therapeutic action of this medication is which of the following?
1. Depresses spinal reflexes
2. Acts directly on the skeletal muscle to relieve spasticity
3. Acts within the spinal cord to suppress hyperactive reflexes
4. Acts on the central nervous system (CNS) to suppress spasms

813. A nurse is reviewing the laboratory studies on a client receiving dantrolene sodium (Dantrium). Which laboratory test would identify an adverse effect associated with the administration of this medication?
1. Creatinine
2. Liver function tests
3. Blood urea nitrogen
4. Hematological function tests

814. A nurse is reviewing the record of a client who has been prescribed baclofen (Lioresal). Which of the following disorders, if noted in the client's history, would alert the nurse to contact the physician?
1. Seizure disorders
2. Hyperthyroidism
3. Diabetes mellitus
4. Coronary artery disease

815. Cyclobenzaprine (Flexeril) is prescribed for a client to treat muscle spasms, and the nurse is reviewing the client's record. Which of the following disorders, if noted in the client's record, would indicate a need to contact the physician regarding the administration of this medication?
1. Glaucoma
2. Emphysema
3. Hyperthyroidism
4. Diabetes mellitus

816. A client receives a prescription for methocarbamol (Robaxin) and the nurse provides instructions to the client regarding the medication. Which client statement would indicate a need for further instructions?
1. "My urine may turn brown or green."
2. "This medication is prescribed to help relieve my muscle spasms."
3. "If my vision becomes blurred, I don't need to be concerned about it."
4. "I need to call my doctor if I experience nasal congestion from this medication."

817. The client has been on treatment for rheumatoid arthritis for 3 weeks. During to the administration of Etanercept (Enbrel), it is most important for the nurse to assess:
1. The injection site for itching and edema
2. The white blood cell counts and platelet counts
3. If the client is experiencing fatigue and joint pain
4. A metallic taste in the mouth with a loss of appetite

818. Alendronate (Fosamax) is prescribed for a client with osteoporosis. The nurse instructs the client to:
1. Take the medication at bedtime.
2. Take the medication in the morning with breakfast.
3. Lie down for 30 minutes after taking the medication.
4. Take the medication with a full glass of water after rising in the morning.

819. A nurse is caring for a client who is taking allopurinol (Zyloprim). Which of the following medications, if prescribed for the client, would the nurse question?
1. Baclofen (Lioresal)
2. Pentazocine (Talwin)
3. Mebendazole (Vermox)
4. Warfarin sodium (Coumadin)

820. A nurse prepares to provide instructions to a client who is taking allopurinol (Zyloprim). The nurse plans to include which of the following in the instructions?
1. Instruct the client to drink 3000 mL of fluid per day.
2. Instruct the client to take the medication on an empty stomach.
3. Inform the client that the effect of the medication will occur immediately.
4. Instruct the client that, if swelling of the lips occurs, this is a normal expected response.

821. Colchicine is prescribed for a client with a diagnosis of gout. The nurse reviews the client's medical history in the health record, knowing that the medication would be contraindicated in which disorder?
1. Myxedema
2. Renal failure
3. Hypothyroidism
4. Diabetes mellitus

ALTERNATE ITEM FORMAT: MULTIPLE RESPONSE

822. In monitoring a client's response to disease-modifying antirheumatic drugs (DMARDs), which findings would the nurse interpret as acceptable responses? Select all that apply.
☐ 1. Symptom control during periods of emotional stress
☐ 2. Normal white blood cell counts, platelet, and neutrophil counts
☐ 3. Radiological findings that show nonprogression of joint degeneration
☐ 4. An increased range of motion in the affected joints 3 months into therapy
☐ 5. Inflammation and irritation at the injection site 3 days after injection is given
☐ 6. A low-grade temperature upon rising in the morning that remains throughout the day

ANSWERS

808. **2**

Rationale: Baclofen is a skeletal muscle relaxant and central nervous system depressant and acts at the spinal cord level to decrease the frequency and amplitude of muscle spasms in clients with spinal cord injuries or diseases and in clients with multiple sclerosis. Options 1, 3, and 4 are incorrect.

Test-Taking Strategy: Focus on the client's diagnosis. Recalling the action of this medication will direct you to option 2. Review this medication if you had difficulty with this question.

Level of Cognitive Ability: Analysis
Client Needs: Physiological Integrity
Integrated Process: Nursing Process/Planning
Content Area: Pharmacology
Reference: Skidmore-Roth, L. (2008). *2008 Mosby's nursing drug reference* (21st ed., p. 171). St. Louis: Mosby.

809. **3**

Rationale: Baclofen is a central nervous system (CNS) depressant and frequently causes drowsiness, dizziness, weakness, and fatigue. It can also cause nausea, constipation, and urinary retention. Clients should be warned about the possible reactions. Options 1, 2, and 4 are not side effects.

Test-Taking Strategy: Use the process of elimination. Recalling that baclofen is a CNS depressant used to treat muscle spasticity will direct you to option 3. If you had difficulty with this question, review the side effects of this medication.

Level of Cognitive Ability: Analysis
Client Needs: Physiological Integrity
Integrated Process: Nursing Process/Data Collection
Content Area: Pharmacology
Reference: Skidmore-Roth, L. (2008). *2008 Mosby's nursing drug reference* (21st ed., pp. 171-172). St. Louis: Mosby.

810. **2**

Rationale: Baclofen is a central nervous system (CNS) depressant. The client should be cautioned against the use of alcohol and other CNS depressants, because baclofen potentiates the depressant activity of these agents. Constipation rather than diarrhea is an adverse effect of baclofen. It is not necessary to restrict fluids, but the client should be warned that urinary retention can occur. Fatigue is related to a CNS effect that is most intense during the early phase of therapy and diminishes with continued medication use. It is not necessary that the client notify the physician if fatigue occurs.

Test-Taking Strategy: Recalling that baclofen is a CNS depressant will direct you to option 2. If you were unsure of the correct option, use general principles related to medication administration. Alcohol should be avoided with the use of medications. Review this medication if you had difficulty with this question.

Level of Cognitive Ability: Application
Client Needs: Physiological Integrity
Integrated Process: Teaching and Learning
Content Area: Pharmacology
Reference: Skidmore-Roth, L. (2008). *2008 Mosby's nursing drug reference* (21st ed., p. 172). St. Louis: Mosby.

811. **4**

Rationale: The client should be instructed that symptoms such as drowsiness, weakness, and fatigue are more intense in the early phase of therapy and diminish with continued medication use. The client should be instructed never to withdraw or stop the medication abruptly since abrupt withdrawal can cause visual hallucinations, paranoid ideation, and seizures. It is best for the nurse to inform the client that these symptoms will subside and encourage the client to continue the use of the medication.

Test-Taking Strategy: Use the process of elimination. Eliminate option 1 first because it is a rather extreme nursing response. Next, eliminate options 2 and 3 because these responses do not represent the scope of nursing practice or nursing actions. Review this medication if you had difficulty with this question

Level of Cognitive Ability: Application
Client Needs: Physiological Integrity
Integrated Process: Communication and Documentation
Content Area: Pharmacology
Reference: Skidmore-Roth, L. (2008). *2008 Mosby's nursing drug reference* (21st ed., p. 172). St. Louis: Mosby.

812. **2**

Rationale: Dantrium acts directly on skeletal muscle to relieve muscle spasticity. The primary action is the suppression of calcium release from the sarcoplasmic reticulum. This in turn decreases the ability of the skeletal muscle to contract. Options 1, 3, and 4 are not actions of the medication.

Test-Taking Strategy: Use the process of elimination. Options 1, 3, and 4 are all comparable or alike in that they address CNS suppression and the depression of reflexes. Therefore, eliminate these options. Review this medication if you had difficulty with this question.

Level of Cognitive Ability: Application
Client Needs: Physiological Integrity
Integrated Process: Nursing Process/Implementation
Content Area: Pharmacology
Reference: Skidmore-Roth, L. (2008). *2008 Mosby's nursing drug reference* (21st ed., pp. 328-329). St. Louis: Mosby.

813. **2**

Rationale: Dose-related liver damage is the most serious adverse effect of dantrolene. To reduce the risk of liver damage, liver function tests should be performed before treatment and periodically throughout the treatment course. It is administered in the lowest effective dosage for the shortest time necessary.

Test-Taking Strategy: Use the process of elimination. Eliminate options 1 and 3 because these tests both assess kidney function. From the remaining options, it is necessary to recall that this medication affects liver function. Review this medication if you had difficulty with this question.

Level of Cognitive Ability: Analysis
Client Needs: Physiological Integrity
Integrated Process: Nursing Process/Data Collection
Content Area: Pharmacology
Reference: Skidmore-Roth, L. (2008). *2008 Mosby's nursing drug reference* (21st ed., p. 329). St. Louis: Mosby.

814. **1**

Rationale: Clients with seizure disorders may have a lowered seizure threshold when baclofen is administered. Concurrent therapy may require an increase in the anticonvulsive medication. The disorders in options 3, 3, and 4 are not a concern when the client is taking baclofen.

Test-Taking Strategy: Knowledge regarding the contraindications and the cautions associated with the administration of baclofen is required to answer this question. Remember, a lowered seizure threshold can occur when baclofen is administered. If you are unfamiliar with these contraindications and cautions, review this content.

Level of Cognitive Ability: Analysis
Client Needs: Safe and Effective Care Environment
Integrated Process: Nursing Process/Data Collection
Content Area: Pharmacology
Reference: Skidmore-Roth, L. (2008). *2008 Mosby's nursing drug reference* (21st ed., p. 172). St. Louis: Mosby.

815. 1

Rationale: Because this medication has anticholinergic effects, it should be used with caution in clients with a history of urinary retention, angle-closure glaucoma, and increased intraocular pressure. Cyclobenzaprine hydrochloride should be used only for short-term 2- to 3-week therapy.

Test-Taking Strategy: Recalling that this medication has anticholinergic effects will assist in directing you to option 1. If you are unfamiliar with this medication and the contraindications associated with its administration, review this content.

Level of Cognitive Ability: Analysis
Client Needs: Safe and Effective Care Environment
Integrated Process: Nursing Process/Data Collection
Content Area: Pharmacology
References: Kee, J., Hayes, E., & McCuistion, L. (2006). *Pharmacology: A nursing process approach* (5th ed., p. 370). Philadelphia: Saunders.
Lehne, R. (2007). *Pharmacology for nursing care* (6th ed., pp. 240-241). Philadelphia: Saunders.

816. 3

Rationale: The client needs to be told that the urine may turn brown, black, or green. Other adverse effects include blurred vision, nasal congestion, urticaria, and rash. The client needs to be instructed that, if these adverse effects occur, the physician needs to be notified. The medication is used to relieve muscle spasms.

Test-Taking Strategy: Note the strategic words "need for further instructions." These words indicate a negative event query and the need to select the incorrect client statement. Recalling the adverse effects of this medication will direct you to option 3. If you had difficulty with this question, review this medication.

Level of Cognitive Ability: Analysis
Client Needs: Physiological Integrity
Integrated Process: Teaching and Learning
Content Area: Pharmacology
References: Kee, J., Hayes, E., & McCuistion, L. (2006). *Pharmacology: A nursing process approach* (5th ed., pp. 369-370). Philadelphia: Saunders.
Skidmore-Roth, L. (2008). *2008 Mosby's nursing drug reference* (21st ed., pp. 654-655). St. Louis: Mosby.

817. 2

Rationale: Infection and pancytopenia are side effects of etanercept (Enbrel). Laboratory studies are performed prior to and

during drug treatment. The appearance of abnormal white blood cell counts and abnormal platelet counts can alert the nurse to a potential life-threatening infection. Injection site itching is a common occurrences following administration of the medication. A metallic taste with loss of appetite are not common signs of side effects of this medication.

Test-Taking Strategy: Use the process of elimination. Option 4 can be eliminated since this is not a common side effect. In early treatment, residual fatigue and joint pain may still be apparent. Option 2 monitors for a hematologic disorder, which could indicate a reason for discontinuing this medication and should be reported. Review this medication if you had difficulty with this question.

Level of Cognitive Ability: Analysis
Client Needs: Physiological Integrity
Integrated Process: Nursing Process/Data Collection
Content Area: Pharmacology
Reference: Ignatavicius, D., & Workman, M. (2006). *Medical-surgical nursing: Critical thinking for collaborative care* (5th ed., p. 405). Philadelphia: Saunders.

818. 4

Rationale: Precautions need to be taken with administration of alendronate to prevent gastrointestinal side effects (especially esophageal irritation) and to increase absorption of the medication. The medication needs to be taken with a full glass of water after rising in the morning. The client should not eat or drink anything for 30 minutes following administration and should not lie down after taking the medication.

Test-Taking Strategy: Knowledge regarding the administration of alendronate is needed to answer this question. Recalling that this medication can cause esophageal irritation will direct you to option 4. Review this medication if you had difficulty with this question.

Level of Cognitive Ability: Application
Client Needs: Physiological Integrity
Integrated Process: Teaching and Learning
Content Area: Pharmacology
References: Ignatavicius, D., & Workman, M. (2006). *Medical-surgical nursing: Critical thinking for collaborative care* (5th ed., p. 1167). Philadelphia: Saunders.
Lewis, S., Heitkemper, M., & Dirksen, S. (2004). *Medical-surgical nursing: Assessment and management of clinical problems* (6th ed., p. 1711). St. Louis: Mosby.

819. 4

Rationale: Allopurinol is an antigout medication that may increase the effect of oral anticoagulants. Warfarin sodium (Coumadin) is an anticoagulant, and if this medication was prescribed for the client, the nurse would question the order. Baclofen is a skeletal muscle relaxant. Pentazocine is an opioid analgesic. Mebendazole is an anthelmintic.

Test-Taking Strategy: Knowledge regarding the medication interactions related to allopurinol is needed to answer this question. Remember, allopurinol will increase the effect of oral anticoagulants. If you had difficulty with this question, review the interactions associated with this medication.

Level of Cognitive Ability: Analysis
Client Needs: Safe and Effective Care Environment
Integrated Process: Nursing Process/Implementation
Content Area: Pharmacology

Reference: Lilley, L., Harrington, S., & Snyder, J. (2007). *Pharmacology and the nursing process* (5th ed., pp. 683; 688). St. Louis: Mosby.

820. 1

Rationale: Clients taking allopurinol are encouraged to drink 3000 mL of fluid a day. A full therapeutic effect may take 1 week or longer. Allopurinol is to be given with or immediately following meals or milk to prevent gastrointestinal irritation. If the client develops a rash, irritation of the eyes, or swelling of the lips or mouth, he or she should contact the physician since this may indicate hypersensitivity.

Test-Taking Strategy: Use the process of elimination. Option 4 can be eliminated first because it indicates a hypersensitivity, which is not a normal expected response. From the remaining options, recalling that this medication is used to treat gout will direct you to option 1. If you had difficulty with this question, review client instructions related to allopurinol.

Level of Cognitive Ability: Application
Client Needs: Physiological Integrity
Integrated Process: Nursing Process/Planning
Content Area: Pharmacology
Reference: Lilley, L., Harrington, S., & Snyder, J. (2007). *Pharmacology and the nursing process* (5th ed., p. 688). St. Louis: Mosby.

821. 2

Rationale: Colchicine is contraindicated in clients with severe gastrointestinal, renal, hepatic or cardiac disorders, or with blood dyscrasias. Clients with impaired renal function may exhibit myopathy and neuropathy manifested as generalized weakness. This medication should be used with caution in clients with impaired hepatic function, older clients, and debilitated clients.

Test-Taking Strategy: Use the process of elimination. Note that options 1, 3, and 4 are all endocrine-related disorders.

Option 2, the correct option, is different from the others. Review this medication if you had difficulty with this question.

Level of Cognitive Ability: Analysis
Client Needs: Physiological Integrity
Integrated Process: Nursing Process/Data Collection
Content Area: Pharmacology
Reference: Skidmore-Roth, L. (2008). *2008 Mosby's nursing drug reference* (21st ed., pp. 300-301). St. Louis: Mosby.

ALTERNATE ITEM FORMAT: MULTIPLE RESPONSE

822. 1, 2, 3, 4

Rationale: Because emotional stress frequently exacerbates the symptoms of rheumatoid arthritis, the absence of symptoms is a positive finding. DMARDs are given to slow progression of joint degeneration. In addition, the improvement in the range of motion after 3 months of therapy with normal blood work is a positive finding. Temperature elevation and inflammation and irritation at the medication injection site could indicate signs of infection.

Test-Taking Strategy: Use the process of elimination and focus on the subject—acceptable responses to therapy. Recalling that signs of an infection can indicate an unexpected finding will assist in eliminating options 5 and 6. Review the expected effects of this medication if you had difficulty with this question.

Level of Cognitive Ability: Analysis
Client Needs: Physiological Integrity
Integrated Process: Nursing Process/Data Collection
Content Area: Pharmacology
Reference: Lilley, L., Harrington, S., & Snyder, J. (2005). *Pharmacology and the nursing process* (4th ed., pp. 822-826). St Louis: Mosby.

REFERENCES

Ignatavicius, D., & Workman, M. (2006). *Medical-surgical nursing: Critical thinking for collaborative care* (5th ed.). Philadelphia: Saunders.

Kee, J., Hayes, E., & McCuistion, L. (2006). *Pharmacology: A nursing process approach* (5th ed.). Philadelphia: Saunders.

Lehne, R. (2007). *Pharmacology for nursing care* (6th ed.). Philadelphia: Saunders.

Lewis, S., Heitkemper, M., & Dirksen, S. (2004). *Medical-surgical nursing: Assessment and management of clinical problems* (6th ed.). St. Louis: Mosby.

Lilley, L., Harrington, S., & Snyder, J. (2007). *Pharmacology and the nursing process* (5th ed.). St. Louis: Mosby.

Linton, A., & Maebius, N. (2007). *Introduction to medical-surgical nursing* (4th ed.). Philadelphia: Saunders.

McKenry, L., Tessier, E., & Hogan, M. (2006). *Mosby's pharmacology in nursing* (22nd ed.). St. Louis: Mosby.

Skidmore-Roth, L. (2008). *2008 Mosby's nursing drug reference* (21st ed.). St. Louis: Mosby.

The Adult Client With an Immune Disorder

PYRAMID TERMS

acquired immunodeficiency syndrome a chronic illness caused by the human immunodeficiency virus (HIV) and characterized by the breakdown of the immune system

acquired immunity Immunity received passively from the mother's antibodies, animal serum, or production of antibodies in response to a disease; immunization produces active acquired immunity

allergy An abnormal, individual response to certain substances that normally do not trigger such an exaggerated reaction

cellular response A delayed response against slowly developing bacterial infections; also called delayed hypersensitivity

human immunodeficiency virus (HIV) A life-threatening virus that is transmitted from one person to another through blood and body fluids

humoral response An immediate response that provides protection against acute, rapidly developing bacterial and viral infections

immunodeficiency The absence or inadequate production of immune bodies

natural immunity Also called innate immunity; present at birth

Kaposi's sarcoma Skin lesions that occur in individuals with a compromised immune system

Lyme disease An infection acquired from a tick bite; ticks live in wooded areas and survive by attaching to a host

▲ PYRAMID TO SUCCESS

Pyramid points focus on the effects of and complications associated with an immune deficiency. Specific focus relates to the nursing care related to the disorder, the impact of the treatment or disorder, and client adaptation. Acquired immunodeficiency syndrome is a pyramid focus, along with protecting the client from infection, and preventing the transmission of infection to other individuals. Psychosocial issues relate to social isolation and the body-image disturbances that can occur as a result of the immune disorder. The Integrated Processes addressed in this unit include Caring, Clinical Problem-Solving Process (Nursing Process), Communication and Documentation, and Teaching and Learning.

CLIENT NEEDS

Safe and Effective Care Environment

Acting as an advocate related to the client's decisions
Addressing advance directives
Consulting with members of the health care team
Establishing priorities
Handling hazardous and infectious materials safely
Implementing standard and other precautions
Maintaining asepsis
Maintaining confidentiality regarding diagnosis
Obtaining informed consent for treatments and
    procedures
Preventing infection
Upholding client rights

Health Promotion and Maintenance

Ensuring that the client receives recommended
    immunizations
Implementing health screening measures
Monitoring for expected body-image changes
Preventing disease related to infection
Providing health promotion programs
Respecting client lifestyle choices

Psychosocial Integrity

Assisting in mobilizing appropriate support and
    resource systems
Assisting the client and family to cope
Assisting the client to cope, adapt, and problem-solve
    during illness or stressful events
Considering religious, spiritual, and cultural preferences

Discussing grief and loss related to death and the dying process

Promoting a positive environment to maintain optimal quality of life

Physiological Integrity

Managing pain

Managing medical emergencies

Monitoring for the expected and unexpected responses to treatments

Promoting nutrition

Protecting the client from infection

Providing basic care and comfort

Reviewing diagnostic test and laboratory test results

REFERENCES

Black, J., & Hawks, J. (2005). *Medical-surgical nursing: Clinical management for positive outcomes* (7th ed.). Philadelphia: Saunders.

Chernecky, C., & Berger, B. (2008). *Laboratory tests and diagnostic procedures* (5th ed.). Philadelphia: Saunders.

Christensen, B., & Kockrow, E. (2006). *Adult health nursing* (5th ed.). St. Louis: Mosby.

Christensen, B., & Kockrow, E. (2006). *Foundations of nursing* (5th ed.). St. Louis: Mosby.

deWit, S. (2009). *Medical-surgical nursing: Concepts & practice*. Philadelphia: Saunders.

Hodgson, B., & Kizior, R. (2008). *Saunders nursing drug handbook 2008*. Philadelphia: Saunders.

Ignatavicius, D., & Workman, M. (2006). *Medical-surgical nursing: Critical thinking for collaborative care* (5th ed.). Philadelphia: Saunders.

Kee, J., Hayes, E., & McCuistion, L. (2006). *Pharmacology: A nursing process approach* (5th ed.). Philadelphia: Saunders.

Lehne, R. (2007). *Pharmacology for nursing care* (6th ed.). Philadelphia: Saunders.

Lewis, S., Heitkemper, M., Dirksen, S., & Bucher, L. (2007). *Medical-surgical nursing: Assessment and management of clinical problems* (7th ed.). St. Louis: Mosby.

Linton, A., & Maebius, N. (2007). *Introduction to medical-surgical nursing* (4th ed.). Philadelphia: Saunders.

McKenry, L., Tessier, E., & Hogan, M. (2006). *Mosby's pharmacology in nursing* (22nd ed.). St. Louis: Mosby.

Monahan, F., Sands, J., Neighbors, M., Marek, J., Green, C. (2007). *Phipps' medical-surgical nursing: Health and illness perspectives* (8th ed.). St. Louis: Mosby.

National Council of State Boards of Nursing (eds.) (2008). *2008 Detailed Test Plan for the NCLEX-PN® Examination, National Council of State Boards of Nursing*. Chicago: Author.

National Council of State Boards of Nursing, Inc. Web site: http://www.ncsbn.org.

Perry, A., & Potter, P. (2006). *Clinical nursing skills & techniques* (6th ed.). St. Louis: Mosby.

Skidmore-Roth, L. (2008). *2008 Mosby's nursing drug reference* (21st ed.). St. Louis: Mosby.

CHAPTER 60

Immune Disorders

I. FUNCTIONS OF THE IMMUNE SYSTEM
A. The immune system provides protection against invasion from microorganisms from outside the body
B. The immune system protects the body from internal threats and maintains the internal environment by removing dead or damaged cells

II. IMMUNE RESPONSE
A. T- and B-cells
1. Lymphocytes migrate to lymphoid tissue where they wait to form sensitized lymphocytes for cellular immunity or antibodies for humoral immunity
2. Some B-cells lie dormant until a specific antigen enters the body, at which time they greatly increase in number and are available for defense
3. T-cells are responsible for rejection of transplanted tissue
4. T- and B-cells are necessary for a normal immune response
B. **Humoral response**
1. **Humoral response** is immediate
2. This type of response provides protection against acute, rapidly developing bacterial and viral infections
C. **Cellular response**
1. **Cellular response** is delayed and is called delayed hypersensitivity
2. This type of response is active against slowly developing bacterial infections and is involved in autoimmune response, some allergic reactions, and rejection of foreign cells

III. IMMUNITY
A. Natural immunity
1. Also called **innate** or native **immunity**
2. Present at birth and includes biochemical, physical, and mechanical barriers of defense as well as the inflammatory response
B. **Acquired immunity**
1. **Acquired** or adaptive **immunity** is received passively from the mother's antibodies, animal serum, or from the production of antibodies in response to a disease

2. Immunization produces active **acquired immunity**

IV. IMMUNIZATIONS (Refer to Chapter 38 for information about immunizations)

V. LABORATORY STUDIES
A. Antinuclear antibody (ANA) titer
1. ANA titer is a blood test used in the differential diagnosis of rheumatic diseases and to detect antinucleoprotein factors and patterns associated with certain autoimmune diseases
2. The test is positive at a titer of 1:20 or 1:40, depending on the laboratory
3. A positive result does not necessarily confirm a disease
4. The ANA titer is positive in most individuals diagnosed with systemic lupus erythematosus (SLE)
5. An ANA titer can be false positive in a small proportion of the normal population
B. Anti–double-stranded DNA (dsDNA) antibody test
1. The anti-dsDNA antibody test is a blood test done specifically to identify or differentiate DNA antibodies found in SLE
2. The test supports a diagnosis, monitors disease activity and response to therapy, and establishes a prognosis for SLE
3. Values
a. Negative: less than 70 units by enzyme-linked immunosorbent assay (ELISA)
b. Borderline: 70 to 200 units
c. Positive: greater than 200 units
C. Refer to Chapter 11 for testing related to **acquired immunodeficiency syndrome (AIDS)**
D. Skin testing
1. Description
a. The administration of an allergen to the surface of the skin or into the dermis
b. Administered by patch, scratch, or intradermal techniques
2. Interventions preprocedure
a. Discontinue systemic corticosteroids or antihistamine therapy 5 days before the test as prescribed

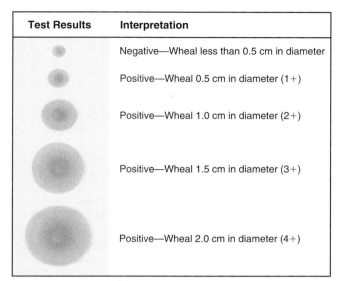

Test Results	Interpretation
	Negative—Wheal less than 0.5 cm in diameter
	Positive—Wheal 0.5 cm in diameter (1+)
	Positive—Wheal 1.0 cm in diameter (2+)
	Positive—Wheal 1.5 cm in diameter (3+)
	Positive—Wheal 2.0 cm in diameter (4+)

FIG. 60-1 Interpretation of intradermal allergy test results based on size of wheal after 15 to 30 minutes. (From Monahan, F., Sands, J., Neighbors, M., et al. [2007]. *Phipps' medical-surgical nursing: Concepts and clinical practice* [8th ed.]. St. Louis: Mosby.)

b. Obtain informed consent
c. Have resuscitation equipment available if a scratch test is performed since it may induce an anaphylactic reaction
3. Interventions postprocedure
a. Record the site, date, and time of the test
b. Record the date and the time for follow-up site reading
c. Inspect the site for erythema, papules, vesicles, edema and wheal (Figure 60-1)
d. Measure wheal and document size and other findings
e. Provide the client with a list of potential allergens, if identified

VI. IMMUNE DEFICIENCY
A. Description
1. **Immune deficiency** is the absence or inadequate production of immune bodies
2. The disorder can be congenital (primary) or acquired (secondary)
3. Treatment depends on the inadequacy of immune bodies and its primary cause
B. Data collection
1. Factors that decrease immune function
2. Frequent infections
3. Nutritional status
4. Medication history, such as use of corticosteroids for long periods
5. History of alcohol or drug abuse
C. Interventions
1. Protect the client from infection
2. Promote a balanced diet with adequate nutrition

3. Use strict aseptic technique for all procedures
4. Provide psychosocial care regarding lifestyle changes and role changes
5. Instruct the client in measures to prevent infection

VII. HYPERSENSITIVITY AND ALLERGY
A. Description
1. An **allergy** is an abnormal, individual response to certain substances that normally do not trigger such an exaggerated reaction
2. In some types of allergies, a reaction occurs on a second and subsequent contact with the allergen
3. Skin testing may be done to determine the allergen
4. Types of hypersensitivity reactions (Table 60-1)
B. Data collection
1. History of exposure to allergens
2. Itching, tearing, and burning of eyes and skin
3. Rashes
4. Nose twitching and nasal stuffiness
C. Interventions
1. Identification of the specific allergen
2. Management of the symptoms with antihistamines, anti-inflammatory agents, or corticosteroids
3. Ointments, creams, wet compresses, and soothing baths for local reactions
4. Desensitization programs may be recommended

VIII. ANAPHYLAXIS
A. Description
1. Anaphylaxis is a serious and immediate hypersensitivity reaction with the release of histamine from the damaged cells
2. Anaphylaxis can be systemic or cutaneous (localized)
B. Data collection (Figure 60-2)
C. Interventions
1. Establish a patent airway
2. Prepare for the administration of epinephrine (Adrenalin), diphenhydramine hydrochloride (Benadryl), or corticosteroids
3. Provide measures to control shock
4. Provide emotional support
5. Instruct the client to wear a Medic-Alert bracelet prior to discharge from emergent care
6. Instruct the client on the use of prescribed medication such as epinephrine (EpiPen) for immediate treatment of a future reaction

IX. LATEX ALLERGY
A. Description
1. Latex **allergy** is a hypersensitivity to latex
2. The source of the allergic reaction is thought to be due to the proteins in the natural rubber latex or the various chemicals used in the manufacturing process of latex gloves

TABLE 60-1   Types of Hypersensitivity Reactions

	Type	Causative Component	Pathologic Process	Reaction
I	Immediate/anaphylactic	IgE	Mast cell degranulation ↓ Histamine and leukotriene release	Anaphylaxis Atopic diseases Skin reaction
II	Cytolytic/cytotoxic	IgG IgM Complement	Complement fixation ↓ Cell lysis	ABO incompatibility Drug-induced hemolytic anemia
III	Immune complex	Antigen-antibody complexes	Deposition in vessels and tissue walls ↓ Inflammation	Arthus reaction Serum sickness Systemic lupus erythematosus Acute glomerulonephritis
IV	Cell-mediated/delayed	Sensitized T cells	Lymphokine release	Tuberculosis Contact dermatitis Transplant rejection

IG, Immunoglobulin.
From Black, J., & Hawks, J. (2005). *Medical-surgical nursing: Clinical management for positive outcomes* (7th ed.). Philadelphia: Saunders.

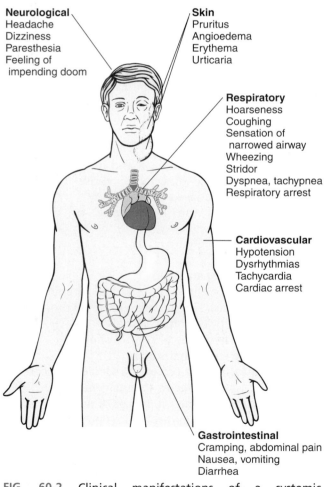

Neurological
Headache
Dizziness
Paresthesia
Feeling of
  impending doom

Skin
Pruritus
Angioedema
Erythema
Urticaria

Respiratory
Hoarseness
Coughing
Sensation of
  narrowed airway
Wheezing
Stridor
Dyspnea, tachypnea
Respiratory arrest

Cardiovascular
Hypotension
Dysrhythmias
Tachycardia
Cardiac arrest

Gastrointestinal
Cramping, abdominal pain
Nausea, vomiting
Diarrhea

FIG. 60-2 Clinical manifestations of a systemic anaphylactic reaction. (From Lewis, S., Heitkemper, M., & Dirksen, S. [2007]. *Medical-surgical nursing: Assessment and management of clinical problems* [7th ed.]. St. Louis: Mosby.)

3. Symptoms of the **allergy** can range from mild contact dermatitis to moderately severe symptoms of rhinitis, conjunctivitis, urticaria, and bronchospasm to severe life-threatening anaphylaxis

B. Common routes of exposure (Box 60-1)
  1. Cutaneous: natural latex gloves and latex balloons
  2. Percutaneous and parenteral: IV lines and catheters; hemodialysis equipment
  3. Mucosal: use of latex condoms, catheters, airways, and nipples
  4. Aerosol: aerosolization of powder from latex gloves can occur when gloves are dispensed from the box or when gloves are removed from the hands

C. At-risk individuals
  1. Health care workers
  2. Individuals who work in the rubber industry
  3. Individuals having multiple surgeries
  4. Individuals with spina bifida
  5. Individuals who wear gloves frequently such as food handlers, hairdressers, and auto mechanics
  6. Individuals allergic to kiwis, bananas, pineapples, tropical fruits, grapes, avocados, potatoes, hazelnuts, and water chestnuts

D. Data collection
  1. Anaphylaxis or Type I Hypersensitivity is a response to natural rubber latex (Figure 60-3; see Figure 60-2)
  2. A delayed Type IV Hypersensitivity can occur within 6 to 48 hours: symptoms of contact dermatitis include pruritus, edema, erythema, vesicles, papules, and crusting and thickening of the skin.

E. Interventions (Box 60-2)

BOX 60-1	**Products That May Contain Natural Rubber Latex**

Ace bandages (brown)
Adhesive or elastic bandages
Ambu Bag
Balloons
Blood pressure cuff (tubing and bladder)
Catheter leg bag straps
Catheters
Condoms
Diaphragms
Elastic pressure stockings
Electrocardiogram pads
Feminine hygiene pads
Gloves
Intravenous catheters, tubing, and rubber injection ports
Levin tubes
Pads for crutches
Prepackaged enema kits
Rubber stoppers on medication vials
Stethoscopes
Syringes

Note: Health care agencies use as many non-latex products as possible and have non-latex supplies available for clients with a latex allergy.

X. AUTOIMMUNE DISEASE

A. Description
 1. Body is unable to recognize its own cells as a part of itself
 2. Autoimmune disease can affect collagenous tissue
B. Systemic lupus erythematosus (SLE)
 1. Description
  a. A chronic progressive systemic inflammatory disease that can cause major organs and systems to fail
  b. Connective tissue and fibrin deposits collect in blood vessels on collagen fibers and on organs
  c. The deposits lead to necrosis and inflammation in blood vessels, lymph nodes, gastrointestinal tract, and pleura
  d. No cure for the disease is known
 2. Causes
  a. The cause of SLE is unknown, and SLE is thought to be due to a defect in the immunological mechanisms and have a genetic origin
  b. Precipitating factors include medications, stress, genetic factors, sunlight or ultraviolet light, and pregnancy
 3. Data collection
  a. Assess for precipitating factors
  b. Butterfly erythema or rash of the face
  c. Dry, scaly, raised rash on the face or upper body
  d. Fever

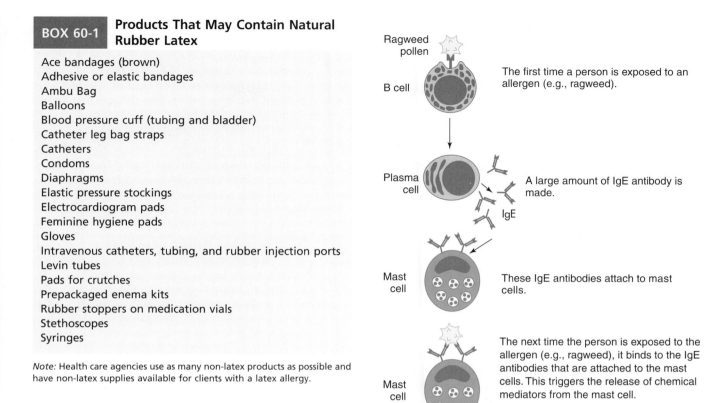

FIG. 60-3 Steps in a type I allergic reaction. (From Lewis, S., Heitkemper, M., & Dirksen, S. [2007]. *Medical-surgical nursing: Assessment and management of clinical problems* [7th ed.]. St. Louis: Mosby.)

BOX 60-2	**Interventions for the Client With a Latex Allergy**

Ask the client about a known allergy to latex when performing the initial assessment.
Identify risk factors to a latex allergy in the client.
Use non-latex gloves and all latex-safe supplies.
Keep a latex-safe supply cart near the client's room.
Apply a cloth barrier to the client's arm under a blood pressure cuff.
Use latex-free syringes, medication containers (glass ampules), and latex-safe intravenous equipment.
Instruct the client to wear a Medic-Alert bracelet.
Instruct the client about the importance of informing health care providers and local and paramedic ambulance companies about the allergy.

e. Weakness, malaise, and fatigue
f. Anorexia
g. Weight loss
h. Photosensitivity
i. Joint pain
j. Erythema of the palms
k. Anemia
l. Positive ANA test and lupus erythematosus (LE) preparation
m. Elevated sedimentation rate and C-reactive protein

4. Interventions
   a. Monitor skin integrity and provide frequent oral care
   b. Instruct the client to clean the skin with a mild soap, avoiding harsh and perfumed substances
   c. Assist with the use of ointments and creams for the rash as prescribed
   d. Identify factors contributing to fatigue
   e. Administer iron, folic acid, or vitamin supplements as prescribed if anemia occurs
   f. Provide a high-vitamin and high-iron diet
   g. Provide a high-protein diet if there is no evidence of kidney disease
   h. Instruct in measures to conserve energy, such as pacing activities and balancing rest with exercise
   i. Administer topical or systemic corticosteroids, salicylates, and nonsteroidal anti-inflammatory drugs as prescribed for pain and inflammation
   j. Administer medications to decrease the inflammatory response as prescribed
   k. Instruct the client to avoid exposure to sunlight and ultraviolet light
   l. Monitor for proteinuria and red blood cell casts in the urine
   m. Monitor for bruising, bleeding, and injury
   n. Assist with plasmapheresis as prescribed to remove autoantibodies and immune complexes from the blood before organ damage occurs
   o. Monitor for signs of organ involvement such as pleuritis, nephritis, pericarditis, coronary artery disease, hypertension, neuritis, anemia, and peritonitis
   p. Note that lupus nephritis occurs early in the disease process
   q. Provide supportive therapy as major organs become affected
   r. Provide emotional support and encourage the client to verbalize feelings
   s. Provide information regarding support groups and encourage the use of community resources

C. Scleroderma (systemic sclerosis)
   1. Description
      a. Scleroderma is a chronic connective tissue disease similar to SLE that is characterized by inflammation, fibrosis, and sclerosis
      b. This disorder affects the connective tissue throughout the body
      c. It causes fibrotic changes involving the skin, synovial membranes, esophagus, heart, lungs, kidneys, and gastrointestinal tract
      d. Treatment is directed toward forcing the disease into remission and slowing its progress
   2. Data collection
      a. Pain
      b. Stiffness and muscle weakness
      c. Pitting edema of the hands and fingers that progresses to the rest of the body
      d. Taut and shiny skin that is free from wrinkles
      e. Skin tissue is tight, hard, and thick, and it loses its elasticity and adheres to underlying structures
      f. Dysphagia
      g. Decreased range of motion
      h. Joint contractures
      i. Inability to perform activities of daily living
   3. Interventions
      a. Encourage activity as tolerated
      b. Maintain a constant room temperature
      c. Provide small frequent meals while eliminating foods that stimulate gastric secretions, such as spicy foods, caffeine, and alcohol
      d. Advise the client to sit up for 1 to 2 hours after meals if esophageal involvement exists
      e. Provide supportive therapy as the major organs become affected
      f. Administer corticosteroids as prescribed for inflammation
      g. Provide emotional support and encourage the use of resources as necessary

D. Polyarteritis nodosa
   1. Description
      a. Polyarteritis nodosa is a collagen disease and a form of systemic vasculitis that causes inflammation of the arteries in visceral organs, brain, and skin
      b. Treatment is similar to the treatment for SLE
      c. Polyarteritis nodosa affects middle-aged men
      d. The cause is unknown, and the prognosis is poor
      e. Renal disorders and cardiac involvement are the most frequent causes of death
   2. Data collection
      a. Malaise and weakness

b. Low-grade fever
c. Severe abdominal pain
d. Bloody diarrhea
e. Weight loss
f. Elevated sedimentation rate
3. Interventions
a. Provide supportive care as required
b. Provide a well-balanced diet
c. Administer corticosteroids and analgesics to control pain and inflammation
d. Provide emotional support and encourage the client to verbalize feelings
e. Initiate support services for the client
E. Pemphigus
1. Description
a. A group of related disorders including vulgaris, vegetans, foliaceus, and erythematosus
b. Pemphigus is a rare autoimmune disease that occurs predominately between middle and old age
c. The cause is unknown, and the disorder is potentially fatal
d. Treatment is aimed at suppressing the immune response that causes blister formation
2. Data collection
a. Lesions that appear as fragile flaccid bullae
b. Partial-thickness wounds that bleed, weep, and form crusts when bullae are disrupted
c. Debilitation, malaise, and pain
d. Chewing and swallowing difficulties
e. Nikolsky's sign: separation of the epidermis caused by rubbing the skin
f. Leukocytosis, eosinophilia, foul-smelling discharge from skin
3. Interventions
a. Provide supportive care
b. Provide oral hygiene and increase fluid intake
c. Soothe oral lesions
d. Assist with oatmeal or potassium permanganate baths or other soothing baths as prescribed for relief of symptoms
e. Administer topical or systemic antibiotics as prescribed for secondary infections
f. Administer corticosteroids and cytotoxic agents as prescribed to bring about remission
XI. GOODPASTURE'S SYNDROME
A. Description
1. Goodpasture's syndrome is an autoimmune disorder; autoantibodies are made against the glomerular basement membrane and alveolar basement membrane
2. Goodpasture's syndrome is most common in males and young adults that smoke, and the exact cause is unknown

3. The lungs and the kidneys are affected primarily, and the disorder is usually not diagnosed until significant pulmonary or renal involvement occurs
B. Data collection
1. Clinical manifestations indicating pulmonary and renal involvement
2. Shortness of breath
3. Hemoptysis
4. Decreased urine output
5. Edema and weight gain
6. Hypertension and tachycardia
C. Interventions
1. Focus on suppressing the autoimmune response with medications such as corticosteroids and with plasmapheresis (filtration of the plasma to remove some proteins) to remove the autoantibodies
2. Provide supportive therapy for pulmonary and renal involvement
XII. LYME DISEASE
A. Description
1. **Lyme disease** is an infection caused by the spirochete *Borrelia burgdorferi*, acquired from a tick bite (ticks live in wooded areas and survive by attaching to a host)
2. Infection with the spirochete stimulates inflammatory cytokines and autoimmune mechanisms
B. Data collection (Box 60-3)
C. Interventions
1. Gently remove the tick with tweezers, wash skin with antiseptic, and dispose of the tick by flushing it down the toilet; the tick may also be disposed of by placing it in a sealed jar so that the health care provider can inspect it and determine its type

---

BOX 60-3 Data Collection and Stages of Lyme Disease

First Stage
Symptoms can occur several days to months following the bite
A small red pimple develops that spreads into a ring-shaped rash.
Rash may be large or small or may not occur at all
Flu-like symptoms occur, such as headaches, stiff neck, muscle aches, and fatigue
Second Stage
This stage occurs several weeks following the bite
Joint pain occurs
Neurological complications occur
Cardiac complications occur
Third Stage
Large joints become involved
Arthritis progresses

2. Obtain a blood test 4 to 6 weeks after a bite to detect the presence of the disease (testing before this time is not reliable)
3. Instruct the client in the administration of antibiotics as prescribed if the disease is confirmed
4. Instruct the client to avoid areas that contain ticks, such as wooded grassy areas, especially in the summer months
5. Instruct the client to wear long-sleeved tops, long pants, closed shoes, and hats while outside
6. Instruct the client to spray the body with tick repellent before going outside
7. Instruct the client to examine the body when returning inside for the presence of ticks

XIII. **IMMUNODEFICIENCY SYNDROMES**
A. **Acquired Immunodeficiency Syndrome (AIDS)**
1. **AIDS** is a viral disease caused by **human immunodeficiency virus (HIV)** that destroys T cells, thereby, increasing susceptibility to infection and malignancy (Figure 60-4)
2. The syndrome is manifested clinically by opportunistic infection and unusual neoplasms
3. **AIDS** is considered a chronic illness
4. The disease has a long incubation period, sometimes up to 10 years or more
5. Manifestations may not appear until late in the infection

B. Diagnosis and monitoring the client with **AIDS**
1. Refer to Chapter 11 for diagnostic tests
2. Refer to Box 60-4 for tests used to evaluate the progression of **HIV** infection
C. High-risk groups
1. Heterosexual or homosexual contact with high-risk individuals
2. IV drug abusers
3. Persons receiving blood products
4. Health care workers
5. Babies born to infected mothers
D. Data collection
1. Malaise, fever, anorexia, weight loss, influenza-like symptoms
2. Lymphadenopathy of at least 3 months
3. Leukopenia
4. Diarrhea
5. Fatigue
6. Night sweats
7. Presence of opportunistic infections
8. Protozoal infections (*P. jiroveci* pneumonia [major source of mortality])
9. Neoplasms (**Kaposi's sarcoma**: purplish/red lesions of internal organs and skin), B-cell non-Hodgkin's lymphoma, cervical cancer
10. Fungal infections (candidiasis, histoplasmosis)
11. Viral infections (cytomegalovirus, herpes simplex)
12. Bacterial infections

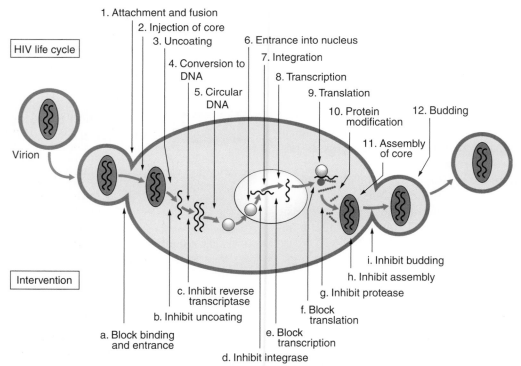

FIG. 60-4   The life cycle of HIV. (From Ignatavicius, D. & Workman, M. [2006]. *Medical surgical nursing: Critical thinking for collaborative care* [5th ed.]. Philadelphia: Saunders.)

E. Interventions
1. Provide respiratory support
2. Administer oxygen and respiratory treatments as prescribed
3. Provide psychosocial support as needed
4. Maintain fluid and electrolyte balance
5. Monitor for signs of infection
6. Prevent the spread of infection
7. Initiate standard precautions
8. Provide comfort as necessary
9. Provide meticulous skin care
10. Provide adequate nutritional support as prescribed
11. Refer to Chapters 22 and 38 for additional information on **AIDS**

F. **Kaposi's sarcoma**
1. Description: skin lesions that occur primarily in individuals with a compromised immune system
2. Data collection
   a. **Kaposi's sarcoma** is a slow-growing tumor that appears as a raised, oblong, purplish/reddish-brown lesion, and that may or may not be tender
   b. Organ involvement includes the lymph nodes, airways, or lungs, or any part of the gastrointestinal tract from the mouth to anus
3. Interventions
   a. Maintain standard precautions
   b. Provide protective isolation if the immune system is depressed
   c. Prepare the client for radiation therapy or chemotherapy as prescribed
   d. Administer immunotherapy, as prescribed, to stabilize the immune system

XIV. IMMUNODEFICIENCY POSTTRANSPLANTATION
A. Description
1. Secondary immunodeficiency is immunosuppression caused by therapeutic agents
2. The client must take immunosuppression agents for the rest of his or her life posttransplant to decrease rejection of the transplanted organ or tissue
B. Diagnosis and monitoring of posttransplant clients
1. Check renal and hepatic function
2. Monitor the complete cell count with differential to monitor for signs of infection
3. Assess all body secretions periodically for blood
C. High-risk clients
1. Clients with a history of malignancy or premalignancy have an increased susceptibility to malignancy if immunosuppressed
2. Clients with recent infection or exposure to tuberculosis, herpes zoster, or chickenpox have a high risk for severe generalized disease when on immunosuppressive agents
D. Data collection
1. Assess for signs of opportunistic infections
2. Assess nutritional status
3. Assess for signs of rejection (signs will depend on the organ or tissue transplant)
E. Interventions
1. Strict aseptic technique is necessary
2. Provide teaching regarding asepsis and the signs of infection and rejection
3. Provide psychosocial support as needed
4. Provide client teaching about immunosuppressants

BOX 60-4	Tests Used to Evaluate HIV Progression

Complete Blood Cell Count
WBC count normal to decreased
Lymphopenia (<30% of the normal number of WBCs)
Thrombocytopenia (decreased platelet count)
Lymphocyte Screen
Reduced CD4+/CD8+ T-cell ratio
CD4+ (helper) lymphocytes decreased
CD8+ lymphocytes increased
Quantitative Immunoglobin
IgG increased
IgA frequently increased
Chemistry Panel
Lactate dehydrogenase increased (all fractions)
Serum albumin decreased
Total protein increased
Cholesterol decreased
AST and ALT elevated
Anergy Panel
Nonreactive (anergic) or poorly reactive to infectious agents or environmental materials (e.g., pokeweed, phytohemagglutinin mitogens and antigens, mumps, *Candida*)
Hepatitis B Surface Antigen
To detect the presence of hepatitis C
Blood Cultures
To detect septicemia
Chest Radiograph
To detect *Pneumocystis jiroveci* infection or tuberculosis

ALT, Alanine aminotransferase; *AST*, aspartate aminotransferase; immunoglobulin; *WBC*, white blood cell.
From Copstead, L. & Banasik, J. (2005). *Pathophysiology* (3rd ed.). St. Louis: Mosby.

PRACTICE QUESTIONS

More questions on the companion CD!

823. Which of the following individuals is least likely at risk for the development of Kaposi's sarcoma?
1. A kidney transplant client
2. A male with a history of same-sex partners
3. A client receiving antineoplastic medications

4. An individual working in an environment where exposure to asbestos exists

824. The nurse prepares to give a bath and change the bed linens on a client with cutaneous Kaposi's sarcoma lesions. The lesions are open and draining a scant amount of serous fluid. Which of the following would the nurse incorporate in the plan during the bathing of this client?
1. Wearing gloves
2. Wearing a gown and gloves
3. Wearing a gown, gloves, and a mask
4. Wear a gown and gloves to change the bed linens and gloves only for the bath

825. A client is suspected of having systemic lupus erythematous. The nurse monitors the client, knowing that which of the following is one of the initial characteristic sign of systemic lupus erythematous?
1. Weight gain
2. Subnormal temperature
3. Elevated red blood cell count
4. Rash on the face across the bridge of the nose and on the cheeks

826. A client with pemphigus is being seen in the clinic regularly. The nurse plans care based on which of the following descriptions of this condition?
1. The presence of tiny red vesicles
2. An autoimmune disease that causes blistering in the epidermis
3. The presence of skin vesicles found along the nerve caused by a virus
4. The presence of red, raised papules and large plaques covered by silvery scales

827. The client is brought to the emergency department and is experiencing an anaphylaxis reaction from eating shellfish. The nurse implements which immediate action?
1. Maintaining a patent airway
2. Administering a corticosteroid
3. Administering epinephrine (Adrenalin)
4. Instructing the client on the importance of obtaining a Medic-Alert bracelet

828. The nurse is assisting in planning care for a client with a diagnosis of immune deficiency. The nurse would incorporate which of the following as a priority in the plan of care?
1. Protecting the client from infection
2. Providing emotional support to decrease fear
3. Encouraging discussion about lifestyle changes
4. Identifying factors that decreased the immune function

829. A client calls the nurse in the emergency department and tells the nurse that he was just stung by a bumblebee while gardening. The client is afraid of a severe reaction because the client's neighbor experienced such a reaction just 1 week ago. The appropriate nursing action is to:

1. Advise the client to soak the site in hydrogen peroxide.
2. Ask the client if he ever sustained a bee sting in the past.
3. Tell the client to call an ambulance for transport to the emergency room.
4. Tell the client not to worry about the sting unless difficulty with breathing occurs.

830. The nurse is assisting in administering immunizations at a health care clinic. The nurse understands that an immunization will provide
1. Protection from all diseases
2. Innate immunity from disease
3. Natural immunity from disease
4. Acquired immunity from disease

831. The nurse is assigned to care for a client with systemic lupus erythematosus (SLE). The nurse plans care knowing that this disorder is:
1. A local rash that occurs as a result of allergy
2. A disease caused by overexposure to sunlight
3. An inflammatory disease of collagen contained in connective tissue
4. A disease caused by the continuous release of histamine in the body

832. The nurse is assigned to care for a client admitted to the hospital with a diagnosis of systemic lupus erythematosus (SLE). The nurse reviews the physician's orders, expecting to note that which medication is prescribed?
1. Antibiotic
2. Antidiarrheal
3. Corticosteroid
4. Opioid analgesic

833. The community health nurse is conducting a research study and is identifying clients in the community at risk for latex allergy. Which client population is at most risk for developing this type of allergy?
1. Hairdressers
2. The homeless
3. Children in day care centers
4. Individuals living in a group home

834. The home care nurse is collecting data from a client who has been diagnosed with an allergy to latex. In determining the client's risk factors associated with the allergy, the nurse questions the client about an allergy to which food item?
1. Eggs
2. Milk
3. Yogurt
4. Bananas

835. A nurse is assigned to care for a client who returned home from the emergency department following treatment for a sprained ankle. The nurse notes that the client was sent home with crutches that have rubber axillary pads and needs instructions regarding crutch walking. On

data collection, the nurse discovers that the client has an allergy to latex. Before providing instructions regarding crutch walking, the nurse should:
1. Contact the physician.
2. Cover the crutch pads with cloth.
3. Call the local medical supply store and ask for a cane to be delivered.
4. Tell the client that the crutches must be removed from the house immediately.

836. The home care nurse is ordering dressing supplies for a client who has an allergy to latex. The nurse asks the medical supply personnel to deliver which of the following?
1. Elastic bandages
2. Adhesive bandages
3. Brown Ace bandages
4. Cotton pads and silk tape

837. The camp nurse prepares to instruct a group of children about Lyme disease. Which of the following information would the nurse include in the instructions?
1. Lyme disease is caused by a tick carried by deer.
2. Lyme disease is caused by contamination from cat feces.
3. Lyme disease can be contagious by skin contact with an infected individual.
4. Lyme disease can be caused by the inhalation of spores from bird droppings.

838. The client is diagnosed with stage I of Lyme disease. The nurse assesses the client for which characteristic of this stage?
1. Arthralgias
2. Flu-like symptoms
3. Enlarged and inflamed joints
4. Signs of neurological disorders

839. A female client arrives at the health care clinic and tells the nurse that she was just bitten by a tick and would like to be tested for Lyme disease. The client tells the nurse that she removed the tick and flushed it down the toilet. Which of the following nursing actions is most appropriate?
1. Refer the client for a blood test immediately.
2. Inform the client that there is not a test available for Lyme disease.
3. Tell the client that testing is not necessary unless arthralgia develops.
4. Instruct the client to return in 4 to 6 weeks to be tested because testing before this time is not reliable.

840. A Cub Scout leader who is a nurse is preparing a group of Cub Scouts for an overnight camping trip and instructs the scouts about the methods to prevent Lyme disease. Which statement by one of the Cub Scouts indicates a need for further instructions?
1. "I need to bring a hat to wear during the trip."
2. "I should wear long-sleeved tops and long pants."
3. "I should not use insect repellents because it will attract the ticks."
4. "I need to wear closed shoes and socks that can be pulled up over my pants."

841. The client with acquired immunodeficiency syndrome is diagnosed with cutaneous Kaposi's sarcoma. Based on this diagnosis, the nurse understands that this has been confirmed by which of the following?
1. Swelling in the genital area
2. Swelling in the lower extremities
3. Punch biopsy of the cutaneous lesions
4. Appearance of reddish-blue lesions on the skin

ALTERNATE ITEM FORMAT: MULTIPLE RESPONSE

842. Select the interventions that would apply in the care of a client at high risk for an allergic response to a latex allergy. Select all that apply.
☐ 1. Use non-latex gloves.
☐ 2. Use medications from glass ampules.
☐ 3. Place the client in a private room only.
☐ 4. Do not puncture rubber stoppers with needles.
☐ 5. Keep a latex-safe supply cart available in the client's area.
☐ 6. Use a blood pressure cuff from an electronic device only to measure the blood pressure.

ANSWERS
823. **4**
Rationale: Kaposi's sarcoma is a vascular malignancy that presents as a skin disorder and is a common acquired immunodeficiency syndrome indicator. It is seen frequently in men with a history of same-sex partners. Although the cause of Kaposi's sarcoma is not known, it is considered to be due to an alteration or failure in the immune system. The renal transplant client and the client receiving antineoplastic medications are at risk for immunosuppression.

Exposure to asbestos is not related to the development of Kaposi's sarcoma.
Test-Taking Strategy: Use the process of elimination. Note the strategic words "least likely at risk." Option 2 can be eliminated easily. Note that options 1 and 3 are comparable or alike. These clients are at risk for immunosuppression. With this in mind, these options can be eliminated. If you had difficulty with this question, review the risk factors associated with Kaposi's sarcoma.
Level of Cognitive Ability: Analysis

Client Needs: Physiological Integrity
Integrated Process: Nursing Process/Data Collection
Content Area: Adult Health/Immune
Reference: Black, J., & Hawks, J. (2005). *Medical-surgical nursing: Clinical management for positive outcomes.* (7th ed., p. 2393). Philadelphia: Saunders.

824. **2**
Rationale: Gowns and gloves are required if the nurse anticipates contact with soiled items, such as wound drainage, or while caring for a client who is incontinent with diarrhea or a client who has an ileostomy or colostomy. Masks are not required unless droplet or airborne precautions are necessary. Regardless of the amount of wound drainage, a gown and gloves must be worn.
Test-Taking Strategy: Use the process of elimination and think about the method of transmission of infection when answering a question of this type. Read the question, noting the task that is presented in this case is bathing and changing linens. Eliminate option 3 because the method of transmission is not respiratory. Eliminate options 1 and 4 because neither provides adequate protection based on the method of transmission. If you had difficulty with this question, review standard and transmission-based precautions.
Level of Cognitive Ability: Application
Client Needs: Safe and Effective Care Environment
Integrated Process: Nursing Process/Planning
Content Area: Adult Health/Immune
Reference: Potter, P., & Perry, A. (2005) *Fundamentals of nursing* (6th ed., p. 797). St. Louis: Mosby.

825. **4**
Rationale: Skin lesions or rash on the face across the bridge of the nose and on the cheeks is an initial characteristic sign of systemic lupus erythematosus (SLE). Fever and weight loss may also occur. Anemia is most likely to occur later in SLE.
Test-Taking Strategy: Use the process of elimination and note the strategic words "characteristic sign." Recalling the characteristic butterfly rash associated with SLE will direct you to option 4. If you are unfamiliar with this disorder, review this content.
Level of Cognitive Ability: Analysis
Client Needs: Physiological Integrity
Integrated Process: Nursing Process/Data Collection
Content Area: Adult Health/Immune
Reference: Linton, A., & Maebius, N. (2007). *Introduction to medical-surgical nursing* (4th ed., p. 607). Philadelphia: Saunders.

826. **2**
Rationale: Pemphigus is an autoimmune disease that causes blistering in the epidermis. The client has large flaccid blisters (bullae). Because the blisters are in the epidermis, they have a thin covering of skin and break easily, leaving large denuded areas of skin. On initial examination, clients may have crusting areas instead of intact blisters. Option 1 describes eczema, option 3 describes herpes zoster, and option 4 describes psoriasis.
Test-Taking Strategy: Use the process of elimination. Recalling that pemphigus vulgaris is an autoimmune disorder

will direct you easily to option 2. If you had difficulty with this question, review the characteristics of this disorder.
Level of Cognitive Ability: Comprehension
Client Needs: Physiological Integrity
Integrated Process: Nursing Process/Planning
Content Area: Adult Health/Immune
Reference: Linton, A., & Maebius, N. (2007). *Introduction to medical-surgical nursing* (4th ed., p. 1142). Philadelphia: Saunders.

827. **1**
Rationale: If the client experiences an anaphylactic reaction, the immediate action would be to maintain a patent airway. The client then would receive epinephrine. Corticosteroids may also be prescribed. The client will need to be instructed about obtaining and wearing a Medic-Alert bracelet, but this is not the immediate action.
Test-Taking Strategy: Focus on the strategic word "immediate." This strategic word tells you that you need to prioritize your nursing actions. Use the ABCs—airway, breathing, and circulation—to answer the question. Airway is always the priority. Review care to the client experiencing an anaphylactic reaction if you had difficulty with this question.
Level of Cognitive Ability: Application
Client Needs: Physiological Integrity
Integrated Process: Nursing Process/Implementation
Content Area: Delegating/Prioritizing
Reference: Christensen, B., & Kockrow, E. (2006). *Adult health nursing* (5th ed., p. 762). St. Louis: Mosby.

828. **1**
Rationale: The client with immune deficiency has inadequate or absence of immune bodies and is at risk for infection. The priority nursing intervention would be to protect the client from infection. Options 2, 3, and 4 may be components of care but are not the priority.
Test-Taking Strategy: Use Maslow's hierarchy of needs theory to answer the question. Remember that physiological needs are the priority. This will direct you to option 1. Review the care of a client with immune deficiency if you had difficulty with this question.
Level of Cognitive Ability: Application
Client Needs: Physiological Integrity
Integrated Process: Nursing Process/Planning
Content Area: Delegating/Prioritizing
Reference: Linton, A., & Maebius, N. (2007). *Introduction to medical-surgical nursing* (4th ed., p. 174). Philadelphia: Saunders.

829. **2**
Rationale: In some types of allergies, a reaction occurs only on second and subsequent contacts with the allergen. Therefore, the appropriate action would be to ask the client if he ever received a bee sting in the past. Option 1 is not appropriate advice. Option 3 is unnecessary. The client should not be told "not to worry."
Test-Taking Strategy: Use the steps of the nursing process to answer the question. Option 2 is the only option that addresses data collection. Review information related to allergic reactions if you had difficulty with this question.
Level of Cognitive Ability: Application

Client Needs: Physiological Integrity
Integrated Process: Nursing Process/Implementation
Content Area: Adult Health/Immune
Reference: Lewis, S., Heitkemper, M., Dirksen, S., & Bucher, L. (2007). *Medical-surgical nursing: Assessment and management of clinical problems* (7th ed., p. 1834). St. Louis: Mosby.

830. **4**

Rationale: Acquired immunity can occur by receiving an immunization that causes antibodies to a specific pathogen to form. Natural (innate) immunity is present at birth. No immunization protects the client from all diseases.
Test-Taking Strategy: Use the process of elimination and knowledge regarding immunity to disease to answer the question. Eliminate option 1 first because of the close-ended word "all." Next eliminate options 2 and 3 because they are comparable or alike. Review natural and acquired immunity if you had difficulty with this question.
Level of Cognitive Ability: Comprehension
Client Needs: Health Promotion and Maintenance
Integrated Process: Nursing Process/Implementation
Content Area: Adult Health/Immune
Reference: Linton, A., & Maebius, N. (2007). *Introduction to medical-surgical nursing* (4th ed., pp. 174-175, 594). Philadelphia: Saunders.

831. **3**

Rationale: SLE is an inflammatory disease of collagen contained in connective tissue. Options 1, 2, and 4 are not associated with this disease.
Test-Taking Strategy: Use the process of elimination. Eliminate option 1 because SLE is a systemic disorder, not a local one. Next eliminate option 4 because of its similarity to option 1. From the remaining options, select option 3 because of its systemic characteristic. If you are unfamiliar with this disorder, review its characteristics.
Level of Cognitive Ability: Comprehension
Client Needs: Physiological Integrity
Integrated Process: Nursing Process/Planning
Content Area: Adult Health/Immune
Reference: Christensen, B., & Kockrow, E. (2006). *Adult health nursing* (5th ed., p. 94). St. Louis: Mosby.

832. **3**

Rationale: Treatment of SLE is based on the systems involved and symptoms. Treatment normally consists of anti-inflammatory drugs, corticosteroids, and immunosuppressants. Options 1, 2, and 4 are not a standard component of medication therapy.
Test-Taking Strategy: Use the process of elimination. Recalling that SLE is an inflammatory disorder will direct you to option 3. If you are unfamiliar with the treatments normally prescribed in this disease, review this content.
Level of Cognitive Ability: Comprehension
Client Needs: Physiological Integrity
Integrated Process: Nursing Process/Planning
Content Area: Adult Health/Immune
Reference: Black, J., & Hawks, J. (2005). *Medical-surgical nursing: Clinical management for positive outcomes* (7th ed., p. 2355). Philadelphia: Saunders.

833. **1**

Rationale: Individuals at risk for developing a latex allergy include health care workers; individuals who work in the rubber industry; individuals having multiple surgeries; individuals with spina bifida; individuals who wear gloves frequently such as food handlers, hairdressers, and auto mechanics; and individuals allergic to kiwis, bananas, pineapples, tropical fruits, grapes, avocados, potatoes, hazelnuts, and water chestnuts.
Test-Taking Strategy: Focus on the subject—a latex allergy. Recalling the cause and the source of the allergic reaction will direct you easily to option 1. Review the cause of this type of allergy and the individuals at risk if you had difficulty with this question.
Level of Cognitive Ability: Comprehension
Client Needs: Health Promotion and Maintenance
Integrated Process: Nursing Process/Data Collection
Content Area: Adult Health/Immune
Reference: Ignatavicius, D., & Workman, M. (2006). *Medical-surgical nursing: Critical thinking for collaborative care* (5th ed., p. 461). Philadelphia: Saunders.

834. **4**

Rationale: Individuals who are allergic to kiwis, bananas, pineapples, tropical fruits, grapes, avocados, potatoes, hazelnuts, and water chestnuts are at risk for developing a latex allergy. This is thought to be due to a possible cross-reaction between the food and the latex allergen. Options 1, 2, and 3 are unrelated to latex allergy.
Test-Taking Strategy: Use the process of elimination and knowledge regarding the food items related to a latex allergy. Eliminate options 1, 2, and 3 because they are comparable or alike and relate to dairy products. Review the food items that are associated with a risk for latex allergy if you had difficulty with this question.
Level of Cognitive Ability: Comprehension
Client Needs: Physiological Integrity
Integrated Process: Nursing Process/Data Collection
Content Area: Adult Health/Immune
Reference: Christensen, B., & Kockrow, E. (2006). *Adult health nursing* (5th ed., p. 763). St. Louis: Mosby.

835. **2**

Rationale: The rubber pads used on crutches may contain latex. If the client requires the use of crutches, the nurse can cover the pads with a cloth to prevent cutaneous contact. Option 4 is inappropriate and may alarm the client. The nurse cannot order a cane for a client. In addition, this type of assistive device may not be appropriate considering this client's injury. No reason exists to contact the physician at this time.
Test-Taking Strategy: Use the process of elimination and knowledge regarding the alternative resources for a client with an allergy to latex. No data in the question support the need to contact the physician. The nurse should not prescribe assistive devices for the client. Option 4 is not a therapeutic action. Review care to the client with a latex allergy if you had difficulty with this question.
Level of Cognitive Ability: Application
Client Needs: Physiological Integrity

Integrated Process: Nursing Process/Implementation
Content Area: Adult Health/Immune
Reference: Lewis, S., Heitkemper, M., Dirksen, S., & Bucher, L., (2007). *Medical-surgical nursing: Assessment and management of clinical problems* (7th ed., p. 232). St. Louis: Mosby.

836. **4**

Rationale: Cotton pads and plastic or silk tape are latex-free products. The items identified in options 1, 2, and 3 are products that contain latex.
Test-Taking Strategy: Use the process of elimination and knowledge regarding the products that contain latex to answer this question. Eliminate options 1 and 3 first because they are comparable or alike. Noting the strategic words "cotton" and "silk" in option 4 will assist in answering correctly from the remaining options. Review the list of products that contain latex if you had difficulty with this question.
Level of Cognitive Ability: Application
Client Needs: Physiological Integrity
Integrated Process: Nursing Process/Implementation
Content Area: Adult Health/Immune
Reference: Ignatavicius, D., & Workman, M. (2006). *Medical-surgical nursing: Critical thinking for collaborative care* (5th ed., p. 461). Philadelphia: Saunders.

837. **1**

Rationale: Lyme disease is a multisystem infection that results from a bite by a tick carried by several species of deer. Persons bitten by *Ixodes* ticks can be infected with the spirochete *Borrelia burgdorferi*. Lyme disease cannot be transmitted from one person to another. Histoplasmosis is caused by the inhalation of spores from bat or bird droppings. Toxoplasmosis is caused from the ingestion of cysts from contaminated cat feces.
Test-Taking Strategy: Use the process of elimination. Recalling that this disease is caused by a bite will assist in eliminating the incorrect options. If you had difficulty with this question, review the cause of Lyme disease.
Level of Cognitive Ability: Application
Client Needs: Health Promotion and Maintenance
Integrated Process: Teaching and Learning
Content Area: Adult Health/Immune
Reference: Ignatavicius, D., & Workman, M. (2006). *Medical-surgical nursing: Critical thinking for collaborative care* (5th ed., p. 418). Philadelphia: Saunders.

838. **2**

Rationale: The hallmark of stage I is the development of a skin rash within 2 to 30 days of infection, generally at the site of the tick bite. The rash develops into a concentric ring, giving it a bull's-eye appearance. The lesion enlarges up to 50 to 60 cm, and smaller lesions develop farther away from the original tick bite. In stage I, most infected persons develop flu-like symptoms that last 7 to 10 days; these symptoms may reoccur later. Neurological deficits occur in stage II. Arthralgias and joint enlargements are most likely to occur in stage III.
Test-Taking Strategy: Use the process of elimination and eliminate options 1 and 3 first because they are comparable or alike. Next, note that the question asks for the characteristic of

stage I. From the remaining two options, select the least serious one because the subject of the question relates to stage I. Expect neurological disorders to occur with progression of the disease. If you had difficulty with this question, review the stages of Lyme disease.
Level of Cognitive Ability: Comprehension
Client Needs: Physiological Integrity
Integrated Process: Nursing Process/Data Collection
Content Area: Adult Health/Immune
Reference: Ignatavicius, D., & Workman, M. (2006). *Medical-surgical nursing: Critical thinking for collaborative care* (5th ed., p. 418). Philadelphia: Saunders.

839. **4**

Rationale: A blood test is available to detect Lyme disease; however, the test is not reliable if performed before 4 to 6 weeks following the tick bite. Antibody formation takes place in the following manner: immunoglobulin M is detected 3 to 4 weeks after Lyme disease onset, peaks at 6 to 8 weeks, and then gradually disappears; immunoglobulin G is detected 2 to 3 months after infection and may remain elevated for years. Options 1, 2, and 3 are incorrect.
Test-Taking Strategy: Use the process of elimination. Eliminate option 1 first. The word "immediately" should indicate that this is potentially an incorrect option. A blood test is available; therefore, eliminate option 2. Eliminate option 3 because treatment should begin before the arthralgia develops. If you had difficulty with this question, review the method of diagnosing Lyme disease.
Level of Cognitive Ability: Application
Client Needs: Physiological Integrity
Integrated Process: Nursing Process/Implementation
Content Area: Adult Health/Immune
Reference: Ignatavicius, D., & Workman, M. (2006). *Medical-surgical nursing: Critical thinking for collaborative care* (5th ed., p. 418). Philadelphia: Saunders.

840. **3**

Rationale: In the prevention of Lyme disease, individuals need to be instructed to use an insect repellent on the skin and clothes when in an area where ticks are likely to be found. Long-sleeve tops and long pants, closed shoes, and a hat or cap should be worn. If possible, one should avoid heavily wooded areas or areas with thick underbrush. Socks can be pulled up and over the pant legs to prevent ticks from entering under clothing.
Test-Taking Strategy: Use the process of elimination and note the strategic words "need for further instructions." These words indicate a negative event query and ask you to select an option that is an incorrect statement. Note that option 3 uses the words "should not." Reading carefully will assist in directing you to this option. If you had difficulty with this question, review the measures to prevent contact with ticks.
Level of Cognitive Ability: Analysis
Client Needs: Safe and Effective Care Environment
Integrated Process: Teaching and Learning
Content Area: Adult Health/Immune
Reference: Ignatavicius, D., & Workman, M. (2006). *Medical-surgical nursing: Critical thinking for collaborative care* (5th ed., p. 418). Philadelphia: Saunders.

841. 3

Rationale: Kaposi's sarcoma lesions begin as red, dark blue, or purple macules on the lower legs that change into plaques. These large plaques ulcerate or open and drain. The lesions spread by metastasis through the upper body and then to the face and oral mucosa. They can move to the lymphatic system, lungs, and gastrointestinal tract. Late disease results in swelling and pain in the lower extremities, penis, scrotum, or face. Diagnosis is made by punch biopsy of cutaneous lesions and biopsy of pulmonary and gastrointestinal lesions.

Test-Taking Strategy: Use the process of elimination. Eliminate options 1 and 2 first because these symptoms occur late in the development of Kaposi's sarcoma. From the remaining options, note the strategic word "confirmed." This strategic word will assist in directing you to the option that will confirm the diagnosis: the biopsy of the lesions. Review diagnostic measures for Kaposi's sarcoma if you had difficulty with this question.

Level of Cognitive Ability: Analysis
Client Needs: Physiological Integrity
Integrated Process: Nursing Process/Data Collection
Content Area: Adult Health/Immune
References: Black, J., & Hawks, J. (2005). *Medical-surgical nursing: Clinical management for positive outcomes* (7th ed., p. 2393). Philadelphia: Saunders.
Huether, S., & McCance, K. (2004). *Understanding pathophysiology* (3rd ed., p. 1157). St. Louis: Mosby.

ALTERNATE ITEM FORMAT: MULTIPLE RESPONSE

842. **1, 2, 4, 5**

Rationale: If a client is allergic to latex and is at high risk for an allergic response, the nurse would use non-latex gloves and latex-safe supplies and would keep a latex-safe supply cart available in the client's area. Any supplies or materials that contain latex would be avoided. These include blood pressure cuffs, medications with a rubber stopper that requires puncture with a needle, latex-safe syringes, and latex-safe intravenous tubing. It is not necessary to place the client in a private room.

Test-Taking Strategy: Focus on the subject—the client is at high risk for an allergic response to a latex allergy. Recalling that items that contain rubber are likely to contain latex will direct you to the correct interventions. Also noting the close-ended word "only" in options 3 and 6 will assist in eliminating these options. Review care to the client with a latex allergy if you had difficulty with this question.

Level of Cognitive Ability: Application
Client Needs: Safe and Effective Care Environment
Integrated Process: Nursing Process/Implementation
Content Area: Adult Health/Immune
Reference: Harkreader, H., & Hogan, M.A. (2004). *Fundamentals of nursing: caring and clinical judgment* (2nd ed., p. 1221). Philadelphia: Saunders.

REFERENCES

Black, J., & Hawks, J. (2005). *Medical-surgical nursing: Clinical management for positive outcomes* (7th ed.). Philadelphia: Saunders.

Christensen, B., & Kockrow, E. (2006). *Adult health nursing* (5th ed.). St. Louis: Mosby.

Harkreader, H., & Hogan, M.A. (2004). *Fundamentals of nursing: Caring and clinical judgment* (2nd ed.). Philadelphia: Saunders.

Huether, S., & McCance, K. (2004). *Understanding pathophysiology* (3rd ed.). St. Louis: Mosby.

Ignatavicius, D., & Workman, M. (2006). *Medical-surgical nursing: Critical thinking for collaborative care* (5th ed.). Philadelphia: Saunders.

Lewis, S., Heitkemper, M., Dirksen, S., & Bucher, L. (2007). *Medical-surgical nursing: Assessment and management of clinical problems* (7th ed.). St. Louis: Mosby.

Linton, A., & Maebius, N. (2007). *Introduction to medical-surgical nursing* (4th ed.). Philadelphia: Saunders.

Potter, P., & Perry, A. (2005). *Fundamentals of nursing* (6th ed.). St. Louis: Mosby.

Immunological Medications

I. HUMAN IMMUNODEFICIENCY VIRUS (HIV) AND ACQUIRED IMMUNODEFICIENCY SYNDROME (AIDS)

A. Medications include nucleoside/nucleotide reverse transcriptase inhibitors, non-nucleoside reverse transcriptase inhibitors, protease inhibitors, and fusion inhibitors (Box 61-1 and Figure 61-1).

B. Nucleoside/nucleotide reverse transcriptase inhibitors and non-nucleoside reverse transcriptase inhibitors work by inhibiting the activity of reverse transcriptase

C. Protease inhibitors work by interfering with the activity of the enzyme protease

D. Fusion inhibitors work by inhibiting the binding of **human immunodeficiency virus (HIV)** to cells

E. Standard treatment consists of using three or four medications in regimens known as highly active antiretroviral therapy (HAART); this therapy is not curative but can delay or reverse loss of immune function, preserve health, and prolong life

F. Example of a recommended regimen for initial therapy of established HIV infection (Box 61-2)

G. Other medications include those that are used to treat complications or opportunistic infections that develop (see Box 61-1).

H. Nucleoside/nucleotide reverse transcriptase inhibitors

1. Abacavir (Ziagen): can cause nausea; monitor for hypersensitivity reaction, including fever, nausea, vomiting, diarrhea, lethargy, malaise, sore throat, shortness of breath, cough, and rash

2. Abacavir/lamivudine (Epzicom): in addition to the effects that can occur from abacavir and lamivudine, hypersensitivity reactions, lactic acidosis, and severe hepatomegaly can occur

3. Didanosine (Videx): can cause nausea, diarrhea, peripheral neuropathy, hepatotoxicity, and pancreatitis

4. Emtricitabine (Emtriva): can cause headache, diarrhea, nausea, rash, hyperpigmentation of the palms and soles, lactic acidosis, and severe hepatomegaly

---

BOX 61-1 Medications for HIV and AIDS

Nucleoside/Nucleotide Reverse Transcriptase Inhibitors
Abacavir (Ziagen)
Abacavir/lamivudine (Epzicom)
Didanosine (Videx)
Emtricitabine (Emtriva)
Emtricitabine/tenofovir (Truvada)
Lamivudine (Epivir)
Lamivudine/zidovudine (Combivir)
Lamivudine/zidovudine/abacavir (Trizivir)
Stavudine (d4t, Zerit)
Tenofovir (Viread)
Zalcitabine (ddC, HIVID)
Zidovudine (Retrovir, Azidothymidine, AZT, ZDV)

Non-Nucleoside Reverse Transcriptase Inhibitors
Delavirdine (Rescriptor)
Efavirenz (Sustiva)
Nevirapine (Viramune)

Protease Inhibitors
Amprenavir (Agenerase)
Atazanavir (Reyataz)
Fosamprenavir (Lexiva)
Indinavir (Crixivan)
Lopinavir/ritonavir (Kaletra)
Nelfinavir (Viracept)
Ritonavir (Norvir)
Saquinavir (Invirase)
Tipranavir (Aptivus)

Fusion Inhibitor
Enfuvirtide (Fuzeon)

Anti-inflammatory Medication
Sulfasalazine (Azulfidine)

Anti-infective Medications
Atovaquone (Mepron)
Metronidazole (Flagyl)
Pentamidine isethionate (Pentam 300)
Sulfamethoxazole/Trimethoprim (Bactrim)

Antifungal Medications
Amphotericin B (Fungizone)
Fluconazole (Diflucan)
Ketoconazole (Nizoral)

Antiviral Medications
Acyclovir (Zovirax)
Foscarnet (Foscavir)
Ganciclovir (Cytovene)

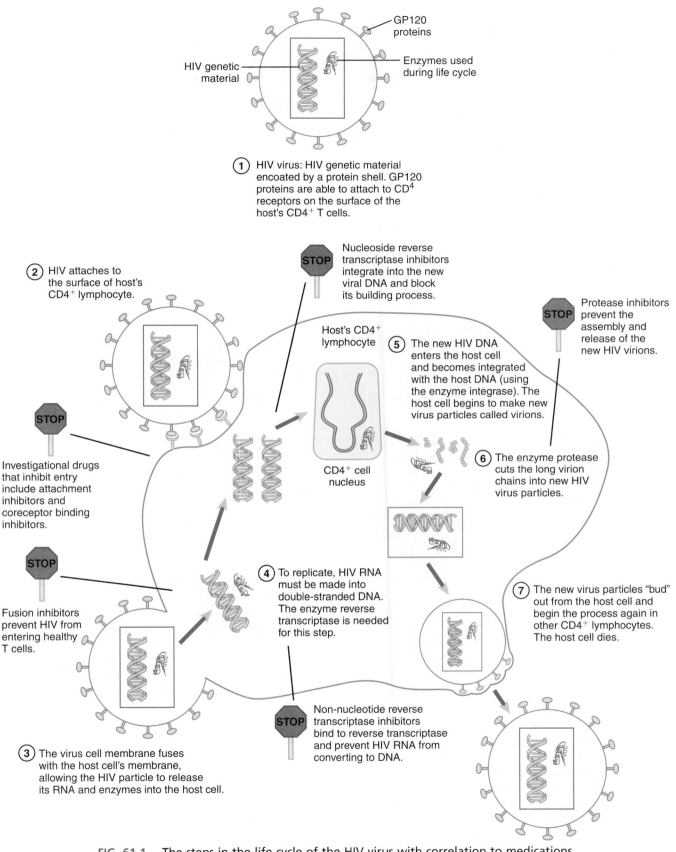

① HIV virus: HIV genetic material encoated by a protein shell. GP120 proteins are able to attach to CD⁴ receptors on the surface of the host's CD4⁺ T cells.

GP120 proteins

HIV genetic material

Enzymes used during life cycle

② HIV attaches to the surface of host's CD4⁺ lymphocyte.

STOP Nucleoside reverse transcriptase inhibitors integrate into the new viral DNA and block its building process.

STOP Protease inhibitors prevent the assembly and release of the new HIV virions.

Host's CD4⁺ lymphocyte

⑤ The new HIV DNA enters the host cell and becomes integrated with the host DNA (using the enzyme integrase). The host cell begins to make new virus particles called virions.

STOP Investigational drugs that inhibit entry include attachment inhibitors and coreceptor binding inhibitors.

CD4⁺ cell nucleus

⑥ The enzyme protease cuts the long virion chains into new HIV virus particles.

STOP Fusion inhibitors prevent HIV from entering healthy T cells.

④ To replicate, HIV RNA must be made into double-stranded DNA. The enzyme reverse transcriptase is needed for this step.

⑦ The new virus particles "bud" out from the host cell and begin the process again in other CD4⁺ lymphocytes. The host cell dies.

STOP Non-nucleotide reverse transcriptase inhibitors bind to reverse transcriptase and prevent HIV RNA from converting to DNA.

③ The virus cell membrane fuses with the host cell's membrane, allowing the HIV particle to release its RNA and enzymes into the host cell.

FIG. 61-1   The steps in the life cycle of the HIV virus with correlation to medications. (From Black, J., & Hawks, J. [2009]. *Medical-surgical nursing: Clinical management for positive outcomes* [8th ed.]. Philadelphia: Saunders.)

Regimens for Initial Therapy of Established HIV Infection

All regimens contain three antiretroviral drugs: NNRTI-based regimens contain an NNRTI combined with 2 NRTIs; PI-based regimens contain a PI combined with 2 NRTIs; and one regimen contains 3 NRTIs.

Preferred Regimens
NNRTI-Based
Efavirenz* + (lamivudine or emtricitabine) + (zidovudine or tenofovir)
PI-Based
Lopinavir/ritonavir [Kaletra]†+ (lamivudine or emtricitabine) + zidovudine

Alternative Regimens
NNRTI-Based
Efavirenz* + (lamivudine or emtricitabine) + (abacavir, didanosine, or stavudine)
Nevirapine + (lamivudine or emtricitabine) + (abacavir, didanosine, stavudine, tenofovir, or zidovudine)
PI-Based
Atazanavir + (lamivudine or emtricitabine) + (abacavir, didanosine, stavudine, or zidovudine) or (tenofovir + ritonavir, 100 mg/day)
Fosamprenavir + (lamivudine or emtricitabine) + (abacavir, didanosine, stavudine, tenofovir, or zidovudine)
Fosamprenavir/ritonavir†+ (lamivudine or emtricitabine) + (abacavir, didanosine, stavudine, tenofovir, or zidovudine)
Indinavir/ritonavir†+ (lamivudine or emtricitabine) + (abacavir, didanosine, stavudine, tenofovir, or zidovudine)
Lopinavir/ritonavir [Kaletra]†+ (lamivudine or emtricitabine) + (abacavir, stavudine, tenofovir, or zidovudine)
Nelfinavir + (lamivudine or emtricitabine) + (abacavir, didanosine, stavudine, tenofovir, or zidovudine)
Saquinavir/ritonavir†+ (lamivudine or emtricitabine) + (abacavir, didanosine, stavudine, tenofovir, or zidovudine)
3 NRTI-Based‡
Abacavir + lamivudine + zidovudine

NNRTI, Non-nucleoside reverse transcriptase inhibitor; *NRTI*, nucleoside/nucleotide reverse transcriptase inhibitor; *PI*, protease inhibitor.
*Efavirenz is not recommended for use in the first trimester of pregnancy or by women with a high pregnancy potential.
†The purpose of ritonavir in this combination is to inhibit metabolism of the other PI, and hence ritonavir dosage is low.
‡Use only when other options cannot or should not be used.
From Lehne, R. (2007). *Pharmacology for nursing care* (7th ed.). Philadelphia: Saunders.

5. Emtricitabine/tenofovir (Truvada): in addition to the effects that can occur from emtricitabine and tenofovir, lactic acidosis and severe hepatomegaly can occur
6. Lamivudine (Epivir): causes nausea and nasal congestion
7. Lamivudine/zidovudine (Combivir): can cause anemia and neutropenia and lactic acidosis with hepatomegaly

8. Lamivudine/zidovudine/abacavir (Trizivir): in addition to the effects that can occur from lamivudine, zidovudine, and abacavir, the following can also occur: hypersensitivity reactions, anemia, neutropenia, lactic acidosis, and severe hepatomegaly
9. Stavudine (d4t, Zerit): can cause peripheral neuropathy and pancreatitis
10. Tenofovir (Viread): can cause nausea and vomiting
11. Zalcitabine (ddC, HIVID) can cause oral ulcers, peripheral neuropathy, hepatotoxicity, and pancreatitis
12. Zidovudine (Retrovir, Azidothymidine, AZT, ZDV): can cause nausea, vomiting, anemia, leukopenia, myopathy, fatigue, and headache

I. Non-nucleoside reverse transcriptase inhibitors
1. Delavirdine (Rescriptor): can cause rash, liver function changes, and pruritus
2. Efavirenz (Sustiva): can cause rash, dizziness, confusion, difficulty concentrating, dreams, and encephalopathy
3. Nevirapine (Viramune): can cause rash, Stevens-Johnson syndrome, hepatitis, and increased transaminase levels

J. Protease inhibitors
1. Amprenavir (Agenerase)
   a. Can cause nausea, vomiting, headache, altered taste sensations, perioral paresthesia, rashes, and increased liver function studies
   b. Oral solution contains an alcohol that can interact with metronidazole (Flagyl) and can cause feelings of inebriation
2. Atazanavir (Reyataz): can cause nausea, headache, infection, vomiting, diarrhea, drowsiness, insomnia, fever, hyperglycemia, hyperlipidemia, and increased bleeding in clients with hemophilia
3. Fosamprenavir (Lexiva): similar to amprenavir; can cause nausea, vomiting, headache, altered taste sensations, perioral paresthesia, rashes, and increased liver function studies
4. Indinavir (Crixivan): can cause nausea, diarrhea, hyperbilirubinemia, nephritis, and kidney stones
5. Lopinavir/ritonavir combination (Kaletra): can cause nausea, diarrhea, altered taste sensations, circumoral paresthesia, and hepatitis
6. Nelfinavir (Viracept): can cause nausea, flatulence, and diarrhea
7. Ritonavir (Norvir): can cause nausea, vomiting, diarrhea, altered taste sensations, circumoral paresthesia, hepatitis, and increased triglyceride levels
8. Saquinavir (Invirase): can cause nausea, diarrhea, photosensitivity, and headache
9. Tipranavir (Aptivus): hepatotoxicity (liver damage); can also cause nausea, vomiting, diarrhea, headache, and fatigue

BOX 61-3 Immunosuppressants

Calcineurin Inhibitors
Cyclosporine (Sandimmune, Gengraf, Neoral)
Tacrolimus (Prograf)
Cytotoxic Medications
Azathioprine (Imuran)
Cyclophosphamide (Cytoxan, Neosar)
Methotrexate (Rheumatrex, Trexall)
Mycophenolate mofetil (CellCept)
Mycophenolic acid (Myfortic)
Antibodies
Basiliximab (Simulect)
Daclizumab (Zenapax)
Lymphocyte Immune Globulin, Antithymocyte
   Globulin (Equine)
Muromonab-CD3 (Orthoclone OKT3)
RH₀(D) immune globulin (RhoGAM)
Other
Sirolimus (Rapamune)
Glucocorticoids (see Chapter 45)

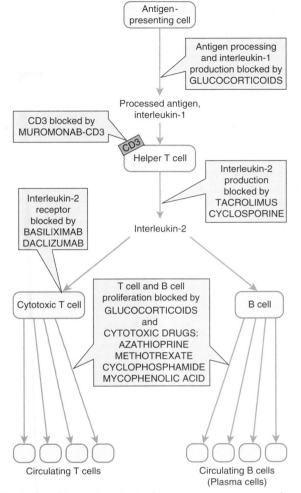

FIG. 61-2 Sites of action of immunosuppressant drugs. (From Lehne, R. [2007]. *Pharmacology for nursing care* [6th ed.]. Philadelphia: Saunders.)

K. Fusion inhibitor: enfuvirtide (Fuzeon) can cause skin irritation at injection site, fatigue, nausea, insomnia, and peripheral neuropathy

L. Anti-infective medications: used to treat opportunistic infections such as *Pneumocystic jiroveci* pneumonia; *Toxoplasma* encephalitis is treated with sulfamethoxazole/trimethoprim (Bactrim) (see Box 61-1)

M. Antifungal medications: used to treat candidiasis, cryptococcal meningitis (see Box 61-1)

N. Antiviral medications: used to treat cytomegalovirus retinitis, herpes simplex, varicella-zoster virus (see Box 61-1)

II. **IMMUNOSUPPRESSANTS** (Box 61-3 and Figure 61-2)

A. Description: immunosuppressants are used for transplant clients to prevent organ or tissue rejection and to treat autoimmune disorders such as systemic lupus erythematosus

B. Cyclosporine (Sandimmune, Gengraf, Neoral)
   1. Used for prevention of rejection following allogenic organ transplant
   2. Usually administered with a glucocorticoid and another immunosuppressant
   3. Most common adverse effects are nephrotoxicity, infection, hypertension, and hirsutism

C. Tacrolimus (Prograf)
   1. Used for prevention of rejection following liver or kidney transplant
   2. Adverse effects include nephrotoxicity, neurotoxicity, gastrointestinal effects, hypertension, hyperkalemia, hyperglycemia, hirsutism, and gum hyperplasia

D. Azathioprine (Imuran)
   1. Generally used with renal transplant clients
   2. Can cause neutropenia and thrombocytopenia

E. Cyclosphosphamide (Cytoxan, Neosar)
   1. Used for its immunosuppresant action to treat autoimmune disorders
   2. Can cause neutropenia and hemorrhagic cystitis

F. Methotrexate (Rheumatrex, Trexall)
   1. Used for its immunosuppresant action to treat autoimmune disorders
   2. Can cause hepatic fibrosis and cirrhosis, bone marrow suppression, ulcerative stomatitis, and renal damage

G. Mycophenolate mofetil (CellCept) and mycophenolic acid (Myfortic)
   1. Used to prevent rejection following kidney, heart, and liver transplants
   2. Can cause diarrhea, vomiting, neutropenia, sepsis; increased risk of infection and malignancies, especially lymphomas

H. Basiliximab (Simulect) and Daclizumab (Zenapax)
   1. Used to prevent rejection following kidney transplants.
   2. Can cause severe acute hypersensitivity reactions, including anaphylaxis

---

BOX 61-4 Antibiotics

Aminoglycosides
Amikacin (Amikin)
Gentamicin (Garamycin)
Kanamycin (Kantrex)
Neomycin (Neo-Fradin)
Streptomycin (Streptomycin)
Tobramycin (Nebcin)
Cephalosporins
Cefaclor (Ceclor)
Cefadroxil (Duricef)
Cefazolin (Ancef, Kefzol)
Cefdinir (Omnicef)
Cefditoren (Spectracef)
Cefepime (Maxipime)
Cefotaxime (Claforan)
Cefotetan (Cefotan)
Cefoxitin (Mefoxin)
Cefpodoxime (Vantin)
Cefprozil (Cefzil)
Ceftazidime (Ceptaz, Fortaz, Tazicef)
Ceftibuten (Cedax)
Ceftizoxime (Cefizox)
Ceftriaxone (Rocephin)
Cefuroxime (Ceftin)
Cephalexin (Keflex)
Loracarbef (Lorabid)

Fluoroquinolones
Ciprofloxacin (Cipro)
Gatifloxacin (Tequin)
Gemifloxacin (Factive)
Levofloxacin (Levaquin)
Lomefloxacin (Maxaquin)
Moxifloxacin (Avelox)
Norfloxacin (Noroxin)
Ofloxacin (Floxin)
Trovafloxacin (Trovan)
Macrolides
Azithromycin (Zithromax)
Clarithromycin (Biaxin)
Dirithromycin (Dynabac)
Erythromycin
Lincosamides
Clindamycin (Cleocin)
Lincomycin (Lincocin)
Monobactam
Aztreonam (Azactam)
Penicillins
Amoxicillin (Amoxil)
Ampicillin (Principen)
Carbenicillin (Geocillin)
Penicillin G (Bicillin, Permapen,
    Pfizerpen, Wycillin)

Penicillin V (Veetids)
Piperacillin
Ticarcillin (Ticar)
Penicillinase-Resistant
Dicloxacillin
Nafcillin
Oxacillin
Sulfonamides
Sulfamethoxazole
Sulfadiazine
Sulfasalazine
Sulfisoxazole
Trimethoprim (TMP) and Sulfamethoxazole
    (SMZ) (Bactrim, Cotrim, Septra)
Tetracyclines
Demeclocycline (Declomycin)
Doxycycline (Vibramycin)
Minocycline (Minocin)
Oxytetracycline (Terramycin)
Tetracycline (Sumycin)
Antimycobacterials
Antituberculosis (refer to Chapter 49)
Leprostatics: clofazimine (Lamprene
    and dapsone

I. Lymphocyte immune globulin, antithymocyte globulin (Equine)
   1. Used to prevent rejection following kidney, heart, liver, and bone marrow transplants
   2. Side effects include fever, chills, leukopenia, and skin reactions
   3. Can cause anaphylactoid reactions
J. Muromonab-CD3 (Orthoclone OKT3)
   1. Used to prevent rejection following kidney, heart, and liver transplants.
   2. Side effects include fever, chills, dyspnea, chest pain, nausea, vomiting
   3. Can cause anaphylactoid reactions
▲ K. RH₀(D) immune globulin (refer to Chapter 26)
   L. Sirolimus (Rapamune)
   1. Used to prevent renal transplant rejection
   2. Increases the risk of infection, raises cholesterol and triglyceride levels, and can cause renal injury
   3. Other side effects include rash, acne, anemia, thrombocytopenia, joint pain, diarrhea, and hypokalemia
▲ III. IMMUNIZATIONS (refer to Chapter 38)
▲ IV. ANTIBIOTICS (Box 61-4)
   A. Inhibit the growth of bacteria
   B. Include medication classifications of aminoglycosides, cephalosporins, fluoroquinolones, macrolides, lincosamides, monobactam, penicillins and penicillinase-resistant, sulfonamides, tetracyclines, and antimycobacterials (see Box 61-4)

C. Adverse effects (Table 61-1)
D. Nursing considerations
   1. Assess for allergies
   2. Monitor appropriate laboratory values before therapy as appropriate and during therapy to assess for adverse effects
   3. Monitor for adverse effects and report to physician if any occur
   4. Determine appropriate method of administration and provide instructions to the client
   5. Monitor intake and output
   6. Encourage fluid intake (unless contraindicated)
   7. Initiate safety precautions because of possible central nervous system effects
   8. Teach the client about the medication and how to take the medication and emphasize the importance of completing the full prescribed course

PRACTICE QUESTIONS

More questions on the companion CD!

843. The client who is human immunodeficiency virus seropositive has been taking Stavudine (d4t, Zerit). The nurse monitors which of the following most closely while the client is taking this medication?
   1. Gait
   2. Appetite
   3. Level of consciousness
   4. Hemoglobin and hematocrit blood levels

TABLE 61-1	Antibiotics and Their Adverse Effects		
Classification	**Adverse Effects**	**Classification**	**Adverse Effects**
Aminoglycosides	Ototoxicity	Monobactam	Gastrointestinal effects
	Confusion, disorientation		Hepatotoxicity
	Renal toxicity		Allergic reactions
	Gastrointestinal irritation	Penicillins and	Gastrointestinal effects including sore
	Palpitations, blood pressure changes	penicillinase-	mouth and furry tongue
	Hypersensitivity reactions	resistant	Superinfections
Cephalosporins	Gastrointestinal disturbances		Hypersensitivity reactions including
	Pseudomembranous colitis		anaphylaxis
	Headache, dizziness, lethargy,	Sulfonamides	Gastrointestinal effects
	paresthesias		Hepatotoxicity
	Nephrotoxicity		Nephrotoxicity
	Superinfections		Bone marrow depression
Fluoroquinolones	Headache, dizziness, insomnia,		Dermatological effects including
	depression		hypersensitivity and
	Gastrointestinal effects		photosensitivity
	Bone marrow depression		Headache, dizziness, vertigo, ataxia,
	Fever, rash, photosensitivity		depression, seizures
Macrolides	Gastrointestinal effects	Tetracyclines	Gastrointestinal effects
	Pseudomembranous colitis		Hepatotoxicity
	Confusion, abnormal thinking		Teeth (staining) and bone damage
	Superinfections		Superinfections
	Hypersensitivity reactions		Dermatological reactions including
Lincosamides	Gastrointestinal effects		rash and photosensitivity
	Pseudomembranous colitis		Hypersensitivity reactions
	Bone marrow depression	Antimycobacterials:	Gastrointestinal effects
		Leprostatics	Neuritis, dizziness, headache, malaise,
			drowsiness, hallucinations

844. The client with acquired immunodeficiency syndrome has begun therapy with zidovudine (Retrovir, Azidothymidine, AZT, ZDV). The nurse carefully monitors which of the following laboratory results during treatment with this medication?
    1. Blood culture
    2. Blood glucose level
    3. Blood urea nitrogen
    4. Complete blood count

845. The nurse is reviewing the results of serum laboratory studies drawn on a client with acquired immunodeficiency syndrome who is receiving didanosine (Videx). The nurse interprets that the client may have the medication discontinued by the physician if which of the following significantly elevated results is noted?
    1. Serum protein
    2. Blood glucose
    3. Serum amylase
    4. Serum creatinine

846. The nurse is caring for a postrenal transplant client taking cyclosporine (Sandimmune, Gengraf, Neoral). The nurse notes an increase in one of the client's vital signs, and the client is complaining of a headache. What is the vital sign that is most likely increased?

    1. Pulse
    2. Respirations
    3. Blood pressure
    4. Pulse oximetry

847. Amikacin (Amikin) is prescribed for a client with a bacterial infection. The nurse instructs the client to contact the physician immediately if which of the following occurs?
    1. Nausea
    2. Lethargy
    3. Hearing loss
    4. Muscle aches

848. The client who is human immunodeficiency virus seropositive has been taking zalcitabine (ddC, HIVID) as a component of treatment. The nurse plans to monitor which of the following most closely while the client is taking this medication?
    1. Glucose level
    2. Platelet count
    3. Red blood cell count
    4. Liver function studies

849. The nurse is assigned to care for a client with cytomegalovirus retinitis and acquired immunodeficiency syndrome who is receiving foscarnet (Foscavir), an antiviral. The nurse checks the

latest results of which of the following laboratory studies while the client is taking this medication?
1. CD4 cell count
2. Serum albumin
3. Serum creatinine
4. Lymphocyte count

850. The client with acquired immunodeficiency syndrome and *Pneumocystis jiroveci* infection has been receiving pentamidine (Pentam 300). The client develops a temperature of 101° F. The nurse does further monitoring of the client, knowing that this sign would most likely indicate:
1. The dose of the medication is too low.
2. The client is experiencing toxic effects of the medication.
3. The client has developed inadequacy of thermoregulation.
4. The result of another infection caused by leukopenic effects of the medication.

851. Saquinavir (Invirase) is prescribed for the client who is human immunodeficiency virus seropositive. The nurse reinforces medication instructions and tells the client to:

1. Avoid sun exposure.
2. Eat low-calorie foods.
3. Eat foods that are low in fat.
4. Take the medication on an empty stomach.

ALTERNATE ITEM FORMAT: MULTIPLE RESPONSE

852. Ketoconazole (Nizoral) is prescribed for a client with a diagnosis of candidiasis. Select the interventions that the nurse includes when administering this medication.
☐ 1. Restrict fluid intake.
☐ 2. Instruct the client to avoid alcohol.
☐ 3. Monitor hepatic and liver function studies.
☐ 4. Administer the medication with an antacid.
☐ 5. Instruct the client to avoid exposure to the sun.
☐ 6. Administer the medication on an empty stomach.

ANSWERS

843. 1
Rationale: Stavudine (d4t, Zerit) is an antiretroviral used to manage human immunodeficiency virus infection in clients who do not respond to or who cannot tolerate conventional therapy. The medication can cause peripheral neuropathy, and the nurse should monitor the client's gait closely and ask the client about paresthesia. Options 2, 3, and 4 are unrelated to the use of the medication.
Test-Taking Strategy: Focus on the name of the medication. Recalling that this medication causes peripheral neuropathy will direct you to option 1. If you are not familiar with this medication and the important assessment measures, review this content.
Level of Cognitive Ability: Application
Client Needs: Physiological Integrity
Integrated Process: Nursing Process/Data Collection
Content Area: Adult Health/Immune
Reference: Hodgson, B., & Kizior, R. (2007). *Saunders nursing drug handbook 2007* (p. 1077). Philadelphia: Saunders.

844. 4
Rationale: A common side effect of this medication therapy is leukopenia and anemia. The nurse monitors the complete blood count results for these changes. Options 1, 2, and 3 are unrelated to the use of this medication.
Test-Taking Strategy: Focus on the name of the medication. Recalling that zidovudine causes leukopenia and anemia will direct you to option 4. Review this medication if you had difficulty with this question.
Level of Cognitive Ability: Analysis
Client Needs: Physiological Integrity
Integrated Process: Nursing Process/Data Collection

Content Area: Adult Health/Immune
Reference: Hodgson, B., & Kizior, R. (2007). *Saunders nursing drug handbook 2007* (p. 1231). Philadelphia: Saunders.

845. 3
Rationale: Didanosine (Videx) can cause pancreatitis. A serum amylase level that is increased 1.5 to 2 times normal may signify pancreatitis in the client with acquired immunodeficiency syndrome and is potentially fatal. The medication may have to be discontinued. The medication is also hepatotoxic and can result in liver failure.
Test-Taking Strategy: Focus on the name of the medication. Recalling that this medication can cause damage to the pancreas and is hepatotoxic will direct you to the correct option. Review this medication if you had difficulty with this question.
Level of Cognitive Ability: Analysis
Client Needs: Physiological Integrity
Integrated Process: Nursing Process/Data Collection
Content Area: Adult Health/Immune
Reference: Hodgson, B., & Kizior, R. (2007). *Saunders nursing drug handbook 2007* (p. 354). Philadelphia: Saunders.

846. 3
Rationale: Hypertension can occur in a client taking cyclosporine (Sandimmune,Gengraf, Neoral), and since this client is also complaining of a headache, the blood pressure is the vital sign to be monitoring most closely. Other adverse effects include infection, nephrotoxicity, and hirsutism. Options 1, 2, and 4 are unrelated to the use of this medication.
Test-Taking Strategy: Focus on the name of the medication and the data in the question, and recall that this medication can cause hypertension. Review the adverse effects of this medication if you had difficulty with this question.

Level of Cognitive Ability: Analysis
Client Needs: Physiological Integrity
Integrated Process: Nursing Process/Data Collection
Content Area: Adult Health/Immune
Reference: Lehne, R. (2007). *Pharmacology for nursing care* (6th ed., pp. 795-797). Philadelphia: Saunders.

847. 3
Rationale: Amikacin (Amikin) is an aminoglycoside. Adverse effects of aminoglycosides include ototoxicity (hearing problems), confusion, disorientation, gastrointestinal irritation, palpitations, blood pressure changes, nephrotoxicity, and hypersensitivity. The nurse instructs the client to report hearing loss to the physician immediately. Lethargy and muscle aches are not associated with the use of this medication. It is not necessary to contact the physician immediately if nausea occurs. If nausea persists or results in vomiting, the physician should be notified.
Test-Taking Strategy: Note the strategic words "contact the physician immediately." Recalling that this medication is an aminoglycoside (most aminoglycoside medication names end in the letters *-cin*) and that aminogylcosides are ototoxic will direct you to the correct option. Review the adverse effects of aminoglycosides if you had difficulty with this question.
Level of Cognitive Ability: Application
Client Needs: Physiological Integrity
Integrated Process: Teaching and Learning
Content Area: Adult Health/Immune
Reference: Lehne, R. (2007). *Pharmacology for nursing care* (6th ed., p. 999). Philadelphia: Saunders.

848. 4
Rationale: Zalcitabine (ddC, HIVID) is an antiretroviral (nucleoside reverse transcriptase inhibitor) used to manage human immunodeficiency virus infection with other antiretrovirals. Zalcitabine has also been used as a single agent in clients who are intolerant of other regimens. Zalcitabine can cause serious liver damage, and liver function studies should be monitored closely. Options 1, 2, and 3 are not associated specifically with the use of this medication.
Test-Taking Strategy: Focus on the name of the medication. Recalling that this medication is hepatotoxic will direct you to option 4. If you are unfamiliar with this medication, review this content.
Level of Cognitive Ability: Application
Client Needs: Physiological Integrity
Integrated Process: Nursing Process/Data Collection
Content Area: Adult Health/Immune
Reference: Skidmore-Roth, L. (2007). *2007 Mosby's nursing drug reference* (20th ed., p. 1050). St. Louis: Mosby.

849. 3
Rationale: Foscarnet (Foscavir) is toxic to the kidneys. Serum creatinine is monitored before therapy, two to three times per week during induction therapy, and at least weekly during maintenance therapy. Foscarnet may also cause decreased levels of calcium, magnesium, phosphorus, and potassium. Thus these levels are also measured with the same frequency.
Test-Taking Strategy: Use the process of elimination. Recalling that this medication is nephrotoxic will direct you easily

to option 3. Review this medication if you are unfamiliar with it.
Level of Cognitive Ability: Application
Client Needs: Physiological Integrity
Integrated Process: Nursing Process/Data Collection
Content Area: Adult Health/Immune
Reference: Hodgson, B., & Kizior, R. (2007). *Saunders nursing drug handbook 2007* (p. 516). Philadelphia: Saunders.

850. 4
Rationale: Frequent side effects of this medication include leukopenia, thrombocytopenia, and anemia. The client should be monitored routinely for signs and symptoms of infection. Options 1, 2, and 3 are inaccurate interpretations.
Test-Taking Strategy: Use the process of elimination focusing on the strategic words "develops a temperature." Note the relationship between these strategic words and option 4. Review the side effects of this medication if you had difficulty with this question.
Level of Cognitive Ability: Analysis
Client Needs: Physiological Integrity
Integrated Process: Nursing Process/Data Collection
Content Area: Adult Health/Immune
Reference: Hodgson, B., & Kizior, R. (2007). *Saunders nursing drug handbook 2007* (p. 913). Philadelphia: Saunders,

851. 1
Rationale: Saquinavir (Invirase) is an antiretroviral (protease inhibitor) used with other antiretroviral medications to manage human immunodeficiency virus infection. Saquinavir is administered with meals and is best absorbed if the client consumes high-calorie, high-fat meals. Saquinavir can cause photosensitivity, and the nurse should instruct the client to avoid sun exposure.
Test-Taking Strategy: Use the process of elimination. Options 2 and 3 can be eliminated first, knowing that these dietary measures would not likely be prescribed for this client. From the remaining options, you must know that this medication can cause photosensitivity. Review this medication if you had difficulty with this question.
Level of Cognitive Ability: Application
Client Needs: Physiological Integrity
Integrated Process: Teaching and Learning
Content Area: Adult Health/Immune
Reference: Hodgson, B., & Kizior, R. (2007). *Saunders nursing drug handbook 2007* (p. 1043). Philadelphia: Saunders.

ALTERNATE ITEM FORMAT: MULTIPLE RESPONSE

852. 2, 3, 5
Rationale: Ketoconazole (Nizoral) is an antifungal medication. It is administered with food (not on an empty stomach) and antacids are avoided for 2 hours after taking the medication to ensure absorption. The medication is hepatotoxic and the nurse monitors liver function studies. The client is instructed to avoid exposure to the sun because the medication increases photosensitivity. The client is also instructed to avoid alcohol. There is no reason for the client to restrict fluid intake. In fact, this could be harmful to the client.

Test-Taking Strategy: Use general medication guidelines to assist in selecting the correct interventions. Also remember that this medication is administered with food and that it is hepatotoxic. Review this medication if you had difficulty with this question.
Level of Cognitive Ability: Application

Client Needs: Physiological Integrity
Integrated Process: Nursing Process/Implementation
Content Area: Adult Health/Immune
Reference: Hodgson, B., & Kizior, R. (2007). *Saunders nursing drug handbook 2007* (p. 654). Philadelphia: Saunders.

REFERENCES

Black, J., & Hawks, J. (2005). *Medical-surgical nursing: Clinical management for positive outcomes* (7th ed.). Philadelphia: Saunders.

Hodgson, B., & Kizior, R. (2007). *Saunders nursing drug handbook 2007*. Philadelphia: Saunders.

Lehne, R. (2007). *Pharmacology for nursing care* (6th ed.). Philadelphia: Saunders.

Skidmore-Roth, L. (2007). *2007 Mosby's nursing drug reference* (20th ed.). St. Louis: Mosby.

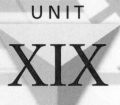

The Adult Client With a Mental Health Disorder

PYRAMID TERMS

abuse An act of misuse, deceit, or exploitation; a wrong or improper use or action toward another individual that results in injury, damage, maltreatment, or corruption

addiction Also known as drug dependence; incorporates the concepts of loss of control with respect to the use of a drug, taking the drug despite related problems and complications, and a tendency to relapse

coping mechanisms Methods of adjusting to environmental stress without altering one's own goals or purposes; can include both conscious and unconscious mechanisms

crisis A temporary state of disequilibrium in which an individual's usual coping mechanisms or problem-solving methods fail; it can result in personality growth or personality disorganization

defense mechanisms A coping mechanism (protective defense) of the ego that attempts to protect the individual from feelings of inadequacy and worthlessness and prevent awareness of anxiety; when anxiety is too painful, the individual copes by using defense mechanisms to protect the ego and decrease anxiety

milieu The physical and social environment in which an individual lives; milieu therapy focuses on positive physical and social environmental manipulation to produce positive change

rape-trauma syndrome A syndrome characterized by an acute phase and a long-term reorganization process that occurs after an actual or attempted sexual assault; each phase has separate symptoms

restraints (security devices) Physical restraints include any manual method or mechanical device, material, or equipment that inhibits free movement; chemical restraints include the administration of medications for the specific purpose of inhibiting a specific behavior or movement

seclusion Placing a client alone in a specially designed room for protection and close supervision; it is the last measure in a process to maximize safety to the client and others

suicide The ultimate act of self-destruction in which an individual purposefully ends his or her own life

suicide attempt Any willful, self inflicted, or life-threatening attempt by an individual that has not led to death

PYRAMID TO SUCCESS

The Pyramid to Success focuses on the therapeutic nurse-client relationship, client rights, hospital admission procedures, ethical and legal issues related to the care of the client with a mental health disorder, grief and loss, and end-of-life issues. Pyramid points focus on the use of restraints, seclusion, and electroconvulsive therapy (ECT). Focus on care of the client with an addiction, such as an eating disorder or drug or alcohol disorder. Additional focus areas include anxiety, depression, suicide, abuse and violence, rape crisis interventions, post-traumatic stress disorders, obsessive-compulsive disorders, schizophrenia, and bipolar disorders. Pyramid points address the use of medications prescribed for the client with a mental health disorder, particularly lithium and the benzodiazepines. The Integrated Processes addressed in this unit include: Caring, the Clinical Problem-Solving Process (Nursing Process), Communication and Documentation, and Teaching and Learning.

CLIENT NEEDS

Safe and Effective Care Environment

Ensuring client advocacy

Implementing legal responsibilities related to reporting incidences of violence and abuse

Maintaining confidentiality

Obtaining informed consent related to treatments, such as restraints, seclusion, and electroconvulsive therapy (ECT)

Providing psychiatric consultations and referrals

Providing safety to client and others

Upholding client rights

Using restraints and seclusion appropriately and safely

Health Promotion and Maintenance

Identifying individual lifestyle choices

Performing psychosocial assessment techniques

Providing health promotion programs related to addictions

Psychosocial Integrity

Monitoring for abuse/neglect situations

Monitoring for chemical dependency

Monitoring for domestic violence

Addressing grief and loss and end-of-life issues

Caring for the client who has been sexually abused or raped

Considering religious, cultural, and spiritual influences on health

Developing a therapeutic nurse-client relationship

Identifying appropriate counseling techniques

Identifying coping mechanisms

Identifying support systems

Implementing behavioral interventions

Providing crisis intervention

Providing a therapeutic milieu

Teaching stress management techniques

Physiological Integrity

Administering medications as prescribed

Assessing for abusive and self-destructive behavior

Monitoring elimination patterns

Monitoring for alterations in body systems related to addictions

Monitoring for expected and untoward effects of medications

Monitoring for potential complications related to medications and electroconvulsive therapy

Monitoring laboratory values related to medication therapy

Monitoring rest and sleep patterns

Providing adequate nutrition

Providing personal hygiene measures

REFERENCES

Chernecky, C., & Berger, B. (2008). *Laboratory tests and diagnostic procedures* (5th ed.). St. Louis: Saunders.

Fortinash, K., & Holoday-Worret, P. (2008). *Psychiatric mental health nursing* (4th ed.). St. Louis: Mosby.

Harkreader, H., Hogan, M.A., & Thobaben, M. (2007). *Fundamentals of nursing: Caring and clinical judgment* (3rd ed.). St. Louis: Saunders.

Hodgson, B., & Kizior, R. (2008). *Saunders nursing drug handbook 2008*. Philadelphia: Saunders.

Ignatavicius, D., & Workman, M. (2006). *Medical surgical nursing: Critical thinking for collaborative care* (5th ed.). St. Louis: Saunders.

Keltner, N., Schwecke, L., & Bostrom, C. (2007). *Psychiatric nursing* (5th ed.). St. Louis: Mosby.

Lehne, R. (2007). *Pharmacology for nursing care* (6th ed.). Philadelphia: Saunders.

Lewis, S.L., Heitkemper, M.M., & Dirksen, S.R., et al. (2007). *Medical-surgical nursing: Assessment and management of clinical problems* (7th ed.). St. Louis: Mosby.

Lilley, L., Harrington, S., & Snyder, J. (2007). *Pharmacology and the nursing process* (5th ed.). St. Louis: Mosby.

McKenry, L., Tessier, E., & Hogan, M. (2006). *Mosby's pharmacology in nursing* (22nd ed.). St. Louis: Mosby.

Monahan, F., Sands, J., Neighbors, M., Marek, J., & Green, C. (2007). *Phipps' medical-surgical nursing: Health and illness perspectives* (8th ed.). St. Louis: Mosby.

Morrison-Valfre, M. (2005). *Foundations of mental health care* (3rd ed.). St. Louis: Mosby.

National Council of State Boards of Nursing, (eds.) (2008). *2008 Detailed Test Plan for the NCLEX-PN Examination, National Council of State Boards of Nursing*. Chicago: Author.

National Council of State Boards of Nursing, Inc. Web site: www.ncsbn.org.

Stuart, G., & Laraia, M. (2005). *Principles and practice of psychiatric nursing* (8th ed.). St. Louis: Mosby.

Varcarolis, E., Carlson, V., & Shoemaker, N. (2006). *Foundations of psychiatric mental health nursing* (5th ed.). Philadelphia: Saunders.

Foundations of Psychiatric Mental Health Nursing

I. THE NURSE-CLIENT RELATIONSHIP

A. Principles
1. Genuineness, respect, and empathic understanding are characteristics important to the development of a therapeutic nurse-client relationship
2. The client should be cared for in a holistic manner
3. The nurse considers the religious and spiritual practices of the client and whether these practices may give the client hope, comfort, and support while healing
4. The nurse considers the client's cultural beliefs and values in assessing the client's response to the nurse-client relationship and his or her adaptation to stressors
5. Appropriate limits and boundaries define and facilitate a therapeutic nurse-client relationship
6. Honest and open communication is an important cornerstone for the development of trust—an underpinning of the therapeutic nurse-client relationship
7. The nurse uses therapeutic communication techniques to encourage the client to express thoughts and feelings as they address identified problem areas
8. The nurse respects the client's confidentiality and limits discussion of the client to members of the treatment team
9. The goal of the nurse-client relationship is to assist the client to develop problem-solving and **coping mechanisms**

B. Phases of a therapeutic nurse-client relationship
1. Preinteraction phase
   a. The preinteraction phase begins before the nurse's first contact with the client
   b. The nurse's task in the preinteraction phase is to explore any preconceived ideas, stereotypes, biases, and values that may impinge on the nurse-client relationship
2. Orientation or introductory phase
   a. Acceptance, trust, and boundaries are established
   b. Expectations and the time frame of the relationship are identified (establishing a contract)
   c. Client-centered goals are defined
   d. The termination of the relationship and the ensuing separation are discussed in anticipation of the time-limited nature of the relationship
3. Working phase
   a. An attitude of acceptance and active listening assists the client to express thoughts and feelings and to learn about his or her **coping mechanisms**
   b. Identifying themes and patterns of behavior promotes insight into problem-solving and **coping mechanisms**
   c. Encouraging independence in the client facilitates recovery and leads to readiness for termination
4. Termination or separation phase
   a. Prepare the client for termination and separation on initial contact
   b. Evaluate progress and achievement of goals
   c. Identify responses related to termination and separation, such as anger, distancing from the relationship, a return of symptoms, and dependency
   d. Encourage the client to express feelings about termination
   e. Identify the client's strengths and anticipated needs for follow-up care.
   f. Refer the client to other support systems

II. THERAPEUTIC COMMUNICATION PROCESS

A. Principles
1. Communication includes verbal and nonverbal expression (Figure 62-1)
2. Successful communication includes appropriateness, efficiency, flexibility, and feedback
3. Anxiety in the nurse or client impedes communication
4. Communication needs to be goal directed within a professional framework

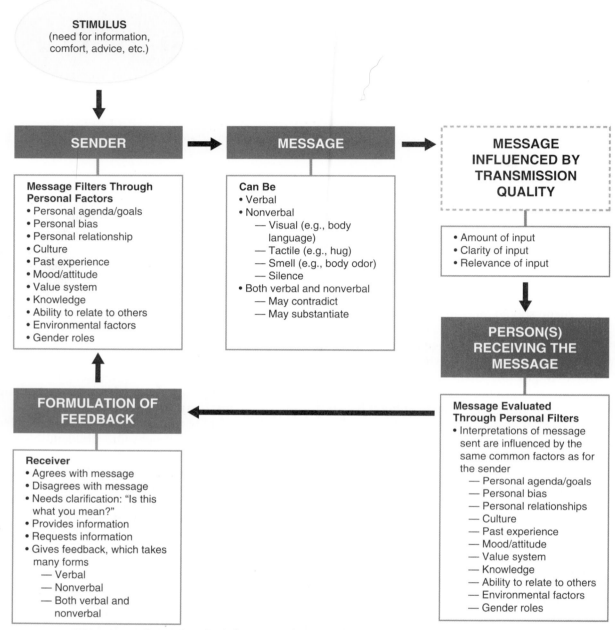

FIG. 62-1 Operational definition of communication. (Data from Ellis, R., & McClintock, A. [1990]. *If you take my meaning*. London: Arnold.)

B. Therapeutic and nontherapeutic communication techniques (Box 62-1)

III. MENTAL HEALTH

A. Mental health is a lifelong process of successful adaptation to a changing internal and external environment

B. The mentally healthy individual is *in contact with reality*, is able to relate to people and situations in their environment, and can resolve conflicts within a problem-solving framework

C. The mentally healthy individual has psychobiological resilience

IV. PSYCHIATRIC/MENTAL HEALTH ILLNESS

A. Description

1. Psychiatric illness is the loss of ability to respond to the environment in ways that are in harmony with oneself or the expectations of society

2. Psychiatric illness is characterized by thought or behavior patterns that impair functioning and cause distress

B. Personality characteristics

1. Self-concept is distorted

2. Perception of strengths and weaknesses is not realistic

BOX 62-1	Therapeutic and Nontherapeutic Communication Techniques

Therapeutic Techniques
Clarifying and validating
Encouraging formulation of a plan of action
Focusing and refocusing
Giving information and presenting reality
Listening
Maintaining neutral responses
Maintaining silence
Providing acknowledgment and feedback
Providing nonverbal encouragement
Reflecting
Restating
Sharing perceptions
Summarizing
Using broad openings and open-ended questions
Nontherapeutic Techniques
Asking the client "Why?"
Being defensive or challenging the client
Changing the subject
Giving advice or approval or disapproval
Making stereotypical comments
Making value judgments
Placing the client's feelings on hold
Providing false reassurance

3. Thoughts and perceptions may not be reality based
4. The ability to find meaning and purpose in life may be impaired
5. Life direction and productivity may be disturbed
6. Meeting one's own needs may be problematic
7. Excessive reliance or preoccupation on the thoughts, opinions, and actions of self or others may be present

C. Adaptations to stress
   1. The individual's sense of self-control and environmental mastery may be affected
   2. Perception of the environment may be distorted
   3. **Coping mechanisms** may be ineffective or nonexistent

D. Interpersonal relationships
   1. Interpersonal relationships may suffer or even be minimally existent
   2. The ability to enjoy sustained intimacy in relationships is impaired

V. COPING AND DEFENSE MECHANISMS
A. **Coping mechanisms**
   1. Coping involves any effort to decrease anxiety
   2. **Coping mechanisms** can be constructive or destructive, task oriented in relation to direct problem-solving, or defense oriented and regulating the response to protect oneself

B. Defense mechanisms
   1. As anxiety increases, the individual copes by using **defense mechanisms**
   2. A defense mechanism is a coping mechanism used in an effort to protect the individual from feelings of anxiety (Box 62-2)

C. Interventions
   1. Assist the client to identify the source of anxiety
   2. Assist the client to explore methods to reduce anxiety
   3. Assess the client's use of **defense mechanisms**
   4. Facilitate appropriate use of **defense mechanisms**
   5. Determine whether the **defense mechanisms** used by the client are effective for him or her or create additional distress
   6. Avoid criticizing the behavior and use of **defense mechanisms**

VI. DIAGNOSTIC AND STATISTICAL MANUAL OF MENTAL HEALTH DISORDERS
A. The Diagnostic and Statistical Manual of Mental Health Disorders (DSMIV-TR) classifies psychiatric diagnoses according to the American Psychiatric Association
B. The manual is a system used in clinical, research, and educational settings, in which diagnostic criteria are included for each diagnosis
C. The manual includes a list of culture-bound syndromes that may be associated with a particular diagnostic category
D. Knowledge of the characteristics of a particular psychiatric diagnosis will assist the nurse in assessing the client's nursing care needs

VII. TYPES OF MENTAL HEALTH ADMISSIONS AND DISCHARGES
A. Voluntary admission
   1. The client (or the client's guardian) seeks admission for care
   2. The voluntary client is free to sign out of the hospital with physician notification and order
   3. Detaining a voluntary client against his or her will is termed false imprisonment
   4. Civil rights are retained fully by the client (Box 62-3)

B. Right to Confidentiality
   1. A client has a right to confidentiality of his or her medical information; Health Insurance Portability and Accountability Act (HIPAA) of 1996 ensures client confidentiality with regard to release and electronic transmission of data
   2. Client information can only be released by the client's informed consent, which specifies the information that can be released and the time frame the release is valid
   3. Information sometimes must be released in life-threatening situations without the client's consent

BOX 62-2 **Types of Defense Mechanisms**

Compensation: Putting forth extra effort to achieve in areas where one has a real or imagined deficiency

Conversion: The expression of emotional conflicts through physical symptoms

Denial: Disowning consciously intolerable thoughts and impulses

Displacement: Feelings toward one person are directed to another who is less threatening, thereby satisfying an impulse with a substitute object

Dissociation: The blocking off of an anxiety-provoking event or period of time from the conscious mind

Fantasy: Gratification by imaginary achievements and wishful thinking

Fixation: Never advancing to the next level of emotional development and organization; the persistence in later life of interests and behavior patterns appropriate to an earlier age

Identification: The unconscious attempt to change oneself to resemble an admired person

Insulation: Withdrawing into passivity and becoming inaccessible in order to avoid further threatening situations

Intellectualization: Excessive reasoning to avoid feelings; the thinking is disconnected from feelings, and situations are dealt with at a cognitive level

Introjection: A type of identification in which the individual incorporates the traits or values of another into self

Isolation: Response in which a person blocks feelings associated with an unpleasant experience

Projection: Transferring one's internal feelings, thoughts, and unacceptable ideas and traits to someone else

Rationalization: An attempt to make unacceptable feelings and behaviors acceptable by justifying the behavior

Reaction formation: Developing conscious attitudes and behaviors and acting out behaviors opposite to what one really feels

Regression: Returning to an earlier developmental stage to express an impulse to deal with reality

Repression: An unconscious process in which the client blocks undesirable and unacceptable thoughts from conscious expression

Sublimation: Replacement of an unacceptable need, attitude, or emotion with one more socially acceptable

Substitution: The replacement of a valued unacceptable object with an object that is more acceptable to the ego

Suppression: The conscious, deliberate forgetting of unacceptable or painful thoughts, ideas, and feelings

Symbolization: The conscious use of an idea or object to represent another actual event or object; many times the meaning is not clear because the symbol may be representative of something unconscious

Undoing: Engaging in behavior that is considered to be opposite of a previous unacceptable behavior, thought, or feeling

BOX 62-3 **Client Rights**

Right to accessible health care
Right to coordination and continuity of health care
Right to courteous and individualized health care
Right to information about the qualifications, names, and titles of personnel delivering care
Right to refuse observation by those not directly involved in care
Right to privacy and confidentiality
Right to informed consent
Right to treatment and to refuse treatment
Right to treatment in the least restrictive setting
Right not to be subjected to unnecessary restraints
Right to habeas corpus; may request a hearing at any time to be released from the hospital
Right to information about diagnosis, prognosis, and treatment
Right to information on the charges of service
Right to communicate with people outside the hospital through written correspondence, telephone, and personal visits
Right to keep clothing and personal effects
Right to be employed
Right to religious freedom
Right to execute wills
Right to retain licenses, privileges, or permits established by the law, such as a driver's or professional license

Modified from Stuart, G., & Laraia, M. (2005). *Principles and practice of psychiatric nursing* (8th ed.). St. Louis: Mosby.

4. In the event of a specific threat against an identified individual, the health care professional has a legal obligation to warn intended victim(s) of a client's threats of harm

C. Involuntary admission
1. Involuntary admission may be necessary when a person is mentally ill, is a danger to self or others, or is in need of psychiatric treatment or physical care
2. Involuntary admission occurs when a client is admitted or detained involuntarily for mental health treatment because of actual or imminent danger to self or others
3. The client who is admitted involuntarily retains his or her right for informed consent
4. The client retains the right to refuse treatments, including medications, unless a separate and specific treatment order is obtained from the court
5. The client loses the right to refuse treatment when the client poses an immediate danger to self or others, requiring immediate action by the health care team
6. An order from a judge is required for involuntary admissions except in the case of emergency, which allows time to obtain the necessary order from a judge; in the case of all involuntary admissions, legal counsel must be provided for the client

7. A court hearing is held by a judge within a specified time for clients admitted involuntarily; the specific time varies by state
8. In most states, the client can institute a court hearing to seek an expedient judicial discharge (a writ of habeas corpus)
9. At the court hearing, a determination is made as to whether the client may be released from the hospital or detained for further treatment and evaluation or committed to a mental health facility for an undetermined time
10. The client has the right to treatment in the least restrictive treatment environment (if treatment objectives can be achieved, for example, by court-ordered treatment to an outpatient facility as opposed to an inpatient facility, the client has the right to be treated in the former setting)
11. The client is considered legally competent unless he or she has been declared incompetent through a legal hearing separate from the involuntary commitment hearing
12. In the course of providing nursing care and carrying out medical orders, if the nurse believes that a client lacks competency to make informed decisions, action should be initiated to determine if a legal guardian needs to be appointed by the court

D. Release from the hospital
1. Description
   a. A client may be released voluntarily, against medical advice, or with conditions (conditional release)
   b. The client who sought voluntary admission has the right to demand to be released
2. Voluntary release
   a. In the absence of an act of self-harm or danger to others, a voluntary client should never be detained
   b. If a voluntary client wishes to be discharged from treatment but is considered potentially dangerous to self or others, the physician can order the client to be detained while legal proceedings for involuntary status are sought
   c. Some states provide for conditional release of involuntarily hospitalized clients; this enables the treating physician to order continued treatment on an outpatient basis as opposed to discharging the client to follow-up on his or her own initiative
   d. Conditional release usually involves outpatient treatment for a specified period to determine the client's compliance with medication protocol, ability to meet basic needs, and ability to reintegrate into the community
   e. An involuntary client who is released conditionally may be reinstitutionalized while the commitment is still in effect without

recommencement of formal admission procedures
3. Discharge planning and follow-up care
   a. Discharge (unconditional release) is the termination of the client-institution relationship
   b. This release may be ordered by the psychiatrist, court, or administration for involuntarily admitted clients and may be requested by voluntary clients at any time
   c. In most states, the client can institute a court hearing to seek an expedient judicial discharge (writ of habeas corpus)
   d. Discharge planning and follow-up care are important for the continued well-being of the client with a mental health disorder
   e. After-care case managers are used to facilitate the client's adaptation back into the community and to provide early referral if the treatment plan is not successful

VIII. MILIEU THERAPY
A. Description
1. The **milieu** refers to the physical and social environment in which an individual is receiving treatment
2. **Milieu** therapy uses a safe environment to meet the individual client's treatment needs
3. Safety is the number one priority in managing the **milieu**
4. **Milieu** therapy is staffed by persons educated to provide support, understanding, and individual attention; all encounters with the client have the goal of being "therapeutic"
5. All members of the treatment team contribute to the planning and functioning of the **milieu**; the team generally includes the registered nurse, social worker, exercise therapist, recreational therapist, psychologist, psychiatrist, occupational therapist, clinical nurse specialist, or nurse practitioner
6. All treatment team members are viewed as significant and valuable to the client's successful treatment outcomes
B. Focus of **milieu** therapy
1. To use the physical and social environment to effect a positive change directed toward accomplishing the client's treatment goals
2. To empower the client through involvement in setting his or her own goals and develop purposeful relations with the staff to assist in meeting these goals
3. To use community meetings, activity groups, social skills groups, and physical exercise programs to accomplish treatment goals.
4. To have one-to-one relationships with staff to examine client behaviors, feelings, and interactions within the context of the therapeutic group activities

IX. INTERPERSONAL PSYCHOTHERAPY

A. Description
1. A treatment modality that uses a therapeutic relationship to modify the client's feelings, attitudes, and behaviors
2. Therapeutic communication forms the foundation of the therapist-client relationship

B. Focus of interpersonal psychotherapy
1. To establish a contract, clarify roles, and work within an agreed-upon time frame toward meeting the client's goals
2. Focusing on the therapist-client relationship is used as a way for clients to examine other relationships in his or her life

C. Levels of psychotherapy (Box 62-4)
1. Supportive therapy
   a. Allows the client to express feelings, explore alternatives, and make decisions in a safe, caring environment
   b. May be needed briefly or over a period of years
   c. No plan exists to introduce new methods of coping; instead, the therapist reinforces the client's existing **coping mechanisms**
2. Re-educative therapy
   a. Involves learning new ways of perceiving and behaving
   b. The client explores alternatives in a planned, systematic way and requires a longer period of therapy than supportive therapy
   c. The client enters into a contract that specifies desired changes of behavior
   d. May include short-term psychotherapy, reality therapy, cognitive restructuring, behavior modification, and the development of coping skills
3. Reconstructive therapy
   a. Involves the use of psychotherapy or psychoanalysis to make major changes in the client's life
   b. May require several years of therapy and focuses on all aspects of the client's life
   c. Emotional and cognitive restructuring of self takes place
   d. Positive outcomes include a greater understanding of self and others, more emotional freedom, and the development of potential abilities

X. BEHAVIOR THERAPY

A. A treatment approach that uses the principles of Skinnerian (operant conditioning) or Pavlovian (classical conditioning) behavior theory to bring about behavioral change
B. The belief is that most behaviors are learned
C. Operant conditioning refers to the manipulation of selected reinforcers to elicit and strengthen desired behavioral responses; the reinforcer refers to the consequence of the behavior, which is defined as anything that increases the occurrence of a behavior (Figure 62-2)
D. In classical conditioning (respondent conditioning) the individual responds to a stimulus but is basically a passive agent (see Figure 62-2)
E. Desensitization is a form of behavior therapy by which exposure to increasing increments of a feared stimulus paired with increasing levels of relaxation helps to reduce the intensity of fear to a more tolerable level
F. Aversion therapy is a form of behavior therapy by which negative reinforcement is used to change behavior; for example, a stimulus *attractive* to the client is paired with an *unpleasant* event in hopes of endowing the stimulus with negative properties, thereby dissuading the behavior
G. Modeling is behavioral therapy whereby the therapist acts as a role model for specific identified behaviors so that the client learns through imitation

XI. COGNITIVE THERAPY

A. An active, directive, time-limited, structured approach used to treat a variety of disorders including anxiety, depression, and phobias
B. Based on the principle that how an individual feels and behaves is determined by the way in which he or she thinks about the world and his or her place in it; the individual's cognitions are based on the attitudes or assumptions developed from previous experiences.
C. Therapeutic techniques are designed to identify, reality test, and correct distorted conceptualizations and the dysfunctional beliefs underlying these cognitions

---

BOX 62-4   Levels of Psychotherapy

Supportive therapy
Re-educative therapy
Reconstructive therapy

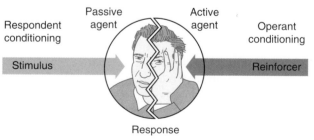

FIG. 62-2 Respondent versus operant conditioning. (From Carson, V. [2000]. *Mental health nursing: The nurse-patient journey* [2nd ed.]. Philadelphia: Saunders.)

D. The therapist helps the individual to change the way he or she thinks, thereby reducing symptoms

▲ XII. GROUP DEVELOPMENT AND GROUP THERAPY

A. Description: group therapy involves a therapist and ideally five to eight members working on his or her individual goals within the context of a group, which presumably increases the opportunity for feedback and support

▲ B. Stages of group development (Box 62-5)
▲ 1. Initial stage
   a. During this stage, group development involves superficial rather than open and trusting communication
   b. Members become acquainted with each other and search for similarity between themselves and other group members
   c. Members may be unclear about the purpose or goals of the group
   d. Group norms, roles, and responsibilities are established
▲ 2. Working stage
   a. During this stage, the real work of the group is accomplished
   b. Members are familiar with each other, the group leader, and the group roles, and they feel free to address and attempt to solve their problem
   c. Both conflict and cooperation surface during the group's work as the members learn to work with each other
▲ 3. Termination stage
   a. Members' feelings are explored regarding their accomplishments and the impending termination of the group
   b. The termination stage provides an opportunity for members to learn to deal more realistically and comfortably with this normal part of human experience

C. Group therapy models (note: these models apply to individual or group psychotherapy)
   1. Psychoanalytical group psychotherapy
      a. The therapist holds a main position
      b. Each client in the group has a relationship with the therapist
      c. Communication is focused on three levels: unconscious, semiconscious, and conscious information

2. Transactional analysis
   a. The three ego states of the individual are examined
   b. The goal is for individuals in the group to communicate from the proper ego states for the situation and responses of others, thereby lessening conflict and promoting mature relationships
3. Rational emotive therapy is a kind of cognitive therapy in which the therapist focuses on how irrational beliefs and thoughts contribute to psychological distress
4. Rogerian therapy
   a. The therapist's goal is to help the members express their feelings toward one another during group sessions
   b. The therapist's role is one of encouraging the expression of feelings, clarifying these feelings with clients, and accepting clients and their feelings nonjudgmentally
5. Gestalt therapy
   a. Emphasis is on the "here and now"
   b. Emphasizes self-expression, self-exploration, and self-awareness in the present
   c. The client and therapist focus on everyday problems and try to solve them
   d. The individual becomes aware of the total self and the surrounding environment
   e. Awareness of the problem renders the client capable of change
   f. The therapist's role is to help the members express their feelings and grow from their experiences
6. Interpersonal group therapy: promotes the individual's comfort with others in the group, which then transfers to other relationships
7. Self-help or support groups (Box 62-6)   ▲
   a. Support groups are based on the premise that persons who have experienced a similar problem are able to help others who have the same problem
   b. A prototype support group would be Alcoholics Anonymous, where alcoholics work together to support each other's recovery through member-run group meetings

XIII. FAMILY THERAPY

A. Family therapy is a specific intervention mode based on the premise that the member who has the presenting symptoms will signal the presence of problems in the entire family; this premise also assumes that a change in one member will bring about changes in other members

B. The therapist works to assist family members to identify and express their thoughts and feelings; define family roles and rules; try new, more productive styles of relating; and restore strength to the family

BOX 62-5 **Stages of Group Development**

Initial stage
Working stage
Termination stage

BOX 62-6	Examples of Self-help or Support Groups

Adult Children of Alcoholics
Al-Anon
Alcoholics Anonymous
Co-dependents Anonymous
Gamblers Anonymous
Narcotics Anonymous
Overeaters Anonymous
Cancer Support
Mental Illness support groups
Bereavement groups
Parents without partners
Recovery groups, such as for those who have experienced trauma
Smoking cessation
Unexpected body-image changes, such as mastectomy or colostomy

PRACTICE QUESTIONS

More questions on the companion CD!

853. A nurse is assigned to care for a client who is experiencing disturbed thought processes. The nurse is told that the client believes that the food is being poisoned. Which communication technique does the nurse plan to use to encourage the client to eat?
   1. Open-ended questions and silence
   2. Focusing on self-disclosure regarding food preferences
   3. Stating the reasons that the client may not want to eat
   4. Offering opinions about the necessity of adequate nutrition

854. A nurse is assigned to care for a client admitted to the hospital after sustaining an injury from a house fire. The client attempted to save a neighbor involved in the fire but, in spite of the client's efforts, the neighbor died. Which action would the nurse take to enable the client to work through the meaning of the crisis?
   1. Identifying the client's ability to function
   2. Identifying the client's potential for self-harm
   3. Inquiring about the client's feelings that may affect coping
   4. Inquiring about the client's perception of the cause of the neighbor's death

855. A nurse is assisting with the data collection on a client admitted to the psychiatric unit. The nurse reviews the data obtained and identifies which of the following as a priority concern?
   1. The client's report of suicidal thoughts
   2. The client's report of not eating or sleeping
   3. The presence of bruises on the client's body
   4. The family member is disapproving of the treatment

856. Laboratory work is prescribed for a client who has been experiencing delusions. When the laboratory technician approaches the client to obtain a specimen of the client's blood, the client begins to shout, "You're all vampires. Let me out of here!" The nurse who is present at the time should respond by stating which of the following?
   1. "The technician will leave and come back later for your blood."
   2. "What makes you think that the technician is out to hurt you?"
   3. "Are you fearful and think that others may want to hurt you?"
   4. "The technician is not going to hurt you, but is going to help you!"

857. An inebriated client is brought to the emergency department by the local police. The client is told that the physician will be in to see the client in about 30 minutes. The client becomes very loud and offensive and wants to be seen by the physician immediately. The nurse assisting to care for the client would plan for which appropriate nursing intervention?
   1. Watch the behavior escalate before intervening.
   2. Attempt to talk with the client to de-escalate the behavior.
   3. Offer to take the client to an examination room until he or she can be treated.
   4. Inform the client that he or she will be asked to leave if the behavior continues.

858. A client is admitted to a psychiatric unit for treatment of psychotic behavior. The client is at the locked exit door and is shouting, "Let me out. There's nothing wrong with me. I don't belong here." The nurse identifies this behavior as:
   1. Denial
   2. Projection
   3. Regression
   4. Rationalization

859. A client says to the nurse, "I'm going to die, and I wish my family would stop hoping for a 'cure'! I get so angry when they carry on like this! After all, I'm the one who's dying." The therapeutic response by the nurse is:
   1. "Have you shared your feelings with your family?"
   2. "I think we should talk more about your anger with your family."
   3. "You're feeling angry that your family continues to hope for you to be 'cured'?"
   4. "Well, it sounds like you're being pretty pessimistic. After all, years ago people died of pneumonia."

860. A nurse in a psychiatric unit is assigned to care for a client admitted to the unit 2 days ago. On review of the client's record, the nurse notes that the

admission was a voluntary admission. Based on this type of admission, the nurse would expect which of the following?
1. The client will be angry and will refuse care.
2. The client will participate in the treatment plan.
3. The client will be very resistant to treatment measures.
4. The client's family will be very resistant to treatment measures.

861. A licensed practical nurse (LPN) enters a client's room, and the client is demanding release from the hospital. The LPN reviews the client's record and notes that the client was admitted 2 days ago for treatment of an anxiety disorder, and that the admission was a voluntary admission. The LPN reports the findings to the registered nurse (RN) and expects that the RN will take which of the following actions?
1. Contact the physician.
2. Call the client's family.
3. Persuade the client to stay a few more days.
4. Tell the client that discharge is not possible at this time.

862. A client is admitted to the psychiatric nursing unit. When collecting data from the client, the nurse notes that the client was admitted by involuntary status. Based on this type of admission, the nurse likely expects that the client:
1. Presents a harm to self
2. Requested the admission
3. Consented to the admission
4. Provided written application to the facility for admission

863. Following a group therapy session, a client approaches the licensed practical nurse (LPN) and verbalizes a need for seclusion because of uncontrollable feelings. The LPN reports the findings to the registered nurse (RN) and expects that the RN will take which of the following actions?
1. Call the client's family.
2. Place the client in seclusion immediately.
3. Inform the client that seclusion has not been prescribed.
4. Get a written order from the doctor and obtain an informed consent.

864. A nurse is providing care to a client admitted to the hospital with a diagnosis of anxiety disorder. The nurse is talking with the client and the client says, "I have a secret that I want to tell you. You won't tell anyone about it, will you?" The appropriate nursing response is which of the following?
1. "No, I won't tell anyone."
2. "I cannot promise to keep a secret."

3. "If you tell me the secret, I will tell it to your doctor."
4. "If you tell me the secret, I will need to document it in your record."

865. A psychiatric nurse is greeted by a neighbor in a local grocery store. The neighbor says to the nurse, "How is Carol doing? She is my best friend and is seen at your clinic every week." The appropriate nursing response is which of the following?
1. "I cannot discuss any client situation with you."
2. "I'm not supposed to discuss this, but since you are my neighbor, I can tell you that she is doing great!"
3. "You may want to know about Carol, so you need to ask her yourself so you can get the story firsthand."
4. "I'm not supposed to discuss this, but since you are my neighbor, I can tell you that she really has some problems!"

866. A nurse is preparing a client for the termination phase of the nurse-client relationship. Which nursing task would the nurse appropriately plan for this phase?
1. Plan short-term goals.
2. Identify expected outcomes.
3. Assist in making appropriate referrals.
4. Assist in developing realistic solutions.

867. During the termination phase of the nurse-client relationship, the clinic nurse observes that the client continuously demonstrates bursts of anger. The appropriate interpretation of the behavior is that the client:
1. Needs to be admitted to the hospital
2. Needs to be referred to the psychiatrist as soon as possible
3. Requires further treatment and is not ready to be discharged
4. Is displaying typical behaviors that can occur during termination

868. Therapy that involves pairing a stimulus attractive to the client with an unpleasant event is known as which of the following?
1. Milieu therapy
2. Desensitization
3. Aversion therapy
4. Self-control therapy

869. A nurse informs a client with an eating disorder about group meetings with Overeaters Anonymous. Which statement by the client indicates the need for additional information about this self-help group?
1. "The leader of this self-help group is a nurse or psychiatrist."
2. "The members of this self-help group provide support to each other."

3. "This self-help group is designed to serve people who have a common problem."

4. "In this self-help group, people who have a similar problem are able to help others."

870. A client is attending a Gamblers Anonymous meeting for the first time. The model used by this group is the 12-step program developed by Alcoholics Anonymous. The nurse understands that the first step in the 12-step program is which of the following?

1. Admitting to having a problem
2. Substituting gambling for other activities
3. Stating that the gambling will be stopped
4. Discontinuing relationships with friends who are gamblers

871. A nurse is assisting in conducting a group therapy session and a client with a manic disorder is monopolizing the group. The appropriate nursing action is which of the following?

1. Ask the client to leave.
2. Refer the client to another group.
3. Tell the client to stop monopolizing the group.
4. Suggest that the client stop talking and try listening to others.

872. A nurse is assisting in a group therapy session. During this session, the members are identifying tasks and boundaries. The nurse understands that these activities are characteristic of which stage of group development?

1. Middle stage
2. Beginning stage
3. Termination stage
4. Self-awareness stage

873. A nurse assists in planning care for a client scheduled to be discharged from a mental health clinic. The nurse understands that the client's unresolved feelings related to loss may resurface during which phase of the therapeutic nurse-client relationship?

1. Trusting phase
2. Working phase
3. Orientation phase
4. Termination phase

874. A client with depression who has attempted suicide says to the nurse, "I should have died. I've always been a failure. Nothing ever goes right for me." The nurse makes which therapeutic response to the client?

1. "I don't see you as a failure."
2. "You have everything to live for."
3. "Feeling like this is all part of being ill."
4. "You've been feeling like a failure for a while?"

875. The nurse is collecting data from a client and is attempting to obtain subjective data regarding the client's sexual reproductive status. The client states, "I don't want to discuss this; it's private and personal." Which statement by the nurse indicates a therapeutic response?

1. "I hate being asked these sorts of questions too."
2. "I am a nurse and as such I'll have you know that all information is kept confidential."
3. "I know that some of these questions are difficult for you, but as a nurse, I must legally respect your confidentiality."
4. "This is difficult for you to speak about, but I am trying to perform a complete data collection and I need this information."

876. A nurse is caring for a client who says, "I don't want you to touch me. I'll take care of myself!" The nurse should make which therapeutic response to the client?

1. "If you didn't want our care, why did you come here?"
2. "Why are you being so difficult? I only want to help you."
3. "Sounds like you're feeling pretty troubled by all of us. Let's work together so you can do everything for yourself as you request."
4. "I will respect your feelings. I'll just leave this cup for you to collect your urine in. After breakfast, I will take more blood from you."

ALTERNATE ITEM FORMAT: MULTIPLE RESPONSE

877. The nurse in the mental health unit reviews the therapeutic and nontherapeutic communication techniques with a nursing student. Select all therapeutic communication techniques.

☐ 1. Restating
☐ 2. Listening
☐ 3. Asking the client, "Why?"
☐ 4. Maintaining neutral responses
☐ 5. Giving advice or approval or disapproval
☐ 6. Providing acknowledgment and feedback

ANSWERS

853. **1**

Rationale: Open-ended questions and silence are strategies used to encourage clients to discuss their problem. Options 3 and 4 do not encourage the client to express feelings. The nurse should not offer opinions and should not state the reasons but should encourage the client to identify the reasons for the behavior. Option 2 is not a client-centered intervention.

Test-Taking Strategy: Use the process of elimination. Eliminate options 3 and 4 first, because they do not support client expression of feelings. Eliminate option 2 next, because it is not a client-centered intervention. Focusing on the client's feelings will direct you to option 1. Review therapeutic communication techniques if you had difficulty with this question.

Level of Cognitive Ability: Application

Client Needs: Psychosocial Integrity
Integrated Process: Caring
Content Area: Mental Health
Reference: Keltner, N., Schwecke, L., & Bostrom, C. (2007). *Psychiatric nursing* (5th ed., pp. 90-92, 566-567). St. Louis: Mosby.

854. **3**
Rationale: The client must first deal with feelings and negative responses before the client is able to work through the meaning of the crisis. Option 3 pertains directly to the client's feelings. Options 1, 2, and 4 do not directly address the client's feelings.
Test-Taking Strategy: Use the process of elimination. Focusing on the feelings of the client will direct you to option 3. Review the nurse's actions in a crisis situation if you had difficulty with this question.
Level of Cognitive Ability: Application
Client Needs: Psychosocial Integrity
Integrated Process: Nursing Process/Implementation
Content Area: Mental Health
References: Fortinash, K., & Holoday-Worret, P. (2008). *Psychiatric mental health nursing* (4th ed., pp. 457-459). St. Louis: Mosby.
Morrison-Valfre, M. (2005). *Foundations of mental health care* (3rd ed., pp. 23, 90-91). St. Louis: Mosby.

855. **1**
Rationale: The client's thoughts are extremely important when verbalized. Suicidal thoughts are the highest priority. Options 2, 3, and 4 will all affect the treatment of the client but are not of greatest importance at this time.
Test-Taking Strategy: The client is the focus of the question; therefore, eliminate option 4. Focus on the strategic words "priority concern" and use prioritizing skills. Remember, if the client verbalizes suicidal thoughts, it is a priority concern. Review data collection techniques related to the suicidal client if you had difficulty with this question.
Level of Cognitive Ability: Analysis
Client Needs: Psychosocial Integrity
Integrated Process: Nursing Process/Data Collection
Content Area: Mental Health
References: Keltner, N., Schwecke, L., & Bostrom, C. (2007). *Psychiatric nursing* (5th ed., p. 385). St. Louis: Mosby.
Morrison-Valfre, M. (2005). *Foundations of mental health care* (3rd ed., pp. 283, 287). St. Louis: Mosby.

856. **1**
Rationale: Option 3 is the only option that recognizes the client's need. This response helps the client focus on the emotion underlying the delusion but does not argue with it. If the nurse attempts to change the client's mind, the delusion may, in fact, be even more strongly held. Options 1, 2, and 4 do not focus on the client's feelings
Test-Taking Strategy: Use therapeutic communication techniques and knowledge regarding the dynamics of delusions and how delusions meet the client's underlying needs. This will direct you to option 3. In addition, option 3 focuses on the client's feelings. Review therapeutic communication techniques if you had difficulty with this question.

Level of Cognitive Ability: Application
Client Needs: Psychosocial Integrity
Integrated Process: Communication and Documentation
Content Area: Mental Health
References: Keltner, N., Schwecke, L., & Bostrom, C. (2007). *Psychiatric nursing* (5th ed., pp. 90-92, 361). St. Louis: Mosby.
Morrison-Valfre, M. (2005). *Foundations of mental health care* (3rd ed., p. 328). St. Louis: Mosby.

857. **3**
Rationale: Safety of the client, other clients, and staff is of prime concern. When dealing with an impaired individual, trying to talk may be out of the question. Waiting to intervene could cause the client to become even more agitated and a threat to others. Option 4 would only further aggravate an already agitated individual. Option 3 is in effect an isolation technique that allows for separation from others and provides a less stimulating environment, where the client can maintain dignity.
Test-Taking Strategy: Focus on the subject of the question and use the process of elimination. Noting that the client is inebriated will assist in directing you to option 3. Option 3 most directly addresses the situation and the behavior and feelings of the client. Review nursing interventions for a client who is inebriated if you had difficulty with this question.
Level of Cognitive Ability: Application
Client Needs: Psychosocial Integrity
Integrated Process: Nursing Process/Planning
Content Area: Mental Health
References: Fortinash, K., & Holoday-Worret, P. (2008). *Psychiatric mental health nursing* (4th ed., pp. 30-31, 521). St. Louis: Mosby.
Morrison-Valfre, M. (2005). *Foundations of mental health care* (3rd ed., pp. 71, 116). St. Louis: Mosby.

858. **1**
Rationale: Denial is refusal to admit to a painful reality and is treated as if it does not exist. In projection, a person unconsciously rejects emotionally unacceptable features and attributes them to other people, objects, or situations. In regression, the client returns to an earlier, more comforting, although less mature way of behaving. Rationalization is justifying the unacceptable attributes about oneself.
Test-Taking Strategy: Use the process of elimination. Note the strategic words, "There's nothing wrong with me." Select the option that recognizes the client's attempt to avoid looking at the reality of the situation. If you had difficulty with this question, review defense mechanisms.
Level of Cognitive Ability: Comprehension
Client Needs: Psychosocial Integrity
Integrated Process: Nursing Process/Data Collection
Content Area: Mental Health
References: Keltner, N., Schwecke, L., & Bostrom, C. (2007). *Psychiatric nursing* (5th ed., pp.106-107). St. Louis: Mosby.
Morrison-Valfre, M. (2005). *Foundations of mental health care* (3rd ed., p. 70). St. Louis: Mosby.

859. **3**
Rationale: Reflection is the therapeutic communication technique that redirects the client's feelings back to validate what the client is saying. In option 2, the nurse attempts to use

focusing, but the attempt to discuss central issues seems premature. In option 4, the nurse makes a judgment and is nontherapeutic in the one-on-one relationship. In option 1, the nurse is attempting to assess the client's ability to openly discuss feelings with family members. Although this may be appropriate, the timing is somewhat premature and closes off facilitation of the client's feelings.

Test-Taking Strategy: Use therapeutic communication techniques. Note that option 3 uses the therapeutic technique of reflection and focuses on the client's feelings. Options 1, 2, and 4 are nontherapeutic at this time. Review therapeutic communication techniques if you had difficulty with this question.

Level of Cognitive Ability: Application
Client Needs: Psychosocial Integrity
Integrated Process: Communication and Documentation
Content Area: Mental Health
References: Fortinash, K., & Holoday-Worret, P. (2008). *Psychiatric mental health nursing* (4th ed., p. 72). St. Louis: Mosby.
Keltner, N., Schwecke, L., & Bostrom, C. (2007). *Psychiatric nursing* (5th ed., pp. 90-92). St. Louis: Mosby.
Morrison-Valfre, M. (2005). *Foundations of mental health care* (3rd ed., p. 88). St. Louis: Mosby.

860. **2**
Rationale: Generally, voluntary admission is sought by the client or client's guardian. If the client seeks voluntary admission, the most likely expectation is that the client will participate in the treatment program.
Test-Taking Strategy: Use the process of elimination. Note the strategic words "voluntary admission." This will direct you to option 2. In addition, note that options 1, 3, and 4 are comparable or alike. Review the various types of hospital admission processes if you had difficulty with this question.
Level of Cognitive Ability: Comprehension
Client Needs: Psychosocial Integrity
Integrated Process: Nursing Process/Planning
Content Area: Mental Health
References: Fortinash, K., & Holoday-Worret, P. (2008). *Psychiatric mental health nursing* (4th ed., p. 157). St. Louis: Mosby.
Morrison-Valfre, M. (2005). *Foundations of mental health care* (3rd ed., p. 23). St. Louis: Mosby.

861. **1**
Rationale: Generally, voluntary admission is sought by the client or client's guardian. Voluntary clients have the right to demand and obtain release. The best nursing action is to contact the physician.
Test-Taking Strategy: Use the process of elimination. Noting the type of hospital admission will assist in eliminating option 4. It is inappropriate to "persuade" a client to stay in the hospital. Option 2 should be eliminated simply based on the issue of client rights and the issue of confidentiality. Review the various types of hospital admission and discharge processes if you had difficulty with this question.
Level of Cognitive Ability: Application
Client Needs: Safe and Effective Care Environment
Integrated Process: Nursing Process/Implementation
Content Area: Mental Health

References: Keltner, N., Schwecke, L., & Bostrom, C. (2007). *Psychiatric nursing* (5th ed., p. 58). St. Louis: Mosby.
Morrison-Valfre, M. (2005). *Foundations of mental health care* (3rd ed., p. 23). St. Louis: Mosby.

862. **1**
Rationale: Involuntary admission is made without the client's consent. Involuntary admission is necessary when a person is a danger to self or others or is in need of psychiatric treatment or physical care. Options 2, 3, and 4 describe the process of voluntary admission.
Test-Taking Strategy: Use the process of elimination. Note the strategic words "involuntary status." This should direct you to option 1. Also, note that options 2, 3, and 4 are comparable or alike. Review the process of involuntary admission if you had difficulty with this question.
Level of Cognitive Ability: Comprehension
Client Needs: Psychosocial Integrity
Integrated Process: Nursing Process/Planning
Content Area: Mental Health
Reference: Keltner, N., Schwecke, L., & Bostrom, C. (2007). *Psychiatric nursing* (5th ed., p. 58). St. Louis: Mosby.

863. **4**
Rationale: A client may request to be secluded or restrained. Federal laws require the consent of the client, unless an emergency situation exists in which an immediate risk to the client or others can be documented. The use of seclusion and restraint is permitted only on the written order of a physician, which must be reviewed and renewed every 24 hours; it must also specify the type of restraint to be used.
Test-Taking Strategy: Use the process of elimination. There is no reason to call the family at this time; therefore, eliminate option 1. Knowing that a physician's written order is necessary in this situation will assist in eliminating option 2. Option 3 is not the best choice because this information, if given to a client experiencing uncontrollable feelings, may cause escalation of the feelings. Review the procedures for seclusion if you had difficulty with this question.
Level of Cognitive Ability: Application
Client Needs: Safe and Effective Care Environment
Integrated Process: Nursing Process/Implementation
Content Area: Mental Health
References: Keltner, N., Schwecke, L., & Bostrom, C. (2007). *Psychiatric nursing* (5th ed., p. 137). St. Louis: Mosby.
Morrison-Valfre, M. (2005). *Foundations of mental health care* (3rd ed., pp. 25, 262-263). St. Louis: Mosby.

864. **2**
Rationale: The nurse should never promise to keep a secret. Secrets are appropriate in a social relationship, but not in a therapeutic one. The nurse needs to be honest with the client and tell the client that a promise cannot be made to keep the secret.
Test-Taking Strategy: Use the process of elimination and knowledge of therapeutic communication techniques. Option 1 can be eliminated because it is inappropriate. Also, options 3 and 4 are not only inappropriate, but are threatening to an extent and may even block further communication. Review the principles related to a therapeutic nurse-client relationship if you had difficulty with this question.

Level of Cognitive Ability: Application
Client Needs: Psychosocial Integrity
Integrated Process: Communication and Documentation
Content Area: Mental Health
References: Fortinash, K., & Holoday-Worret, P. (2008). *Psychiatric mental health nursing* (4th ed., pp. 26, 75-78). St. Louis: Mosby.
Morrison-Valfre, M. (2005). *Foundations of mental health care* (3rd ed., p. 185). St. Louis: Mosby.

865. **1**
Rationale: A nurse is required to maintain confidentiality regarding clients and their care. Confidentiality is basic to the therapeutic relationship and is a client's right. Option 3 is correct in a sense; however, it is a rather blunt statement. Both options 2 and 4 identify statements that do not maintain client confidentiality.
Test-Taking Strategy: Use the process of elimination. Focus on the subject of the question—maintaining confidentiality. This should assist in eliminating options 2 and 4. From the remaining options, select option 1 over option 3 because it is most direct and correct. Option 3 is a rather blunt and somewhat rude statement. Review confidentiality issues if you had difficulty with this question.
Level of Cognitive Ability: Application
Client Needs: Safe and Effective Care Environment
Integrated Process: Communication and Documentation
Content Area: Mental Health
References: Keltner, N., Schwecke, L., & Bostrom, C. (2007). *Psychiatric nursing* (5th ed., p. 54). St. Louis: Mosby.
Morrison-Valfre, M. (2005). *Foundations of mental health care* (3rd ed., p. 21). St. Louis: Mosby.

866. **3**
Rationale: Tasks of the termination phase include evaluating client performance, evaluating achievement of expected outcomes, evaluating future needs, making appropriate referrals, and dealing with the common behaviors associated with termination. Options 1, 2, and 4 identify the tasks of the working phase of the relationship.
Test-Taking Strategy: Noting the strategic words "termination phase" should direct you to option 3. If you are unfamiliar with the appropriate tasks of the phases of the nurse-client relationship, review this content.
Level of Cognitive Ability: Application
Client Needs: Psychosocial Integrity
Integrated Process: Nursing Process/Planning
Content Area: Mental Health
Reference: Keltner, N., Schwecke, L., & Bostrom, C. (2007). *Psychiatric nursing* (5th ed., p. 104). St. Louis: Mosby.

867. **4**
Rationale: In the termination phase of a relationship, it is normal for a client to demonstrate a number of regressive behaviors. Typical behaviors include return of symptoms, anger, withdrawal, and minimizing the relationship. The anger that the client is experiencing is a normal behavior during the termination phase and does not necessarily indicate the need for hospitalization or treatment.
Test-Taking Strategy: Use the process of elimination. Note the strategic words "termination phase." This alone may assist in

directing you to option 4. In addition, note the similarity among options 1, 2, and 3. These options address the need for further supervised treatment. If you are unfamiliar with the client behaviors associated with the termination phase, review this content.
Level of Cognitive Ability: Analysis
Client Needs: Psychosocial Integrity
Integrated Process: Nursing Process/Evaluation
Content Area: Mental Health
References: Keltner, N., Schwecke, L., & Bostrom, C. (2007). *Psychiatric nursing* (5th ed., p. 104). St. Louis: Mosby.
Morrison-Valfre, M. (2005). *Foundations of mental health care* (3rd ed., p. 107). St. Louis: Mosby.

868. **3**
Rationale: Aversion therapy, also known as aversion conditioning or negative reinforcement, is a technique used to change behavior. In this therapy, a stimulus attractive to the client is paired with an unpleasant event in hopes of associating the stimulus with negative properties. Desensitization is the reduction of intense reactions to a stimulus by repeated exposure to the stimulus in a weaker and milder form. Milieu therapy provides positive environmental manipulation, both physical and social, to effect a positive change in the client. Self-control therapy combines cognitive and behavioral approaches and is useful to deal with stress.
Test-Taking Strategy: Focus on the information in the question. Recalling that aversion therapy is a form of negative reinforcement will direct you to the correct option. If you had difficulty with this question, review this form of therapy.
Level of Cognitive Ability: Comprehension
Client Needs: Psychosocial Integrity
Integrated Process: Nursing Process/Implementation
Content Area: Mental Health
Reference: Fortinash, K., & Holoday-Worret, P. (2008). *Psychiatric mental health nursing* (4th ed., p. 516). St. Louis: Mosby.

869. **1**
Rationale: The leader of a self-help group is an experienced member of the group. A nurse or psychiatrist may be asked by the group to serve as a resource but would not be the leader of the group. Options 2, 3, and 4 are characteristics of a self-help group.
Test-Taking Strategy: Use the process of elimination and note the strategic words "need for additional information" in the query of the question. Note that options 2, 3, and 4 are comparable or alike. This should direct you to option 1. Review the characteristics of a self-help group if you had difficulty with this question.
Level of Cognitive Ability: Comprehension
Client Needs: Psychosocial Integrity
Integrated Process: Nursing Process/Evaluation
Content Area: Mental Health
References: Keltner, N., Schwecke, L., & Bostrom, C. (2007). *Psychiatric nursing* (5th ed., pp. 146-147). St. Louis: Mosby.
Morrison-Valfre, M. (2005). *Foundations of mental health care* (3rd ed., p. 49). St. Louis: Mosby.

870. **1**
Rationale: The first step in the 12-step program is to admit that a problem exists. Options 3 and 4 are unrealistic as a first

step in the process to recovery. Although option 2 may be a strategy, it is not the first step.
Test-Taking Strategy: Note the strategic words "first step" in the question. This will assist in directing you to option 1. If you are unfamiliar with the 12-step program, review this content.
Level of Cognitive Ability: Comprehension
Client Needs: Psychosocial Integrity
Integrated Process: Nursing Process/Implementation
Content Area: Mental Health
References: Fortinash, K., & Holoday-Worret, P. (2008). *Psychiatric mental health nursing* (4th ed., p. 334). St. Louis: Mosby.
Stuart, G., & Laraia, M. (2005). *Principles and practice of psychiatric nursing* (8th ed., pp. 506-507). St. Louis: Mosby.

871. **4**
Rationale: If a client is monopolizing the group, it is important that the nurse be direct and decisive. The best action is to suggest that the client stop talking and try listening to others. Although option 3 may be a direct response, option 4 is the most therapeutic direct statement. Options 1 and 2 are inappropriate.
Test-Taking Strategy: Use the process of elimination. Eliminate options 1 and 2 first because they are comparable or alike. Use therapeutic communication techniques to assist in directing you to option 4. If you had difficulty with this question, review therapeutic communication techniques.
Level of Cognitive Ability: Application
Client Needs: Psychosocial Integrity
Integrated Process: Nursing Process/Implementation
Content Area: Mental Health
References: Fortinash, K., & Holoday-Worret, P. (2008). *Psychiatric mental health nursing* (4th ed., pp 220-221). St. Louis: Mosby.
Keltner, N., Schwecke, L., & Bostrom, C. (2007). *Psychiatric nursing* (5th ed., pp. 90-92). St. Louis: Mosby.

872. **2**
Rationale: In the beginning or initial stage, the members are identifying tasks and boundaries. Information is given and group norms are established. In the middle stage, members are confronting each other, groups develop cohesiveness, and a sense of trust is established. The termination stage is where members may leave the group abruptly, the group decides that its work is done, and the group members feel that they have met their goals. There is no such stage of group development called the self-awareness stage.
Test-Taking Strategy: Use the process of elimination. Note the strategic word "identifying" in the question. This word should assist in directing you to option 2. If you had difficulty with this question, review the stages of group development.
Level of Cognitive Ability: Comprehension
Client Needs: Psychosocial Integrity
Integrated Process: Nursing Process/Implementation
Content Area: Mental Health
Reference: Stuart, G., & Laraia, M. (2005). *Principles and practice of psychiatric nursing* (8th ed., p. 672). St. Louis: Mosby.

873. **4**
Rationale: In the termination phase, the relationship comes to a close. Ending treatment may sometimes be traumatic for clients who have come to value the relationship and the help. Because loss is an issue, any unresolved feelings related to loss may resurface during this phase. Options 1, 2, and 3 are incorrect.
Test-Taking Strategy: Note the strategic words "unresolved" and "loss" in the question. Consider the phases of the therapeutic nurse-client relationship to direct you to option 4. Review these phases and the nursing implications if you had difficulty with this question.
Level of Cognitive Ability: Comprehension
Client Needs: Psychosocial Integrity
Integrated Process: Caring
Content Area: Mental Health
References: Keltner, N., Schwecke, L., & Bostrom, C. (2007). *Psychiatric nursing* (5th ed., p. 104). St. Louis: Mosby.
Morrison-Valfre, M. (2005). *Foundations of mental health care* (3rd ed., pp. 105-107). St. Louis: Mosby.

874. **4**
Rationale: Responding to the feelings expressed by a client is an effective therapeutic communication technique. The correct option is an example of the use of restating. Options 1, 2, and 3 block communication because they minimize the client's feelings and do not facilitate exploration of the client's expressed feelings.
Test-Taking Strategy: Use therapeutic communication techniques. Select the option that directly addresses the client's feelings and concerns. Option 4 is the only option that is stated in the form of a question and is open-ended; therefore, it will encourage the verbalization of feelings. Review these techniques if you had difficulty with this question.
Level of Cognitive Ability: Application
Client Needs: Psychosocial Integrity
Integrated Process: Communication and Documentation
Content Area: Mental Health
References: Keltner, N., Schwecke, L., & Bostrom, C. (2007). *Psychiatric nursing* (5th ed., pp. 90-92, 385-386). St. Louis: Mosby.
Morrison-Valfre, M. (2005). *Foundations of mental health care* (3rd ed., p. 88). St. Louis: Mosby

875. **3**
Rationale: Option 3 is the only option that identifies a therapeutic response. In option 1, the nurse's feelings are the focus. This response clearly ignores the fact that the issue is about the client and the client's discomfort, not about the nurse. In option 2, the nurse becomes pompous and a little angry and supercilious, which is not therapeutic. In option 4, the nurse begins correctly with an empathetic stance but then becomes demanding.
Test-Taking Strategy: Using the process of elimination and therapeutic communication techniques will easily direct you to option 3. Review therapeutic communication techniques if you had difficulty with this question.
Level of Cognitive Ability: Analysis
Client Needs: Psychosocial Integrity
Integrated Process: Communication and Documentation
Content Area: Mental Health
References: Keltner, N., Schwecke, L., & Bostrom, C. (2007). *Psychiatric nursing* (5th ed., pp. 115-116). St. Louis: Mosby.
Morrison-Valfre, M. (2005). *Foundations of mental health care* (3rd ed., p. 88). St. Louis: Mosby.

876. **3**

Rationale: The therapeutic response is the one that reflects the client's feelings and offers the client control of care. In option 4, the nurse uses avoidance and gives information. Option 1 is an aggressive and nontherapeutic communication technique. Option 2 is social and nontherapeutic, because it labels the client's behavior and is likely to provoke anger from the client.

Test-Taking Strategy: Focus on the client's statement and use therapeutic communication techniques. Option 3 is the only option that addresses the client's statement. Review therapeutic communication techniques if you had difficulty with this question.

Level of Cognitive Ability: Application
Client Needs: Psychosocial Integrity
Integrated Process: Communication and Documentation
Content Area: Mental Health
Reference: Keltner, N., Schwecke, L., & Bostrom, C. (2007). *Psychiatric nursing* (5th ed., pp. 90-92). St. Louis: Mosby.

ALTERNATE ITEM FORMAT: MULTIPLE RESPONSE

877. **1, 2, 4, 6**

Rationale: Some of the therapeutic communication techniques include listening, maintaining silence, maintaining neutral responses, using broad openings and open-ended questions, focusing and refocusing, restating, clarifying and validating, sharing perceptions, reflecting, providing acknowledgment and feedback, giving information and presenting reality, encouraging formulation of a plan of action, providing nonverbal encouragement, and summarizing.

Test-Taking Strategy: Focus on the subject—therapeutic communication techniques. This will assist you in selecting the correct answers. Review therapeutic and nontherapeutic techniques if you had difficulty with this question.

Level of Cognitive Ability: Comprehension
Client Needs: Psychosocial Integrity
Integrated Process: Teaching and Learning
Content Area: Mental Health
Reference: Keltner, N., Schwecke, L., & Bostrom, C. (2007). *Psychiatric nursing* (5th ed., pp. 90-92). St. Louis: Mosby.

REFERENCES

Fortinash, K., & Holoday-Worret, P. (2008). *Psychiatric mental health nursing* (4th ed.). St. Louis: Mosby.

Keltner, N., Schwecke, L., & Bostrom, C. (2007). *Psychiatric nursing* (5th ed.). St. Louis: Mosby.

Morrison-Valfre, M. (2005). *Foundations of mental health care* (3rd ed.). St. Louis: Mosby.

Stuart, G., & Laraia, M. (2005). *Principles and practice of psychiatric nursing* (8th ed.). St. Louis: Mosby.

Mental Health Disorders

I. ANXIETY

A. Description
1. Anxiety is a normal response to stress
2. A subjective experience that includes feelings of apprehension, uneasiness, uncertainty, or dread
3. Occurs as a result of threats that may be misperceived or misinterpreted or as a result of a threat to identity or self-esteem
4. May result when values are threatened or preceding new experiences

B. Types of anxiety
1. Normal: a healthy type of anxiety
2. Acute: precipitated by imminent loss or change that threatens one's sense of security
3. Chronic: anxiety that persists as a characteristic response to daily activities

C. Levels of anxiety
1. Mild
   a. Associated with the tension of everyday life
   b. The individual is alert
   c. The perceptual field is increased
   d. Mild anxiety can be motivating, produce growth, enhance creativity, and increase learning
2. Moderate
   a. The focus is on immediate concerns
   b. Moderate anxiety narrows the perceptual field
   c. Selective inattentiveness occurs
   d. Learning and problem-solving still take place
3. Severe
   a. Severe anxiety is a feeling that something bad is about to happen
   b. A significant narrowing in the perceptual field occurs
   c. Focus is on minute or scattered details
   d. All behavior is directed at relieving the anxiety
   e. Learning and problem-solving are not possible
   f. The individual needs direction to focus

4. Panic
   a. Panic is associated with dread and terror and a sense of impending doom
   b. The personality is disorganized
   c. The individual is unable to communicate or function effectively
   d. Increased motor activity occurs
   e. Loss of rational thoughts with distorted perception occurs
   f. Inability to concentrate occurs
   g. If prolonged, panic can lead to exhaustion and death

D. Interventions: general nursing measures
1. Recognize the anxiety
2. Establish trust
3. Protect the client
4. Do not criticize **coping mechanisms**
5. Do not force the client into situations that provoke anxiety
6. Decrease stimulation in the environment
7. Modify the environment by setting limits or limiting interaction with others
8. Provide creative outlets
9. Provide activities that limit the amount of time for destructive behavior
10. Promote relaxation techniques such as breathing exercises or guided imagery
11. Monitor vital signs and administer antianxiety medications as prescribed

E. Interventions: mild to moderate levels
1. Help the client identify the anxiety
2. Encourage the client to talk about feelings and concerns
3. Help the client identify thoughts and feelings that occurred before the onset of anxiety
4. Encourage problem-solving
5. Encourage gross motor exercise

F. Interventions: severe to panic levels
1. Reduce the anxiety quickly
2. Use a calm manner
3. Always remain with the client
4. Minimize environmental stimuli
5. Provide clear, simple statements

6. Use a low-pitched voice
7. Attend to the physical needs of the client
8. Provide gross motor activity
9. Administer antianxiety medications as prescribed

II. **GENERALIZED ANXIETY DISORDER**
A. Description
   1. Generalized anxiety disorder is an unrealistic anxiety about everyday worries that persist over time and is not associated with another psychiatric or medical disorder
   2. Physical symptoms occur
B. Data collection
   1. Restlessness and inability to relax
   2. Episodes of trembling and shakiness
   3. Chronic muscular tension
   4. Dizziness
   5. Inability to concentrate
   6. Chronic fatigue and sleep problems
   7. Inability to recognize the connection between the anxiety and physical symptoms
   8. Client is focused on the physical discomfort
C. Panic disorder
   1. Description
      a. Panic disorder produces a sudden onset of feelings of intense apprehension and dread
      b. The cause usually cannot be identified
      c. Severe, recurrent, intermittent anxiety attacks occur, lasting 5 to 30 minutes
   2. Data collection
      a. Choking sensation
      b. Labored breathing
      c. Pounding heart
      d. Chest pain
      e. Dizziness
      f. Nausea
      g. Blurred vision
      h. Numbness or tingling of the extremities
      i. A sense of unreality and helplessness
      j. A fear of being trapped
      k. A fear of dying
   3. Interventions
      a. Remain with the client
      b. Attend to physical symptoms
      c. Assist the client to identify the thoughts that aroused the anxiety and to identify the basis for these thoughts
      d. Assist the client to change the unrealistic thoughts to more realistic thoughts
      e. Use cognitive restructuring to replace distorted thinking
      f. Administer antianxiety medications if prescribed

III. **POSTTRAUMATIC STRESS DISORDER**
A. Description: after experiencing a psychologically traumatic event, the individual is prone to reexperience the event and have recurrent and intrusive dreams or flashbacks

B. Stressors
   1. A natural disaster
   2. A terrorist attack
   3. Combat experiences
   4. Accidents
   5. Victim of rape
   6. Victim of crime or violence
   7. Victim of sexual, physical, and emotional **abuse**
   8. Reexperiencing the event as flashbacks
C. Data collection
   1. Emotional numbness
   2. Detachment
   3. Depression
   4. Anxiety
   5. Sleep disturbances and nightmares
   6. Flashbacks of the event
   7. Hypervigilance
   8. Guilt about surviving the event
   9. Poor concentration and avoidance of activities that trigger the memory of the event
D. Interventions (Box 63-1)

IV. **PHOBIAS**
A. Description
   1. An irrational fear of an object or situation that persists although the person may recognize it as unreasonable
   2. Is associated with panic level anxiety if the object, situation, or activity cannot be avoided
   3. **Defense mechanisms** commonly used include repression and displacement
B. Types (Box 63-2)
C. Interventions
   1. Stay with the client when the anxiety is high to promote safety and security
   2. Identify the basis of the anxiety

BOX 63-1 | **Interventions for Posttraumatic Stress Disorder**

Be nonjudgmental and supportive.
Assure the client that his or her feelings and behaviors are normal reactions.
Assist the client to recognize the association between his or her feelings and behaviors and the trauma experience.
Encourage the client to express his or her feelings; provide individual therapy that addresses loss of control or anger issues.
Assist the client to develop adaptive coping mechanisms and to use relaxation techniques.
Encourage the use of support groups.
Facilitate a progressive review of the trauma experience.
Encourage the client to establish and reestablish relationships.
Inform the client that hypnotherapy or systematic desensitization may be used as a form of treatment.

BOX 63-2 Types of Phobias

Acrophobia: fear of heights
Agoraphobia: fear of open spaces
Astraphobia: fear of electrical storms
Claustrophobia: fear of closed spaces
Hematophobia: fear of blood
Hydrophobia: fear of water
Monophobia: fear of being alone
Mysophobia: fear of dirt or germs
Nyctophobia: fear of darkness
Pyrophobia: fear of fires
Social phobia: fear of situations in which one might be
  embarrassed or criticized and the fear of making
  a fool of oneself
Xenophobia: fear of strangers
Zoophobia: fear of animals

3. Allow the client to verbalize feelings about the anxiety-producing object or situation; frequently talking about the feared object is the first step in the desensitization process
4. Teach relaxation techniques such as breathing exercises, muscle relaxation exercises, and visualization of pleasant situations
5. Promote desensitization by gradually introducing the individual to the feared object or situation in small doses
6. Do not force the client to have contact with the phobic object or situation

V. **OBSESSIVE-COMPULSIVE DISORDER**
A. Obsessions: preoccupation with persistent intrusive thoughts and ideas
B. Compulsion
  1. A compulsion is the performance of rituals or repetitive behaviors designed to prevent some event, divert unacceptable thoughts, and decrease anxiety
  2. Obsessions and compulsions often occur together and can disrupt normal daily activities
  3. Anxiety occurs when one resists obsessions or compulsions, and from being powerless to resist the thoughts or rituals
  4. Obsessive thoughts can involve issues of violence, aggression, sexual behavior, orderliness, or religion and can uncontrollably interrupt conscious thoughts and the ability to function
C. Compulsive behavior patterns (behaviors or rituals)
  1. Compulsive behavior patterns decrease the anxiety
  2. The patterns are associated with the obsessive thoughts
  3. The patterns neutralize the thought
  4. During stressful times, the ritualistic behavior increases
  5. **Defense mechanisms** include repression, displacement, and undoing
D. Interventions (Box 63-3)

BOX 63-3 Interventions for Obsessive-Compulsive Disorder

Ensure that basic needs (food, rest, grooming) are met.
Identify the situations that precipitate the compulsive behavior; encourage the client to verbalize concerns and feelings.
Be empathetic toward the client, and be aware of his or her need to perform the compulsive behavior.
Do not interrupt the compulsive behaviors unless they jeopardize the safety of the client or others (provide for client safety related to the behavior).
Allow time for the client to perform the compulsive behavior but set limits on behaviors that may interfere with the client's physical well-being in order to protect the client from physical harm.
Implement a schedule for the client that distracts from the behaviors (structure simple activities, games, or tasks for the client).
Establish a written contract that will assist the client to decrease the frequency of compulsive behaviors gradually.
Recognize and reinforce positive nonritualistic behaviors.

BOX 63-4 Types of Somatoform Disorders

Conversion disorder
Hypochondriasis
Somatization disorder

VI. **SOMATOFORM DISORDERS**
A. Description (Box 63-4)
  1. Somatoform disorders are characterized by persistent worry or complaints regarding physical illness without supporting physical findings
  2. The client focuses on the physical signs and symptoms and is unable to control the signs and symptoms
  3. The physical signs and symptoms increase with psychosocial stressors
  4. The anxiety is redirected into a somatic concern
  5. The client may unconsciously use somatization for secondary gains such as increased attention and decreased responsibilities
B. Conversion disorder
  1. Description
    a. A physical symptom or a deficit suggesting loss or altered body function related to psychological conflict or a neurological disorder
    b. Conversion disorder is an expression of a psychological conflict or need
    c. The most common conversion symptoms are blindness, deafness, paralysis, and the inability to talk
    d. Conversion disorder has no organic cause

e. Symptoms are beyond the conscious control of the client and are directly related to conflict

f. The development of physical symptoms reduces anxiety

2. Data collection

a. "La belle indifference": unconcerned with symptoms

b. Physical limitation or disability

c. Feelings of guilt, anxiety, or frustration

d. Low self-esteem and feelings of inadequacy

e. Unexpressed anger or conflict

f. Secondary gain

C. Hypochondriasis

1. Description

a. The preoccupation with fears of having a serious disease

b. No evidence of physical illness exists

c. Hypochondriasis significantly impairs social and occupational functioning

2. Data collection

a. Preoccupation with physical functioning

b. Frequent somatic complaints

c. Complaints of fatigue and insomnia

d. Anxiety

e. Difficulty expressing feelings

f. Extensive use of home remedies or nonprescription medications

g. Repeatedly visiting the doctor in spite of repeated reassurance and test results that are normal

h. Secondary gain

D. Somatization disorder

1. Description

a. The client has multiple physical complaints involving multiple body systems

b. The etiology of these complaints is presumed to be psychological

2. Data collection

a. Physical complaints of pain, denial of emotional problems, and signs of anxiety, fear, and low self-esteem may be present

b. Secondary gain: the client may unconsciously use somatization for secondary gains such as increased attention and decreased responsibilities

E. Interventions

1. Obtain a nursing history and assess for physical problems

2. Discourage verbalization about physical symptoms by not responding with positive reinforcement

3. Allow a specific time period to discuss physical complaints because the client will feel less threatened if this behavior is limited rather than stopped completely

4. Explore with the client the needs being met by the physical symptoms

5. Assist the client to identify alternative ways of meeting needs

6. Assist the client to relate feelings and conflicts to the physical symptoms

7. Convey understanding that the physical symptoms are real to the client

8. Assure the client that physical illness has been ruled out

9. Explore the source of anxiety and stimulate verbalization of anxiety

10. Encourage the use of relaxation techniques as the anxiety increases

11. Use a pain assessment scale if the client complains of pain, and implement pain-reduction measures as required.

12. Report and assess any new physical complaint

13. Encourage diversional activities

14. Provide positive feedback

15. Assist the client in recognizing his or her own feelings and emotions

16. Administer antianxiety medications if prescribed

VII. DISSOCIATIVE DISORDER

A. Description

1. Dissociative disorder is a disruption in integrative functions of memory, consciousness, or identity

2. Dissociative disorder is associated with exposure to an extremely traumatic event

B. Dissociative identity disorder (multiple personality)

1. Description

a. Two or more fully developed distinct and unique personalities exist within the person

b. The host is the primary personality and the other personalities are referred to as alters

c. Alter personalities may take full control of the client, one at a time, and may or may not be aware of each other

d. The alters may be aware of the host but the host is not usually aware of the alter(s)

2. Data collection

a. The client may have an inability to recall important information (unrelated to ordinary forgetfulness)

b. Transition from one personality to the other is related to stress or a traumatic event and is sudden

c. Dissociation is used as a method of distancing and defending one's self from anxiety and traumatizing experiences

C. Dissociative amnesia

1. Description

a. The inability to remember important personal information because it is anxiety provoking

b. Memory impairment may range from partial to almost complete

2. Data collection
   a. Localized: the client blocks out all memories about a specified period
   b. Selective: the client recalls some but not all memories about a specified period
   c. Generalized: the client has a loss of all memory about past life

D. Dissociative fugue
   1. Description
      a. The client assumes a new identity in a new environment
      b. The disorder may occur suddenly
   2. Data collection
      a. The client may drift from place to place
      b. The client develops few social relationships
      c. When the fugue lifts, the client returns home and is unable to recall the fugue state

E. Depersonalization disorder
   1. Description: an altered self-perception in which one's own reality is temporarily lost or changed
   2. Data collection
      a. Feelings of detachment
      b. Intact reality testing

F. Interventions
   1. Develop a trusting relationship with the client
   2. Encourage verbal expression of painful experiences, anxieties, and concerns
   3. Explore methods of coping
   4. Identify sources of conflict
   5. Focus on the client's strengths and skills
   6. Orient the client
   7. Provide nondemanding simple routines
   8. Allow the client to progress at his or her own pace
   9. Implement stress-reduction techniques
   10. Plan for individual, group, and/or family psychotherapy to integrate dissociated aspects of personality or memory and to expand self-awareness

▲ VIII. MOOD DISORDERS
A. Bipolar disorder
   1. Description (Box 63-5)
      a. Bipolar disorder is characterized by episodes of mania and depression with periods of normal mood and activity in between
      b. The medication of choice has traditionally been lithium carbonate, which can be toxic and therefore requires the regular monitoring of serum lithium levels
      c. Other medications such as divalproex (Valproate), olanzapine (Zyprexa), and carbamazepine (Tegretol) may also be prescribed to reduce the symptoms of acute bipolar manic episodes

---

BOX 63-5 Data Collection: Bipolar Disorder

Mania
Becomes angry quickly
Delusional self-confidence
Distracted by environmental stimuli
Extroverted personality
Flight of ideas
Grandiose and persecutory delusions
High and unstable affect
Inability to eat or sleep because of involvement in more important things
Inability to sleep yet still active
Inappropriate affect
Inappropriate dress
Initiation of activity
Pressured speech
Restlessness
Sexually promiscuous
Significant decrease in appetite
Unlimited energy
Urgent motor activity

Depression
Increased or decreased appetite
Decrease in activities of daily living
Decreased emotion and physical activity
Easily fatigued
Inability to make decisions
Poor concentration
Internalizing hostility
Introverted personality
Social isolation and withdrawn from groups
Lack of energy
Lack of initiative
Lack of self-confidence and low self-esteem
Lack of sexual interest
Psychomotor retardation
Suicidal thinking

---

2. Interventions for mania (Box 63-6)   ▲
   a. Remove hazardous objects from the environment
   b. Assess the client closely for fatigue
   c. Use comfort measures to promote sleep
   d. Provide frequent rest periods
   e. Monitor the client's sleep patterns
   f. Provide a private room if possible
   g. Administer a hypnotic or sedative medication as prescribed
   h. Encourage the client to ventilate feelings
   i. Use calm, slow interactions
   j. Help the client focus on one topic during the conversation
   k. Ignore or distract the client from grandiose thinking
   l. Present reality to the client
   m. Do not argue with the client
   n. Limit group activities and assess the client's tolerance level

BOX 63-6 Dealing With Inappropriate Behaviors Associated With Bipolar Disorder

Aggressive Behavior
Assist the client in identifying feelings of frustration and aggression.
Encourage the client to talk out instead of acting out feelings of frustration.
Assist the client in identifying precipitating events or situations that lead to aggressive behavior.
Describe the consequences of the behavior on self and others.
Assist in identifying previous coping mechanisms.
Assist the client in problem-solving techniques to cope with frustration or aggression.

De-Escalation Techniques
Maintain safety for the client, other clients, and self.
Maintain a large personal space and use a nonaggressive posture.
Use a calm approach and communicate with a calm, clear tone of voice (be assertive, not aggressive).
Determine what the client considers to be his or her need.
Avoid verbal struggles.
Provide the client with clear options that deal with the client's behavior.
Assist the client with problem-solving and decision-making regarding the options.

Manipulative Behavior
Set clear, consistent, realistic, and enforceable limits, and communicate expected behaviors.
Be clear about the consequences associated with exceeding set limits and follow through with the consequences in a nonpunitive manner if necessary.
Discuss the client's behavior in a nonjudgmental and nonthreatening manner.
Avoid power struggles with the client (avoid arguing with the client).
Assist the client in developing means of setting limits on personal behavior.

o. Provide high-calorie finger foods and fluids
p. Supervise the client's choice of clothing
q. Reduce environmental stimuli
r. Set limits on inappropriate behaviors
s. Provide physical activities and outlets for tension
t. Avoid competitive games
u. Provide gross motor activities such as walking and writing
v. Provide structured activities or one-to-one activities with the nurse
w. Provide simple and direct explanations for routine procedures
x. Supervise the administration of medication
3. Major depressive disorder
   a. Data collection (see Box 63-5)
   b. Interventions for depressed clients (Box 63-7)

BOX 63-7 Interventions for Depressed Clients

Assess for suicidal ideation.
Provide safety from suicidal actions.
Assist with activities of daily living.
Use gentle encouragement to participate in activities of daily living and unit therapies.
Do not push decision-making or making complex choices; make decisions that the client is not ready to make.
Monitor sleep patterns.
Monitor nutritional intake and weight.
Provide achievable activities in which the client can achieve success (focus on strengths).
Remind the client of times when he or she felt better and was successful.
Spend time with the client to communicate the client's value.
Respond to anger therapeutically.

IX. SCHIZOPHRENIA
A. Description
   1. Schizophrenia is a group of mental disorders characterized by psychotic features (hallucinations and delusions), disordered thought processes, and disrupted interpersonal relationships
   2. Disturbances in affect, mood, behavior, and thought processes occur
B. Data collection (Figure 63-1)
   1. Physical characteristics
      a. Unkempt appearance
      b. Body image distortions
      c. May be preoccupied with somatic complaints
      d. May neglect hygiene, eating, sleeping, and elimination
   2. Motor activity (Box 63-8)
      a. Catatonic posturing: holding bizarre postures for long periods
      b. Catatonic excitement: moving excitedly with no environmental stimuli present
      c. Possible total immobilization
      d. Inability to respond to commands or responding only to commands
      e. Waxy flexibility
      f. Repetitive or stereotyped movements
      g. Motor activity that may be increased as evidenced by agitation, pacing, inability to sleep, loss of appetite and weight, and impulsiveness
      h. Possible inability to initiate activity (anergia)
   3. Emotional characteristics
      a. Mistrust may be present
      b. View of the world as threatening and unsafe
      c. Affect may be blunted, flat, or inappropriate
      d. May display feelings ambivalence, helplessness, anxiety, anger, guilt, or depression in response to hallucinations, delusions, or as a result of the grief related to losses imposed by this illness

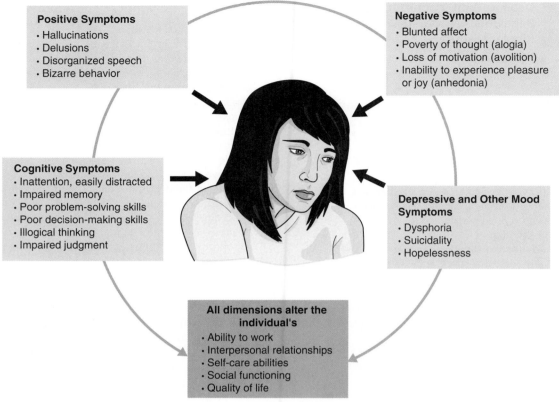

Positive Symptoms
- Hallucinations
- Delusions
- Disorganized speech
- Bizarre behavior

Negative Symptoms
- Blunted affect
- Poverty of thought (alogia)
- Loss of motivation (avolition)
- Inability to experience pleasure or joy (anhedonia)

Cognitive Symptoms
- Inattention, easily distracted
- Impaired memory
- Poor problem-solving skills
- Poor decision-making skills
- Illogical thinking
- Impaired judgment

Depressive and Other Mood Symptoms
- Dysphoria
- Suicidality
- Hopelessness

All dimensions alter the individual's
- Ability to work
- Interpersonal relationships
- Self-care abilities
- Social functioning
- Quality of life

FIG. 63-1 Treatment-relevant dimensions of schizophrenia. (From Varcarolis, C., & Shoemaker, V. [2006]. *Foundations of psychiatric mental health nursing* [5th ed.]. Philadelphia: Saunders.)

BOX 63-8 **Abnormal Motor Behaviors**

Description
Abnormal motor behavior or activity displayed by the mentally ill client and occurring as a result of a psychiatric disorder

Types of Abnormal Motor Behaviors

Echolalia
Repeating the speech of another person

Echopraxia
Repeating the movements of another person

Waxy Flexibility
Having one's arms or legs placed in a certain position and holding that same position for hours

---

4. Compulsive rituals: performed as an attempt to solve conflicting feelings by constant, repetitive activity
5. Overcompliance: attempt to deny responsibility for any action by doing only what another exactly instructs
6. Affective disturbances
   a. Flat or incongruent affect or inappropriate affect
   b. Altered thought processes
7. Thought processes (Box 63-9)

a. Impaired reality testing
b. Fragmentation of thoughts
c. Thought blocking
d. Loose associations
e. Echolalia
f. Distorted perception of the environment
g. Neologisms
h. Magical thinking
i. Inability to conceptualize meaning in words or thoughts
j. Inability to organize facts logically
k. Delusions associated with thought processes or content

8. Types of delusions (Box 63-10)
   a. Loss of reference in which the client believes that certain events, situations, or interactions are related directly to self
   b. Delusions of persecution in which the client believes that he or she is being harassed, threatened, or persecuted by some powerful force
   c. Delusions of grandeur in which the client attaches special significance to self in relation to others or the universe and has an exaggerated sense of self that has no basis in reality

BOX 63-9 Abnormal Thought Processes

Description
Abnormal thought processes displayed by the mentally ill client and occurring as a result of a psychiatric disorder

Circumstantiality
Before getting to the point or answering a question, the individual gets caught up in countless details and explanations

Confabulation
Filling a memory gap with detailed fantasy believed by the teller; the purpose of confabulation is to maintain self-esteem; seen in organic conditions such as Korsakoff's psychosis

Flight of Ideas
A constant flow of speech in which the individual jumps from one topic to another in rapid succession; a connection between topics exists, although it is sometimes difficult to identify; seen in manic states

Looseness of Association
Haphazard, illogical, and confused thinking and interrupted connections in thought; seen mostly in schizophrenic disorders

Neologisms
Words that an individual makes up that only have meaning for the individual; often part of a delusional system

Thought Blocking
A sudden cessation of a thought in the middle of a sentence; the client is unable to continue the train of thought; often sudden new thoughts come up unrelated to the topic

Word Salad
A mixture of words and phrases that have no meaning

BOX 63-10 Delusions

Description
A false belief held to be true even when there is evidence to the contrary

Types
Grandeur
The false belief that one is a powerful and important person

Jealousy
The false belief that one's partner or mate is going out with other persons

Persecution
The thought that one is being singled out for harm by others

Interventions
Ask the client to describe the delusion.
Be open and honest in interactions to reduce suspiciousness.
Focus the conversation on reality-based topics rather than on the delusion.
Encourage the client to express feelings and focus on the feelings that the delusions generate.
If the client obsesses on the delusion, set firm limits on the amount of time for talking about the delusion.
Do not dispute with the client or try to convince the client that the delusions are false.
Validate if part of the delusion is real.

BOX 63-11 Hallucinations

Description
A sense (occurs with one of the five senses) perception for which no external stimuli exist; can have an organic or functional cause

Types
Auditory
Hearing voices when none are present
Gustatory
Experiencing taste in the absence of stimuli
Olfactory
Smelling smells that do not exist
Tactile
Feeling touch sensations in the absence of stimuli
Visual
Seeing things that are not there

Interventions
Ask the client directly about the hallucination.
Avoid reacting to the hallucination as if it were real.
Decrease stimuli or move the client to another area.
Do not negate the client's experience.
Focus on reality-based topics.
Attempt to engage the client's attention through a concrete activity.
Respond verbally to anything real that the client talks about.
Avoid touching the client.
Monitor for signs of increasing anxiety or agitation, which may indicate that the hallucinations are increasing.

---

     d. Somatic delusions in which the client believes that his or her body is changing or responding in an unusual way, which has no basis in reality

9. Perceptual distortions
     a. Illusions that may be brief experiences with a misinterpretation or misperception of reality
     b. Hallucinations (five senses) such as perceiving objects, sensations, or images with no basis in reality (Box 63-11)

10. Language and communication disturbances (Box 63-12)
     a. Related to disorders in thought process
     b. Inability to organize language
     c. Difficulty communicating clearly
     d. Inappropriate responses to a situation
     e. A single word or phrase that may represent the whole meaning of the conversation such that the client may feel that he or she has communicated adequately
     f. Development of a private language

BOX 63-12 **Language and Communication Disturbances**

Clang association: Repetition of words or phrases that are similar in sound but in no other way

Echolalia: Repetition of words or phrases heard from another person

Mutism: Absence of verbal speech

Neologism: A new word devised that has special meaning only to the client

Pressured speech: Speaking as if the words are being forced out quickly

Verbigeration: Purposeless repetition of words or phrases

Word salad: Form of speech in which words or phrases are connected meaninglessly

---

BOX 63-13 **Types of Schizophrenia**

Catatonic
Disorganized
Paranoid
Residual
Undifferentiated

C. Types of schizophrenia (Box 63-13)
  1. Paranoid schizophrenia
    a. Suspiciousness
    b. Hostility
    c. Delusions
    d. Auditory hallucinations
    e. Anxiety and anger
    f. Aloofness
    g. Persecutory themes
    h. Violence
  2. Disorganized schizophrenia
    a. Extreme social withdrawal
    b. Disorganized speech or behavior
    c. Flat or inappropriate affect
    d. Silliness unrelated to speech
    e. Stereotyped behaviors
    f. Grimacing mannerisms
    g. Inability to perform activities of daily living
  3. Catatonic schizophrenia
    a. Psychomotor disturbances
    b. Immobility
    c. Stupor
    d. Waxy flexibility
    e. Excessive purposeless motor activity
    f. Echolalia
    g. Automatic obedience
    h. Stereotyped or repetitive behavior
  4. Undifferentiated schizophrenia
    a. Undifferentiated schizophrenia does not meet the criteria for paranoid, disorganized, or catatonic schizophrenia
    b. Delusions and hallucinations

c. Disorganized speech
    d. Disorganized or catatonic behavior
    e. Flat affect
    f. Social withdrawal
  5. Residual schizophrenia
    a. Diagnosed as schizophrenic in the past
    b. Time limited between attacks but may last for many years
    c. The client exhibits considerable social isolation and withdrawal and impaired role functioning
D. Interventions (Box 63-14)
E. Interventions: active hallucinations
  1. Monitor for hallucination cues and assess content of hallucinations; safety first: ensure that the client does not have an auditory command telling him or her to harm self or others
  2. Intervene with one-on-one contact
  3. Decrease stimuli or move the client to another area
  4. Avoid conveying to the client that others are also experiencing the hallucination
  5. Respond verbally to anything real that the client talks about
  6. Avoid touching the client
  7. Encourage the client to express feelings
  8. During a hallucination, attempt to engage the client's attention through a concrete activity
  9. Accept and do not joke about or judge the client's behavior
  10. Provide easy activities and a structured environment with routine activities of daily living
  11. Monitor for signs of increasing fear, anxiety, or agitation
  12. Decrease stimuli as needed
  13. Administer medications as prescribed
F. Interventions: delusions
  1. Interact based on reality
  2. Encourage the client to express feelings
  3. Do not dispute the client or try to convince the client that delusions are false
  4. In the beginning, initiate activities on a one-on-one basis
  5. Alter hospital routines as necessary, such as using canned or packaged food or food from home
  6. Recognize accomplishments and provide positive feedback for successes
X. **PARANOID DISORDERS**
A. Description
  1. Paranoid disorder is a concrete, pervasive delusional system characterized by persecutory and grandiose beliefs
  2. The client demonstrates suspiciousness and mistrust of others
  3. The client is often viewed by others as hostile, stubborn, and defensive

BOX 63-14   Interventions for Schizophrenia

Assess the client's physical needs.
Set limits on the client's behaviors when it interferes with others and becomes disruptive.
Maintain a safe environment.
Initiate one-on-one interaction and progress to small groups as tolerated.
Spend time with the client even if the client is unable to respond.
Monitor for altered thought processes.
Maintain ego boundaries and avoid touching the client.
Limit the time of interaction with the client.
Avoid an overly warm approach; a neutral approach is less threatening.
Do not make promises to the client that cannot be kept.
Establish daily routines.
Assist the client to improve grooming and accept responsibility for personal care.
Sit with the client in silence if necessary.
Provide brief and frequent contact with the client.
Tell the client when you are leaving.
Tell the client when you do not understand.
Do not "go along" with the client's delusions or hallucinations.

Provide simple, concrete activities, such as puzzles or word games.
Reorient the client as necessary.
Help the client establish what is real and unreal.
Stay with the client if the client is frightened.
Speak to the client in a simple, direct, and concise manner.
Reassure the client that the environment is safe.
Remove the client from group situations if the client's behavior is too bizarre, disturbing, or dangerous to others.
Set realistic goals.
Initially, do not offer choices to the client, and gradually assist the client in making decisions.
Use canned or packaged food, especially with the paranoid schizophrenic client.
Provide a radio or tape player at night for insomnia.
Explain to the client everything that is being done.
Set limits on the client's behavior if the client cannot.
Decrease excessive stimuli in the environment.
Monitor for suicide risk.
Assist the client to use alternative means to express feelings through music or art therapy or writing.

BOX 63-15   Types of Paranoid Disorders

Paranoid personality
Paranoid state
Paranoia
Paranoid schizophrenia

▲ B. Behaviors
    1. Suspicious and mistrustful
    2. Emotionally distant
    3. Distortion of reality
    4. Poor insight and poor judgments
    5. Hypervigilance
    6. Low self-esteem
    7. Highly sensitive, difficulty in admitting own error, and taking pride in being correct
    8. Hypercritical and intolerant of others
    9. Hostile, aggressive, and quarrelsome
    10. Evasive
    11. Concrete thinking
▲ C. Delusions
    1. Delusions serve a purpose in establishing identity and self-esteem
    2. Client may have grandiose and persecutory delusions
    3. Process of delusion includes denial, projection, and rationalization
    4. As trust in others increases, the need for delusions decreases

D. Types of paranoid disorders (Box 63-15)
    1. Paranoid personality disorder
        a. Suspicious
        b. Nonpsychotic
        c. No hallucinations or delusions
        d. No symptoms of schizophrenia
    2. Paranoid induced state
        a. Abrupt onset in response to stress and subsides when stress decreases
        b. No hallucinations but experiences paranoid delusions
        c. May be sensitive and suspicious before the development of delusions
        d. No symptoms of schizophrenia
    3. Paranoia
        a. Exhibits an organized delusional system
        b. No hallucinations
        c. Reserved and sensitive before onset
        d. Psychotic state
        e. No symptoms of schizophrenia
    4. Paranoid schizophrenia
        a. Before onset, the client becomes cold, withdrawn, distrustful, resentful, argumentative, sarcastic, and defiant
        b. Bizarre, numerous, and changeable delusions occur
        c. Delusions become less logical as the client becomes more disorganized
        d. Persecutory hallucinations occur
        e. Psychotic state ensues
        f. All symptoms of schizophrenia are present
E. Interventions (Box 63-16)

BOX 63-16	Interventions for Paranoid Disorders

Assess for suicide risk.
Diminish suspicious behavior.
Avoid direct eye contact.
Establish a trusting relationship.
Promote increased self-esteem.
Remain calm, nonthreatening, and nonjudgmental.
Provide continuity of care.
Respond honestly to the client.
Follow through on commitments made to the client.
Acknowledge the client's feelings, but tell the client that you do not share the client's interpretation of an event.
Provide a daily schedule of activities.
Assist the client to identify diversionary activities.
Gradually introduce the client to groups.
Refocus conversation to reality-based topics.
Use role playing to help the client identify thoughts and feelings.
Provide positive reinforcement for successes.
Do not argue with delusions.
Use concrete, specific words.
Do not be secretive with the client.
Do not whisper in the client's presence.
Assure the client that he or she will be safe.
Involve the client in noncompetitive tasks.
Provide the client opportunity to complete small tasks.
Monitor eating, drinking, sleeping, and elimination patterns.
Limit physical contact.
Monitor for agitation and decrease stimuli as needed.

XI. PERSONALITY DISORDERS

A. Description
1. Personality disorders include various inflexible maladaptive behavior patterns or traits that may impair functioning and relationships
2. The individual usually remains in touch with reality and typically has a lack of insight into his or her behavior
3. Stress exacerbates manifestations of the personality disorder
4. In severe cases the personality disorder may deteriorate to a psychotic state

B. Characteristics
1. Poor impulse control
    a. Acting out to manage internal pain
    b. Forms of acting out include physical and verbal attacks (such as yelling and swearing, and self-injurious behaviors such as cutting own skin, banging the head, punching self), manipulation, substance **abuse,** promiscuous sexual behaviors, and **suicide attempts**
    c. Client may be preoccupied with self, religion, or sex

2. Mood characteristics
    a. May experience abandonment and depression
    b. Moods may include rage, guilt, fear, and emptiness
3. Impaired judgment
    a. Difficulty with problem-solving
    b. Inability to perceive the consequences of behavior
4. Impaired reality testing: distortion of reality and often projection of own feelings onto others
5. Impaired object relations: rigid and inflexible, with difficulty in intimate relationships
6. Impaired self-perception: distorted self-perception and experience of self-hate or self-idealization
7. Impaired thought processes
    a. Concrete or diffuse thinking
    b. Difficulty concentrating
    c. Impaired memory
8. Impaired stimulus barrier
    a. Inability to regulate incoming sensory stimuli
    b. Increased excitability
    c. Excessive response to noise and light
    d. Poor attention span
    e. Agitated
    f. Insomnia

C. Cluster A Personality Disorder types include the odd/eccentric types: Schizoid, Schizotypal, and Paranoid
1. Schizoid personality disorder is characterized by an inability to form warm, close social relationships
    a. Social detachment and lack of close relationships
    b. Interest in solitary activities
    c. Aloof and indifferent
    d. Restricted expression of emotions
    e. Lack of interest in others
2. Schizotypal personality disorder is characterized by the display of abnormal or highly unusual thoughts, perceptions, speech, and behavior patterns
    a. Suspicious
    b. Paranoia
    c. Magical thinking
    d. Odd thinking and speech
    e. Relationship deficits
3. Paranoid personality disorder is characterized by suspiciousness and mistrust of others
    a. May be argumentative
    b. May be hostile, aloof
    c. May be rigid, critical, and controlling of others
    d. May have thoughts of grandiosity

D. Cluster B Personality Disorders include the over-emotional, erratic types: histrionic, narcissistic, borderline, and antisocial
1. Histrionic personality disorder is characterized by overly dramatic and intensely expressive behavior
   a. Lively and dramatic and enjoys being the center of attention
   b. Has poor and shallow interpersonal relations
   c. May be sexually seductive or provocative
   d. Dramatizes their life and may appear theatrical
   e. Overly concerned with appearance
   f. Easily bored
2. Narcissistic personality disorder is characterized by an increased sense of self-importance, preoccupation with fantasies and a sense of unlimited success
   a. Need for admiration and inflation of accomplishments
   b. Overestimation of abilities and underestimation of contributions of others
   c. Lack of empathy and sensitivity to needs of others
3. Antisocial personality disorder is comprised of a pattern of irresponsible and antisocial behavior, selfishness, an inability to maintain lasting relationships, poor sexual adjustment, a failure to accept social norms, and a tendency toward irritability and aggressiveness
   a. Perceives the world as hostile
   b. Superficial charm and hostility
   c. No shame or guilt
   d. Self-centered
   e. Unreliable
   f. Easily bored
   g. Poor work history
   h. Inability to tolerate frustration
   i. Views others as objects to be manipulated
   j. Poor judgment
   k. Impulsive
4. Borderline personality disorder is characterized by instability in interpersonal relationships, unstable mood and self-image, and impulsive and unpredictable behavior.
   a. Unclear identity
   b. Unstable and intense
   c. Extreme shifts in mood
   d. Easily angered
   e. Easily bored
   f. Argumentative
   g. Depression
   h. Self-destructive behavior
   i. Manipulation
   j. Inability to tolerate anxiety
   k. Chronic feelings of emptiness and fear of being alone

   l. Splitting (sees others as all good or all bad; creates conflict between individuals by playing one person against another)
E. Cluster C Personality Disorders include the anxious, fearful types of personality disorders: obsessive-compulsive personality, avoidant and dependence
1. Obsessive-compulsive personality disorder is characterized by difficulty expressing warm and tender emotions, perfectionism, stubbornness, the need to control others, and a devotion to work
   a. Overly conscientious
   b. Inflexible and preoccupied with details and rules
   c. Extreme devotion to work to the exclusion of leisure activities and friendships
   d. Miserly and stubborn
   e. Hoarding behavior
   f. Engages in rituals
2. Avoidant personality disorder is characterized by social withdrawal and extreme sensitivity to potential rejection
   a. Feelings of inadequacy
   b. Hypersensitive to reactions of others and poor reaction to criticism
   c. Social isolation
   d. Lack of support system
3. Dependent personality disorder is characterized by intense lack of self-confidence and low self-esteem, and lack of ability to function independently, such that the individual passively allows others to make decisions and assume responsibility for major areas in the person's life; the dependent client has great difficulty making decisions
F. General interventions for the client with a personality disorder
1. Maintain safety against behaviors that are self-destructive
2. Allow the client to make choices and be as independent as possible
3. Encourage the client to discuss feelings rather than act them out
4. Provide consistency in response to the client's acting-out behaviors
5. Discuss expectations and responsibilities with the client
6. Discuss the consequences that will follow certain behaviors
7. Inform the client that harm to self, others, and property is unacceptable
8. Identify splitting behavior
9. Assist the client to deal directly with anger
10. Develop a written safety and/or behavioral contract with the client
11. Encourage the client to keep a journal recording daily feelings

12. Encourage the client to participate in group activities, and praise nonmanipulative behavior
13. Set and maintain limits to decrease manipulative behavior
14. Remove the client from group situations in which attention-seeking behaviors occur
15. Provide realistic praise for positive behaviors in social situations

XII. COGNITIVE IMPAIRMENT DISORDERS

A. Autism: refer to Chapter 30
B. Attention deficit hyperactivity disorder: refer to Chapter 30
C. Dementia and Alzheimer's disease
   1. Dementia
      a. Dementia is a syndrome with progressive deterioration in intellectual functioning; secondary to structural or functional changes
      b. Long- and short-term memory loss occurs with impairment in judgment, abstract thinking, problem-solving ability, and behavior
      c. Dementia results in a self-care deficit
      d. The most common type of dementia is Alzheimer's disease
   2. Alzheimer's disease (Box 63-17)
      a. Alzheimer's disease is an irreversible form of senile dementia from nerve cell deterioration
      b. Individuals with Alzheimer's disease experience cognitive deterioration and progressive loss of ability to carry out activities of daily living
      c. The client experiences a steady decline in physical and mental functioning and usually requires long-term care facility placement in the final stages of the illness
   3. Interventions
      a. Identify and reinforce retained skills
      b. Provide continuity of care
      c. Orient the client to the environment
      d. Furnish the environment with familiar possessions
      e. Acknowledge the client's feelings
      f. Help the client and family members manage memory deficits and behavior changes
      g. Encourage the family members to express feelings about caregiving
      h. Provide the caregiver support and identify the resources and support groups available

---

BOX 63-17 **Alzheimer's Disease**

Agnosia: Failure to recognize or identify objects despite intact sensory function
Amnesia: Loss of memory caused by brain degeneration
Aphasia: Language disturbance in understanding and expressing the spoken word
Apraxia: Inability to perform motor activities despite intact motor function

---

   i. Monitor activities of daily living
   j. Remind the client how to perform self-care activities
   k. Maintain independence
   l. Provide consistent routines
   m. Provide exercise such as walking with an escort
   n. Avoid activities that tax the memory
   o. Allow plenty of time to complete a task
   p. Use constant encouragement in a simple step-by-step approach
   q. Provide activities that distract and occupy time, such as listening to music, coloring, and watching television
   r. Provide mental stimulation with simple games or activities
4. Wandering
   a. Provide a safe environment
   b. Prevent unsafe wandering
   c. Provide close supervision
   d. Close and secure doors
   e. Use identification bracelets and electronic surveillance
5. Communication
   a. Adapt to the communication level of the client
   b. Use a firm volume and a low-pitched voice to communicate
   c. Stand directly in front of the client and maintain eye contact
   d. Call the client by name and identify self; wait for a response
   e. Use a calm and reassuring voice
   f. Use pantomime gestures if the client is unable to understand spoken words
   g. Speak slowly and clearly, using short words and simple sentences
   h. Ask only one question at a time and give one direction at a time
   i. Repeat questions if necessary but do not rephrase
6. Impaired judgment
   a. Remove throw rugs, toxic substances, and dangerous electrical appliances from the environment
   b. Reduce hot water heater temperature
7. Altered thought processes
   a. Call the client by name
   b. Orient the client frequently
   c. Use familiar objects in the room
   d. Place a calendar and clock in a visible place
   e. Maintain familiar routines
   f. Allow the client to reminisce
   g. Make tasks simple
   h. Allow time for the client to complete a task
   i. Provide positive reinforcement for positive behaviors

8. Altered sleep patterns
   a. Allow the client to wander in a safe place until the client becomes tired
   b. Prevent shadows in the room by using indirect light
   c. Avoid the use of hypnotics since they cause confusion and aggravate the sundown effect

9. Agitation
   a. Assess the precipitant of the agitation
   b. Reassure the client
   c. Remove items that can be hazardous during the time of agitation
   d. Approach the client slowly and calmly from the front, and then speak, gesture, and move slowly
   e. Remove client to a less stressful environment
   f. Use touch gently
   g. Do not argue with the client or force the client

XIII. PSYCHOSEXUAL ALTERATIONS

A. Sexuality
   1. One's sense of being a sexual individual
   2. Includes how one looks, behaves, and relates to others
B. Sexual expression (Box 63-18)
C. Alterations in sexual behavior
   1. Transsexualism: feeling that one's sex is inappropriate and desiring to acquire sexual characteristics of the opposite sex
   2. Exhibitionism: sexual urges and fantasies and exposure of genitals to strangers to bring sexual gratification and/or arousal
   3. Fetishism: using nonliving objects for sexual gratification
   4. Pedophilia: desiring sexual activity with a child under age 13
   5. Sexual masochism: sexual gratification that involves receiving pain
   6. Sexual sadism: sexual gratification that involves inflicting pain
   7. Voyeurism: sexual gratification through observing others disrobing or engaging in sexual activity
   8. Zoophilia: intense sexual arousal or desire for sexual contact with animals
   9. Frotteurism: intense sexual arousal or desire when rubbing against a nonconsenting person

---

BOX 63-18 **Sexual Expression**

Bisexuality: Sexual attraction to and activity with both sexes
Heterosexuality: Male-female sexual relationships
Homosexuality: Sexual attraction to a member of the same sex
Transvestism: Obsession with wearing clothing of the opposite sex

---

D. Interventions
   1. Assess sexual history, history of trauma or **abuse,** and precipitating event for the sexual disorder
   2. Encourage the client to explore personal beliefs
   3. Provide a nonjudgmental attitude
   4. Provide supportive psychotherapy

PRACTICE QUESTIONS

More questions on the companion CD!

878. A male client with delirium becomes agitated and confused in his room at night. The best initial intervention by the nurse is to:
   1. Move the client next to the nurse's station.
   2. Use a night light and turn off the television.
   3. Keep the television and a soft light on during the night.
   4. Play soft music during the night and maintain a well-lit room.

879. A nurse is collecting data on a client who is actively hallucinating. Which nursing statement would be therapeutic at this time?
   1. "I know you feel 'they are out to get you,' but it's not true."
   2. "I can hear the voice and she wants you to come to dinner."
   3. "Sometimes people hear things or voices others can't hear."
   4. "I talked to the voices you're hearing and they won't hurt you now."

880. A nurse is caring for a client with a diagnosis of depression. The nurse monitors for signs of constipation and urinary retention, knowing that these problems are likely caused by:
   1. Poor dietary choices
   2. Lack of exercise and poor diet
   3. Inadequate dietary intake and dehydration
   4. Psychomotor retardation and side effects of medication

881. A client is admitted to the in-patient unit and is being considered for electroconvulsive therapy (ECT). The client appears calm, but the family is hypervigilant and anxious. The client's mother begins to cry and states, "My son's brain will be destroyed. How can the doctor do this to him?" The nurse makes which therapeutic response?
   1. "It sounds as though you need to speak to the psychiatrist."
   2. "Perhaps you'd like to see the ECT room and speak to the staff."
   3. "Your son has decided to have this treatment. You should be supportive of him."
   4. "It sounds as though you have some concerns about the ECT procedure. Why don't we sit down together and discuss any concerns you may have?"

882. A client who is diagnosed with pedophilia and has been recently paroled as a sex offender says, "I'm in treatment and I have served my time. Now this group has posters of me all over the neighborhood telling about me with my picture on it." Which of the following is an appropriate response by the nurse?
    1. "When children are hurt as you hurt them, people want you isolated."
    2. "You're lucky it doesn't escalate into something pretty scary after your crime."
    3. "You understand that people fear for their children, but you're feeling unfairly treated?"
    4. "You seem angry, but you have committed serious crimes against several children, so your neighbors are frightened."

883. A nurse is preparing for the hospital discharge of a client with a history of command hallucinations to harm self or others. The nurse instructs the client about interventions for hallucinations and anxiety and determines that the client understands the interventions when the client states:
    1. "My medications won't make me anxious."
    2. "I'll go to a support group and talk so that I won't hurt anyone."
    3. "I won't get anxious or hear things if I get enough sleep and eat well."
    4. "I can call my therapist when I'm hallucinating so that I can talk about my feelings and plans and not hurt anyone."

884. A nurse observes that a client is psychotic, pacing, and agitated and is making aggressive gestures. The client's speech pattern is rapid and the client's affect is belligerent. Based on these observations, the nurse's immediate priority of care is to:
    1. Provide safety for the client and other clients on the unit.
    2. Provide the clients on the unit with a sense of comfort and safety.
    3. Assist the staff in caring for the client in a controlled environment.
    4. Offer the client a less-stimulated area to calm down and gain control.

885. A nurse is caring for a client diagnosed with catatonic stupor. The client is lying on the bed, with the body pulled into a fetal position. The appropriate nursing intervention is which of the following?
    1. Ask direct questions to encourage talking.
    2. Leave the client alone and intermittently check on him.
    3. Sit beside the client in silence and verbalize occasional open-ended questions.
    4. Take the client into the dayroom with other clients so they can help watch him.

886. A mother of a teenage client with an anxiety disorder is concerned about her daughter's progress on discharge. She states that her daughter "stashes food, eats all the wrong things that make her hyperactive," and "hangs out with the wrong crowd." In helping the mother prepare for her daughter's discharge, the nurse suggests that the mother:
    1. Restrict the daughter's socializing time with her friends.
    2. Restrict the amount of chocolate and caffeine products in the home.
    3. Keep her daughter out of school until she can adjust to the school environment.
    4. Consider taking time from work to help her daughter readjust to the home environment.

887. A client is unwilling to go out of the house for fear of "doing something crazy in public." Because of this fear, the client remains homebound except when accompanied outside by the spouse. The nurse determines that the client has:
    1. Agoraphobia
    2. Hematophobia
    3. Claustrophobia
    4. Hypochondriasis

888. A client has reported that crying spells have been a major problem over the past several weeks, and that the doctor said that depression is probably the reason. The nurse observes that the client is sitting slumped in the chair and the clothes that the client is wearing don't fit well. The nurse interprets that further data collection should focus on:
    1. Weight loss
    2. Sleep patterns
    3. Medication compliance
    4. Onset of the crying spells

889. A client was admitted to a medical unit with acute blindness. Many tests are performed and there seems to be no organic reason why this client cannot see. The nurse later learns that the client became blind after witnessing a hit-and-run car crash, in which a family of three was killed. The nurse suspects that the client may be experiencing a:
    1. Psychosis
    2. Repression
    3. Conversion disorder
    4. Dissociative disorder

890. A manic client announces to everyone in the dayroom that a stripper is coming to perform that evening. When the psychiatric nurse's aide firmly states that the client's behavior is not appropriate, the manic client becomes verbally abusive and threatens physical violence to the nurse's aide. Based on the analysis of this

situation, the nurse determines that the appropriate action would be to:
1. Escort the manic client to his or her room.
2. Orient the client to time, person, and place.
3. Tell the client that the behavior is not appropriate.
4. Tell the client that smoking privileges are revoked for 24 hours.

891. A nurse notes documentation in a client's record that the client is experiencing delusions of persecution. The nurse understands that these types of delusions are characteristic of which of the following?
1. The false belief that one is a very powerful person
2. The false belief that one is a very important person
3. The false belief that one is being singled out for harm by others
4. The false belief that one's partner is going out with other people

892. A nurse collects data on a client with a diagnosis of bipolar affective disorder–mania. The finding that requires the nurse's immediate intervention is:
1. The client's outlandish behaviors and inappropriate dress
2. The client's nonstop physical activity and poor nutritional intake
3. The client's grandiose delusions of being a royal descendant of King Arthur
4. The client's constant, incessant talking that includes sexual innuendoes and teasing the staff

893. A client in a manic state emerges from her room. She is topless and is making sexual remarks and gestures toward staff and peers. The appropriate nursing action is to:
1. Approach the client in the hallway and insist that she go to her room.
2. Quietly approach the client, escort her to her room, and assist her in getting dressed.
3. Ask the other clients to ignore her behavior; eventually she will return to her room.
4. Confront the client on the inappropriateness of her behaviors and offer her a time-out.

894. A nurse reviews the activity schedule for the day and determines that the best activity that the manic client could participate in is:

1. Ping-pong
2. A paint-by-number activity
3. A brown bag lunch and a book review
4. A deep breathing and progressive relaxation group

895. A client who is delusional says to the nurse, "The federal guards were sent to kill me." The nurse should make which appropriate response to the client?
1. "I don't believe this is true."
2. "The guards are not out to kill you."
3. "What makes you think the guards were sent to hurt you?"
4. "I don't know anything about the guards. Do you feel afraid that people are trying to hurt you?"

896. A woman comes into the emergency department in a severe state of anxiety following a car accident. The most important nursing intervention is to:
1. Remain with the client.
2. Put the client in a quiet room.
3. Teach the client deep breathing.
4. Encourage the client to talk about her feelings and concerns.

ALTERNATE ITEM FORMAT: MULTIPLE RESPONSE

897. Choose all nursing interventions for a hospitalized client with mania who is exhibiting manipulative behavior. Select all that apply.
☐ 1. Communicate expected behaviors to the client.
☐ 2. Ensure that the client knows that he or she is not in charge of the nursing unit.
☐ 3. Assist the client in developing means of setting limits on personal behavior.
☐ 4. Follow through about the consequences of behavior in a nonpunitive manner.
☐ 5. Enforce rules and inform the client that he or she will not be allowed to attend therapy groups.
☐ 6. Be clear with the client regarding the consequences of exceeding limits set regarding behavior.

ANSWERS

878. **2**
Rationale: It is important to provide a consistent daily routine and a low-stimulation environment when the client is agitated and confused. Noise levels including a radio and television may add to the confusion and disorientation. Moving the client next to the nurses' station is not the initial intervention. *Test-Taking Strategy:* Use the process of elimination and note the strategic word "initial" in the question. Eliminate options

3 and 4 first because they are comparable or alike. From the remaining options, recalling that a low-stimulation environment is best will direct you to option 2. Review measures related to the client with agitation and confusion if you had difficulty with this question.*Level of Cognitive Ability:* Application
Client Needs: Psychosocial Integrity
Integrated Process: Nursing Process/Implementation
Content Area: Mental Health

References: Keltner, N., Schwecke, L., & Bostrom, C. (2007). *Psychiatric nursing* (5th ed., p. 445). St. Louis: Mosby. Morrison-Valfre, M. (2005). *Foundations of mental health care* (3rd ed., pp. 168-169). St. Louis: Mosby.

879. 3

Rationale: It is important for the nurse to reinforce reality with the client. Options 1, 2, and 4 do not reinforce reality but reinforce the hallucination that the voices are real.

Test-Taking Strategy: Use the process of elimination. Note that options 1, 2, and 4 all indicate reinforcement to the client that the voices are real. Option 3 is the only statement that indicates reality. Review nursing interventions related to the client who is hallucinating if you had difficulty with this question.

Level of Cognitive Ability: Application

Client Needs: Psychosocial Integrity

Integrated Process: Communication and Documentation

Content Area: Mental Health

References: Keltner, N., Schwecke, L., & Bostrom, C. (2007). *Psychiatric nursing* (5th ed., pp. 90-92, 105). St. Louis: Mosby. Morrison-Valfre, M. (2005). *Foundations of mental health care* (3rd ed., pp. 88, 328). St. Louis: Mosby.

880. 4

Rationale: Constipation can be related to inadequate food intake, lack of exercise, and poor diet. In this situation, urinary retention is most likely due to medications. Option 4 is the only option that addresses both constipation and urinary retention.

Test-Taking Strategy: Use the process of elimination and focus on the data in the question. Options 1, 2, and 3 are all comparable or alike and address diet. Option 4 addresses both concerns of constipation and urinary retention. If you had difficulty with this question, review the interventions for a client with depression and the effects of medications prescribed for this disorder.

Level of Cognitive Ability: Analysis

Client Needs: Physiological Integrity

Integrated Process: Nursing Process/Data Collection

Content Area: Mental Health

References: Keltner, N., Schwecke, L., & Bostrom, C. (2007). *Psychiatric nursing* (5th ed., pp. 383-384). St. Louis: Mosby. Morrison-Valfre, M. (2005). *Foundations of mental health care* (3rd ed., pp. 220, 336). St. Louis: Mosby.

881. 4

Rationale: The nurse needs to encourage the family and client to verbalize their fears and concerns. Option 4 is the only option that encourages verbalization. Options 1, 2, and 3 avoid dealing with the client or family concerns.

Test-Taking Strategy: Use therapeutic communication techniques and focus on the client's and family's feelings and concerns. This will direct you to option 4. Review these techniques if you had difficulty with this question.

Level of Cognitive Ability: Application

Client Needs: Psychosocial Integrity

Integrated Process: Nursing Process/Implementation

Content Area: Mental Health

References: Morrison-Valfre, M. (2005). *Foundations of mental health care* (3rd ed., pp. 88, 218). St. Louis: Mosby.

Stuart, G., & Laraia, M. (2005). *Principles & practice of psychiatric nursing* (8th ed., p. 605). St. Louis: Mosby.

882. 3

Rationale: Focusing and verbalizing the implied concern is the therapeutic response because it assists the client to clarify thinking and re-examine what the client is really saying. Option 3 is the only option that reflects the use of this therapeutic communication technique. Option 1 is insensitive and anxiety-provoking. Option 4 does not facilitate the client's expression of feelings. Option 2 gives advice and does not facilitate the client's expression of feelings.

Test-Taking Strategy: Use therapeutic communication techniques to answer the question. Remembering to focus on the client's feelings and concerns will direct you to option 3. Review these techniques if you had difficulty with this question.

Level of Cognitive Ability: Application

Client Needs: Psychosocial Integrity

Integrated Process: Communication and Documentation

Content Area: Mental Health

Reference: Keltner, N., Schwecke, L., & Bostrom, C. (2007). *Psychiatric nursing* (5th ed., pp. 90-92, 487-488). St. Louis: Mosby.

883. 4

Rationale: There may be an increased risk for impulsive and/or aggressive behavior if a client is receiving command hallucinations to harm self or others. Talking about the auditory hallucinations can interfere with the subvocal muscular activity associated with a hallucination. Option 4 is a specific agreement to seek help and evidences self-responsible commitment and control over his or her own behavior.

Test-Taking Strategy: Use the process of elimination. Note the relation between the word "hallucinations" in the question and in the correct option. Review care of the client with command hallucinations if you had difficulty with this question.

Level of Cognitive Ability: Comprehension

Client Needs: Psychosocial Integrity

Integrated Process: Nursing Process/Evaluation

Content Area: Mental Health

Reference: Stuart, G., & Laraia, M. (2005). *Principles & practice of psychiatric nursing* (8th ed., pp. 462-463). St. Louis: Mosby.

884. 1

Rationale: Safety to the client and other clients is the priority. Option 1 is the only option that addresses the client and other clients' safety needs. Option 4 addresses the client's needs. Option 2 addresses other clients' needs. Option 3 is not client centered.

Test-Taking Strategy: Use the process of elimination and focus on the subject—safety. Option 1 is the umbrella option and addresses the safety of all. Review care of the psychotic client if you had difficulty with this question.

Level of Cognitive Ability: Application

Client Needs: Safe and Effective Care Environment

Integrated Process: Nursing Process/Implementation

Content Area: Mental Health *References:* Fortinash, K., & Holoday-Worret, P. (2008). *Psychiatric mental health nursing* (4th ed., pp. 521, 657). St. Louis: Mosby. Morrison-Valfre, M. (2005). *Foundations of mental health care* (3rd ed., p. 116). St. Louis: Mosby.

885. 3

Rationale: Clients with catatonic stupor may be immobile and mute and may require consistent, repeated approaches. The nurse facilitates communication with the client by sitting in silence, asking open-ended questions, and pausing to provide opportunities for the client to respond. The nurse would not leave the client alone. Option 4 relies on other clients to care for this client, and this is an inappropriate expectation. Asking direct questions of this client is not therapeutic. Option 3 is the best action since it provides for client supervision and communication as appropriate.

Test-Taking Strategy: Use the process of elimination. Eliminate option 2 since the nurse would not leave the client alone. Eliminate option 4 next since this action relies on other clients to care for this client. Eliminate option 1 since asking direct questions of this client is not therapeutic. Review care of the client with catatonic stupor if you had difficulty with this question.

Level of Cognitive Ability: Application
Client Needs: Psychosocial Integrity
Integrated Process: Nursing Process/Implementation
Content Area: Mental Health
Reference: Varcarolis, E., Carlson, V., & Shoemaker, N. (2006). *Foundations of psychiatric mental health nursing* (5th ed., p. 414). Philadelphia: Saunders.

886. 2

Rationale: Clients with anxiety disorder should abstain from or limit their intake of caffeine, chocolate, and alcohol. These products have the potential of increasing anxiety. Options 1 and 3 are unreasonable and are an unhealthy approach. It may not be realistic for a family member to take time away from work.

Test-Taking Strategy: Use the process of elimination. Options 1, 3, and 4 are comparable or alike and are concerned with monitoring or curtailing the client's physical activities. Option 2 addresses preparation of the client's environment and focuses on the concern or subject expressed in the question. Review discharge planning for the client with anxiety disorder if you had difficulty with this question.

Level of Cognitive Ability: Application
Client Needs: Psychosocial Integrity
Integrated Process: Teaching and Learning
Content Area: Mental Health
Reference: Stuart, G., & Laraia, M. (2005). *Principles and practice of psychiatric nursing* (8th ed., pp. 266, 487). St. Louis: Mosby.

887. 1

Rationale: Agoraphobia is a fear of being alone in open or public places where escape might be difficult. Agoraphobia includes experiencing fear or a sense of helplessness or embarrassment if a phobic attack occurs. Avoidance of such situations usually results in the reduction of social and professional interactions. Hematophobia is the fear of blood. Claustrophobia is a fear of closed-in places. Clients with hypochondriacal symptoms focus their anxiety on physical complaints and are preoccupied with their health.

Test-Taking Strategy: Use the process of elimination and focus on the data in the question. Recalling the specific types of phobias and associated client behaviors will direct you to

option 1. If you had difficulty with this question, review phobia types and associated client behaviors.

Level of Cognitive Ability: Comprehension
Client Needs: Psychosocial Integrity
Integrated Process: Nursing Process/Data Collection
Content Area: Mental Health
References: Fortinash, K., & Holoday-Worret, P. (2008). *Psychiatric mental health nursing* (4th ed., p. 183). St. Louis: Mosby.
Morrison-Valfre, M. (2005). *Foundations of mental health care* (3rd ed., pp. 185-186). St. Louis: Mosby.

888. 1

Rationale: All the options are possible issues to address; however, the weight loss is the first item that needs further data collection because ill-fitting clothing could indicate a problem with nutrition. The client has already told the nurse that the crying spells have been a problem. Medication or sleep patterns are not mentioned or addressed in the question.

Test-Taking Strategy: Use the process of elimination and Maslow's Hierarchy of Needs theory to answer the question. Focusing on the data in the question will assist in eliminating options 2, 3, and 4. Review the priorities of care for a client with depression if you had difficulty with this question.

Level of Cognitive Ability: Analysis
Client Needs: Physiological Integrity
Integrated Process: Nursing Process/Data Collection
Content Area: Mental Health
References: Keltner, N., Schwecke, L., & Bostrom, C. (2007). *Psychiatric nursing* (5th ed., p. 384). St. Louis: Mosby.
Morrison-Valfre, M. (2005). *Foundations of mental health care* (3rd ed., p. 215). St. Louis: Mosby.

889. 3

Rationale: A conversion disorder is the alteration or loss of a physical function that cannot be explained by any known pathophysiological mechanism. It is thought to be an expression of a psychological need or conflict. In this situation, the client witnessed an accident that was so psychologically painful that the client became blind. A dissociative disorder is a disturbance or alteration in the normally integrative functions of identity, memory, or consciousness. Psychosis is a state in which a person's mental capacity to recognize reality, communicate, and relate to others is impaired, thus interfering with the person's capacity to deal with life's demands. Repression is a coping mechanism in which unacceptable feelings are kept out of awareness.

Test-Taking Strategy: Use the process of elimination. Noting that the client evidences no organic reason to account for the blindness will direct you to option 3. If you had difficulty with this question, review conversion disorders and defense mechanisms.

Level of Cognitive Ability: Comprehension
Client Needs: Psychosocial Integrity
Integrated Process: Nursing Process/Data Collection*Content Area:* Mental Health
References: Fortinash, K., & Holoday-Worret, P. (2008). *Psychiatric mental health nursing* (4th ed., pp. 198-199). St. Louis: Mosby.

Morrison-Valfre, M. (2005). *Foundations of mental health care* (3rd ed., pp. 229-230). St. Louis: Mosby.

890. **1**
Rationale: The client is at risk for injury to self and others and therefore should be escorted out of the dayroom. Option 4 may increase the agitation that already exists in this client. Orientation will not halt the behavior. Telling the client that the behavior is not appropriate has already been attempted by the psychiatric nurse's aide.
Test-Taking Strategy: Use the process of elimination and therapeutic interventions for the manic client. Options 2, 3, and 4 will not de-escalate the client's agitation. If you had difficulty with this question, review the appropriate interventions in dealing with a manic client.
Level of Cognitive Ability: Application
Client Needs: Psychosocial Integrity
Integrated Process: Nursing Process/Implementation
Content Area: Mental Health
References: Keltner, N., Schwecke, L., & Bostrom, C. (2007). *Psychiatric nursing* (5th ed., pp. 400-401). St. Louis: Mosby. Stuart, G., & Laraia, M. (2005). *Principles and practice of psychiatric nursing* (8th ed., p. 351). St. Louis: Mosby.

891. **3**
Rationale: A delusion is a false belief held to be true even when there is evidence to the contrary. A delusion of persecution is the thought that one is being singled out for harm by others. A delusion of grandeur is the false belief that he or she is a very powerful and important person. A delusion of jealousy is the false belief that one's partner is going out with other people.
Test-Taking Strategy: Use the process of elimination. Eliminate options 1 and 2 first since they are comparable or alike. From the remaining options, note the relationship between the word "persecution" in the question and the description in option 3. Review the description of the types of delusions if you had difficulty with this question.
Level of Cognitive Ability: Comprehension
Client Needs: Psychosocial Integrity
Integrated Process: Nursing Process/Data Collection
Content Area: Mental Health
References: Fortinash, K., & Holoday-Worret, P. (2008). *Psychiatric mental health nursing* (4th ed., p. 260). St. Louis: Mosby.
Stuart, G., & Laraia, M. (2005). *Principles & practice of psychiatric nursing* (8th ed., p. 112). St. Louis: Mosby.

892. **2**
Rationale: Mania is a mood characterized by excitement, euphoria, hyperactivity, excessive energy, decreased need for sleep, and impaired ability to concentrate or complete a single train of thought. It is a period when the mood is predominantly elevated, expansive, or irritable. Option 2 identifies a physiological need requiring immediate intervention.
Test-Taking Strategy: Use the process of elimination and note the strategic words "immediate intervention." Use Maslow's Hierarchy of Needs theory to assist in answering the question. Option 2 indicates a potential disruption in the client's physiological status. Review care of the client with mania if you had difficulty with this question.
Level of Cognitive Ability: Comprehension

Client Needs: Psychosocial Integrity
Integrated Process: Nursing Process/Data Collection
Content Area: Mental Health
References: Keltner, N., Schwecke, L., & Bostrom, C. (2007). *Psychiatric nursing* (5th ed., pp 405-407). St. Louis: Mosby. Morrison-Valfre, M. (2005). *Foundations of mental health care* (3rd ed., pp. 214-215). St. Louis: Mosby.

893. **2**
Rationale: A person who is experiencing mania lacks insight and judgment, has poor impulse control, and is highly excitable. The nurse must take control without creating increased stress or anxiety in the client. A quiet, firm approach while distracting the client (walking her to her room and assisting her to get dressed) achieves the goal of having her being dressed appropriately and preserving her psychosocial integrity. Option 3 is inappropriate. "Insisting" that the client go to her room may meet with a great deal of resistance. Confronting the client and offering her a consequence of "time-out" may be meaningless to her.
Test-Taking Strategy: Use the process of elimination and focus on the subject of the question. Noting that the subject relates to having the client dress appropriately will direct you to option 2. Review care of the client with mania if you had difficulty with this question.
Level of Cognitive Ability: Application
Client Needs: Psychosocial Integrity
Integrated Process: Nursing Process/Implementation
Content Area: Mental Health
References: Keltner, N., Schwecke, L., & Bostrom, C. (2007). *Psychiatric nursing* (5th ed., pp. 404-405). St. Louis: Mosby. Morrison-Valfre, M. (2005). *Foundations of mental health care* (3rd ed., p. 221). St. Louis: Mosby.

894. **1**
Rationale: A person who is experiencing mania is overactive, full of energy, lacks concentration, and has poor impulse control. The client needs an activity that will allow him or her to use excess energy but not endanger others during the process. Options 2, 3, and 4 are relatively sedate activities that require concentration, a quality that is lacking in the manic state. Such activities may lead to increased frustration and anxiety for the client. Ping-pong is an activity that will help to expend the increased energy this client is experiencing.
Test-Taking Strategy: Use the process of elimination. Note that options 2, 3, and 4 are comparable or alike in that they are relatively sedate activities that require concentration. Review the appropriate interventions for a manic client if you had difficulty with this question.
Level of Cognitive Ability: Application
Client Needs: Psychosocial Integrity
Integrated Process: Nursing Process/Implementation
Content Area: Mental Health
Reference: Stuart, G., & Laraia, M. (2005). *Principles and practice of psychiatric nursing* (8th ed., p. 355). St. Louis: Mosby.

895. **4**
Rationale: Disagreeing with delusions may make the client more defensive, and the client may cling to the delusions even more. It is most therapeutic for the nurse to empathize with the client's experience. Options 1 and 2 are

statements that disagree with the client. Option 3 encourages discussion regarding the delusion.

Test-Taking Strategy: Use therapeutic communication techniques for the client experiencing delusions. Eliminate options 1 and 2 because they are comparable or alike and are statements that disagree with the client. Option 3 encourages discussion regarding the delusion. Review communication techniques for the client experiencing delusions if you had difficulty with this question.

Level of Cognitive Ability: Application
Client Needs: Psychosocial Integrity
Integrated Process: Communication and Documentation
Content Area: Mental Health
References: Keltner, N., Schwecke, L., & Bostrom, C. (2007). *Psychiatric nursing* (5th ed., pp. 90-92). St. Louis: Mosby. Morrison-Valfre, M. (2005). *Foundations of mental health care* (3rd ed., pp. 88, 100). St. Louis: Mosby.

896. **1**
Rationale: If a client is left alone with severe anxiety, he or she may feel abandoned and become overwhelmed. Placing the client in a quiet room is also indicated, but the nurse must stay with the client. It is not possible to teach the client deep breathing until the anxiety decreases. Encouraging the client to discuss concerns and feelings would not take place until the anxiety has decreased.

Test-Taking Strategy: Use the process of elimination. Note the strategic words "severe" and "most important nursing intervention." Eliminate options 3 and 4 first, knowing that these actions are not possible when the client is in a severe state of anxiety. From the remaining options, remember the most important intervention is to remain with the client. Review care of the client with severe anxiety if you had difficulty with this question.

Level of Cognitive Ability: Application

Client Needs: Psychosocial Integrity
Integrated Process: Nursing Process/Implementation
Content Area: Mental Health
Reference: Varcarolis, E., Carlson, V., & Shoemaker, N. (2006). *Foundations of psychiatric mental health nursing* (5th ed., p. 216). Philadelphia: Saunders.

ALTERNATE ITEM FORMAT: MULTIPLE RESPONSE

897. **1, 3, 4, 6**
Rationale: Interventions for dealing with the client exhibiting manipulative behavior include setting clear, consistent, and enforceable limits on manipulative behaviors; being clear with the client regarding the consequences of exceeding limits set; following through with the consequences in a nonpunitive manner; and assisting the client in developing means of setting limits on personal behaviors. Enforcing rules and informing the client that he or she will not be allowed to attend therapy groups is a violation of a client's rights. Ensuring that the client knows that he or she is not in charge of the nursing unit is inappropriate; power struggles need to be avoided.

Test-Taking Strategy: Focus on the subject—manipulative behavior. Recalling clients' rights and that power struggles need to be avoided will assist in selecting the correct interventions. Review care to the client with manipulative behavior if you had difficulty with this question.

Level of Cognitive Ability: Application
Client Needs: Psychosocial Integrity
Integrated Process: Nursing Process/Implementation
Content Area: Mental Health
Reference: Varcarolis, E., Carlson, V., & Shoemaker, N. (2006). *Foundations of psychiatric mental health nursing* (5th ed., pp. 367-368). Philadelphia: Saunders.

REFERENCES

Fortinash, K., & Holoday-Worret, P. (2008). *Psychiatric mental health nursing* (4th ed.). St. Louis: Mosby.

Keltner, N., Schwecke, L., & Bostrom, C. (2007). *Psychiatric nursing* (5th ed.). St. Louis: Mosby.

Morrison-Valfre, M. (2005). *Foundations of mental health care* (3rd ed.). St. Louis: Mosby.

Stuart, G., & Laraia, M. (2005). *Principles & practice of psychiatric nursing* (8th ed.). St. Louis: Mosby.

Varcarolis, E., Carlson, V., & Shoemaker, N. (2006). *Foundations of psychiatric mental health nursing* (5th ed.). Philadelphia: Saunders.

CHAPTER

64

Addictions

I. EATING DISORDERS

A. Description: eating disorders are characterized by uncertain self-identification and grossly disturbed eating habits (Figure 64-1)

B. Compulsive overeating
   1. Compulsive overeating is binge-like overeating without purging
   2. Food consumption is out of the individual's control and occurs in a stereotyped fashion
   3. Client may be repulsed by eating, and the eating relieves tension but does not produce pleasure
   4. Client is aware that eating patterns are abnormal and feels depressed after eating
   5. Client eats secretly during a binge and consumes high-calorie and easily digestible food
   6. Client repeatedly tries to diet but without success
   7. Client feels helpless and hopeless about weight
   8. When experiencing guilt, anger, depression, boredom, loneliness, inadequacy, or ambivalence, client responds by eating

C. Anorexia nervosa
   1. Description
      a. The onset often is associated with a stressful life event
      b. The client intensely fears obesity
      c. Body image is distorted, and the client has a disturbed self-concept
      d. Client is preoccupied with foods that prevent weight gain and has a phobia against foods that produce weight gain
      e. The eating disorder can be life-threatening
      f. Death can occur from starvation, **suicide**, cardiomyopathies, or electrolyte imbalance
   2. Data collection
      a. Refusal to eat and appetite loss
      b. Appetite denial
      c. Feelings of lack of control
      d. Self-induced vomiting and self-administered enemas
      e. Compulsive exercising

   f. Overachiever and perfectionist
   g. Decreased temperature, pulse, and blood pressure
   h. Weight loss
   i. Gastrointestinal disturbances
   j. Constipation
   k. Electrolyte imbalances
   l. Scaly, dry skin
   m. Presence of lanugo on extremities
   n. Sleep disturbances
   o. Hormone deficiencies
   p. Amenorrhea for at least three consecutive menstrual periods
   q. Teeth and gum deterioration
   r. Cyanosis and numbness of extremities
   s. Esophageal varices from vomiting
   t. Bone degeneration

D. Bulimia nervosa
   1. Description
      a. The client indulges in eating binges followed by purging behaviors
      b. Most clients remain within a normal weight range but feel that their lives are dominated by the eating-related conflict
   2. Data collection
      a. Preoccupied with body shape and weight
      b. Consumption of high-calorie food in secret; guilt about secretive eating
      c. Binge and purge syndrome
      d. Attempts to lose weight through diets, vomiting, enemas, cathartics, and amphetamines or diuretics
      e. Has need for control yet experiences feelings of powerlessness or loss of control
      f. Low self-esteem
      g. Poor interpersonal relationships
      h. Decreased or absence of interest in sex
      i. Mood swings
      j. Electrolyte imbalances
      k. Loss of tooth enamel and dental decay
      l. Stomach ulcers and rectal bleeding
      m. Esophageal varices from vomiting
      n. Cardiac disease and hypertension

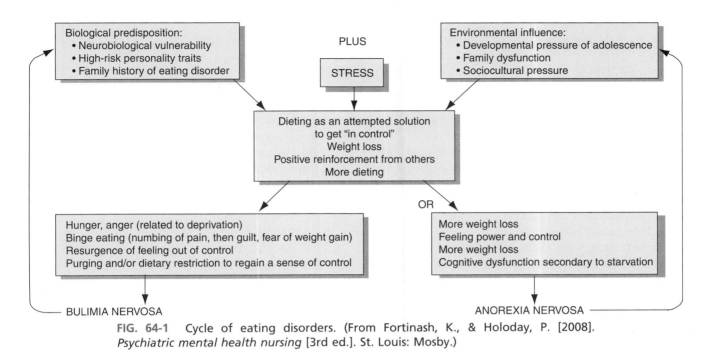

FIG. 64-1 Cycle of eating disorders. (From Fortinash, K., & Holoday, P. [2008]. *Psychiatric mental health nursing* [3rd ed.]. St. Louis: Mosby.)

E. Interventions: clients with an eating disorder
1. Assess the client's nutritional status and the severity of any medical problems
2. Establish a one-to-one therapeutic relationship with the client; the nurse needs to establish trust and recognize any client reluctance to establish a relationship
3. Establish a contract with the client concerning the nutritional plan for the day
4. Assist the client to identify precipitants to the eating disorder
5. Encourage the client to express feelings about the eating behavior
6. Be accepting and nonjudgmental
7. Work with the client on exploring self-concept and establishing identity
8. Implement behavior modification techniques
9. Supervise the client during mealtimes and for a specified period after meals
10. Set a time limit for each meal
11. Provide a pleasant, relaxed environment for eating
12. Monitor for signs of physical complications related to the eating disorder
13. Record intake and output (I&O)
14. Weigh the client daily at the same time, using the same scale, after the client voids
15. When weighing the client, ensure that the client is wearing the same clothing as when the previous weight was taken
16. Monitor and restore fluid and electrolyte balance
17. Monitor elimination patterns
18. Assess and limit the client's activity level

BOX 64-1 CAGE Screening Test

C: Have you ever felt the need to cut down on your drinking/drug use?
A: Have you ever been annoyed at criticism of your drinking/drug use?
G: Have you ever felt guilty about something you have done when you have been drinking or taking drugs?
E: Have you ever had an eye opener: drinking or taking drugs first thing in the morning to get going or to avoid withdrawal symptoms?

19. Encourage the client to participate in diversional activities
20. Assess the client's suicidal potential
21. Administer antidepressant medication if prescribed
22. Encourage psychotherapy
23. Refer the client to support groups

II. **SUBSTANCE ABUSE DISORDERS**
A. Description: Substance **abuse** disorders cause behavioral and physiological changes
B. CAGE Screening test (Box 64-1)
C. Substance dependence
1. Substance dependence is a pattern of repeated use of a substance, which usually results in tolerance, withdrawal, and compulsive drug-taking behavior
2. The client takes substances in larger amounts and over longer periods than was intended
3. The client has the desire to cut down but has unsuccessful efforts to decrease or discontinue use
4. Daily activities revolve around the use of a substance

D. Substance tolerance is the need for increased amounts of the substance to achieve the desired effect

E. Substance **abuse**
1. Client recurrently uses substances
2. Client experiences recurrent, significant harmful consequences related to the use of substances
3. Client may have legal issues to resolve, and involvement with the legal system is not uncommon

F. Substance withdrawal
1. Physiological and substance-specific cognitive symptoms occur
2. Substance withdrawal occurs when an individual experiences a decrease in blood levels of a substance to which they are physiologically dependent

G. Other factors to consider in the client with a substance-related disorder
1. Rebellion and peer group pressure in adolescence may contribute to the onset of substance use
2. Substance use may become a coping mechanism for decreasing physical and emotional pain
3. Depression may precede or occur as a result of or in association with substance use
4. Grief and loss may be associated with substance use

H. Dysfunctional behaviors related to substance **abuse**
1. Preoccupation with obtaining and using substance
2. Manipulation to avoid consequences of behavior.
3. Impulsiveness
4. Anger, including physical and verbal **abuse**
5. Avoidance of relationships
6. Sense of self-importance
7. Denial; blaming everything but the substance use for his or her problems
8. Uses rationalization and projection to justify unacceptable behavior
9. Likely to be involved in codependent relationships whereby a significant other also unknowingly serves as a significant enabler
10. Low self-esteem
11. Depression

III. ALCOHOL ABUSE
A. Description
1. Alcohol is a central nervous system (CNS) depressant affecting all body tissues
2. Physical dependence is a biological need for alcohol to avoid physical withdrawal symptoms, whereas psychological dependence refers to craving for the subjective effect of alcohol.

B. Risk factors
1. Biological predisposition; genetic and familial predisposition may be a risk factor
2. Depressed and highly anxious characteristics
3. Low self-esteem
4. Poor self-control
5. History of rebelliousness, poor school performance, or delinquency
6. Poor parental relationships

C. Data collection
1. Slurred speech
2. Uncoordinated movements
3. Unsteady gait
4. Restlessness
5. Belligerence
6. Confusion
7. Sneaking drinks, drinking in the morning, and experiencing blackouts
8. Binge drinking
9. Arguments about drinking
10. Missing work
11. Increased tolerance to alcohol
12. Intoxication, with blood alcohol levels of 0.1% (100 mg alcohol per deciliter of blood) or higher

D. Psychological symptoms
1. Depression
2. Hostility
3. Suspiciousness
4. Rationalization
5. Irritability
6. Isolation
7. Decrease in inhibitions
8. Decrease in self-esteem
9. Denial that a problem exists

E. Complications associated with chronic alcohol use
1. Vitamin deficiencies
   a. Vitamin B deficiency causing peripheral neuropathies
   b. Thiamine deficiency causing Korsakoff's syndrome (a form of amnesia)
2. Alcohol-induced persistent amnesic disorder causing severe memory problems
3. Wernicke's encephalopathy (degenerative condition of the brain) causing confusion, ataxia, and abnormal eye movements
4. Hepatitis; cirrhosis of the liver
5. Esophagitis and gastritis
6. Pancreatitis
7. Anemias
8. Immune system dysfunctions
9. Brain damage
10. Peripheral neuropathy
11. Cardiac disorders

IV. ALCOHOL WITHDRAWAL
A. Description
1. Early signs develop within a few hours after cessation of alcohol intake

BOX 64-2 **Early Signs of Alcohol Withdrawal**

Anorexia (nausea and vomiting may occur)
Anxiety
Easily startled
Hyperalertness
Hypertension
Insomnia
Irritability
Jerky movements
Possibly experiences hallucinations, illusions, or vivid nightmares
Possibly reports a feeling of "shaking inside"
Seizures (usually appear 7-48 hours after cessation of alcohol)
Tachycardia
Tremors

BOX 64-3 **Manifestations of Alcohol Withdrawal Delirium**

Agitation
Anorexia
Anxiety
Delirium
Diaphoresis
Disorientation with fluctuating levels of consciousness
Fever (temperature of 100° to 103° F)
Hallucinations and delusions
Insomnia
Tachycardia and hypertension

2. These signs peak after 24 to 48 hours and then rapidly disappear, unless the withdrawal progresses to alcohol withdrawal delirium
3. At the onset of withdrawal (Box 64-2), follow agency protocol using specified withdrawal assessment scales as indicated by unit or agency policy
4. Chlordiazepoxide (Librium) is the most commonly prescribed medication for acute alcohol withdrawal and is usually given orally unless a more immediate onset is required (any benzodiazepine will decrease the withdrawal symptoms because of cross tolerance) (see Chapter 66 for a list of benzodiazepines)
5. An intramuscular injection of vitamin B_1 (thiamine) followed by several days of oral administration is administered to prevent Wernicke-Korsakoff's syndrome
B. Withdrawal (see Box 64-2)
C. Withdrawal delirium (Box 64-3)
   1. Withdrawal delirium is a medical emergency
   2. Death can occur from myocardial infarction, fat emboli, peripheral vascular collapse, electrolyte imbalance, aspiration pneumonia, or **suicide**
   3. The state of delirium usually peaks 48 to 72 hours after cessation or reduction of intake (although can occur later) and lasts 2 to 3 days
D. Interventions
   1. Provide care in a nonjudgmental manner
   2. Check the client frequently
   3. Monitor vital signs and neurological signs (as often as every 15 minutes) and provide one-to-one supervision
   4. Provide a quiet, nonstimulating environment; encourage a family member (one at a time) to stay with the client to minimize anxiety

5. Orient the client frequently
6. Explain all treatments and procedures in a quiet and simple manner
7. Initiate seizure precautions
8. Administer sedating or anticonvulsant medication as prescribed
9. Provide small, frequent, high-carbohydrate foods (administer antiemetic before meals as needed)
10. Monitor I&O
11. Administer vitamins (multivitamin, vitamin B complex [including thiamine], and vitamin C)
12. Assist client with activities of daily living and assist with ambulation if stable
13. Allow client to express fears
E. Disulfiram (Antabuse) therapy
   1. Description
      a. Disulfiram is an alcohol deterrent used for alcoholic dependence
      b. The medication sensitizes the client to alcohol, so a disulfiram-alcohol reaction occurs if alcohol is ingested
      c. The client must abstain from alcohol for at least 12 hours before the initial dose is administered
      d. Adverse effects usually begin within minutes to a half hour after consuming alcohol and may last 30 to 120 minutes
      e. Alcohol consumption for up to 14 days after disulfiram therapy has been discontinued; places the client at risk for disulfiram-alcohol reaction
   2. Adverse reactions
      a. Facial flushing
      b. Sweating
      c. Throbbing headache
      d. Neck pain
      e. Nausea and vomiting
      f. Hypotension
      g. Tachycardia
      h. Respiratory distress

3. Client education
    a. Educate as to the effects of the medication
    b. Ensure that the client agrees to abstain from alcohol and any substances that contain alcohol
    c. Instruct the client that the effects of the medication may occur for several days after discontinuance
    d. Instruct the client to avoid the use of substances that contain alcohol, such as cough medicines, rubbing compounds, vinegar, mouthwashes, and aftershave lotions
    e. Other medications used to assist with cravings include acamprosate calcium (Campral) and naltrexone (ReVia)
F. Dealing with the client who **abuses** alcohol (Boxes 64-4 and 64-5)
V. **DRUG DEPENDENCY**
A. CNS depressants
    1. CNS depressants can include alcohol, benzodiazepines, and barbiturates, and they act as a depressant, sedative, and hypnotic
    2. Intoxication (Box 64-6)
    3. Overdose can produce cardiovascular or respiratory depression, coma, shock, convulsions, and death

4. Overdose: if the client is awake, vomiting is induced and activated charcoal is administered; if the client is comatose, airway establishment and maintenance and gastric lavage with activated charcoal are the priorities; seizure precautions are indicated
5. Flumazenil (Romazicon) intravenously may be used in benzodiazepine overdose to reverse the effects
6. Withdrawal effects include nausea, vomiting, tachycardia, diaphoresis, irritability, tremors, insomnia, and seizures; withdrawal must be treated with a carefully titrated similar drug (abrupt withdrawal can lead to death)
7. Withdrawal from CNS depressants such as barbiturates is generally treated with a barbiturate such as phenobarbital or a long-acting benzodiazepine
B. CNS stimulants
    1. CNS stimulants can include amphetamines, cocaine, and crack
    2. Intoxication (Box 64-7)
    3. Overdose can produce respiratory distress, ataxia, hyperpyrexia, seizures, coma, brain attack (stroke), myocardial infarction, and death
    4. Overdose is treated with antipsychotics and management of associated effects
    5. Withdrawal effects include fatigue, depression, agitation, apathy, anxiety, insomnia, disorientation, lethargy, and craving

---

BOX 64-4 **Dealing With the Client Who Abuses Alcohol**

Direct the client's focus to the substance abuse problem.
Identify with the client those situations that precipitate angry feelings.
Set limits on manipulative behavior and verbal and physical abuse.
Hold the client firmly to reasonable limits, consistently reinforcing rules, with reasonable consequences for breaking rules.
Hold the client accountable for all behaviors.
Assist the client to explore strengths and weaknesses.
Encourage focusing on strengths if the client is losing control.
Encourage the client to participate in group therapy and support groups.

BOX 64-5 **Therapies for Substance Abuse Clients and Their Families**

Behavior therapy, aversion conditioning with disulfiram (Antabuse), or another medication
Hospitalization
Psychotherapy (individual, group, family)
Support groups such as Alcoholics Anonymous; Narcotics Anonymous; Pills Anonymous; Al-Anon, Al-a-Teen, or Narc-Anon (for family members and friends of alcoholics or addicts); and Adult Children of Alcoholics
Transitional living programs (halfway houses)

BOX 64-6 **Intoxication: Central Nervous System Depressants**

Drowsiness
Hypotension
Impairment of memory, attention, judgment, and social or occupational functioning
Incoordination and unsteady gait
Irritability
Slurred speech

BOX 64-7 **Intoxication: Central Nervous System Stimulants**

Dilated pupils
Euphoria
Hypertension
Impairment of judgment and social or occupational functioning
Insomnia
Nausea and vomiting
Paranoia, delusions, or hallucinations
Potential for violence
Tachycardia

6. Withdrawal is treated with antidepressants, a dopamine agonist, or bromocriptine (Parlodel); withdrawal is primarily supportive, particularly when dealing with the severe depression and suicidal ideation that accompanies stimulant withdrawal

C. Opioids

1. Opioids can include opium, heroin, meperidine (Demerol), morphine sulfate, codeine sulfate, methadone (Dolophine), hydromorphone (Dilaudid), and fentanyl (Sublimaze)
2. Intoxication (Box 64-8)
3. Overdose can produce respiratory depression, coma, shock, seizures, and death
4. Overdose is treated with an opioid antagonist such as naloxone (Narcan)
5. Withdrawal effects include yawning, insomnia, irritability, rhinorrhea, diaphoresis, cramps, nausea and vomiting, muscle aches, chills, fever, lacrimation, and diarrhea
6. Withdrawal may be treated by methadone detoxification or tapering dosage with other opioids
7. Clonidine (Catapres) as an α-adrenergic blocker assists in reducing the severity of sympathetic nervous system–generated withdrawal discomfort
8. Specific symptom management measures may also be used (e.g., bismuth subsalicylate [Kaopectate] for diarrhea, acetaminophen [Tylenol] for muscle aches)

D. Hallucinogens

1. Hallucinogens can include lysergic acid diethylamide (LSD), mescaline (peyote), psilocybin (mushrooms), or phencyclidine (PCP)
2. Intoxication (Box 64-9)
3. Overdose effects of LSD, peyote, and psilocybin include psychosis, brain damage, and death; effects of PCP include psychosis, hypertensive crisis, hyperthermia, seizures, and respiratory arrest
4. Treatment (LSD, peyote, psilocybin) involves low environmental stimuli (speak slowly, clearly, and in a low voice) and medications to treat anxiety

5. Treatment (PCP) involves possible gastric lavage (if alert), acidifying urine to assist in excreting drug, and interventions to treat behavioral disturbances, hyperthermia, hypertension, and respiratory distress
6. Withdrawal is primarily supportive and may include medications to target particular problem behaviors, such as agitation

E. Inhalants

1. Inhalants can include gases or liquids such as butane, paint thinner, paint and wax removers, airplane glue, nail polish remover, and nitrous oxide
2. Intoxication (Box 64-10)
3. Overdose can cause damage to the nervous system and death
4. Withdrawal management is mainly supportive including treating affected body systems

F. Marijuana (*Cannabis*)

1. Marijuana generally is smoked but can be ingested
2. Marijuana causes euphoria, detachment, relaxation, talkativeness, slowed perception of time, anxiety, or paranoia
3. Long-term dependence can result in lethargy, difficulty concentrating, memory loss, and possibly chronic respiratory disorders
4. Withdrawal management is mainly supportive

BOX 64-9 **Intoxication: Hallucinogens**

Agitation and belligerence
Anxiety and depression
Bizarre behavior, regressive behavior, or violent behavior
Blank stare
Diaphoresis
Dilated pupils
Elevated vital signs including blood pressure
Hallucinations
Impairment of judgment and social and occupational functioning
Incoordination
Muscular rigidity and chronic jerking
Paranoia
Seizures
Tachycardia
Tremors

BOX 64-8 **Intoxication: Opioids**

Constricted pupils
Decreased respirations
Drowsiness
Euphoria
Hypotension
Impairment of memory, attention, and judgment
Psychomotor retardation
Slurred speech

BOX 64-10 **Intoxication: Inhalants**

Enhancement of sexual pleasure
Euphoria
Excitation followed by drowsiness, lightheadedness, disinhibition, and agitation
Giggling and laughter

G. Other recreational and club drugs
1. Other recreational drugs include ecstasy, (methylenedioxymethamphetamine) GHB (gamma-hydroxybutyrate), methamphetamine (crank, meth, and other slang names), and ketamine
2. Effects include euphoria, increased energy, increased self-confidence, and increased sociability
3. Adverse effects include hyperthermia, rhabdomyolysis, renal failure, hepatotoxicity, depression, panic attacks, psychosis, cardiovascular collapse, and death
4. The use of over-the-counter medications containing ephedrine or pseudoephedrine to manufacture illegal supplies of methamphetamine has led many states to adopt laws requiring limited sales and signatures for the purchase of these medications
5. Programs for **addiction** also address nicotine withdrawal and the pharmacologic and psychotherapeutic interventions for this problem, such as nicotine patches, nicotine inhalers, and bupropion (Zyban) for the reduction of withdrawal and cravings
6. Anabolic steroids have also gained increased attention as increasing adverse events, including death, have become more present in the public media
H. Interventions: withdrawal
1. Initiate seizure precautions
2. Hydrate the client
3. Monitor vital signs every hour
4. Monitor I&O
5. Orient client frequently
6. Maintain minimal stimuli
7. Approach client in an accepting and nonjudgmental manner
8. Direct client's focus to the substance **abuse** problem
9. Assist the client with identifying situations that precipitate angry feelings
10. Assist the client to deal with emotions
11. Limit the client's blame-placing or rationalizing to explain the substance **abuse** problem
12. Assist the client to use assertive techniques rather than manipulation to meet needs
13. Set limits on manipulative behavior and verbal and physical **abuse**
14. Maintain firm and reasonable limits, consistently reinforcing rules, with reasonable consequences for breaking rules
15. Hold the client accountable for all behaviors
16. Assist the client to explore strengths and weaknesses
17. Encourage focusing on strengths if the client is losing control

---

BOX 64-11 Withdrawal: Nursing Care

Obtain information regarding the drug type and amount consumed.
Assess vital signs.
Remove unnecessary objects from the environment.
Provide one-to-one supervision if necessary.
Provide a quiet, calm environment with minimal stimuli.
Maintain client orientation.
Ensure client's safety by implementing seizure precautions.
Use restraints, if necessary and prescribed, to prevent the client from harming self and others.
Provide for physical needs.
Provide food and fluids as tolerated.
Administer medications as prescribed to decrease withdrawal symptoms.
Collect blood and urine samples for drug screening.

---

18. Encourage the client to participate in unit activities
19. Encourage the client to participate in group therapy and support groups
20. Box 64-11 delineates nursing care for clients
I. Dual diagnoses
1. Sometimes the use of alcohol and drugs masks underlying psychiatric pathology
2. Psychiatric pathology may also be precipitated by substance use and **abuse**
3. When psychiatric disorders and substance **abuse** are both present, it is often referred to as dual diagnosis
4. Separating out psychiatric diagnosis and substance dependence can only be done over time following a sustained period of abstinence
J. **Addiction** and **abuse** in health care professionals: suspicious signs
1. Frequently reporting that drugs have been wasted without being witnessed by another nurse
2. Administering maximum dosages of controlled substances when other nurses do not
3. A variance in usual pain relief in the absence of a change in dosage or frequency in their clients
4. Work patterns include the following: always volunteering to carry opioid (narcotic) drug cabinet or drawer keys, choosing shifts where less supervision is present, choosing work areas where the use of controlled substances is high, such as critical care units, operating room, anesthesia, and trauma units
5. Nurses have a professional and ethical obligation to report impaired co-workers
6. The majority of impaired nurses are able to return to work through the State Board of Nursing assistance and monitoring programs; such programs usually require strict adherence

to clearly stated rules and regular reports and drug screens

K. Codependency issues

1. Codependency refers to the presence of coexisting behaviors present in a significant other, which serves to enable the addict or alcoholic to continue the irresponsible patterns of use without experiencing consequences

2. Examples of codependency: paying bills the addict or alcoholic is responsible for; bailing the addict or alcoholic out of jail, helping the addict or alcoholic to call in sick

3. It is important to address codependency issues with the family to maximize the chance for recovery of both the client with the **addiction** and the person with codependent behaviors.

PRACTICE QUESTIONS

More questions on the companion CD!

898. A nurse is caring for a female client who was recently admitted to the hospital for anorexia nervosa. The nurse enters the client's room and notes that the client is doing vigorous push-ups. Which nursing action is appropriate?
    1. Interrupt the client and weigh her immediately.
    2. Interrupt the client and offer to take her for a walk.
    3. Allow the client to complete her exercise program.
    4. Tell the client that she is not allowed to exercise vigorously.

899. A nurse is caring for a client with anorexia nervosa. The nurse is monitoring the behavior of the client and understands that the client with anorexia nervosa manages anxiety by:
    1. Engaging in immoral acts
    2. Always reinforcing self-approval
    3. Observing rigid rules and regulations
    4. Having the need to always make the right decision

900. A nursing student is developing a plan of care for the hospitalized client with bulimia nervosa. The nursing instructor intervenes if the student documents which incorrect intervention in the plan?
    1. Monitor I&O.
    2. Monitor electrolyte levels.
    3. Observe for excessive exercise.
    4. Monitor for the use of laxatives and diuretics.

901. A nurse is monitoring a client who abuses alcohol for signs of alcohol withdrawal delirium. The nurse monitors for which of the following?
    1. Hypotension, ataxia, vomiting
    2. Stupor, agitation, muscular rigidity
    3. Hypotension, bradycardia, agitation
    4. Hypertension, disorientation, hallucinations

902. The spouse of a client admitted to the hospital for alcohol withdrawal says to the nurse, "I should get out of this bad situation." The most helpful response by the nurse would be:
    1. "Why don't you tell your husband about this?"
    2. "This is not the best time to make that decision."
    3. "What do you find difficult about this situation?"
    4. "I agree with you. You should get out of this situation."

903. A nurse is caring for a client who is suspected of being dependent on drugs. Which question would be appropriate for the nurse to ask when collecting data from the client regarding drug abuse?
    1. "Why did you get started on these drugs?"
    2. "How much do you use and what effect does it have on you?"
    3. "How long did you think you could take these drugs without someone finding out?"
    4. The nurse does not ask any questions because of fear that the client is in denial and will throw the nurse out of the room.

904. A client who has been drinking alcohol on a regular basis admits to having "a problem" and is asking for assistance with the problem. The nurse would encourage the client to attend which of the following community groups?
    1. Al-Anon
    2. Fresh Start
    3. Families Anonymous
    4. Alcoholics Anonymous

905. A client with a diagnosis of anorexia nervosa, who is in a state of starvation, is in a two-bed hospital room. A newly admitted client will be assigned to this client's room. Which client would be an appropriate choice as this client's roommate?
    1. A client with pneumonia
    2. A client receiving diagnostic tests
    3. A client who thrives on managing others
    4. A client who could benefit from the client's assistance at mealtime

906. A nurse is assigned to care for a client at risk for alcohol withdrawal. The nurse monitors the client, knowing that the early signs of withdrawal will usually develop within how much time after cessation or reduction of alcohol intake?
    1. In 7 days
    2. In 14 days
    3. In 21 days
    4. Within a few hours

907. A nurse determines that the wife of an alcoholic client is benefiting from attending an Al-Anon group when the nurse hears the wife say:
    1. "I no longer feel that I deserve the beatings my husband inflicts on me."

2. "My attendance at the meetings has helped me to see that I provoke my husband's violence."
3. "I enjoy attending the meetings because they get me out of the house and away from my husband."
4. "I can tolerate my husband's destructive behaviors now that I know they are common in alcoholics."

908. A female client with anorexia nervosa is a member of a support group. The client has verbalized that she would like to buy some new clothes but her finances are limited. Group members have brought some used clothes for the client to replace her old clothes. The client believes that the new clothes were much too tight, so she has reduced her calorie intake to 800 calories daily. The nurse identifies this behavior as:
1. Normal
2. Regression
3. Indicative of the client's ambivalence
4. Evidence of the client's altered and distorted body image

909. A hospitalized client with a history of alcohol abuse tells the nurse, "I am leaving now. I have to go. I don't want any more treatment. I have things that I have to do right away." The client has not been discharged. In fact, the client is scheduled for an important diagnostic test to be performed in 1 hour. After the nurse discusses the client's concerns with the client, the client dresses and begins to walk out of the hospital room. The appropriate nursing action is to:
1. Call the nursing supervisor
2. Call security to block all exit areas
3. Restrain the client until the physician can be reached

4. Tell the client that she cannot return to this hospital again if she leaves now

910. A nursing student is asked to identify the characteristics of bulimia nervosa. Which response by the student indicates a need to further research the disorder?
1. Dental erosion
2. Electrolyte imbalances
3. Enlarged parotid glands
4. Body weight well below ideal range

911. A nurse is caring for a client who has a history of opioid abuse and is monitoring the client for signs of withdrawal. Which clinical manifestations are specifically associated with withdrawal from opioids?
1. Dilated pupils, tachycardia, and diaphoresis
2. Yawning, irritability, diaphoresis, cramps, and diarrhea
3. Tachycardia, hypertension, sweating, and marked tremors
4. Depressed feelings, high drug craving, fatigue, and agitation

ALTERNATE ITEM FORMAT: MULTIPLE RESPONSE

912. Choose the appropriate interventions for caring for the client in alcohol withdrawal. Select all that apply.
☐ 1. Monitor vital signs
☐ 2. Maintain an NPO status
☐ 3. Provide a safe environment
☐ 4. Address hallucinations therapeutically
☐ 5. Provide stimulation in the environment
☐ 6. Provide reality orientation as appropriate

ANSWERS

898. 2
Rationale: Clients with anorexia nervosa are frequently preoccupied with vigorous exercise and push themselves beyond normal limits to work off caloric intake. The nurse must provide for appropriate exercise as well as place limits on vigorous activities. Options 1, 3, and 4 are inappropriate nursing actions.
Test-Taking Strategy: Use the process of elimination. Recalling that the nurse needs to set firm limits with clients who have this disorder will direct you to option 2. If you had difficulty with this question, review interventions for the client with anorexia nervosa.
Level of Cognitive Ability: Application
Client Needs: Physiological Integrity
Integrated Process: Nursing Process/Implementation
Content Area: Mental Health
References: Fortinash, K., & Holoday-Worret, P. (2008). *Psychiatric mental health nursing* (4th ed., p. 400). St. Louis: Mosby.

Keltner, N., Schwecke, L., & Bostrom, C. (2007) *Psychiatric nursing* (5th ed., p. 555). St. Louis: Mosby.
Morrison-Valfre, M. (2005). *Foundations of mental health care* (3rd ed., pp. 240-241). St. Louis: Mosby.

899. 3
Rationale: Clients with anorexia nervosa have the desire to please others. Their need to be correct or perfect interferes with rational decision-making processes. These clients are moralistic. Rules and rituals help the clients manage their anxiety. Options 1, 2, and 4 are incorrect.
Test-Taking Strategy: Use the process of elimination and focus on the subject—managing anxiety. Eliminate options 2 and 4 because of the close-ended word "always." Eliminate option 1 because it is not characteristic of the client with anorexia. Review the characteristics associated with this disorder if you had difficulty with this question.
Level of Cognitive Ability: Comprehension
Client Needs: Psychosocial Integrity
Integrated Process: Nursing Process/Data Collection

Content Area: Mental Health
References: Keltner, N., Schwecke, L., & Bostrom, C. (2007). *Psychiatric nursing* (5th ed., p. 548). St. Louis: Mosby.
Morrison-Valfre, M. (2005). *Foundations of mental health care* (3rd ed., p. 235). St. Louis: Mosby.

900. 3
Rationale: Excessive exercise is a characteristic of anorexia nervosa, not bulimia nervosa. Frequent vomiting, in addition to laxative and diuretic abuse, may lead to dehydration and electrolyte imbalance. Monitoring for dehydration and electrolyte imbalance are important nursing actions. Option 3 is the only option that is not associated with care of the client with bulimia.
Test-Taking Strategy: Note the strategic word "incorrect" in the question. This word indicates a negative event query and the need to select the incorrect intervention. Options 1, 2, and 4 are comparable or alike and directly or indirectly infer concern about fluid and electrolyte balance. Option 3 is different from the other options. Review the characteristics associated with bulimia nervosa if you had difficulty with this question.
Level of Cognitive Ability: Analysis
Client Needs: Physiological Integrity
Integrated Process: Nursing Process/Planning
Content Area: Mental Health
References: Keltner, N., Schwecke, L., & Bostrom, C. (2007). *Psychiatric nursing* (5th ed., p. 549). St. Louis: Mosby.
Morrison-Valfre, M. (2005). *Foundations of mental health care* (3rd ed., pp. 237-238). St. Louis: Mosby.

901. 4
Rationale: The symptoms associated with alcohol withdrawal delirium typically are anxiety, insomnia, anorexia, hypertension, disorientation, visual or tactile hallucinations, agitation, fever, and delusions.
Test-Taking Strategy: Use the process of elimination. Review each option carefully to ensure that all the symptoms are contained in the correct option. Eliminate options 1 and 3 first, knowing that hypertension rather than hypotension occurs. From the remaining options, recalling that the client who is stuporous is not likely to exhibit agitation will direct you to option 4. Review the symptoms associated with alcohol withdrawal if you had difficulty with this question.
Level of Cognitive Ability: Analysis
Client Needs: Physiological Integrity
Integrated Process: Nursing Process/Data Collection
Content Area: Mental Health
References: Keltner, N., Schwecke, L., & Bostrom, C. (2007). *Psychiatric nursing* (5th ed., p. 509). St. Louis: Mosby.
Stuart, G., & Laraia, M. (2005). *Principles and practice of psychiatric nursing* (8th ed., p. 491). St. Louis: Mosby.

902. 3
Rationale: The most helpful response is the one that encourages the client to problem-solve. Giving advice implies that the nurse knows what is best and can also foster dependency. The nurse should not agree with the client nor should the nurse request that the client provide explanations.
Test-Taking Strategy: Use therapeutic communication techniques. Eliminate option 1 because of the word "Why," which should be avoided in communication. Eliminate

option 4 because the nurse is agreeing with the client. Eliminate option 2 because this option places the client's feelings on hold. Option 3 is the only option that addresses the client's feelings. Review therapeutic communication techniques if you had difficulty with this question.
Level of Cognitive Ability: Application
Client Needs: Psychosocial Integrity
Integrated Process: Communication and Documentation
Content Area: Mental Health
References: Fortinash, K., & Holoday-Worret, P. (2008). *Psychiatric mental health nursing* (4th ed., p. 329). St. Louis: Mosby.
Keltner, N., Schwecke, L., & Bostrom, C. (2007). *Psychiatric nursing* (5th ed., pp. 90-92). St. Louis: Mosby.
Morrison-Valfre, M. (2005). *Foundations of mental health care* (3rd ed., p. 88). St. Louis: Mosby.

903. 2
Rationale: Whenever the nurse collects data from a client who is dependent on drugs, it is best for the nurse to attempt to elicit information by being nonjudgmental and direct. Option 1 is incorrect because it is judgmental, off focus, and reflects the nurse's bias. Option 3 is incorrect because it is judgmental, insensitive, and aggressive, which is nontherapeutic. Option 4 is incorrect because it indicates passivity on the nurse's part and uses rationalization to avoid the therapeutic nursing intervention.
Test-Taking Strategy: Use the process of elimination and therapeutic communication techniques to answer the question. Option 2 is the statement that is nonjudgmental and direct. Review data collection of a client who is a drug abuser if you had difficulty with this question.
Level of Cognitive Ability: Application
Client Needs: Psychosocial Integrity
Integrated Process: Nursing Process/Data Collection
Content Area: Mental Health
References: Keltner, N., Schwecke, L., & Bostrom, C. (2007). *Psychiatric nursing* (5th ed., pp. 90-92, 110). St. Louis: Mosby.
Morrison-Valfre, M. (2005). *Foundations of mental health care* (3rd ed., pp. 298-299). St. Louis: Mosby.

904. 4
Rationale: Alcoholics Anonymous is a major self-help organization for the treatment of alcoholism. Option 1 is a group for families of alcoholics. Option 3 is for parents of children who abuse substances. Option 2 is for nicotine addicts.
Test-Taking Strategy: Use the process of elimination. If you are unfamiliar with these support groups, note the relation between "drinking" in the question and "Alcoholics" in the correct option. Familiarize yourself with the purposes of specific support groups if you had difficulty with this question.
Level of Cognitive Ability: Application
Client Needs: Safe and Effective Care Environment
Integrated Process: Nursing Process/Implementation
Content Area: Mental Health
References: Fortinash, K., & Holoday-Worret, P. (2008). *Psychiatric mental health nursing* (4th ed., p. 334). St. Louis: Mosby.
Morrison-Valfre, M. (2005). *Foundations of mental health care* (3rd ed., p. 299). St. Louis: Mosby.

905. 2

Rationale: The client receiving diagnostic tests is an appropriate roommate. The client with anorexia is most likely experiencing hematological complications, such as leukopenia. Having a roommate with pneumonia would place the client with anorexia nervosa at risk for infection. The client with anorexia nervosa should not be put in a situation in which he or she can focus on the nutritional needs of others or be managed by others, because this may contribute to sublimation and suppression of their own hunger.

Test-Taking Strategy: Use the process of elimination and note the strategic words "in a state of starvation." Recalling the characteristics and complications associated with anorexia nervosa will direct you to option 2. Review care of the client with anorexia nervosa if you have difficulty with this question.

Level of Cognitive Ability: Analysis
Client Needs: Safe and Effective Care Environment
Integrated Process: Nursing Process/Planning
Content Area: Mental Health
References: Keltner, N., Schwecke, L., & Bostrom, C. (2007). *Psychiatric nursing* (5th ed., p. 561). St. Louis: Mosby.
Morrison-Valfre, M. (2005). *Foundations of mental health care* (3rd ed., p. 236). St. Louis: Mosby.
Stuart, G., & Laraia, M. (2005). *Principles & practice of psychiatric nursing* (8th ed., p. 532). St. Louis: Mosby.

906. 4

Rationale: Early signs of alcohol withdrawal develop within a few hours after cessation or reduction of alcohol and peak after 24 to 48 hours.

Test-Taking Strategy: Use the process of elimination and note the strategic words "early" and "usually develop." This will assist in directing you to option 4. If you are unfamiliar with the manifestations associated with alcohol withdrawal, review this content.

Level of Cognitive Ability: Comprehension
Client Needs: Physiological Integrity
Integrated Process: Nursing Process/Data Collection
Content Area: Mental Health
Reference: Fortinash, K., & Holoday-Worret, P. (2008). *Psychiatric mental health nursing* (4th ed., p. 329). St. Louis: Mosby.

907. 1

Rationale: Al-Anon support groups are a protected, supportive opportunity for spouses and significant others to learn what to expect and to obtain suggestions about successful behavioral changes. Option 1 is the healthiest response, because it exemplifies an understanding that the alcoholic partner is responsible for his behavior and cannot be allowed to blame family members for loss of control. The nonalcoholic partner should not feel responsible when the spouse loses control (option 2). Option 4 indicates that the wife remains codependent. Option 3 indicates that the group is being seen as an escape, not a place to work on issues.

Test-Taking Strategy: Use the process of elimination and focus on the subject of the question—benefiting from attending an Al-Anon group. This will direct you to option 1. Review the purpose of this type of support group if you had difficulty with this question.

Level of Cognitive Ability: Analysis
Client Needs: Psychosocial Integrity
Integrated Process: Nursing Process/Evaluation
Content Area: Mental Health
Reference: Fortinash, K., & Holoday-Worret, P. (2008). *Psychiatric mental health nursing* (4th ed., p. 334). St. Louis: Mosby.

908. 4

Rationale: Altered or distorted body image is a concern with clients with anorexia nervosa. Although the client may struggle with ambivalence and present with regressed behavior, the client's coping pattern relates to the basic issue of distorted body image. The client's behavior is not normal.

Test-Taking Strategy: Use the process of elimination. Focus on the information provided in the question to determine that the subject relates to a distorted body image. This will direct you to option 4. If you had difficulty with this question, review the characteristics associated with the client with anorexia nervosa.

Level of Cognitive Ability: Comprehension
Client Needs: Psychosocial Integrity
Integrated Process: Nursing Process/Data Collection
Content Area: Mental Health
Reference: Fortinash, K., & Holoday-Worret, P. (2008). *Psychiatric mental health nursing* (4th ed., p. 396). St. Louis: Mosby.

909. 1

Rationale: A nurse can be charged with false imprisonment if a client is made to wrongfully believe that he or she cannot leave the hospital. Most health care facilities have documents that the client is asked to sign, which relate to the client's responsibilities when they leave against medical advice (AMA). The client should be asked to sign this document before leaving. The nurse should request that the client wait to speak to the physician before leaving, but, if the client refuses to do so, the nurse cannot hold the client against his or her will. Restraining the client and calling security to block exits constitutes false imprisonment. Any client has a right to health care (option 4) and cannot be told otherwise.

Test-Taking Strategy: Use the process of elimination. Keeping the concept of false imprisonment in mind, eliminate options 2 and 3 because they are comparable or alike. Eliminate option 4, knowing that any client has a right to health care. Review the points related to false imprisonment if you had difficulty with this question.

Level of Cognitive Ability: Application
Client Needs: Safe and Effective Care Environment
Integrated Process: Nursing Process/Implementation
Content Area: Mental Health
References: Keltner, N., Schwecke, L., & Bostrom, C. (2007). *Psychiatric nursing* (5th ed., p. 57). St. Louis: Mosby.
Morrison-Valfre, M. (2005). *Foundations of mental health care* (3rd ed., pp. 24-25). St. Louis: Mosby.

910. 4

Rationale: Clients with bulimia nervosa may not initially appear to be physically or emotionally ill. They are often at or slightly below ideal body weight. On further inspection, the client demonstrates enlargement of the parotid glands

with dental erosion and caries if the client has been inducing vomiting. Electrolyte imbalances are present.
Test-Taking Strategy: Use the process of elimination and note the strategic words "need to further research." Focusing on the client's diagnosis will direct you to option 4. Option 4 is a characteristic sign of anorexia nervosa, not bulimia nervosa. Review the characteristics of these disorders if you had difficulty with this question.
Level of Cognitive Ability: Comprehension
Client Needs: Physiological Integrity
Integrated Process: Teaching and Learning
Content Area: Mental Health
References: Fortinash, K., & Holoday-Worret, P. (2008). *Psychiatric mental health nursing* (4th ed., p. 397). St. Louis: Mosby.
Keltner, N., Schwecke, L., & Bostrom, C. (2007). *Psychiatric nursing* (5th ed., p. 552). St. Louis: Mosby.
Morrison-Valfre, M. (2005). *Foundations of mental health care* (3rd ed., p. 237). St. Louis: Mosby.

911. **2**
Rationale: Opioids are central nervous system (CNS) depressants. Withdrawal effects include yawning, insomnia, irritability, rhinorrhea, diaphoresis, cramps, nausea and vomiting, muscle aches, chills, fever, lacrimation, and diarrhea. Withdrawal is treated by methadone tapering or medication detoxification. Option 2 identifies the clinical manifestations associated with withdrawal from opioids. Option 3 describes withdrawal from alcohol. Option 1 describes intoxication from hallucinogens. Option 4 describes withdrawal from cocaine.
Test-Taking Strategy: Focus on the subject of the question—the clinical manifestations associated with withdrawal from opioids. Recalling that opioids are CNS depressants will

direct you to option 2. If you had difficulty with this question, review the manifestations associated with opioid withdrawal.
Level of Cognitive Ability: Analysis
Client Needs: Physiological Integrity
Integrated Process: Nursing Process/Data Collection
Content Area: Mental Health
Reference: Fortinash, K., & Holoday-Worret, P. (2008). *Psychiatric mental health nursing* (4th ed., p. 329). St. Louis: Mosby.

ALTERNATE ITEM FORMAT: MULTIPLE RESPONSE

912. **1, 3, 4, 6**
Rationale: When the client is experiencing withdrawal from alcohol, the priority for care is to prevent the client from harming himself or herself or others. The nurse would provide a low stimulating environment to maintain the client in as calm a state as possible. The nurse would monitor the vital signs closely and report abnormal findings. The nurse would frequently reorient the client to reality and would address hallucinations therapeutically. Adequate nutritional and fluid intake needs to be maintained.
Test-Taking Strategy: Use therapeutic communication techniques to assist in selecting the correct interventions. Also, recalling the characteristics associated with alcohol withdrawal will assist in answering correctly. Review these interventions if you had difficulty with this question.
Level of Cognitive Ability: Application
Client Needs: Psychosocial Integrity
Integrated Process: Nursing Process/Implementation
Content Area: Mental Health
Reference: Keltner, N., Schwecke, L., & Bostrom, C. (2007). *Psychiatric nursing* (5th ed., pp. 506-507). St. Louis: Mosby.

REFERENCES

Fortinash, K., & Holoday-Worret, P. (2008). *Psychiatric mental health nursing* (4th ed.). St. Louis: Mosby.
Keltner, N., Schwecke, L., & Bostrom, C. (2007). *Psychiatric nursing* (5th ed.). St. Louis: Mosby.

Morrison-Valfre, M. (2005). *Foundations of mental health care* (3rd ed.). St. Louis: Mosby.
Stuart, G., & Laraia, M. (2005). *Principles & practice of psychiatric nursing* (8th ed.). St. Louis: Mosby.

Crisis Theory and Intervention

I. CRISIS INTERVENTION

A. Description
1. **Crisis** is a temporary state of severe emotional disorganization caused by failure of **coping mechanisms** and lack of support
2. Decision-making and problem-solving are inadequate
3. Treatment is aimed at assisting the client and the family through the stressful situation

B. Phases of a **crisis**
1. Phase 1: external precipitating event
2. Phase 2
   a. Perception of the threat
   b. Increase in anxiety
   c. Client may cope or resolve the **crisis**
3. Phase 3
   a. Failure of coping
   b. Increasing disorganization
   c. Emergence of physical symptoms
   d. Relationship problems
4. Phase 4
   a. Mobilization of internal and external resources
   b. Goal is to return the individual to at least a precrisis level of functioning

C. Types of crises (Box 65-1)

D. **Crisis** intervention
1. Treatment is immediate, supportive, and directly responsive to the immediate **crisis**
2. Interventions are goal directed
3. Feelings of the client are acknowledged
4. Intervention provides opportunities for expression and validation of feelings
5. Connections are made between the meaning of the event and the **crisis**
6. Client explores alternative **coping mechanisms** and tries out new behaviors

II. GRIEF

A. Grief is a natural emotional response to loss that individuals must experience as they attempt to accept the loss

B. Grief usually involves moving through a series of stages or tasks to help resolve the grief (Box 65-2)

C. Feelings associated with grief can include anger, frustration, loneliness, sadness, guilt, regret, or peace

D. Healing can occur when the pain of the loss has lessened and the survivor has adapted to life without the deceased; the survivor will continue to experience memories of the deceased

E. Types of grief
1. Normal grief: physical, emotional, cognitive, or behavioral reactions can occur; the process of resolution can take months to years
2. Anticipatory grief occurs before the loss and is associated with an acute, chronic, or terminal illness
3. Disenfranchised grief occurs when a loss is experienced and cannot be acknowledged openly (societal norms do not define the loss as a loss within its traditional definition)
4. Dysfunctional grief occurs with prolonged emotional instability and a lack of progression to successful coping with the loss
5. Children's grief is based on their developmental level (Box 65-3)

III. LOSS

A. Loss is the absence of something desired or previously thought to be available

B. Actual loss can be identified by others and can arise in response to or in anticipation of a situation

C. Perceived loss is experienced by one person and cannot be verified by others

D. Anticipatory loss is experienced before the loss occurs

E. Mourning
1. The outward and social expression of loss
2. May be dictated by cultural and religious beliefs

F. Bereavement
1. Includes the inner feelings and the outward reactions of the survivor
2. Includes grief and mourning

IV. NURSE'S ROLE: GRIEF AND LOSS

A. The nurse's role includes communicating with the client, family members, and significant other (Box 65-4)

BOX 65-1 Types of Crises

Maturational Crisis
Relates to developmental stages and associated role changes; examples include marriage, birth of a child, and retirement

Situational Crisis
Arises from an external source, is often unanticipated, and is associated with a life event that upsets an individual or a group's psychological equilibrium; examples include loss of a job or a change in job, a change in financial status, death of a loved one, divorce, abortion, and severe physical or mental illness

Adventitious Crisis
Relates to a crisis of disaster or an event that is not a part of everyday life and is unplanned and accidental; this type of crisis may result from a natural disaster such as a flood, earthquake, hurricane, fire, or tornado; a national disaster such as war, riots, acts of terrorism; or a crime of violence such as rape, assault, murder, spousal or child abuse

BOX 65-2 The Grief Response

Stage 1: Shock and Disbelief
Survivor may have feelings of numbness, difficulties with decision-making, emotional outbursts, denial, and isolation.

Stage 2: Experiencing the Loss
Survivor may feel angry at the loved one who died or may feel guilt about the death.
Bargaining and or depression may also occur in this stage.

Stage 3: Reintegration
Survivor begins to reorganize his or her life and accepts the reality of the loss.

BOX 65-3 Children's Grief

Birth to 1 Year
Infant has no concept of death.
Infant reacts to the loss of mother or caregiver.

1 to 2 Years
Child may see death as reversible.
Grief response occurs only to the death of the significant person in the child's life.
Child may scream, withdraw, or become disinterested in the environment.

2 to 5 Years
Child may see death as reversible.
Child has a sense of loss and is concerned about who will provide care.
Regression or aggressive behavior may occur.

5 to 9 Years
Child begins to see death as permanent.
Child may feel responsible for the occurrence.
Child has difficulty concentrating.

Preadolescent Through Adolescence
Adolescent sees death as permanent.
Adolescent experiences a strong emotional reaction.
Adolescent may regress.

BOX 65-4 Communication Process

Determine how much the client and family want to know.
Determine whether there is a spokesperson for the family.
Be aware of cultural and religious beliefs and how they may affect the communication process; consider personal space issues, eye contact, and touch.
Obtain an interpreter if necessary.
Allow opportunity for informed choices.
Assist with the decision-making process if asked; use problem-solving to assist in decision-making, and avoid interjecting personal views or opinions.
Encourage expression of feelings, concerns, and fears.
Be honest and truthful, and let the client and family know that you will not abandon them.
Ask the client and family about their expectations and needs.
Be a sensitive listener; sit in silence if necessary and appropriate.
Extend touch and hold the client's or family member's hand if appropriate.
Encourage reminiscing.
If you do not know what to do in a particular situation, seek assistance.
If you do not know what to say to a client or family who is talking about death, listen attentively and use therapeutic communication techniques such as open-ended questions or reflection.
Acknowledge your own feelings; let the client and family know that the topic of conversation is a difficult one and that you do not know what to say.
Realize that it is acceptable to cry with the client and family during the grief process.

B. Allow ongoing opportunities for fully informed choices.
C. Facilitate the grief process; assess grief and assist the survivor to feel the loss and complete the tasks of the grief process
D. Consider the survivor's culture, religion, family structure, individual life experiences, coping skills, and support systems
E. Grief affects survivors physically, psychologically, socially, and spiritually; therefore, a multidisciplinary team approach including a bereavement specialist facilitates the grief process

▲ V. END OF LIFE
A. Description: end of life refers to issues related to death and dying
B. Cultural and religious issues (refer to Chapter 6 and Box 6-4 for information regarding cultural and religious issues)

C. Legal and ethical issues
 1. Outcomes related to care during illness and the dying experience should be based on the client's wishes
 2. Issues for consideration may include organ and tissue donations, advance directives or other legal documents, withholding or withdrawing treatment, and cardiopulmonary resuscitation
D. Palliative care
 1. Palliative care focuses on caring interventions and symptom management rather than cure for diseases that no longer respond to treatment
 2. A pain- and symptom-controlled environment is established (the dying client should be as pain free and as comfortable as possible)
 3. Hospice care provides support and care for clients in the last phases of incurable diseases so that they might live as fully and as comfortable as possible; client and family needs are the focus of any intervention
E. Near-death physiological manifestations
 1. As death approaches, metabolism is reduced and the body gradually slows down until all function ends
 2. Sensory: client experiences blurred vision, decreased sense of taste and smell, decreased pain and touch perception, and loss of blink reflex; the client also appears to stare (hearing is believed to be the last sense lost)
 3. Respirations
  a. Respirations may be rapid, slow, shallow, and irregular
  b. Respirations may be noisy and wet sounding (death rattle)
  c. Cheyne-Stokes respiration is alternating periods of apnea and deep, rapid breathing
 4. Circulation
  a. Heart rate slows, and blood pressure falls progressively
  b. Skin is cool to touch, and the extremities become pale, mottled, and cyanotic
  c. Skin is wax-like very near death
 5. Urinary output gradually decreases; incontinence may occur
 6. Gastrointestinal motility and peristalsis diminish, leading to constipation, gas accumulation, and distention; a bowel movement may occur before death or at the time of death
 7. Musculoskeletal system: client gradually loses ability to move, has difficulty speaking and swallowing, and loses the gag reflex
F. Death
 1. Death occurs when all vital organs and body systems cease to function
 2. Generally respirations cease first, and then the heart beat stops a few minutes thereafter

---

BOX 65-5 **Physical Care to the Dying Client**

Pain
Administer pain medication.
Do not delay or deny pain medication.
Dyspnea
Elevate the head of the bed or position on the side.
Administer supplemental oxygen.
Suction fluids from the airway as needed.
Skin
Assess color and temperature.
Assess for breakdown.
Implement measures to prevent breakdown.
Dehydration
Maintain regular oral care.
Encourage taking ice chips and sips of fluid.
Do not force the client to eat or drink.
Use moist cloths to provide moisture to the mouth.
Apply lubricant to the lips and oral mucous membranes.
Anorexia, Nausea, and Vomiting
Provide antiemetics before meals.
Have family members provide the client's favorite foods.
Provide frequent small portions of favorite foods.
Elimination
Monitor urinary and bowel elimination.
Place absorbent pads under the client and check frequently.
Weakness and Fatigue
Provide rest periods.
Assess tolerance for activities.
Provide assistance and support as needed for maintaining bed or chair positions.
Restlessness
Maintain a calm soothing environment.
Do not restrain.
Limit the number of visitors at the client's bedside.
Allow a family member to stay with the client.

G. Brain death occurs when the cerebral cortex stops functioning or is irreversibly damaged
H. Nursing care
 1. Assessment of the client; avoid repeated, unnecessary assessments on the dying client
  a. Assessment should be limited to obtaining essential data
  b. Frequency of assessment depends on the client's stability (at least every 8 hours); as changes occur, assessment needs to be done more frequently
 2. Physical care (Box 65-5)
 3. Psychosocial care
  a. Monitor for anxiety and depression
  b. Monitor for fear (Box 65-6)
  c. Encourage the client and family to express feelings
  d. Provide support and advocacy for the client and family
  e. Provide privacy for the client and family
  f. Provide a private room for the client

BOX 65-6   **Fear Associated With Dying**

Fear of Pain
Fear of pain may occur based on anxieties related to dying.
Do not delay or deny pain relief measures to a
   terminally ill client.
Fear of Loneliness and Abandonment
Allow family members to stay with the client.
Holding hands and touching (if culturally acceptable)
   and listening to the client are important.
Fear of Being Meaningless
Client may feel hopeless and powerless.
Encourage life reviews and focus on the client's positive
   aspects of his or her life.

Modified from Lewis, S., Heitkemper, M., & Dirksen, S. (2004). *Medical-surgical nursing: Assessment and management of clinical problems* (6th ed.). St. Louis: Mosby.

BOX 65-7   **General Postmortem Procedures**

Close the client's eyes.
Replace dentures.
Wash the body.
Place pads under the perineum.
Remove tubes and dressings.
Straighten the body and place a pillow under the head
   in preparation for family viewing.

   4. Postmortem care (Box 65-7)
      a. Maintain respect and dignity for the client
      b. Determine whether the client is an organ donor; if so, follow appropriate procedures related to the donation
      c. Consider cultural rituals, state laws, and agency procedures when performing postmortem care
      d. Prepare the body for immediate viewing by the family
      e. Provide privacy and time for the family to be with the deceased person
▲ VI. **DEPRESSION**
   A. Description (refer to Chapter 63)
      1. Depression affects feelings, thoughts, and behaviors
      2. It can occur after a loss, including loss of self-esteem, the end of a significant relationship, the death of a loved one, or a traumatic event
      3. The loss is followed by grief and mourning; if this process does not resolve, depression results
      4. Depression may be mild, moderate, or severe
      5. Treatment includes counseling, antidepressant medication, and electroconvulsive therapy (ECT)
▲ B. Mild depression
      1. Triggered by an external event, and the experience follows the normal grief reaction
      2. Lasts less than 2 weeks

   3. Feeling sad
   4. Feeling let down or disappointed
   5. Mild alterations in sleep patterns
   6. Feeling less alert
   7. Irritability
   8. Disinterested in spending time with others
   9. Increased use of alcohol or drugs
C. Moderate depression
   1. Persists over time
   2. The person experiences a sense of change and often seeks help
   3. Despondent and gloomy
   4. Dejected
   5. Low self-esteem
   6. Helplessness and powerlessness
   7. May experience intense anxiety and anger
   8. Diurnal variation: the person may feel better at a certain time of the day, such as in the morning
   9. Slow thought processes and difficulty in concentrating
   10. Rumination: persistent thinking about and discussion of a particular subject
   11. Negative thinking and suicidal thoughts
   12. Sleep disturbances
   13. Social withdrawal
   14. Anorexia, weight loss, and fatigue
   15. Somatic complaints
   16. Menstrual changes
   17. Increased use of alcohol or drugs
D. Severe depression
   1. Intense and pervasive
   2. Despair and hopelessness
   3. Guilt and worthlessness
   4. Flat affect
   5. May show agitation and pace about
   6. Poor posture and unkempt appearance
   7. Decreased speech
   8. Self-destructive thoughts; however, the client may lack energy to act on the thought
   9. Social withdrawal
   10. Poor concentration and overwhelmed by simple tasks
   11. Severe psychomotor retardation
   12. Anorexia and considerable weight loss
   13. Constipation and urinary retention
   14. Lack of sexual interest
   15. Terminal insomnia
   16. Diurnal variation: the person feels worse in the morning and better as the day goes on
   17. Delusions and hallucinations
E. Interventions
   1. Altered thought processes
      a. Encourage the client to discuss losses or changes in the life situation
      b. Encourage the client to express sadness or anger and allow adequate time for verbal responses

c. Assist the client in developing short-term goals
d. Encourage the use of problem-solving and positive thinking
e. Limit decision-making
f. Spend short periods throughout the day with the client
g. Be on time when a schedule is planned with the client
h. Sit in silence with the client who is not verbalizing
i. Use simple, concrete words when communicating
j. Avoid a cheerful attitude

2. Risk for self-harm
   a. Assess for **suicide** clues and intervene to provide safety precautions as necessary
   b. Ask the client directly, "Have you thought of hurting yourself?"
   c. Assess lethality of plans
   d. Do not leave the client alone for extended periods
   e. If the client has a suicidal plan, place on a one-to-one supervision
   f. Form a suicidal contract with the client

3. Activity intolerance
   a. Encourage daily exercise.
   b. Assist with activities of daily living if the client is unable to perform them
   c. Begin with one-to-one activities
   d. Provide activities for easy mastery to increase self-esteem and assist to alleviate guilt feelings
   e. Provide activities that do not require a great deal of concentration (simple card games, drawing)
   f. Engage in gross motor activities (walking)
   g. Eventually bring the client into small group activities and then large groups

4. Altered nutrition
   a. Ensure adequate nutrition
   b. Offer small, high-calorie, high-protein snacks, and fluids throughout the day
   c. Stay with the client during meals
   d. Weigh the client weekly
   e. Assess bowel patterns for constipation

5. Sleep pattern disturbance
   a. Ensure adequate sleep
   b. Provide rest periods after activities
   c. Encourage the client to dress and stay out of bed during the day
   d. Provide relaxation measures at bedtime
   e. Decrease environmental stimuli at bedtime
   f. Spend time with the client before bedtime

VII. ELECTROCONVULSIVE THERAPY (ECT)
A. Description
   1. An effective treatment for depression that consists of inducing a grand mal (tonic-clonic) seizure by passing an electrical current through electrodes that are attached to the temples
   2. The administration of a muscle relaxant minimizes seizure activity, preventing damage to long bones and cervical vertebrae
   3. The usual course is 6 to 12 treatments given two to three times per week
   4. Maintenance ECT once a month may help to decrease the relapse rate for the client with recurrent depression
   5. ECT is not a permanent cure
   6. Not necessarily effective in the client with dysthymic depression or the client with depression and personality disorders, those with drug dependence, or those with depression as a result of situational or social difficulties
   7. Possible contraindications include recent myocardial infarction, brain attack (stroke) or cerebral vascular malformation, or clients with intracranial mass lesions

B. Uses
   1. Clients with major depressive and bipolar-depressive disorders, especially when psychotic symptoms are present, such as delusions of guilt, somatic delusions, and delusions of infidelity
   2. Clients who have depression with marked psychomotor retardation and stupor
   3. Manic clients whose conditions are resistant to lithium and antipsychotic medications and in clients who are rapid cyclers (a client with a bipolar disorder who has many episodes of mood swings close together)
   4. Clients with schizophrenia (especially catatonia), those with schizoaffective syndromes, and psychotic clients

C. Indications for use (Box 65-8)
D. Preprocedure
   1. Explain the procedure to the client
   2. Encourage the client to discuss feelings, including myths regarding ECT
   3. Teach the client and family what to expect

BOX 65-8 Electroconvulsive Therapy (ECT): Indications for Use

When antidepressant medications have no effect
When there is a need for a rapid definitive response such as when a client is suicidal or homicidal
The client is in extreme agitation or stupor
The risks of other treatments outweigh the risk of ECT
The client has a history of poor medication response, a history of good ECT response, or both
The client prefers ECT as a treatment

4. Informed consent must be obtained when voluntary clients are being treated
5. For involuntary clients, when informed consent cannot be obtained, permission may be obtained from the next of kin, although in some states the permission for ECT must be obtained from the court
6. NPO after midnight or at least 4 hours prior to treatment
7. Take baseline vital signs
8. Ask the client to void
9. Remove hairpins, contact lenses, and dentures
10. Administer preoperative medication if prescribed; glycopyrrolate (Robinul) or atropine sulfate may be prescribed to prevent the potential for aspiration and to minimize bradydysrhythmias in response to electrical stimulus

E. During the procedure
1. Place a blood pressure cuff on one of the client's arms
2. An IV line is inserted and EEG and ECG electrodes are attached
3. A pulse oximeter is placed onto the client's finger
4. Blood pressure is monitored throughout the treatment
5. Medications administered may include a short-acting anesthetic such as methohexital sodium (Brevital Sodium), thiopental sodium (Pentothal), and a muscle relaxant such as succinylcholine (Anectine)
6. 100% oxygen by mask via positive pressure is administered throughout the procedure
7. An airway or bite block is placed to prevent biting the tongue
8. Electrical stimulus is administered and the seizure should last 30 to 60 seconds

F. Postprocedure
1. The client will be transported to a recovery room with the blood pressure cuff and oximeter in place, where oxygen, suction, and other emergency equipment is available
2. Once the client is awake, talk to the client and take vital signs
3. The client may be confused; provide frequent orientation (brief, distinct, and simple) and reassurance
4. The client returns to the nursing unit when at least a 90% oxygen saturation level is maintained, vital signs are stable, and mental status is satisfactory
5. Assess the gag reflex before giving the client fluids, food, or medication

G. Potential side effects
1. Major side effects include confusion, disorientation, and short-term memory loss

2. The client may be confused and disorientated upon awakening
3. Memory deficits may occur, but memory usually recovers completely, although some clients have memory loss lasting up to 6 months

VIII. SUICIDAL BEHAVIOR
A. Description
1. Suicidal clients characteristically have feelings of worthlessness, guilt, and hopelessness that are so overwhelming that they feel unable to go on with life and feel unfit to live
2. The nurse caring for a depressed client always considers the possibility of **suicide**
B. High-risk groups
1. Those with a history of previous **suicide attempts**
2. Family history of **suicide attempts**
3. Adolescents
4. Older clients
5. Disabled or terminally ill adults
6. Clients with personality disorders
7. Clients with organic brain syndrome or dementia
8. Depressed or psychotic clients
9. Substance abusers
C. Clues (Box 65-9)
D. Data collection (Box 65-10)
E. Interventions
1. Initiate **suicide** precautions
2. Remove harmful objects
3. Do not leave the client alone
4. Provide one-to-one supervision at all times
5. Provide a nonjudgmental, caring attitude
6. Develop a contract that is written, dated, and signed and that indicates alternative behavior at times of suicidal thoughts
7. Encourage the client to talk about feelings and to identify positive aspects about self

---

BOX 65-9 **Suicidal Clues**

Giving away personal, special, and prized possessions
Canceling social engagements
Making out or changing a will
Taking out or changing insurance policies
Positive or negative changes in behavior
Poor appetite
Sleeping difficulties
Feelings of hopelessness
Difficulty in concentrating
Loss of interest in activities
Client statements that indicate an intent to attempt suicide
Sudden calmness or improvement in a depressed client
Client questions about poisons, guns, or other lethal objects

BOX 65-10 **Suicidal Client: Data Collection**

The Plan
Does the client have a plan?
What is the plan, how lethal is the plan, and how likely is death to occur?
Does the client have the means to carry out the plan?

Client History of Attempts
What suicide attempts occurred in the past and what were the outcomes (i.e., physiological injuries)?
Was the client accidentally rescued?
Have the past attempts and methods been the same, or have methods increased in lethality?

Psychosocial
Is the client alone or alienated from others?
Is hostility or depression present?
Do hallucinations exist?
Is substance abuse present?
Has client had any recent losses or physical illness?
Has client had any environmental or lifestyle changes?

8. Encourage active participation in own care
9. Keep the client active by assigning achievable tasks
10. Check that visitors do not leave harmful objects in the client's room
11. Identify support systems
12. Do not allow the client to leave the unit unless accompanied by a staff member
13. Continue to assess the client's **suicide** potential

IX. **ABUSIVE BEHAVIORS**

A. Anger
  1. A feeling of annoyance that may be displaced onto an object or person
  2. Used to avoid anxiety and gives a feeling of power in situations in which the person feels out of control
B. Aggression can be harmful and destructive when not controlled
C. Violence is the physical force that is threatening to the safety of self and others
D. Data collection
  1. History of violence or self-harm
  2. Poor impulse control and low tolerance of frustration
  3. Defiant and argumentative
  4. Raising of voice
  5. Making verbal threats
  6. Pacing and agitation
  7. Muscle rigidity
  8. Flushed face
  9. Glaring at others
E. Interventions
  1. Maintain safety
  2. Use a calm approach and communicate with a calm, clear tone of voice (be assertive but not aggressive, and avoid verbal struggles)

3. Maintain a large personal space and use a non-aggressive posture
4. Listen actively and acknowledge the client's anger
5. Determine what the client considers to be his or her need
6. Provide the client with clear options that deal with the client's behavior, set limits on behavior, and make the client aware of the consequences of anger and violence
7. Discuss the use of **restraints** or **seclusion** if the client is unable to control angry behavior that may lead to violence
8. Assist the client with problem-solving and decision-making regarding the options

F. **Restraints** and **seclusion**
  1. Description
    a. Physical **restraints**: any manual method or mechanical device, material, or equipment that inhibits free movement
    b. **Seclusion**: a process in which a client is placed alone in a specially designed room for protection and close supervision
    c. Chemical **restraints**: medications given for a specific purpose of inhibiting a specific behavior or movement and that have an impact on the client's ability to relate to the environment
  2. Use of **restraints** and **seclusion**
    a. **Restraints** and **seclusion** should never be used as punishment or for the convenience of the health care staff
    b. **Restraints** and **seclusion** are used when behavior is physically harmful to the client or others and when alternative or less restrictive measures are insufficient in protecting the client or others from harm
    c. The nurse must document the behavior leading to the use of **restraints** or **seclusion**
    d. **Restraints** and **seclusion** are used when the client anticipates that a controlled environment would be helpful and requests **seclusion**
    e. **Restraints** require a written order of a physician, which must be reviewed and renewed every 24 hours and which also must specify the type of restraint to be used, the duration of the restraint or **seclusion**, and the criteria for release (agency policy and procedures need to be followed)
    f. In an emergency, the qualified nurse may place a client in **restraints** or **seclusion** and obtain a written or verbal order as soon as possible thereafter
    g. Within 1 hour of the initiation of **restraints** or **seclusion**, the psychiatrist must make a face-to-face assessment and evaluation

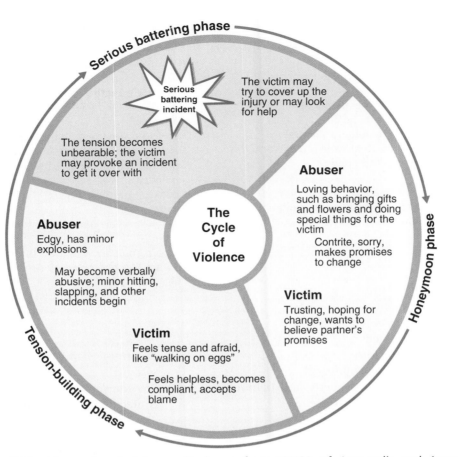

FIG. 65-1 The cycle of violence. (Redrawn from YWCA of Annapolis and Anne Arundel County, 1517 Ritchie Highway, Arnold, MD 21012.)

of the client and must continuously reevaluate the need for continued restraint or **seclusion**

h. While in **restraints** or **seclusion,** the client must be protected from all sources of harm by having one-to-one supervision with a staff member within an arm's length of the client

i. The client in **restraints** or **seclusion** needs constant one-to-one supervision; physical, safety, and comfort needs must be assessed every 15 to 30 minutes, and these observations are also documented (such as food, fluids, bathroom needs, range-of-motion exercise, and ambulation)

▲ **X. FAMILY VIOLENCE**

A. Description (Figure 65-1)

1. The violence begins with threats or verbal or physical minor assaults (tension building), and the victim attempts to comply with the requests of the abuser
2. The abuser loses control and becomes destructive and harmful (acute battering) while the victim attempts to protect himself or herself

3. Following the battering, the abuser then becomes loving and attempts to make peace (calmness and a diffusion of tension)
4. The abuser justifies that violence is normal and the victim is responsible for the **abuse**
5. Outsiders are usually not aware of what is happening in the family
6. Family members are isolated socially and lack autonomy and trust among each other; caring and intimacy in the family are absent
7. Family members expect other members of the family to meet their needs, but none are able to do so
8. The abuser threatens to abandon the family

B. Types of violence (Box 65-11)

C. The vulnerable person

1. The vulnerable person is the one in the family unit against whom violence is perpetrated
2. Those most vulnerable are children and older adults
3. The perpetrator of violence and the person targeted by the violence can be male or female
4. Battering is a crime

BOX 65-11 **Types of Violence**

Physical violence: Infliction of physical pain or bodily harm
Sexual violence: Any form of sexual contact without consent
Emotional violence: Infliction of mental anguish
Physical neglect: Failure to provide health care to prevent or treat physical or emotional illnesses
Developmental neglect: Failure to provide physical and cognitive stimulation needed to prevent developmental deficits
Educational neglect: Depriving a child of education
Economic exploitation: Illegal or improper exploitation of money, funds, or other resources for one's personal gain

BOX 65-12 **Data Collection Questions for Violence and Abuse**

"Has anyone ever touched you in a way that made you uncomfortable?"
"Is anyone hurting you now?"
"How do you and your partner deal with anger (or disagreement)?"
"Has your partner ever hit you?"
"Have you ever been threatened by_____?"
"Does your partner prevent you from seeing family or friends?"
"Does your partner ever use the children to manipulate you?"
"Did (or does) anyone in your family deal with anger by hitting?"
"Who do you play with most often? Is there anyone you do not like playing with? Are there games you don't like playing?"

▲ D. Characteristics of abusers
  1. Impaired self-esteem
  2. Strong dependency needs
  3. Narcissistic and suspicious
  4. History of **abuse** during childhood
  5. Perceive victims as their property and believe that they are entitled to **abuse** them
▲ E. Characteristics of victims
  1. Victims feel trapped, dependent, helpless, and powerless
  2. Victims of **abuse** may become depressed as they are trapped in the abuser's power and control cycle (see Figure 65-1)
  3. As victims' self-esteem becomes diminished with chronic **abuse,** they may blame themselves for the violence and be unable to see a way out of the situation
▲ F. Interventions
  1. Report suspected or actual cases of child **abuse** or **abuse** to the older adult to appropriate authorities (follow state and agency guidelines)
  2. Assess for evidence of physical injuries
  3. Ensure privacy and confidentiality during the assessment and provide a nonjudgmental and empathetic approach to foster trust; reassure the victim that he or she has not done anything wrong (see Box 65-12 for examples of assessment questions)
  4. Assist the victim to develop self-protective abilities and other problem-solving abilities
  5. Even if the victim is not ready to leave the situation, encourage the victim to develop a specific safety plan (a fast escape if the violence returns) and the best place to obtain help (hotlines, safe houses, and shelters); an abused person is usually reluctant to call the police
  6. Assess suicidal potential of the victim
  7. Assess the potential for homicide
  8. Assess for the use of drugs and alcohol
  9. Determine family coping patterns and support systems
  10. Provide support and assistance in coping with contacting the legal system
  11. Assist in resolving family dysfunction with prescribed therapies
  12. Encourage individual therapy for the victim that promotes coping with the trauma and prevents further psychological conflict
  13. Individual therapy that focuses on preventing violent behavior and repairing relationships is encouraged for abusers
  14. Encourage psychotherapy, counseling, group therapy, and support groups to assist family members to develop coping strategies
  15. Assist the family to access community and personal resources
  16. Maintain accurate and thorough medical health records

XI. **CHILD ABUSE** (refer to Chapter 30) ▲
  A. Description: child **abuse** involves physical, emotional, or sexual **abuse** and can involve neglect
  B. Data collection
    1. Physical **abuse**
      a. Unexplained bruises, burns, or fractures
      b. Bald spots on the scalp
      c. Apprehensiveness in the child
      d. Extreme aggressiveness or withdrawal
      e. Fear of parents
      f. Lack of crying when approached by a stranger
    2. Physical neglect
      a. Inadequate weight gain
      b. Poor hygiene
      c. Consistent hunger (begs or steals food)
      d. Inconsistent school attendance

e. Constant fatigue
f. Reports of lack of child supervision
g. Delinquency
3. Emotional **abuse**
   a. Speech disorders
   b. Habit disorders, such as sucking, biting, and rocking
   c. Learning disorders
   d. Self-harm behaviors
4. Sexual **abuse**
   a. Difficulty walking or sitting
   b. Torn, stained, or bloody underclothing
   c. Pain, swelling, or itching of the genitals
   d. Bruises, bleeding, or lacerations in the genital or anal area
   e. Poor peer relations
   f. Delinquency
   g. Changes in sleep patterns
   h. Self-harm behaviors
5. Shaken baby syndrome
   a. **Abuse** can cause intracranial hemorrhage, leading to cerebral edema and death
   b. Baby often has respiratory problems
   c. Nurse would note full bulging fontanels and a head circumference greater than expected
6. Child abduction
   a. Many cases involve abduction by a family member (usually a parent) who takes or keeps the child and violates a custody order
   b. Most vulnerable age for children abduction is less than 6 years of age
   c. Parents at risk for abducting their child include those who have made a prior threat of intent, cases in which there is a suspicion of **abuse** of the child, those wanting the child to grow up in their country of origin, or a parent with a mental illness, especially a sociopathic parent
C. Interventions
1. Assess injuries; support the child during a thorough physical assessment
2. Report cases of suspected **abuse** to appropriate authorities (follow state and agency guidelines); reporting is mandated by federal law
3. The child will likely be removed from the abusive environment to a safe place to prevent further injury while the case is investigated
4. Move slowly and avoid any loud noises when near the child
5. Communicate with the child at the child's eye level
6. Reassure the child that he or she is not "bad" and is not responsible for the abuser's behavior
7. Document accurately and completely all information related to the suspected **abuse**

8. When working with parents in follow-up care or counseling, assist the parents in identifying stressors and alternative ways to express feelings
9. Provide education to the parents, and refer parents to **crisis** hotlines and community support systems such as Parents Anonymous (a group for parents who have abused or fear that they may **abuse** their child physically) or Parents United International, Inc. (a group devoted to helping sexually abused families)
XII. **ABUSE TO THE OLDER ADULT**
A. Description
1. **Abuse** to an older adult involves physical, emotional, or sexual **abuse** and can involve neglect or economic exploitation
2. Individuals at most risk include those who are dependent because of illness, immobility, or altered mental status
3. Factors that contribute to **abuse** and neglect include long-standing family violence, caregiver stress, and the individual's increasing dependence on others
4. Victims may attempt to dismiss injuries as accidental, and abusers may prevent victims from receiving proper medical care to avoid discovery
5. Victims are often isolated socially by their abusers
B. Data collection
1. Physical **abuse**
   a. Sprains, dislocations, or fractures
   b. Abrasions, bruises, or lacerations
   c. Pressure sores
   d. Puncture wounds
   e. Burns
   f. Skin tears
2. Sexual **abuse**
   a. Torn or stained underclothing
   b. Discomfort or bleeding in the genital area
   c. Difficulty in walking or sitting
   d. Unexplained genital infections or disease
3. Emotional **abuse**
   a. Confusion
   b. Fearful and agitated
   c. Changes in appetite and weight
   d. Withdrawn and loss of interest in self and social activities
4. Neglect
   a. Disheveled appearance
   b. Dressed inadequately or inappropriately
   c. Dehydration and malnutrition
   d. Lacking physical needs, such as glasses, hearing aids, and dentures
5. Signs of medication overdose
6. Economic exploitation
   a. Inability to pay bills and fearful when discussing finances

b. Confused, inaccurate, or no knowledge of finances

C. Interventions

1. Assess for and treat physical injuries
2. Report cases of suspected **abuse** to appropriate authorities (follow state and agency guidelines)
3. Separate the older adult from the abusive environment if possible and contact adult protective services for assistance in placement while the **abuse** is investigated
4. Explore alternative living arrangements that are the least restrictive and disruptive to the victim
5. The older adult who has been abused may need assistance for financial or legal matters
6. Provide referrals to emergency community resources
7. When working with caregivers, assess the need for respite care or counseling if needed to deal with caregiver stress

XIII. **RAPE AND SEXUAL ASSAULT**

A. Description

1. Rape is engaging another person in a sexual act and/or sexual intercourse through the use of force and without the consent of the sexual partner
2. The victim is not required by law to report the rape or assault
3. The victim is often blamed by others and often receives no support from significant others
4. Acquaintance rape involves someone known to the victim
5. Statutory rape is the act of sexual intercourse with a person under the age of legal consent, even if the minor consents
6. Marital rape
   a. The belief that marriage bestows rights to sex whenever wanted and without consent of the partner contributes to the occurrence of marital rape
   b. Victims of marital rape describe being forced to perform acts they did not wish to perform and being physically abused during sex

B. Data collection

1. Female client
   a. Obtain the date of the last menstrual period
   b. Determine the form of birth control used and the last act of intercourse before rape
   c. Determine the duration of intercourse, orifices violated, and whether penile penetration occurred
   d. Determine the use of a condom by the perpetrator
2. Shame, embarrassment, and humiliation
3. Anger and revenge
4. Fear of telling others for fear of not being believed

C. It is important to note that males may be sexually abused both as children and as adults and are the usual targeted victim of pedophiles; males may have more difficulty with disclosing their **abuse**

D. Rape trauma syndrome

1. Sleep disturbances and nightmares
2. Loss of appetite
3. Fears, anxiety, phobias, and suspicion
4. Decrease in activities and motivation
5. Disruptions in relationships with partner, family, and friends
6. Self-blame, guilt, and shame
7. Lowered self-esteem and feelings of worthlessness
8. Somatic complaints

E. Interventions

1. Perform data collection in a quiet, private area
2. Stay with the victim
3. Assess the victim's stress level before performing treatments and procedures
4. Victim should not shower, bathe, douche (female), or change clothing until an examination is performed
5. Obtain written consent for the examination, photographs, laboratory tests, release of information, and laboratory samples
6. Assist with the female pelvic examination and obtain specimens to detect semen (the pelvic examination may trigger a flashback of the attack); a shower and fresh clothing should be made available to the client after the examination
7. Preserve any evidence
8. Treat physical injuries and provide client safety
9. Document all events in the care of the victim
10. Reinforce to the victim that surviving the assault is most important; if the victim survived the rape, he or she did exactly what was necessary to stay alive
11. Refer the victim to **crisis** intervention and support groups

PRACTICE QUESTIONS

More questions on the companion CD!

913. A nurse is caring for an older adult client who has recently lost her husband. The client says, "No one cares about me anymore. All the people I loved are dead." Which response by the nurse is therapeutic?
   1. "Right! Why not just 'pack it in'?"
   2. "That seems rather unlikely to me."
   3. "I don't believe that, and neither do you."
   4. "You must be feeling all alone at this point."

914. A nurse is planning care for a client who is being hospitalized because the client has been displaying violent behavior and is at risk for potential

harm to others. The nurse avoids which intervention in the plan of care?
1. Facing the client when providing care
2. Ensuring that a security officer is within the immediate area
3. Keeping the door to the client's room open when with the client
4. Assigning the client to a room at the end of the hall to prevent disturbing the other clients

915. Which behaviors observed by the nurse might lead to the suspicion that a depressed adolescent client could be suicidal?
1. The client gives away a prized CD and a cherished autographed picture of the performer.
2. The client runs out of the therapy group swearing at the group leader and then runs to her room.
3. The client gets angry with her roommate when the roommate borrows her clothes without asking.
4. The client becomes angry while speaking on the telephone and slams the receiver down on the hook.

916. A client is admitted to the psychiatric unit following a serious suicidal attempt by hanging. The nurse's most important aspect of care is to maintain client safety and plans to:
1. Request that a peer remain with the client at all times.
2. Remove the client's clothing and place the client in a hospital gown.
3. Assign a staff member to the client who will remain with the client at all times.
4. Admit the client to a seclusion room where all potentially dangerous articles are removed.

917. The police arrive at the emergency room with a client who has seriously lacerated both wrists. The initial nursing action is to:
1. Administer an antianxiety agent.
2. Examine and treat the wound sites.
3. Secure and record a detailed history.
4. Encourage and assist the client to vent feelings.

918. A nurse is caring for a client with severe depression. Which of the following activities would be appropriate for this client?
1. A puzzle
2. Drawing
3. Checkers
4. Paint by number

919. A client experiencing a severe major depressive episode is unable to address activities of daily living. The appropriate nursing intervention is to:
1. Feed, bathe, and dress the client as needed until the client can perform these activities independently.

2. Offer the client choices and consequences to the failure to comply with the expectation of maintaining activities of daily living.
3. Structure the client's day so that adequate time can be devoted to the client's assuming responsibility for the activities of daily living.
4. Have the client's peers confront the client about how the noncompliance in addressing activities of daily living affects the milieu.

920. An older male client who is a victim of elder abuse and the client's family have been attending weekly counseling sessions. Which statement by the abusive family member would indicate that he or she has learned positive coping skills?
1. "I will be more careful to make sure that my father's needs are met."
2. "Now that my father is moving into my home, I will need to change my ways."
3. "I feel better able to care for my father now that I know where to obtain assistance."
4. "I am so sorry and embarrassed that the abusive event occurred. It won't happen again."

921. A nurse is assisting in planning care for a client being admitted to the nursing unit who has attempted suicide. Which priority nursing intervention will the nurse include in the plan of care?
1. One-to-one suicide precautions
2. Suicide precautions, with 30-minute checks
3. Checking the whereabouts of the client every 15 minutes
4. Asking that the client report suicidal thoughts immediately

922. A nurse is reviewing the health care record of a client admitted to the psychiatric unit. The nurse notes that the admission nurse has documented that the client is experiencing anxiety as a result of a situational crisis. The nurse would determine that this type of crisis could be caused by:
1. Witnessing a murder
2. The death of a loved one
3. A fire that destroyed the client's home
4. A recent rape episode experienced by the client

923. A nurse is gathering data from a client in crisis. When determining the client's perception of the precipitating event that led to the crisis, the most appropriate question to ask is:
1. "With whom do you live?"
2. "Who is available to help you?"
3. "What leads you to seek help now?"
4. "What do you usually do to feel better?"

924. A nurse is assisting in developing a plan of care for the client in a crisis state. When developing the plan, the nurse will consider which of the following?
1. A crisis state indicates that the individual is suffering from a mental illness.

2. A crisis state indicates that the individual is suffering from an emotional illness.

3. Presenting symptoms in a crisis situation are similar for all individuals experiencing a crisis.

4. A client's response to a crisis is individualized, and what constitutes a crisis for one person may not constitute a crisis for another person.

925. A nurse observes that a client with a potential for violence is agitated, pacing up and down in the hallway, and making aggressive and belligerent gestures at other clients. Which statement would be appropriate to make to this client?

1. "You need to stop that behavior now!"
2. "You will need to be placed in seclusion!"
3. "What is causing you to become agitated?"
4. "You will need to be restrained if you do not change your behavior."

926. During a conversation with a depressed client on a psychiatric unit, the client says to the nurse, "My family would be better off without me." The nurse should make which therapeutic response to the client?

1. "Have you talked to your family about this?"
2. "Everyone feels this way when they are depressed."

3. "You will feel better once your medication begins to work."
4. "You sound very upset. Are you thinking of hurting yourself?"

ALTERNATE ITEM FORMAT: MULTIPLE RESPONSE

927. A nurse is preparing to care for a dying client, and several family members are at the client's bedside. Select the therapeutic techniques that the nurse will use when communicating with the family. Select all that apply.

☐ 1. Discourage reminiscing.
☐ 2. Make the decisions for the family.
☐ 3. Encourage expression of feelings, concerns, and fears.
☐ 4. Explain everything that is happening to all family members.
☐ 5. Extend touch and hold the client's or family member's hand if appropriate.
☐ 6. Be honest and truthful and let the client and family know that you will not abandon them.

ANSWERS

913. **4**

Rationale: The client is experiencing loss and is feeling hopeless. The therapeutic response by the nurse is the one that attempts to translate words into feelings. In option 2, the nurse is voicing doubt, which is often used when a client verbalizes delusional ideas. In option 3, the nurse is disagreeing with the client, which implies that the nurse has passed judgment on the client's ideas or opinions. In option 1, the nurse uses sarcasm, which gives advice and is nontherapeutic as a nursing response.

Test-Taking Strategy: Use therapeutic communication techniques. Option 4 is the only option that focuses on the client's feelings. Review therapeutic communication techniques if you had difficulty with this question.

Level of Cognitive Ability: Application
Client Needs: Psychosocial Integrity
Integrated Process: Communication and Documentation
Content Area: Mental Health
References: Fortinash, K., & Holoday-Worret, P. (2008). *Psychiatric mental health nursing* (4th ed., p. 214, 643). St. Louis: Mosby.
Keltner, N., Schwecke, L., & Bostrom, C. (2007). *Psychiatric nursing* (5th ed., pp. 90-92). St. Louis: Mosby.
Morrison-Valfre, M. (2005). *Foundations of mental health care* (3rd ed., pp. 88, 161). St. Louis: Mosby.

914. **4**

Rationale: The client should be placed in a room near the nurses' station and not at the end of a long, relatively unprotected corridor. The nurse should not isolate himself or herself with a potentially violent client. The door to the client's room should be kept open, and the nurse should never turn away

from the client. A security officer or male aide should be within immediate call in case the possibility of violence is suspected.

Test-Taking Strategy: Use the process of elimination and note the strategic word "avoids." This word indicates a negative event query and the need to select the incorrect intervention. Keeping in mind that safety is the subject will direct you to option 4. If you had difficulty with this question, review guidelines for caring for the violent client.

Level of Cognitive Ability: Application
Client Needs: Safe and Effective Care Environment
Integrated Process: Nursing Process/Planning
Content Area: Mental Health
References: Fortinash, K., & Holoday-Worret, P. (2008). *Psychiatric mental health nursing* (4th ed., pp. 278-279). St. Louis: Mosby.
Morrison-Valfre, M. (2005). *Foundations of mental health care* (3rd ed., p. 116). St. Louis: Mosby.

915. **1**

Rationale: A depressed, suicidal client often gives away that which is of value as a way of saying "goodbye" and wanting to be remembered. Options 2, 3, and 4 identify acting-out behaviors.

Test-Taking Strategy: Use the process of elimination. Options 2, 3, and 4 are comparable or alike in that they deal with anger and "acting-out behaviors," which are often typical of some adolescents. Option 1 is different in nature and could indicate that the client may be saying goodbye. Review the clues that indicate suicide if you had difficulty with this question.

Level of Cognitive Ability: Analysis
Client Needs: Psychosocial Integrity

Integrated Process: Nursing Process/Data Collection
Content Area: Mental Health
References: Fortinash, K., & Holoday-Worret, P. (2008). *Psychiatric mental health nursing* (4th ed., p. 469). St. Louis: Mosby.
Stuart, G., & Laraia, M. (2005). *Principles and practice of psychiatric nursing* (8th ed., p. 367). St. Louis: Mosby.

916. **3**
Rationale: Hanging is a serious suicide attempt. The plan of care must reflect action that will promote the client's safety. Constant observation status (one on one) with a staff member who is never less than an arm's length away is the safest intervention.
Test-Taking Strategy: Use the process of elimination. Eliminate option 4 because seclusion should not be the initial intervention. Eliminate option 1 next since the responsibility to safeguard a client is not the peer's responsibility. Eliminate option 2 since removing one's clothing will not maximize all possible safety strategies. Review nursing interventions for the client at risk for suicide if you had difficulty with this question.
Level of Cognitive Ability: Application
Client Needs: Safe and Effective Care Environment
Integrated Process: Nursing Process/Implementation
Content Area: Mental Health
References: Fortinash, K., & Holoday-Worret, P. (2008). *Psychiatric mental health nursing* (4th ed., p. 476). St. Louis: Mosby.
Morrison-Valfre, M. (2005). *Foundations of mental health care* (3rd ed., p. 288). St. Louis: Mosby.

917. **2**
Rationale: The initial nursing action is to examine and treat the self-inflicted injuries. Injuries from lacerated wrists can lead to a life-threatening situation. Other interventions may follow after the client has been treated medically.
Test-Taking Strategy: Use Maslow's Hierarchy of Needs theory to prioritize. Physiological needs come first. Option 2 addresses the physiological need. Review care of the client who has attempted suicide if you had difficulty with this question.
Level of Cognitive Ability: Application
Client Needs: Physiological Integrity
Integrated Process: Nursing Process/Implementation
Content Area: Mental Health
Reference: Varcarolis, E., Carlson, V., & Shoemaker, N. (2006). *Foundations of psychiatric mental health nursing* (5th ed., p. 479). Philadelphia: Saunders.

918. **2**
Rationale: Concentration and memory are poor in a client with severe depression. When a client has a diagnosis of severe depression, the nurse needs to provide activities that require little concentration. Activities that have no right or wrong choices or decisions minimize opportunities for the client to put down himself or herself.
Test-Taking Strategy: Use the process of elimination. Note the that options 1, 3, and 4 are comparable or alike in that they all require concentration. It is important to remember that clients with depression have difficulty concentrating and need activities that require little concentration. Review care of the client with severe depression if you had difficulty with this question.

Level of Cognitive Ability: Application
Client Needs: Psychosocial Integrity
Integrated Process: Nursing Process/Implementation
Content Area: Mental Health
Reference: Fortinash, K., & Holoday-Worret, P. (2008). *Psychiatric mental health nursing* (4th ed., p. 534). St. Louis: Mosby.

919. **1**
Rationale: The client with depression may not have the energy or interest to complete activities of daily living. Often, severely depressed clients are unable to perform even the simplest activities of daily living. The nurse assumes this role and completes these tasks with the client. Options 2 and 3 are incorrect because the client lacks the energy and motivation to perform these tasks independently. Option 4 will increase the client's feelings of poor self-esteem and unworthiness.
Test-Taking Strategy: Use the process of elimination and note the strategic words "severe major depressive episode." Eliminate options 2 and 3 because the client lacks the energy and motivation to do these independently. In addition, option 2 may lead to increased feelings of worthlessness as the client fails to meet expectations. Option 4 will increase the client's feelings of poor self-esteem and unworthiness. Review care of the client with severe depression if you had difficulty with this question.
Level of Cognitive Ability: Application
Client Needs: Physiological Integrity
Integrated Process: Nursing Process/Implementation
Content Area: Mental Health
Reference: Keltner, N., Schwecke, L., & Bostrom, C. (2007). *Psychiatric nursing* (5th ed., pp. 373-374). St. Louis: Mosby.

920. **3**
Rationale: Elder abuse sometimes occurs with family members who are being expected to care for their aging parents. This can cause family members to become overextended, frustrated, or financially depleted. Knowing where in the community to turn for assistance in caring for aging family members can bring much-needed relief. Using these alternatives is a positive alternative coping strategy, which many families use.
Test-Taking Strategy: Use the process of elimination and focus on the subject—a coping strategy. Only option 3 identifies a means of coping with the subjects. The other options are statements of good faith or promises, which may or may not be kept in the future. Option 3 outlines a definitive plan for how to handle the pressure associated with the father's care. Review effective coping strategies if you had difficulty with this question.
Level of Cognitive Ability: Analysis
Client Needs: Psychosocial Integrity
Integrated Process: Nursing Process/Evaluation
Content Area: Mental Health
Reference: Fortinash, K., & Holoday-Worret, P. (2008). *Psychiatric mental health nursing* (4th ed., pp. 503-504). St. Louis: Mosby.

921. **1**
Rationale: One-to-one suicide precautions are required for the client who has attempted suicide. Options 2 and 3 are not appropriate, considering the situation. Option 4 may be an

appropriate nursing intervention, but the priority is stated in option 1. The best option is constant supervision so that the nurse may intervene as needed if the client attempts to cause harm to himself or herself.
Test-Taking Strategy: Use the process of elimination and note the strategic word "priority." Recalling that one-to-one suicide precautions are the priority in caring for a suicidal client will direct you to option 1. Review interventions for the suicidal client if you had difficulty with this question.
Level of Cognitive Ability: Application
Client Needs: Safe and Effective Care Environment
Integrated Process: Nursing Process/Implementation
Content Area: Mental Health
Reference: Varcarolis, E., Carlson, V., & Shoemaker, N. (2006). *Foundations of psychiatric mental health nursing* (5th ed., p. 481). Philadelphia: Saunders.

922. 2
Rationale: A situational crisis is associated with a life event. External situations that could precipitate a situational crisis include loss or change of a job, the death of a loved one, abortion, change in financial status, divorce, and severe illness. Options 1, 3, and 4 identify adventitious crises. An adventitious crisis relates to a crises, disaster, or event that is not a part of everyday life, is unplanned, and is accidental.
Test-Taking Strategy: Use the process of elimination and focus on the strategic words "situational crisis." This will assist in eliminating options 1, 3, and 4 because they are comparable or alike. If you had difficulty with this question, review the types of crisis.
Level of Cognitive Ability: Comprehension
Client Needs: Psychosocial Integrity
Integrated Process: Nursing Process/Data Collection
Content Area: Mental Health
Reference: Fortinash, K., & Holoday-Worret, P. (2008). *Psychiatric mental health nursing* (4th ed., p. 452). St. Louis: Mosby.

923. 3
Rationale: A nurse's initial task when gathering data from a client in crisis is to assess the individual or family and the problem. The more clearly the problem can be defined, the better the chance a solution can be found. Option 3 will assist in determining data related to the precipitating event that led to the crisis. Options 1 and 2 identify situational supports. Option 4 identifies personal coping skills.
Test-Taking Strategy: Use the process of elimination and note the strategic words "precipitating event." Focus on these strategic words when selecting the correct option. Eliminate options 1 and 2, because these data will determine support systems. Eliminate option 4, because this question would be asked when determining coping skills. Review data collection methods for a client in crisis if you had difficulty with this question.
Level of Cognitive Ability: Application
Client Needs: Psychosocial Integrity
Integrated Process: Nursing Process/Data Collection
Content Area: Mental Health
Reference: Keltner, N., Schwecke, L., & Bostrom, C. (2007). *Psychiatric nursing* (5th ed., pp. 125-126). St. Louis: Mosby.

924. 4
Rationale: Although each crisis response can be described in similar terms as far as presenting symptoms are concerned, what constitutes a crisis for one person may not constitute a crisis for another person, because each is a unique individual. Being in a crisis state does not mean that the client is suffering from an emotional or mental illness.
Test-Taking Strategy: Use the process of elimination. Eliminate option 3 because of the close-ended word "all." Next, eliminate options 1 and 2 because a crisis does not indicate "illness." Review the characteristics of a crisis state if you had difficulty with this question.
Level of Cognitive Ability: Comprehension
Client Needs: Psychosocial Integrity
Integrated Process: Nursing Process/Data Collection
Content Area: Mental Health
References: Fortinash, K., & Holoday-Worret, P. (2008). *Psychiatric mental health nursing* (4th ed., p. 457). St. Louis: Mosby.
Morrison-Valfre, M. (2005). *Foundations of mental health care* (3rd ed., pp. 69-71). St. Louis: Mosby.

925. 3
Rationale: The best statement is to ask the client what is causing the agitation. This will assist the client to become aware of the behavior and will assist the nurse in planning appropriate interventions for the client. Option 1 is demanding behavior, which could cause increased agitation in the client. Options 2 and 4 are threats to the client and are inappropriate.
Test-Taking Strategy: Use the process of elimination. Eliminate option 1 because of the demand that it places on the client. Eliminate options 2 and 4 because they indicate threats to the client. Review appropriate nursing interventions for the agitated client if you had difficulty with this question.
Level of Cognitive Ability: Application
Client Needs: Psychosocial Integrity
Integrated Process: Communication and Documentation
Content Area: Mental Health
References: Fortinash, K., & Holoday-Worret, P. (2008). *Psychiatric mental health nursing* (4th ed., p. 279). St. Louis: Mosby.
Keltner, N., Schwecke, L., & Bostrom, C. (2007). *Psychiatric nursing* (5th ed., pp. 90-92). St. Louis: Mosby.
Morrison-Valfre, M. (2005). *Foundations of mental health care* (3rd ed., pp. 88, 226). St. Louis: Mosby.

926. 4
Rationale: Clients who are depressed may be at risk for suicide. It is critical for the nurse to assess suicidal ideation and plan. The client should be directly asked if a plan for self-harm exists. Options 1, 2, and 3 are not therapeutic responses.
Test-Taking Strategy: Use therapeutic communication techniques. Option 4 is the only option that deals directly with the client's feelings. Additionally, clients at risk for suicide need to be directly assessed regarding the potential for self-harm. Review data collection techniques for the depressed client if you had difficulty with this question.
Level of Cognitive Ability: Application
Client Needs: Psychosocial Integrity
Integrated Process: Nursing Process/Data Collection
Content Area: Mental Health

Reference: Keltner, N., Schwecke, L., & Bostrom, C. (2007). *Psychiatric nursing* (5th ed., pp. 90-92, 385). St. Louis: Mosby.

ALTERNATE ITEM FORMAT: MULTIPLE RESPONSE

927. **3, 5, 6**

Rationale: The nurse must determine whether there is a spokesperson for the family and how much the client and family want to know. The nurse needs to allow the family and client the opportunity for informed choices and assist with the decision-making process if asked. The nurse should encourage expression of feelings, concerns, and fears, as well as reminiscing. The nurse needs to be honest and truthful and let the client and family know that they will not be abandoned. It is important to extend touch and hold the client's or family member's hand if appropriate.

Test-Taking Strategy: Recalling therapeutic communication techniques and client and family rights will assist you in answering this question. Review these techniques and care to the dying client if you had difficulty with this question.

Level of Cognitive Ability: Application
Client Needs: Psychosocial Integrity
Integrated Process: Caring
Content Area: Mental Health
References: Keltner, N., Schwecke, L., & Bostrom, C. (2007). *Psychiatric nursing* (5th ed., pp. 90-92, 183). St. Louis: Mosby.
Potter, P., & Perry, A. (2005) *Fundamentals of nursing* (6th ed., pp. 586-587). St. Louis: Mosby.
Varcarolis, E., Carlson, V., & Shoemaker, N. (2006) *Foundations of psychiatric mental health nursing* (5th ed., p. 606). Philadelphia: Saunders.

REFERENCES

Fortinash, K., & Holoday-Worret, P. (2008). *Psychiatric mental health nursing* (4th ed.). St. Louis: Mosby.

Keltner, N., Schwecke, L., & Bostrom, C. (2007). *Psychiatric nursing* (5th ed.). St. Louis: Mosby.

Morrison-Valfre, M. (2005). *Foundations of mental health care* (3rd ed.). St. Louis: Mosby.

Potter, P., & Perry, A. (2005). *Fundamentals of nursing* (6th ed.). St. Louis: Mosby.

Varcarolis, E., Carlson, V., & Shoemaker, N. (2006). *Foundations of psychiatric mental health nursing* (5th ed.). Philadelphia: Saunders.

CHAPTER 66

Psychiatric Medications

I. SELECTIVE SEROTONIN REUPTAKE INHIBITORS (SSRIs) (Box 66-1)

A. Description
   1. Inhibit serotonin uptake and elicit an antidepressant response
   2. The potential for medication interactions is high, and complete medication assessments must be obtained and evaluated; inquire about the use of herbal therapies, especially St. John's wort

B. Side effects
   1. Nausea, vomiting, cramping, and diarrhea
   2. Dry mouth
   3. Central nervous system (CNS) stimulation, including akathisia (restlessness, agitation)
   4. Photosensitivity
   5. Insomnia/somnolence (sleepy, drowsy)
   6. Nervousness
   7. Headache, dizziness
   8. Seizure activity
   9. Weight loss or gain
   10. Decreased libido
   11. Apathy
   12. Tremors
   13. Increased sweating

C. Interventions
   1. SSRIs interact with a number of medications
   2. Monitor vital signs since SSRIs can potentially lower or elevate blood pressure
   3. Monitor weight
   4. Initiate safety precautions, particularly if dizziness occurs
   5. Instruct the client to avoid alcohol
   6. Administer with a snack or meal to reduce the risk of dizziness and lightheadedness
   7. Monitor the suicidal client, especially during improved mood and increased energy levels
   8. Instruct the client taking fluoxetine (Prozac) and bupropion (Wellbutrin) to take the medication early in the day to prevent interference with sleep
   9. For the client on long-term therapy, monitor liver and renal function tests; altered values may occur, requiring dosage adjustments
   10. Monitor white blood cell and neutrophil counts; the medication may be discontinued if levels fall below normal
   11. If priapism (painful, prolonged penile erection) occurs, the medication is withheld and the physician is notified
   12. Inform the client about the possibility of decreased libido
   13. Instruct the client to change positions slowly to avoid a hypotensive effect
   14. Instruct the client to report any visual changes to the physician
   15. Educate the client about the potential for a discontinuation syndrome if medication is stopped abruptly rather than tapered; the syndrome is characterized by gastrointestinal (GI) distress, behavioral or perceptual oddities, movement problems, and sleep disturbances
   16. Be aware of the potential for serotonin syndrome characterized by elevated temperature, muscle rigidity, and elevated CPK levels; this risk is greatly increased when SSRIs are given with monoamine oxidase inhibitors (MAOIs), and thus this medication combination needs to be avoided
   17. Instruct the client that over-the-counter (OTC) cold medicines can increase the likelihood of serotonin syndrome
   18. In pregnancy, consultation with an obstetrician regarding taking these medications is recommended
   19. Monitor the medication response in children, adolescents, and older clients since the response may be different than in an adult client
   20. Encourage psychotherapy

II. TRICYCLIC ANTIDEPRESSANTS (TCAs) (Box 66-2)

A. Description
   1. Block the reuptake of norepinephrine (and serotonin) at the presynaptic neuron and are used to treat depression
   2. May reduce seizure threshold

BOX 66-1 **Reuptake Inhibitors**

Selective Serotonin Reuptake Inhibitors
Citalopram (Celexa)
Escitalopram (Lexapro)
Fluoxetine (Prozac)
Fluvoxamine
Paroxetine hydrochloride (Paxil, Pexeva)
Sertraline hydrochloride (Zoloft)
Serotonin/Norepinephrine Reuptake Inhibitors
Venlafaxine (Effexor)
Duloxetine
Atypical Antidepressants
Amoxapine
Bupropion hydrochloride (Wellbutrin)
Mirtazapine (Remeron)
Nefazodone
Reboxetine (Vestra)
Trazodone (Desyrel)

BOX 66-2 **Tricyclic Antidepressants**

Amitriptyline hydrochloride
Clomipramine (Anafranil)
Desipramine hydrochloride (Norpramin)
Doxepin hydrochloride (Sinequan)
Imipramine hydrochloride (Tofranil)
Maprotiline
Nortriptyline hydrochloride (Aventyl, Pamelor)
Protriptyline hydrochloride (Vivactil)
Trimipramine maleate (Surmontil)

3. May reduce effectiveness of antihypertensive agents
4. Concurrent use with alcohol or antihistamines can cause CNS depression
5. Concurrent use with MAOIs can cause hypertensive crisis
6. Cardiac toxicity can occur and all clients should undergo electrocardiographic (ECG) evaluation prior to treatment and periodically thereafter
7. Overdose is life-threatening, necessitating immediate treatment (Box 66-3)
8. The tricyclic antidepressant clomipramine (Anafranil) may be used to treat obsessive-compulsive disorder

B. Side effects
1. Anticholinergic effects: dry mouth, difficulty voiding, dilated pupils and blurred vision, decreased GI motility, and constipation
2. Photosensitivity
3. Cardiovascular disturbances such as tachycardia and dysrhythmias
4. Orthostatic hypotension
5. Sedation
6. Weight gain
7. Anxiety, restlessness, and irritability
8. Decreased or increased libido with ejaculatory and erection disturbances

BOX 66-3 **Symptoms and Interventions for Tricyclic Antidepressant Overdose**

Symptoms
Dysrhythmias, including tachycardia, intraventricular blocks, complete atrioventricular block, and ventricular fibrillation
Hypothermia
Flushing
Dry mouth
Dilation of the pupils
Confusion, agitation, and hallucinations
Seizures followed by coma
Interventions
Maintain a patent airway
Monitor vital signs
Obtain an ECG
Gastric lavage with activated charcoal to prevent further medication absorption
Physostigmine (a cholinesterase inhibitor) to counteract anticholinergic actions
Antidysrhythmic medications

C. Interventions
1. Instruct the client that the medication may take several weeks to produce the desired effect (client response may not occur until 2-4 weeks after the first dose)
2. Monitor the suicidal client, especially during improved mood and increased energy levels
3. Instruct the client to change positions slowly to avoid a hypotensive effect
4. Monitor pattern of daily bowel activity
5. Assess for urinary retention
6. For the client on long-term therapy, monitor liver and renal function tests
7. Administer with food or milk if GI distress occurs
8. Administer the entire daily oral dose at one time, preferably at bedtime
9. Instruct the client to avoid alcohol and nonprescription medications to prevent adverse medication interactions
10. Instruct the client to avoid driving and other activities requiring alertness until the response is known; sedation is expected in early therapy and may subside with time
11. When the medication is discontinued by the physician, it should be tapered gradually
12. The potential for medication interactions with OTC cold medication exists
13. Caution the client about photosensitivity and to take measures to prevent exposure to sunlight
14. Encourage oral hygiene and the use of hard candies and mouth rinses to relieve dry mouth
15. Encourage psychotherapy

BOX 66-4 **Monoamine Oxidase Inhibitors**

Isocarboxazid (Marplan)
Phenelzine sulfate (Nardil)
Tranylcypromine sulfate (Parnate)
Moclobemide

BOX 66-5 **Foods to Avoid That Contain Tyramine**

Avocados
Bananas
Beef or chicken liver
Brewer's yeast
Broad beans
Caffeine such as coffee, tea, or chocolate
Cheese, especially aged, except cottage cheese
Figs
Meat extracts and tenderizers
Overripe fruit
Papaya
Pickled herring
Raisins
Red wine, beer, and sherry
Sausage, bologna, pepperoni, and salami
Sour cream
Soy sauce
Yogurt

III. MONOAMINE OXIDASE INHIBITORS (MOAIS) (Box 66-4)

A. Description
1. Inhibit the enzyme monoamine oxidase, which is present in the brain, blood platelets, liver, spleen, and kidneys
2. Monoamine oxidase metabolizes amines, norepinephrine, and serotonin; the concentration of these amines increases with MAOIs
3. Used for depression in the client who has not responded to other antidepressant therapies, including electroconvulsive therapy
4. Concurrent use with amphetamines, other antidepressants, dopamine, epinephrine, guanethidine, levodopa, methyldopa, nasal decongestants, norepinephrine, reserpine, tyramine-containing foods, and vasoconstrictors may cause hypertensive crisis
5. Concurrent use with opioid analgesics may cause hypertension, hypotension, coma, or seizures

B. Side effects
1. Orthostatic hypotension
2. Restlessness
3. Insomnia
4. Dizziness
5. Weakness and lethargy
6. GI upset
7. Dry mouth
8. Weight gain
9. Peripheral edema
10. Anticholinergic effects
11. CNS stimulation, including anxiety, agitation, and mania
12. Delay in ejaculation

C. Hypertensive crisis
1. Hypertension
2. Occipital headache radiating frontally
3. Neck stiffness and soreness
4. Nausea and vomiting
5. Sweating
6. Fever and chills
7. Clammy skin
8. Dilated pupils
9. Palpitations, tachycardia, or bradycardia
10. Constricting chest pain
11. Antidote for hypertensive crisis: 5 to 10 mg phentolamine IV injection

D. Interventions
1. Monitor blood pressure frequently for hypertension
2. Monitor for signs of hypertensive crisis
3. If palpitations or frequent headaches occur, withhold the medication and notify the physician
4. Administer with food if GI distress occurs
5. Instruct the client that the medication effect may be noted during the first week of therapy, but maximum benefit may take up to 3 weeks
6. Instruct the client to report headache, neck stiffness, or neck soreness immediately
7. Instruct the client to change positions slowly to prevent orthostatic hypotension
8. Instruct the client to avoid caffeine or OTC preparations such as weight-reducing pills or medications for hay fever and colds
9. Monitor for client compliance with medication administration
10. Instruct the client to carry a Medic-Alert card indicating that an MAOI medication is taken
11. Avoid administering the medication in the evening because insomnia may result
12. When the medication is discontinued by the physician, it should be discontinued gradually
13. Instruct the client to avoid foods that require bacteria/molds for their preparation/preservation or those that contain tyramine (Box 66-5 and Figure 66-1)

IV. MOOD STABILIZERS (Box 66-6)

A. Description: affect cellular transport mechanism and enhance serotonin and/or gamma-aminobutyric acid (GABA) functioning, which are associated with mood

Influence of Dietary Tyramine in the Absence of MAO Inhibitors

Influence of Dietary Tyramine in the Presence of MAO Inhitbitors

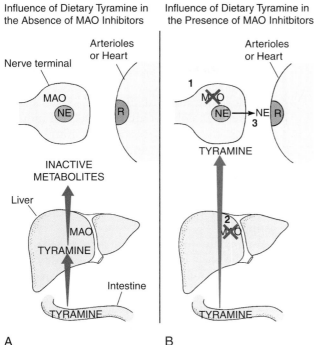

A   B

FIG. 66-1 A, Interaction between dietary tyramine and monoamine oxidase inhibitors (MAOIs). In the absence of MAOIs, dietary tyramine is absorbed from the intestine, transported to the liver, and then immediately inactivated by hepatic MAO. No tyramine reaches the general circulation. **B,** Three events occur in the presence of MAOIs: (1) Inhibition of neuronal MAO raises the levels of norepinephrine (NE) in sympathetic nerve terminals. (2) Inhibition of hepatic MAO allows dietary tyramine to pass through the liver and enter the systemic circulation intact. (3) Upon reaching peripheral sympathetic nerve terminals, tyramine promotes the release of accumulated NE stores, thereby causing massive vasoconstriction and excessive stimulation of the heart. *MAO,* Monoamine oxidase; *NE,* norepinephrine; *R,* receptor for norepinephrine. (From Lehne, R. [2007]. Pharmacology for nursing care [6th ed.]. Philadelphia: Saunders.)

B. Lithium
  1. Concurrent use with diuretics, fluoxetine (Prozac), methyldopa, or nonsteroidal antiinflammatory medications increases lithium reabsorption by the kidney or inhibits lithium excretion, either of which increases the risk of lithium toxicity
  2. Acetazolamide (Diamox), aminophylline, phenothiazines, or sodium bicarbonate may increase renal excretion of lithium, reducing its effectiveness
  3. The therapeutic dose is only slightly less than the amount producing toxicity
  4. The therapeutic drug serum level of lithium is 0.6 to 1.2 mEq/L; the actual dose at which the therapeutic effect is achieved and the levels at which toxicity appears are highly variable among individuals

BOX 66-6 Mood Stabilizers

Lithium Preparations
Lithium carbonate (Eskalith, Lithobid)
Lithium citrate
Other Mood Stabilizers
Aripiprazole (Abilify)
Carbamazepine (Tegretol)
Gabapentin (Neurontin)
Lamotrigine (Lamictal)
Olanzapine (Zyprexa)
Olanzapine/fluoxetine (Symbyax)
Oxcarbazepine (Trileptal)
Quetiapine (Seroquel)
Risperidone (Risperdal)
Valproic acid (Depakene, Depakote, Depacon)
Ziprasidone (Geodon)

  5. The causes of an increase in the lithium level include decreased sodium intake; fluid and electrolyte loss associated with severe sweating, dehydration, diarrhea, or diuretic therapy; and illness or overdose
  6. Serum lithium levels should be checked every 1 to 2 months or whenever any behavioral change suggests an altered serum level
  7. Blood samples to check serum lithium levels should be drawn in the morning, 12 hours after the last dose was taken
C. Side effects
  1. Polyuria
  2. Polydipsia
  3. Anorexia, nausea
  4. Dry mouth
  5. Mild thirst
  6. Weight gain
  7. Abdominal bloating
  8. Soft stools or diarrhea
  9. Fine hand tremors
  10. Inability to concentrate
  11. Muscle weakness
  12. Lethargy
  13. Fatigue
  14. Headache
  15. Hair loss
  16. Hypothyroidism
D. Interventions
  1. Monitor the suicidal client, especially during improved mood and increased energy levels
  2. Administer the medication with food to minimize GI irritation
  3. Instruct the client to maintain a fluid intake of six to eight glasses of water a day
  4. Instruct the client to avoid excessive amounts of coffee, tea, or cola, which have a diuretic effect
  5. Instruct the client to maintain an adequate salt intake

6. Do not administer diuretics while the client is taking lithium
7. Instruct the client to avoid alcohol
8. Instruct the client to avoid OTC medications
9. Instruct the client that he or she may take a missed dose within 2 hours of the scheduled time; otherwise, the client should skip the missed dose and take the next dose at the scheduled time
10. Instruct the client not to adjust the dosage without consulting the physician since lithium should be tapered and not discontinued abruptly
11. Instruct the client about the signs and symptoms of lithium toxicity
12. Instruct the client to notify the physician if polyuria, prolonged vomiting, diarrhea, or fever occur
13. Instruct the client that the therapeutic response to the medication will be noted in 1 to 3 weeks
14. Monitor ECG, renal function tests, and thyroid tests (ensure that these tests are obtained before the start of therapy)
15. Monitor weight

E. Lithium toxicity
   1. Description
      a. Occurs when ingested lithium cannot be detoxified and excreted by the kidneys
      b. Symptoms of toxicity begin to appear when the serum lithium level is at 1.5 to 2 mEq/L
   2. Mild toxicity
      a. Serum lithium level at 1.5 mEq/L
      b. Apathy
      c. Lethargy
      d. Diminished concentration
      e. Mild ataxia
      f. Coarse hand tremors
      g. Slight muscle weakness
   3. Moderate toxicity
      a. Serum lithium level between 1.5 and 2.5 mEq/L
      b. Nausea, vomiting
      c. Severe diarrhea
      d. Mild to moderate ataxia and incoordination
      e. Slurred speech
      f. Tinnitus
      g. Blurred vision
      h. Muscle twitching
      i. Irregular tremor
   4. Severe toxicity
      a. Serum lithium level above 2.5 mEq/L
      b. Nystagmus
      c. Muscle fasciculations
      d. Deep tendon hyperreflexia
      e. Visual or tactile hallucinations
      f. Oliguria or anuria
      g. Impaired level of consciousness

      h. Tonic-clonic seizures or coma leading to death
   5. Interventions for lithium toxicity
      a. Withhold lithium and notify the physician
      b. Monitor vital signs and level of consciousness
      c. Monitor cardiac status
      d. Prepare to obtain lithium levels for monitoring; electrolytes, blood urea nitrogen, and creatinine level; and complete blood cell count
      e. Monitor for suicidal tendencies and institute **suicide** precautions

V. ANTIANXIETY OR ANXIOLYTIC MEDICATIONS
A. Description
   1. Antianxiety medications depress the CNS, thereby increasing the effects of GABA, which produces relaxation and may depress the limbic system
   2. Benzodiazepines have anxiety-reducing (anxiolytic), sedative-hypnotic, muscle-relaxing, and anticonvulsant actions (Box 66-7)
   3. Benzodiazepines are contraindicated in clients with acute narrow-angle glaucoma and should be used cautiously in children and the older client
   4. Benzodiazepines interact with other CNS medications, producing an additive effect
   5. Abrupt withdrawal of benzodiazepines can be potentially life threatening and withdrawal should be done only under medical supervision
B. Side effects
   1. Daytime sedation
   2. Ataxia
   3. Dizziness
   4. Headaches
   5. Blurred or double vision
   6. Hypotension
   7. Tremor
   8. Amnesia
   9. Slurred speech
   10. Urinary incontinence
   11. Constipation
   12. Paradoxical CNS excitement
   13. Lethargy
   14. Behavioral change
C. Acute toxicity
   1. Somnolence
   2. Confusion
   3. Diminished reflexes and coma
   4. Flumazenil (Romazicon), a benzodiazepine antagonist administered intravenously, will reverse benzodiazepine intoxication in 5 minutes
   5. The client being treated for an overdose of a benzodiazepine may experience agitation, restlessness, discomfort, and anxiety

---

BOX 66-7 Benzodiazepines

Alprazolam (Xanax, Niravam)
Chlordiazepoxide (Librium)
Clonazepam (Klonopin)
Clorazepate (Tranxene)
Diazepam (Valium)
Estazolam (ProSom)
Flurazepam (Dalmane)
Lorazepam (Ativan)
Midazolam (Versed)
Oxazepam (Serax)
Quazepam (Doral)
Temazepam (Restoril)
Triazolam (Halcion)
Nonbenzodiazepine Anxiolytics
Buspirone (BuSpar)

BOX 66-8 Barbiturates and Sedative Hypnotics

Barbiturates
Amobarbital (Amytal)
Butabarbital (Butisol)
Pentobarbital (Nembutal)
Phenobarbital (Luminal)
Secobarbital (Seconal)
Sedative Hypnotics
Chloral hydrate (Aquachloral Supprettes, Somnote)
Eszopiclone (Lunesta)
Meprobamate (Miltown)
Paraldehyde (Paral)
Ramelteon (Rozerem)
Zaleplon (Sonata)
Zolpidem (Ambien)

D. Interventions
1. Monitor for motor responses such as agitation, trembling, and tension
2. Monitor for autonomic responses such as cold clammy hands and sweating
3. Monitor for paradoxical CNS excitement during early therapy, particularly in older and debilitated individuals
4. Monitor for visual disturbances since the medications can worsen glaucoma
5. Monitor liver and renal function tests and complete blood cell counts
6. Reduce the medication dose as prescribed for the older adult client and for the client with impaired liver function
7. Initiate safety precautions because the older adult client is at risk for falling when taking the medication for sleep or anxiety
8. Assist with ambulation if drowsiness or light-headedness occurs
9. Instruct the client that drowsiness usually disappears during continued therapy
10. Instruct the client to avoid tasks that require alertness until the response to the medication is established
11. Instruct the client to avoid alcohol
12. Instruct the client not to take other medications without consulting the physician
13. Instruct the client not to stop the medication abruptly (can result in seizure activity)

E. Withdrawal
1. To lessen withdrawal symptoms, the dosage of a benzodiazepine should be tapered gradually over 2 to 6 weeks
2. Abrupt or too rapid withdrawal results in the following symptoms
   a. Restlessness
   b. Irritability
   c. Insomnia
   d. Hand tremors

   e. Abdominal or muscle cramps
   f. Sweating
   g. Vomiting
   h. Seizures

VI. BARBITURATES AND SEDATIVE HYPNOTICS (Box 66-8)
A. Description
1. These medications depress the reticular activating system by promoting the inhibitory synaptic action of the neurotransmitter GABA
2. These medications are used for short-term treatment of insomnia or for sedation to relieve anxiety, tension, and apprehension

B. Side effects
1. Dizziness and drowsiness
2. Confusion
3. Irritability
4. Allergic reactions
5. Agranulocytosis
6. Thrombocytopenia purpura
7. Megaloblastic anemia

C. Overdose
1. Tachycardia
2. Hypotension
3. Cold and clammy skin
4. Dilated pupils
5. Weak and rapid pulse
6. Signs of shock
7. Depressed respirations
8. Absent reflexes
9. Coma and death may result from respiratory and cardiovascular collapse

D. Withdrawal
1. Severe withdrawal symptoms begin within 24 hours after the medication is discontinued in an individual with severe medication dependence
2. Gradual withdrawal is used to detoxify a dependent person
3. Anxiety

4. Insomnia
5. Nightmares
6. Daytime agitation
7. Tremors
8. Delirium
9. Seizures
10. Behavioral changes

E. Interventions
   1. Administer lower doses as prescribed for the older client
   2. Medications should be used with caution in the client who has suicidal tendencies or has a history of drug addiction
   3. Maintain safety by supervising ambulation and using side rails at night
   4. Instruct the client to take the medication as directed
   5. Instruct the client to avoid driving or operating hazardous equipment if drowsiness, dizziness, or unsteadiness occurs
   6. Instruct the client to avoid alcohol
   7. For insomnia, instruct the client to take the medication 30 minutes before bedtime; avoid taking with a heavy meal to help absorption
   8. Instruct the client that a hangover effect may occur in the morning
   9. Instruct the client not to discontinue the medication abruptly
   10. Instruct the client taking chloral hydrate to take the medication with food and a full glass of water, fruit juice, or ginger ale to prevent gastric irritation

VII. ANTIPSYCHOTIC MEDICATIONS (Box 66-9)
A. Description
   1. Improve the thought processes and the behavior of the client with psychotic symptoms, especially the client with schizophrenia
   2. Affect dopamine receptors in the brain, thereby reducing the psychotic symptoms

---

BOX 66-9   **Antipsychotic Medications**

Typical Antipsychotics
Chlorpromazine hydrochloride (Thorazine)
Fluphenazine decanoate (Prolixin decanoate)
Haloperidol decanoate (Haldol)
Loxapine (Loxitane)
Molindone hydrochloride (Moban)
Pimozide (Orap)
Thiothixene hydrochloride (Navane)
Trifluoperazine
Atypical Antipsychotics
Aripiprazole (Abilify)
Clozapine (Clozaril)
Olanzapine (Zyprexa)
Quetiapine (Seroquel)
Risperidone (Risperdal)
Ziprasidone (Geodon)

---

3. Typical antipsychotics are more effective for positive symptoms of schizophrenia such as hallucinations, aggression, and delusions; typical antipsychotic medications also block the chemoreceptor trigger zone and vomiting center in the brain, producing an antiemetic effect
4. Atypical antipsychotics are more effective for the negative symptoms of schizophrenia, such as avolition, apathy, and alogia
5. The effects of antipsychotic medications will be potentiated when given with other CNS-acting medications

B. Side effects (Box 66-10)
C. Interventions
   1. Monitor vital signs
   2. Monitor for extrapyramidal side effects
   3. Monitor for symptoms of neuroleptic malignant syndrome
   4. Monitor urine output

BOX 66-10   **Side Effects of Antipsychotic Medications**

Anticholinergic Effects
Dry mouth
Increased heart rate
Urinary retention
Constipation
Hypotension
Extrapyramidal Side Effects
Parkinsonism
Tremors
Mask-like facies
Rigidity
Shuffling gait
Dysphagia
Drooling
Dystonias
Abnormal or involuntary eye movements, including oculogyric crisis
Facial grimacing
Twisting of the torso or other muscle groups
Akathisia
Restlessness
Agitation
Tardive dyskinesia
Protrusion of the tongue
Chewing motion
Involuntary movement of the body and extremities
Other Side Effects
Drowsiness
Blood dyscrasias
Pruritus
Photosensitivity
Elevated blood glucose
Increased weight
Impaired body temperature regulation
Gynecomastia
Lactation

5. Monitor serum glucose
6. Note that the client taking an antipsychotic medication may require long-term medication for parkinsonian symptoms
7. Administer the medication with food or milk to decrease gastric irritation
8. For oral use, the liquid form might be preferred because some clients hide tablets to avoid taking them
9. Note that the absorption rate is faster with the liquid form of oral medication
10. Avoid skin contact with the liquid concentrate to prevent contact dermatitis
11. Protect the liquid concentrate from light
12. Dilute the liquid concentrate with fruit juice
13. Inform the client that a full therapeutic effect of the medication may not be evident for 3 to 6 weeks following initiation of therapy; however, an observable therapeutic response may be apparent after 7 to 10 days
14. Inform the client that some medications may cause a harmless change in urine color to pinkish to red-brown
15. Instruct the client to use sunscreen, hats, and protective clothing when outdoors
16. Instruct the client to avoid alcohol or other CNS depressants
17. Instruct the client to change positions slowly to avoid orthostatic hypotension
18. Instruct the client to report signs of agranulocytosis, including sore throat, fever, and malaise
19. Instruct the client to report signs of liver dysfunction, including jaundice, malaise, fever, and right upper abdominal pain
20. When discontinuing antipsychotics, the medication dosage should be reduced gradually to avoid sudden reoccurrence of psychotic symptoms

▲ VIII. NEUROLEPTIC MALIGNANT SYNDROME
A. Description
1. A potentially fatal syndrome that may occur at any time during therapy with neuroleptic medications (antipsychotic medications)
2. Although rare, neuroleptic malignant syndrome more commonly occurs at the initiation of therapy, after the client is changed from one medication to another, after a dosage increase, or when a combination of medications is used
B. Data collection
1. Dyspnea or tachypnea
2. Tachycardia or irregular pulse rate
3. Fever
4. High or low blood pressure
5. Increased sweating
6. Loss of bladder control
7. Skeletal muscle rigidity
8. Pale skin

9. Excessive weakness or fatigue
10. Altered level of consciousness
11. Seizures
12. Severe extrapyramidal side effects
13. Difficulty swallowing
14. Excessive salivation
15. Oculogyric crisis
16. Dyskinesia
17. Elevated white blood cell count, liver function results, and creatinine phosphokinase level
C. Interventions
1. Notify the physician
2. Monitor vital signs
3. Initiate safety and seizure precautions
4. Prepare to discontinue the medication
5. Monitor level of consciousness
6. Administer antipyretics as prescribed
7. Use a cooling blanket to lower the body temperature
8. Monitor electrolytes and administer fluids intravenously as prescribed

IX. MEDICATIONS TO TREAT ATTENTION DEFICIT HYPERACTIVITY DISORDER (ADHD) (Box 66-11)
A. Children with attention deficit hyperactivity disorder may require medication to reduce hyperactive behavior and lengthen attention span
B. Medications that are most effective in controlling this disorder are CNS stimulants
C. CNS stimulants, which increase agitation and activity in adults, have a calming effect on children with ADHD and increase alertness and sensitivity to stimuli
D. Side effects
1. Tachycardia
2. Anorexia and weight loss
3. Elevated blood pressure
4. Dizziness
5. Agitation
E. Interventions
1. Monitor for CNS side effects
2. Obtain a baseline ECG
3. Monitor the blood pressure
4. Instruct the child/parents that OTC medications need to be avoided

BOX 66-11	**Medications to Treat Attention Deficit Hyperactivity Disorder**

Amphetamine
Atomoxetine (Strattera)
Dexmethylphenidate (Focalin)
Dextroamphetamine (Dexedrine)
Dextroamphetamine and amphetamine (Adderall XR)
Methamphetamine (Desoxyn)
Methylphenidate (Ritalin, Concerta, Metadate, Methylin)
Pemoline (Cylert)

5. Instruct the child/parents that the last dose of the day should be taken at least 6 hours before bedtime (14 hours for extended-released forms) to prevent insomnia
6. Monitor height and weight (particularly in children)
7. Reinforce that several weeks of therapy may be necessary before the therapeutic effect is noted
8. Instruct the client/parents that a drug-free period may be prescribed to allow growth of the child if the medication has caused growth retardation

X. **MEDICATIONS TO TREAT ALZHEIMER'S DISEASE** (Box 66-12)
A. Acetylcholinesterase inhibitors may be used to treat Alzheimer's disease to improve cognitive functions in the early stages
B. Donepezil (Aricept)
   1. An inhibitor of acetylcholinesterase used to treat mild to moderate dementia of Alzheimer's disease
   2. Common side effects include nausea and diarrhea
   3. Donepezil can slow the heart rate through its vagotonic effect
C. Galantamine (Razadyne)
   1. An inhibitor of cholinesterase used to treat mild to moderate dementia of Alzheimer's disease
   2. Side effects include nausea, vomiting, diarrhea, anorexia, and weight loss
   3. Can cause bronchoconstriction and is used with caution in clients with asthma and chronic obstructive pulmonary disease
D. Memantine (Namenda)
   1. An NMDA (*N*-methyl-D-aspartate receptor antagonist) indicated for moderate to severe Alzheimer's disease
   2. Side effects include dizziness, headache, confusion, and constipation
   3. Should not be used in combination with other NMDA antagonists such as amantadine (Symmetrel) or ketamine (Ketalar); such combinations produce undesirable additive effects
   4. Sodium bicarbonate and other medications that alkalinize the urine can decrease renal excretion of memantine; accumulation to toxic levels can result
E. Rivastigmine (Exelon)
   1. An inhibitor of cholinesterase used to treat mild to moderate dementia of Alzheimer's disease
   2. Side effects include nausea, vomiting, diarrhea, abdominal pain, and anorexia
   3. Used with caution in clients with peptic ulcer disease, bradycardia, sick sinus syndrome, urinary obstruction, and lung disease because it enhances cholinergic transmission, thus intensifying symptoms of the diseases

BOX 66-12	Medications to Treat Alzheimer's Disease

Donepezil (Aricept)
Galantamine (Razadyne)
Memantine (Namenda)
Rivastigimine (Exelon)
Tacrine (Cognex)

F. Tacrine (Cognex)
   1. A centrally acting cholinesterase inhibitor used to treat mild to moderate dementia of Alzheimer's disease
   2. Side effects include ataxia, loss of appetite, nausea, vomiting, and diarrhea
   3. An adverse effect is hepatotoxicity; liver function studies need to be monitored

PRACTICE QUESTIONS

More questions on the companion CD!

928. A nurse is caring for a hospitalized client who has been taking clozapine (Clozaril) for the treatment of a schizophrenic disorder. Which laboratory study prescribed for the client will the nurse specifically review to monitor for an adverse effect associated with the use of this medication?
1. Platelet count
2. Cholesterol level
3. White blood cell count
4. Blood urea nitrogen level

929. Disulfiram (Antabuse) is prescribed for a client who is seen in the psychiatric health care clinic. The nurse is collecting data on the client and is providing instructions regarding the use of this medication. Which is most important for the nurse to determine before administration of this medication?
1. A history of hyperthyroidism
2. A history of diabetes insipidus
3. When the last full meal was consumed
4. When the last alcoholic drink was consumed

930. A nurse is collecting data from a client and the client's spouse reports that the client is taking donepezil hydrochloride (Aricept). Which disorder would the nurse suspect that this client may have based on the use of this medication?
1. Dementia
2. Schizophrenia
3. Seizure disorder
4. Obsessive-compulsive disorder

931. Fluoxetine (Prozac) is prescribed for the client. The nurse provides instructions to the client

regarding the administration of the medication. Which statement by the client indicates an understanding about administration of the medication?
1. "I should take the medication with my evening meal."
2. "I should take the medication at noon with an antacid."
3. "I should take the medication in the morning when I first arise."
4. "I should take the medication right before bedtime with a snack."

932. A client receiving a tricyclic antidepressant arrives at the mental health clinic. Which observation indicates that the client is correctly following the medication plan?
1. Reports not going to work for this past week
2. Complains of not being able to "do anything" anymore
3. Arrives at the clinic neat and appropriate in appearance
4. Reports sleeping 12 hours per night and 3 to 4 hours during the day

933. A nurse is performing a follow-up teaching session with a client discharged 1 month ago who is taking fluoxetine (Prozac). What information would be important for the nurse to gather regarding the adverse effects related to the medication?
1. Cardiovascular symptoms
2. Gastrointestinal dysfunctions
3. Problems with mouth dryness
4. Problems with excessive sweating

934. A client taking buspirone (BuSpar) for 1 month returns to the clinic for a follow-up visit. Which of the following would indicate medication effectiveness?
1. No rapid heartbeats or anxiety
2. No paranoid thought processes
3. No thought broadcasting or delusions
4. No reports of alcohol withdrawal symptoms

935. A client taking lithium carbonate (Eskalith) reports vomiting, abdominal pain, diarrhea, blurred vision, tinnitus, and tremors. The lithium level is checked as a part of the routine follow-up and the level is 3.0 mEq/L. The nurse knows that this level is:
1. Toxic
2. Normal
3. Slightly above normal
4. Excessively below normal

936. A client arrives at the health care clinic and tells the nurse that he has been doubling his daily dosage of bupropion hydrochloride (Wellbutrin) to help him get better faster. The nurse understands that the client is now at risk for which of the following?

1. Insomnia
2. Weight gain
3. Seizure activity
4. Orthostatic hypotension

937. Immediately after taking a routine evening dose of alprazolam (Xanax), a client says, "I'm not sure I should have taken that stuff." The nurse makes which appropriate statement to the client?
1. "Let's talk about how you feel about Xanax for a while."
2. "Anxiety is to be expected with any new experience."
3. "You are afraid of the media claims about this medication."
4. "Your depression will fade once the medication begins to work."

938. A client is scheduled for discharge and will be taking phenobarbital (Luminal) for an extended period. The nurse would place highest priority on teaching the client which of the following points that directly relates to client safety?
1. Take the medication only with meals.
2. Take medication at the same time each day.
3. Avoid drinking alcohol while taking this medication.
4. Always use a dose container to help prevent missed doses.

939. A depressed client who is on tranylcypromine sulfate (Parnate) has been instructed on diet. The nurse feels confident that the client understands the diet when given a choice of restaurant foods if the client selects:
1. Pepperoni pizza, salad, and cola
2. Pickled herring, French fries, and milk
3. Fried haddock, baked potato, and cola
4. Roasted chicken, roasted potatoes, and beer

940. A nurse provides medication instructions to a client who is taking lithium carbonate (Eskalith). The nurse determines that the client needs additional instructions if the client states that he or she will:
1. Take the lithium with meals.
2. Monitor lithium blood levels very closely.
3. Decrease fluid intake while taking the lithium.
4. Contact the physician if excessive diarrhea, vomiting, or diaphoresis occurs.

941. Buspirone (BuSpar) is prescribed for a client with an anxiety disorder. The nurse instructs the client regarding the medication and informs the client that which of the following is a characteristic of this medication?
1. The medication is addicting.
2. Dizziness and headaches may occur.
3. Tolerance can occur with the medication.
4. The medication can produce a sedating effect.

ALTERNATE ITEM FORMAT: MULTIPLE RESPONSE

942. A hospitalized client is started on phenelzine sulfate (Nardil) for the treatment of depression. The nurse instructs the client to avoid consuming which foods while taking this medication? Select all that apply.

☐ **1.** Figs
☐ **2.** Yogurt
☐ **3.** Crackers
☐ **4.** Aged cheese
☐ **5.** Tossed salad
☐ **6.** Oatmeal cookies

ANSWERS

928. 3
Rationale: Hematological reactions can occur in the client taking clozapine and include agranulocytosis and mild leukopenia. The white blood cell count should be checked before initiating treatment and should be monitored closely during the use of this medication. The client should also be monitored for signs indicating agranulocytosis, which may include sore throat, malaise, and fever. Options 1, 2, and 4 are unrelated to this medication.
Test-Taking Strategy: Knowledge regarding the adverse effects that can occur in association with the use of clozapine is required to answer this question. Remember, clozapine can cause agranulocytosis and mild leukopenia. If you are unfamiliar with these adverse effects and the laboratory studies that need to be monitored, review this content.
Level of Cognitive Ability: Analysis
Client Needs: Physiological Integrity
Integrated Process: Nursing Process/Data Collection
Content Area: Pharmacology
Reference: Hodgson, B., & Kizior, R. (2008). *Saunders nursing drug handbook 2008* (p. 281). Philadelphia: Saunders.

929. 4
Rationale: Disulfiram is used as an adjunct treatment for selected clients with chronic alcoholism who want to remain in a state of enforced sobriety. Clients must abstain from alcohol intake for at least 12 hours before the initial dose of the medication is administered. The most important data are to determine when the last alcoholic drink was consumed. The medication is used with caution in clients with diabetes mellitus, hypothyroidism, epilepsy, cerebral damage, nephritis, and hepatic disease. It is also contraindicated in severe heart disease, psychosis, or hypersensitivity related to the medication.
Test-Taking Strategy: Use the process of elimination, recalling that the medication is used as an adjunct treatment for selected clients with chronic alcoholism. This will assist in directing you to option 4. Review this medication if you had difficulty with this question.
Level of Cognitive Ability: Analysis
Client Needs: Physiological Integrity
Integrated Process: Nursing Process/Data Collection
Content Area: Pharmacology
Reference: Lilley, L., Harrington, S., & Snyder J. (2007). *Pharmacology and the nursing process* (5th ed., p. 91). St. Louis: Mosby.

930. 1
Rationale: Donepezil hydrochloride is a cholinergic agent used in the treatment of mild to moderate dementia of the Alzheimer type. It enhances cholinergic functions by increasing the concentration of acetylcholine. It slows the progression of Alzheimer's disease. Options 2, 3, and 4 are incorrect.

Test-Taking Strategy: Knowledge regarding the use of donepezil hydrochloride is needed to answer this question. Remember, this medication is used to treat mild to moderate dementia. Review this medication if you had difficulty with this question.
Level of Cognitive Ability: Analysis
Client Needs: Physiological Integrity
Integrated Process: Nursing Process/Data Collection
Content Area: Pharmacology
Reference: Hodgson, B., & Kizior, R. (2008). *Saunders nursing drug handbook 2008* (pp. 383-384). Philadelphia: Saunders.

931. 3
Rationale: Fluoxetine hydrochloride is administered in the early morning without consideration to meals. Options 1, 2, and 4 are incorrect.
Test-Taking Strategy: Use the process of elimination. Eliminate options 1, 2, and 4 because they are comparable or alike and indicate taking the medication with an antacid or food. If you are unfamiliar with the use of this medication and the client-teaching points, review this content.
Level of Cognitive Ability: Analysis
Client Needs: Physiological Integrity
Integrated Process: Nursing Process/Evaluation
Content Area: Pharmacology
Reference: Lehne, R. (2007). *Pharmacology for nursing care* (6th ed., p. 351). Philadelphia: Saunders.

932. 3
Rationale: Depressed individuals will sleep for long periods, are not able to go to work, and feel as if they cannot "do anything." Once they have had some therapeutic effect from their medication, they will report resolution of many of these complaints as well as demonstrate an improvement in their appearance.
Test-Taking Strategy: Use the process of elimination. The observations identified in options 1, 2, and 4 are all symptoms of depression. The improvement in appearance indicates a therapeutic response to the medication, thus indicating compliance with the medication regimen. Review the expected effects of tricyclic antidepressants if you had difficulty with this question.
Level of Cognitive Ability: Analysis
Client Needs: Physiological Integrity
Integrated Process: Nursing Process/Evaluation
Content Area: Pharmacology
Reference: Lehne, R. (2007). *Pharmacology for nursing care* (6th ed., p. 333). Philadelphia: Saunders.

933. 2
Rationale: The most common adverse effects related to fluoxetine include central nervous system (CNS) and gastrointestinal

(GI) system dysfunction. This medication affects the GI system by causing nausea and vomiting, cramping, and diarrhea. Options 1, 3, and 4 are not adverse effects of this medication.
Test-Taking Strategy: Knowledge regarding the adverse effects related to fluoxetine is required to answer this question. Remember that this medication causes CNS and GI system dysfunction. Review these side effects and adverse reactions if you had difficulty with this question.
Level of Cognitive Ability: Analysis
Client Needs: Physiological Integrity
Integrated Process: Nursing Process/Data Collection
Content Area: Pharmacology
Reference: Lehne, R. (2007). *Pharmacology for nursing care* (6th ed., p. 351). Philadelphia: Saunders.

934. 1
Rationale: Buspirone hydrochloride is not recommended for the treatment of drug or alcohol withdrawal, paranoid thought disorders, or schizophrenia (thought broadcasting or delusions). Buspirone hydrochloride is most often indicated for the treatment of anxiety and aggression.
Test-Taking Strategy: Knowledge regarding the use of buspirone hydrochloride will direct you to the correct option. Recalling that this medication is an antianxiety drug will direct you to option 1. Review this medication if you had difficulty with this question.
Level of Cognitive Ability: Analysis
Client Needs: Physiological Integrity
Integrated Process: Nursing Process/Evaluation
Content Area: Pharmacology
Reference: Hodgson, B., & Kizior, R. (2008). *Saunders nursing drug handbook 2008* (p. 167). Philadelphia: Saunders.

935. 1
Rationale: The therapeutic serum level of lithium is 0.6 to 1.2 mEq/L. A level of 3 mEq/L indicates toxicity.
Test-Taking Strategy: Knowledge regarding the therapeutic serum level of lithium will direct you to option 1. Remember the therapeutic level is 0.6 to1.2 mEq/L. Review this level if you had difficulty with this question.
Level of Cognitive Ability: Comprehension
Client Needs: Physiological Integrity
Integrated Process: Nursing Process/Data Collection
Content Area: Pharmacology
Reference: Keltner, N., Schwecke, L. & Bostrom, C. (2007). *Psychiatric nursing* (5th ed., p. 257). St. Louis: Mosby.

936. 3
Rationale: Bupropion does not cause significant orthostatic blood pressure changes. Seizure activity is common in dosages greater than 450 mg daily. Bupropion frequently causes a drop in body weight. Insomnia is a side effect, but seizure activity causes a greater client risk.
Test-Taking Strategy: Use the process of elimination. Noting that the client has been doubling the medication dose and recalling that seizure activity can occur with higher-than-recommended doses will direct you to option 3. Review this medication if you had difficulty with this question.
Level of Cognitive Ability: Analysis
Client Needs: Physiological Integrity

Integrated Process: Nursing Process/Data Collection
Content Area: Pharmacology
Reference: Hodgson, B., & Kizior, R. (2008). *Saunders nursing drug handbook 2008* (p. 165). Philadelphia: Saunders.

937. 1
Rationale: The nurse should focus on determining the reason for the client's concern. The nurse would add anxiety to the client by mentioning media concerns. Alprazolam is used to treat anxiety, not depression. Cliché responses (option 2) do not express concern.
Test-Taking Strategy: Use therapeutic communication techniques. Remembering to address the client's feelings will direct you to option 1. Review these techniques if you had difficulty with this question.
Level of Cognitive Ability: Application
Client Needs: Psychosocial Integrity
Integrated Process: Communication and Documentation
Content Area: Pharmacology
Reference: Lilley, L., Harrington, S., & Snyder, J. (2007). *Pharmacology and the nursing process* (5th ed., p. 232). St. Louis: Mosby.

938. 3
Rationale: Phenobarbital is an anticonvulsant and a hypnotic agent. The client should avoid taking any other central nervous system depressants (such as alcohol) while taking this medication. The medication may be given without regard to meals. Taking the medication at the same time each day enhances compliance and maintains more stable blood levels of the medication. Using a dose container or "pillbox" may be helpful for some clients.
Test-Taking Strategy: Use the process of elimination. Focus on the subject, client safety, and note the strategic words "highest priority." This tells you that more than one or all of the options may be partially or totally correct and that you must prioritize your answer. Eliminate options 1 and 4 because of the close-ended words "only" and "always" in these options. Also, remember that alcohol should not be consumed when taking hypnotics. Review client-teaching points related to this medication if you had difficulty with this question.
Level of Cognitive Ability: Application
Client Needs: Safe and Effective Care Environment
Integrated Process: Teaching and Learning
Content Area: Pharmacology
Reference: Hodgson, B., & Kizior, R. (2008). *Saunders nursing drug handbook 2008* (p. 930). Philadelphia: Saunders.

939. 3
Rationale: Tranylcypromine sulfate is a monoamine oxidase inhibitor (MAOI) used to treat depression. A tyramine-restricted diet is required while on this medication to avoid hypertensive crisis, a life-threatening side effect of the medication. Foods to be avoided are meats prepared with tenderizer, smoked or pickled fish, beef or chicken liver, and dry sausage (salami, pepperoni, bologna). In addition, figs; bananas; aged cheese; yogurt; sour cream; beer; red wine; sherry, soy sauce; yeast extract; chocolate; caffeine; and aged, pickled, fermented, or smoked foods need to be avoided. Many over-the-counter medications also contain tyramine and must be

avoided as well.
Test-Taking Strategy: Knowledge that tranylcypromine sulfate is an MAOI medication and that tyramine-containing foods need to be avoided with these medications is necessary to answer this question. Review these foods if you had difficulty with this question.
Level of Cognitive Ability: Analysis
Client Needs: Physiological Integrity
Integrated Process: Nursing Process/Evaluation
Content Area: Pharmacology
Reference: Lilley, L., Harrington, S., & Snyder, J. (2007). *Pharmacology and the nursing process* (5th ed., p. 237). St. Louis: Mosby.

940. **3**
Rationale: Because therapeutic and toxic dosage ranges are so close, lithium blood levels must be monitored very closely, more frequently at first and then once every several months. The client should be instructed to contact the physician if excessive diarrhea, vomiting, or diaphoresis occurs. Lithium is irritating to the gastric mucosa; therefore, lithium should be taken with meals. A normal diet and normal salt and fluid intake (1500-3000 mL/day) should be maintained, since lithium decreases sodium reabsorption by the renal tubules, which could cause sodium depletion. A low sodium intake causes lithium retention and could lead to toxicity.
Test-Taking Strategy: Use the process of elimination and note the strategic words "needs additional instructions." These words indicate a negative event query and the need to select the incorrect client statement. Remember that, generally, it is important that clients be taught to maintain an adequate fluid intake. This principle will direct you to option 3. Review the client teaching points related to the administration of this medication if you had difficulty with this question.
Level of Cognitive Ability: Comprehension
Client Needs: Physiological Integrity
Integrated Process: Teaching and Learning
Content Area: Pharmacology
Reference: Hodgson, B., & Kizior, R. (2008). *Saunders nursing drug handbook 2008* (p. 699). Philadelphia: Saunders.

941. **2**
Rationale: Buspirone is used in the management of anxiety disorders. The advantages of this medication are that it is not sedating, tolerance does not develop, and it is not addicting. Dizziness, nausea, headaches, nervousness, lightheadedness, and excitement, which generally are not major problems, are side effects of the medication.
Test-Taking Strategy: Knowledge regarding the side effects and the advantages of buspirone is needed to answer this question. Remember, this medication is not sedating or addicting, and tolerance does not develop with its use. Review this medication and its use if you had difficulty with this question.
Level of Cognitive Ability: Application
Client Needs: Physiological Integrity
Integrated Process: Nursing Process/Implementation
Content Area: Pharmacology
Reference: Hodgson, B., & Kizior, R. (2008). *Saunders nursing drug handbook 2008* (p. 167). Philadelphia: Saunders.

ALTERNATE ITEM FORMAT: MULTIPLE RESPONSE
942. **1, 2, 4**
Rationale: Phenelzine sulfate (Nardil) is a monoamine oxidase inhibitor. The client should avoid taking in foods that are high in tyramine. Use of these foods could trigger a potentially fatal hypertensive crisis. Some foods to avoid include yogurt, aged cheeses, smoked or processed meats, red wines, and fruits such as avocados, raisins, and figs.
Test-Taking Strategy: Recall that phenelzine sulfate is a monoamine oxidase inhibitor and that foods high in tyramine needed to be avoided. Next, from the food items listed in the question, identify the food that contains tyramine. Review the food items to avoid with monoamine oxidase inhibitors if you had difficulty with this question.
Level of Cognitive Ability: Application
Client Needs: Physiological Integrity
Integrated Process: Nursing Process/Implementation
Content Area: Pharmacology
Reference: Lilley, L., Harrington, S., & Snyder, J. (2007). *Pharmacology and the nursing process* (5th ed., p. 237). St. Louis: Mosby.

References

Fortinash, K., & Holoday-Worret, P. (2008). *Psychiatric mental health nursing* (4th ed.). St. Louis: Mosby.
Hodgson, B., & Kizior, R. (2008). *Saunders nursing drug handbook 2008*. Philadelphia: Saunders.
Kee, J., Hayes, E., & McCuistion, L. (2006). *Pharmacology: A nursing process approach* (5th ed.). Philadelphia: Saunders.
Keltner, N., Schwecke, L., & Bostrom, C. (2007). *Psychiatric nursing* (5th ed.). St. Louis: Mosby.
Lehne, R. (2007). *Pharmacology for nursing care* (6th ed.). Philadelphia: Saunders.
Lilley, L., Harrington, S., & Snyder, J. (2007). *Pharmacology and the nursing process* (5th ed.). St. Louis: Mosby.
McKenry, L., Tessier, E., & Hogan, M. (2006). *Mosby's pharmacology in nursing* (22nd ed.). St. Louis: Mosby.
Monahan, F., Sands, J., Neighbors, M., Marek, J., & Green, C. (2007). *Phipps' medical-surgical nursing: Health and illness perspectives* (8th ed.). St. Louis: Mosby.

Comprehensive Test

QUESTIONS

More questions on the companion CD!

943. A nurse reinforces home care instructions to the parents of a child hospitalized with pertussis. The child is in the convalescent stage and is being prepared for discharge. Which statement by the parents indicates a need for further instructions?
   1. "We need to encourage adequate fluid intake."
   2. "Coughing spells may be triggered by dust or smoke."
   3. "We need to maintain respiratory precautions and a quiet environment for at least 2 weeks."
   4. "Good hand-washing techniques need to be instituted to prevent spreading the disease to others."

944. A client enters the emergency room confused, twitching, and having seizures. His family states he recently was placed on corticosteroids for arthritis and was feeling better and exercising daily. Upon assessment, he has flushed skin, dry mucous membranes, an elevated temperature, and poor skin turgor. His serum sodium level is 172 mEq/L. Choose the interventions that the physician would likely prescribe. Select all that apply.
   □ 1. Monitor I&O.
   □ 2. Monitor vital signs.
   □ 3. Monitor electrolyte levels.
   □ 4. Increase water intake orally.
   □ 5. Provide sodium-reduced diet.
   □ 6. Administer sodium replacements.

945. A nurse is monitoring a client receiving glipizide (Glucotrol). Which outcome indicates an ineffective response from the medication?
   1. A decrease in polyuria

   2. A decrease in polyphagia
   3. A fasting plasma glucose of 100 mg/dL
   4. A glycosylated hemoglobin level of 12%

946. A nurse is reinforcing discharge instructions to a client receiving sulfisoxazole. Which of the following would be included in the plan of care for instructions?
   1. Maintain a high fluid intake.
   2. Discontinue the medication when feeling better.
   3. If the urine turns dark brown, call the physician immediately.
   4. Decrease the dosage when symptoms are improving to prevent an allergic response.

947. Before administering an intermittent tube feeding through a nasogastric tube, the nurse checks for gastric residual volume. The nurse understands that the rationale for checking gastric residual volume before administering the tube feeding is to:
   1. Observe the digestion of formula.
   2. Check fluid and electrolyte status.
   3. Evaluate absorption of the last feeding.
   4. Confirm proper nasogastric tube placement.

948. A postoperative client requests medication for flatulence (gas pains). Which medication from the following PRN list should the nurse administer to this client?
   1. Droperidol (Inapsine)
   2. Simethicone (Mylicon)
   3. Acetaminophen (Tylenol)
   4. Magnesium hydroxide (milk of magnesia, MOM)

949. A client is admitted to the hospital with a diagnosis of major depression. During the admission

interview, the nurse determines that a major concern is the client's altered nutrition related to poor nutritional intake. The appropriate initial nursing intervention related to this concern is:
1. Weigh the client three times per week, before breakfast.
2. Explain to the client the importance of a good nutritional intake.
3. Report the nutritional concern to the psychiatrist and obtain a nutritional consult as soon as possible.
4. Offer the client several small, frequent meals daily, and schedule brief nursing interactions with the client during these times.

950. A client received 20 units of NPH insulin subcutaneously at 8:00 AM. The nurse should check the client for a potential hypoglycemic reaction at what time?
1. 5:00 PM
2. 10:00 AM
3. 11:00 AM
4. 11:00 PM

951. A nurse assists in developing a plan of care for a client with hyperparathyroidism receiving calcitonin-human (Cibacalcin). Which outcome has the highest priority regarding this medication?
1. Relief of pain
2. Absence of side effects
3. Reaching normal serum calcium levels
4. Verbalization of appropriate medication knowledge

952. A nursing instructor asks a nursing student about the cause of hemophilia. The student correctly responds by telling the instructor that:
1. Hemophilia is a Y-linked hereditary disorder.
2. A splenectomy resolves the bleeding disorders.
3. Hemophilia A results from deficiency of factor VIII.
4. A bone marrow transplant is the treatment of choice.

953. A 4-year-old child is admitted to the hospital with suspected acute lymphocytic leukemia (ALL). The nurse understands that which diagnostic study will confirm this diagnosis?
1. A platelet count
2. A lumbar puncture
3. Bone marrow biopsy
4. White blood cell (WBC) count

954. A child with leukemia is experiencing nausea related to medication therapy. The nurse, concerned about the child's nutritional status, should offer which of the following during this episode of nausea?
1. Low-calorie foods
2. Cool, clear liquids
3. Low-protein foods
4. The child's favorite foods

955. To ensure a safe environment for a child admitted to the hospital for a craniotomy to remove a brain tumor, the nurse should include which of the following in the plan of care?
1. Initiating seizure precautions
2. Using a wheelchair for out-of-bed activities
3. Assisting the child with ambulation at all times
4. Avoiding contact with other children on the nursing unit

956. A nurse is preparing to suction an adult client through the client's tracheostomy tube. Select all interventions that the nurse would perform for this procedure.
☐ 1. Apply suction for up to 10 to 15 seconds.
☐ 2. Hyperoxygenate the client before suctioning.
☐ 3. Set the wall suction unit pressure at 160 mm Hg.
☐ 4. Apply suction while gently inserting the catheter.
☐ 5. Apply intermittent suction while rotating and withdrawing the catheter.
☐ 6. Advance the catheter until resistance is met and then pull the catheter back 1 cm.

957. A nurse is assisting in caring for a client who has a placenta previa. The nurse understands that a cervical examination will not be performed on the client primarily because it could do which of the following?
1. Initiate premature labor
2. Cause profound hemorrhage
3. Rupture the fetal membranes
4. Increase the chance of infection

958. A mother is breast-feeding her newborn infant. The mother complains to the nurse that she is experiencing severe nipple soreness. The nurse should provide which of the following suggestions to the client?
1. Avoid rotating breast-feeding positions so that the nipple will toughen.
2. Stop nursing during the period of nipple soreness to allow the nipples to heal.
3. Nurse the newborn infant less frequently and substitute a bottle-feeding until the nipples become less sore.
4. Position the newborn infant with the ear, shoulder, and hip in straight alignment and with the baby's stomach against the mother's.

959. Which behavior should the nurse expect a client diagnosed with agoraphobia to describe when discussing the disorder?
1. A fear of leaving the house
2. A fear of riding in elevators
3. A fear of speaking in public
4. A need to wash hands several times before eating a meal

960. A nurse checks the food on a tray delivered for an Orthodox Jewish client and notes that the client has received a roast beef dinner with whole milk as a beverage. Which action should the nurse take?
    1. Deliver the food tray to the client.
    2. Replace the whole milk with fat-free milk.
    3. Call the dietary department and ask for a different meal.
    4. Ask the dietary department to replace the roast beef with pork.

961. A client is brought to the emergency department by the ambulance team following collapse at home. Cardiopulmonary resuscitation is attempted but is unsuccessful. The wife of the client tells the nurse that the client is an organ donor and that his eyes are to be donated. Which action should the nurse take next?
    1. Place dry, sterile dressings over the eyes of the deceased.
    2. Call the National Donor Association to confirm that the client is a donor.
    3. Close the eyes, elevate the head of the bed, and place a small ice pack on the eyes.
    4. Ask the wife to obtain the legal documents regarding organ donation from the lawyer.

962. A nurse administers a dose of scopolamine (Transderm-Scop) to a postoperative client. The nurse tells the client to expect which of the following side effects of this medication?
    1. Dry mouth
    2. Diaphoresis
    3. Excessive urination
    4. Pupillary constriction

963. A nurse is caring for a child diagnosed with Down syndrome. In describing the disorder to the parents, the nurse bases the explanation on the fact that Down syndrome is a:
    1. Condition characterized by above-average intellectual functioning with deficits in adaptive behavior
    2. Condition characterized by average intellectual functioning and the absence of deficits in adaptive behavior
    3. Condition characterized by subaverage intellectual functioning with the absence of deficits in adaptive behavior
    4. Congenital condition that results in moderate to severe retardation and has been linked to an extra chromosome 21 (group G)

964. A client with a diagnosis of major depression becomes more anxious, reports sleeping poorly, and seems to display increased anger. The nurse interprets the client's behavior as:
    1. The client is at increased risk for suicide.
    2. The client is dealing with pertinent issues.
    3. The client may need some time off the unit.
    4. The client is responding normally to hospitalization.

965. Which of the following electrocardiogram changes should the nurse note on the cardiac monitor with a client whose potassium (K^+) level is 3.2 mEq/L?
    1. U waves
    2. Flat P waves
    3. Elevated T waves
    4. Prolonged PR interval

966. An adult client with hepatic encephalopathy has a serum ammonia level of 95 mcg/dL and receives treatment with lactulose (Chronulac) syrup. The nurse determines that the client has the best and most optimal response if the level changes to which of the following after medication administration?
    1. 5 mcg/dL
    2. 10 mcg/dL
    3. 40 mcg/dL
    4. 80 mcg/dL

967. A nurse assists in developing a plan of care for the child with meningitis. What is the priority nursing diagnosis for this child?
    1. Acute pain
    2. Parental knowledge deficit
    3. Dysfunctional family process
    4. Ineffective cerebral tissue perfusion

968. A nurse is caring for a postoperative client who has been NPO, and the physician has prescribed a clear liquid diet. In planning to initiate this diet, which priority item should the nurse place at the client's bedside?
    1. A straw
    2. Code cart
    3. Cardiac monitor
    4. Suction equipment

969. A nurse has given the client taking ethambutol (Myambutol) information about the medication. The nurse determines that the client understands the instructions if he or she immediately reports:
    1. Impaired sense of hearing
    2. Distressing gastrointestinal side effects
    3. Orange-red discoloration of body secretions
    4. Difficulty discriminating the color red from green

970. A nurse is caring for an older client with a diagnosis of myasthenia gravis and has provided self-care instructions. Which statement by the client indicates that further teaching is necessary?
    1. "I rest each afternoon after my walk."
    2. "I cough and deep breathe many times during the day."
    3. "If I get abdominal cramps and diarrhea, I should call my doctor."
    4. "I can change the time of my medication on the mornings that I feel strong."

971. Select all interventions that apply to the care of a child who is having a seizure.
    ☐ **1.** Time the seizure.
    ☐ **2.** Restrain the child.
    ☐ **3.** Stay with the child.
    ☐ **4.** Insert an oral airway.
    ☐ **5.** Place the child in a supine position.
    ☐ **6.** Loosen clothing around the child's neck.

972. A nurse is preparing to administer a prescribed intramuscular (IM) dose of meperidine hydrochloride (Demerol), 35 mg, to a client. The medication label reads meperidine hydrochloride, 50 mg/mL. How many milliliters will the nurse administer to the client?
    Answer: _____ mL

973. A nurse is calculating a client's 24-hour fluid intake. The client consumed coffee (8 oz), water (8 oz), and orange juice (6 oz) for breakfast; soup (4 oz) and iced tea (8 oz) for lunch; and milk (10 oz), tea (8 oz), and water (8 oz) for dinner. The client also consumed 24 oz of water during the day. How many milliliters of fluid did the client consume in the 24-hour period?
    Answer: _____mL

974. A client with diabetes mellitus who has been controlled with daily insulin has been placed on atenolol (Tenormin) for the control of angina pectoris. Because of the effects of atenolol, the nurse determines that which of the following is the most reliable indicator of hypoglycemia?
    1. Sweating
    2. Tachycardia
    3. Nervousness
    4. Low blood glucose level

975. A nurse is asked to regulate the flow rate of an intravenous (IV) solution being administered to a client. The IV bag contains 50 mL of solution and the solution is to be administered over 30 minutes. The administration set has a drop factor of 10 drops (gtt)/mL. The nurse should regulate the roller clamp on the infusion set to deliver how many drops per minute? (Round to the nearest whole number.)
    Answer: _____ gtt/minute

976. Which data would indicate a potential complication associated with age-related changes in the musculoskeletal system?
    1. Decrease in height
    2. Overall sclerotic lesions
    3. Diminished lean body mass
    4. Changes in structural bone tissue

977. A nurse provides home care instructions to the mother of a child recovering from Reye's syndrome. Which statement by the mother indicates a need for further instruction?
    1. "I need to check for jaundiced skin and eyes every day."

2. "I need to have my child nap during the day to provide rest."
3. "I need to decrease the stimuli at home to prevent intracranial pressure."
4. "I need to give frequent, small, nutritious meals if my child starts to vomit."

978. A physician orders potassium chloride (KCl) elixir, 20 mEq orally twice daily. The medication label states potassium chloride (KCl), 30 mEq/15 mL. The nurse prepares to administer the morning dose. How many milliliters will the nurse prepare to administer one dose?
    Answer: _____ mL

979. A nurse provides medication instructions to a client with peptic ulcer disease. Which statement by the client indicates the best understanding of the medication therapy?
    1. "Antacids will coat my stomach."
    2. "Omeprazole (Prilosec) will coat the ulcer and help it heal."
    3. "Sucralfate (Carafate) will change the fluid in my stomach."
    4. "The nizatidine (Axid) will cause me to produce less stomach acid."

980. In planning activities for the depressed client, especially during the early stages of hospitalization, which of the following is best?
    1. Plan nothing until the client asks to participate in the milieu.
    2. Encourage the client to participate in a structured daily program of activities.
    3. Give the client a menu of daily activities and insist that the client participate in all activities offered.
    4. Provide an activity that is quiet and solitary in nature to avoid increased fatigue, such as working on a puzzle or reading a book.

981. A nurse is assisting in preparing a plan of care for a 4-year-old child hospitalized with nephrotic syndrome. Which dietary intervention is most appropriate for this child?
    1. Provide a high-salt diet.
    2. Provide a high-protein diet.
    3. Discourage visitors at mealtimes.
    4. Encourage the child to eat in the playroom.

982. A nursing instructor asks a student to describe the pathophysiology that occurs in Cushing's disease. Which statement by the student indicates an accurate understanding of this disorder?
    1. "Cushing's disease is characterized by an oversecretion of insulin."
    2. "Cushing's disease is characterized by an oversecretion of glucocorticoid hormones."
    3. "Cushing's disease is characterized by an undersecretion of corticotropic hormones."
    4. "Cushing's disease is characterized by an undersecretion of glucocorticoid hormones."

983. The nursing instructor asks the nursing student about the physiology related to the cessation of ovulation that occurs during pregnancy. Which response by the student indicates an understanding of this physiological process?
    1. "Ovulation ceases during pregnancy because the circulating levels of estrogen and progesterone are high."
    2. "Ovulation ceases during pregnancy because the circulating levels of estrogen and progesterone are low."
    3. "The low levels of estrogen and progesterone increase the release of follicle-stimulating hormone and luteinizing hormone."
    4. "The high levels of estrogen and progesterone promote the release of follicle-stimulating hormone and luteinizing hormone."

984. A nurse is assisting in collecting data on a child with seizures. The nurse is interviewing the child's parents to establish their adjustment to caring for their child with a chronic illness. Which statement by a parent would indicate a need for further teaching?
    1. "Our child sleeps in our bedroom at night."
    2. "We worry about injuries when our child has a seizure."
    3. "Our child is involved in a swim program with neighbors and friends."
    4. "Our babysitter just completed cardiopulmonary resuscitation (CPR) training."

985. A client is taking lansoprazole (Prevacid) for the chronic management of Zollinger-Ellison syndrome. The nurse advises the client to take which of the following products if needed for a headache?
    1. Naprosyn (Aleve)
    2. Ibuprofen (Motrin)
    3. Acetaminophen (Tylenol)
    4. Acetylsalicylic acid (aspirin)

986. A depressed client verbalizes feelings of low self-esteem and self-worth typified by statements such as, "I'm such a failure. I can't do anything right!" The best nursing action would be to:
    1. Tell the client that this is not true, and that we all have a purpose in life.
    2. Remain with the client and sit in silence until the client verbalizes feelings.
    3. Identify recent behaviors or accomplishments that demonstrate skill or ability.
    4. Reassure the client that you know how the client is feeling and that things will get better.

987. A nurse is assigned to care for an infant with cryptorchidism. The nurse anticipates that diagnostic studies will be prescribed to evaluate:
    1. DNA synthesis
    2. Babinski reflex
    3. Kidney function
    4. Chromosomal analysis

988. A nurse is caring for a client with a diagnosis of pemphigus. The nurse understands that a hallmark sign characteristic of this condition is:
    1. Homans' sign
    2. Chvostek's sign
    3. Nikolsky's sign
    4. Trousseau's sign

989. A client asks the nurse about the causes of acne. The nurse most appropriately responds by telling the client:
    1. "It is caused by oily skin."
    2. "The exact cause of acne is not known."
    3. "It is caused as a result of exposure to heat and humidity."
    4. "Acne is caused by eating chocolate, nuts, and fatty foods."

990. In performing cardiopulmonary resuscitation (CPR), the nurse would use the method shown in the figure below to open the airway in which of the following situations?

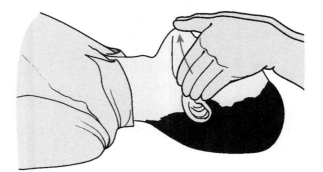

From Harkreader, H., Hogan, M., & Thobaden, M. [2007]. *Fundamentals of nursing: Caring and clinical judgment* [3rd ed.]. Philadelphia: Saunders.

    1. If the client is unconscious
    2. If neck trauma is suspected
    3. In all situations requiring CPR
    4. If the client has a history of headaches

991. The nurse is reviewing the health record of a pregnant client at 16 weeks' gestation. The nurse should expect to note documentation that the fundus of the uterus is located at which of the following areas?
    1. At the umbilicus
    2. Just above the symphysis pubis
    3. At the level of the xiphoid process
    4. Midway between the symphysis pubis and the umbilicus

992. A nurse is assigned to care for a child with a compound (open) fracture of the arm that occurred as a result of a fall. The nurse plans care, knowing that this type of fracture involves:
    1. The entire bone fractured straight across
    2. A greater risk of infection than a simple fracture
    3. One side of the bone being broken and the other side being bent

4. The bone being fractured but not producing a break in the skin

993. A nursing student is asked to discuss the topic of clubfoot at a clinical conference. The student plans to tell the group that clubfoot:
   1. Is a congenital anomaly
   2. Always occurs bilaterally
   3. Affects girls more often than boys
   4. Is a rare deformity of the skeletal system

994. A client with type 1 diabetes mellitus is to begin an exercise program, and the nurse is providing instructions to the client regarding the program. Which of the following should the nurse include in the teaching plan?
   1. Try to exercise prior to mealtime.
   2. Administer insulin after exercising.
   3. Take a blood glucose test before exercising.
   4. Exercise should be performed during peak times of insulin.

995. A nurse is caring for an older client who is terminally ill. Which of the following signs indicates to the nurse that death may be imminent?
   1. Rubor and paresthesias
   2. Eupnea and normal body temperature
   3. Irregular, noisy breathing and cold, clammy skin
   4. Presence of swallowing reflex and active bowel sounds

996. A nurse has given the client with tuberculosis instructions for proper handling and disposal of respiratory secretions. The nurse determines that the client understands the instructions if the client verbalizes which of the following?
   1. Discard used tissues in a plastic bag.
   2. Wash hands at least four times a day.
   3. Brush teeth and rinse the mouth once a day.
   4. Turn the head to the side if coughing or sneezing.

997. A client who has been taking isoniazid (INH) for 1½ months complains to the nurse about numbness, paresthesias, and tingling in the extremities. The nurse interprets that the client is experiencing:
   1. Hypercalcemia
   2. Peripheral neuritis
   3. Small blood vessel spasm
   4. Impaired peripheral circulation

998. A nurse is preparing a 2-year-old child with suspected nephrotic syndrome for a renal biopsy to confirm the diagnosis. The mother asks the nurse, "Will my child ever look thin again?" The nurse appropriately responds by saying:
   1. "Do you feel guilty because you didn't notice the weight gain?"
   2. "In most cases, medication and diet will control fluid retention."
   3. "Wearing loose-fitting clothing should help conceal the extra weight."
   4. "When children are little, it's expected that they'll look a little chubby."

999. A nurse is caring for a client hospitalized with acute exacerbation of chronic obstructive pulmonary disease (COPD). Which of the following would the nurse expect to note in this client?
   1. Hypocapnia
   2. Dyspnea on exertion
   3. Increased oxygen saturation with exercise
   4. A shortened expiratory phase of respiration

1000. A nurse is preparing to administer an enema to an adult client. Choose the interventions that the nurse would perform for this procedure. Select all that apply.
   ☐ 1. Apply disposable gloves.
   ☐ 2. Place the client in the right Sims' position.
   ☐ 3. Lubricate the enema tube and insert it approximately 4 inches.
   ☐ 4. Clamp the tubing if the client expresses discomfort during the procedure.
   ☐ 5. Hang the container containing the enema solution 24 inches above the client's anus.
   ☐ 6. Ensure that the temperature of the solution is between 100° F (37.8° C) and 105° F (40.5° C).

1001. A nurse is assigned to care for an adult client who had a brain attack (stroke) and is aphasic. Choose the appropriate interventions for communicating with the client. Select all that apply.
   ☐ 1. Face the client when talking.
   ☐ 2. Speak slowly and maintain eye contact.
   ☐ 3. Use gestures when talking to enhance words.
   ☐ 4. Avoid the use of body language when talking to the client.
   ☐ 5. Give the client directions using short phrases and simple terms.
   ☐ 6. Phrase what was said differently the second time, if there is a need to repeat it.

1002. The nurse observes that a client with a nasogastric tube connected to continuous gastric suction is mouth breathing, has dry mucous membranes, and has a foul breath odor. In planning care, which nursing intervention would be best to maintain the integrity of this client's oral mucosa?
   1. Offer small sips of water frequently.
   2. Encourage the client to suck on sour, hard candy.
   3. Use lemon glycerin swabs to provide oral hygiene.
   4. Brush the client's teeth frequently; use diluted mouthwash and water to rinse the mouth.

1003. A client is admitted to the hospital with possible rheumatic endocarditis. The nurse would check the client for signs and symptoms of concurrent:
   1. Viral infection

2. Yeast infection
3. Streptococcal infection
4. Staphylococcal infection

1004. A client who is taking hydrochlorothiazide (HydroDIURIL, HCTZ) has been started on triamterene (Dyrenium) as well. The client asks the nurse why both medications are required. The nurse formulates a response, based on the understanding that:
1. Both are weak potassium-losing diuretics.
2. The combination of these medications prevents renal toxicity.
3. Hydrochlorothiazide is an expensive medication, so using a combination of diuretics is cost-effective.
4. Triamterene is a potassium-sparing diuretic, whereas hydrochlorothiazide is a potassium-losing diuretic.

1005. A client who has begun taking fosinopril (Monopril) is very distressed, telling the nurse that he cannot taste food normally since beginning the medication 2 weeks ago. The nurse provides the best support to the client by:
1. Telling the client not to take the medication with food
2. Suggesting that the client taper the dose until taste returns to normal
3. Informing the client that impaired taste is expected and generally disappears in 2 to 3 months
4. Requesting that the physician change the order to another brand of angiotensin-converting enzyme (ACE) inhibitor

1006. A nurse is planning to administer amlodipine (Norvasc) to a client. The nurse plans to check which of the following before giving the medication?
1. Respiratory rate
2. Blood pressure and heart rate
3. Heart rate and respiratory rate
4. Level of consciousness and blood pressure

1007. A client had an aortic valve replacement 2 days ago. This morning, the client says to the nurse, "I don't feel any better than I did before surgery." The appropriate response by the nurse is:
1. "You will feel better in a week or two."
2. "It's only the second day post-op. Cheer up."
3. "This is a normal frustration; it'll get better."
4. "You are concerned that you don't feel any better after surgery."

1008. A nurse is preparing a list of home care instructions regarding stoma and laryngectomy care to a client who had a laryngectomy. Choose the instructions that would be included in the list. Select all that apply.
☐ 1. Restrict fluid intake.
☐ 2. Obtain a Medic-Alert bracelet.
☐ 3. Keep the humidity in the home low.
☐ 4. Prevent debris from entering the stoma.
☐ 5. Avoid exposure to people with infections.
☐ 6. Avoid swimming and use care when showering.

1009. A nurse administers an injection to a client with a diagnosis of acquired immunodeficiency syndrome (AIDS). After administering the medication, the nurse disposes of the used needle by:
1. Asking the client to recap the needle
2. Placing the needle and syringe in a puncture-resistant container
3. Recapping the needle before placing it in a puncture-resistant container
4. Laying the needle and syringe on the bedside table and carefully recapping the needle

1010. A nurse is identifying clients in the community at risk for latex allergy. Which client population is most at risk for developing this type of allergy?
1. Children in day care centers
2. Individuals with spina bifidia
3. Individuals with cardiac disease
4. Individuals living in a group home

1011. A client has just had a cast removed and the underlying skin is yellow-brown and crusted. The nurse determines that further skin care instructions are required when the client states:
1. "I will soak the skin and then wash it gently."
2. "I need to scrub the skin vigorously with soap and water."
3. "I need to apply an emollient lotion to enhance softening."
4. "I need to use a sunscreen on the skin if it's exposed for a period of time."

1012. A client has had skeletal traction applied to the right leg and has an overhead trapeze available for use. The nurse should monitor which of the following as a high-risk area for pressure and breakdown?
1. Scapulae
2. Left heel
3. Right heel
4. Back of the head

1013. A client has been placed in Buck's extension traction. The nurse can provide for countertraction by:
1. Using a footboard
2. Providing an overhead trapeze
3. Slightly elevating the foot of the bed
4. Slightly elevating the head of the bed

1014. A nurse would include which interventions in the plan of care for a client with hypothyroidism (myxedema)? Select all that apply.
☐ 1. Provide a cool environment for the client.
☐ 2. Instruct the client to consume a high-fat diet.

☐ 3. Instruct the client about thyroid replacement therapy.

☐ 4. Encourage the client to consume fluids and high-fiber foods in the diet.

☐ 5. Instruct the client to contact the physician if episodes of chest pain occur.

☐ 6. Inform the client that iodine preparations will be prescribed to treat the disorder.

1015. A nurse is admitting a client with Guillain-Barré syndrome to the nursing unit. The client has an ascending paralysis to the level of the waist. Knowing the complications of the disorder, the nurse brings which of the following items into the client's room?
1. Nebulizer and pulse oximeter
2. Blood pressure cuff and flashlight
3. Flashlight and incentive spirometer
4. Electrocardiographic monitoring electrodes and intubation tray

1016. A client with chronic renal failure is receiving ferrous sulfate (Feosol). The nurse monitors the client for which common side effect associated with this medication?
1. Diarrhea
2. Weakness
3. Headache
4. Constipation

1017. A nurse is attempting to communicate with a hearing-impaired client. Which of the following strategies by the nurse would be least helpful when talking to this client?
1. Reducing any background noise
2. Smiling continuously during conversation
3. Facing the client so that there is light on the nurse's face
4. Avoiding showing frustration through facial expression

1018. A nurse is preparing to administer digoxin (Lanoxin), 0.125 mg orally, to a client with heart failure. Which vital sign is most important for the nurse to check before administering the medication?
1. Heart rate
2. Temperature
3. Respirations
4. Blood pressure

1019. A postoperative client has an order to receive an intravenous (IV) infusion of 1000 mL normal saline solution over a period of 10 hours. The drop (gtt) factor for the IV infusion set is 15 gtt/mL. The nurse sets the flow rate at how many drops per minute?

Answer: _____ gtt/minute

1020. A nurse is preparing to set up a sterile field using the principles of aseptic technique to perform a dressing change. Select all appropriate interventions.

☐ 1. Use a dry table that is below waist level.

☐ 2. Open the distal flap of a sterile package first.

☐ 3. Prepare the sterile field just before the planned procedure.

☐ 4. Don clean gloves before touching items on the sterile field.

☐ 5. Place the sterile field 1 foot behind the working area and out of view of the client.

☐ 6. Avoid placing items within 1 inch of any area surrounding the outer edge of the sterile field.

1021. A nurse is performing nasotracheal suctioning of a client. The nurse interprets that the client is adequately tolerating the procedure if which of the following observations is made?
1. Skin color becomes cyanotic.
2. Secretions are becoming bloody.
3. Coughing occurs with suctioning.
4. Heart rate decreases from 78 to 54 beats/minute.

1022. A nurse inspects the oral cavity of a client with cancer and notes white patches on the mucous membranes. The nurse determines that this occurrence:
1. Is common
2. Suggests that the client is anemic
3. Is characteristic of a thrush infection
4. Is indicative that oral hygiene needs to be improved

1023. A nurse is monitoring the laboratory results of a client preparing to receive chemotherapy. The nurse determines that the white blood cell count (WBC) is normal if which of the following results were present?
1. $2000/mm^3$
2. $3000/mm^3$
3. $5000/mm^3$
4. $15,000/mm^3$

1024. A nurse instructs the client in breast self-examination (BSE). The nurse instructs the client to lie down and to examine the left breast. The nurse instructs the client that while examining the left breast, to place a pillow:
1. Under the left shoulder
2. Under the right scapula
3. Under the right shoulder
4. Under the small of the back

1025. A client suspected of having an abdominal tumor is scheduled for a computerized tomography (CT) scan with dye injection. The nurse tells the client which of the following about the test?
1. The test may be painful.
2. The test takes approximately 2 to 3 hours.
3. Fluids will be restricted following the test.
4. The dye injected may cause a warm, flushing sensation.

1026. A nurse is caring for a client dying of ovarian cancer. During care, the client states, "If I can just live long enough to attend my daughter's graduation, I'll be ready to die." Which phase of coping is this client experiencing?
   1. Anger
   2. Denial
   3. Bargaining
   4. Depression

1027. A nurse is reviewing the health record of a client with laryngeal cancer. The nurse would expect to note which most common risk factor for this type of cancer documented in the record?
   1. Urban living
   2. Alcohol abuse
   3. Cigarette smoking
   4. Use of chewing tobacco

ANSWERS

943. 3
Rationale: Pertussis is transmitted by direct contact or respiratory droplets from coughing. The communicable period occurs primarily during the catarrhal stage. Respiratory precautions are not required during the convalescent phase. Options 1, 2, and 4 are components of home care instructions.
Test-Taking Strategy: Note the strategic words "convalescent" and "need for further instructions." These words indicate a negative event query and the need to select the incorrect statement. Options 1 and 4 can be easily eliminated since they are general interventions associated with convalescence. Knowing that coughing spells are associated with pertussis will assist in directing you to option 3 from the remaining options. In addition, a 2-week period of respiratory precautions is not required. If you had difficulty with this question, review home care instructions for the child with pertussis.
Level of Cognitive Ability: Comprehension
Client Needs: Health Promotion and Maintenance
Integrated Process: Teaching and Learning
Content Area: Child Health
Reference: Hockenberry, M. & Wilson, D. (2007). *Nursing care of infants and children* (8th ed., pp. 672-673). St. Louis: Mosby.

944. 1, 2, 3, 4, 5
Rationale: Hypernatremia is described as having a serum sodium level that exceeds 145 mEq/L. Signs and symptoms would include dry mucous membranes, loss of skin turgor, thirst, flushed skin, elevated temperature, oliguria, muscle twitching, fatigue, confusion, and seizures. Interventions include monitoring fluid balance, monitoring vital signs, reducing dietary intake of sodium, monitoring electrolyte levels, and increasing oral intake of water. Sodium replacement therapy would not be prescribed for a client with hypernatremia.
Test-Taking Strategy: Focus on the data in the question. Noting that a sodium level of 172 mEq/L is elevated will direct you to the correct options. If you had difficulty with this question, review the care for the client experiencing hypernatremia.
Level of Cognitive Ability: Analysis
Client Needs: Physiological Integrity
Integrated Process: Nursing Process/Planning
Content Area: Fundamental Skills
Reference: Linton, A., & Maebius, N. (2007). *Introduction to medical-surgical nursing* (4th ed., pp. 160-161). Philadelphia: Saunders.

945. 4
Rationale: Glipizide (Glucotrol) is an oral hypoglycemic agent administered to decrease the serum glucose level and the signs and symptoms of hyperglycemia. Therefore, a decrease in both polyuria and polyphagia would indicate a therapeutic response. Laboratory values are also used to assess a client's response to treatment. A fasting blood glucose level of 100 mg/dL is within normal limits. However, a glycosylated hemoglobin of 12% indicates poor glycemic control.
Test-Taking Strategy: Note the strategic words "ineffective response." Recalling that glipizide is an oral hypoglycemic agent tells you to look for an option that would indicate hyperglycemia (lack of response to the medication). Options 1 and 2 are comparable or alike and are eliminated first. Next, eliminate option 3 since it is a normal blood glucose level. Review this medication if you had difficulty with this question.
Level of Cognitive Ability: Analysis
Client Needs: Physiological Integrity
Integrated Process: Nursing Process/Evaluation
Content Area: Adult Health/Endocrine
References: Chernecky, C., & Berger, B. (2008). *Laboratory tests and diagnostic procedures* (5th ed., p. 594). Philadelphia: Saunders.
Lehne, R. (2007). *Pharmacology for nursing care* (6th ed., p. 661). Philadelphia: Saunders.

946. 1
Rationale: Each dose of sulfisoxazole should be administered with a full glass of water, and the client should maintain a high fluid intake. The medication is more soluble in alkaline urine. The client should not be instructed to taper or discontinue the dose. Some forms of sulfisoxazole cause the urine to turn dark brown or red. This does not indicate the need to notify the physician.
Test-Taking Strategy: Use the process of elimination. General principles related to medication administration will assist in eliminating options 2 and 4. From the remaining options, recalling that this medication is a sulfonamide will direct you to option 1. Review this medication if you had difficulty with this question.
Level of Cognitive Ability: Application
Client Needs: Physiological Integrity
Integrated Process: Teaching and Learning
Content Area: Pharmacology
References: Kee, J., Hayes, E., & McCuistion, L. (2006). *Pharmacology: A nursing process approach* (5th ed., p. 456). Philadelphia: Saunders.
Lehne, R. (2007). *Pharmacology for nursing care* (6th ed., p. 1007). Philadelphia: Saunders.

947. **3**
Rationale: All the stomach contents are aspirated and measured before administering a tube feeding. This procedure measures the gastric residual volume. The gastric residual volume is checked to confirm whether undigested formula from a previous feeding remains, and thereby evaluates the absorption of the last feeding. It is important to check the gastric residual before administration of a tube feeding. A full stomach could result in overdistention, thus predisposing the client to regurgitation and possible aspiration. If residual feeding is obtained, the health care provider's order and agency policy is checked to determine the course of action (hold or reduce the volume of the intermittent tube feeding).
Test-Taking Strategy: Note that the subject of the question is the purpose of checking residual volume. Focusing on this subject should direct you to option 3. Review this procedure if you had difficulty with this question.
Level of Cognitive Ability: Comprehension
Client Needs: Physiological Integrity
Integrated Process: Nursing Process/Data Collection
Content Area: Adult Health/Gastrointestinal
Reference: Christensen, B., & Kockrow, E. (2006). *Adult health nursing* (5th ed., p. 653). St. Louis: Mosby.

948. **2**
Rationale: Simethicone is an antiflatulent used in the relief of pain cause by excessive gas in the gastrointestinal tract. Droperidol is used to treat postoperative nausea and vomiting. Acetaminophen is a non-opioid analgesic. Magnesium hydroxide is an antacid and laxative.
Test-Taking Strategy: Use the process of elimination and note the strategic words "flatulence (gas pains)." Recalling the classifications of the medications in the options will direct you to option 2. If this question was difficult, review this medication.
Level of Cognitive Ability: Application
Client Needs: Physiological Integrity
Integrated Process: Nursing Process/Implementation
Content Area: Pharmacology
Reference: Hodgson, B., & Kizior, R. (2008). *Saunders nursing drug handbook 2008* (pp. 1062-1063). Philadelphia: Saunders.

949. **4**
Rationale: Change in appetite is one of the major symptoms of depression. Offering the client several small, frequent meals and the nurse's presence at that time to support, encourage, or perhaps even feed the client is the most appropriate intervention. A client with depression experiences poor concentration and will not understand the importance of an adequate nutritional intake. Weighing the client does not address how to increase nutritional intake. Reporting the nutritional problems to the psychiatrist is correct to some degree, but doesn't address how one might increase food intake.
Test-Taking Strategy: Note the strategic word "initial" and focus on the subject—the poor nutritional intake. Option 4 is the only option that addresses the altered nutrition concretely and designs a method in which the client will feasibly increase the nutritional intake. Review care of the client with depression if you had difficulty with this question.
Level of Cognitive Ability: Application
Client Needs: Physiological Integrity

Integrated Process: Nursing Process/Implementation
Content Area: Mental Health
References: Keltner, N., Schwecke, L. & Bostrom, C. (2007). *Psychiatric nursing* (5th ed., p. 384). St. Louis: Mosby. Varcarolis, E., Carlson, V., Shoemaker, N. (2006). *Foundations of psychiatric mental health nursing: A clinical approach* (5th ed., pp. 341). Philadelphia: Saunders.

950. **1**
Rationale: NPH is an intermediate-acting insulin. Its onset of action is 1 to 2½ hours, it peaks in 4 to 12 hours, and its duration of action is 24 hours. Hypoglycemic reactions most likely occur during peak time.
Test-Taking Strategy: Focus on the subject—NPH insulin. Recalling that peak action is between 4 and 12 hours will direct you to option 1. Review the characteristics of NPH insulin if you had difficulty with this question.
Level of Cognitive Ability: Application
Client Needs: Physiological Integrity
Integrated Process: Nursing Process/Implementation
Content Area: Pharmacology
Reference: Lehne, R. (2007). *Pharmacology for nursing care* (6th ed., p. 652). Philadelphia: Saunders.

951. **3**
Rationale: Hypercalcemia can occur in clients with hyperparathyroidism, and calcitonin is used to lower plasma calcium level. The highest priority outcome in this client situation would be a reduction in serum calcium level. Option 1 is unrelated to this medication. Although options 2 and 4 are expected outcomes, they are not the highest priority for administering this medication.
Test-Taking Strategy: Use the process of elimination. Noting the client diagnosis will assist in directing you to option 3. In addition, note the relation between the name of the medication and the word "calcium" in option 3. Review this medication if you had difficulty with this question.
Level of Cognitive Ability: Analysis
Client Needs: Physiological Integrity
Integrated Process: Nursing Process/Evaluation
Content Area: Adult Health/Endocrine
References: Hodgson, B., & Kizior, R. (2008). *Saunders nursing drug handbook 2008* (pp. 173-175). Philadelphia: Saunders. Skidmore-Roth, L. (2007). *Mosby's nursing drug reference* (20th ed., p. 208). St. Louis: Mosby.

952. **3**
Rationale: The term hemophilia refers to a group of bleeding disorders. The identification of the specific factor deficiencies allows for definitive treatment with replacement agents. Hemophilia A results from a deficiency of factor VIII. Hemophilia B (Christmas disease) is a deficiency of factor IX. Hemophilia is inherited in a recessive manner via a genetic defect on the X chromosome, not the Y chromosome. Neither a bone marrow transplant nor a splenectomy are used to treat this disorder.
Test-Taking Strategy: Knowledge regarding hemophilia and related causes and treatment is needed to answer the question. Remember, hemophilia A results from a deficiency of factor VIII. Review this disorder if you had difficulty with this question.
Level of Cognitive Ability: Comprehension

Client Needs: Physiological Integrity
Integrated Process: Teaching and Learning
Content Area: Child Health
References: Price, D., & Gwin, J. (2008). *Pediatric nursing: An introductory text* (10th ed., pp. 245-246). St. Louis: Saunders. Wong, D., Perry, S., Hockenberry, M., Lowdermilk, D., & Wilson, D. (2006). *Maternal child nursing care* (3rd ed. p. 1614). St. Louis: Mosby.

953. **3**

Rationale: The confirmatory test for leukemia is microscopic examination of bone marrow obtained by bone marrow aspirate and biopsy. The WBC count may be high or low in leukemia. A lumbar puncture may be done to look for blast cells in the spinal fluid that are indicative of central nervous system disease. An altered platelet count occurs as a result of chemotherapy.
Test-Taking Strategy: Use the process of elimination and note the strategic word "confirm." This strategic word and recalling that the bone marrow is affected in leukemia will direct you to option 3. Review diagnostic studies related to leukemia if you had difficulty with this question.
Level of Cognitive Ability: Comprehension
Client Needs: Physiological Integrity
Integrated Process: Nursing Process/Planning
Content Area: Child Health
References: Price, D., & Gwin, J. (2008). *Pediatric nursing: An introductory text* (10th ed., p. 242). St. Louis: Saunders. Wong, D., Perry, S., Hockenberry, M., Lowdermilk, D., & Wilson, D. (2006). *Maternal child nursing care* (3rd ed., pp. 1620-1621). St. Louis: Mosby.

954. **2**

Rationale: When the child is nauseated, it is best to offer frequent intake of cool, clear liquids in small amounts because small portions are usually better tolerated. Cool, clear fluids are also soothing and better tolerated when a client is nauseated. It is best not to offer favorite foods when the child is nauseated because foods eaten during times of nausea will be associated with being sick. It is best to offer small, frequent meals of high-protein and high-calorie content once the nausea has been controlled with medication or has subsided
Test-Taking Strategy: The subject of the question relates to nutritional status in a child with nausea. You should easily be able to eliminate options 1 and 3 because of the word "low" in these options. From the remaining options, recalling that the subject is related to nausea will assist in directing you to option 2. Review interventions related to relieving nausea if you had difficulty with this question.
Level of Cognitive Ability: Application
Client Needs: Physiological Integrity
Integrated Process: Nursing Process/Implementation
Content Area: Child Health
References: Price, D., & Gwin, J. (2008). *Pediatric nursing: An introductory text* (10th ed., pp. 163, 245). St. Louis: Saunders. Wong, D., Perry, S., Hockenberry, M., Lowdermilk, D., & Wilson, D. (2006). *Maternal child nursing care* (3rd ed. p. 1628). St. Louis: Mosby.

955. **1**

Rationale: Safety of the child is the nursing priority. Seizure precautions should be implemented for any child with a brain tumor, both preoperatively and postoperatively. A thorough neurological assessment should be performed on the child, and the child's safety should be assessed before allowing the child to get out of bed without help. Assessment of the child's gait should be assessed daily. However, options 2 and 3 are not required unless functional deficits exist. Isolating the child, option 4, is not necessary.
Test-Taking Strategy: Use the process of elimination and note the strategic words "safe environment." Eliminate options 2 and 3 first because they are comparable or alike. In addition, note the close-ended word "all" in option 3. Eliminate option 4 because it is unnecessary. Review care of the child with a brain tumor if you had difficulty with this question.
Level of Cognitive Ability: Application
Client Needs: Safe and Effective Care Environment
Integrated Process: Nursing Process/Planning
Content Area: Child Health
References: Price, D., & Gwin, J. (2008). *Pediatric nursing: An introductory text* (10th ed., pp. 318-319). St. Louis: Saunders. Wong, D., Perry, S., Hockenberry, M., Lowdermilk, D., & Wilson, D. (2006). *Maternal child nursing care* (3rd ed. p. 1694). St. Louis: Mosby.

956. **1, 2, 5, 6**

Rationale: Intermittent suction is applied while rotating the catheter for 10 to 15 seconds. The nurse should hyperoxygenate the client with a resuscitator bag/Ambu-bag connected to an oxygen source before suctioning because suction depletes the client's oxygen supply (option 2). The catheter should be inserted quickly and gently until resistance is met or the client coughs; then pulled back 1 cm or ½ inch. Intermittent suction is applied while rotating and withdrawing the catheter. Option 3 is incorrect because wall suction should be set to 80 to 120 mm Hg. Pressure set at a higher level can cause trauma to respiratory tract tissues. Strict asepsis needs to be maintained, and the nurse would wear sterile gloves to perform this procedure. Suction is never applied when inserting the catheter because it will deplete oxygen and can traumatize tissues.
Test-Taking Strategy: Focus on the subject—suctioning procedure through a tracheostomy. The priority issues to think about when answering this question include maintaining oxygenation, maintaining asepsis, and preventing tissue trauma. This will assist in selecting the correct interventions. Review suctioning procedure if you had difficulty with this question.
Level of Cognitive Ability: Application
Client Needs: Physiological Integrity
Integrated Process: Nursing Process/Implementation
Content Area: Adult Health/Respiratory
References: deWit, S. (2009). *Medical-surgical nursing: Concepts & practice* (pp. 310-312). St. Louis: Saunders. Potter, P., & Perry, A. (2005). *Fundamentals of nursing* (6th ed., pp. 1101-1108). St. Louis: Mosby.

957. **2**

Rationale: Because the placenta is implanted low in the uterus, cervical examination could cause the disruption of the placenta and initiate profound hemorrhage. The other options are also correct, but the profound hemorrhage is of the greatest concern in this case.

Test-Taking Strategy: Use the process of elimination and note the strategic word "primarily." Recalling that bleeding is a primary concern will direct you to option 2. Review care of the client with placenta previa if you had difficulty with this question.
Level of Cognitive Ability: Comprehension
Client Needs: Physiological Integrity
Integrated Process: Nursing Process/Implementation
Content Area: Maternity/Antepartum
References: Leifer, G. (2007). *Introduction to maternity and pediatric nursing* (5th ed., pp. 87-88). Philadelphia: Saunders.
Wong, D., Perry, S., Hockenberry, M., Lowdermilk, D., & Wilson, D. (2006). *Maternal child nursing care* (3rd ed., p. 402). St. Louis: Mosby.

958. **4**
Rationale: Severe nipple soreness most often occurs as a result of poor positioning, incorrect latch-on, improper suck, or monilial infection. Comfort measures for nipple soreness include positioning the newborn with the ear, shoulder, and hip in straight alignment and with the baby's stomach against the mother's. Options 1, 2, and 3 do not identify measures that will alleviate the nipple soreness.
Test-Taking Strategy: Use the process of elimination to answer the question. Eliminate options 2 and 3 because they are comparable or alike. From the remaining options, careful reading of option 1 will assist in eliminating this option. Review these measures if you had difficulty with this question.
Level of Cognitive Ability: Application
Client Needs: Health Promotion and Maintenance
Integrated Process: Teaching and Learning
Content Area: Maternity/Postpartum
References: Leifer, G. (2008). *Maternity nursing: An introductory text* (10th ed., p. 219). Philadelphia: Saunders.
Wong, D., Perry, S., Hockenberry, M., Lowdermilk, D., & Wilson, D. (2006). *Maternal child nursing care* (3rd ed., p. 784). St. Louis: Mosby.

959. **1**
Rationale: Agoraphobia is a fear of open spaces (i.e., leaving the house); panic attacks may occur when doing so. Option 2 describes a fear of closed spaces (claustrophobia). Option 3 describes a fear of public speaking (social phobia). Option 4 describes an obsessive-compulsive behavior.
Test-Taking Strategy: Use the process of elimination and focus on the strategic word "agoraphobia." Recalling the definition of agoraphobia will assist in directing you to option 1. If you had difficulty with this question, review the various types of phobias.
Level of Cognitive Ability: Comprehension
Client Needs: Psychosocial Integrity
Integrated Process: Nursing Process/Data Collection
Content Area: Mental Health
References: Keltner, N., Schwecke, L., & Bostrom, C. (2007). *Psychiatric nursing* (5th ed., p. 416). St. Louis: Mosby.
Varcarolis, E., Carlson, V., Shoemaker, N. (2006). *Foundations of psychiatric mental health nursing: A clinical approach* (5th ed., p. 234). Philadelphia: Saunders.

960. **3**
Rationale: In the Orthodox Jewish tradition, members avoid meat from carnivores, pork products, and certain fish.

The nurse would not deliver the food tray to the client and would ask the dietary department to deliver a different meal. Meat and dairy are served separately, thus the dairy-meat combination is not acceptable, making option 2 incorrect. Option 4 is incorrect as pork and pork products are also not allowed in the diet.
Test-Taking Strategy: Use the process of elimination. Recalling that the dairy-meat combination is not acceptable in the Orthodox Jewish tradition will direct you to option 3. Review the dietary rules of this religious group if you had difficulty with this question.
Level of Cognitive Ability: Application
Client Needs: Psychosocial Integrity
Integrated Process: Nursing Process/Implementation
Content Area: Fundamental Skills
References: Nix, S. (2005). *Williams' basic nutrition and diet therapy* (12th ed., p. 249). St. Louis: Mosby.
Potter, P., & Perry, A. (2005). *Fundamentals of nursing* (6th ed., pp. 132-133). St. Louis: Mosby.
Schlenker, E. & Long, S. (2007). *Williams' essentials of nutrition & diet therapy* (9th ed., p. 6). St. Louis: Mosby.

961. **3**
Rationale: When a corneal donor dies, antibiotic eye drops, such as Neosporin or tobramycin may be prescribed and instilled. The eyes are closed and a small ice pack is placed on the closed eyes. The head of the bed is raised to 30 degrees. Within 2 to 4 hours, the eyes are enucleated. The cornea is usually transplanted within 24 to 48 hours. Option 1 is incorrect because dry dressings are not applied. Some organ donation protocols indicate using normal saline moistened gauze. Option 2 is not an immediate action. In addition, the client should have a signed donor card, living will, or an organ donor—identified driver's license stating his or her wishes. Additional legal documentation should not be required.
Test-Taking Strategy: Use the process of elimination. Note that the subject relates to preservation of the corneas and donation of the eyes. This should assist in eliminating options 2 and 4. From the remaining options, recalling that the head of the bed should be elevated will direct you to option 3. Review this procedure if you had difficulty with the question.
Level of Cognitive Ability: Application
Client Needs: Safe and Effective Care Environment
Integrated Process: Nursing Process/Implementation
Content Area: Fundamental Skills
Reference: Ignatavicius, D., & Workman, M.L. (2006). *Medical-surgical nursing: Critical thinking for collaborative care* (5th ed., p. 1092). St. Louis: Saunders.

962. **1**
Rationale: Scopolamine is an anticholinergic medication that causes the frequent side effects of dry mouth, urinary retention, decreased sweating, and dilation of the pupils. The other options describe the opposite effects of cholinergic-blocking agents and therefore are incorrect.
Test-Taking Strategy: Use the process of elimination. Recalling that this medication is an anticholinergic will direct you to option 1. If this medication is unfamiliar to you, review the side effects associated with anticholinergics.
Level of Cognitive Ability: Application

Client Needs: Physiological Integrity
Integrated Process: Nursing Process/Implementation
Content Area: Pharmacology
Reference: Lilley, L., Harrington, S., & Snyder J. (2007). *Pharmacology and the nursing process* (5th ed., pp. 818-819). St. Louis: Mosby.

963. **4**
Rationale: Down syndrome is a form of mental retardation. It is a congenital condition that results in moderate to severe mental retardation. The syndrome has been linked to an extra group G chromosome, chromosome 21 (trisomy 21). Options 1, 2, and 3 are incorrect descriptions.
Test-Taking Strategy: Use the process of elimination. Eliminate options 1 and 2 first because average and above-average intelligence are not associated with this disorder. Eliminate option 3 because deficits in adaptive behavior do occur with Down syndrome. Also, recalling that Down syndrome is associated with an extra chromosome will help direct you to the correct option. Review the characteristics of this syndrome if you had difficulty with this question.
Level of Cognitive Ability: Comprehension
Client Needs: Physiological Integrity
Integrated Process: Nursing Process/Implementation
Content Area: Child Health
References: Price, D., & Gwin, J. (2008). *Pediatric nursing: An introductory text* (10th ed., pp. 109-110). St. Louis: Saunders. Wong, D., Perry, S., Hockenberry, M., Lowdermilk, D., & Wilson, D. (2006). *Maternal child nursing care* (3rd ed., pp. 1259-1260). St. Louis: Mosby.

964. **1**
Rationale: The behaviors identified in the question may be manifested by the client who is contemplating suicide. In client's who are depressed, anger may be self-directed in the form of suicide. Many of these symptoms are those of the depressed client; however, with this client, these behaviors have increased. Hospitalization may actually lessen these symptoms in the depressed client, because a feeling of hope or relief may occur once treatment begins. Dealing with pertinent issues may be traumatic, but this is not the best interpretation of the behavior. Time off the unit for this client could put the client at risk for injury.
Test-Taking Strategy: Use the process of elimination and focus on the client behaviors addressed in the question. Noting the client's diagnosis and the words "becomes more anxious" will direct you to option 1. If you had difficulty with this question, review the characteristics and client behaviors related to suicide.
Level of Cognitive Ability: Analysis
Client Needs: Psychosocial Integrity
Integrated Process: Nursing Process/Data Collection
Content Area: Mental Health
References: Keltner, N., Schwecke, L., & Bostrom, C. (2007). *Psychiatric nursing* (5th ed., pp. 379;385). St. Louis: Mosby. Varcarolis, E., Carlson, V., Shoemaker, N. (2006). *Foundations of psychiatric mental health nursing: A clinical approach* (5th ed., pp. 335-336). St. Louis: Saunders.

965. **1**
Rationale: A serum potassium level below 3.5 mEq/L is indicative of hypokalemia. Potassium deficit is the most common

electrolyte imbalance and is potentially life-threatening. Cardiac changes with hypokalemia may include peaked P waves, flattened T waves, depressed ST segment, and the presence of U waves.
Test-Taking Strategy: Use the process of elimination. From the information in the question, you need to determine that this client is experiencing hypokalemia. From this point, it is necessary to know the cardiac changes that are expected when hypokalemia exists. Options 2, 3, and 4 are all characteristic cardiac changes noted with hyperkalemia. Review these cardiac effects if you had difficulty with this question.
Level of Cognitive Ability: Analysis
Client Needs: Physiological Integrity
Integrated Process: Nursing Process/Data Collection
Content Area: Fundamental Skills
References: deWit, S. (2009). *Medical-surgical nursing: Concepts & practice* (pp. 46;48). St. Louis: Saunders.
Monahan, F., Sands, J., Marek, J., Neighbors, M., Marek, J., & Green, C. (2007). *Phipps' medical-surgical nursing: Health and illness perspectives* (8th ed., p. 376). St. Louis: Mosby.

966. **3**
Rationale: The normal serum ammonia level is 35 to 65 mcg/dL. In the client with hepatic encephalopathy, the serum level is not likely to drop below normal. The most optimal yet realistic change from the options provided would be to 40 mcg/dL, which falls in the normal range. A level of 80 mcg/dL represents an insufficient effect of the medication. Lactulose is administered for its hyperosmotic laxative effect, thus removing ammonia from the colon. The client should also be monitored for hypokalemia due to the severe purging lactulose causes.
Test-Taking Strategy: Familiarity with the normal serum ammonia level is needed to answer this question. It is also necessary to understand the association between hepatic encephalopathy and this laboratory value. Recalling that the normal level is 35 to 65 mcg/dL will direct you to option 3. Review this test and the desirable effects of this medication if you had difficulty with this question.
Level of Cognitive Ability: Analysis
Client Needs: Physiological Integrity
Integrated Process: Nursing Process/Data Collection
Content Area: Adult Health/Gastrointestinal
Reference: Pagana, K., & Pagana, T. (2005). *Mosby's diagnostic and laboratory test reference* (7th ed., pp. 52-53). St. Louis: Mosby.

967. **4**
Rationale: Ineffective cerebral tissue perfusion is the priority problem for the child with meningitis. Pain related to meningeal irritation may also be an appropriate problem, but is not the priority. There are no data in the question to indicate that options 2 and 3 are a problem.
Test-Taking Strategy: Use Maslow's Hierarchy of Needs theory to assist in eliminating options 2 and 3 because they are psychosocial problems. Next, use the ABCs—airway, breathing, and circulation—to direct you to option 4. Tissue perfusion relates to circulation. Review care of the child with meningitis if you had difficulty with this question.
Level of Cognitive Ability: Analysis
Client Needs: Physiological Integrity

Integrated Process: Nursing Process/Planning
Content Area: Child Health
References: Leifer, G. (2007). *Introduction to maternity and pediatric nursing* (5th ed., pp. 530-531). Philadelphia: Saunders. Wong, D., Perry, S., Hockenberry, M., Lowdermilk, D., & Wilson, D. (2006). *Maternal child nursing care* (3rd ed., p. 1699). St. Louis: Mosby.

968. 4
Rationale: In a postoperative client, a concern related to initiating a diet is aspiration. Initiating postoperative oral fluids may lead to distention and vomiting. Suction equipment must be available. A cardiac monitor and a code cart are unnecessary. A straw may help the client sip fluids, but is not necessary.
Test-Taking Strategy: Note the strategic words "postoperative" and "priority." Use the ABCs—airway, breathing, and circulation—to answer this question. Option 4 will maintain airway clearance. If you had difficulty with this question, review care to the postoperative client.
Level of Cognitive Ability: Application
Client Needs: Physiological Integrity
Integrated Process: Nursing Process/Planning
Content Area: Fundamental Skills
References: deWit, S. (2009). *Medical-surgical nursing: Concepts & practice* (pp. 94-95). St. Louis: Saunders. Potter, P., & Perry, A. (2005). *Fundamentals of nursing* (6th ed., p. 1640). St. Louis: Mosby.

969. 4
Rationale: Ethambutol causes optic neuritis, which decreases visual acuity and the ability to discriminate between the colors red and green. This poses a potential safety hazard when driving a motor vehicle. The client is taught to report this symptom immediately. The client is also taught to take the medication with food if gastrointestinal upset occurs. Impaired hearing results from antitubercular therapy with streptomycin. Orange-red discoloration of secretions occurs with rifampin (Rifadin).
Test-Taking Strategy: Use the process of elimination. Option 2 is the least likely symptom to report; rather, it should be managed by taking the medication with food. Thus, this option can be eliminated first. From the remaining options, it is necessary to know that ethambutol may cause optic neuritis and difficulty with red-green discrimination. If this question was difficult, review the side effects of this medication.
Level of Cognitive Ability: Analysis
Client Needs: Physiological Integrity
Integrated Process: Nursing Process/Evaluation
Content Area: Adult Health/Respiratory
References: Hodgson, B., & Kizior, R. (2008). *Saunders nursing drug handbook 2008* (pp. 453-454). Philadelphia: Saunders. Lehne, R. (2007). *Pharmacology for nursing care* (6th ed., p. 1028). Philadelphia: Saunders.

970. 4
Rationale: The client with myasthenia gravis should be taught that timing of anticholinesterase medication is critical. It is important to instruct the client to administer the medication on time to maintain a chemical balance at the neuromuscular junction. If not given on time, the client may become too

weak to swallow. Options 1, 2, and 3 include the necessary information that the client needs to understand to maintain health with this neurological degenerative disease.
Test-Taking Strategy: Use the process of elimination and note the strategic words "further teaching is necessary." These words indicate a negative event query and the need to select the incorrect client statement. Basic principles related to medication administration will direct you to option 4. Remember, clients should not adjust dosage and medication times. If you had difficulty with this question, review the guidelines related to medication administration.
Level of Cognitive Ability: Analysis
Client Needs: Physiological Integrity
Integrated Process: Teaching and Learning
Content Area: Adult Health/Neurological
References: deWit, S. (2009). *Medical-surgical nursing: Concepts & practice* (p. 607). St. Louis: Saunders. Ignatavicius, D., & Workman, M.L. (2006). *Medical-surgical nursing: Critical thinking for collaborative care* (5th ed., p. 1017). Philadelphia: Saunders. Wold, G. (2008). *Basic geriatric nursing* (4th ed.. pp. 120-123). St. Louis: Mosby.

971. 1, 3, 6
Rationale: During a seizure, the child is placed on his or her side in a lateral position. Positioning on the side will prevent aspiration because saliva will drain out of the corner of the child's mouth. The child is not restrained because this could cause injury to the child. The nurse would loosen clothing around the child's neck and ensure a patent airway. Nothing is placed into the child's mouth during a seizure because this action may cause injury to the child's mouth, gums, or teeth. The nurse would stay with the child to reduce the risk of injury and allow for observation and timing of the seizure.
Test-Taking Strategy: Visualize this clinical situation. Recalling that airway patency and safety is the priority will assist in determining the appropriate interventions. Review care for the child experiencing a seizure if you had difficulty with this question.
Level of Cognitive Ability: Application
Client Needs: Physiological Integrity
Integrated Process: Nursing Process/Implementation
Content Area: Child Health
Reference: Price, D., & Gwin, J. (2008). *Pediatric nursing: An introductory text* (10th ed., p. 252). St. Louis: Saunders.

972. 0.7
Rationale: Use the medication calculation formula and note the prescribed (35 mg) and available doses (50 mg/mL). Formula:

$$\frac{\text{Desired}}{\text{Available}} \times 1\,\text{mL} = \text{mL per dose}$$

$$\frac{35\,\text{mg}}{50\,\text{mg}} \times 1\,\text{mL} = 0.7\,\text{mL}$$

Test-Taking Strategy: Follow the formula for the calculation of the correct dose, noting the prescribed dose and the available dose. Note that the prescribed dose is a smaller amount than the dose available. This indicates that the

amount to be given will be less than 1 mL. Once you have done the calculation, use a calculator to verify the answer. If you had difficulty with this question, review medication calculation problems.
Level of Cognitive Ability: Application
Client Needs: Physiological Integrity
Integrated Process: Nursing Process/Implementation
Content Area: Fundamental Skills
Reference: Ogden, S. J. (2007). *Calculation of drug dosages* (8th ed., pp. 265-266). St. Louis: Mosby.

973. **2520**
Rationale: The client consumed a total of 84 oz of fluid. Because 1 oz is equal to 30 mL, multiply 84 oz by 30 mL/oz. This yields 2520 mL.
Test-Taking Strategy: Focus on the subject—the total milliliters that the client consumed in a 24-hour period. Recalling that 1 oz equals 30 mL will assist in answering the question. Use a calculator to verify the amount. Review the procedure for changing ounces to milliliters if you had difficulty with this question.
Level of Cognitive Ability: Comprehension
Client Needs: Physiological Integrity
Integrated Process: Nursing Process/Data Collection
Content Area: Fundamental Skills
References: Ogden, S. J. (2007). *Calculation of drug dosages* (8th ed., p. 125). St. Louis: Mosby.
Potter, P., & Perry, A. (2005). *Fundamentals of nursing* (6th ed., pp. 1149-1152). St. Louis: Mosby.

974. **4**
Rationale: β-Adrenergic blocking agents, such as atenolol, inhibit the appearance of signs and symptoms of acute hypoglycemia, which would include nervousness, increased heart rate, and sweating. Therefore, the client receiving this medication should adhere to the therapeutic regimen and monitor blood glucose levels carefully. Option 4 is the most reliable indicator of hypoglycemia.
Test-Taking Strategy: Note the strategic words "most reliable" in the question. This indicates that more than one option could be partially or completely correct. Each option is, in fact, an indicator of hypoglycemia. Recalling the masking effects of β-adrenergic blocking agents helps you to choose the blood glucose level as the most reliable indicator. Review this medication if you had difficulty with this question.
Level of Cognitive Ability: Comprehension
Client Needs: Physiological Integrity
Integrated Process: Nursing Process/Data Collection
Content Area: Pharmacology
Reference: Hodgson, B., & Kizior, R. (2008). *Saunders nursing drug handbook 2008* (p. 32). Philadelphia: Saunders.

975. **17**
Rationale: The formula and calculation for this IV flow rate is:

$$gtt/minute = \frac{Volume\,(mL) \times drop\,factor\,(gtt/mL)}{Time\,(in\,minutes)}$$
$$= \frac{50\,mL \times 10\,gtt/mL}{30\,minutes} = \frac{500}{30} = 16.66, \text{ or } 17\,gtt/minute$$

Test-Taking Strategy: To calculate the answer to this question correctly, you must be familiar with the standard formula for calculating IV flow rates. Use the formula and check your answer with a calculator. Remember to round to the nearest whole number. Review this formula if you had difficulty with this question.
Level of Cognitive Ability: Application
Client Needs: Physiological Integrity
Integrated Process: Nursing Process/Implementation
Content Area: Fundamental Skills
Reference: Ogden, S. J. (2007). *Calculation of drug dosages* (8th ed., p. 346). St. Louis: Mosby.

976. **2**
Rationale: Sclerotic lesions occur as bone resorption increases and results in replacement of original bone with fibrous material. This condition occurs in Paget's disease, an age-related disorder. Options 1, 3, and 4 identify normal age-related changes in the musculoskeletal system.
Test-Taking Strategy: Use the process of elimination. Note the strategic words "potential complication." Recalling the normal age-related musculoskeletal findings will assist in directing you to the correct option. Review these normal findings and those that indicate a complication if you had difficulty with this question.
Level of Cognitive Ability: Comprehension
Client Needs: Physiological Integrity
Integrated Process: Nursing Process/Data Collection
Content Area: Adult Health/Musculoskeletal
Reference: Wold, G. (2008). *Basic geriatric nursing* (4th ed., pp. 36-37). St. Louis: Mosby.

977. **4**
Rationale: The vomiting that occurs in Reye's syndrome is caused by cerebral edema and is a symptom of intracranial pressure. Small, frequent meals will not affect the amount of vomiting, and the physician is notified if vomiting occurs. Options 1, 2, and 3 are all correct statements. Decreasing stimuli and providing rest decrease stress on the brain tissue. Checking for jaundice will assist in identifying the presence of liver complications, which are characteristic of Reye's syndrome.
Test-Taking Strategy: Note the strategic words "need for further instruction." These words indicate a negative event query and the need to select the incorrect client statement. Recalling the causes of vomiting with Reye's syndrome will direct you to option 4. Review the pathophysiology associated with Reye's syndrome if you had difficulty with this question.
Level of Cognitive Ability: Comprehension
Client Needs: Physiological Integrity
Integrated Process: Teaching and Learning
Content Area: Child Health
References: Price, D., & Gwin, J. (2008). *Pediatric nursing: An introductory text* (10th ed., p. 163). St. Louis: Saunders.
Wong, D., Perry, S., Hockenberry, M., Lowdermilk, D., & Wilson, D. (2006). *Maternal child nursing care* (3rd ed. pp. 1701-1702). St. Louis: Mosby.

978. **10**
Rationale: Follow the formula for dosage calculation.
Formula:

$$\frac{Desired}{Available} \times mL = mL\,per\,dose$$
$$\frac{20\,mEq}{30\,mEq} \times 15\,mL = 10\,mL$$

Test-Taking Strategy: Follow the formula for the calculation of the correct dose and focus on the key information, 30 mEq/15 mL. Verify the answer with a calculator. Review medication calculations if you had difficulty with this question.
Level of Cognitive Ability: Application
Client Needs: Physiological Integrity
Integrated Process: Nursing Process/Planning
Content Area: Fundamental Skills
Reference: Ogden, S. J. (2007). *Calculation of drug dosages* (8th ed. p. 346). St. Louis: Mosby.

979. 4
Rationale: Nizatidine, a histamine H_2-receptor blocker, is frequently used in the management of peptic ulcer disease. Histamine H_2-receptor blockers decrease the secretion of gastric acid (HCL). Antacids are used as adjunct therapy and neutralize acid in the stomach. Omeprazole is a proton pump inhibitor. Sucralfate (Carafate) promotes healing by covering the ulcer, thus protecting it from erosion caused by gastric acids.
Test-Taking Strategy: Focus on the pathophysiology associated with peptic ulcer disease. Next, recalling the actions of the medications in the options will direct you to option 4. If you are unfamiliar with these medications or their actions, review this content.
Level of Cognitive Ability: Analysis
Client Needs: Physiological Integrity
Integrated Process: Nursing Process/Evaluation
Content Area: Adult Health/Gastrointestinal
Reference: Linton, A., & Maebius, N. (2007). *Introduction to medical-surgical nursing* (4th ed., p. 766). Philadelphia: Saunders.

980. 2
Rationale: A depressed person suffers with depressed mood and is often withdrawn. Also, the person experiences difficulty concentrating, loss of interest or pleasure, low energy, fatigue, and feelings of worthlessness and poor self-esteem. The plan of care needs to provide successful experiences in a stimulating yet structured environment.
Test-Taking Strategy: Use the process of elimination. Options 1 and 4 are eliminated first because they are too restrictive and offer little or no structure and stimulation. Option 3 is eliminated next because of the word "insist" and the close-ended word "all" in this option. Review care of the client with depression if you had difficulty with this question.
Level of Cognitive Ability: Application
Client Needs: Psychosocial Integrity
Integrated Process: Nursing Process/Planning
Content Area: Mental Health
References: Fortinash, K., & Holoday-Worret, P. (2008). *Psychiatric mental health nursing* (4th ed., p. 357). St. Louis: Mosby.
Stuart, G., & Laraia, M. (2005). *Principles and practice of psychiatric nursing* (8th ed., p. 351). St. Louis: Mosby.

981. 4
Rationale: Mealtimes should center on pleasurable socialization. The child should be encouraged to eat meals with other children on the unit. A diet that is normal in protein with a sodium restriction is normally prescribed for a child with nephrotic syndrome. Parents or other family members should be encouraged to be present at mealtimes with a hospitalized child.
Test-Taking Strategy: Use the process of elimination. Eliminate options 1 and 2 first. A diet that is normal in protein with a sodium restriction is normally prescribed. Option 3 diminishes the importance of socialization at mealtime. This leaves option 4 as the correct option. Review dietary recommendations for the child with nephrotic syndrome if you had difficulty with this question.
Level of Cognitive Ability: Application
Client Needs: Physiological Integrity
Integrated Process: Nursing Process/Planning
Content Area: Child Health
References: Price, D., & Gwin, J. (2008). *Pediatric nursing: An introductory text* (10th ed., p. 259). St. Louis: Saunders.
Wong, D., Perry, S., Hockenberry, M., Lowdermilk, D., & Wilson, D. (2006). *Maternal child nursing care* (3rd ed., pp. 1372-1373). St. Louis: Mosby.

982. 2
Rationale: Cushing's syndrome is characterized by an oversecretion of glucocorticoid hormones. Addison's disease is characterized by the failure of the adrenal cortex to produce and secrete adrenocortical hormones. Options 1 and 4 are inaccurate regarding Cushing's syndrome.
Test-Taking Strategy: Use the process of elimination. Options 1 and 4 can be eliminated first because they are not associated with Cushing's syndrome. Remembering that in Cushing's ("u" as in "up") syndrome there is an oversecretion and in Addison's ("d" as in "down") there is an undersecretion will direct you to option 2. Review this disorder if you had difficulty with this question.
Level of Cognitive Ability: Comprehension
Client Needs: Physiological Integrity
Integrated Process: Teaching and Learning
Content Area: Adult Health/Endocrine
Reference: Linton, A., & Maebius, N. (2007). *Introduction to medical-surgical nursing* (4th ed., p. 973). Philadelphia: Saunders.

983. 1
Rationale: Ovulation ceases during pregnancy because the circulating levels of estrogen and progesterone are high, thus inhibiting the release of follicle-stimulating hormone and luteinizing hormone, which are necessary for ovulation. Options 2, 3, and 4 are incorrect.
Test-Taking Strategy: Knowledge regarding the hormonal changes that occur during the menstrual cycle and during pregnancy is required to answer this question. Remember, ovulation ceases during pregnancy because the circulating levels of estrogen and progesterone are high. Review these hormonal changes if you had difficulty with this question.
Level of Cognitive Ability: Comprehension
Client Needs: Physiological Integrity
Integrated Process: Teaching and Learning
Content Area: Maternity/Antepartum
References: Leifer, G. (2007). *Introduction to maternity and pediatric nursing* (5th ed., p. 51). Philadelphia: Saunders.
Wong, D., Perry, S., Hockenberry, M., Lowdermilk, D., & Wilson, D. (2006). *Maternal child nursing care* (3rd ed., p. 238). St. Louis: Mosby.

984. 1

Rationale: Parents are especially concerned about seizures that might go undetected at night time. The nurse should suggest a baby monitor. Reassurance by the nurse should ensure parental confidence and decrease parental overprotection. Option 2 is a common concern. Options 3 and 4 demonstrate the parents' ability to choose respite care and activities appropriately. The parents need to be reminded that, as the child grows, they cannot always observe their child, but that their knowledge of seizure activity and care are appropriate to minimize complications.

Test-Taking Strategy: Use the process of elimination and note the strategic words "need for further teaching." These words indicate a negative event query and the need to select the incorrect client statement. Option 1 identifies a need to provide the parents with an alternative method to monitor for night seizures. Review parent teaching regarding seizures if you had difficulty with this question.

Level of Cognitive Ability: Comprehension
Client Needs: Psychosocial Integrity
Integrated Process: Teaching and Learning
Content Area: Child Health
References: Price, D., & Gwin, J. (2008). *Pediatric nursing: An introductory text* (10th ed., p. 256). St. Louis: Saunders.
Wong, D., Perry, S., Hockenberry, M., Lowdermilk, D., & Wilson, D. (2006). *Maternal child nursing care* (3rd ed., pp. 1710-1711). St. Louis: Mosby.

985. 3

Rationale: Zollinger-Ellison syndrome is a hypersecretory condition of the stomach. The client should avoid taking medications that are irritating to the stomach lining. Irritants would include aspirin and nonsteroidal anti-inflammatory drugs (Naprosyn, ibuprofen). The client should be advised to take acetaminophen for headache.

Test-Taking Strategy: Use the process of elimination. Remember that options that are comparable or alike are not likely to be correct. With this in mind, eliminate options 1 and 2 first. Choose acetaminophen over aspirin because it is least irritating to the stomach. Review this medication and this disorder if you had difficulty with this question.

Level of Cognitive Ability: Application
Client Needs: Physiological Integrity
Integrated Process: Nursing Process/Implementation
Content Area: Pharmacology
Reference: Lehne, R. (2007). *Pharmacology for nursing care* (6th ed., p. 902). Philadelphia: Saunders.

986. 3

Rationale: Feelings of low self-esteem and worthlessness are common symptoms of the depressed client. An effective plan of care is to provide successful experiences for the client that are challenging but will not be met with failure to enhance the client's personal self-esteem. Reminders of the client's past accomplishments or personal successes are ways to interrupt the client's negative self-talk and distorted cognitive view of themselves. Options 1 and 4 offer false reassurance. Option 2 is not a therapeutic intervention with a depressed client.

Test-Taking Strategy: Use the process of elimination and therapeutic communication techniques. Eliminate options

1 and 4 because the nurse is offering an opinion and false reassurance. Eliminate option 2 because, in this situation, silence can be interpreted as agreeing with the client's feelings. Review care of the client with depression if you had difficulty with this question.

Level of Cognitive Ability: Application
Client Needs: Psychosocial Integrity
Integrated Process: Nursing Process/Implementation
Content Area: Mental Health
References: Fortinash, K., & Holoday-Worret, P. (2008). *Psychiatric mental health nursing* (4th ed., p. 358). St. Louis: Mosby.
Varcarolis, E., Carlson, V., & Shoemaker, N. (2006). *Foundations of psychiatric mental health nursing: A clinical approach* (5th ed., p. 340). St. Louis: Saunders.

987. 3

Rationale: Cryptorchidism may be the result of hormone deficiency, intrinsic abnormality of a testis, or a structural problem. Diagnostic tests would assess kidney function, because the kidneys and testes arise from the same germ tissue. Babinski's reflex tests neurological function and is unrelated to this diagnosis. DNA synthesis and a chromosomal analysis are also unrelated to this diagnosis.

Test-Taking Strategy: Use the process of elimination and knowledge regarding the anatomical occurrence of cryptorchidism. Cryptorchidism, undescended or hidden testicles, relates to the genitourinary system. Option 2 relates to neurological function. Options 1 and 4 relate to the structure of cells. Option 3 is the only option that relates to the genitourinary system. Review this disorder if you had difficulty with this question.

Level of Cognitive Ability: Comprehension
Client Needs: Physiological Integrity
Integrated Process: Nursing Process/Planning
Content Area: Child Health
References: Leifer, G. (2007). *Introduction to maternity and pediatric nursing* (5th ed., pp. 671-672). Philadelphia: Saunders.
Wong, D., Perry, S., Hockenberry, M., Lowdermilk, D., & Wilson, D. (2006). *Maternal child nursing care* (3rd ed. p. 1653). St. Louis: Mosby.

988. 3

Rationale: A hallmark sign of pemphigus is Nikolsky's sign. Nikolsky's sign is when the epidermis can be rubbed off by slight friction or injury. Homans' sign, a sign of thrombosis in the leg, is discomfort in the calf on forced dorsiflexion of the foot. Chvostek's sign, seen in tetany, is a spasm of the facial muscles elicited by tapping the facial nerve in the region of the parotid gland. Trousseau's sign is a sign for tetany, in which carpal spasm can be elicited by compressing the upper arm and causing ischemia to the nerves distally.

Test-Taking Strategy: Use the process of elimination. If you knew that Homans' sign was related to thrombophlebitis and that Chvostek's sign and Trousseau's sign are related to tetany, then, by the process of elimination, you would select option 3. If you had difficulty with this question, review these various signs.

Level of Cognitive Ability: Comprehension
Client Needs: Physiological Integrity
Integrated Process: Nursing Process/Data Collection
Content Area: Adult Health/Integumentary
Reference: Monahan, F., Sands, J., Neighbors, M., Marek, J., & Green, C. (2007). *Phipps' medical-surgical nursing: Health and illness perspectives* (8th ed., p. 1890). St. Louis: Mosby.

989. 2
Rationale: The exact cause of acne is unknown. Exacerbations that coincide with the menstrual cycle result from hormonal activity. Oily skin alone is not the cause of acne. Heat, humidity, and excessive perspiration also play a role in exacerbation of acne. There is no evidence that consumption of foods such as chocolate, nuts, or fatty foods affects acne.
Test-Taking Strategy: Use the process of elimination. Note the strategic words, "most appropriately" and focus on the subject—the causes of acne. Options 1, 3, and 4 are not causes of acne. Review this disorder and its causes if you had difficulty with this question.
Level of Cognitive Ability: Application
Client Needs: Physiological Integrity
Integrated Process: Nursing Process/Implementation
Content Area: Adult Health/Integumentary
Reference: Christensen, B., & Kockrow, E. (2006). *Adult health nursing* (5th ed., p. 90). St. Louis: Mosby.

990. 2
Rationale: The jaw thrust without the head-tilt maneuver is used when neck trauma is suspected. This maneuver opens the airway while maintaining proper head and neck alignment, thus reducing the risk of further damage to the neck. Option 1 is incorrect. In situations requiring CPR, the client will be unconscious. Option 4 is also incorrect. In addition, it is unlikely that the nurse will be able to obtain these data.
Test-Taking Strategy: Focus on the data in the question. Eliminate option 3 because of the close-ended word "all." Noting that the client requires CPR will assist in eliminating options 1 and 4. Review CPR guidelines and the various test-taking strategies if you had difficulty with this question.
Level of Cognitive Ability: Application
Client Needs: Physiological Integrity
Integrated Process: Nursing Process/Implementation
Content Area: Adult Health/Cardiovascular
Reference: deWit, S. (2009). *Medical-surgical nursing: Concepts & practice* (pp. 1086-1087). St. Louis: Saunders.

991. 4
Rationale: At 12 weeks' gestation, the uterus extends out of the maternal pelvis and can be palpated above the symphysis pubis. At 16 weeks, the fundus reaches midway between the symphysis pubis and the umbilicus. At 20 weeks, the fundus is located at the umbilicus. By 36 weeks, the fundus reaches its highest level at the xiphoid process.
Test-Taking Strategy: Knowledge regarding the patterns of uterine growth is required to answer this question. Focus on the weeks of gestation identified in the question to assist in directing you to the correct option. Review this uterine growth pattern if you had difficulty with this question.
Level of Cognitive Ability: Comprehension
Client Needs: Physiological Integrity

Integrated Process: Nursing Process/Data Collection
Content Area: Maternity/Antepartum
References: Leifer, G. (2007). *Introduction to maternity and pediatric nursing* (5th ed., p. 80). Philadelphia: Saunders.
Wong, D., Perry, S., Hockenberry, M., Lowdermilk, D., & Wilson, D. (2006). *Maternal child nursing care* (3rd ed., p. 238). St. Louis: Mosby.

992. 2
Rationale: In a compound (open) fracture, a wound in the skin leads to the broken bone, and there is an added danger of infection. Option 1 describes a transverse fracture. Option 3 describes a greenstick fracture. Option 4 describes a closed or simple fracture.
Test-Taking Strategy: Use the process of elimination. Noting the strategic word "open" will assist in directing you to option 2. Review the various types of fractures if you had difficulty with this question.
Level of Cognitive Ability: Comprehension
Client Needs: Physiological Integrity
Integrated Process: Nursing Process/Planning
Content Area: Child Health
References: Price, D., & Gwin, J. (2008). *Pediatric nursing: An introductory text* (10th ed., p. 202). St. Louis: Saunders.
Wong, D., Perry, S., Hockenberry, M., Lowdermilk, D., & Wilson, D. (2006). *Maternal child nursing care* (3rd ed. p. 1807). St. Louis: Mosby.

993. 1
Rationale: Clubfoot, one of the most common deformities of the skeletal system, is a congenital anomaly characterized by a foot that has been twisted inward or outward. The condition generally affects both feet, and boys are affected twice as often as girls.
Test-Taking Strategy: Use the process of elimination. Eliminate option 4 because of the word "rare" and option 2 because of the word "always." From the remaining options, it is necessary to know that this disorder is a congenital anomaly. Review this disorder if you had difficulty with this question.
Level of Cognitive Ability: Comprehension
Client Needs: Physiological Integrity
Integrated Process: Nursing Process/Planning
Content Area: Child Health
References: Price, D., & Gwin, J. (2008). *Pediatric nursing: An introductory text* (10th ed., pp. 106-107). St. Louis: Saunders.
Wong, D., Perry, S., Hockenberry, M., Lowdermilk, D., & Wilson, D. (2006). *Maternal child nursing care* (3rd ed., p. 1820). St. Louis: Mosby.

994. 3
Rationale: A blood glucose test performed before exercising provides information to the client regarding the need to eat a snack first. Exercising during the peak times of insulin effect or prior to mealtime places the client at risk for hypoglycemia. Insulin should be administered as prescribed.
Test-Taking Strategy: The subject of the question relates to the occurrence of a hypoglycemic reaction. Use the process of elimination, keeping in mind this subject and the effects of insulin and exercise on the blood glucose level. You should easily be able to eliminate options 1, 2, and 4. Review the effects of exercise if you had difficulty with this question.

Level of Cognitive Ability: Application
Client Needs: Health Promotion and Maintenance
Integrated Process: Teaching and Learning
Content Area: Adult Health/Endocrine
Reference: Linton, A., & Maebius, N. (2007). *Introduction to medical-surgical nursing* (4th ed., pp. 1010-1011). Philadelphia: Saunders.

995. 3
Rationale: The clinical signs of impending or approaching death include inability to swallow; pitting edema; decreased gastrointestinal and urinary tract activity; bowel and bladder incontinence; loss of motion, sensation, and reflexes; cold or clammy skin; cyanosis; lowered blood pressure; noisy or irregular respiration; and Cheyne-Stokes respirations.
Test-Taking Strategy: Use the process of elimination and eliminate options 2 and 4 because these identify normal findings. Eliminate option 1 because it does not identify signs of approaching death. If you had difficulty with this question, review the signs associated with impending or approaching death.
Level of Cognitive Ability: Comprehension
Client Needs: Physiological Integrity
Integrated Process: Nursing Process/Data Collection
Content Area: Fundamental Skills
Reference: Wold, G. (2008). *Basic geriatric nursing* (4th ed., p. 240). St. Louis: Mosby.

996. 1
Rationale: Used tissues are discarded in a plastic bag, so contaminated respiratory secretions can be contained. The client with tuberculosis should wash hands carefully after each contact with respiratory secretions. Oral care should be performed more than once a day. The client should be instructed to cover the mouth and nose when laughing, sneezing, or coughing and to wear a mask when in contact with others until drug therapy suppresses the infection.
Test-Taking Strategy: Use the process of elimination. Note that the question specifically relates to information about handling and disposal of secretions. The only options that address this topic directly are options 1 and 4. Because turning the head to the side for coughing and sneezing does not specifically address the handling of secretions, eliminate option 4. Disposal of tissues in a plastic bag is correct. Review home care instructions related to tuberculosis if you had difficulty with this question.
Level of Cognitive Ability: Comprehension
Client Needs: Safe and Effective Care Environment
Integrated Process: Nursing Process/Evaluation
Content Area: Adult Health/Respiratory
References: deWit, S. (2009). *Medical-surgical nursing: Concepts & practice* (p. 327). St. Louis: Saunders.
Ignatavicius, D., & Workman, M.L. (2006). *Medical-surgical nursing: Critical thinking for collaborative care* (5th ed., p. 644). Philadelphia: Saunders.

997. 2
Rationale: A common side effect of INH is peripheral neuritis. This is manifested by numbness, tingling, and paresthesias in the extremities. This side effect can be minimized with pyridoxine (vitamin B_6) intake.

Test-Taking Strategy: Use the process of elimination. Options 3 and 4 would not cause the signs and symptoms presented in the question, but instead would be manifested by pallor and coolness. Thus, options 3 and 4 can be eliminated first. From the remaining options, it is necessary to know either that peripheral neuritis is a side effect of the medication or that these signs and symptoms do not correlate with hypercalcemia. Review the side effects associated with isoniazid if you had difficulty with this question.
Level of Cognitive Ability: Analysis
Client Needs: Physiological Integrity
Integrated Process: Nursing Process/Data Collection
Content Area: Adult Health/Respiratory
Reference: Lehne, R. (2007). *Pharmacology for nursing care* (6th ed., p. 1020). Philadelphia: Saunders.

998. 2
Rationale: It is important to give the mother information that addresses the issue that is the parent's concern. Most children experience remission with treatment. Options 1 and 3 are nontherapeutic and may add to the mother's guilt. Option 4 does not acknowledge the concern and is a stereotypical response.
Test-Taking Strategy: Use therapeutic communication techniques and focus on the mother's concern. Options 1, 3, and 4 do not address the mother's concern and are inappropriate and nontherapeutic responses. Remember, always address the mother's feelings and concerns. Review this disorder and therapeutic communication techniques if you had difficulty with this question.
Level of Cognitive Ability: Application
Client Needs: Physiological Integrity
Integrated Process: Communication and Documentation
Content Area: Child Health
References: Price, D., & Gwin, J. (2008). *Pediatric nursing: An introductory text* (10th ed., pp. 259-260). St. Louis: Saunders. Wong, D., Perry, S., Hockenberry, M., Lowdermilk, D., & Wilson, D. (2006). *Maternal child nursing care* (3rd ed., p. 1655). St. Louis: Mosby.

999. 2
Rationale: Clinical manifestations of COPD include hypoxemia, hypercapnia, dyspnea on exertion and at rest, oxygen desaturation with exercise, use of accessory muscles of respiration, and a prolonged expiratory phase of respiration. The chest x-ray will reveal a hyperinflated chest and a flattened diaphragm if the disease is advanced.
Test-Taking Strategy: Use the process of elimination. Eliminate option 3 because oxygen desaturation rather than saturation would occur. Next, eliminate option 4 because, in the client with COPD, a prolonged expiratory phase of respiration would be noted. From the remaining options, reading carefully will assist in directing you to option 2 as the correct option. If you are unfamiliar with the manifestations associated with COPD, review this content.
Level of Cognitive Ability: Comprehension
Client Needs: Physiological Integrity
Integrated Process: Nursing Process/Data Collection
Content Area: Adult Health/Respiratory
References: Ignatavicius, D., & Workman, M. L. (2006). *Medical-surgical nursing: Critical thinking for collaborative care* (5th ed., pp. 596-598). Philadelphia: Saunders.

Linton, A., & Maebius, N. (2007). *Introduction to medical-surgical nursing* (4th ed., pp. 558-559). Philadelphia: Saunders.

1000. 1, 3, 4, 6
Rationale: The administration of an enema is a clean procedure and standard precautions must be used. The nurse applies disposable gloves when administering an enema to prevent the transfer of microorganisms. To administer an enema, the nurse places the client in the left Sims' position because the enema solution will flow downward by gravity along the natural curve of the sigmoid colon and rectum, improving retention of the enema solution. The tube is lubricated for easy insertion and is inserted approximately 3 to 4 inches in an adult. If the client complains of cramping or discomfort during the procedure, the nurse clamps the tubing until the discomfort subsides. The container containing the enema solution is hung about 12 to 18 inches above the client's anus. A flow of solution that is too forceful can damage the bowel. The temperature of the solution should be between 100° F (37.8° C) and 105° F (40.5° C). Solution that is too hot will burn the client, and solution that is too cool will cause cramping.
Test-Taking Strategy: Visualize the procedure for administering an enema. Thinking about the anatomy of the bowel and the precautions that need to be taken to prevent trauma to rectal tissue will assist in identifying the correct interventions. Review the procedure for administering an enema if you had difficulty with this question.
Level of Cognitive Ability: Application
Client Needs: Physiological Integrity
Integrated Process: Nursing Process/Implementation
Content Area: Fundamental Skills
References: Christensen, B., & Kockrow, E. (2006). *Foundations of nursing* (5th ed., pp. 598-599). St. Louis: Mosby.
Potter, P., & Perry, A. (2005). *Fundamentals of nursing* (6th ed., pp. 1399-1402). St. Louis: Mosby.

1001. 1, 2, 3, 5
Rationale: A client who is aphasic has difficulty expressing or understanding language. The nurse would face the client when talking, establish and maintain eye contact, and speak slowly and distinctly. The nurse should use gestures and pantomime when talking to enhance words and use body language to enhance the message. The nurse would give the client directions using short phrases and simple terms, and phrase questions so that they can be answered with a yes or no. If there is a need to repeat something, the nurse should use the same words a second time.
Test-Taking Strategy: Recall that a client who is aphasic has difficulty expressing or understanding language. Using the principles related to communicating to a hearing-impaired client will assist in identifying the correct interventions. Review the guidelines for communicating with an aphasic client if you had difficulty with this question.
Level of Cognitive Ability: Application
Client Needs: Physiological Integrity
Integrated Process: Communication and Documentation
Content Area: Fundamental Skills
References: Ignatavicius, D., & Workman, M. L. (2006). *Medical-surgical nursing: Critical thinking for collaborative care* (5th ed., p. 1042). Philadelphia: Saunders.

Linton, A., & Maebius, N. (2007). *Introduction to medical-surgical nursing* (4th ed., pp. 478;480). Philadelphia: Saunders.
Potter, P., & Perry, A. (2005). *Fundamentals of nursing* (6th ed., p. 1585). St. Louis: Mosby.

1002. 4
Rationale: After the nasogastric tube is in place, mouth care is extremely important. With one naris occluded, the client tends to mouth breathe, drying the mucous membranes. Frequent oral hygiene may be required to prevent or care for dry, irritated mucous membranes. Frequent small sips of water would be contraindicated when the client is on gastric suction. The hard candy would increase the salivation but would not be useful in cleaning the oral cavity. Lemon glycerin swabs have a drying or irritating effect on the mucous membranes.
Test-Taking Strategy: Note the strategic word "best" and focus on the subject—to maintain the integrity of the oral mucosa. Recalling that a client on gastric suction will be NPO and swallowing water or other liquids would be prohibited will assist in eliminating options 1 and 2. From the remaining options, eliminate option 3 because lemon glycerin swabs are drying to the mucosa. Review care of the client with a nasogastric tube if you had difficulty with this question.
Level of Cognitive Ability: Application
Client Needs: Physiological Integrity
Integrated Process: Nursing Process/Implementation
Content Area: Adult Health/Gastrointestinal
References: Linton, A., & Maebius, N. (2007). *Introduction to medical-surgical nursing* (4th ed., p. 743). Philadelphia: Saunders.
Potter, P., & Perry, A. (2005). *Fundamentals of nursing* (6th ed., p. 1408). St. Louis: Mosby.

1003. 3
Rationale: Rheumatic endocarditis, also called rheumatic carditis, is a major indicator of rheumatic fever, which is a complication of infection with group A β-hemolytic streptococcal infections. It is frequently triggered by streptococcal pharyngitis. Options 1, 2, and 4 are incorrect.
Test-Taking Strategy: Use the process of elimination. Recalling that streptococcal infections are largely responsible for rheumatic heart disease will direct you to option 3. Review the causes of endocarditis if you had difficulty with this question.
Level of Cognitive Ability: Application
Client Needs: Physiological Integrity
Integrated Process: Nursing Process/Data Collection
Content Area: Adult Health/Cardiovascular
References: Christensen, B., & Kockrow, E. (2006). *Adult health nursing* (5th ed., pp. 372-373). St. Louis: Mosby.
Ignatavicius, D., & Workman, M. L. (2006). *Medical-surgical nursing: Critical thinking for collaborative care* (5th ed., p. 771). St. Louis: Saunders.

1004. 4
Rationale: Potassium-sparing diuretics include amiloride (Midamor), spironolactone (Aldactone), and triamterene (Dyrenium). They are weak diuretics that are used in combination with potassium-losing diuretics. This combination is

useful when medication and dietary supplement of potassium is not appropriate. The use of two different diuretics does not prevent renal toxicity. Hydrochlorothiazide is an effective and inexpensive generic form of the thiazide classification of diuretics.
Test-Taking Strategy: It is especially helpful to remember that hydrochlorothiazide is a potassium-losing diuretic and triamterene is a potassium-sparing diuretic; thus, option 1 can be eliminated. Toxicity from these medications is the result of fluid and electrolyte imbalances, so option 2 can be eliminated. Hydrochlorothiazide is a common and inexpensive diuretic, so option 3 can be eliminated. Review the action ans uses of these medications if you had difficulty with this question.
Level of Cognitive Ability: Comprehension
Client Needs: Physiological Integrity
Integrated Process: Nursing Process/Implementation
Content Area: Pharmacology
Reference: Hodgson, B., & Kizior, R. (2008). *Saunders nursing drug handbook 2008* (pp. 1180-1182). Philadelphia: Saunders.

1005. **3**
Rationale: ACE inhibitors, such as fosinopril, cause temporary impairment of taste (dysgeusia). The nurse can tell the client that this effect usually disappears in 2 to 3 months, even with continued therapy, and provide nutritional counseling if appropriate to avoid weight loss. Options 1, 2, and 4 are inappropriate actions. Taking this medication with or without food does not affect absorption and action. The dosage should never be tapered without physician approval and the medication should never be stopped abruptly.
Test-Taking Strategy: Use the process of elimination. Eliminate option 2 first because it is an inappropriate nursing action. The nurse does not advise the client to make dosage changes for any prescribed medication. Taking the medication with or without food is not going to change the taste of the food, so option 1 can be eliminated next. From the remaining options, you need to know that this effect occurs with medications in the ACE inhibitor group. Thus, you are left with the correct option, which is informing the client that impaired taste is expected. Review the effects of ACE inhibitors if you had difficulty with this question.
Level of Cognitive Ability: Application
Client Needs: Psychosocial Integrity
Integrated Process: Nursing Process/Implementation
Content Area: Pharmacology
Reference: Kee, J., Hayes, E., & McCuistion, L. (2006). *Pharmacology: A nursing process approach* (5th ed., p. 652). Philadelphia: Saunders.

1006. **2**
Rationale: Amlodipine is a calcium channel blocker. This medication decreases the rate and force of cardiac contraction. Prior to administering a calcium channel blocking agent, the nurse should check the blood pressure and heart rate, which could both decrease in response to the action of this medication. This action will help to prevent or identify early problems related to decreased cardiac contractility, decreased heart rate, and decreased conduction.
Test-Taking Strategy: To answer this question, you must know that amlodipine is a calcium channel blocker, and

that this group of medications decreases the rate and force of cardiac contraction. This in turn lowers the pulse rate and blood pressure. Option 1 can be eliminated first because it is unrelated to the medication. With options 3 and 4, note that only half of the option is correct. When answering questions such as these, with two items per option, both of the items must be correct for that option to be correct. Review this medication if you had difficulty with this question.
Level of Cognitive Ability: Application
Client Needs: Physiological Integrity
Integrated Process: Nursing Process/Data Collection
Content Area: Pharmacology
Reference: Hodgson, B., & Kizior, R. (2008). *Saunders nursing drug handbook 2008* (p. 63). Philadelphia: Saunders.

1007. **4**
Rationale: Paraphrasing is restating the client's message in the nurse's own words. Option 4 uses the therapeutic communication technique of paraphrasing. The client is frustrated and is searching for understanding. Options 1, 2, and 3 are inappropriate communication techniques. Option 1 belittles the client's concerns. Options 2 and 3 offer false reassurance by the nurse.
Test-Taking Strategy: Use therapeutic communication techniques to answer the question. Option 4 focuses on the client's feelings. Review therapeutic communication techniques if you had difficulty with this question.
Level of Cognitive Ability: Application
Client Needs: Psychosocial Integrity
Integrated Process: Communication and Documentation
Content Area: Adult Health/Cardiovascular
References: Christensen, B., & Kockrow, E. (2006). *Foundations of nursing* (5th ed.,pp. 39-42). St. Louis: Mosby.
Linton, A., & Maebius, N. (2007). *Introduction to medical-surgical nursing* (4th ed., p. 628). Philadelphia: Saunders.

1008. **2, 4, 5, 6**
Rationale: The nurse would teach the client how to care for the stoma depending on the type of laryngectomy performed. Most interventions focus on protection of the stoma and the prevention of infection. Interventions include avoiding swimming and using caution when showering, avoiding exposure to people with infections, preventing debris from entering the stoma, and obtaining a Medic-Alert bracelet. Additional interventions include wearing a stoma guard or high-collar clothing to cover the stoma, increasing the humidity in the home, and increasing fluid intake to 3000 mL/day to keep the secretions thin.
Test-Taking Strategy: Recalling that most interventions focus on protection of the stoma and the prevention of infection will assist in identifying the client instructions for home care. Review these instructions if you had difficulty with this question.
Level of Cognitive Ability: Application
Client Needs: Physiological Integrity
Integrated Process: Teaching and Learning
Content Area: Adult Health/Oncology
Reference: Ignatavicius, D., & Workman, M. (2006). *Medical-surgical nursing: Critical thinking for collaborative care* (5th ed., pp. 575, 580-581). Philadelphia: Saunders.

1009. 2

Rationale: The correct procedure for needle disposal is to discard uncapped needles and sharps in a hard-walled, puncture-resistant, leak-proof container immediately after use. Discarding the uncapped needle and attached syringe in a designated sharps container prevents injury to the client and health care personnel. Recapping needles increases the risk of needle-stick injury. Options 1, 3, and 4 are unsafe actions.

Test-Taking Strategy: Use the process of elimination and principles related to the safe disposal of needles and syringes to answer the question. Note that options 1, 3, and 4 are comparable or alike in that they all address recapping the needle. Review these principles if you had difficulty with this question.

Level of Cognitive Ability: Application
Client Needs: Safe and Effective Care Environment
Integrated Process: Nursing Process/Implementation
Content Area: Fundamental Skills
Reference: Christensen, B., & Kockrow, E. (2006). *Foundations of nursing* (5th ed., p. 275). St. Louis: Mosby.

1010. 2

Rationale: Individuals at risk for developing a latex allergy include health care workers; individuals who work with manufacturing latex products; individuals with spina bifida; individuals who wear gloves frequently such as food handlers, hairdressers, and auto mechanics; and individuals allergic to kiwis, bananas, pineapples, passion fruit, avocados, and chestnuts.

Test-Taking Strategy: Focus on the subject—a latex allergy. Recalling the cause and the source of the allergic reaction will easily direct you to option 2. Review the cause of this type of allergy and the individuals at risk if you had difficulty with this question.

Level of Cognitive Ability: Analysis
Client Needs: Health Promotion and Maintenance
Integrated Process: Nursing Process/Data Collection
Content Area: Adult Health/Immune
References: Christensen, B., & Kockrow, E. (2006). *Adult health nursing* (5th ed., p. 763). St. Louis: Mosby.
Ignatavicius, D., & Workman, M. L. (2006). *Medical-surgical nursing: Critical thinking for collaborative care* (5th ed., pp. 461, 512). Philadelphia: Saunders.

1011. 2

Rationale: The skin under a casted area may be discolored and crusted with dead skin layers. The client should gently soak and wash the skin for the first few days. The skin should be patted dry, and a lubricating lotion should be applied. Clients often want to scrub the dead skin away, which irritates the skin. The client should avoid overexposing the skin to the sunlight.

Test-Taking Strategy: Note the strategic words "further skin care instructions are required." Option 3 is obviously helpful, and therefore cannot be the answer to the question as stated. Option 4 is good advice and is eliminated next. Options 1 and 2 seem to oppose each other, making it likely that one of them is correct. Because vigorous scrubbing is more likely to be irritating than providing a gentle wash, it is the most likely choice as the answer to the question. Review skin care measures following cast removal if you had difficulty with this question.

Level of Cognitive Ability: Comprehension
Client Needs: Physiological Integrity
Integrated Process: Teaching and Learning
Content Area: Adult Health/Musculoskeletal
References: Christensen, B., & Kockrow, E. (2006). *Adult health nursing* (5th ed., p.173). St. Louis: Mosby.
Ignatavicius, D., & Workman, M. L. (2006) *Medical-surgical nursing: Critical thinking for collaborative care* (5th ed., p. 1205). Philadelphia: Saunders.

1012. 2

Rationale: Common areas that are under pressure and are at risk for breakdown include the elbows (if they are used for repositioning instead of a trapeze) and the heel of the good leg (which is used as a brace when pushing up in bed). Other pressure points caused by the traction include the ischial tuberosity, popliteal space, and Achilles tendon.

Test-Taking Strategy: Note the strategic words "high-risk area." Thus, you would compare each of the options in terms of their relative risk, and choose the one that is highest. The right heel is eliminated first because it is off the bed in the traction setup. The overhead trapeze would diminish the likelihood that the scapulae and back of the head would be immobile. This leaves the left heel as the answer. This makes sense, given that the client would use the unaffected heel to push into the mattress during repositioning. With repeated use, this could cause the left heel to become reddened and break down. Review the complications of skeletal traction if you had difficulty with this question.

Level of Cognitive Ability: Application
Client Needs: Physiological Integrity
Integrated Process: Nursing Process/Data Collection
Content Area: Adult Health/Musculoskeletal
References: Christensen, B., & Kockrow, E. (2006). *Adult health nursing* (5th ed., p. 175). St. Louis: Mosby.
Monahan, F., Sands, J., Neighbors, M., Marek, J., & Green, C. (2007). *Phipps' medical-surgical nursing: Health and illness perspectives* (8th ed., p.1535). St. Louis: Mosby.

1013. 3

Rationale: The part of the bed under an area in traction is usually elevated to aid in countertraction. For the client in Buck's extension traction (which is applied to a leg), the foot of the bed is elevated.

Test-Taking Strategy: To answer this question correctly, you need to understand the principles of traction and countertraction and be familiar with Buck's extension traction. Option 2 is not used for the purpose of countertraction and is eliminated first. Knowing that Buck's extension traction is applied to the leg helps you eliminate option 4. Of the two remaining choices, option 1 places undue pressure on the client's unaffected foot. Furthermore, a footboard is not used for the purpose of providing countertraction. Option 3 provides a force that opposes the traction force effectively without harming the client. Review care of the client in Buck's extension traction if you had difficulty with this question.

Level of Cognitive Ability: Application
Client Needs: Physiological Integrity
Integrated Process: Nursing Process/Implementation
Content Area: Adult Health/Musculoskeletal

Reference: deWit, S. (2009). *Medical-surgical nursing: Concepts & practice* (p. 793). St. Louis: Saunders.

1014. 3, 4, 5
Rationale: The clinical manifestations of hypothyroidism are the result of decreased metabolism from low levels of thyroid hormone. Interventions are aimed at replacement of the hormones and providing measures to support the signs and symptoms related to a decreased metabolism. The nurse encourages the client to consume a well-balanced diet that is low in fat for weight reduction and high in fluids and high-fiber foods to prevent constipation. The client often has cold intolerance and requires a warm environment. The client would notify the physician if chest pain occurs since it could be an indication of overreplacement of thyroid hormone. Iodine preparations are used to treat hyperthyroidism. These medications decrease blood flow through the thyroid gland and reduce the production and release of thyroid hormone.
Test-Taking Strategy: Focus on the client's diagnosis—hypothyroidism. Recalling that the client has a decreased metabolic rate in this disorder will assist in determining the appropriate interventions. Review interventions for the client with hypothyroidism and hyperthyroidism if you had difficulty with this question.
Level of Cognitive Ability: Application
Client Needs: Physiological Integrity
Integrated Process: Nursing Process/Implementation
Content Area: Adult Health/Endocrine
Reference: Ignatavicius, D., & Workman, M. (2006). *Medical-surgical nursing: Critical thinking for collaborative care* (5th ed., pp. 1491-1492). Philadelphia: Saunders.

1015. 4
Rationale: The client with Guillain-Barré syndrome is at risk for respiratory failure because of ascending paralysis. An intubation tray should be available for use. Another complication of this syndrome is cardiac dysrhythmia, which necessitates the use of ECG monitoring. Because the client is immobilized, the nurse should routinely assess for deep vein thrombosis and pulmonary embolism.
Test-Taking Strategy: Use the process of elimination and the ABCs — airway, breathing, and circulation. With an ascending paralysis, the client is at risk for involvement of respiratory muscles and subsequent respiratory failure. This knowledge makes you look for an option that coincides with this line of thought. Option 4 is the only option that includes an intubation tray, which would be needed if the client's status deteriorated to needing intubation and mechanical ventilation. It also addresses cardiac monitoring. This option most directly addresses the ABCs. Review care of the client with Guillain-Barré syndrome if you had difficulty with this question.
Level of Cognitive Ability: Application
Client Needs: Physiological Integrity
Integrated Process: Nursing Process/Implementation
Content Area: Adult Health/Neurological
References: Christensen, B., & Kockrow, E. (2006). *Adult health nursing* (5th ed., pp. 736-737). St. Louis: Mosby.
Ignatavicius, D., & Workman, M. L. (2006) *Medical-surgical nursing: Critical thinking for collaborative care* (5th ed., pp. 1009-1010). Philadelphia: Saunders.

1016. 4
Rationale: Feosol is an iron supplement used to treat anemia. Constipation is a frequent and uncomfortable side effect associated with the administration of oral iron supplements. Stool softeners are often prescribed to prevent constipation. Options 1, 2, and 3 are not associated with this medication.
Test-Taking Strategy: Focus on the name of the medication. Recalling that oral iron can cause constipation will easily direct you to option 4. If you had difficulty with this question, review the side effects of ferrous sulfate.
Level of Cognitive Ability: Comprehension
Client Needs: Physiological Integrity
Integrated Process: Nursing Process/Data Collection
Content Area: Pharmacology
Reference: Hodgson, B., & Kizior, R. (2008). *Saunders nursing drug handbook 2008* (pp. 478-479). Philadelphia: Saunders.

1017. 2
Rationale: Hearing-impaired clients rely on visual cues to help them comprehend the conversation of others. Smiling continuously is the least helpful strategy, since the smile distorts the appearance of the mouth if the client is trying to read lips. When beginning the conversation, it helps to reduce background noise such as turning off or lowering the volume of the television. Facing the client and standing so that there is light on the nurse's face are helpful strategies, since it assists the client to lip read. Taking care not to show frustration or annoyance with the client's impairment is also helpful to preserve the client's self-esteem.
Test-Taking Strategy: Note the strategic words "least helpful." Noting the words "smiling continuously" in option 2 will direct you to this option. If this question was difficult, review these communication strategies.
Level of Cognitive Ability: Application
Client Needs: Psychosocial Integrity
Integrated Process: Communication and Documentation
Content Area: Adult Health/Ear
References: deWit, S. (2009). *Medical-surgical nursing: Concepts & practice* (p. 630). St. Louis: Saunders.
Potter, P., & Perry, A. (2005). *Fundamentals of nursing* (6th ed., p. 1585). St. Louis: Mosby.

1018. 1
Rationale: Digoxin is a cardiac glycoside that is used to treat heart failure and acts by increasing the force of myocardial contraction. Because bradycardia may be a clinical sign of toxicity, the nurse counts the apical heart rate for 1 full minute before administering the medication. If the pulse rate is below 60 beats/minute in an adult client, the nurse would withhold the medication and report the pulse rate to the registered nurse, who would then contact the physician.
Test-Taking Strategy: Noting that the client has heart failure and recalling the action and nursing interventions related to administering this medication will assist in answering this question. Remember that bradycardia is a sign of toxicity. Review nursing interventions related to the administration of digoxin if you had difficulty with this question.
Level of Cognitive Ability: Application
Client Needs: Physiological Integrity
Integrated Process: Nursing Process/Implementation
Content Area: Pharmacology

References: Hodgson, B., & Kizior, R. (2008). *Saunders nursing drug handbook 2008* (p. 363). Philadelphia: Saunders.
Skidmore-Roth, L. (2007). *Mosby's nursing drug reference* (20th ed., p. 361) St. Louis: Mosby.

1019. 25
Rationale: Use the formula for calculating IV flow rates. Formula:

$$\frac{\text{Total volume to infuse} \times \text{gtt factor}}{\text{Time in minutes}} = \text{gtt/minute}$$

$$\frac{1000\,\text{mL} \times 15\,\text{gtt/mL}}{10\,\text{hours} \times 60\,\text{minutes}} = \frac{15,000}{600} = 25\,\text{gtt/min}$$

Test-Taking Strategy: Follow the formula for calculating an IV flow rate and remember to change hours to minutes. Once you have done the calculation, recheck your work using a calculator and make sure that the answer makes sense. If you had difficulty with this question, review IV flow rates.
Level of Cognitive Ability: Application
Client Needs: Physiological Integrity
Integrated Process: Nursing Process/Implementation
Content Area: Fundamental Skills
Reference: Potter, P., & Perry, A. (2005). *Fundamentals of nursing* (6th ed., p. 1176). St. Louis: Mosby.

1020. 2, 3, 6
Rationale: Sterile packages are opened away from the nurse's body, and the distal flap of a sterile package is opened first. This prevents contaminating the pack by reaching over the exposed sterile contents after the other flaps are opened (option 2). To avoid contamination, the sterile field should be prepared just prior to the planned procedure, and supplies should be used immediately (option 3). The outer 1-inch border of the sterile field must be considered unsterile, and sterile items are not placed within this 1-inch area (option 6). A dry table that is above waist level is used to set up a sterile field. Moisture will contaminate the sterile field and anything below waist level is considered contaminated, according to the principles of surgical asepsis. The sterile field must be kept in sight at all times, and the nurse should not turn away from it. If this happens, the nurse cannot be sure that it is still sterile. Sterile gloves, not clean gloves, are used. An unsterile item touching a sterile item contaminates the sterile item.
Test-Taking Strategy: Focus on the subject—the principles of aseptic technique. Thinking about these principles and visualizing each intervention will assist in identifying those that are appropriate. Review the principles of aseptic technique if you had difficulty with this question.
Level of Cognitive Ability: Application
Client Needs: Safe and Effective Care Environment
Integrated Process: Nursing Process/Implementation
Content Area: Fundamental Skills
References: Christensen, B., & Kockrow, E. (2006). *Foundations of nursing* (5th ed., pp. 297-298). St. Louis: Mosby.
Potter, P., & Perry, A. (2005). *Fundamentals of nursing* (6th ed., pp. 803-807). St. Louis: Mosby.

1021. 3
Rationale: Coughing is a normal response to suctioning for the client with an intact cough reflex, and it is not an indication that the client is not tolerating the procedure. The client should be encouraged to cough to help with removal of secretions from the lungs. The nurse should monitor for the adverse effects of suctioning, which include cyanosis (pulse oximetry falls below 90% or 5% from baseline), excessively rapid or slow heart rate (a 20 beat/minute change), or the sudden development of bloody secretions. If they occur, the nurse stops suctioning, administers oxygen as appropriate, and reports these signs to the physician immediately.
Test-Taking Strategy: Use the process of elimination and note the strategic words "adequately tolerating." Cyanosis (option 1) and bradycardia (option 4) are abnormal findings and are eliminated first. From the remaining options, the use of the word "becoming" in association with bloody secretions tells you that this has not been an ongoing problem, making this an incorrect option. Because the cough reflex is normally present, and suction triggers coughing, option 3 is preferable. Review this procedure if you had difficulty with this question.
Level of Cognitive Ability: Analysis
Client Needs: Physiological Integrity
Integrated Process: Nursing Process/Evaluation
Content Area: Adult Health/Respiratory
References: deWit, S. (2009). *Medical-surgical nursing: Concepts & practice* (p. 312). St. Louis: Saunders.
Perry, A., & Potter, P. (2006). *Clinical nursing skills & techniques* (6th ed., p. 822). St. Louis: Mosby.

1022. 3
Rationale: Candidiasis is a fungal infection caused by *Candida albicans*. When it occurs in the mouth, it is called thrush and appears as white plaques. Although it can occur in an immunocompromised client, it is not considered to be common. Options 2 and 4 are not accurate regarding this infection.
Test-Taking Strategy: Use the process of elimination. Options 1 and 4 can be eliminated first. Recalling that the anemic client is more likely to exhibit pallor will assist in eliminating option 2 and will direct you to option 3. If you are unfamiliar with the manifestations associated with thrush, review this content.
Level of Cognitive Ability: Comprehension
Client Needs: Physiological Integrity
Integrated Process: Nursing Process/Data Collection
Content Area: Adult Health/Oncology
Reference: Linton, A., & Maebius, N. (2007). *Introduction to medical-surgical nursing* (4th ed., p. 752). Philadelphia: Saunders.

1023. 3
Rationale: The normal WBC count ranges from 4500 to 11,000/mm³. Options 1 and 2 identify values lower than normal. Option 4 identifies a value higher than normal.
Test-Taking Strategy: Recalling the normal WBC count will direct you to the correct option. Remember the normal WBC count ranges from 4500 to 11,000/mm³. Review the normal WBC count if you had difficulty with this question.
Level of Cognitive Ability: Comprehension

Client Needs: Physiological Integrity
Integrated Process: Nursing Process/Data Collection
Content Area: Adult Health/Oncology
References: Linton, A., & Maebius, N. (2007). *Introduction to medical-surgical nursing* (4th ed., p. 640). Philadelphia: Saunders.
Pagana, K., & Pagana, T. (2005). *Mosby's diagnostic and laboratory test reference* (7th ed., p. 994). St. Louis: Mosby.

1024. **1**
Rationale: The nurse would instruct the client to lie down and place a towel or pillow under the shoulder on the side of the breast to be examined. If the left breast is to be examined, the pillow would be placed under the left shoulder. Options 2 and 4 are incorrect.
Test-Taking Strategy: Visualize this procedure to select the correct option. Remember, to examine the left breast, the pillow is placed under the left shoulder; to examine the right breast, the pillow is placed under the right shoulder. If you are unfamiliar with the procedure for performing BSE, review this self-examination.
Level of Cognitive Ability: Application
Client Needs: Health Promotion and Maintenance
Integrated Process: Teaching and Learning
Content Area: Adult Health/Oncology
References: Christensen, B., & Kockrow, E. (2006). *Adult health nursing* (5th ed., pp. 821-822). St. Louis: Mosby.
Linton, A., & Maebius, N. (2007). *Introduction to medical-surgical nursing* (4th ed., p. 1038). Philadelphia: Saunders.
Potter, P., & Perry, A. (2005). *Fundamentals of nursing* (6th ed., p. 736). St. Louis: Mosby.

1025. **4**
Rationale: The CT scan causes no pain and takes about 15 to 60 minutes to perform. The dye may cause a warm flushing sensation when injected. Fluids are encouraged following the procedure. If an iodine dye is used, the client should be asked about allergies to seafood or iodine.
Test-Taking Strategy: Use the process of elimination and note the strategic words "dye injection." Noting the relationship between these strategic words and option 4 will assist in answering the question. Review this diagnostic test if you had difficulty with this question.
Level of Cognitive Ability: Comprehension
Client Needs: Physiological Integrity
Integrated Process: Nursing Process/Implementation
Content Area: Adult Health/Oncology
Reference: Pagana, K., & Pagana, T. (2005). *Mosby's diagnostic and laboratory test reference* (7th ed., p. 298). St. Louis: Mosby.

1026. **3**
Rationale: Denial, bargaining, anger, depression, and acceptance are recognized stages that a person experiences when facing a life-threatening illness experiences. The client's statement is indicative of bargaining. Denial is expressed as shock and disbelief and may be the first response to hearing bad news. Depression may be manifested by hopelessness, weeping openly, or remaining quiet or withdrawn. Anger may also be a first response to upsetting news and the predominant theme is "Why me?" or the blaming of others.
Test-Taking Strategy: Focus on the client's statement as identified in the question to assist in selecting the correct option. From this point, you should be able to eliminate options 1, 2, and 4. Review these stages if you had difficulty with this question.
Level of Cognitive Ability: Analysis
Client Needs: Psychosocial Integrity
Integrated Process: Nursing Process/Data Collection
Content Area: Adult Health/Oncology
References: Christensen, B., & Kockrow, E. (2006). *Foundations of nursing* (5th ed., pp. 1133-1134). St. Louis: Mosby.
Linton, A., & Maebius, N. (2007). *Introduction to medical-surgical nursing* (4th ed., pp. 386-387, 1242). Philadelphia: Saunders.

1027. **3**
Rationale: The most common risk factor associated with laryngeal cancer is cigarette smoking. Alcohol abuse may have a synergistic effect with cigarette smoking. Air pollution is also a contributing cause, as well as chronic laryngitis and consistent voice strain.
Test-Taking Strategy: Use the process of elimination and note the strategic words "most common." Begin to answer this question by eliminating options 1 and 2. Because cancer of the upper and lower airway is most often related to tobacco, these are the options that are most likely correct. From the remaining options, recalling that cigarettes are the most harmful guides you to choose this option over the option of chewing tobacco. Review these risk factors if you had difficulty with this question.
Level of Cognitive Ability: Comprehension
Client Needs: Health Promotion and Maintenance
Integrated Process: Nursing Process/Data Collection
Content Area: Adult Health/Oncology
Reference: Linton, A., & Maebius, N. (2007). *Introduction to medical-surgical nursing* (4th ed., p. 756). Philadelphia: Saunders.

REFERENCES

Chernecky, C., & Berger, B. (2008). *Laboratory tests and diagnostic procedures* (5th ed.). Philadelphia: Saunders.
Christensen, B., & Kockrow, E. (2006). *Adult health nursing* (5th ed.). St. Louis: Mosby.
Christensen, B., & Kockrow, E. (2006). *Foundations of nursing* (5th ed.). St. Louis: Mosby.
deWit, S. (2009). *Medical-surgical nursing: Concepts & practice.* St. Louis: Saunders.
Fortinash, K., & Holoday-Worret, P. (2008). *Psychiatric mental health nursing* (4th ed.). St. Louis: Mosby.

Hockenberry, M., & Wilson, D. (2007). *Nursing care of infants and children* (8th ed.). St. Louis: Mosby.
Hodgson, B., & Kizior, R. (2008). *Saunders nursing drug handbook 2008.* Philadelphia: Saunders.
Ignatavicius, D., & Workman, M. (2006). *Medical-surgical nursing: Critical thinking for collaborative care* (5th ed.). Philadelphia: Saunders.
Kee, J., Hayes, E., & McCuistion, L. (2006). *Pharmacology: A nursing process approach* (5th ed.). Philadelphia: Saunders.
Keltner, N., Schwecke, L., & Bostrom, C. (2007). *Psychiatric nursing* (5th ed.). St. Louis: Mosby.

Lehne, R. (2007). *Pharmacology for nursing care* (6th ed.). Philadelphia: Saunders.

Leifer, G. (2007). *Introduction to maternity and pediatric nursing* (5th ed.). Philadelphia: Saunders.

Lilley, L., Harrington, S., & Snyder, J. (2007). *Pharmacology and the nursing process* (5th ed.). St. Louis: Mosby.

Linton, A., & Maebius, N. (2007). *Introduction to medical-surgical nursing* (4th ed.). Philadelphia: Saunders.

Monahan, F., Sands, J., & Marek, J., Neighbors, M., Marek, J., & Green, C. (2007). *Phipps' medical-surgical nursing: Health and illness perspectives* (8th ed.). St. Louis: Mosby.

Nix, S. (2005). *Williams' basic nutrition and diet therapy* (12th ed.). St. Louis: Mosby.

Ogden, S. J. (2007). *Calculation of drug dosages* (8th ed.). St. Louis: Mosby.

Pagana, K., & Pagana, T. (2005). *Mosby's diagnostic and laboratory test reference* (7th ed.). St. Louis: Mosby.

Perry, A., & Potter, P. (2006). *Clinical nursing skills & techniques* (6th ed.). St. Louis: Mosby.

Potter, P., & Perry, A. (2005). *Fundamentals of nursing* (6th ed.). St. Louis: Mosby.

Price, D., & Gwin, J. (2008). *Pediatric nursing: An introductory text* (10th ed.). St. Louis: Saunders.

Schlenker, E., & Long, S. (2007). *Williams' essentials of nutrition & diet therapy* (9th ed.). St. Louis: Mosby.

Skidmore-Roth, L. (2007). *Mosby's nursing drug reference* (20th ed.). St. Louis: Mosby.

Stuart, G., & Laraia, M. (2005). *Principles and practice of psychiatric nursing* (8th ed.). St. Louis: Mosby.

Varcarolis, E., Carlson, V., & Shoemaker, N. (2006). *Foundations of psychiatric mental health nursing* (5th ed.). St. Louis: Saunders.

Wold, G. (2008). *Basic geriatric nursing* (4th ed.). St. Louis: Mosby.

Wong, D., Perry, S., Hockenberry, M., Lowdermilk, D., & Wilson, D. (2006). *Maternal child nursing care* (3rd ed.). St. Louis: Mosby.

Index

Note: Page numbers foiiowed by f indicate figures; those followed by t indicate tables; those followed by b indicate boxed material.

Nasal flaring, 358
cardiovascular defect and, 378b
definition of, 342
Nasal stuffiness, pregnancy and, 232
Nasogastric tube
medication via, 201-202
placement and irrigation of, 201
positioning and, 193
types and routes of, 199
Nasotracheal tube, 204
National Council Licensure Examination for
Practical/Vocational Nurses (NCLEX-PN)
authorization to test form, 8-9
examination process, 2-3
Pyramid to Success, 1
registering for, 8, 14-15
rescheduling/canceling, 9
test plan, 3
National Council of State Boards of Nursing, 11,
12
National Patient Safety Goals, 143b
Native American, 35, 38
Natulan (Procarbazine), 535b
Natural disaster, 66b
Natural immunity, 886, 888
Nausea
near-death care and, 962b
pregnancy and, 231
Near-death physiological manifestations, 962
Near drowning, 345
Nearsightedness, 773
Neck
burn to, 469
of newborn, 283
Necrosis, 855
Necrotizing enterocolitis, 291
Nedocromil (Tilade), 650b
Needle aspiration, of thyroid tissue, 544
Needle biopsy, 500
Negative event query, 24b
Negative feedback loop, 542
Neglect
of child, 350-351
of older adult, 336-337
Neglect syndrome, 824b
Negligence
definition of, 44
malpractice and, 46
Neisseria gonorrhoeae, 286
Nelfinavir, 904b
Nelfinavir (Viracept), 904
Neobladder, creation of, 517
Neologism, 935b, 936b
Neonatal death, 276-277
Neonate
definition of, 214
eye prophylaxis and, 306
HIV and, 237-238
postpartum period and, 272
size and gestational age, 289-290
tuberculosis and, 247-248
Neoplasm
AIDS and, 894
definition of, 496
Neoral (Cyclosporine)
for HIV/AIDS, 905
for rheumatoid arthritis, 880
Nephrectomy, 748
Nephroblastoma (Wilms' tumor), 437
Nephrolithiasis, 721, 745
Nephrolithotomy, 748
Nephron, 723
Nephrostomy, percutaneous, 517
Nephrostomy tube, 204, 517
Nephrotic syndrome, 408-409, 409b
Nephrotoxicity
capreomycin and, 657
organ rejection medication and, 761-762
streptomycin and, 659b
Nephrotoxic substance, 728b
Nerve tract, 807
Neupogen (Filgrastim), 535b
Neuroblastoma, 437-438
Neurogenic hyperventilation, 812b
Neuroleptic malignant syndrome, 983
Neurological disorder, 344-351
in adult, 805-806
Neurological manifestation
of chronic renal failure, 730b, 733
magnesium and, 5b
Neurological medication
antimyasthenic, 838, 839b
antiparkinsonian, 838

Neurological system
anaphylactic reaction and, 890f
anatomy and physiology of, 807-808
data collection and, 810-813
diagnostic testing and, 808-810
immediate postoperative care of, 178
intermediate postoperative care of, 180
newborn and, 286-287
in older adult, 334
positioning and, 194
Neuromuscular blockade, 657
Neuromuscular system, 819
Neuron, 808
Neurotoxicity
isoniazid and, 654
streptomycin and, 659b
Neurotransmitter, 808
Neutrophil, 108t
Nevirapine (Viramune), 904, 904b
Newborn
AIDS and, 294
care of, 282, 288-289
definition of, 214
of diabetic mother, 294-295
fencing position of, 287
gonorrhea and, 247
Hirschsprung's disease in, 396f, 397
physical examination of, 282
postpartum period and, 272
as postterm, 289
as preterm, 289
safety of, 288
substance abuse and, 226
substance addiction in, 293
transient tachypnea of, 290
tuberculosis and, 248
as uncircumcised, 289
Niacin, 117b
Nice girl-good boy orientation, moral development
and, 315b
Nicotine withdrawal, 954
Nifedipine, for preterm labor, 303t
Nightly peritoneal dialysis, 739b
Nipple, cracked, 274
Nitrate, 682, 712-713
Nitrazine test, 235
Nitrofurazone (Furacin), 490
Nitrogen mustard, 531b
Nitroglycerin, 682, 684
Nitrosource, 531b
Nix (Permethrin)
for pediculosis capitis, 417t
for scabies, 418t
Nizatidine (Axid), 615
Nizoral (Ketoconazole), 653
N-methyl-D-aspartate receptor antagonist (NMDA
antagonist), 984
Nomogram chart, 457b, 457f
Nonadherent dressing, for skin, 488
Nonbenzodiazepine anxiolytic, 981b
Noncommunicating hydrocele, 399
Noncommunicating hydrocephalus, 345b
Noncontact tonometry measurement, 773
Nongerminal tumor, 506b
Noninvasive transcutaneous pacing, 680
Nonmaleficence, 44b
Non-nucleoside reverse transcriptase inhibitor,
902b, 904
Non-opioid analgesic
NSAIDs as, 843-844
types of, 843b
Non-opioid antitussive, 652b
Non-rebreather mask, 630, 630f
Nonselective beta-adrenergic blocker, 714b
Nonsteroidal anti-inflammatory drug (NSAID)
for eyes, 797b
for juvenile idiopathic rheumatoid arthritis, 426b
as nephrotoxic substance, 728b
overview of, 843-844
for rheumatoid arthritis, 879
side effects of, 843b
types of, 843b
Nonstress test, 235b
Nontherapeutic communication technique, 915b
Nonurgent priority 3, in ER triage system, 69b
Normal grief, 960
Normal sinus rhythm, 676, 676f, 677f
Normothermia, 815
Norpace (disopyramide phosphate), 654
Norvir (Ritonavir), 904
Nose
of newborn, 283
physiology of, 624

Nosebleed
intervention for, 358
pregnancy and, 232
Nuchal rigidity
definition of, 805
encephalitis and, 829
meningitis and, 830
stroke and, 824
Nuclear cardiology, 671
Nucleoside/nucleotide reverse transcriptase
inhibitor, 902, 902b
Nucleus, 808
Nullipara, 224
Nurse
client confidentiality and, 50
disaster planning and, 68
disciplinary action against, 46
floating and, 46
reporting responsibility of, 53
responsibilities of, 61-62
role of, 62
Nurse-client relationship, 913
Nurse licensure compact, 10
Nurse practice act, 45
Nurse practitioner, 62
Nursing
cultural diversity and, 39
testing knowledge of, 13, 14
Nursing assistant
delegatable tasks for, 65b
role of, 63
Nursing care. See Perioperative nursing care
Nursing care plan, 60
Nursing delivery system, 61
Nursing practice, regulation of, 45-46
Nursing process
data collection and, 26b
evaluation and, 27b
implementation and, 27b
planning and, 26b
steps of, 26
Nutrient
definition of, 115
types of, 116-117
Nutrition
adolescence and, 329
burn and, 473
child and, 328
crisis intervention and, 964
cultural diversity and, 33
infant and, 323-324
with leukemia, 434-436
postpartum period and, 273
pregnancy and, 235-236
preoperative care and, 174
preschooler and, 326
toddler and, 325
Nutritionist, 63
Nyctophobia, 930b
Nydrazid (INH, Isonazid), 653-655

O

Oat cell carcinoma, 512
Obedience-punishment orientation, moral
development and, 315b
Obesity, 169
Objective, of organization, 60
Object relations, personality disorder and, 938
Oblique muscle, 771
Obsession, 930
Obsessive-compulsive disorder
characteristics of, 939
intervention for, 930b
overview of, 930
Occipital lobe, 808b
Occupational lung disease, 638
Occupational Safety and Health Act, 53
Occupational therapist, 63
Octreotide acetate (Sandostatin), 569t
Ocular disorder, 655
Ocular irritation, CRF and, 733
Ocular melanoma, 777
Oculomotor nerve, 771
Oculovestibular reflex (caloric testing), 810
Ocusert system, 799
Oddi, sphincter of, 587
Older adult
abuse of, 336-337
care of, 334-337
Olfactory hallucination, 935
Oliguria
definition of, 721
radical nephrectomy and, 748-749